Psychiatric Nursing

in the Hospital and the Community

WITHDRAWN

5TH EDITION

Ann Wolbert Burgess, R.N., C.S., D.N.Sc.
van Ameringen Professor of Psychiatric Mental Health Nursing
University of Pennsylvania School of Nursing
Philadelphia, Pennsylvania

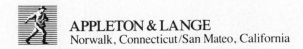
APPLETON & LANGE
Norwalk, Connecticut/San Mateo, California

0-8385-8008-4

Notice: Our knowledge in clinical sciences is constantly changing. As new information becomes available, changes in treatment and in the use of drugs become necessary. The author and the publisher of this volume have taken care to make certain that the doses of drugs and schedules of treatment are correct and compatible with the standards generally accepted at the time of publication. The reader is advised to consult carefully the instruction and information material included in the package insert of each drug or therapeutic agent before administration. This advice is especially important when using new or infrequently used drugs.

Prentice Hall International (UK) Limited, *London*
Prentice Hall of Australia Pty. Limited, *Sydney*
Prentice Hall Canada, Inc., *Toronto*
Prentice Hall Hispanoamericana, S.A., *Mexico*
Prentice Hall of India Private Limited, *New Delhi*
Prentice Hall of Japan, Inc., *Tokyo*
Simon & Prentice Asia Pte. Ltd., *Singapore*
Editora Prentice Hall do Brasil Ltda., *Rio de Janeiro*
Prentice Hall, *Englewood Cliffs, New Jersey*

Library of Congress Cataloging-in-Publication Data

Burgess, Ann Wolbert
    Psychiatric nursing in the hospital and
the community.

    Rev. ed. of: Psychiatric nursing in the hospital and
the community. 4th ed. c1985.
    Includes bibliographies and index.
    1. Psychiatric nursing.   I. Burgess, Ann Wolbert.
Psychiatric nursing in the hospital and the community.
II. Title. [DNLM: 1. Community Mental Health Services.
2. Psychiatric Nursing. WY 160 B955p]
RC440.B89   1989   610.73'68   89-6619
ISBN 0-8385-8008-4

Acquisitions Editor: Marion Kalstein-Welch
Production Editor: Christopher J. Bacich
Designer: Steven M. Byrum

PRINTED IN THE UNITED STATES OF AMERICA

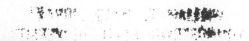

To the memory of my parents
Anna Kehrli Wolbert
John Norman Wolbert

Contributing Authors

Gerald Bennett, R.N., Ph.D.
Chairperson and Association Professor
Department of Psychiatric Mental Health
  Nursing
Medical College of Georgia
Augusta, Georgia

Ann Wolbert Burgess, R.N., C.S., D.N.Sc.
van Ameringen Professor of Psychiatric
  Mental Health Nursing
University of Pennsylvania School of Nursing
Philadelphia, Pennsylvania

Constance M. Carino, R.N., D.N.Sc., C.S.
Clinical Director, Psychiatric Nursing
Hospital of the University of Pennsylvania
Clinical Educator
School of Nursing and School of Medicine
University of Pennsylvania
Philadelphia, Pennsylvania

Patricia Chmelko, R.N., B.S.
In-Patient Psychiatric Service
Hospital of the University of Pennsylvania
Philadelphia, Pennsylvania

Ann Bertrand-Clark, R.N., M.S.
Graduate Student, School of Nursing
University of Pennsylvania
Philadelphia, Pennsylvania

Janis Davidson, R.N., Ph.D.
Department of Adult Health and Illness
School of Nursing
University of Pennsylvania
Philadelphia, Pennsylvania

Christine A. Grant, R.N., Ph.D.
Research Associate
School of Nursing
University of Pennsylvania
Philadelphia, Pennsylvania

Karla J. Hannibal, R.N., B.S.N.
Graduate Student
School of Nursing
University of Cincinnati
Cincinnati, Ohio

Carol R. Hartman, R.N., D.N.Sc., C.S.
Professor of Psychiatric Mental Health
  Nursing
Boston College
Chestnut Hill, Massachusetts

Mary H. Hennessey, R.N., M.S.
Department of Nursing
University of Massachusetts at Boston
Boston, Massachusetts

Barbara J. Holder, R.N., Ph.D.
Department of Psychiatric Mental
  Health Nursing
School of Nursing
University of Pennsylvania
Philadelphia, Pennsylvania

Selina Kassels, Ph.D.
Clinical Psychologist
Newton-Wellesley Hospital
Newton, Massachusetts

Margaret Knight, R.N., M.S.
Department of Nursing
MacLean Hospital
Belmont, Massachusetts

Santa J. Kozak, R.N.
Hanna Pavilion
University Hospitals of Cleveland
Cleveland, Ohio

Joyce Kemp Laben, R.N., M.S., J.D.
Professor of Nursing
Vanderbilt University
Nashville, Tennessee

Colleen Powell MacLean, J.D.
Private Practice
Nashville, Tennessee

Maureen P. McCausland, R.N., D.N.Sc., C.N.A.A.
Associate Vice President for Nursing
Beth Israel Hospital
Boston, Massachusetts

Marita Prater, R.N., M.S.
Department of Nursing
Massachusetts Bay Community College
Wellesley, Massachusetts

Eileen E. Rinear, R.N., Ph.D., C.S.
Private Practice
Southampton, Pennsylvania

Gloria Edelhauser Shapiro, R.N., M.S.
Clinical Specialist in Psychiatry
University Hospital
Boston, Massachusetts

Eunice M. Shishmanian, R.N., M.S.
Director of Nursing Program
Development Evaluation Clinic
Children's Hospital
Boston, Massachusetts

Nancy R. Starefos, R.N., M.S.
Mohegan Community College
Norwich, Connecticut

Marcia A. Ullman, R.N., M.S.
Assistant Professor of Nursing
State University of New York
Brockport, New York

Christine Vourakis, D.N.Sc., R.N.
Doctoral Fellow, Alcohol Research Group
University of California Berkeley
Berkeley, California

Nancy Worley, R.N., Ph.D.
Department of Psychiatric Mental Health Nursing
School of Nursing
University of Pennsylvania
Philadelphia, Pennsylvania

Contents

About the Author

Dr. Ann Wolbert Burgess, pioneer in the field of victimology and psychiatric mental health nursing, received her B.S. and D.N.Sc. degrees from Boston University and her M.S. from the University of Maryland. She was appointed the first van Ameringen Professor of Psychiatric Mental Health Nursing in 1983 at the University of Pennsylvania School of Nursing, the first endowed chair in psychiatric mental health nursing in the country, which was established by the van Ameringen Foundation of New York. Prior to the appointment she served as Chairperson and Professor of the Department of Nursing, Graduate School of Arts and Sciences, Boston College, and Professor and Director of Research at Boston University School of Nursing.

Dr. Burgess's work with rape and child abuse prevention has brought together the judiciary, law enforcement agencies, and health professions in the design and implementation of the victim assistance programs nationwide. Her numerous publications on the subject are used extensively in the training of criminal justice professionals and counselors throughout the United States and abroad.

Dr. Burgess is a fellow in the American Academy of Nursing and past member of the American Nurses' Association's Cabinet on Nursing Research. She has served on the Board of Directors of the American Orthopsychiatric Association, the National Organization for Victim Assistance, the American Professional Society on the Abuse of Children and the Society for Traumatic Stress Studies. She was the first chairperson of the Advisory Committee to the National Center for Rape Prevention and Control of the United States Department of Health and Human Services, a member of the Task Force for the American Bar Association's Criminal Justice Mental Health Standards Project, a member of the 1984 United States Attorney General's Task Force on Family Violence, the 1985 Surgeon General's Symposium on Violence, and a charter member of the National Center for Nursing Research Advisory Council of the National Institutes of Health. She is also certified as a clinical specialist in psychiatric mental health nursing, has a private practice, and testifies as an expert witness in criminal and civil judicial proceedings.

Dr. Burgess received the 1979 Current Impact on Research and Scholarship award of the American Nurses Association Council of Specialists in Psychiatric Mental Health Nursing, the 1980 Massachusetts Nurses Association General Award in Nursing, and the 1982 American Nurses Association Honorary Nursing Practice Award.

Foreword

If this book surprises some teachers of psychiatric mental health nursing, it is because it is not a cookbook presentation with multiple recipes for the quick and sure approach to the mentally ill. It is also not a Rand McNally guide to the intricacies of the diagnostic nomenclature with the entire clinical entities neatly mapped out. It presents, rather, an exciting way to think and to be concerned about those human beings who are suffering and at times dying from emotional illness. The text stimulates us to become involved, yet helps us to remain objective. It not only calls upon us to understand, but demands an empathetic acceptance of the patients with all their hurts no matter how frightened we may be. Its major purpose is clear: to motivate nurses as human beings to acknowledge and respond to another human in a way that is therapeutic. It demonstrates a catalytic approach where the nurse catalysts are intimately involved yet ultimately themselves and not part of the pathological process.

Although the focus is the student in the psychiatric setting, the principles are clearly applicable to all areas of nursing and indeed often to situations outside of the profession.

The author has devoted attention to stalls in the therapeutic process. How often in the past have students felt they were the only ones who experienced no movement in their relationships? How reassuring to learn otherwise. The text strips away the facade of detached omnipotence behind which the nurse, in the past, could safely hide. It identifies the pitfalls in relationships that are universal and tells us how to heal ourselves after traumatic encounters.

GERTRUDE E. FLYNN, R.N., D.N.Sc.
Consultant in Psychiatric Mental Health Nursing
Keene, New Hampshire

Preface

The fifth edition of *Psychiatric Nursing in the Hospital and the Community** addresses itself to students and practitioners of psychiatric mental health nursing. Psychiatric mental health nursing has placed a primary emphasis on theoretical frameworks and clinical modalities in its practice and on the process of communication. In addition, key beliefs and values regarding the individual have contributed to the success of many psychiatric nurse clinicians. Their practices have respected the uniqueness of the individual. Recent multidisciplinary efforts at therapeutic interventions have cast more light on the communication process as the major vehicle for change. This edition directs attention to the expanding knowledge base in the the science of psychiatric mental health nursing and to the processes involved in communication, that is, the generating, exchanging, and interpreting of information. Since communication is essential to growth and development, delving into the intricacies of communication provides critical information as to how life is influenced and changed.

A continued focus of this book is on the human dimension in psychiatric mental health nursing. Patients matter as people. They must be seen as individuals who are suffering in their behaviors, in their thoughts, and especially in their feelings. Mental illness represents the patients' attempts to cope with overwhelming experiences. It is their way of making the best out of a bad situation.

By the human dimension, we also mean that nurses matter as people. Their discomfort with patients represents not a treatment failure but a diagnostic clue that there is a subtle and complicated clinical situation to be understood. The nurses' feelings must be attended to by themselves, their colleagues, and their supervisors if nurses are to fully develop their skills as clinicians.

The 1970s saw an increase in the need for the delivery of mental health services to individual citizens, the family, and the community. The early 1980s identified the need for services to the unserved and the underserved. In order to meet the requests for services, psychiatric nursing expanded its practice in scope and direction. The mid-1980s witnessed the impact of economic constraints on mental health services and the shortcomings of deinstitutionalization. The challenge as we approach the 21st century is for psychiatric mental health nursing to incorporate research findings from the cognitive and biological sciences especially as they relate to symptom management and reduction, information processing, and communication. Psychiatric nursing has the opportunity to provide leadership through its role as a generalist in traditional service institutions, creative units of services such as nursing clinics and centers, and through its role as a clinical specialist in practice, research, and consultation. This fifth edition is presented with the following objectives in mind:

1. Integrate research contributions from the sociocultural, neurobiological, behavioral

---

* NOTE TO INSTRUCTORS: A Testbank and Teacher's Manual is available for this edition of *Psychiatric Nursing in the Hospital and Community*. Please contact Appleton & Lange if you are interested in obtaining these aids.

and cognitive sciences into a theoretical framework for practice.

2. Emphasize the role of information processing, communication, and psychiatric mental health nursing practice.

3. Present new clinical techniques useful in patient situations for nurses to add to their nursing practice in general and which are based on the ANA Division of Psychiatric Mental Health Nursing Statement on Practice and 1982 Standards of Psychiatric Mental Health Nursing Practice.

4. Integrate psychiatric nursing diagnoses and the *DSM-III-R* through clinical case examples.

5. Present clinical nursing research for integration into nursing practice.

6. Respond to the comments and suggestions recommended by instructors and students who have reviewed and studied from the fourth edition of this text.

PART ONE, "Introduction" includes two chapters that apply the humanistic perspective to both student and patient. We first make nurses aware of the subjective experiences of their predecessors in order for them to appreciate that their anxieties are understandable. The subjective experiences of patients are then presented to keep in sight from the very beginning that patients are real, live persons with extraordinary capacities to sense what is going on around them. The content for both chapters is derived from a research model in which a group is gathered to discuss a specific topic, the data is recorded and reduced, and the themes conceptualized for transfer back to a general audience. New to this section is childrens' responses to being hospitalized on an in-patient child and adolescent psychiatric unit.

PART TWO, "Theoretical Frameworks in Psychiatric Mental Health Nursing," has expanded the knowledge base that nurses bring with them to psychiatric mental health nursing. The concept of psychological equilibrium and mental health helps students to begin to appreciate the overall focus of the book—that is, the distress experienced by a person when his or her emotional status is disrupted. New chapters include Barbara J. Holder's "Sociocultural Issues of Mental Illness" that contributes to the influence of sociocultural components in understanding human behavior. Other new chapters include the contributions of the neurobiological sciences, the behavioral and cognitive sciences,

theories of personality, and life-span developmental theory. An updated chapter on assessing ego functions, self-representation, and mechanisms of defense provides a basis for understanding an individual's demeanor and personality style. Carol R. Hartman's chapter on "Communication Theory" completes the section for formulating a therapeutic communication model for psychiatric nursing practice.

PART THREE, "The Nursing Process in Psychiatric Mental Health Nursing," provides additional depth for understanding the basis for psychiatric mental health nursing practice. A chapter on psychiatric mental health nursing as an art and a science traces the roots of the discipline and confronts contemporary issues of defining the essence of psychiatric nursing from other mental health professions. A new chapter on "Assessment Protocols in Psychiatric Mental Health Nursing" by Ann W. Burgess and Carol R. Hartman provides protocols starting at the patient's point of entry into the health care system as well as assessing functional health status and the mental status examination. A new chapter on "Nursing Diagnosis" by Santa J. Kozak and Karla J. Hannibal incorporates the history and implementation of nursing diagnosis within the framework of case examples and nursing care plans. Updated chapters include Eileen E. Rinear's chapter on "Spiritual Dimensions of Psychiatric Mental Health Nursing," Carol R. Hartman's chapter on "Communication and the Therapeutic Process," and Joyce Kemp Laben and Colleen Powell MacLean's chapter on "Legal Aspects of Psychiatric Mental Health Nursing."

We attempt to conceptualize the therapeutic process in a way that enables nurses to maximize their individual human styles. Formulations and intellectualizations, which separate the nurse from the patient, are avoided. Subsequent chapters include techniques that facilitate the humanistic process and a description of stall factors that might impede the process.

PART FOUR, "Clinical Modalities in Psychiatric Mental Health Nursing," focuses on specific types of practice. A new chapter on the evolution of nursing thought traces the development of nursing and its convergence with an articulated framework for practice. The chapter on conceptual models of psychiatric nursing care helps the student understand the theoretical basis for the clinical modality in order to be able to practice the therapy. Carol R. Hartman and Margaret Knight have updated the "Pharmacotherapy" chapter to include current research in drug education, management, and treatment. A new chapter by Ann Bertrand-Clark on "Milieu Management" describes the history and role of the psychiatric nurse in this model of care. Updated chapters include "Individual Psychotherapies" and "Crisis Theory and Intervention" by Ann W. Burgess. A new chapter by Ann W. Burgess and Carol R. Hartman on "Trauma Therapy" implements a conceptual framework drawn from the cognitive sciences of information processing theory to a case of child abuse. Gloria E. Shapiro's updated chapter on "Family Work in Nursing Practice," Ann W. Burgess' updated chapters on "Working with Groups" and "Liaison Consultation and Community Mental Health Practice," and Selina Kassels' expanded chapter on "Psychological Testing and Psychological Measurement" complete this section.

PART FIVE, "Clinical Syndromes and Human Responses," applies what has been learned thus far to the various syndromes that are encountered in clinical practice. Some persons believe that psyhiatric diagnostic categories are not relevant to the practice of psychiatric-mental health practice. Although there are limitations to the use of psychiatric diagnostic categories, we believe the historically derived syndromes do lend themselves to study of the human dimension. Concurrently we also present, from the nursing perspective, a human response to actual or potential problems. Thus, the first chapter in this part integrates psychiatric diagnoses from the *DSM-III-R* and nursing diagnoses. This view values interdisciplinary collaboration between nursing and psychiatry and conceptualizes each syndrome as a complex of feelings, thoughts, and behaviors, all of which represent ways of coping with human miseries. In this way, clinical pathology may be treated independent of psychiatric diagnosis. Clinicians with special areas of expertise have contributed to these chapters: "Childhood Disorders" and "Adolescent Disorders" include updated content by Maureen P. McCausland; "Eating Disorders" includes updated content by Constance M. Cariono and Patricia Chmelko; "Treating the Drug Abuser" includes updated content by Christine Vourakis and Gerald Bennett; "Alcoholism: A Treatable Disease" includes updated content by Mary H. Hennessey; "Sexual Disorders" includes updated content by Ann W. Burgess, Carol R. Hartman, and Christine A. Grant; "Stress Response and Physical Illness" includes updated content by Nancy R. Starefos and Marita Prater; and "Developmental

Disabilities" includes updated content by Eunice Shishmanian. Also included in this section are updated chapters on organic mental disorders, schizophrenic disorders, delusional disorders, mood disorders, anxiety disorders, somatoform disorders, and dissociative disorders.

PART SIX, "Special Populations," includes several new chapters related to client groups needing priority visibility. Maureen P. McCausland and Ann W. Burgess write on "Child Abuse and Neglect and Sexual Victimization"; Nancy Worley writes on "The Chronically Mentally Ill"; Marcia A. Ullman writes on "Aging and Mental Health"; and Janis Davidson writes on "The Psychosocial Issues Concerning AIDS." Also included in this section are updated chapters on the suicidal patient, a new chapter on the combative patient, and updated content related to victims of rape and family violence.

This book addresses itself to the increasing clinical responsibilities of psychiatric mental health nurses, who, in many situations, have become primary caretakers. Because nurses are often the first ones to see a patient (and sometimes the only ones) it is necessary for psychiatric mental health nurses to become general practitioners of psychiatric mental health care, and possess a broad range of information that will enable them to determine which specialists, if any, need to be called upon.

In summary, the emphasis of this text is on communicating with patients and on understanding their humanism within a theoretical framework. Psychiatric nursing's commitment to a model of communication which supports the healing processes of the individual, family, and community, and to raising the human dimension of patienthood to its proper perspective, provides a solid basis for optimal treatment to be possible in the delivery of mental health care services. I wish to thank Elizabeth Jane Burgess, Margaret Smith Hamilton, Carol R. Hartman, Anna Melone Pollack, Eleanor Rosenwald, Gloria Edelhauser Shapiro, Carolyn J. Thomas, Dawn Huber Warrington, and graduate students at the University of Pennsylvania School of Nursing for contributions of clinical examples cited in the book.

My warmest thanks go to Elizabeth, Benton, Clayton, and Sarah Burgess, and above all, I owe a special debt to Allen G. Burgess for computer programming assistance and suggestions through all phases of the manuscript revision.

A. W. B.
Boston and Philadelphia

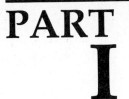

PART I

Introduction

The Introduction helps the reader to develop an attitude of involvement with the human dimension. To do this, students must perceive patients as they really are, regardless of the particular setting in which they are found, and must at the same time understand their own reactions to these patients

CHAPTER 1: STUDENT REACTION TO PSYCHIATRIC NURSING

Being aware of their own thoughts, feelings, and actions in the beginning of the psychiatric nursing experience facilitates the students' understanding of the human dimension.

CHAPTER 2: THROUGH THE EYES OF THE PATIENT

Knowledge of the thoughts, feelings, and actions of the child and adult patient also facilitates the students' understanding of the human dimension.

Chapter 1

Student Reaction to Psychiatric Nursing

Ann Wolbert Burgess

Chapter Objectives

The students successfully attaining the goals of this chapter will be able to:

- Examine their own subjective feelings and reactions to beginning a clinical experience in psychiatric nursing.
- Compare their own feelings to other students' reactions, noting where possible the reasons for these feelings.
- Resolve past nursing experiences before beginning a new nursing experience in order to ensure a strong commitment to the new experience.
- Identify their own behavior as a basis for understanding the behavior of other people.
- Acknowledge that anxieties are understandable when starting a new clinical experience.
- Discuss *autognosis* as a self-assessment concept essential for humanistic nursing practice.
- Identify the content in this chapter as a descriptive research approach to conceptualizing student reactions to psychiatric nursing.

One's initial experience in a new setting can trigger a broad spectrum of human responses. Consider the following statement.

. . . terror, that was what I felt. My legs literally wobbled as I walked down the corridor. I couldn't even remember the name of the person I was looking for. . . . Then I looked and saw her . . . sitting at the table with a knife in her hand. She was sitting there peeling apples. . . . I just wished she would hurry up and run out of apples or finish the pie or that three o'clock would come. I was afraid to say anything; afraid to talk. . . . What if she asked me a question? What would I say? I thought the id in my mind would come out and say something.

The feelings described above are those of a nursing student on her first day on a psychiatric ward. She is concerned that her fears are unique

NOTE: This chapter has been adapted from Chapter 1 of A. W. Burgess, *Psychiatric Nursing in the Hospital and the Community,* 4th ed. (Englewood Cliffs, N.J.: Prentice-Hall, Inc., 1981).

to her and that they symbolize her inability to function effectively as a psychiatric nurse. This student's reaction in anticipating her first psychiatric contact is, in fact, quite normal.

In this chapter, we will first describe a wide range of normal questions, worries, and fears experienced by beginners in psychiatric nursing. The authors gathered this material during group discussions with nursing students who had just completed their second visit to a psychiatric ward, and through informal discussions with students who had completed outpatient and community rotations. Second, we will discuss the difference between the role-appropriate and the subjective (idiosyncratic) feelings and reactions of the nurse. Finally, we will discuss *autognosis*, the process whereby nurses learn to understand the clinical situation by observing their own feelings and reactions to patients.

SPECIFIC REACTIONS TO PSYCHIATRIC PATIENTS

Feeling Anxious before the First Interview

1. I have a friend who is in a psychiatric hospital—locked up and bars on the windows. He was having problems with drugs. I thought the hospital would be like that one.

2. I went in blank, not knowing what to expect. You hear stories about keys and locked doors. I didn't know what to talk to my patient about. Mental hospitals are so stereotyped—set up on a hill.

3. I was looking forward to this experience till the first class, and then I began to wonder how I was going to react to my patient. I was really shaking on the bus going over. I didn't know what I'd find there. Then my patient talked to me and told me how scared she was, and I forgot how scared I was listening to *her*.

4. In every phase of nursing I'm ready to jump in and love it. Each new experience is something different and I'm looking forward to it. But the psychiatric hospital wasn't a situation I automatically jumped into. The whole six-week vacation before this experience I thought about how I'd feel when I came here. But this is another part of nursing, and I want to do well in all parts of nursing. But psychiatric nursing scares you and bothers you—just knowing you have to go into the hospital and talk with a patient. I'm the type who talks a lot and when I got to my patient's door, I couldn't even say her

name. When her roommate said she wasn't there, I was so relieved. But then I knew I would have another day to wait, and the other students had already talked to their patients. . . . I just hope I get along with this patient and that I don't chatter a lot.

In anticipating the first interview the student commonly feels frightened and inadequate to the task. As it is with many new ventures, we have fantasies about the very worst happening. These fantasies can come from past experience (see statement 1), from stories or stereotypes (see statement 2), or from the depths of our imaginations. It would be most unusual for the student to feel calm and assured before a first interview.

Feeling Useless and Appearing like a Beginner

5. I was excited this summer, thinking of coming to the psychiatric hospital, because I think the mind is very important—maybe even more so than the body in terms of feeling well. I had visions of really helping the patients—really trying and being able to do something. But when I got there, I had the feeling that I'm not as intelligent as a doctor and maybe I won't really be able to get into this as I want. I began to worry that I'd be failing at this, and that I wouldn't have enough knowledge to help this person.

6. I wondered what good I could be to someone; I have no knowledge of psychological problems.

7. I remember being told in Fundamentals if a patient asked us if this was our first time doing a dressing, to look rather indignant. I was trying to think how I could look like this wasn't the first time I had even been in a place like this . . . how I could look like this was something I had done before.

The major theme of statements 5 and 6 is the lack of enough knowledge to be helpful to the patient. If students do not know how to help, they are in the awkward situation of looking like beginners (see statement 7).

The students' feelings and concerns are normal and understandable. They are beginners. They do not know what to do and must learn to deal with the uncertainty of a first experience.

In another sense, students in psychiatric nursing are never beginners. They have spent years talking with and listening to people. Many nonpatients (friends and relatives) have turned to them for psychological help in time of trouble. Even more important, they have undoubtedly experienced their own personal problems and sometimes shared them with others. The students certainly have a great deal to learn about listening and talking, but they already have a good start.

Will the Patient Talk?

Many students voiced concern over whether or not the patient would talk.

8. When the patient saw me, she got right on the phone and stayed there for 30 minutes. She wouldn't even talk to me.
9. I was afraid the patient wouldn't talk, but she is talking really well and I feel extremely lucky.
10. My patient doesn't talk. She said it's because she doesn't trust anyone. It seems everyone else's patient is talking to them, so I feel it must be something wrong with me.

It certainly is easier for beginning students, who are understandably anxious, to work with verbal patients. If patients speak little or are mute, students feel compelled to speak, although they are unsure of whether or not this will be helpful to the patient. Students must remember, however, that it is the patient's problem—not the student's—that the patient is not verbal. Students should not begin by assuming that they are failing. Instead, they should ask themselves what it is about the patient's past experience and present illness that leads to the current state of mental functioning. What the student can do to help may then become more apparent.

It may be appropriate to ask patients why they are silent. It also may be useful to sit with the patient in silence. It may even be therapeutic to leave the patient. Which course of action makes most sense will depend on the assessment of the individual patient.

Wanting to Know the Patient's History before the Interview

Whether it is necessary or useful to have background information about the patient before the first interview is a controversial issue. Sentiments reflecting different points of view are described below.

11. What confuses me is that the patient knows what he is there for, and we walk in and say we are students. The patients know we're to ask them about their illness and they know what they are there for, but we are out in the cold because we know little about them.
12. I would like to have the patient's family background and environmental background. We were just told the bare essentials like age, sex, religion, and diagnosis, and that was it; then we had to go and talk to our patients. . . . I'd like to know what got my patient so upset. When my patient told me about her family, it was all very new and I didn't know how to react. I had no idea what in the environment had upset her so much, and therefore I had trouble saying anything. . . . With a physical disease or an operation, if you know what they have, you know how to deal with them.
13. I don't agree. You can read a chart and prejudge patients. We're here to listen and understand them and help them communicate. If you know the background, what's the sense of talking to them? You're trying to find out what's troubling them and if you already know, they can probably sense this . . . and with emotional illness, it isn't so clear-cut. It's not like the patient has this symptom and this is the way she'll act.

If it is thought best to learn by not having the history prior to the interview, the student need not be concerned. The patient does not necessarily expect that the student will have read the chart. He might even resent the student's knowing more about him than he was willing to reveal himself.

On the other hand, it may be that the student's desire to know the historical details before meeting the patient reflects understandable anxiety over making contact with the patient. Knowing the history may allow the student to feel more in control of the situation and therefore less anxious.

Some Unpleasant Reactions to the First Interview

The Patient Rejects the Student

14. My patient rejected having any student nurse. Before seeing her, I had tried to build up my self-confidence. I walked in and told her who I was, and she said she didn't want anything to do with a student nurse. I could feel my self-confidence slipping away. I tried to think that she doesn't know us and it must be from past

experiences. She kept saying that she had no intention of being talked to by a student nurse.

15. My patient was hiding from me. She'd make all kinds of excuses not to see me, like she had to put her makeup on or go to lunch or something. I looked one whole hour for her; all I'm doing is chasing her. She makes me feel like a jerk.

16. My patient immediately told me she only told her doctor about her problem and she had no intention of telling me. She just talked about superficial things.

The patient's rejection of the student nurse during the initial interview is not uncommon. In statement 14, the student made the astute observation that the patient did not know anything about the students. Therefore, the patient must be reacting to her own past experience. One can only speculate what that experience might have been. Perhaps a previous student was not helpful. More likely the patient has recently "lost" a student through graduation or the completion of training. The patient still misses the student, is angry about the termination, and refuses to establish a new relationship. (If the new student learns that this is why the patient is resisting the new relationship, a supervisor should offer some techniques for establishing a working relationship with the patient.) The patient's statement that she did not want to be "talked to" by a student nurse may indicate the patient's misunderstanding of the nurse–patient relationship. It is to be hoped that the patient will be listened to and be engaged in dialogue rather than be "talked to."

There are many other reasons why a patient rejects a student. For example, the patient may prefer to keep all personal material between herself and her therapist. The patient may have a child who is close in age to the student and she cannot tell her new "child" certain personal problems. The patient may be angry at her therapist; and the anger is then displaced onto the next person who enters the room—the student nurse.

The Student Becomes Depressed

17. I had a patient who has been depressed for years. It was hard to set a goal with her. I wanted to bring her out of depression, but I knew I couldn't. She told me everything she had done in life was a failure; she didn't like herself; she wanted me to take her down to the railroad tracks. . . . It's depressing.

18. This experience is depressing me beyond words. I was sitting listening to the social worker talk to us and I almost fell asleep. And I know I wasn't tired. I knew I had to go up and talk to my patient after the class. While I was seeing her, I couldn't wait to get out of there. This had something to do with my having to talk with her.

Although there are many reasons why the student may feel depressed, one of the most common reasons is the student's feeling of helplessness, a normal reaction, especially for the beginner. This feeling diminishes considerably once the student becomes better acquainted with the tools of psychiatric nursing. The patient who is depressed often communicates his mood to the nurse (or to anyone who listens). One may say that the patient's feelings are contagious. In this situation the nurse's depression tells us more about the patient than about the nurse.

The Student Is Overwhelmed

19. I wasn't looking forward to this experience at all. Walking into this hospital and seeing the group of patients who just haven't made it floored me.

This student came to the psychiatric experience with more negative feelings than most beginners; she did not look forward "at all" to this experience. Feeling overwhelmed by seeing patients who "just haven't made it" may be a result of several factors, such as discomfort over relatives or friends suffering from mental illness or the student's own concerns about "making it."

The Student Is "Strained"

20. My patient just sits there and I feel like I have to pull the information from her. It's such a strain and I feel like I am talking to a wall.

The experience of having to "pull the information" is common in certain patient groups such as those suffering from depression. The experience of the "strain" is most probably related to the clinical situation and not to the specific characteristics of the student.

The Student Is Interviewed by the Patient

21. My patient completely reversed the situation and asked me all about myself. She was very

good at questioning me, and I had to stop and realize what was going on.

The experience of being interviewed by the patient is related more to the style of the patient than to the specific characteristics of the student. The patient who attempts to interview the helper wants to be in control of the situation and is having a difficult time being a patient. The student took the proper first step by stopping to realize what was going on.

The Student Is Angered by the Patient

22. I was surprised at my reaction of anger when I talked to a group of patients. It seemed they were indulging themselves in their depression. It was as if they were each trying to say their own depression was the worst.

The Patient Attempts to Embarrass the Student

23. The first time I went to see my patient, he said, "Well, here's the zoo and here's the animals in it, and now you've observed it and you can go back and tell everyone about it." I told him it wasn't a zoo and he was a human being.

The patient feels like he is an animal in a zoo. He then projects his feelings onto the student, whom he accuses of seeing him as an animal in a zoo. The patient, feeling uncomfortable, tries to make the student uncomfortable. The student handled the situation superbly by respectfully pointing out the reality of the situation to him. The student does not share the patient's view of himself as an animal but perceives him as a human being.

The Students' Concern about Their Own Mental Health

A common concern of student nurses and others beginning their training in psychiatric nursing is the fear that they will discover mental illness in themselves. In addition, there is also the concern that they will "catch" the illness from the patient or that the patient will drive them crazy.

24. I was riding the subway the other day and looking around. I saw lots of people that should have been in this hospital. There's such a thin line.

25. I'm afraid I'll be left here.

26. We've all been aware of certain phrases like, "It's driving me crazy or whacky or nuts."

27. I wonder how stable everyone is. At what point do people lose their ability to cope?

28. My patient said she was afraid of driving in New York City, and I cut her short and changed the subject because that is a problem I have and it bothered me to hear her say it. I have all the problems my patient has and I think I should stay here.

The student is correct in observing similarities between the patient and herself. This observation is a result of the health of the patient rather than any sickness of the student. Hospitalized psychiatric patients are healthy in many ways. Their area of illness often encompasses only a small aspect of their total personality.

Students may also be concerned about their own phobias, minor mood swings, and idiosyncrasies. They should bear in mind that these symptoms and aspects of their own personalities are commonly found in normal populations. Illness is measured less by what one thinks and feels than by how one functions.

The Concern That the Patient Will Demand Too Much

29. I was told before seeing the patient that the last nurse had helped him so much that he developed a mother complex or Oedipus complex toward her. Now I don't know if I want to be a mother to him, and I don't know how to avoid this.

30. First thing my patient did was to ask me to bring her a candy bar, which I did. The second meeting she immediately asked if I brought the candy bar—didn't even say good morning or anything. I think this was a test to see if I would bring it, but it is to the point where she'll ask other things of me like when she gets privileges, she wants me to go down town shopping with her. I don't know how I'll react to the situation.

In statement 29 the student was concerned that the patient would expect her to be a mother or a lover. In statement 30 the patient was already expecting that the student would be more than a nurse.

Patients often have expectations of the students (and other therapeutic personnel) above and beyond their designated professional roles.

Students need to understand that these needs and wishes are the patient's problem. They must set the proper limits on the relationship without offending the patient. The student will often need supervisory assistance with many patients who present such requests as described above.

The Fear of Hurting the Patient

Hurting the patient is a common fear of students.

31. If the patient isn't there the second day, I have the fear that I drove him away.

32. I felt it was my fault when the patient walked away from me. I didn't know what to do.

33. I was afraid I'd make my patient feel on display; like making her feel she was different and that was why I was there to see her.

34. My patient started crying and talking about suicide right away. I didn't know what to do. I felt if she went home and committed suicide, it would be my fault because I didn't know what to say to her.

35. Most of us are afraid of saying something wrong. We don't want to harm the patient. I think these patients are very sensitive to what we say. I was afraid to ask the patient about her illness, afraid it would upset her. I couldn't see what good I'd do as a nursing student.

Patients are stronger than we often give them credit for. Furthermore, they are forgiving even when we do make a clumsy statement.

The patient in statement 34 who started crying and talking of suicide was merely responding with what was on her mind to an interested student. The student did not cause the patient to feel suicidal. Of course, the student should report this information to someone on the staff. If the student listens with respect and is appropriately supportive in asking questions, the patient will not be hurt.

The Fear of Being Hurt by the Patient

The students often bring to the patient contact some fears of being physically or psychologically hurt by the patient.

36. I had a fear of being clobbered. I knew it wouldn't really happen, but somehow the feeling was there. While talking with this one patient, I knew he felt closed in and at times banged his fist against the wall. I had the thought, What if he banged his fist on my head?

37. After the first day I was anxious to hear how everyone else's day went, and I'd ask classmates how their day went and they would ask me back. I wanted to know if my day was like theirs. I had fears because of the stories I had heard, like getting physically hurt, the stories of broken jaws and murders. But I wasn't thinking too much about it till I was late for class and I went to open the door to go out and it was locked. Suddenly it came to me that I was on a psychiatric ward with the door locked and no one around to let me out. I knew a moment of pure panic.

38. I was afraid the patient would yell at me if I said the wrong thing.

Although it is common for the student to fear being hurt by the patient, it is quite improbable that such an event will ever occur.

Being Honest

39. I told my patient who I was and this was part of my nursing training and I wanted to talk with her and would she mind. She asked if she had to talk with me and I said no, so she said she'd talk and she sure did. I didn't expect that.

This statement illustrates how a simple direct statement together with an attitude of respect can be effective in beginning a therapeutic encounter.

Differences between Psychiatric and Medical-Surgical Nursing

The nursing students discussed several aspects in which they felt psychiatric nursing differs from medical-surgical nursing.

40. We just came from medical-surgical nursing where we seemed to be able to do things for the patients. Now as I sit with my patient, I wonder what good I can be to her. By my patient's telling me of her experiences, I don't feel I am accomplishing anything.

41. In a medical problem you can always do something to make the patients feel better. You can rub their backs, for instance. You are touching them and making them feel better. You cannot do that in psychiatric nursing.

These sentiments express the subjective sense of uselessness and lack of accomplishment in psychiatric nursing in contrast to the feeling of being able to do something in medical-surgical nursing. It is true that one does more for a patient in a physical way in medical-surgical nursing. Physical efforts prove to students that they are working and accomplishing something. In psychiatric nursing one has to be psychologically active but physically passive much of the time. It takes some time to realize that listening to what aches in the hearts of patients may touch them more profoundly than a back rub.

42. Each experience is so new each time. After the first day I went to my text, but I couldn't find my patient anywhere in the book; she wasn't written up.

The Student in the Community and Other Ambulatory Settings

43. Some of the families with whom I worked had numerous "helpers"—social workers, school counselors, ministers, child protection workers, etc. Sometimes in working with these families and all of the agencies I felt fragmented and confused. I wondered if these families ever felt confused by dealing with so many people— all of them trying to be helpful, yet all seeing the problem from different perspectives. One day I realized that the best way to be helpful to these families was to attempt to coordinate all of their helping systems into a cohesive whole. With the help of their primary welfare workers, I was able to decrease some of the confusion among the helpers. Sometimes when you're the primary nurse-therapist, you have to create a helping system for the client.

The nurse's experience in the community and in other ambulatory settings often elicits a set of questions, concerns, and feelings quite different from those aroused during inpatient services.

1. The nurse may feel like an alien intruder as she enters the patient's world, often a racially or ethnically homogeneous community different from her own. As a result, she may feel anxious over her separateness, embarrassed by her newly discovered prejudices, and confused over whether the patient's behavior is psychopathology or just cultural style.
2. Working with ambulatory patients com-

monly leads to two additional areas of concern. First, the problems of the outpatient may seem so subtle (as compared to inpatients) that the student wonders why he (the outpatient) is seeking help. Second, outpatients usually return home after seeing just one clinician, in contrast to inpatients who remain hospitalized in the care of many clinicians. As a result, the student is apt to experience a sense of anxiety, uncertainty, and undue responsibility in the early days of the outpatient rotation.

ROLE-APPROPRIATE VERSUS SUBJECTIVE (IDIOSYNCRATIC) FEELINGS AND REACTIONS

Role-appropriate feelings and reactions are those that are understandable, normal, and natural for a given situation. For example, it is appropriate for a boxer to strike his opponent in the boxing arena, for an actor to embrace a strange actress in a screen play, for an auto mechanic to lie on his back dirtying his hands in a garage, for a surgeon to open someone's abdomen in the operating room, for a physician or nurse to examine a nude body in the hospital. Yet these specific behaviors, appropriate in the contexts described above, are obviously inappropriate in almost all other situations.

It is often an unsettling experience when one moves into a role in which new and strange feelings and behaviors become appropriate— the medical student making an incision into a cadaver, the soldier firing his weapon during battle, the nursing student listening to a patient's most intimate personal details during a nursing interview.

Under the circumstances of assuming a new role, the students' reactions described in the preceding pages are for the most part appropriate. The students feel anxious because they do not know what will happen; they fear the worst—that they will hurt or be hurt by the patients, they will "catch" the patients' illnesses, that they will reject or be rejected by the patients, or that the patients will demand too much of them, or that the patients will recognize them as beginners. The students are unsure of how to say "hello" and "good-bye"; they do not know if they should be honest with the patients or if they should learn the patients' histories ahead of time.

After the initial experiences, the students often feel strained, angered, embarrassed, or depressed; it seems that all their fears have been confirmed. However, as they become more experienced and less overwhelmed by the unpleasant worries of the beginner, the therapeutic feelings of caring, concern, compassion, sensitivity, and understanding become stronger.

Whereas role-appropriate feelings and reactions are natural and understandable for given situations, subjective (or idiosyncratic) feelings and reactions have more to do with the special characteristics of the student. In other words, each student may react to a patient in a slightly different way because of her special personality and past experiences.

For example, the student who has a father suffering from alcoholism might put forth special therapeutic energies or feel disgust and hostility in caring for an alcoholic patient. The student may also react to a patient on the basis of a physical resemblance to a friend or relative. Again, depending on the relationship, the student may react to the patient in an authoritarian, competitive, seductive, helpless, punitive, or protective manner—as if the patient were a friend or relative.

The students' reactions to patients, whether appropriate to the situation or based on their subjective reactions, may either facilitate or stall the therapeutic process.

The following are examples of therapeutic responses.

1. The student or nurse in the role of a helping, caring person communicates this attitude to the patient, who then feels supported and reassured.

2. The students who have had positive relationships with their grandparents may react subjectively in an unusually supportive and respectful manner to older patients.

The following are examples of reactions that stall the therapeutic process.

1. Students in their normal concern over being a beginner make several clumsy remarks that make the patient more anxious.

2. Students in treating patients who resemble their

own formidable fathers feel intimidated in their therapeutic attempts with older men.

AUTOGNOSIS

Therapeutic skill is rooted in a nurse's mastery of both technical and personal aspects of intervention. Clinical training is an intensive learning process undertaken to develop the professional skills and competence of a nursing student. It is the bridge that enables and enhances the application of academic and theoretical concepts to the specific nurse within the context of actual nursing intervention. Within the field of psychiatric nursing, a plethora of models and beliefs about human behavior and change exist as well as an abundance of training interventions and strategies. However, there is one element that is common to every training model: interventions are conducted by people within an interpersonal situation. Consequently, the common thread between training programs is the "self" of the nurse in a relationship with a patient. Despite process recordings or tape recorders, it is a human person who is alone in a room with the patient or a family. In the therapeutic setting, the individual nurse uses his or her expertise and knowledge, as well as personal life experiences and value system, to engage with patients in ways that will improve the quality of the patients' lives.

The critical question emerges and challenges the beginning student: how to develop the competency of the "self" in the nurse? The answer includes the need to tune into one's internal processes, or autognosis.

Positive Use of Autognosis

Autognosis (auto-diagnosis) is the process by which nurses can diagnose and understand a clinical situation by paying acute attention to their own feelings, thoughts, and behaviors toward patients. In order to develop and make use of this exquisitely sensitive clinical tool, nurses must first get accustomed to and comfortable with the ideas that (1) they respond to various patients with a complexity of feelings—both negative and positive; (2) such subjective responses to patients are universal; and (3) the presence of negative subjective feelings, if not acted upon, does no harm to the patient.

Nurses may react to patients in a variety of subjective ways. They may feel warmth, caring, or sexual arousal, leading to the wish to nurture, hold, cradle, cling, understand, invite to dinner, or approach sexually. On the other hand, they also may feel disgust, rejection, abuse, or fear, leading to the desire to reject, assault, or abandon.

As nurses discuss these feelings with their peers, they will learn that certain feelings are fairly predictable given the clinical situation. For example, a strong, young, psychotic male generally elicits some anxiety in most clinicians. On the other hand, certain feelings are specific reactions to a particular nurse's prior experience. Regardless of whether nurses' subjective responses are common or unusual, they can learn to count on having similar responses whenever such a clinical situation arises. Therein lies its diagnostic value. For instance, if I always feel restless and annoyed in a particular way whenever a patient becomes manipulative, I can use this very sense of restlessness and annoyance as a diagnostic clue that some manipulation is occurring, even when it is not obvious.

In addition to autognosis being used to diagnose clinical conditions, it can be helpful in diagnosing stalls or clinical impasses. For instance, when things are not going well clinically, nurses can realize that they are being affected by the patient in an unusual way, such as when they find themselves coming late, dreaming about the patient, thinking incessantly about the patient, behaving in unusual ways toward the patient, or being excessively pessimistic or optimistic. These autognostic clues alert nurses that they are being affected by the patient in a specific way that requires further exploration.

Increasing Self-awareness

How do nurses enhance their self-awareness as a clinical tool? There are several ways in which nurses can explore their responses to patients and, in turn, increase their self-awareness. Hartman outlines three routes to self-awareness as (1) involvement in relationships; (2) reading; and (3) writing.[1]

Communication with others and involvement in relationships is an important way to learn about oneself. One's first social network—the family—is a primary learning arena. Family relationships provide some of the most enduring lessons in self-awareness. The second social network system—school—provides additional lessons through relationships with teachers. Teachers usually assume positions of influence to the degree that the student allows the influence process to develop. In nursing, the student–supervisor relationship can be an influential avenue for self-awareness. The relationship with a mentor is another valuable and influential one. A mentor, writes Hartman, is a guide who provides a relationship in which the intellectual and career development of another person is supported, facilitated, and promoted.[2] Sometimes an instructor or supervisor becomes a mentor. The mentor's expertise and caring are a powerful combination in guiding the nurse's growth in self-knowledge. Lessons learned in these various relationships are modified by subsequent life experiences that usually include additional deep and lasting relationships.

Counseling and therapy are additional ways to learn about oneself. If the nurse happens to be in therapy or counseling, s/he has a ready-made situation in which to learn autognosis. Or nursing students may elect to work with a therapist as a route to learning how to be more effective in therapeutic relationships with patients. Through this exchange, the nurse creates an opportunity to gain greater self-awareness, a more positive regard for the self, and personal characteristics that increase effectiveness in working with patients.

Reading is a second route to self-awareness. Through the formal study of psychiatric mental health nursing, students are exposed to written ideas about clinical practice. The habit of reading should always be encouraged. Reading fiction and nonfiction helps one learn about human nature as well as about oneself. Books portray human lives in terms of human struggles and emotions and the ways in which people relate themselves to others. Autobiographies are rich sources of detail about the personal experiences of people. One nursing text, *Perspectives on Nursing Theory*, employs a modified autobiographical style. This text edited by Leslie Nicoll[3] includes both a collection of seminal articles on the critical thinking in the nursing theory-development movement and each author's autobiographical sketch and comments on the context and purposes that stimulated the original creation of the papers. The comments not only enhance the value and understanding of the individual's thinking but also give insights into the continuities and changes in thinking during the evolution of theory and research development in nursing.

The third route for enhancing self-awareness is writing in a diary, journal, or log. The student can write notes in a completely unstructured style as sporadically or regularly as desired to gain the most benefit from this personal experience.

Process recording is a more formal method of writing that helps students deal more effectively with patients. Process recordings are descriptions and analyses of interactions with patients. Various formats can be used, but the record usually includes a verbatim account of the nurse–patient communication. Process recordings contribute to the effectiveness of clinical supervision. Over time, at regular intervals, the process recordings can be reviewed and summarized to document major patterns or themes and overall progress of the nurse–patient interaction.

As nurses develop greater comfort and skill in autognosis, they will (1) become more effective as diagnosticians of patients and clinical processes and (2) be better able to reverse therapeutic stalls and avoid acting on feelings and impulses that would be detrimental to patient care.

Application of Self-awareness

The application of self-awareness and ways of developing the nurse into an effective healer is addressed by Beck, Rawlins, and Williams.[4] They placed particular emphasis on characteristics that are inherent in the nurses' self-awareness: awareness of self-regard, of beliefs and values, and of problems in living. In addition, the authors discuss self-awareness in five dimensions: physical, emotional, intellectual, social, and spiritual.

Awareness of Self-regard. Self-regard, in particular, thinking well of oneself, can have an important effect on the nurse's therapeutic effectiveness. Maintaining a positive self-regard for oneself while evaluating one's behavior and its impact on others enables the nurse to demonstrate creative and purposeful behavioral flexibility. Positive self-regard and flexibility free the nurse to use a greater range of choices in the therapeutic work.[5]

Awareness of Beliefs and Values. Beliefs and values strongly influence perceptions and interpersonal relationships. Some values have powerful effects, leading to rejection of involvement with others who have different beliefs. Other values matter to some degree but do not prevent interaction. Still others seem to matter little if at all in the course of relationships. The more optimistic the values and beliefs of the nurse, the more opportunities for the growth of others and oneself.

Awareness of Problems in Living. Nurses can experience problems in living similar to those that their patients experience. The therapeutic effectiveness of the nurse is enhanced by (1) acknowledgment of problems in living as opposed to denial of the problems; (2) an underlying optimism that the difficulties can be resolved and a higher level of health restored; and (3) a nonjudgmental attitude toward oneself or the client for having the problems in living.

Self-awareness in Five Dimensions. The nurse's physical being is a filter through which information about herself and the external world is exchanged. Self-awareness can be examined in the emotional dimension, which includes a sensitivity to feelings and mood states. Self-awareness in the intellectual dimension involves an understanding of thoughts and the impact of discussions and readings on one's inner state. Self-awareness in the social dimension requires attention to activities that are engaged in or rejected and the reason for doing so. Self-awareness in the value and spiritual dimension includes a sorting of key beliefs and presuppositions that are highly regarded.[6]

The growth of the self, observes Mauksch, is fostered through education, guidance, encouragement, and above all, through respectful recognition and support.[7] It is not enough to learn only theory, skills, and techniques. Learning about the self is extremely delicate, because such skills and sensitivities are difficult to define in conventional terms.

The development of the self of the nurse must be a continuous and ongoing process. Although the foregoing statement seems obvious, it is easy to fall into a daily routine that denies the time and energy needed for the nurturing of the self. When nurses ignore the development of the internal processes that enable them to recognize and deal with various interpersonal elements, they are unable to model for patients the integration of wellness or positive growth processes that are at the heart of the therapeutic process.[8] An alive and vibrant self is a source of energy and creativity that is of benefit to the therapeutic encounter as well as to the well-being of the nurse. The nurses maintain direct one-to-one contact with patients, their energies are renewed, and the danger of burnout is lessened.[9]

As nurses develop greater comfort and skill in autognosis, (1) they will become more effective as diagnosticians of patients and clinical processes; and (2) they will be better able to reverse therapeutic stalls and avoid acting on feelings and impulses that would be detrimental to patient care.[10]

Summary

There is a wide range of unpleasant but normal feelings, worries, and concerns that the nursing student experiences at the beginning of her psychiatric nursing work. A series of verbatim statements taken from a group discussion of students beginning the psychiatric nursing experience was presented to exemplify what neophytes in this clinical specialty area typically experience.

Almost all these feelings and reactions are role appropriate because they are normal or typical for the situation. If students are aware that these feelings are appropriate, they can be more comfortable with themselves and more therapeutic with patients.

In addition to role-appropriate feelings, there are subjective (idiosyncratic) reactions to the patient that are based more on the student's past experience than on the student's objectivity with the situation. Subjective feelings and reactions, like role-appropriate feelings, may be psychotherapeutic or may stall the therapeutic relationship.

In order to understand the feelings and reactions to clinical situations that stall the therapeutic process, students must develop the art of autognosis—the ability to understand the patient by identifying and describing their own thoughts and feelings. By doing so, students gain perspective and control of the situation. Making the unknown known reduces the mystique, the fear, and the insecurity that the feeling evokes. The nurse is then free to be therapeutic.

Questions

1. Define and give three examples of autognosis from your first days in psychiatric nursing.
2. List four comparable feelings between your own reactions to psychiatric nursing and another student's reactions.
3. Identify a nursing approach from a past nursing experience that you used to handle silence during an interview.
4. Differentiate between a previous nursing experience and the psychiatric nursing experience and analyze your reactions using the autognosis concept.
5. Discuss the research approach used to develop the content for this chapter.
6. Report on your experience in increasing self-awareness using one of the suggested methods.

REFERENCES AND SUGGESTED READINGS

1. Hartman, C. R. Developing a therapeutic relationship. In C. M. Beck, R. P. Rawlins, & S. R. Williams (Eds.), *Mental Health-Psychiatric Nursing*. St. Louis: C. V. Mosby, 1984.
2. Ibid.
3. Nicoll, L. H. (Ed.). *Perspectives on Nursing Theory*. Boston: Little, Brown, 1986.
4. Beck, C. M., Rawlins, R. P., & Williams, S. R., (Eds.), *Mental Health Psychiatric Nursing*. St. Louis: C. V. Mosby, 1984, pp. 162–165.
5. Hartman, op. cit., p. 165.
6. Ibid., p. 166.
7. Mauksch, H. O. Use of self: Towards a technology of helping. Unpublished manuscript, 1986.
8. Luthman, S. G., & Kirschenbaum, M. *The Dynamic Family*. Palo Alto, Calif.: Science and Behavior Books, 1974.
9. Baldwin, M., & Satir, V. (Eds.). The use of self in therapy. *Journal of Psychotherapy and the Family*, 1987, 3(1), p. 155.
10. Messner, E. Autognosis: Diagnosis by the use of the self. In A. Lazare (Ed.). *Outpatient Psychiatry*. Baltimore: Williams & Wilkins, 1979.

Chapter *2*

Through the Eyes of the Patient

Ann Wolbert Burgess and Ann Bertrand-Clark

Chapter Objectives

The students successfully attaining the goals of this chapter will be able to:

- Recognize a descriptive clinical research approach to conceptualizing child and adult reactions to becoming a psychiatric patient.
- Identify three reactions noted by individuals when they became psychiatric patients.
- Differentiate between role-appropriate and subjective feelings and reactions of child and adult patients.
- Identify seven areas where patients have advised that nurses might improve their clinical care.
- Compare and contrast patient concerns in institutional settings versus community and ambulatory settings.

Just as students experience a wide range of intense emotional reactions as they begin to work with psychiatric patients, the person designated "patient" also undergoes considerable emotional upheaval. Being unable to cope with the emotional problems of his daily life is painful enough. Now he carries the added burden of being considered (or considering himself) a psychiatric patient. He worries about his current feelings about himself and other people's reac-

NOTE: This chapter has been adapted from Chapter 2 of A. W. Burgess, *Psychiatric Nursing in the Hospital and the Community*, 4th ed. (Englewood Cliffs, N.J.: Prentice-Hall, Inc., 1981).

tions to him. As if that were not enough, he now has to contemplate what it will be like to be a patient in a psychiatric hospital.

The nurse must have some sense of the inner experience of the patient in order to be therapeutic. If the patient is frightened, the nurse can be therapeutic only if she knows that he is experiencing fear or anxiety, even if he gives the appearance of being brave. If the patient is sad, the nurse must respond to the sadness, even though the patient may conceal his sadness and attempt to amuse the staff.

To help the student understand the worries, fears, and wishes of the psychiatric patient,

15

the authors met with two groups of patients on a psychiatric ward in a general hospital. The patients were asked how they felt about coming to the hospital, how they felt nurses were helpful, and how they felt nurses could be more helpful.

After commenting on the various patient responses, we will discuss the distinction between role-appropriate and subjective feelings and reactions of the patient. Role-appropriate feelings are a direct result of patienthood and are shared by many patients. Subjective feelings, as we will describe, are determined by very special personal experiences from the patient's past.

ADULT PATIENT RESPONSES

Reactions to Becoming a Patient

The Patient is "Scared"

1. Felt very scared when my brother left and I was all alone in the hospital.
2. I was scared stiff coming in, but the staff reassured me and I took their word. I'm in a strange town and this is a strange hospital. I've never experienced something like this.
3. My fear is frustration and fright and pain—that is how I feel in this hospital.
4. I asked to be put here to get help. I'm nervous and get excited over small things. I've never been in a place like this.
5. I was scared to death when I came in here.
6. I felt parachuted into the middle of nowhere.

The above statements illustrate the fear, nervousness, and scared feelings that characterize almost all patients who enter a psychiatric hospital. Statements 2, 4, and 6 vividly illustrate the profound sense of being in a strange place—"something never before experienced," "parachuted into the middle of nowhere." Somewhere related to the strangeness is the sense of aloneness (see statement 1). Statement 4 illustrates the point that the patient is already troubled and nervous. As if that were not enough, she is then put "in a place like this."

These reactions to hospitalization are observed in all clinical settings: small and large wards, organized and disorganized hospitals, private and state hospitals. It is important to recognize the universality of these reactions because the nurse might attribute the patient's discomfort to the setting of a large, unpleasant ward and therefore feel there is no way that she can help.

Statement 2 indicates what the nurse can do. The supportive relationship of the nurse can be and often is everything to the new patient.

The Patient is Relieved

7. Home was such hell; this place is like heaven; it's no hassle.
8. I felt exhausted when I came in, physically and mentally. I was shot.
9. I came here to unwind.

Some patients are so overwhelmed by their life situations that the psychiatric ward is experienced more as a relief than a source of anxiety. These patients often elicit the reaction in staff that they are malingering, lazy, or indifferent. The nurse must keep in mind that the outside situation must have been desperate to warrant psychiatric hospitalization.

These patients may appear relatively comfortable throughout the hospitalization—until the discharge approaches. Then, as they face the return to the situation that overwhelmed them, all the anxiety that initially led to the hospitalization is reawakened. For this reason it is essential to deal with the outside situation before discharge.

Feelings about a Previous Hospitalization

The patient's reaction is often colored by his experience during a previous hospitalization.

10. I was here before. I didn't have much choice over coming. It was here or the other hospital and that place is awful. I didn't want to be put back here and I don't want to stay.
11. I spent six months in a violent ward. I remember another patient slugging me. It was scary and I thought this place might be the same way.
12. I feel like a failure when I have to come back here. To reenter the hospital every few years is something I can't cope with. When I come back, I know I haven't made it.

The patient may behave as if something terrible will happen to him because something terrible may have happened to him in the past. Once the nurse learns about these past experiences, they can be discussed and be put into proper perspective.

Statement 12 illustrates the patient's feelings of failure on having to return. This feeling is certainly understandable. Often the staff also feels a sense of disappointment and failure on seeing a former patient return. This staff reaction must be guarded against so that the patient's sense of failure is not intensified. The nurse must understand that some psychiatric illnesses are chronic as are certain kinds of medical illness. That some patients need *only* to be hospitalized intermittently, not continuously, is a tribute to current methods of treatment.

Patients' Advice to Nurses

The patient is an acute observer of the clinical situation. We have all been a patient at some time, either in a hospital or in a doctor's office or clinic. In this situation many of us feel that if only someone would listen, we could improve clinical care.

Don't Avoid Human Contact

13. Please talk to me rather than go to that staff meeting or into the nurse's office. When you reach out to a person at a certain moment, to another human being for help, you reach out in that moment and it becomes so important to reach out. Then to have some mundane type of staff meeting become more important than a human being. . . .

14. Don't you get sick of having to do all the clerical work of writing notes and reports?

Although the nurse must write reports and attend conferences, it is important to understand that these activities may be perceived by the patients as devices to avoid contact. In fact, nurses will acknowledge that they do use the nurse's office and the clerical work to avoid patients when they feel psychologically exhausted or repulsed by particular patients.

Don't Depersonalize the Patient

15. Please avoid labels, all labels in all forms: the white uniform, the secretary at the desk. No labels! That helped me break through a lot of inhibitions. I don't think I would have made it had I been put into a hospital bed somewhere, with the white sheets, white pillowcase, very antiseptic with a tray and the bed rolled up and the white sheet closing around it, everything white. I might have been rested but not helped with my problems. I merely would have been

brought back to a state where I'd previously been treated for exhaustion and nothing more.

The patient is asking for the staff to treat him personally, to interact with him, to provide more than a sterile rest.

16. Nurses come in and immediately I am scared of a needle. Sometimes they don't use psychology; they just stick that needle in your arm like it was a piece of meat. Nothing about it; that's just it; no technique. Maybe if they came in with a green needle or a joke, it would help. I had blood taken and the nurse hardly said hello.

The patient is asking, among other things, to be treated not like a piece of meat but like a human being.

Don't be Snide

17. I'll tell you what turns me off—Someone cracking a joke that you can take either way. Not a "ha ha" joke but a snide joke like, "Why don't you get out of bed? You spend all your time in bed. The only time you get up is to take your pills." Nurses should come on with a positive remark instead of trying to be smart or funny about it.

Don't be Bubbly

18. You don't have to come on as Susy Goodshoes and laugh and be bubbly all the time.

Don't Break Promises

19. I hate to be told someone will talk to me later, then never does. I won't go up and mention that they promised to come and talk. Patients hate to keep after the nurses for things.

20. I get upset when I tell a nurse something and nothing seems to be done about it, and I hate to repeat myself a second time. I figure if they didn't take care of it the first time, I am making a nuisance of myself to repeat it.

Clarify the Communication

21. How do things get communicated about what is told? I know the nurse and social worker talked with my boss, and I'd like to know what was said before I go in to work. I might make a damn fool out of myself if I don't know what is going on.

22. I'd like to know who tells who what. I tell the nurse I have a certain pain or feeling, and then

when I ask the doctor, he said he hadn't heard about it. How do you know what is important?

The patient makes an excellent point. It is the responsibility of the staff to clarify the communications among themselves.

Don't Put Me Down

23. The nurses showed no compassion. It never occurred to them that I was scared of the place. They thought, "Why, he's just trying to be difficult," and they were thoroughly rotten about the whole thing. I wanted someone to be concerned as to why I was scared. I was in severe pain and at the same time pretty well unhinged, and they kept saying, "Oh, come on, at your age, scared of hospitals. Ha! Ha! Ha!" They must have thought I was an overgrown baby, but I was scared.

24. When you say "Hi" to someone and they give you a cold shoulder, it makes you feel bad. I don't like cold people and I think it is harmful.

25. Sometimes after I talk with a nurse I get this feeling, and I won't talk with them again. I feel they just talk with me so that they can go out and make a joke.

26. Last Friday night I was upset and frightened and wanted to go in the quiet room. One of the staff came in and said, "There's a $20 extra charge for this room." She should have asked me what was the matter. I felt put down and won't ever talk to her again. There was a reason for my being there; I felt bad. She should have asked to talk about my fright. She wasn't the least bit sympathetic; she thought I was being capricious.

Don't Overmedicate the Patient

27. Too many medications are given out. Patients are "zonked out."

The "zonked out" or drugged appearance of the patient is an important clinical observation. Although this drugged appearance may be an unfortunate side effect of a therapeutic dosage of medication, it may in some clinical instances be a sign that the dosage should be lowered.

The patients' advice described in statements 13 through 27 is reasonable and profound: Don't avoid me; *talk to me*. Don't depersonalize me; *treat me as a human being*. Don't be smart or funny; *take me seriously*. Don't be bubbly; *be yourself*. Don't break promises; *do what you say you will do*. Don't "put me down;" *show*

compassion, be friendly, trust me, have understanding.

In general, critical remarks of patients should be taken seriously. There are times, however, when because of the patient's hypersensitivity or distortion of reality his critical remarks must be placed in the broader perspective of his clinical condition.

How can we account for the fact that a bright and sensitive group of nurses can be perceived in the negative terms described above? We believe that nurses will give these impressions to patients when they do not understand the patient and when they are hindered by their own discomfort (exhaustion, for example) in the clinical situation. When these two problems are solved, the nurse can be free to give what is in her to give.

Concerns about Confidentiality

28. I'm afraid people will talk about me. Do nurses have to take an oath like the doctors do? I'm afraid I might get blackmailed after I get out of here.

Although paranoid patients may have an extraordinary distrust of staff and other patients, almost all patients have an understandable concern about confidentiality. This concern is intensified in community mental health centers in which neighbors are admitted to the same ward. In another sense, when a patient is talking about confidentiality, she may be asking whether she can trust the nurse. When trust develops in the therapeutic relationship, concerns about confidentiality usually lessen.

How Nurses Help

29. The nurses are the shrinks around here. The doctors zip in and out. They come in for a minute to ask how you are, and then you don't see them for a week. The nurses have to let the doctors know how we are doing.

30. I've had more contact with nurses this past year than I have ever had in my entire life (77 years old). I've learned you can say anything to a nurse—no matter what—it is safe.

31. I can only rap with certain nurses about what really bugs me. You have to find one person to rap with or you can't stay here. You need one person to bleed on. It's a personality thing as to whom you can get along with.

32. They listen. They don't interrupt you. They hear you out no matter how hard it is.
33. They try to help.
34. They give you medication.
35. They will talk to you.
36. They are there when you need them.

Statements 29 and 36 indicate the importance of the consistency and availability of the nurse. Statements 30, 31, and 32 illustrate the importance of the nurse's listening, no matter what the content. Statement 33 and others point to the importance of the attitude of wanting to help.

Patients' Discussion about Student Nurses

PATIENT TRASK: I think they should go through the experience of being a patient; to be on the other side of the white uniform. I'd grab them out of class one day and throw them in a state hospital and tell them they were committed.

PATIENT CRANE: I don't think they would go into psychiatric nursing if you did that.

PATIENT TRASK: They would understand their own little hang-ups and those of others. They'd have to look inward and be able to tell what was an idiosyncrasy and what was a major hang-up.

PATIENT ALLEN: If the students love people, they will go into psychiatric nursing.

Patient Reactions in Community and Ambulatory Settings

Adult patients in community and ambulatory settings may have concerns and perspectives that differ from those of inpatients. For example, they may have particular concerns over confidentiality because neighbors and members of their community may work at the health center. They may wonder whether the student will appreciate the cultural style of the community. They may want the student to intervene to change other people (i.e., spouse or parents), whereas inpatients are more apt to want symptom relief.

THROUGH THE EYES OF THE CHILD

There has been an increasing need for psychiatric and mental health services for children.

Consequently, beginning students in psychiatric nursing need to be sensitive to the subjective responses of children hospitalized for a mental health problem.

Reaction to Becoming a Patient

A group of children and adolescents on the inpatient psychiatric unit of a teaching hospital in a mid-Atlantic city were interviewed by a psychiatric nurse clinician in order to understand how they perceived their hospitalization experience. They were asked how they felt and what they thought about being in the hospital, how nurses helped them, and what advice they would like to give to nurses. The following comments were elicited in a community meeting and during informal conversations over a period of several months.

The Child is "Scared"
1. I was okay until my parents left; then I was scared.
2. I didn't know what would happen to me, or if the other kids would be tough, or if the staff would be mean.
3. When I saw that the doors were locked, I figured that they didn't want anybody to know what went on. I thought it was so bad that people tried to escape.
4. The nurse was nice, but I wondered if she was going to be nice after my Mom left.
5. My parents kept telling me that if I kept it up, they were going to have to put me in the hospital. I figured the hospital would be pretty bad.

These statements reflect the anxiety and fears of children entering a locked psychiatric unit. Statements 1 and 4 convey the nervousness and alarm the child experiences when parents leave the unit: "I was okay until my parents left"; would the nurse "be nice after my Mom left"? To these children, their parents' departure meant that they were alone and unprotected in this strange new environment. The experience of encountering locked doors triggers a frightening image—"they didn't want anybody to know what went on" and "it was so bad that people tried to escape." In statement 5, the threat of hospitalization has become a reality. This 10-year-old boy had been told repeatedly that if his behavior continued, his parents "were going to have to" admit him to the hospital. He sensed his parents' ambivalence and deduced that the reason for it was that the experience would be "pretty bad." Statement 2 illustrates the 15-year-old's fear of loss of control ("what would happen to me") and fear of harm ("if the other kids would be tough, or if the staff would be mean").

The Child Feels Abandoned

6. I miss my mom and my brother and sisters. I'm never going to see them again.
7. I hate being in here, and now I have to go to another hospital. My Mom just wants to get rid of me.
8. My Mom put me in here 'cause I was always in trouble, so she got rid of me. I was so bad she had to go to Florida to rest her nerves.
9. The social worker brung [sic] me 'cause my Ma had to work. I hope my Ma will come, but she might not 'cause I'm so much trouble.

Statement 6 is an undeniable cry from the heart of a sad 5-year-old who has been hospitalized. He believes that he has lost his family forever ("I'm never going to see them again."). Even the brother and sisters with whom he "fights" are missed; as far as he is concerned, his family has deserted him. Statements 7 and 8 reflect the sense of loss and anger experienced by two 11-year-old boys. Not only has the boy in statement 7 been hospitalized, which he "hates," but now he is going to "another hospital" for continued treatment. The only explanation is that his mother "just wants to get rid of" him. The second boy believes that he too has been hospitalized because he was "always in trouble." In fact, his behavior has been extreme enough to send his mother away "to rest her nerves." His unspoken fear is that she may not want him back when she returns. Statement 9 reflects the ambivalence a 15-year-old experiences after an angry outburst to her mother preceding her hospitalization. She had told her mother that she "never" wanted to see her again. Her social worker brought her to the hospital because of her mother's work schedule; however, she is not sure that her mother will come at all "'cause I'm so much trouble."

The Child Feels Lonely

10. I miss my friends.
11. I miss my room and my dog and my family.
12. It's okay, but I just want to go home. I miss my toys.

These statements reflect the feelings of younger children. In statement 10 the 8-year-old expressed the sense of loss she is feeling during her hospitalization. For the school-aged child the loss of peer group is almost as difficult as the loss of family since, developmentally, children between the ages of 6 and 18 years consider peers to be their primary reference group. The 9-year-old in statement 11 misses his room, which has been a kind of sanctuary for him away from the difficulties of school, "hassles" with peers and siblings, and his parents' violent arguments. However, he too misses his family. During a later discussion of feelings, this boy expressed great loneliness without the constant companionship of his dog; "he's just there . . . he stays with me when I feel bad; it's good to have him around. . . . Here I'm always by myself." Statement 12 sums up the feelings of a homesick 6-year-old girl.

The Child Feels Punished

13. They put me in here 'cause I kept running away.
14. If they'll just let me come home, I'll be good.
15. If you work on people's nerves too much, they lock you up.

Hospitalization may sometimes be perceived as a penalty for unacceptable behavior. For example, the 14-year-old in statement 13 believed that the primary reason for her hospitalization was "running away." The fact that she had attempted suicide was unimportant; "the hospital is sort of like 'juvy' (the juvenile detention center) except nicer." Running away isn't "against the law; it's a problem for my parents . . . but I don't see why they should lock me up for trying to kill myself." Statement 14 presents evidence that some children equate hospitalization with punishment. The 9-year-old boy who made this statement was hospitalized for setting fires. He experiences hospitalization and its regimentation as punishment for his behavior. The last statement (15) underscores the feeling of an 8-year-old boy that he has gone way beyond the limits since he is now "locked up."

The Child Feels Blamed

16. I like it here except for family meetings. My family says everything is my fault, but they don't tell about the things that they do.
17. I thought things were going to get better at first, but my family and everybody keeps tell-

ing me I got to work on my problems. Well, they've got problems too.
18. I feel like this is all my fault.

Statement 16 manifests the feelings of a 13-year-old girl who has been hospitalized for continuing problems at home and at school. She feels that her family blames her for "everything"; in fact, during family sessions, this family did tend to "scapegoat" the girl for many issues including the parents' marital conflicts. Her present hospitalization underscored the blame she already felt. Statement 17 displays a similar sense of blame on the part of an 11-year-old girl who acknowledged that she did have "problems" to work on, but who was seeking the same kind of acknowledgment from her family. Finally, statement 18 provides evidence of a 16-year-old abuse victim's feelings that she is responsible for the discord and polarization in her family since her abuse was revealed. The remark accentuates the degree to which she has accepted the onus and the shame of the incestuous relationship.

The Child Is Relieved
19. I like it here better than at home. I don't have to listen to my parents fight, or watch my old man get drunk.
20. It's not so bad here. I don't have to do so much stuff here—all the housework and my school work and watching my little sister.
21. I like being in the hospital because everybody comes and stays for awhile, and they bring me presents and money. How long do you think I'll stay?

Sometimes children, like adults, find hospitalization to be a relief from their lives. The 14-year-old boy in statement 19 lives with an alcoholic family in which there is much violence. His parents "fight"; there is little positive interaction with his parents. The "best times" are when his father gets "really drunk" and goes to sleep. His mother "nags all the time" at his father, himself, and his brother. By contrast, life on the unit is "pretty quiet." The 12-year-old girl in statement 20 is also from an alcoholic family, but there is only one parent—her mother—at home. Her mother works during the day, and she is out drinking many nights as well. The girl has been the primary caretaker for her younger sister and responsible for the household chores. Although she continued to "worry" about her sister, the girl was able to concentrate on her

own problems and family issues in a less pressured atmosphere. The 11-year-old girl in statement 21 enjoyed the attention that she received from her family while on the unit. She described her pleasure at spending time with "everybody" and with the "presents and money" they brought. When asked to explain how this was different, she described seeing her father sporadically (her parents were divorced) and her grandparents only occasionally. Her mother worked, and when she was off, she was often "too tired" to spend time with the girl. Thus, hospitalization brought "friends, things to do" and much desired attention from her family.

The Child "Wonders if I'm Crazy"
22. I don't mind it here too much, but visitors and sometimes your family act like everybody up here is crazy. Maybe you too.
23. If I call my friends and tell them where I am, they'll think I'm crazy. I don't want to feel like that.
24. I guess I'm here 'cause they think I'm crazy, but I'm not.

These statements reflect the concerns of hospitalized children and adolescents about their "craziness." Statement 22 reveals the 13-year-old boy's thoughts about how visitors and "sometimes" his family act toward him and his peers. Visitors and hospital staff who don't work on the child and adolescent unit are often curious about the reasons for children's hospitalization. Sometimes, their behavior communicates fear or apprehension—especially if they have witnessed angry outbursts or bizarre behavior. However, visitors to locked psychiatric units sometimes respond negatively to the experience of encountering locked doors. They may wonder—as some of the children quoted here did—why locked doors are necessary or what happens once the doors are locked behind them. Statement 23 demonstrates the hesitation some children and adolescents feel about revealing their hospitalization to friends. This 14-year-old girl is concerned about her friends' response to her being on a "mental unit"; her anxiety prevents her from maintaining contact with them. Unfortunately, her lack of peer contact increased the sense of isolation she experienced while hospitalized. The 9-year-old boy in statement 24 expressed his complete rejection of the idea that he is "crazy"; however, his words suggest that he has considered the possibility. He also may be feeling anxious about how this may affect his life in the future.

The Child Is Angry

25. I hate being in here. You can't do anything except think about your problems and feel awful.
26. There are more rules here than at home. My Ma doesn't bug me all the time, and if she does, I just split. I can't do that here.
27. I hate it here. People keep asking me why I tried to kill myself. I get embarrassed when I tell them the reason.

All of these statements reveal the anger which many children feel about being hospitalized even though the reasons are diverse. In statement 25, the 17-year-old girl feels cornered; "you can't do anything except think about your problems and feel awful." When she was asked what she did when she felt "awful," she explained "I get high," or "I take off and do something fun." The 13-year-old boy in statement 26 is encountering the frustration of "rules" that he is unable to ignore without consequences. Further, there are expectations from staff that he will abide by the rules as his peers do. He feels blocked by not being able to "split" when he feels tense or disagrees with set limits. The 15-year-old girl in statement 27 is "embarrassed" about her recent suicide attempt and the reason for it. The experience of having to talk about her feelings and thoughts as opposed to acting on them is a new one for her. Further, "every time" she talks about the events which led to her hospitalization, she feels "like it's happening all over again."

How Nurses Help

28. They talk to you when you have a problem.
29. They listen to you.
30. They stay with you when you're scared.
31. They hug you when you're feeling miserable.
32. They teach you how to play games.
33. Some of them are nice; they make you feel like they care about you.
34. Nurses give you medicine when you feel sick.

Children's Advice to Nurses

35. Give us a reason for doing something instead of saying "just do it."

36. Don't say we can talk later or play a game later and then not do it.
37. Let the older kids have more privileges.
38. Don't laugh at us.
39. Listen to us more.

It appears that children and adolescents share adult patients' thoughts on advice to nurses. It is important to note some issues specific to this population. Giving directions to this group is as frequent an activity as setting limits. However, "giving a reason" can sometimes be a complicated business. Sometimes it's easy to give one; sometimes it's not so simple. For example, if there is an emergency or a need to have something done quickly, it may not be feasible to give a reason at that moment, but once things settle down, a brief explanation can be given. At other times, giving a reason is simpler: "Jumping on the furniture can cause damage," or "you may fall off and hurt yourself." Other times, "just do it," as most parents know, is sometimes shorthand for either not repeating an explanation that has been given already or an imperative to listen. Statement 37 is a helpful reminder to recognize developmental differences. On a child and adolescent unit where there is a wide age range, it may be necessary to "shift gears" when dealing with children of different ages or developmental levels.

ROLE-APPROPRIATE VERSUS SUBJECTIVE (IDIOSYNCRATIC) FEELINGS AND REACTIONS

The role-appropriate feelings of the child and adult psychiatric patient have been described in the previous pages. They include feeling scared, alone, frustrated, nervous, suspicious, violated, out of control, empty, and relieved. These feelings are so common that the nurse should assume that they are probably being experienced by each new patient. With this index of suspicion, the nurse is ready to respond in a supportive fashion to an otherwise difficult patient. For instance, if a patient refuses to speak and appears to be frightened, the nurse might say, "You seem terribly frightened." If the nurse were correct about the patient's feelings, these four words would be extraordinarily supportive, for now the patient would know that in this lonely and frightening place someone understands.

Subjective feelings and reactions of the child and adult patient, analogous to those feelings of the nurse, are idiosyncratic responses to the current situation based on personal experiences of the patient in the past. In practice, the patient may respond to the nurse with a variety of subjective feelings of different intensity. He may be very angry at the nurse or be very fond of her. He may want to control her or be controlled by her. He may want to inappropriately care for her or be cared for by her. These reactions may appear at any time during the course of treatment, and they may change from day to day.

It is important for the nurse to identify these subjective reactions of the patient so that she will not be overwhelmed by them. She must remind herself that these feelings are not real in that they are directed by the patient not toward her but toward someone else in the patient's life. Fortified with this knowledge, the nurse need not reject the patient because of her own anxiety. She can continue to communicate her concern for his emotional well-being.

Summary

The patient's reaction to hospitalization covers a wide range of human emotions. Some patients feel scared, alone, frustrated, and nervous to be in a psychiatric setting. These feelings are similar to those of the student beginning her psychiatric rotation and are not necessarily a part of the psychiatric illness.

The patient's reactions may be based on his feelings about previous hospitalizations, fear of physical harm from other patients, and a fear of failure on having to reenter the hospital.

Patients have made suggestions to student nurses for improving psychiatric care: Do not avoid patients by staying in the nurse's station to write reports and by attending meetings; do not depersonalize patients by labeling them; do not be snide in your comments; do not be bubbly; do not break promises; do not "put them down"; clarify communication lines between staff; do not give too much medication.

The patients stated the ways that the nurses help them: talking with them; giving them their time; listening; giving medication; being available when needed; hearing about their pain.

Role-appropriate and subjective feelings of the patient were distinguished. Role-appropriate feelings are usual, normal, and appropriate for someone with an emotional disorder who has recently been admitted to a psychiatric hospital. In contrast, subjective feelings are idiosyncratic and not appropriate to the situation, having their origins in the patient's past. Understanding both kinds of feelings frees the student to be more therapeutic.

Questions

1. How could you collect data on patient feelings and reactions in other than psychiatric nursing settings?
2. What feelings and reactions do psychiatric patients have in common with patients you have previously cared for or interviewed?
3. What questions would you ask clients in an ambulatory setting regarding their feelings about psychiatric care?
4. How can the nurse ensure confidentiality for a client in an ambulatory setting?
5. How important do you believe attending to client feelings about being a psychiatric patient is in comparison to other patient settings?

REFERENCES AND SUGGESTED READINGS

Kauffman, M. Sharing the patient's experience. *American Journal of Nursing*, 1978, *78*, 860–861.

Levinson, D., Merrifield, J., & Berg, K. Becoming a mental patient. *Archives of General Psychiatry*, 1967, *17*, 385–406.

Olds, J. The inpatient treatment of adolescents in a milieu including younger children. *Adolescent Psychiatry*, 1982, *10*, 373–381.

Plath, S. *The Bell Jar*. New York: Harper & Row, 1971.

Reilly, E. Sylvia Plath: Talented poet, tortured woman. *Perspectives in Psychiatric Care*, 1978, *16*(3), 129–136.

Sebastian, L. Psychiatric hospital admissions: Assessing patients' perceptions. *Journal of Psychosocial Nursing and Mental Health Services*, 1987, *25*(6), 25–28.

Sweeney, L. J. Psychiatric patients' perceptions of their milieu therapy program. *Journal of Psychosocial Nursing and Mental Health Services*, 1978, *16*(8), 28–32.

Templin, H. E. The system and the patient. *American Journal of Nursing*, 1982, *82*, 108–111.

Vonnegut, M. *The Eden Express*. New York: Bantam, 1976.

Worth, B. Reflections of a psychiatric nurse–patient relationship. *Perspectives in Psychiatric Care*, 1969, *7*(2), 73–75.

PART II

Theoretical Frameworks in Psychiatric Mental Health Nursing

A theoretical framework is presented in order to add to the knowledge base that nurses bring with them to psychiatric mental health nursing. An overview of mental health functioning and dysfunctioning and the sociocultural issues of mental illness will help the nurse to focus on the area of study. In addition, the nurse is introduced to current research contributions from the sociocultural, neurobiological, behavioral, and cognitive sciences, theories of personality, and developments in psychological defense styles of patients. Current thinking on life-span developmental theory and communication theory, especially neurolinguistic programming, is included. In this latter type of communication theory, understanding how people think, that is, their cognitions, assists in understanding how they behave and ultimately provides suggestion for ways of intervening to help change behavior to adaptive methods for coping.

CHAPTER 3: MENTAL HEALTH FUNCTIONS AND DYSFUNCTIONS

The discipline of mental health and psychiatric nursing has a long history of practice, and thus a view of conceptualizing mental functioning as well as mental health disturbances and dysfunctioning is presented.

CHAPTER 4: SOCIOCULTURAL ISSUES OF MENTAL ILLNESS

The influence of the sociocultural issues in understanding human behavior is presented in terms of historical antecedents as well as current social beliefs and patterns. The psychiatric nursing implications are outlined.

CHAPTER 5: CONTRIBUTIONS OF THE NEUROBIOLOGICAL SCIENCES

The recent findings from brain research that have increased our understanding of the role of biologic dynamics in human behavior are presented, including the science basis for psychopharmacology, the functioning of the brain, circadian rhythms, sleep, and genetics.

CHAPTER 6: CONTRIBUTIONS OF THE BEHAVIORAL AND COGNITIVE SCIENCES

The history of the recent cognitive revolution is presented to illustrate the contributions to our understanding of intellectual integration in addition to contributions from learning and motivation theory.

CHAPTER 7: THEORIES OF PERSONALITY

Psychiatric mental health nursing derives many of its concepts for practice from personality theory. A comparative approach is taken to examine the major schools of thought proposed by personologists.

CHAPTER 8: EGO FUNCTIONS, SELF-REPRESENTATION, AND MECHANISMS OF DEFENSE

Knowledge of the current research on ego functioning and self-representation systems provides an understanding for working with the psychological defensive styles of people under stress.

CHAPTER 9: LIFE-SPAN DEVELOPMENTAL THEORY

The course of a person's life has qualitatively different phases, which are presented in this chapter and include an emphasis on the second half of the life cycle.

CHAPTER 10: COMMUNICATION THEORY

Psychiatric mental health nursing practice has been built on the process of communication. This process is recommended as a vehicle for assisting in helping people to change their behavior.

Chapter 3

Mental Health Functions and Dysfunctions

Ann Wolbert Burgess

Chapter Objectives

The students successfully attaining the goals of this chapter will be able to:

- Explain the meaning of mental health and give characteristics of a psychologically healthy individual.
- Identify three criteria of mental dysfunction and give examples of each.
- Explain the relationship of psychological equilibrium and psychological conflicts.

Mental health as a concept is an elusive term. Psychological health deals with an individual's ability to cope with mental stress, much in the way that physical health deals with an individual's ability to deal with physiological stress. In a very simplistic manner, normality or psychological health may be conceptualized as involving an individual's success in negotiating and resolving psychological conflict in order to live with what is or cannot be psychologically settled or resolved. The other side of the coin—mental disorder or mental illness—has a common denominator of an acute or chronic surrender to psychological conflict and the resultant blow to self-esteem that this surrender inevitably entails.[1]

PSYCHOLOGICAL EQUILIBRIUM THEORY

Equilibrium theory views health as a balance of the process in which humans interact with their environment. This process is constantly being influenced by factors that may also be varying. As long as the process remains in balance, the person is viewed as being healthy. An imbalance of these factors reflects a failure of the body's adaptive, self-regulating powers to maintain internal balance in the face of external stressors. This theory considers health to be a dynamic process rather than something static and unchanging. The healthy individual is reacting constantly to the stimuli of the environment and adjusting to them and maintaining equilibrium through various coping mechanisms and strategies.

Nurses speak of mental health in terms of equilibrium theory when they speak of balancing all the various factors—biological, psychological, social, cultural, economic, and educational—in our society. The psychologically normal person, although believed to be mythical by many authorities, may be defined in equilibria terms as one who is able to achieve biopsychosocial stability in spite of the various stresses and conflicting forces that are inherent in living in our society. Psychiatrist John Nemiah identifies four human characteristics that he believes are components of this normal psychological equilibrium.[2]

1. Behaving in a realistic and responsive manner to the world around you.
2. Being capable of experiencing a wide range of feelings.
3. Entering into lasting and satisfying human relationships.
4. Working creatively and effectively.

In addition, this person achieves a balance of his inner emotional state and is goal-directed without being constricted, warped, or stunted psychologically. Balance is achieved among the various psychological elements, and flexibility maintains equilibrium or facilitates a prompt restitution in the face of emotional stress.

CONCEPT OF MENTAL HEALTH

Mental Health

Mental health is a term that is used daily. Yet, what does it mean to be mentally healthy or mentally unhealthy? The answer to this question is not simply given, and a completely adequate and universally applicable or acceptable definition is highly elusive.

Mental health, as a concept, gained steadily in acceptance after the founding of the National Association for Mental Health by Clifford Beers in 1909. Attention is continually being focused on the relative definitions of the normal personality and of mental health. It appears that one of the major difficulties in adequately defining mental health is that to a certain extent, the con-cept of mental health varies with each individual person rather than having specific scientific guidelines.

Definitions of mental health may range from one end of the spectrum to the other. In actual practice, such as in criminal court proceedings, psychiatrists will differ in their evaluation as to whether a defendant is sane or insane. In operational terms, the dictionary defines *mental* as "pertaining to the mind" and in the broadest sense, refers to the "integrated activity of the organism." The definition of health formulated by the World Health Organization, states that health is not merely the absence of disease or infirmity.

The President's Commission on Mental Health printed a letter after the commission was first formed that implied the universality of mental health[3]:

Mental health . . . affects every one of us—depression, marital problems, drugs- and alcohol-related problems, inability to cope as the result of a death or serious accident, low self-esteem, social maladjustment problems, dealing with delinquent children, and so many more situations.

The report also stated that the letter was a reminder that almost all Americans encounter these problems, either in themselves or in their families or among their neighbors and friends. Given the official statement of mental health in America, the concept of psychological equilibrium becomes essential to understand.

HEALTH BALANCING FACTORS

The classical disease-entity conception of mental illness is excessively static and does not hold up under scrutiny in the light of clinical reality. In illness the organism is not invaded passively by a foreign influence, except possibly in the case of trauma. Throughout life, the organism continuously and actively adapts to changes in both the internal and the external milieu. Through this process of adaptation, the organism achieves a dynamic steady state in which the variables necessary for its continued existence in those altered circumstances are optimized as far as possible. Acute illness can be thought of as the transition from a previous steady state to a new steady state in response to a change in the milieu. The total adaptive success of the new steady state may fail to equal the previous level of adaptation, and this failure represents a cost borne by the organism through a residual adaptive deficit. Additional changes in the milieu may require further alterations of the organism to achieve a new adaptation. For example, the clinical reality is that the mental disorder, schizophrenia, presents precisely this variable picture. The thought disorder that is manifest in one statement is absent in the next. The hallucinations are intermittent. In fact, the schizophrenic syndrome can be thought of as an effort to adapt to a highly altered experience of both inner and outer reality.

It has been as difficult to define mental illness as it has been mental health. Herman Melville provides a literary insight from a passage in *Billy Budd*:

Who in the rainbow can draw the line where the violet tint ends and the orange tint begins. Distinctly we see the difference of the color, but where exactly does the first one visibly enter into the other? So with sanity and insanity. In pronounced cases there is no question about them . . . there are instances where it is next to impossible to determine whether a man is sane or beginning to be otherwise.

In order to manage a balance between mental health and mental illness, certain balancing factors are believed to play an important role. These factors may be discussed in terms of defense mechanisms, e.g., a buffer to reject disequilibrium, or as health-promoting factors to balance health and ill health. Two such factors under study are those of hardiness and humor.

Hardiness

The personality characteristic of hardiness, comprising control, commitment, and challenge, was identified by psychologist Suzanne Kobassa in the late 1970s and is viewed as "an inherent health-promoting factor in a stress-laden human environment."[4] Primarily investigated as a buffer between stress and illness, hardiness has direct relevance to nursing practice. Through identification of those individuals who (1) do not feel that they can control or influence the events in their lives; (2) do not feel deeply involved in or committed to the activities in their lives; or (3) do not anticipate change as an exciting challenge to further development, nurses can im-

plement stress-reducing interventions to aid in preventing stress-related illness.[5]

In conceptualizing hardiness, Kobassa built on existentialist formulations of the strenuousness of authentic living, of competence, appropriate striving, goal-oriented productivity, and the hypothesis that persons who experience high degrees of stress without falling ill have a personality structure that differentiates them from persons who become ill under stress.[6] The concept of hardiness has been deductively derived from existential psychology through Maddi's fulfillment theories and conceptually developed as a personality-based trait.[7,8]

Hardiness is defined as a composite of commitment, control, and challenge.[9,10] These three existential concepts Kobassa recognizes as being especially relevant to the ability to rise to the challenges of the environment and turn stressful life events into possibilities or opportunities for personal growth and benefit.[11] Lack of these three dimensions of hardiness describes burnout.

Each of the three components of hardiness has been contrasted with other personality characteristics. Commitment has been viewed as the opposite of alienation; control has been viewed as the opposite to powerlessness; and challenge as the opposite to vegetativeness.

Although hardiness may represent only one aspect of stress resistance, the implications of understanding this personality characteristic and style are numerous.[12] Lambert and Lambert suggest that once the scientific community is able to determine from where it comes, how it is developed, and/or how it is learned, nurses can begin to test effectively for hardiness in clients who may be faced with stressful life events and can then make appropriate interventions before a low-hardiness individual experiences stress.[13]

Humor

Humor may be viewed as a health-promoting factor. Humor serves as a form of communication, a release of tension and anxiety, as a way of coping with stress, a biologic reflex, a socially acceptable outlet for aggression, a means for social corrections and protections, and as an agent of self-disclosure.[14] McGhee's literature review of the humor response suggests that a theoretical view of humor was first introduced by Freud, who linked the economy of psychic energy with the experience of pleasure or satisfaction. The saving in feeling that characterizes humor is achieved by reducing the seriousness of a situation that would otherwise produce some strong negative emotion. By denying the threat, the individual feels better able to cope with the situation at hand. The consequent saving of energy is discharged as laughter.[15]

The concept of humor discussed by Robinson includes wit, laughter, joking, comedy, kidding, teasing, clowning, mimicking, satire, and freak enjoyment of the imperfect.[16] Humor is contagious and has a circular relationship. People laugh because a story is funny and the story is known to be funny because people laugh.

Humor distorts reality and allows us to see another way, exploding the bonds of logic or social propriety. An example is given of a father reprimanding his son for being rude to the therapist. As the father was saying to the son, "you should show more respect to Dr. . . .," he could not remember the therapist's name. "Just call me Butch," said the therapist. Humor can act as a wonderful enzyme for making the symptoms interpersonal. Shared humor is a self-to-self experience.

Humor is also a way to be insulting without being annihilating. How many nurse–therapists does it take to change a light bulb? Forget the light bulb, let's rewire the house.

Humor is like any spice. It must be infused in the right proportion to improve the taste. Autognosis is essential when using humor to depersonalize therapeutic experience. Nurses need to be aware of their motivation for using humor. A symptom may be the therapist's anxiety mounting before adding humor. In fact, anxiety in the therapist may be a barrier to using humor.

Humor can have a cruel and distancing effect. Much depends on the object of the humor and whether the motive is to discharge aggression. Humor by itself is not sadistic; the person is sadistic. Humor by itself is not distancing; the person is distancing. Sadistic comments can lie beneath the thin veneer of social protocol.

Humor can be useful in therapy. According to Burbridge, humor is a powerful tool that can be used to free patients from imprisoning reality models and opens doors to new cognitive and affective freedom.[17] It does this through reframing so the patient becomes aware of choices open and his ability to choose. Therapeutic humor, observes Burbridge, is shown to involve

disidentification from a limiting self-concept and to bypass defenses by working through paradox and indirection. Expressions of therapeutic humor involve simple joke sharing, humorous reframing, and sophisticated mirroring techniques.[18]

Warner outlines the positive outcomes of humor therapy within a therapeutic milieu as including increased congruence, awareness, catharsis, pleasure, and self-esteem.[19] Humor allows one to risk speaking of anxiety-producing content in a safe, socially accepted way without fear of censure, allows pleasure for self and others, and allows one to rise above and gain a sense of control over a problem area through laughter.

In summary, two health-promoting factors have been identified as hardiness and humor. These attributes should be noted as strengths of a person's personality.

CONCEPT OF MENTAL DISTRESS

The equilibrium theory views an imbalance as a disturbance in equilibria. When the proper balance between an individual and the environment is upset, certain processes come into play with the goal of restoring this balance. Interventions from external areas are directed toward encouraging, nurturing, reinforcing, and strengthening behaviors that will regain the equilibrium.

There are several similarities between the mind's expression of psychological distress and the body's expression of biologic distress. For example, a single manifestation of distress may result from a variety of clinical conditions. In medicine, diarrhea may be a manifestation of infection, ingestion of toxic materials, anxiety, obstruction, or other causes. In psychiatry, anxiety may be a manifestation of schizophrenia, various neurotic conditions, or situational reactions. Another similarity is when both the mind and a particular organ manifest their distress in a limited number of ways, regardless of etiology. For example, pathology in the lower gastrointestinal tract, whether caused by an ulcer, a tumor, inflammation, or trauma, will manifest symptoms in limited ways: pain, bloating, diarrhea, constipation, or bleeding. Psychological distress, as we will show, may be expressed by feelings, thoughts, and behaviors.

Mental distress may be conceptualized as

the mind expressing its discomfort in thoughts, feelings, and behaviors. For instance, a troubled person may feel anxious or depressed, think in an obsessional or psychotic manner, or behave impulsively. Sometimes feelings, thoughts, and behaviors are simultaneous manifestations of psychological distress. Often, however, only one or two of these three dimensions are apparent in a given patient.

Feelings

Feelings, also described as affect, are subjective mood states. They may be pleasant and enjoyable, or they may be painful and uncomfortable. Human feelings are numerous; the differences among them may be subtle. To identify just a few:

Alienation	Helplessness
Anger	Hope
Anxiety	Hopelessness
Caution	Hostility
Contentment	Inadequacy
Delight	Indifference
Disgust	Isolation
Distrust	Joy
Embarrassment	Loneliness
Envy	Love
Exasperation	Resentment
Fear	Respect
Frustration	Sadness
Guilt	Suspicion
Happiness	Worry

In terms of mental health, one looks for the spontaneous availability and expression of a full range of appropriate feelings. The state of mental health includes the capacity to bear and tolerate certain kinds of feelings, even when they are painful or unbearable. When the feeling is unbearable, two situations may occur. First, another feeling may be substituted as an avoidance or defensive technique. For example, anger may be used to avoid feelings of closeness or love; depression may be used to avoid sadness; or elation may be used to avoid anxiety or depression. Second, abnormal states of action or thought function to avoid the genuine affective states. For instance, a patient suffering from overwhelming anxiety may break a window or begin to hallucinate.

What brings a person to seek psychological assistance is usually not the desire to examine

his life, but psychological pain. And the most immediate experience of intrapsychic conflict takes the form of painful affect. The affects include the patient's experience and expression of emotion. Affects can at times be either defended against or can serve defensive purposes; they are functions of the ego. This is more apparent when noting their three basic roles. They are simultaneously:

1. Subjective experiences (conscious perceptions of ourselves),
2. Modes of communication, and
3. States with specific bodily manifestations of the system and skeletal musculature.

The assessment of emotion presents difficulties for the nurse. It is far easier to record the content of a person's dialogue than to chart the affective material of the interview. Such recording includes facial expressions, gestures, characteristics of speech, and all other factors indicating an emotional state. In the final analysis, the nurse should employ empathy in assessing affect.

Ego Affects

The two primary ego affects—anxiety and depression—are found in almost all psychiatric disorders. They are indicators of strain in the psychological structure when it is under stress of a precipitating event. This stress tips the balance between the instinctual drives and the ego-controlling mechanisms.

The ability to tolerate painful affects is especially indicative of ego strength. Anxiety and depression are unavoidable experiences; their absence is remarkable in a person seeking help with a problem. The ability of a healthy ego to tolerate these feelings is impaired in various character styles. For example, some people control anxiety and depression by distancing themselves from affect; others become angry when they feel threatened, humiliated, or thwarted.

Each character type deals with experiences and relationships in one way or another to avoid anxiety and depression. The healthy personality accepts anxiety as a signal of danger and sadness as an appropriate response to loss.

Anxiety

Anxiety is most often described as an uncomfortable feeling state. It is characterized by a subjective sense of impending disaster. The common physical or somatic alterations in the body systems associated with anxiety may be experienced as follows:

- Circulatory system: perspiration, clammy hands, flushing, blushing, feeling hot or cold.
- Respiratory system: heavy breathing, sighing respirations, hyperventilation, dizziness.
- Gastrointestinal system: abdominal pain, anorexia, nausea, dry mouth, diarrhea, constipation, butterflies in the stomach.
- Genitourinary system: urinary frequency, various interferences with sexual function.
- Mental functioning: impaired attention, poor concentration, impairment of memory, changes in outlook and future planning.
- Emotional reaction: irritability, mood change, dream disturbances, changes in relationships with family and friends.

The above symptoms of anxiety are known to all of us. A useful way to judge the normal feeling of anxiety is that it does not involve repression. One can consciously feel and acknowledge it and by so doing, keep it proportionate to the threat.

Neurotic anxiety, however, is a reaction disproportionate to the threat. This kind of anxiety and its results are discussed in Chapter 40.

Anxiety may be regarded as pathological when it is severe and persistent or when it seems to be triggered by some minor cause. Sometimes the individual's previous experiences cause an automatic reaction. To one man the presence of a policeman may provoke an anxious anticipation; to another the same policeman elicits a feeling of protection and safety.

To some students the instructor, when returning an examination paper, incites a feeling of anticipation and curiosity. To other students the action produces fear and anxiety.

Depression

Depression is most often described as an affective state ("I feel depressed"). It is also used to describe a state of the ego ("he is depressed"). Depression may be used to describe a psychiatric disorder such as neurotic or psychiatric disorder such as neurotic or psychotic depression and a characterological state. The core of depres-

sion is a sense of helplessness and disappointment over an actual or perceived loss. The ability to bear the affective state of depression is a sign of mental health, of ego strength. As Binstock states[20]:

Bearing a depression successfully is a maturing experience; it strengthens the ego. In this sense it is true that suffering does build character.

For those persons who cannot bear depression, the presence of a supportive person can help to bear the distressing feelings. This supportive relationship is achieved by the helper understanding what the sufferer feels, why he feels it and conveying this empathy to the sufferer.

Loss is one of the most common precipitants of acute problems leading to mental health assistance. Helping a person to bear the feelings associated with loss (i.e., depression) is emotional first aid that can intervene in the development of additional recurrent symptoms.

Any life event has the potential of being interpreted as a loss. While a developmental step forward may be viewed optimistically, it may alternatively be viewed pessimistically as a loss. To choose is also to lose the rejected alternative. To be a male is to lose the opportunity to be a female; to be an adult is to lose one's childhood; to marry is to lose being single; and to become the supervisor is to lose the goal of becoming the supervisor.

Love and Other Positive Feelings

Love and human closeness may be difficult feelings for many people to bear. In current society, people are frequently more comfortable discussing matters of aggression and sex than matters of love and fondness. Can you imagine a friend coming up to you and saying, "I am very fond of you. You are a very fine person." Almost anyone would become uneasy.

People may avoid being loved by expressing hostility or by withdrawing. In psychiatric nursing the patient commonly explains his fear of closeness as a protection against being rejected or as a protection against his fear of wanting too much.

Anger

Anger may be an appropriate response to a frustrating situation. Some people, however, use the feeling of anger to defend against human closeness. It is paradoxical that those to whom we feel closest often provoke our greatest anger and cause us to behave in unpleasant ways. The important people in our lives evoke both the greatest joy and the strongest anger. Instead of bearing the human feeling of love, people often use defensive techniques. For example, when someone slams a door or berates another person, his behavior may be a response to a critical remark just made by a close friend, an insensitive spouse, or an indifferent parent.

The anger may also be a defense against a real feeling of helplessness. That is, if a person feels weak, ineffective, and overwhelmed by this feeling, it may be easier for him to get angry to show that he is the big tough guy rather than live with the feeling of helplessness. For example, the grade-school bully who goes around pushing other children may really be overcompensating for feelings of helplessness.

Another example is the patient who comes into the hospital ward outraged at how dirty the ward looks or how inefficient the ward seems to be or wanting to know why the staff cannot be therapeutic. That person may be defending against his own feelings of anxiety, helplessness, or insignificance by trying to be critical of the ward.

Guilt and Shame

The feeling of guilt can be understood as the form of anxiety inflicted by a threat from the superego. Shame can be understood as the form of anxiety inflicted by the ego-ideal when one has fallen short of its standards. It is important to remember that the patient's feeling of guilt or shame does not change external reality any more than worry does. To accomplish practical change, one must change one's actions.

Thoughts

The second way the mind may express distress is through thoughts. Thoughts are pathological when they interfere with productive activities and when they defend against normal feeling states. One kind of pathological thought is a wish or fantasy that interferes with a particular feeling, relationship, or goal. For instance, an adolescent may substitute a fantasied love affair with the "perfect girl" rather than risk the threat of rejection by a real girl friend. Another kind of pathological thinking is a psychosis in which the person avoids reality by denying it.

In terms of assessing normal from abnor-

mal, thinking can be divided into five aspects: rate, continuity, control, content, and form.

Rate. Effective communication requires that we maintain a rate of language expression that can be easily understood. The range for this rate varies, but there are two extremes. In slowed or inhibited thinking, the person's language is reduced in rate to the point at which ideas and images present themselves less frequently or sometimes to the point at which there are no images entering the consciousness (i.e., mutism). In rapid thinking, the person's language is increased in rate. The rate may be described as a flight of ideas and may be accompanied by pressured speech. On the other hand, the connections between words and phrases may reflect thought as becoming almost nonsensical as noted in puns or rhymes.

Continuity of Thinking. The train of thinking must be directed and consistent and must stay on track if the person is to make himself understood. Specific disturbances include: **circumstantiality**, in which the person's thinking is overly detailed, intricate, and slowed; **tangentiality**, in which the train of thought is sidetracked and the goal of the thought is not reached; **thought blocking**, in which the person suddenly stops talking and, when he resumes, is on another topic; and **perseveration**, in which the person is unable to move from one track to another, and thus the language becomes repetitive of words, phrases, and questions.

Control of Thinking. Control of thinking means the subjective experience of the degree of self-determination operating in one's thinking and the sense that one's thoughts are one's own. Two varieties of disturbances include: **obsessional thinking**, which refers to a type of experience in which the person cannot be free of certain ideas, fears, images, or impulses that are recognized as senseless; and **thought alienation**, in which the person describes his thoughts as being under the control of someone else or that he is unable to control his thoughts.

Content of Thinking. The major concern regarding content of thinking is the presence of delusions, which is considered one of the most serious disturbances of thinking. Delusions are false, unshakable beliefs that are incommensurate with the person's social and cultural background and cannot be influenced by reason or experience.

Form of Thinking. Form of thinking refers to several features: the logical character of thinking; the abstractability; the connectedness of clauses, phrases, and sentences that permit the person to be understood; and the quality of associations.

Behaviors

In addition to thoughts and feelings, a third way in which people express distress is through their behavior. The normal discharge of actions is through motor activity or goal-directed, problem-solving behavior. For example, if your foot is hot, you take it off the radiator. If you feel you must kick the radiator, you would be overreacting to the situation. Some people use gymnasiums to release tension. Also waiting for a telephone call or a date inspires some people to use motor activity. Other people knit or doodle as a means of handling agitation. These are all normal ways of dealing with feelings through action.

Sometimes the behavior is not productive and does not relieve the tension but instead gets the person into more trouble. The behavior can become pathological. When you are tense, it is not helpful to break a window or door because you generally have to pay a penalty. But if you call someone to tell him what is on your mind, the behavior tends to be more adaptive and corrects the psychological imbalance.

The other extreme may be seen in the bizarre behavior of thought-disordered persons, or the manic behavior of affective disorders, or the antisocial acts of robbery, rape, and murder or alcoholism, suicide, and drug abuse.

An underlying factor influencing behavior is motivation. Situations and factors can increase or decrease motivation. In such situations, the behaviors of hypoactivity (withdrawal), hyperactivity (mania), sexuality, and aggression are commonly seen.

Aggression and Sexuality

The two great themes of human motives are sexuality and aggression. Since it is beyond the scope of this chapter to discuss the complexities of dysfunctional sexual development and since the efforts to account for human aggression and

the distressingly destructive forms it too often takes defy an exposition of any length, we will address the issue under the problem of sadomasochism.

The terms **sadism** and **masochism** were originally applied to the overt infliction of pain as a concomitant of sexual gratification. The psychodynamic model suggests a more widespread phenomenon of destructiveness toward others and the self more distant from immediate bodily sensations of pleasure and pain. There is a profound distinction between aggression expressed in assertiveness or fighting for a constructive goal and cruelty and malice toward others or the self carried on for its own sake. This difference is difficult to capture in theory, but it is unmistakable in clinical encounters.

Sadomasochism is a basic perversion in which sexuality and aggression have fused at a primitive level of development. Assessing how a person handles his sexuality and aggression provides an inventory of the personality. Estimating the degree to which his mental activity is committed to sadomasochistic motives and concerns about defending against the dangers they present provides an index of how ill the person really is.

SYMPTOMS

Symptoms, from a sociocultural perspective, can be understood as a transactional phenomenon. The communication aspects of symptoms merit primary consideration by nurses since they carry valuable information for intervention. To obtain this information, the nurse needs to act as a translator of a "foreign" language. In the analysis of dream content, clinicians aim to decode significant intrapsychic conflicts by searching for wish fulfillment and using the patient as a resource for further exploitation of associated mental events. Thus, in the social analysis of symptoms, the aim is to decode the communication of symptoms from the interpersonal content of the language to arrive at their psychosocial significance. This task is accomplished by looking at data on the individual's relationships to important people in his family as well as at data on his relationships to other significant groups. Further discussion of language as symptom communication is noted in Chapters 10 and 16 on formulating and implementing therapeutic communication strategies in psychiatric mental health nursing.

Symptoms—and their analysis—may be normal or abnormal; they may be used as a defense, and they may impact on the formation of a syndrome.

Normal and Abnormal Symptoms

A symptom, depending on the associated conditions, may be a manifestation of a normal or a pathological state. For example, constipation would be normal if it resulted from a change in diet. It would be abnormal if it resulted from a tumor or an obstruction of the intestinal tract. Intense sadness would be normal following an important loss, and abnormal when there is no good reason for the mood state. Certain symptoms are always abnormal regardless of the associated condition. In general medicine, vomiting blood or passing blood in the urine is always abnormal. In psychiatry, suicidal behavior and visual hallucinations are always abnormal.

Symptoms as a Defense

Symptoms often perform defensive functions. For instance, a fever may be viewed as a defense against an infection in the body. Vomiting following the consumption of contaminated food functions to expel or "defend against" the irritant. Following staphylococcal infection, an abscess functions to wall off the infection.

Similarly, a delusion may be an attempt by the mind to protect itself from something more painful. It may be easier to think unreal thoughts than to face an overwhelming situation. There may be less anxiety in fainting than in facing the fright of an aggressive encounter. It may be easier to develop an obsessional thought than to feel like hitting someone. Or it may be safer to forget to attend class than to tell the instructor the homework was not completed.

Symptom Formation

The process of symptom formation and the onset of psychiatric illness are related to the nature of psychological equilibrium. Essentially, there is a stable balance of psychological factors that persist over time and determine the quality of behavior and the relationships inherent in the individual's unique personality. Under stress, the balance of forces has the potential to be altered and disrupted. Stress may be the result of external or internal factors. Chapter 24 on crisis theory examines more precisely the various stressors that are capable of producing a psychological imbalance. Depending on the nature of the stress, the length of time the stress has existed, and the magnitude of the stress, the stress impacts on the existing psychological equilibrium and has the potential to influence the balance toward pathological psychological equilibrium or psychiatric disorder and symptom formation.

CONCEPT OF MENTAL DYSFUNCTION

The concept of mental dysfunction has a relationship to psychological equilibrium theory. However, what is meant by "abnormal" or "psychopathological" is very difficult to define. The concept of mental dysfunction may be viewed by classifying psychiatric disorders into three categories[21]:

1. Those disorders that cause the individual pain and about which, consequently, she or he complains.
2. Those disorders considered unusual and abnormal by others or by society at large.
3. Those disorders that deviate from a theoretical concept of normal functioning.

These three categories are then further divided according to subjective, normative, and theoretical criteria.

Subjective Criteria

One way to define dysfunction is to let the individual or client decide if he is abnormal or not. This method of defining mental disorder allows the individual who is experiencing the psychological distress to seek out mental health intervention. Although this self-report method is humane and avoids the labeling of an individual, the subjectivity and responsibility involved may miss many people. There are people who would be unwilling or unable to declare themselves mentally ill. For example, a person who rapes would not self-refer to a mental health clinic, realizing that such admission could also lead to criminal charges being filed. Children constitute another population group who would have difficulty self-referring. It would be rare indeed to see a child walk into a psychiatric facility announcing that he or she needs help. And a person who is severely paranoid would not be likely to confide in someone that he was mentally ill and that his belief that he was a spiritual leader was false.

Normative Criteria

Mental health is culturally defined. Although a person may be healthy and normal in that he conforms to the usual patterns of behavior, these patterns may not be considered normal in another culture or even in a different age group or in a particular situation within the same culture. Thus the use of the concept of normal is not especially helpful when discussing or evaluating mental or psychosocial aspects because of the various values and customs of different groups of people.

Cultural factors in a society refer to those aspects or ways of life for a given population that distinguish it from other populations. And the definition of the mentally ill differs from culture to culture. In some cultures, individuals who are mentally ill are thought to be possessed by demons. In other cultures, the mentally ill are thought to be possessed by magic and other special and highly valued powers. In still other cultures, the mentally ill person is the outcast or scapegoat for the community.

The definition of mental disorder can be strongly influenced by such factors as family and social network relationships, child-rearing practices, aging, peer groups, race, migration, socioeconomic status, unemployment, war, and social crises. It should also be noted that different population groups within a society will differ in frequency and kind of mental disorder. Social scientists are trying to discover the reason why some population groups have a higher incidence of mental disorders than other population groups.

A study by August Hollingshead and Frederick Redlich of a representative sample of people living in New Haven, Connecticut, reported that adult deprivation resulting from lower-class position was a determinant in severely disordered psychological functioning.[22] This study further indicated that the lowest status groups show the highest rates of hospitalized psychiatric disorders. Relevant to this is the fact that social and cultural patterns associated with social class status influence diagnostic judgments, that is, the lower the status, the more severe the psychiatric diagnoses.

The individual has a social role expectation as he relates to his family and to his community. These cultural expectations of individuals may be potential stress factors, factors that, in turn, may lead to the breakdown of the individual.

Individuals first learn expected role and attitude behavior in the family group. The socialization process then progresses through schooling and interactions with other groups, for example, peer groups, religious groups, neighbors, and colleagues. How each group views health and illness and the behavior that it allows teaches the individual his or her attitude.

Theoretical Criteria

The definition of mental dysfunction, as a descriptive statistic established through theoretical norms, identifies someone who falls to a certain side of an arbitrarily chosen cut-off point. Deviancy from a norm, however, is not always undesirable. All A's on a scholastic record, a very high salary, and a high IQ are all deviancies from the norm but are not considered undesirable. Evaluative statements are made regarding desirable norms. However, the factor of values becomes an issue. For example, a high IQ in a person and his belief that he is God are two statistically infrequent points. One factor is seen as desirable and one is not. Norms tend to be compounded with implicit values.

The dilemma of wishing to avoid the entanglement of value judgments on what is abnormal or normal has led to operational definitions. One definition is the physical location. That is, the locale should be able to tell who is abnormal and who is not. For example, one might assume that those persons confined to a psychiatric institution can be defined as abnormal. However, a quote from Chapter 6 of Lewis Carroll's *Alice in Wonderland* raises questions for such a criterion:

"We're all mad here. I'm mad. You're mad."
"How do you know I'm mad?" said Alice.

"You must be," said the Cat, "or you wouldn't have come here." Alice didn't think that proved it at all.

Many psychiatric nurses would agree with Alice: all abnormal people are not in psychiatric facilities, and not being in a facility is no guarantee of normality.[23]

In summary, Thoits suggests that any discussion of mental health and mental dysfunction depends heavily on how mental health is conceptualized and measured, with all measures in current use having serious drawbacks.[24] The more interesting and challenging observation is to note the individual's characteristic style or way of being healthy (functional) or dysfunctional, at least by the diagnostic criteria in the Diagnostic and Statistical Manual of Mental Disorders, Revised Third Edition (DSM III-R), published by the American Psychological Association (APA) in 1987.

The terms "mental illness," "mental disorder," and "mental dysfunction" will be used interchangeably in this book for variety in the text. These terms are used to refer to a clinically significant syndrome or pattern that is exhibited by an individual and is typically associated with unpleasant symptoms or with impairment in one or more areas of functioning—consistent with the concept of mental disorder described in DSM-III-R.

Summary

Mental health and mental dysfunction were discussed in terms of psychological equilibrium theory and as a beginning framework to understand normal and abnormal behavior. The health-promoting factors of hardiness and humor suggest areas for assessment of positive strengths for patients.

Questions

1. Define mental health and mental illness.
2. How does a psychological conflict develop?
3. Give two examples of pathological psychological equilibrium.
4. How would you respond to a colleague who observes: crazy talk is funny.
5. Give an example of hardiness.

REFERENCES AND SUGGESTED READINGS

1. Binstock, W. A. The psychodynamic approach. In A. Lazare (Ed.), *Outpatient Psychiatry*. Baltimore: Williams & Wilkins, 1979.
2. Nemiah, J. The dynamic bases of psychopathology. In A. M. Nicholi, Jr. (Ed.), *The Harvard Guide to Modern Psychiatry*. Cambridge, Mass.: Harvard University Press, 1979.
3. President's Commission on Mental Health. *Report to the President* (Vol. 1). Washington, D.C.: U.S. Government Printing Office, 1978.
4. Bigbee, J. Hardiness: A new perspective in health promotion. *Nurse Practitioner*, 1985, *10*(11), 51–56.
5. Lambert, C. E., & Lambert, V. A. Hardiness: Its development and relevance to nursing. *Image*, 1987, *19*(2), 92.
6. Kobassa, S. Stressful life events, personality, and health: An inquiry into hardiness. *Journal of Personality and Social Psychology*, 1979, *37*(1), 1–11.
7. Kobassa, S., & Maddi, S. Hardiness measurement. Unpublished memo, Department of Behavioral Sciences, University of Chicago, 1982.
8. Maddi, S. The existential neurosis. *Journal of Abnormal Psychology*, 1967, *72*(4), 311–325.
9. Kobassa, op. cit.
10. Kobassa and Maddi, op. cit.
11. Kobassa, S. The hardy personality: Toward a social psychology of stress and health. In J. Suls &

G. Sanders (Eds.), *Social Psychology of Health and Illness.* Hillsdale, N.J.: Erlbaum.

12. Bigbee, op. cit.

13. Lambert and Lambert, op. cit.

14. Warner, S. L. Humor and self-disclosure within the milieu. *Journal of Psychosocial Nursing and Mental Health Services*, 1984, 22(4), 16–21.

15. McGhee, P. E. Development of the humor response: A review of the literature. *Psychological Bulletin*, 1971, 76(5), 328–348.

16. Robinson, V. M. Humor in nursing. In C. E. Carlson & B. Blackwell (Eds.), *Behavioral Concepts and Nursing Interventions.* Philadelphia: Lippincott, 1970.

17. Burbridge, R. The nature and potential of therapeutic humor. *Dissertation Abstracts International*, 1978, 39(6–13), 2974.

18. Ibid.

19. Warner, op. cit.

20. Binstock. *Ibid.*, p. 49.

21. Nemiah, op. cit., pp. 165–166.

22. Hollingshead, A. B., & Redlich, F. C. *Social Class and Mental Illness.* New York: Wiley, 1958.

23. Finkel, N. J. *Mental Illness and Health: Its Legacy, Tensions, and Changes.* New York: Macmillan, 1976, pp. 1–2.

24. Thoits, P. Position paper. In A. Eichler & D. L. Parron (Eds.), *Women's Mental Health: Agenda for Research.* Washington, D.C.: National Institute of Mental Health, 1987, p. 84.

Chapter 4

Sociocultural Issues of Mental Illness

Barbara J. Holder

Chapter Objectives:

The students successfully attaining the goals of this chapter will be able to:

- Describe sociocultural concepts affecting ethnicity.
- Describe the sociocultural concept of misdiagnosis.
- Discuss the relationship between ethnicity and psychopharmacology.
- Outline the nursing implications for ethnically different patients.

Cultures vary in their emphasis on social structure, environment, world view, and framework, and these cultural emphases provide clues for mental health services.

SOCIOCULTURAL CONCEPTS

Ethnicity is a crucial process that evolves out of individuals' interactions with their family, their ethnic group, and the larger society. An individual's belief regarding a common ancestry based on shared individual characteristics and shared sociocultural experience with an ethnic group is defined as ethnic identity. Ethnic groups are unique sociocultural groups that have been created, maintained, and defined by

historical and contemporary social conditions and experiences. Members of these ethnic groups share a sense of peoplehood based on assumed or real shared sociocultural experiences and similar physical characteristics. The sociocultural experiences may be religious, racial, national, geographical, oppressive, or historical. The shared physical similarities include race and language. Differences in social class, geographical location or relocation and the degree of urbanization result in variation within ethnic groups.

Ethnicity covertly ensures individuals' historical continuity and overtly influences their thinking, feelings, and behavior. Moreover, individuals' life-styles are determined by ethnicity that provides them with experiences for psychosocial growth and development.[1] Since ethnicity also influences an individual's cognition and emotions and psychological systems important for his mental health, the chapter will focus on sociocultural issues related to ethnicity that affect mental health and the practice of psychiatric mental health nursing.

SOCIOCULTURAL ISSUES AFFECTING ETHNICITY

Migration, life-cycle issues, stereotyping, racism, and communication are sociocultural issues that affect ethnicity.

Migration

Geographical origin has been indicated as a central factor in individuals' ethnic identity and sense of continuity.[2] Cross-cultural research suggests that members of an ethnic group who relocate from one geographical area to another tend to identify strongly with their geographical area of origin.[3,4] The research also suggest that the beliefs, values, and coping ability of these ethnically diverse immigrants were influenced by their cultural experiences before and after relocation to their new environment.

Life-cycle Issues

Life-cycle issues that influence ethnicity include sex, age, and psychosocial experiences related to race, economic status, and the degree of involvement in the larger society. Gender, age, discrimination, and experience with members of other ethnic groups are factors that influence ethnic identity. Suggestions that ethnic identity changes over time and is stronger among males than females have been attributed to differences in experiences and to interaction with members of other ethnic groups. Research concerned with Afro-Americans indicates that, for ethnic minorities, a strong ethnic identity is probably reinforced by the animosity and resentment of members of other ethnic groups, being constantly reminded of their ancestors' oppression, and, for males, the lack of involvement in the larger society's opportunity structure because of racial and economic discrimination.[5]

Ethnicity defines how members of various ethnic groups interact with the larger society.[6] The degree of societal acceptance and integration of various ethnic groups and their members depends upon the degree of their involvement within the larger society. Differences in social class, education, and the degree of contact with other ethnic group members are indicated as responsible for variations in the degree of integration of beliefs and values of ethnic subgroups and the larger society. However, variations in beliefs and values among racially similar yet ethnically different subgroups have been found to persist across social class and gender.[7]

Stereotyping

The phenomenon of stereotyping also influences an individual's ethnic identity. Stereotyping consists of beliefs about the personal attributes such as race, sex, or ethnicity of a group of people. Ganong et al. categorize problems related to stereotyping as cognitive confirming, behavioral confirming, or self-rejecting and self-devaluating.[8] Cognitive-confirming problems result from distorted perceptions that blind the perceiver to behaviors that do not fit stereotypic expectations. The perceiver tends to focus on behaviors congruent with beliefs held about the stereotyped group. Beliefs or myths in this category can lead to communication problems that result in misinterpretation of patient behavior.

Problems resulting from behavioral-confirming stereotypic beliefs are related to behaviors that result in the stereotyped groups being treated differently from other groups of people. Problems related to discrimination or racism fall in this category. Ganong's study on stereotyping showed that nurses on an acute inpatient psychiatric unit made more contacts and spent more time with their favored than with their nonfavored patients. The nurses did give as much attention to the physical needs of their nonfavored patients as to their favored patients. However, the nurses initiated more time with patients that they preferred.[9]

Self-evaluating and self-devaluating problems are due to stereotypic beliefs that influence interaction with members of the group. Problems in this category result from behavior that is elicited by members of the stereotyped group. The behavior confirms the initial stereotype and affects how members of a group perceive and value themselves.

Racism

Racism is described by Brantley as basing of decisions, policies, and behavior on some belief or behavior about an ethnic, sex, or racial group for the purpose of subordinating and maintaining control over that group.[10] Brantley defines racism as a kind of paranoid projection in which one group protects itself from the hostility of another.[11] Based on this definition, racism functions similarly to a delusional system in that the projection of negative impulses is used to maintain a societal standard of subservence of one group to another. Because of its functional limitations, racism is a maladaptive defense that creates problems in nurse–patient interaction in the therapeutic relationship.

Racism may be overt and covert, active and passive, and conscious and unconscious process. Types of racism include individual, institutional, and cultural. Individual racism consists of behavior of individuals that supports beliefs of racial superiority of one or more groups over others. Institutional racism is the systematic oppression of people through institutional policies and practices in order to maintain the status quo for members of the stereotyped groups. Cultural racism occurs when an individual or institution expresses superiority of their cultural heritage over that of another individual's or group's cultural heritage. The occurrence of racism in the therapeutic relationship is a devastating blow to the sense of hope of ethnic minority people and other stereotyped groups.[12] The ability to control one's own destiny is a basic human need. Hostile social environments or circumstances such as institutional racism deprive ethnic minorities and other stereotyped groups of the opportunity to actualize positive and hopeful options that should be available through life. Racist situations are also anxiety producing. Ethnic minorities who are subjected to racist behaviors and concepts often develop negative self-perceptions. Victims of racism often react rapidly to these feelings, develop hostility, and want to retaliate against persons responsible for the racist experience. Racist threats to the ego of ethnic minorities result in negative feelings that are projected in various social situations and result in problems in self-esteem.

Communication

Stereotypic thinking leads to communication problems that affect the nurse–patient relationship. Problems caused by cross-cultural differences between the nurse and patient in language, mannerisms, and styles of relating generally result in misinterpretations that might be labeled as psychopathology.[13] Unfamiliarity with a patient's styles of relating might result in misinterpreting and labeling a patient's emotional expressions as a disturbance of affect. Unfamiliarity with a patient's mannerisms might result in misinterpretation and labeling of being bizarre. Unwillingness might be misinterpreted and labeled as resistance. Misunderstanding of the patient's language might be considered as evidence of a thought disorder.

The inability to empathize or relate to a patient from a different ethnic background in an experiental way can also lead to communication barriers between nurse and patient.[14] A nurse from an ethnic group that values distance who confronts a patient from an intensely interactional culture may interpret the patient's interaction as problematic and attempt inappropriately to control it. On the other hand, a nurse from an intensely interactional culture may become frustrated as she tries to increase her emotional involvement with a family from a reserved culture because of their lack of response. However, when the nurse and client come from similar ethnic backgrounds, problems in communicating are generally related to the nurse's either overidentifying with or denying racial or ethnic identification with the client.

Perceptions of counseling, guidance, or psychiatric service as privileges that are available only to the white middle class, self-perceptions of being suppressed by the larger society, use of unmeaningful communication style or phrases in an unfamiliar way, and blaming the client for not clarifying what he said are communication barriers suggested by Mitchell as interfering with the therapeutic communication between a white mental-health provider and black clients.[14]

SOCIOCULTURAL FACTORS AFFECTING MENTAL HEALTH

Mental health problems can neither be diagnosed nor treated without some understanding of a frame of reference and norms of the person seeking help.[15] Help seeking depends on one's attitude toward the helper. Italians have been described as relying on the family and only using outside helpers as a last resource. Afro-Americans mistrust help from traditional middle-class institutions. Puerto Ricans and Asians appear to somatize when stressed and thus tend to seek medical care rather than mental health care. Norwegians have been reported as converting emotional tension into physical symptoms that are culturally accepted and of seeking help from a surgeon. Iranians have been described as relying on medications and vitamins to treat symptoms. Thus, culture determines not only whether a symptom is labeled a problem but also an individual's help-seeking behavior.

Misdiagnosis

Psychiatry's reliance almost entirely on signs, symptoms, and behaviors is a major drawback in psychiatric diagnosis. Different illnesses may have the same or similar signs, symptoms, and behavior.[16] As previously discussed, symptoms and behaviors are culturally related and thus differ from one ethnic group to another. Certain psychopathologies change diagnostic category entirely in different cultures. Syndromes classified as behavioral problems or psychosomatic syndromes in one culture may mask depression in another culture. The relative distribution of depression, conversion reaction, anxiety, and obsessive-compulsion disorders differs from one culture to another. Alcohol and drug abuse may also be manifested in psychopathology. Societies with high rates of substance abuse have been found to have corresponding low rates of diagnosed neurotic disorders, thereby suggesting that alcoholism and drug abuse may be alternatives to neurotic disorders.

In mental health, misinterpretation and misunderstanding of a symptom presentation occur in three areas—disorder of thought content, disorder of thought process (looseness of association, incomplete thought, and flights of ideas), and cultural distance between patient and therapist (language, behavioral mannerisms, and style of relating).[17] Cultural differences in symptomatology in these three areas can lead to problems in the nurse–patient relationship and to misdiagnosis of patient's symptoms and behaviors.

Misinterpretation of patients' presenting symptomatology may lead to a misdiagnosis of schizophrenia. Schizophrenia is an illness category that inherits whatever is marginal or unclear to the mental health clinician. Unclear and confused clinical pictures tend to be diagnosed as schizophrenia. Jones and Grey suggest that

blacks are overdiagnosed as schizophrenic and underdiagnosed for affective illness. Black and Hispanic bipolar patients are more at risk for being misdiagnosed as schizophrenic, particularly if they are young and experiencing auditory hallucinations during an affective episode, than white patients. Thus, there is a suggestion that race and diagnosis are significantly related to psychiatric misdiagnosis.[18]

The overdiagnosis of blacks as schizophrenic has been attributed to clinicians being impressed by symptoms such as hallucinations.[16] Altered states of consciousness that may appear to be mental illness are encouraged in some cultures. There are universal phenomena that are experienced in a number of forms by all humans (dreams, drug or alcohol intoxication). Less familiar states include trance and possession trance. A trance is generally interpreted as an absence of some kind and is frequently linked to hallucinations or visions. Possession trance involves a belief that the body has been taken over in its function by a spiritual entity. These forms of altered consciousness are generally considered sacred, ritual states and involve cultural patterning influenced by learning, tradition, and culture. The notion of possession is common among American Pentecostal groups, charismatic religious movements in which the Holy Ghost is believed to possess individuals (good possession). From a mental health perspective, a patient indicating that he is possessed by a spirit may be viewed as expressing symptoms of a mental disorder. From a cultural perspective, the patient may be viewed as engaging in normal, culturally sanctioned behavior based on culturally prescribed belief systems.

An understanding of black norms means being aware of a body of adaptive character traits, such as cultural paranoia and a reluctance and hesitancy that have been developed by blacks in response to a particular environment.[19] Cultural paranoia is a protective wariness that is often mistaken for paranoia, symptomatic schizophrenia, especially if the patient is a black male. The reluctance and hesitancy that some blacks manifest in relating to white clinicians is characterized by a strict control over affective response and resistance to establishing rapport and communication. This reluctance and hesitancy is frequently interpreted as dislike and hostility.

Affective disorder is a disorder of mood that constitutes number and type of illnesses. Mood illnesses are distributed across a wide spectrum from mild depression to life-threatening mania. It is often difficult to determine which disorder is present, particularly without knowledge of the patient's past history and previous course of illness. Symptoms are considered related primarily to mood and activity, such as depression and psychomotor retardation or elation and hyperactivity. Affective conditions also incorporate symptoms of thought disorder. Nontreatment can lead to manic states difficult to distinguish from schizophrenia.

The same symptoms may be expressed through a variety of behavioral actions that are culturally determined. Cultural stereotypes such as "blacks are generally happy," "blacks seldom suffer from depression" leads to misdiagnosis of affective disorder in blacks. The lack of a clear distinction of depression and a perception of hyperactive behaviors as normal are other factors that contribute to misdiagnosis in ethnic minorities. Cultural differences in languages, mannerisms, and styles of relating may also be misinterpreted as depression or hypomania if the nurse is unfamiliar with the patient's culture and social actions. Stereotypic thinking such as "depression and mania are upper and middle class illnesses" also contribute to misdiagnosis. Variance in symptom presentation is one factor that contributes to misdiagnosis.[20]

Racism

Racism is devastating to the psychiatric patient who is already vulnerable by weakened coping mechanisms. The patient must use his fragile defensive structure to protect himself from a real external psychological assault on his sense of self. On a conscious level, the patient may react with a greater immediacy. The more direct the racist action, the more difficulty the patient has withholding his antagonistic impulses. Depending on the strength of his ability to cope, the patient may react impulsively and aggressively if the insult is directed at his sense of self and he feels the full impact of the injury to his ego.[21]

ETHNICITY AND PSYCHOPHARMACOLOGY

A review of well-controlled cross-cultural studies of psychotropic drugs by Lin, Pland and

Lesser suggests that responses to dosage requirements and manifestation of drug toxicity vary significantly among patients from different ethnic groups. For example, effective weight-standardized dosages of chlorpromazine are significantly lower for Asian patients than those for white American patients who were matched for age, sex, and diagnosis. Also, the average stabilizing dosage of neuroleptics for Asians patients is reported to be significantly lower than for white and black patients.[22] Furthermore, Asian schizophrenic patients appear to manifest a significantly higher incidence of extrapyramidal reactions to haloperidol than black and white schizophrenic patients. Chinese patients had consistently higher plasma haloperidol levels after 6 weeks of a fixed dose of oral haloperidol treatment. Thus, Chinese, and Asians in general, appear to require significantly lower dosages and to be more sensitive to the effects of neuroleptic drugs than non-Asians.

Other cross-cultural research concerned with lithium carbonate acid suggests that manic patients in Japan and Taiwan are generally treated with lower dosages and have lower plasma levels of lithium than patients in the United States. The reported therapeutic serum lithium levels ranging from 0.4 to 0.8 mEq/L were significantly lower than the therapeutic serum lithium levels of 0.98 mEq/L for white American patients. Lithium doses that were well tolerated by American patients produced intolerable side effects in Japanese and Taiwanese patients. Thus, lower dosage levels of lithium appear to be more effective for Asians patients than for white American patients.[23]

The research suggestion of an effective dosage range of tricyclic antidepressants for Asian patients from 1.4 to 2.7 mg/kg of body weight is half the dosage range, 3.5 mg/kg, required for American patients. The plasma levels for lower oral dosage for Asian patients (100 mg/ml) were also proportionately lower than for American patients (180 mg/ml). Higher plasma levels of clomipramine have also been reported among healthy subjects of Indian or Pakistani origin as compared to English subjects. There are indications that black and Hispanic patients also require a lower therapeutic dosage of tricyclics than white patients. Black depressive patients have been found to have a 50 percent higher plasma level of nortriptyline than white patients in similar circumstances.[24]

Strong evidence suggests that factors such as genetics, environment, diet, and cultural attitudes and beliefs are responsible for ethnic variations in psychotropic drug use. Poor metabolism of certain psychotropic drugs because of genetic factors has been indicated as being responsible for drug side effects in Asians, blacks, and native Americans. Environmental factors such as smoking, alcohol intake, and exposure to drugs and toxins have been attributed to the rapid elimination of psychotropic drugs. A low-protein, high-carbohydrate diet has been attributed to a lower elimination of antipyrine and theophylline in Asian Indians and West Africans. Research indicates that individuals who are action-oriented and have a high need for controlling their surroundings become increasingly agitated and confused by and require a larger amount of sedatives.[25]

NURSING IMPLICATIONS

An effective nurse–patient relationship requires empathy and helpfulness. Nurses must be able to deal with their own conflict about ethnically different patients.

Shared experiences are believed to be catalysts for ethnic minority patients to develop a relationship with the nurse. Typical reasons given for failure in the therapeutic relationship is the nurse's inability to empathize or relate to the patient in an experiential way. However, problems between the nurse and a patient from a similar background have been attributed either to the nurse's overidentification with or denial of racial or ethnic identification with her patients. The impact of either attitude is detrimental to the therapeutic relationship.[26]

Leininger's Sunrise model provides a useful guideline for cross-cultural interviewing.[27] The nurse who listens and is knowledgeable about cultural variations will be able to note these themes during the interview and explicate ideas for therapeutic implications that concern the client. Patients from different cultures use different body language or nonverbal expressions. Verbal and nonverbal communication are both important in assessment and in validating meaning when possible. Body language expressions and vocal tones and intensity can help the nurse grasp the feeling and importance of different elements to the patient's social structure.

The nurse can assist the patient in being an active participant by making him feel valuable and an important partner in the interview process. Allowing the patient to actively participate in the interview process greatly increases his co-

operation and facilitates a productive and qualitatively rich interview. The patient will also feel it is acceptable to share cultural ideas and to have them respected by the interviewer. When the patient is treated as a true participant, he generally shares more detailed cultural information.

Consensus among nursing staff of nursing diagnoses decreases misdiagnosis. Agreement between two or more nurses helps in avoiding many of the communication problems previously outlined. Westermayer notes that diagnostic reliability between two clinicians is higher for organic psychiatric symptoms, intermediate for schizophrenia, and low for depression and affective disorder.[18] Diagnostic discrepancy is greatest with patients who have symptoms and signs that cut across diagnostic categories, such as schizophrenia and depression. The validity of a nursing diagnosis can be assessed by observing treatment variables, studying outcomes, and measuring patient responses to nursing interventions and treatment. The latter also includes monitoring psychotropic drug dosage and side effects.

In patient situations complicated by racism, initial interventions that the nurse can use include exploring with the patient his coping mechanisms and ways of developing more productive avenues for dealing with the anxiety triggered by racism. The patient should be allowed to express frustrations aroused by racial discrimination. This helps the nurse in assessing the impact of the racist event on the patient and helps the patient to increase control over his or her reaction. The nurse should accept the patient's feelings openly and frankly without over- or underidentification to allow the patient to express feelings without judgment from the nurse. Minimization of the racial issue should also be avoided. By using these initial interventions the nurse will assist the patient in coping with the external environmental factors and thus move to deal with other, more internal conflicts and issues. The nurse must be sensitive to race when intervening with a racial or discriminatory issue. Patients who respond in a maladaptive way may also have preexisting difficulties that may require deeper exploration.

Exploration of the patient's reaction to conflicts about race permits less projection and externalization and assists the patient in dealing more effectively with personal conflicts. When possible, this exploration should be separated from the patient's internal struggles. The nurse should also use the therapeutic process to assist patients in exploring their misperceptions of self and to establish a more positive sense of self-worth. By doing this, the irrationality of racism may be revealed and its negative images made more apparent. Failure to address patients' racial questions may result in unsuccessful resolution of these issues and may impede the treat-

ment. The nurse must confront her own stance on racism while simultaneously assisting the patient or she will be unable to hear the importance of the patient's racially related message. The nurse may also try to explain away the patient's responses and may become a participant in the patient's denial system.

Summary

The importance of a knowledge of cultural norms facilitates a positive working relationship between nurses and their patients. This chapter reviews sociocultural concepts of migration, life-cycle, stereotyping, racism, and communication that affect ethnicity.

Questions

1. Autognose your feelings regarding ethnically different patients.
2. Identify five concepts affecting ethnicity.
3. Give an example of sociocultural misdiagnosis.

REFERENCES AND SUGGESTED READINGS

1. McGoldrick, M. Overview: Ethnicity and family therapy. In M. McGoldrick, J. K. Pearse and J. Giordano (Eds.), *Ethnicity and Family Therapy.* New York: Guilford Press, 1982.
2. Ibid.
3. Ballard, A. B. *One More Day's Journey.* New York: McGraw-Hill, 1974.
4. Lewis, J. M., & Looney, J. G. *The Long Struggle, Well-Functioning Working-Class Black Families.* New York: Brunner Mazel, 1983.
5. Ballard, op. cit.
6. McGoldrick, op. cit.
7. Glantz, O. Native sons and immigrants: Some beliefs and values of American-black and West Indian blacks at Brooklyn College. *Ethnicity,* 1978, 5, 189–202.
8. Ganong, L. H., Bzdek, V., & Manderino, M. A. Stereotyping by nurses and nursing students: A critical review of research. *Research in Nursing and Health,* 1978, 10.
9. Ibid.
10. Brantley, T. Racism and its impact on psychotherapy. *American Journal of Psychiatry,* 1983, 140(12).
11. Ibid.
12. Brantley, op. cit.
13. Jones, B., & Grey, B. A. Problems in diagnosing schizophrenia and affective disorders among blacks. *Hospital and Community Psychiatry,* 1986, 37, 1, 61–65.
14. Mitchell, A. C. Barriers to therapeutic communication with black clients. *Nursing Outlook,* 1978, 26(2), 109–112.
15. McGoldrick, op. cit.
16. Westermayer, J. Psychiatric diagnosis across cultural boundaries. *American Journal of Psychiatry,* 1985, 142(7), 798–805.
17. Ibid.
18. Jones and Gray, op. cit.
19. Ibid.
20. Jones and Gray, op. cit.
21. Brantley, op. cit.
22. Lin, K.-M., Pland, R. E., & Lesser, I. M. Ethnicity and psychopharmocology. *Culture, Medicine and Psychiatry,* 1986, 10, 151–165.
23. Ibid.
24. Ibid.
25. Ibid.
26. Brantley, op. cit.
27. Leininger, M. Transcultural interviewing and health assessment. In P. B. Pederson, N. Sartorius, and A. J. Marsella (Eds.), *Mental Health Services, the Cross-Cultural Context.* Beverly Hills, Calif.: Sage Publications, 1984, 109–133.

Chapter 5

Contributions From the Neurobiological Sciences

Ann Wolbert Burgess

Chapter Objectives

The students successfully attaining the goals of this chapter will be able to:

- Define the triune brain.
- Compare and contrast right and left brain hemispheres.
- Describe the history of psychotropic drugs.
- Outline the functioning of the central nervous system and the autonomic nervous system and discuss their relationship to receptor site theory and drugs.
- Define biologic rhythms.
- Outline the function and periods of sleep.

The past two decades has seen a phenomenal increase in research on the brain. Major developments have occurred in the knowledge of neuroanatomy and physiology that help to explain the biologic dynamics that underlie human behavior. Although research on brain behavior has been slow, the developing knowledge helps in understanding normal human functioning and structure of the central nervous system.

This chapter will describe the scientific basis of psychopharmacology and provide an overview of the brain's functioning, biologic rhythms, sleep, and genetics.

SCIENTIFIC BASIS OF PSYCHOPHARMACOLOGY

What is the scientific basis of psychopharmacology? Many disciplines have been involved in the study of the action of psychotropic drugs, including biochemistry, physiology, neuroanatomy, clinical psychiatry, and psychiatric nursing. All these disciplines aid in understanding how drugs act on the mind. In the 30 years since the initiation of vigorous research with psychotropic drugs, it has become evident that the effects of greatest relevance to understanding the clinical actions of the drugs are exerted on neurotransmitter disposition. Accordingly, fundamental understanding of psychopharmacology demands a familiarity with central nervous system (CNS) neurotransmitters, the history of psychotropic drugs, and the regulatory aspects of the brain.

REGULATORY ASPECTS OF THE BRAIN

A basic assumption of mind and body interaction is that the brain is the primary system of behavior regulation.* Therefore, biologic interventions are aimed at regulatory aspects of the brain.

Brain regulatory functioning is usually not obvious to people. However, during illness, this concept is easier to comprehend. For example, when a patient has a high fever, the difficulty the patient has with memory detail or talking can be clinically observed (see Fig. 5-1).

Environmental demands can be physical, social, and psychological, as illustrated in Figure 5-1. For example, excessive cold as a stimulus is perceived through the sense organs and is transmitted to the brain. The result is muscle activity, which moves arms and legs and the person into a sheltered place for warmth. Negative feedback is information processed by special areas of the brain to clarify the danger for other areas of the brain and to initiate actions to move the person closer to heat and safety.

It is more difficult to envision how stimuli originating from a mental stimulus trigger information centers in the brain, for example, one's fear of being alone or the thoughts and memory of a missing loved one. Such stimuli result in sad emotions and a deceleration of physical behavior. What is especially perplexing is the notion that awareness of the sadness and deceleration does not always result in behavior to counteract the deceleration. Rather, the person often seems trapped in remembering thoughts and events. With such an impasse we are confronted with a breakdown of the regulatory functions of the brain. Using a systems approach, the following questions begin to direct the search for the breakdown and a possible point of intervention. Is the impasse in the

* NOTE: This section through page 54 has been prepared by Carol R. Hartman.

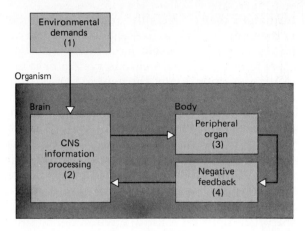

Figure 5-1. The brain as the primary system of behavioral regulation: *Adapted from Gary E. Schwartz, Psychosomatic disorders and biofeedback: A psychobiological model of deregulation. In Psychopathology: Experimental Models, eds. Martin E. P. Selliguran and Jack D. Maswer (San Francisco: W. H. Freeman, 1977).*

source of stimulation, for example, the psychological memories of the deceased? Is there a disruption of brain function? Is there a breakdown in the negative feedback system itself? Is there no information coming through that says, "Stop brooding, you're interrupting your life"?

Figure 5-1 illustrates that mind and body are one when the brain is understood as the primary system of behavioral regulation through a complex system of information feedback. Emphasis is placed on negative feedback because it is the type of information that clues the brain into action to bring stability to the organism. Negative feedback gives the stimulus to the body via the brain to correct the organ behavior that ultimately threatens the existence of the brain itself. For example, heat sensed in the fingertips is returned to the brain as a stimulus. This stimulus is processed in the brain, and information is sent to the fingers to be removed from the hot stove. When the fingers blister and burn, it is the brain that interprets the experience of pain. If the return of information from the fingers is limited or missing (positive feedback), the fingers are not removed despite their blistering. Here we see a breakdown in central nervous system regulation because of a failure of negative feedback.

The model shown in Figure 5-1 recognizes the holistic functioning of psychobiological experiences and establishes a rationale for concentrating on areas of activity that are thought to impede the brain in its primary function of behavioral regulation. Negative feedback is information that corrects the regulating activities of the brain. Failure to use negative feedback can be due to three causes. First, there may be a disease of the central nervous system or failure in the development of the central nervous system as a result of genetics and maturation. The impairment may be such as to alter perceiving and receiving centers, or there may be alterations in the sorting and processing activities. Second, the peripheral organ itself can be damaged, or it may be hyperactive or hypoactive, thus altering information feedback in such a manner that the brain cannot compensate for the organ defect. Or third, environmental stress can be so great it interferes with the receiving of negative feedback. For example, a man runs from a burning car to escape death, not noting pain from a broken leg.

Schwartz's model in Figure 5-1 links brain and body through the important concept of negative feedback. Behavioral conditioning interventions and psychosocial interventions focus on 1, 3, and 4 with the aim of influencing and altering 2 (brain). Biologic interventions most often focus on the brain. Some therapies, such as fever therapy, were thought to influence brain functioning by altering the physical state of an individual. Others, such as electroshock, are meant to alter brain functioning, albeit in a gross manner, by direct action. Today, the most interesting and informative biologic approach has been in the use of drugs that are referred to as psychotropic medications. The history of the discovery of these drugs is interesting since most of them were accidentally discovered to have potent central nervous system effects. The investigation of these effects has resulted in a strong biochemical hypothesis of central nervous system regulation and certain psychiatric disorders. Not only have the findings built strong evidence for this notion but they have become important in redefining psychopathological states.

HISTORY OF PSYCHOTROPIC DRUGS

Present-day psychopharmacology emanates from two important areas: (1) basic research, and (2) fortuitous observations in clinical practice.

Basic Research

Two major contributions of basic research in the area of neurotransmitters include: (1) acetylcho-

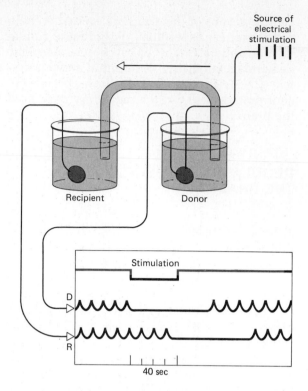

Figure 5-2. Otto Loewi's experiment, 1921. *Adapted from Conan Kornetsky, Pharmacology: Drugs Affecting Behavior, New York: Wiley, 1976, p. 48.*

line and (2) norepinephrine. Otto Loewi first demonstrated experimentally in 1921 that the transmission of nerve impulses was mediated by the release of chemicals into the synaptic cleft.[1] He found that if you stimulated the vagus nerve of a perfused frog heart, a substance was given off that slowed the heart rate of a second perfused frog heart (Fig. 5-2).

Electrical stimulation of the vagus nerve (see Fig. 5-2) in the donor causes a cessation in the heart rate (D). The vagus nerve of the donor heart releases acetylcholine into the bath. The bath solution with acetylcholine crosses over into the bath solution of the recipient heart (R) through the curved tube. There is a small time lag for the crossover of solution, but soon the acetylcholine stimulates the vagus nerve of the recipient heart and the heart rate in (R) stops. Loewi called the substance *vagusstoff*. This substance was later identified as acetylcholine. When Loewi stimulated the sympathetic nerve of the donor heart, he observed the reverse: the heart rate increased. W. B. Cannon and J. E. Uridil studied the effects of stimulating the sympathetic nerve to the liver in 1921.[2] They noted the material released was similar to epinephrine and called it "sympathin." It is thought that this substance was, in fact, norepinephrine.

Clinical Observations

Before 1950, no important chemical agents existed in psychiatric practice except sedatives and amphetamines. These had limited use because of their toxic and addicting effects. Since the 1950s, a remarkable development in behavior intervention has taken place in the area of psychotropic drugs. Drug therapy has been aimed at, and has clarified to an increasing degree, the regulatory functions of the brain. Laboratory disruptions of these functions have been related to certain signs and symptoms associated with mental illness.

Five important clinical observations and discoveries can be identified to provide the foundation of present-day drug intervention. The first discovery was lithium salts made by J. F. J. Cade in Australia. Cade accidentally observed the calming effects of lithium ions in animals.[3] Lithium carbonate is now recognized for its value in the treatment of manic patients.

The second clinical observation raised the possibilities of today's drugs used for the treatment of psychiatric problems. *Rauwolfia serpentina*, which had been used by Hindu physicians for centuries, was introduced to Western medicine in the mid-1940s to treat hypertension. In 1953, R. W. Wilkins and W. E. Judson at Boston University noted its beneficial effect in anxious, tense patients.[4] In 1954, Nathan Kline reported positive results at Rockland State Hospital in New York with disturbed schizophrenic patients.[5] However, continued use with psychiatric patients as well as hypertensive patients demonstrated that the drug causes severe depression. It is thought that either depletion of serotonin or depletion of catecholamines is the cause of the depressive behavior. The drug is not used in psychiatry today. However, its effects are important in nonpsychiatric patients suffering from hypertension.

The third clinical observation was the effect of chlorpromazine on psychiatric problems. Chlorpromazine was synthesized in 1950 at Rhone-Poulenc Laboratories in France. In 1949, H. Laborit discovered the calming effect of this drug on people, and it was originally tested in France as an anesthetic. In 1952 in France, it was first tested for the treatment of schizophrenics.[6]

While chlorpromazine was being discovered in France, meprobamate was being discovered in the United States in 1950 to treat anxiety and neurotic states. Because of its addicting qualities, it is not used today, but other antianxiety drugs have been developed.

Monoamine oxidase inhibitors were the fourth clinical observation. This substance was tested to treat depression. The drugs were discovered by noting that the mood of tuberculosis patients was elevated when they were on new antituberculin drugs, isoniazid and iproniazid (1952). Iproniazid proved to be more useful in the discovery of monoamine oxidase inhibitor than as an antituberculin drug. MAO inhibitors have certain interactive characteristics that caution that they be used carefully in the treatment of depression.

The fifth clinical observation was the discovery of tricyclic antidepressants (imipramine) in 1957. It was only by careful clinical observations that these drugs, which so closely resemble the phenothiazines, were discovered to reduce depressive states but not schizophrenic states.

P. A. Janssen, in the United States in the 1960s, tried to synthesize a drug with morphine-like qualities that was nonaddicting. He discovered a drug that did not have the analgesic effects but did have typical chlorpromazine effects. Thus, the butyrophenones are another group of antipsychotic drugs. The most widely used in the United States is haloperidol.[7] It is interesting to note that most psychotropic drugs were discovered by people pursuing drugs for nonpsychiatric problems, and the discovery of tricyclics was almost missed because the researchers were looking for a drug to treat schizophrenia. Today we have three major groups of psychopharmacologic agents that have replaced, for the most part, the use of sedatives, amphetamines, and *Rauwolfia*. These are antipsychotic, antidepressant, and antianxiety drugs. These drugs have also replaced psychosurgery, hydrotherapy, and insulin coma. Their impact in psychiatry has been equated with the impact of antibiotics in general medicine. Since the 1950s there has been extensive molecular manipulation of the major chemical structures first found useful with psychotic, depressive, and anxious states. Research with these drugs has been most important in gaining an understanding of how drugs work; how the neuroregulatory functions of the brain are affected; and how hypothesized neuroregulators play a critical role in deviant behavior.[8]

DRUG ACTION FRAMEWORK

The concept of neuroreception is central to a framework of drug action. To date, information about what actually occurs in a cell is very limited, and the only experimentally validated neurotransmitter is acetylcholine.[9]

In developing a framework, it is important to distinguish between drug action and drug effect. It is believed that most drugs produce their effect by combining with enzymes, cell membranes, or some other part of the cell.[10] It is also thought that the drug interacts with some component of the cell that starts a sequence of physiological and biochemical events that characterize the pharmacologic effects of the drug. It is the initial result of the drug interaction with the cell that is defined as drug action.[11]

Two Principles of Drug Action

Structure-Activity Relationship

Conan Kornetsky emphasizes two important principles of drug action. One is the structure-activity relationship.[12] This principle underscores that the structure of a drug is closely related to the action of the drug. By investigation of the chemical structure of drugs, we have learned that at times a slight change in the structure of the drug can result in an entirely different drug effect. With other drugs, slight changes in their chemical structure can result in only a slight change in their effect, altering only their potency. Side effects, for example in psychotropic medications, are often reduced through slight molecular alterations. What is perplexing, though, is that sometimes drugs of quite dissimilar structures can have similar effects. Despite this confusing possibility, many drugs have been developed by manipulating their chemical structure and observing their effect. In some cases these manipulations have been most useful in generating important hypotheses of how these drugs act at the cell level. An example is the phenothiazine chlorpromazine (Thorazine) and its subsequent derivatives and the subsequent discovery of imipramine (Tofranil), an antidepressant. Later, this will be discussed in more detail.

Receptor Site Activity

The second principle is that of the *receptor*.[13] It is postulated that the initial action of a drug is at the receptor site of a cell. This postulate is based on anatomic and physiological studies of cells and, in particular, neurons. As noted earlier, Otto Loewi's experiment demonstrated that there was chemical activity involved at the synapse of neurons. What has emerged from experimentation and clinical observation is a theory about receptor site activity.

Assumptions about the receptor site theory are threefold: (1) there are specific receptors for specific chemical structures; (2) the drug receptor interaction is chemical in nature; and (3) this chemical reaction is usually reversible. Kornetsky likens these assumptions to locks (receptor sites) waiting to be fitted by keys (chemical structure of the drug).[14] Drug effects occur either within the cell or at the cell surface.

However, not all drugs enter the human system and fit the receptor like a key. There is a drug–cell action that binds drugs to enzymes, plasma, and cell proteins, where the main function appears to be the biotransmission of drugs. This biotransmission often results in some drugs being broken down into metabolites, whose chemical structures might then act at the receptor sites, be excreted, or participate in other active cellular processes. An example of this is antibiotics.

Drug action at the receptor site is further defined by specific characteristics. When a drug interacts with the receptor and also initiates a drug action, it is called an **agonist**.[15] An **antagonist** is a drug that combines with a receptor and fails to show any action. **Affinity** is shown when a drug combines with the receptor with or without an action. Both antagonist and agonist show an affinity. However, only the drug that combines to have an effect has intrinsic activity or efficacy, and only the agonist has intrinsic activity.[16]

When these assumptions of how a drug interacts at a receptor are used to explain the phenomenon of drug tolerance, an interesting speculation arises. First, drug tolerance has been explained by the notion that drugs that combine, that is, show an affinity but have a decreased intrinsic affinity (effect), remain in the synapse, occupying space, so that additional amounts of the drug cannot combine. New theories suggest that drugs that combine (affinity) without effect may alter the metabolism of neurotransmitters within the presynaptic neuron, as well as within the postsynaptic neuron.[17] This notion opens up a whole new area for understanding drug action. The idea of neurotransmission and drugs acting on this process is at the heart of understanding the efficacy of psychotropic drugs and the biochemistry of behavior and mental disorders.

This new theory of altered metabolic state within neurons and receptor site activity is basic to understanding drug action in psychopharmacology. In order for the presynaptic neuron to produce an impulse in the postsynaptic neuron (receptor), certain events must occur in sequence.[18] The nerve cell must actively pass an electric current via an exchange of sodium (Na+) and potassium (K+) located in the membrane of the nerve cell (presynaptic neuron). When this current readies the storage vesicles, the stored neurotransmitter is released by the process of exocytosis.[19] Following the release from the presynaptic neuron, the neurotransmitter traverses the synaptic cleft, binds briefly to its postsynaptic receptor, and is released back into the synaptic cleft. A process of reabsorption (re-uptake) occurs within the presynaptic neuron. What is left over in the cleft is metabolized by monoamine oxidase (MAO), an enzyme located in the mitochondria of the nerve cell. The remainder of the neurotransmitter is metabolized by a second enzyme in the synaptic cleft, catechol methyltransferase (COMT).[20]

Synaptic Mechanism

The junction between one neuron and the next is called a **synapse**. When an electrical nerve impulse travels from one neuron to the next, the impulse must cross the synaptic cleft, which is a space between the adjoining neurons (Fig. 5-3). When a nerve impulse reaches a presynaptic terminal, electrical stimulation causes the release of an excitatory transmitter substance, e.g., norepinephrine and/or serotonin, among others. The excitatory transmitter substance is stored in the excitatory transmitter vesicles located at the synaptic end of the presynaptic terminal. Simply stated, upon release of the transmitter substance, the electrical nerve impulse is allowed to cross the synapse and eventually evoke a stimulation or response of the central nervous system.

RECEPTOR SITE ACTIVITY AND THE AUTONOMIC AND CENTRAL NERVOUS SYSTEM

Neurons are located throughout the human body. A major theoretical division is made be-

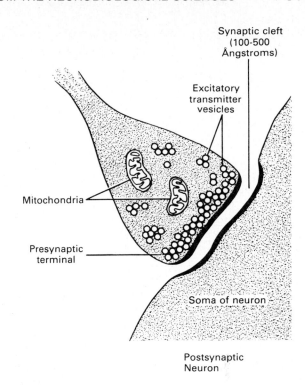

Figure 5-3. Structure-activity relationship. Synaptic exchange.

tween neurons found in the central nervous system and those of the autonomic nervous system. What is known about each system's neuroreceptor transmission activity varies because of the problems of direct access to the physiological functioning of the brain and nerves. The autonomic nervous system is more directly observable from anatomic and physiological perspectives (Fig. 5-4).

Neuroreceptor Transmission

Neurotransmissions within the autonomic nervous system are carried out primarily by acetylcholine and norepinephrine.[21] The two primary neurotransmitters of the autonomic nervous system divide into two major systems. Drugs that have cholinergic actions identify the parasympathetic system. These drugs are called **parasympathomimetic**. Drugs that have adrenergic effects identify the sympathetic system. These drugs are called **sympathomimetic**.[22]

As we trace nerves from the central nervous system and the spinal cord to the major organs and glands, we find that functions of organs and glands are influenced by adrenergic receptors (sympathetic nervous system) and by the ace-

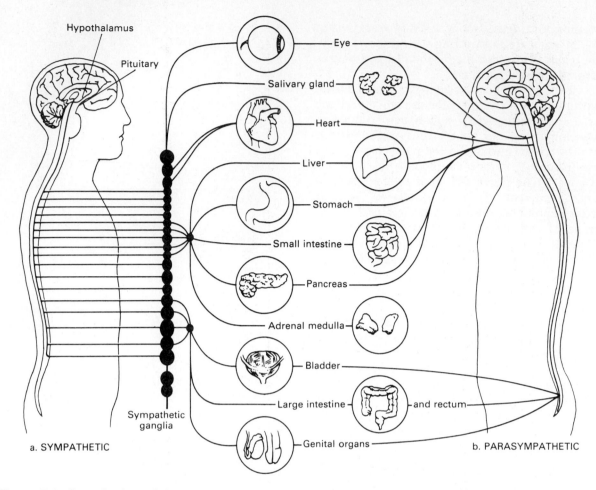

Figure 5-4. Organization of the autonomic nervous system. The sympathetic division functions to arouse the body and speed up its vital processes, whereas the parasympathetic division slows down bodily processes. The two divisions work together to maintain an equilibrium within the body.

tylcholine receptors (parasympathetic nervous system).

Adrenergic Receptors

Adrenergic receptors are of two types: (1) *alpha receptors*, which mediate smooth muscle contractions, resulting in vasoconstriction, increased blood pressure, pupillary dilation, and contraction of the nectating membrane and the splenic capsule; and (2) *beta receptors*, which, when stimulated, result in vasodilation in skeletal muscles, tachycardia, bronchial relaxation, and increased strength of muscular contractions of the heart.[23] It is important to realize that whether the organ function is ultimately influenced by cholinergic receptors or by adrenergic receptors, all neurotransmission in the autonomic nervous system is initially influenced by

cholinergic receptors (preganglionic).[24] In both the parasympathetic and sympathetic systems, nervous tissue comes together in ganglia, from which new networks of nerves (postganglionic) emanate to specific effector organs. Again, the distinction (postganglionic) is made at the receptor site chemical activity level. In the sympathetic system, postganglionic receptor activity is mainly adrenergic, with the exception of cholinergic activity of sweat glands. In the parasympathetic postganglionic chains, receptor site activity is cholinergic. In somatic nerves that emanate from the cranial nerves and the fourth, third, and second sacral regions, which frequently directly innervate effector organs, cholinergic activity dominates.[25] Where there are postganglionic tracks, the receptor site remains cholinergic.

When the autonomic nervous system is

stimulated, the response of the effector organ is shown in Table 5-1.

In investigating drug effect and action, use is made of studying effects at the organ site. Drugs that stimulate the autonomic system result in an excess of organ action described under the parasympathetic (cholinergic) and sympathetic (adrenergic) systems. Blocking drugs result in a reduction of noted action.

Drugs are identified according to their blocking properties. Blocking agents of adrenergic receptors are of two types: alpha and beta blockers. Alpha blocking drugs, for example, result in a lowering of blood pressure, whereas

TABLE 5-1. AUTONOMIC NERVE STIMULATION AND EFFECTOR ORGAN

Effector Organ	Parasympathetic (cholinergic-parasympathetic drug)	Sympathetic (adrenergic-sympathetic drug)
Eye and lacrimal glands	Secretion of tears, miosis of pupil.	Mydriasis of pupil.
Glands of nose, mouth, salivary glands	Vasodilation, profuse watery secretion.	Reduced blood flow to glands and sparse, thick, viscous mucous secretions.
Lungs	Bronchial constriction (bronchi and bronchioles). Increased glandular secretion of these tubes.	Bronchial dilatation of bronchi and bronchioles.
Heart	Bradycardia. Decrease in blood volume. Possible constriction of coronary arteries.	Tachycardia. Increase in blood volume. Dilatation of coronary arteries.
Digestive system	Increased peristalsis. Relaxation of sphincter. Increased secretion of digestive gland, i.e., pancreas.	Decrease in peristalsis. Constriction of sphincter. Inhibition of gastric secretions. Increase in glucose in the bloodstream.
Blood vessels	Dilation of blood vessels in the glands in the head. Dilation of blood vessels in the digestive system. Increased circulation in the erectile tissue of the genital system.	Constriction of vessels to lungs, digestive system, and skin. Dilatation of coronary arteries and arteries of the voluntary muscles.
Sweat glands		Secretions (acetylcholine) to sweat glands control body temperature. However, sweating of palms and soles of feet is seen as adrenergic sweating.
Pilomotor (hair) muscles of the skin		Contraction (piloerection and goose pimples).
Adrenal glands		Secretes epinephrine and norepinephrine.
Genital system	Engorgement of erectile tissue, active secretion of the accessory glands.	Ejaculation of semen by involuntary muscles of genital glands and ducts accompanied by somatic nerve stimulation of the voluntary muscles. Except for the blood vessels, ovaries, testes, and uterus do not respond to autonomic stimuli.

Source: Adapted from Conan Kornetsky, *Pharmacology: Drugs Affecting Behavior* (New York, John Wiley & Sons, Inc., 1976, pp. 52–53).

beta blocking drugs can result in a rise in blood pressure.

Cholinergic Receptors

Cholinergic receptors are activated by acetylcholine. This substance in mammals is usually an excitatory substance. There appear to be two types of cholinergic receptors. They are named muscarinic and nicotinic. The cholinergic receptor sites gain these names because they are stimulated either by the drug muscarine or by nicotine. Cholinergic receptors are basically nicotinic at the autonomic ganglia and at the neuromuscular junctions. Cholinergic receptors of the target organs of the autonomic nervous system are muscarinic. Both types—muscarinic and nicotinic—are found in the central nervous system. The spinal cord contains nicotinic receptors. The brain contains both, but the predominant receptor is nicotinic.[26]

Cholinergic and adrenergic activity is responsible for bodily functioning. Drugs that act as stimulants to these receptors or drugs that have strong anticholinergic properties or adrenergic blocking activity will have a broad range of effect. For example, *C. botulinum* toxin present in poorly preserved food prevents the release of acetylcholine and thus selectively shuts off cholinergic synapses. The venom of a black widow spider, on the other hand, causes the continuous release of acetylcholine into the synaptic cleft. Important groups of psychotropic medications have strong anticholinergic properties, thus affecting the autonomic nervous system as well as the central nervous system.

Considering chemical transmission in the central nervous system, it must be remembered that with the exception of acetylcholine, the role of norepinephrine and other transmitter substances has not been conclusively proven. A schematic review of the major divisions and subdivisions of the brain and their behavioral functions will help as a framework in further understanding the impact of drugs on receptor sites (in this case central nervous system) as interpreted by behavioral changes such as motor activity, thought, and mood.

BRAIN ORGANIZATION

The brain dictates behavior. As such, it provides the vital functions of receiving, processing, eval-

uating, and storing information. Based on the information derived from these processes, the brain then determines the behavioral response. Past experiences, meanings, symbolism, current related emotions and thoughts, as well as a myriad of other factors become critical to this process. An external observer is only able to note a fraction of the variables that the brain evaluates before initiating a behavior response. It is therefore possible to understand why a person's behavior may not be totally explainable to even the most careful observer.[27]

Inputs of external and internal information constantly bombard the brain. These messages are coded according to an electrical frequency. The importance of the message determines the firing rate of the neuronal pathway carrying the message. The electrical code is interrupted by a temporary chemical coding whenever one neuron has to relay the message to another neuron in the sensory pathway. The message is carried across the space, or synapse, between the connecting neurons and coded according to importance by the amount of neurotransmitter released from the presynaptic membrane of the first neuron. The brain receives messages from a variety of locations simultaneously; thus it basically is a frequency analyzer. Stated a different way, the brain receives a large number of stimuli at varying frequency rates. Its task is to make an analysis of the appropriate behavior response. The response usually serves to facilitate survival and to increase meaning, enjoyment, and other behavior luxuries.[28]

The Triune Brain

The overall perspective of the structure and functions of the brain, developed over many years of research by Dr. Paul MacLean[29] and interpreted by nurse-physiologist Margaret E. Armstrong,[30] helps to explain the dynamics of commonly observed behaviors.*

Reptilian Brain

The most basic brain functions are located in the reptilian brain, so named because reptiles have only this brain. It is also referred to as the "survival" brain since it contains all the structures necessary for survival of the organisms includ-

---

* This section through page 59 has been reprinted with permission from M. E. Armstrong, Neurophysiological Theories, pp. 41–48.

ing the brainstem structures and the basal ganglia. With this brain, the individual is able to regulate essential physiological functions such as respiration, blood pressure, and heart rate. Movement regulated by the basal ganglia is needed for seeking food, shelter, and sexual mates. Establishment and defense of territory, grooming, courtship, and mating are all survival functions that may be enacted by this brain. The formation of social groups and creation of a social hierarchy are also included within these functions. This brain may also be called the sensory brain since it provides the entrance pathways for sensory information coming into the brain. Although some preliminary processing of the incoming information may have taken place in the spinal cord and brainstem structures, the individual is not yet consciously aware of the information. The reptilian brain serves to influence physiological functions and relay incoming physiological information. Both processes are normally accomplished without the conscious awareness of the individual.

Emotional Brain

The paleomammalian or emotional brain contains the midbrain limbic structures in addition to the frontal cerebral cortex. The so-called old mammals (e.g., the lemur) have this brain in addition to the first and therefore are capable of processing emotions or feelings about their experiences.

Cognitive Brain

The neomammalian or cognitive brain includes the cerebral and cerebellar cortex. The new mammals, including humans, have this brain as well and are thus able to have thoughts about their experiences. It is believed that the higher cortical centers may serve as a "data bank" for unconscious information while the limbic brain deals with conscious thought and reflection.[31] Further research should help to clarify the anatomy and physiology of thought processes.

The three brains work in concert according to a set of functional principles that provide the three basic components of any life experience: the sensory, emotional, and cognitive aspects. These principles help to explain behavior that may otherwise be puzzling to the observer. For instance, why does the same experience invoke a variety of behaviors among a group of individuals or within the same person from one time to another? Why do we often "fall apart" emotionally after an emergency? Why is the unknown more anxiety-provoking than knowing the worst? When one's survival is threatened, why can one seemingly be overconcerned about simple physical sensation? The answers to these and other behaviors can be explained, at least partially, with the triune brain perspective.

First, all three brains receive information from the internal and external environment. Pathways exist among the three brains for comparison of their reactions to this information. It is as if a message is brought to a room of people who all hear the message and then compare notes as to their sensations, feelings, and thoughts concerning the message. Then, all three brains have the opportunity to contribute to the response to the incoming information. This response takes the form of internal and external behavior on the part of the individual.

There is a hierarchy of control among the three brains. If left on its own, the reptilian brain will act to maintain survival functions. However, the emotional brain can override the functioning of the reptilian brain. This can easily be observed when someone is angry or excited; emotional expression and limbic brain influence take precedence over functions normally controlled by the reptilian brain. Pathways from the frontal cerebral cortex or other structures of the limbic brain have connecting pathways with the autonomic nervous system that affect the functioning of most internal organs such as heart rate, respiratory rate, and blood pressure. In addition, the cognitive brain can attempt to dominate behavior over the emotional and sensory brains. This hierarchy can be altered in some instances, most commonly when structures in one of the brains is already active for some reason. When this occurs, the brain, already active, has the opportunity to dominate behavior.

Although we do not usually see behavior that is wholly enacted by one brain, it is not rare to observe dominance by intellectual, emotional, or survival behaviors, any of which may or may not be appropriate at the time. MacLean's favorite example of reptilian behavior is that which is often seen in committee meetings.[32] When facts are not provided to give the cognitive brain something to deal with and the committee members do not have emotional feelings about the task at hand, the "reptiles" within us are allowed to dominate, with behavioral displays exhibited for the purpose of establishing social hierarchy. (Behaviors for the establishment of a social hierarchy are a function of the reptilian brain.) This example demonstrates that another way to upset the hierarchy of control is to give the two higher brains nothing to deal with, thus leaving the reptilian brain to dominate.

The functional principles of the triune brain, plus the impact of past learning and cultural background, readily explain the variance observed in response to the same input among different people. Depending on the unique aspects of the current situation, the individual may respond to the same experience differently from one time to another. For example, if one is already upset, a seemingly insignificant event, such as breaking a glass, may result in emotionally dominated behavior when, ordinarily, one would not have responded that way.

Another example is that of an emergency. One may function quite well until the emergency situation is over. One then attempts to relax and the cognitive brain no longer dominates behavior, since its work has been completed. Now the emotional brain has the opportunity to respond, and it will automatically do so according to the hierarchy of the three brains. One may experience behaviors such as anxious giggling, trembling, or crying. Such reactions are common to everyone, and it is best to allow this expression to occur rather than inhibit the behavior. With the buildup of emotions waiting to be expressed, the emotional brain is forced to express itself internally or in an inappropriate or excessive manner later. People tend to strive for a sophisticated, intellectual, or "correct" approach to behavior, thereby overriding expression by the other two brains. However, the three brains will influence one's behavior one way or the other at some point in time, with physiological or behavioral pathology as a possible result.

When someone is dealing with the unknown, as in not knowing the cause of an illness, the cognitive brain is left with no facts with which to operate, thereby allowing the emotional brain to dominate behavior. Naturally, a person would be quite anxious in this situation. Even realizing the worst possible cause gives the cognitive brain some information to process. The cognitive brain can then contribute to the person's behavior and can decrease the amount of influence by the emotional brain and, therefore, the extent of anxiety able to be expressed. Thus, cognitive functions may serve to assist in moderating emotions.

When a person's survival is threatened, for example with the awareness that he or she has a terminal disease, health professionals are sometimes surprised that the patient appears overly concerned with physical comfort factors, such as the temperature of the room, rather than expressing emotions about their prognosis. This temporary preoccupation occurs because the threat to survival alerts the reptilian brain structures that also function to relay incoming physical sensations. This increased alertness increases the individual's sensitivity to physical sensations, resulting in behavior that is difficult to understand, given the circumstances.

Awareness of the general organization and functional principles of the triune brain gives the mental health professional a framework to better understand the physiological nature of behavior. Using this information, one can then choose therapeutic approaches to elicit desired behavioral changes. The triune perspective of the brain has similarities to other explanations of how behavior is organized, as in Freud's framework of the id, superego, and ego. Components of both perspectives bear a rough resemblance to each other, with the triune brain adding anatomic and physiological details. Maslow's principles of the hierarchy of needs identifies physiological needs as the most basic and resembles the role of the sensory or reptilian brain. While Freud, Maslow, and MacLean are explaining different processes and functions, they share an assumption of a hierarchy of function with primitive, physiological survival needs being primary. As more is learned about the internal organization of the brain, explanations of behavior will continually be refined. Freud himself predicted that behavioral explanations would eventually be modified by the developing knowledge of neurobiology.[33]

Organization of Brain Structures Relevant to Behavior

Emotions

The limbic brain appears to contain structures designed to process and respond to information from an emotional or feeling perspective. There is a difference in opinion about the structures responsible for these functions, but they generally include the midbrain structures: hypothalamus, thalamus, amygdala, hippocampus, septum, cingulate gyrus, and the frontal portion of the cerebral cortex. The hypothalamus provides the interface between the limbic structures and the autonomic nervous, endocrine, and immunological systems.[34] As a result, a person's, emotional state often affects physiological functioning via pathways to these systems. For example, when one is angry or anxious, physiological functions such as heart and respiratory rates are commonly affected. The specific functions of the frontal lobe are still being defined. Activities such as self-awareness, initiative, and planning are thought possibly to take place in this area.[35]

As more details are clarified as to the pathways and mechanisms involved, there will be a much clearer picture of the complexity of the functioning of the limbic structures. Recently, a pathway was identified that indicates the route through which extreme emotions processed in the frontal cortex affect heart rate.[36] Continued stimulation of this pathway initially increases the heart rate. If stimulation continues, arrythmias occur, then fibrillation and cardiac arrest if stimulation is sufficiently severe or prolonged. Microscopic damage to heart tissue may result. Sudden cardiac arrest and other cardiovascular pathologies may in some instances have their origin in persistent or extremely stressful emotional experiences.

Cognition

Until the past decade, the processes underlying thinking or cognition were shrouded in ambiguity. There is evidence that the ancient Egyptians had a surprisingly accurate understanding of some of the more important cognitive functions, such as speech. However, only recently has the way in which the two cerebral hemispheres process information been even generally understood. For a long time, the left hemisphere was designated as the dominant hemisphere, since in most individuals that side of the brain was responsible for verbal behavior. In the early 1970s, Robert Ornstein demonstrated that one hemisphere was not necessarily dominant over the other. Instead, Ornstein identified that the right and left hemispheres generally process and use incoming information differently. Each provides a unique but helpful perspective to a person's total awareness.[37]

Knowledge concerning the differentiated hemispheric functioning (also called hemispheric lateralization) continues to increase. The left cerebral hemisphere generally organizes inputs in parts or units. This is helpful in activities such as mathematics, logical reasoning, and analytical thinking. In contrast, the right side of the brain generally organizes inputs in patterns or wholes that, in turn, are necessary for creative or intuitive thinking.[38] The right side of the brain is thought to process new or unfamiliar experiences. Once some familiarity is gained, the left side of the brain may then take over that function if appropriate. Handling a particular type of information may change from one hemisphere to the other if the way in which the inputs are processed changes. For example, one may initially process the patterns and rhythms of music according to its parts; the music wil then be processed by the left hemisphere. One can then no longer recall the music selections as easily as a whole.[39]

The right side of the brain is usually listed as the emotional side, meaning that thoughts about emotions are processed in the right hemisphere. It is now believed that this aspect of lateralization is influenced by gender. While most males process both negative and positive emotions in the right hemisphere, most females process negative (anxious) emotions on the right side and positive emotions on the left side of the brain.

Although the reasons are unclear, knowledge is steadily building that there are several other gender differences in hemispheric lateralization. In development, the left side appears to develop more rapidly in females and the right side in males. The causative factor may be testosterone, which is known to slow left hemisphere development.[40] In the adult brain, females seem to be able to use both sides of the cerebrum at the same time more easily than males. This difference may be either an advantage or disadvantage, depending on the case. Females may be more easily distracted from a given task while males may be better able to concentrate on one task at a time. By the same token, females may be better able to attend to different types of cues in the environment at the same time. Thus, when a man and woman compare analyses of someone's behavior, they may find that the woman is more aware than the man of the nonverbal and the verbal behaviors. An anatomic difference may account for this difference in ability. The corpus callosum is a collection of neural pathways that transfers information back and forth between the right and left sides of the brain. Without this transfer of information, as with the split brain, one side does not know what the other side is thinking. The splenium is the portion of the corpus callosum that conveys nonverbal information. It has recently been shown that the splenium is significantly thicker in the female brain. Therefore, the female is anatomically more equipped to process nonverbal information while simultaneously attending to verbal inputs.[41]

This brief description of the lateralization of cognition is true for approximately 85 to 90 percent of the population. Data indicate that the hand position used for writing may give a clear clue to the nature of lateralization in the person being observed.[42] The lateralization described above seems to hold true for right-handed people who write with a straight wrist and those left-handed people who write with a hooked wrist. In contrast, left-handed writers who use a straight wrist and the small minority of right-handed people who write with a hooked wrist seem to have lateralization opposite to that described above. Some people are most plastic in their cognitive functioning, which means that both hemispheres tend to process all information. In these instances, lateralization is not present to any significant degree.

Two types of inhibitions typically occur in cognitive function. Ipsilateral (same side) inhibition occurs when one side of the cerebrum is attending to an input that causes other activities by the same side of the brain to be relatively inhibited during that time. The sayings "I can only think of one thing at a time" and "I have a one track mind" may come from this type of inhibition. Contralateral (opposite side) inhibition occurs when one side of the brain is active and the ability of the opposite side of the brain to attend to inputs is relatively inhibited.

These inhibition mechanisms can be used in a creative fashion by the clinician. For example, when extremely anxious, one may be unable to attend to a therapeutic activity or thought. In this case, it might be helpful to temporarily decrease the anxiety. To accomplish this via the inhibition described above, the clinician may ask the person to attend to rhythmical, happy music. If successful, this activity would use ipsilateral inhibition to take the right brain on a "brief vacation" away from the thoughts that are producing the anxiety. It is easy to see why wearing earphones to listen to music is so popular in these stressful times. If the person is not able to concentrate on the music, the clinician could use contralateral inhibition with the same therapeutic objective in mind. Engaging the person in a conversation that requires sequential thinking, such as relating the details of

a baseball game, would automatically activate the left hemisphere that, by contralateral inhibition, would slow the thinking of the right brain. The better the clinician knows the client, the easier it is to choose an activity that will reach the desired objective. However, application of knowledge related to hemispheric lateralization and inhibition mechanisms can increase the therapeutic options of the psychiatric mental health nurse.

Abnormalities in the lateralization of cognitive functions, as well as handedness, have been implicated in the presenting symptoms and even as part of the etiology of several mental diseases.[43,44] For example, left hemisphere deficit or, in other words, right hemisphere dominance has been studied in relation to schizophrenia.[45] However, the problem may not be of dominance as much as a deficiency in the ability of the corpus callosum to carry information back and forth between the two hemispheres.

Right hemisphere dominance is more common among left-handed people. A number of studies have been done that illuminate the relationship between left-handedness and a number of diseases including schizophrenia, dyslexia, migraine headaches, and a variety of autoimmune disorders.[46,47] Left-handed people have approximately ten times the rate of learning disabilities, three times the rate of autoimmune diseases, and a significantly higher rate of schizophrenia and phobias than the right-handed population. By some unknown mechanism, right hemisphere dominance over the left hemisphere tends to make a person more vulnerable to these conditions.

Testosterone seems to be a common factor in these disorders. Testosterone slows the development of the left hemisphere during fetal development via a mechanism not yet fully understood. Too much testosterone during development of the nervous system contributes to the relative overdevelopment and later dominance of the right hemisphere. Testosterone also alters the expression of the immune system including the thymus gland, site of the production of some types of immune cells. Males tend to have a higher incidence of left-handedness. It is curious that females tend to suffer more from autoimmune diseases until one looks at the results of current research showing that these women seem to metabolize testosterone abnormally. Two new terms have been defined to indicate the clinical relationships describe above: psychoneuroimmunity and neuroimmunoendocrinology.[48] There is much yet to be learned about the effect of hemisphere lateralization on behavior and mental disease; however, the horizon appears to be rich in relevant possibilities.

Learning and Memory

Learning and memory have long eluded explanation; however, current research is helping to clarify the process. Learning has generally been defined as a change in behavior, but somehow this change has to be the result of an anatomic and/or physiological change at the cellular level in the brain. Memory, the retention of learning, has been hypothesized to be an electrical event in the case of short-term memory and a biochemical or structural event for long-term memory. Changes in action potentials, synaptic events and structures, neurotransmitters, dendritic growth, and specialized neuronal circuits have all been studied for the effects on learning and memory.

Current information indicates that synaptic connections are susceptible to strengthening or weakening in response to sensitization and habituation, respectively.[49] Learning may well have an effect on the structure and arrangement of neuronal circuits as they develop, but once the brain is fully formed, those circuits are probably relatively fixed (this idea may change with more research). However, the strength of the connections or synapses between neurons is not as rigid and is thus malleable to experience.

Neurotransmitters, the chemicals that carry information from one neuron to another across the synapse, are released from what are called active zones in the varicosities at the terminal end of the axon of the neuron. Studies of this process have shown the following about the physiology of learning: First, simple learning takes place at synaptic connections. Second, long-term memory occurs via changes in the strength of already-existing change in the amount of neurotransmitter released, thereby changing the strength of the connections between neurons.

When an animal habituates, that is, ceases to pay attention to an input, the number of active zones and thereby the amount of neurotransmitter released decreases. Therefore, the message is slowed or stopped in its transmission along the neuronal pathways. Conversely, when an animal is being sensitized to an input, that is, paying more attention to it, the number of active zones and the amount of neurotrans-

mitter released increases. Thus, both structural and chemical changes take place during learning.

Various forms of therapeutic counseling are based on the premise that learning takes place on the part of the individual in relation to his or her abnormal behavior. Frequently, medications are given as an adjunct to psychotherapy in an attempt to correct excesses or deficits in neurotransmitters and thereby increase the efficacy of the counseling. The assumption is made that the counseling and medications will work together to actualize the same structural and biochemical premises. Ideally, when patterns of behavior occur that indicate that stabilized changes have occurred at the synaptic level, medication and then therapy may be discontinued.

There has also been an interesting development in our understanding of the mechanism by which memories are retained and then recalled at a later time. Memories of events are apparently retained in their full context, that is, both the factual content and the emotional aspects of the experience.[50] The details of the process are not yet well understood, but it appears that when a given memory is recalled, the process is facilitated by remembering both the factual and emotional aspects. Therefore, if one is anxious while in a particular learning situation, the anxiety will be reexperienced when attempting to recall the factual information. This concept has broad implications for the kind of approaches used in education programs, whether they be for students or patients.

An inability to remember and an exaggeration of memories may both play an important role in mental disorders. As one patient with schizophrenia stated, "Recovery comes to the patient if the brain begins to function by trying to remember."[51]

BIOLOGIC RHYTHMS

Inherent components of life are the rhythmic cycles of nature and the universe such as the tides, the seasons of the year, sounds, temperature, and alterations of light and darkness that occur during a 24-hour period. There is a characteristic daily rhythm in the functioning system of the human body, e.g., the sleep–wake cycle, intraocular pressure in the eye, secretion of various hormones, motility of the cilia in the respiratory tract. Wehr and Goodwin noted that although body rhythms are influenced by many factors, when rhythms are studied in constant environmental conditions, they persist, indicating that they are endogenous and self-sustained.[52] In fact, these cyclic changes in the body's internal milieu are noted to constitute a kind of temporal anatomy, suggesting that disturbances in biologic rhythms would be consistent with illness.[53]

A primary focus of chronobiology research has been an intrinsic inner clock system—the circadian 24-hour cycle—that apparently became embedded in human physiology through evolution on a planet that rotates once every 24 hours. This focus reflects the adaptational significance of two important rhythms in nature, the solar day cycle of 24 hours and the gravitational lunar cycle of 24.8 hours.

Healthy persons experience a disruption in their circadian rhythm from airline travel and jet lag. Some flights with time changes disrupt a person for 4 to 5 days with symptoms of fatigue and dysphoric mood as the inner clock system resynchronizes. It is hypothesized that circadian rhythms originate in the hypothalamus by means of at least two oscillators, or biological clocks, and are keyed to the solar day through neural pathways that respond to 24-hour time cues in the environment. Thus, circadian rhythm disturbances could arise from defects in these pacemakers or in the mechanism that keyed the pacemakers to the environment, or from desynchronization in the coupling of the two pacemakers.[53]

People, colloquially described as "night people" and "day people," consistently use different social cues for activity. Many day-active persons have the ability to set an awakening time with their inner biologic clocks, consistently awakening 1 or 2 minutes before their bedside alarm rings. It is not understood at this time whether this capacity is acquired or genetic, but it is believed to be an important variable in evaluating personality style and defense mechanisms used by a person, conceivably correlating with perceptual coping patterns. If a person consciously or unconsciously, because of erratic schedules, stress, or conflict begins to ignore important synchronizing cues, the inner rhythm system may be unconstrained so that the body is prepared for day activity during night and night activity during the day.[54]

Experimental circadian research studies have been conducted to describe the normal circadian rhythm and how it works, to investigate the relationship of circadian disturbances to mood disorders, and to examine how experimental circadian treatments can alter clinical mood states. There are important implications for clinical nursing practice from such research. As observed by Ryan, Montgomery, and Meyers and the circadian rhythm research being conducted at the Clinical Center, National Institute of Mental Health, most nurses are taught to view patients holistically, paying attention to the interactions of mind and body.[55] Thus, the biologic area of circadian rhythms is especially relevant since it is so closely tied with many of nursing's focused areas of concern—sleep, temperature, rest, and activity, as well as mood. Nurses are in a particularly advantageous position to collaborate in this area of study as nurse investigators as well as nurse clinicians.[56]

Evidence is now overwhelming that the body's time structure should be considered as a variable in evaluating many diagnostic and therapeutic procedures. This evaluation would include routine clinical indices, such as mental status and mood ratings, body temperature, urine and serum constituents, and the time of procedures such as psychotherapy. For example, highly significant circadian variation has been demonstrated in time of drug administration, absorption, tissue receptor receptibility, and drug secretion.

SLEEP

Following the invention of the electroencephalogram (EEG) in the 1930s, it soon became clear that sleep was not a single physiological state. Currently, three distinct cyclical stages of sleep are separated from the relaxed waking state and outlined as follows.

- *Relaxed Waking.* The typical adult, eyes closed, relaxed EEG shows epochs of occipital alpha waves intermixed with high-voltage fast activity.
- *Stage 2 Sleep.* (S-Sleep). Sleep is considered present as the EEG desynchronizes and lower amplitude sleep spindles appear, usually accompanied periodically by k-complex activity. Little has been written about stage 2. As sleep is only achieved through stage 2, it cannot be varied independently of total sleep time. Typically, half the night

is occupied by stage 2, although it is elastic. Variations in the time spent in the other two stages are replaced by stage 2 sleep.

- *Delta (Slow Wave) Sleep.* (D-Sleep). After a few minutes of stage 2 sleep, the EEG becomes dominated by large amplitude delta waves. This is deep, physically restorative sleep, and physiological systems are at their most regular and lowest ebb of the 24-hour cycle. In healthy young adults, delta sleep accounts for about a quarter of the night's sleep but occurs exclusively in the first half of the night.[57]

Since 1950, research on sleep has advanced our understanding of this regular, recurrent, easily reversible state.[58] Sleep may be defined as a behavioral state, although it is also a biologic state. Certain EEG and polygraphic characteristics can now be accepted as part of a definition of sleep because of their regular and constant association with the behavior of sleep. The individual EEG changes often considered characteristics of sleep may be deceptive. The deep, slow waves usually associated with sleep, for instance, are also seen during certain phases of anesthesia and coma. Thus, when an EEG tracing is used to make the diagnosis of sleep, the regular cyclic pattern, rather than any single characteristic wave form, is most important.

Nurses are interested in sleep for a number of reasons.

1. Complaints of sleep disturbance are common symptoms among a wide range of persons. It is important to know when a sleep symptom is serious.
2. Sleep symptoms can be important in psychiatric and nursing diagnosis. For example, sleep disturbance is one of the earliest symptoms of depression, suicidal thoughts, and impending psychosis.
3. Sleep complaints may lead to a diagnosis of several distinct sleep illnesses, including sleep apnea. Sleep recordings are necessary for such medical diagnoses.
4. There are theoretical relationships between research in sleep and dreaming and research into mental illness. Immanuel Kant wrote that the psychotic is a waking dreamer; Sigmund Freud pointed out that people are psychotic when dreaming. Ernest Hartmann suggests that the biology of the dreaming state will be informative also about the biology of "primary process" functioning.[59]

Phenomenology of Human Sleep

What occurs during a typical night of sleep in a healthy young adult, that is, information about the phenomenology of sleep, is derived from polygraphic studies. As a person falls asleep, the brain waves undergo certain characteristic changes. Sleep is cyclical, with four or five periods of emergence from the different stages of sleep. When awakened during those periods of emergence, persons frequently—60 to 90 percent of the time—report that they have been dreaming. Such periods are characterized not only by EEG patterns and by rapid eye movements but also by a host of other distinguishing factors, including irregularity in pulse rate, respiratory rate, and blood pressure; the presence of full or partial penile erections, vaginal excitation; and generalized muscular atony interrupted by sporadic movements in small muscle groups. This distinct state of sleep is referred to as D-sleep (Delta, desynchronized, or dreaming sleep) and the remainder of sleep is known as S-sleep (synchronized sleep). These two stages of sleep are also known as rapid eye movement (REM) sleep and nonrapid eye movement (NREM) sleep, as paradoxical sleep and orthodox sleep, and as active sleep and quiet sleep.

The constant and regular characteristics of a night of normal sleep are sensitive indicators of disturbance. Such characteristics can be used to study alterations associated with various forms of mental distress or can be produced by various drugs.[60]

Differences

There are some important differences among the states of waking, S-sleep, and D-sleep. Simple recordings of various physiological measures, such as pulse, blood pressure, respiration, muscle potential, galvanic skin response, and penile erections, reveals certain patterns. In normal persons, S-sleep is a peaceful state. Pulse rate is typically slowed, 5 to 10 beats a minute below the level of restful waking, and the pulse during S-sleep is very regular. Respiration behaves in a similar manner, and blood pressure also tends to be low, with few minute-to-minute variations. Resting muscle potential of body musculature is lower in S-sleep than it is in waking. There are no or few rapid eye movements, and there are seldom any penile erections. Blood flow through most tissues, including cerebral blood flow, is also slightly reduced.

S-sleep is quiet and peaceful sleep; however, the deepest portions of S-sleep are sometimes associated with unusual arousal characteristics. When persons are aroused 30 minutes to 1 hour after sleep onset, they find themselves disoriented and at such a time they would probably do poorly on a formal mental status examination. In certain persons, the disorientation during arousal results in specific problems, including enuresis, somnambulism, and nightmares or night terrors.

D-sleep is considerably different. Many polygraphic measures show irregular patterns resembling aroused waking patterns. If one were not aware of the behavioral state of the person, one would undoubtedly conclude that the person was in an active waking state. Pulse, respiration, and blood pressure are all high during D-sleep—much higher than S-sleep and quite often higher than waking state. Even more striking than the level or rate is the variability from minute to minute. The highest and the lowest pulse and respiratory rates of the night usually occur during D-sleep. D-sleep is also associated with rapid conjugate movements of the eyes and, in the very young, rapid phasic movements of other small muscles. In the human male, as well as in other species, almost every D-period is accompanied by a partial or full penile erection. All that aroused-appearing activity is superimposed on very relaxed muscular state. Essentially, the internal system is in a state of activation and turmoil protected by the superstructure of a relaxed peripheral musculature. It is not surprising, writes Evans, that the highest incidence of several medical crises occurs during REM sleep, including seizures, myocardial infarction, cerebral accidents, asthma, and duodenal ulcer. Patients at risk for such diseases must be carefully withdrawn from any procedure that increases the amount of REM sleep. Withdrawal from alcohol, benzodiazepines, and to lesser degrees many other medications temporarily increases REM time during the night.[61]

As far as the body's physiology is concerned, D-sleep could be called an active and aroused state, but with muscular immobility. That description could also be applied to the psychological state during dreaming; most typ-ical dreams are reported from D-sleep. In a dream, one is conscious and apparently aware—watching things, getting involved, experiencing emotions—and yet everything happens without one being able to move a muscle.

Functions of Sleep

Why do people sleep? As yet, the functions of sleep are not fully understood. Of all the proposed hypotheses, the best accepted one is that it serves a restorative function. Prolonged periods of sleep deprivation sometimes lead to increasing ego disorganization, hallucinations, and delusions. Although it has been widely assumed that periods of sleep deprivation can produce a psychosis in normal persons, research on the problem has not been conducted because of ethical constraints and/or the type of person who would volunteer for such a study.

Studies on sleep requirements have involved long sleepers (more than 9 hours sleep per night) and short sleepers (less than 6 hours sleep per night). Hartmann and colleagues administered psychological tests as well as extensive interviews and reported that short sleepers should be characterized as a group of persons who were generally efficient, energetic, ambitious, socially adept, and satisfied with themselves and their lives. They were relatively free of psychopathology. The short sleepers used defense mechanisms of avoidance, keeping busy, and denial. The long sleepers were a group who had various types of minor psychopathology—usually mild depression, anxiety, or simple shyness; they were also a group of nonconformist thinkers and worriers. In fact, the simplest one-word differentiation of the group was the word "worry." The long sleepers worried about their lives, about the state of the world, about the research study. The short sleepers were strikingly nonworriers, who tended to take the attitude, "Nothing I can do about it so why worry?" In computer terms, the long sleepers could be seen as reprogramming themselves every day and changing their ways of functioning, whereas the short sleepers appeared to be preprogrammed; they had found a way of doing things that they liked, and they kept doing them that way. Such clear-cut differences quite possibly apply only to extreme groups of constant long sleepers and short sleepers. Studies on college freshmen could find no clear-cut psychological differences between the two groups.[62]

GENETICS

Hereditary traits are transmitted from parent to child through specific molecules of deoxyribonucleic acid (DNA). The science of genetics has made major advances in the past decade. Today it unites molecular biology, biochemistry, and cell biology in working toward the goal of explaining the transmission, expression, and variation of gene-coded information in developing organisms. Contributions of genetics to psychiatric nursing and mental health have been slow in realization. Heretofore, the ancient dichotomies of nature–nurture and mind–matter forced mental health professionals to choose between biologic and psychological approaches to etiology and treatment. Particularly in the United States, the biologic and genetic formulations of psychiatrists Kraeplin and Freud were forgotten, and heredity and environmental factors were considered as separate and competing agents.[63]

The past decade has witnessed a gradual shift toward accepting the contributions from the biologic sciences as major advances are noted in cytological, biochemical, and population genetics. Experimental psychology studied individual differences in animals and began to trace these to their genetic constitution, operating in the context of their total milieu. In human development, theories of interaction of genetic and ecological forces became predominant, biologic evolution merging with the study of social evolution in sociology and anthropology.

Mental health professionals, drawing on their clinical experience, have become more aware of the importance of family patterns, individual differences, and metabolic and pharmacologic distinctions. The goal of psychiatric genetics as a science may be considered, in the broadest sense, to be the clarification of the mechanisms of human variation and development not only in psychiatric disorders but also in normal behavior.

Molecular Biochemistry of Genetic Substance

Since Gregor Mendel's observations of the transmission of physical traits from one generation of plants to the next, scientists have struggled to enhance their view of the genetic material of all living organisms. One of the most significant biologic discoveries has been the nature of genetic material, i.e., the molecules coding in every cell the genetic information expressed in development and function as the synthesis of enzymes and other proteins during life and transferred by reproductive cells from generation to generation. By 1952, it had been established that this genetic substance was not protein, as had long been thought, but deoxyribonucleic acid (DNA). The following year, Watson and Crick described the structure of the molecule as two long polynucleotide chains that twisted about each other to form a double helix.[64] The chains are linked at the central axis by hydrogen bonding, which can, however, only take place between adenine on one chain and thymine on the other, or guanine on one chain and cytosine on the other. A gene may consist of hundreds to thousands of such base pairs.

The Watson–Crick model made it possible to explain the main functions of the genetic material: (1) its ability to replicate itself exactly in cell division; and (2) its ability to transmit information to the cytoplasm of the cell to govern the synthesis of unique enzymes and other proteins. Predicted theoretically by the model, these functions have since been verified experimentally, their details have been expounded, and the knowledge has been put to use in hitherto only imagined ways in studying gene localization, in effecting gene transfer, and in establishing a new industry, genetic engineering.[65]

Replication. If the two chains forming the double helix unwind and separate, each half can reform its missing half from the surrounding materials with the aid of specialized enzymes. In so doing, the base pairs—adenine–guanine and cytosine–thymine—must be preserved; hence there result two double-helical chains, each of which is identical in sequence to the original.

Protein Synthesis. The sequence of base pairs in a given gene is of paramount importance because it represents the code that determines the synthesis of a unique protein. Proteins are composed of one or more polypeptide chains; these chains, in turn, are made of long strings of hundreds of amino acids in a particular order. The process begins when a message on a portion of the DNA is copied by a single-stranded molecule, ribonucleic acid (RNA), a step known as transcription. The RNA molecule contains a sequence of nucleotides complementary to that in the DNA, except that thymine is replaced by uracil.

Mutations. Gene mutations represent changes in the genetic instruction, so that new cells produce different substances than do the cells that preceded the mutation. If these mutations take place in germ cells, they may produce a change in the genetic information contained in the zygote and, depending on the locus of the mutation, a resultant enzyme deficiency or disease.

In the context of molecular biology of the gene, a mutation may be thought of as a change in the sequence of base pairs in the DNA. Some of these changes may represent a substitution of one base for another at a given locus, e.g., sickle cell disease. Others may consist of a deletion or rearrangement of large segments of the DNA molecule. Such changes take place through an error in the replication process at the time of cell division, possibly through the action of certain chemicals or as a result of high-energy radiation. If a sufficiently charged message is sent a different enzyme or other protein may be produced. The mutation will be reproduced in all cells formed by divisions of the original cell.

Control of DNA Function. A basic requirement in this picture of gene action and protein synthesis is a mechanism for control or regulations. In each human organism, every somatic cell has the same 46 chromosomes, descendants of the chromosomes in the original fertilized ovum or zygote, but it is clear that cells differentiate and perform different functions, and that no cell is manufacturing its product at all times.[66]

Research on the Human Genome

The 54th meeting of the Advisory Committee to the Director of the National Institutes of Health, James B. Wyngaarden, held in October 1986, focused on both scientific and policy aspects attendant on recent technological developments in molecular genetics as they related to mapping and sequencing the human genome. It was reported that the central endeavor of human molecular biology is to understand the relationships among genes, proteins, and functions. In

many cases, a protein and its function can be related through biochemistry. In other cases, however, availability of the gene coding for a protein is the only way to determine its function. Most of what is known about many human genes comes from the study of lower organisms, as it is easier to obtain mutants from these organisms and they have less DNA to sequence.[67]

Federal support for research on genetics is considerable. In fiscal year 1985, the National Institutes of Health (NIH) spent approximately $213 million on genetic research, with the National Institute of General Medical Sciences alone spending approximately $20 million each year to support projects that are directly related to physically characterizing and sequencing the human genome.[68]

There are more than 3000 known genetic diseases. As knowledge regarding inherited risk factors accumulates, it is becoming increasingly apparent that genetics play an important part in many disease states.

The human genome contains approximately 3 billion base pairs. The dimensions of the effort involved in the contemplated sequencing of the entire human genome involve two separate calculations:

1. The number of human genes already mapped is approximately 1000; the ratio of mapped to unmapped is at least 1:50.
2. The total calculated number of nucleotides in the human genome is about 3 billion; the ratio of sequenced to unsequenced nucleotides is approximately 1:600.

The importance of the research on mapping and sequencing of the human genome to the mental health field is the increasingly observed role of the genetics of psychiatric disorders. For example, in reviewing the status of schizophrenia genetics, it can be argued that the cumulative evidence for a necessary genetic vulnerability is generally accepted. Research designs have included: (1) pedigree analysis; (2) family risk studies: comparison of risk in specified groups of relatives of patients with the general population risk; (3) twin studies; (4) adoption studies; (5) high-risk studies: prospective long-term observation focusing on early differences in children with one or two schizophrenic parents; and (6) biologic studies looking for genetic markers either linked or associated with the condition.[69]

Summary

Many contributions have been made over the past decade from the neurobiological sciences to the understanding of the mind and human behavior. This chapter reviews some of these contributions in terms of receptor site theory and psychotropic drugs, the triune brain, circadian rhythm research, the phenomenology of sleep, and human genetics research.

Questions

1. Identify two important features of the triune brain.
2. What is the role of gender in right and left brain hemispheres?
3. Give two examples of receptor site theory and drug interaction.
4. Why might a heart attack occur during sleep?
5. What mental illnesses have been identified as having a genetic cause?

REFERENCES AND SUGGESTED READINGS

1. Loewi, O. Üeber humoral Üebertragbarkeit der Herneven wirkung. *Pflugers Archiv für die Gesamte Physiologie*, 1921, *189* (Pt. 1), 239–242. Summarized in Hoemstedt & Liljestrand (Eds.), *Readings in Pharmacology*. Elmsford, N.Y.: Pergamon Press, 1963, pp. 190–196.
2. Cannon, W. B., & Uridil, J. E. Studies on the conditions of activity in endocrine glands: VIII. Some effects on the denervated heart of stimulating the nerves of the liver. *American Journal of Physiology*, 1921, *50*, 353–354.
3. Cade, J. F. J. Lithium salts in the treatment of psychotic excitement. *Medical Journal of Australia*, 1944, *36*, 349–352.
4. Wilkins, R. W., & Judson, W. E. The use of *Rauwolfia serpentina* in hypertensive patients. *New England Journal of Medicine*, 1953, *248*, 48–53.
5. Kline, N. *Rauwolfia serpentina* in neuropsychiatric conditions. *Annals of New York Academy of Science*, 1954, *95*, 107–122.
6. Laborit, H. *Acta Chirurgica Belgica*, 1950, *49*, 390.
7. Janssen, P. A., & Van den Eycken, C. A. M. The chemical anatomy of potent morphine-like analgesia. In A. Burger (Ed.), *Medicinal Research* (Vol. 2). New York: Marcel Dekker, 1968.
8. Caldwell, A. E. History of pharmacology. In W. G. Clark & J. del Guidice (Eds.), *Principles of Psychopharmacology*. New York: Academic Press, 1970.
9. Kornetsky, C. *Pharmacology: Drugs Affecting Behavior*. New York: Wiley, 1976, pp. 45–62.
10. Carlson, N. R. *Physiology of Behavior*. Boston: Allyn & Bacon, 1977.
11. Kornetsky, op. cit.
12. Ibid., pp. 6–7.
13. Ibid., pp. 1–22.
14. Ibid.
15. Ibid., pp. 63–80.
16. Ibid.
17. Ibid.
18. Carlson, op. cit., pp. 11–24.
19. Axelrod, J. Amphetamine: Metabolism, physiological disposition and its effects on catecholamine storage. In E. Cast & S. Garattini (Eds.), *Amphetamine and Related Compounds*. New York: Raven Press, 1970, p. 207.
20. Adolphe, A. B. et al. The neuropharmacology of depression. *Diseases of the Nervous System*, 1977, 841–856.
21. Carlson, op. cit., pp. 11–24.
22. Ibid.
23. Ibid., pp. 63–83.
24. Kornetsky, op. cit.
25. Ibid.
26. Ibid.
27. Armstrong, M. E. Neurophysiological theories. In D. L. Critchley & J. T. Maurin (Eds.), *The Clinical Specialist in Psychiatric Mental Health Nursing*. New York: Wiley, 1985, pp. 39–57.
28. Ibid.
29. MacLean, P. *A Triune Concept of Brain and Behavior*. Toronto: Toronto Press, 1975.
30. Armstrong, op. cit.
31. Ferguson, M. New neurobiology era parallels leap in physics. *Brain Mind Bulletin*, October 24, 1983, pp. 1–3.

32. Holden, D. Paul MacLean and the triune brain. *Science*, June 8, 1979, pp. 1066–1068.

33. Trotter, R. J. Psychiatry for the 80's. *Science News*, May 30, 1981, p. 119.

34. Cox, T. *Stress*. Baltimore: University Park Press, 1978.

35. Pines, M. The human differences. *Psychology Today*, September 1983, pp. 62–68.

36. Skinner, J. E. Heart attacks from stress, via brain. *Science News*, November 18, 1978, p. 94.

37. Ornstein, R. E. *The Psychology of Consciousness*. San Francisco: W. H. Freeman, 1972.

38. Springer, S. P., Deutsch, G. *Left Brain Right Brain*. San Francisco: W. H. Freeman, 1981.

39. Bever, T. G., & Chiarello, R. J. Cerebral dominance in musicians and nonmusicians. *Science*, August 9, 1974, pp. 537–539.

40. Durden-Smith, D., & DeSimone, D. Hidden threads of illness. *Science Digest*, January 1984, pp. 51–105.

41. Fackelmann, K. A. Male-female brain anatomy may differ. *Science News*, June 6, 1982, pp. 121; 422.

42. Sibanti, A. The Japanese brain. *Science 80*, December 1980, pp. 22–27.

43. Beale, I. L., & Corballis, M. C. *The Ambivalent Mind: The Neuropsychology of Left and Right*. Chicago: Nelson Hall, 1983.

44. Segalowitz, S. J. *Two Sides of the Brain*. Englewood Cliffs, N.J.: Prentice-Hall, 1983.

45. Magaro, P. A. The paranoid and the schizophrenic: The case for distinct cognitive styles. *Schizophrenia Bulletin*, 1981, 7, 632–661.

46. Durden-Smith & DeSimone, op. cit.

47. Marx, J. L. Autoimmunity in left-handers. *Science News*, July 9, 1982, pp. 141–144.

48. Ader, R. (Ed.). *Psychoneuroimmunity*. New York: Academic Press, 1981.

49. Kandel, E. R. Changes in the brain produced by learning. *The Science of the Brain*. American Psychiatric Association Convention, Smith, Kline, & French, 1982 (Audiocassette).

50. Bower, B. Emotional rescue. *Science News*, April 18, 1981, pp. 253–255.

51. Dawson, D., Blum, H. M., & Bartolucci, G. *Schizophrenia in Focus*. New York: Human Sciences Press, 1983.

52. Wehr, T. A., & Goodwin, F. K. Biological rhythms and psychiatry. In S. Arieti & H. K. H. Brodie (Eds.), *American Handbook of Psychiatry* (2nd ed., Vol. 3). New York: Basic Books, 1981.

53. Ryan, L., Montgomery, A., & Meyers, S. Impact of circadian rhythm research on approaches to affective illness. *Archives of Psychiatric Nursing*, 1987, 1(4), 236–240.

54. Stroebel, C. F. Biological rhythms in psychiatry. In H. I. Kaplan & B. J. Sadock (Eds.), *Comprehensive Textbook of Psychiatry*, 4th ed. Baltimore: Williams & Wilkins, 1985.

55. Ryan, Montgomery, & Meyers, op. cit.

56. Ibid.

57. Evans, F. J. Sleep disorders and insomnia. *Carrier Foundation Letter #129*, November 1987, pp. 1–4.

58. Hartmann, E. L. Sleep. In H. I. Kaplan and B. J. Sadock (Eds.), *Comprehensive Textbook of Psychiatry*, 4th ed. Baltimore: Williams & Wilkins, 1985.

59. Ibid.

60. Ibid.

61. Evans, op. cit.

62. Hartmann, op. cit.

63. Rainer, J. D. Genetics and psychiatry. In H. I. Kaplan & B. J. Sadock (Eds.), *Comprehensive Textbook of Psychiatry*, 4th ed. Baltimore: Williams & Wilkins, 1985.

64. Lewin, B. *Genes*. New York: Wiley, 1983.

65. Ibid.

66. Rainer, op. cit.

67. Proceedings of the 54th Meeting of the Advisory Committee to the Director, National Institutes of Health, Bethesda, Md. October 16–17, 1986, pp. 1–34.

68. Ibid.

69. Ibid.

Chapter 6

Contributions of the Behavioral and Cognitive Sciences

Ann Wolbert Burgess

Chapter Objectives

The students successfully attaining the goals of this chapter will be able to:

- Discuss motivation as a critical issue in nursing practice.
- Give an example of machine emulation of the brain.
- Give an example of human information processing and an example of a barrier to information processing.

The scientific investigation of behavior has a long history of more than a century of experimental studies of both normal and abnormal behavior. For example, psychology has traditionally been involved with methods of researching the mind. The concept of introspection has always been employed, but more recently other disciplines of the behavioral and cognitive sciences have provided methods for measurable observation of behavior.

For the student of psychiatric nursing this means that one is not only a student of human behavior but of that unit of the organism that regulates and organizes behavior, i.e., the brain or, in psychological terminology, the mind. What we have gained from the various sciences for application in nursing practice are propositions, theories, and models that relate to brain, to mind, and to social interaction. What is pre-sented in this chapter are highlights of some of the theoretical categories developed over the years to understand the function of the mind, including humanistic and motivational, factor, and learning theories.

HUMANISTIC AND MOTIVATION THEORIES

Humanistic theory is primarily concerned with what is unique and distinctive about human behavior and experience. Gordon Allport (1897–1967), a personality theorist, envisioned personality as an open system in constant interaction with its environment. He suggested that motivation may be, and usually is in healthy personalities, independent in its origins. Traits—

TABLE 6-1. MAJOR APPROACHES TO MOTIVATION

Approach	Theories	Primary Concern
1. Content	Need hierarchy theory	*What* motivates people
2. Process	Reinforcement theory	*How* people are motivated

generalized predispositions to behavior—provide the basis for personality description.

Abraham Maslow (1908–1970) developed a theory of psychic health rather than psychic illness. The theory presents a hierarchy of needs underlying human motivation, starting with basic physiological needs and extending to the highest order of spiritual and esthetic needs. The self-actualized individual who fully uses all his potential and capacity is central to the theory. In treatment, Maslow focused on increasing self-knowledge and understanding and mobilizing the resources of the person toward greater self-realization.

Motivation is a critical issue in the nursing care of people. The question of how to motivate people has been philosophically and practically posed in many fields. The many theories that have been advanced to answer this question can be grouped into two motivational approaches: content and process. These approaches and major theories of motivation with which they are associated are summarized in Table 6-1 and form the basis for the following discussion.

Content Approach

The content approach to motivation is concerned with what within people motivates them to behave in a certain way, attempting to answer such questions as "What forces prompt people to behave as they do?" If you want to understand what motivates people, you must identify their needs. The needs for security and recognition are just two examples of forces that may motivate people and determine their actions. The two content theories that have generated the most interest are Maslow's need hierarchy theory and Herzberg's two-factor theory.

Maslow's Need Hierarchy Theory

Abraham Maslow's need hierarchy theory is one of the most popular and widely known theories

of motivation.[1] According to Maslow, people are motivated to satisfy five categories of needs:

1. Physiological needs, including the need for food, water, air, and sex.
2. Safety needs, or the need for security, stability, and freedom from fear of threat.
3. Social needs, including the need for friendship, affection, acceptance, and interaction with others.
4. Esteem needs, including both a need for personal feelings of achievement or self-esteem and a need for recognition or respect from others.
5. Self-actualization needs, a feeling of self-fulfillment or the realization of one's potential.

Maslow held that these needs are arranged in a hierarchy of ascending importance, from low to high. He contended that a "lower" need must be satisfied before the next "higher" need could motivate behavior. For example, a person's safety needs would have to be satisfied before the next level of need (social) could motivate behavior. Thus, the strength of any need is determined by its position in the hierarchy and by the degree to which it and all lower needs have been satisfied. Satisfaction of a need, however, triggers dissatisfaction at the next higher level. This sequence of "increased satisfaction, decreased importance, increased importance of the next higher need" repeats itself until the highest level of the hierarchy (self-actualization) is reached.

Maslow suggested that a person could progress down as well as up the various need levels. If a lower-level need (safety, for instance) were threatened at some later point in time, it again would become dominant and assume an important position in a person's total motivational system. Thus, sudden unemployment or loss of a loved one could shift one's concern from a pursuit of personal recognition to a preoccupation with providing for home and family.

Critics of Maslow's theory focus their comments in two areas. First, research has been unable to reproduce the five need levels Maslow proposed, suggesting instead that there are no more than two or three levels. Second, although people do generally place a great deal of emphasis on satisfying their lower-level needs (for example, hunger, thirst, sex), research suggests that once these needs are satisfied most people do not climb Maslow's need hierarchy in the proposed manner. Indeed, there appears to be no particular pattern governing which needs will become dominant once a person's lower-level needs are satisfied.

Nursing Implications. Despite the criticism of it, Maslow's need hierarchy theory continues to exert a significant influence on current thinking about motivation. Perhaps its greatest value lies in its numerous nursing implications, especially for patient teaching.

1. Nurses should bear in mind that motivation is generally determined by multiple needs. The belief that one, and only one, factor accounts for motivation is usually an oversimplification.
2. Nurses must identify their patients' most important needs and link need satisfaction to desired outcome. For example, symptom reduction (less anxiety) or function improvement (clearer thinking) can be built-in incentives. Recognition of the patient's successful completion of a health promotion course can be the listing of the name with others.
3. Nurses need to be aware that what motivates one person may not motivate another. Different people want different things. Nurses must be sensitive to differences in reward preferences.

Process Approach

As we have noted, the content approach is concerned with what within people motivates them to behave in a certain way. In contrast, the process approach is concerned with how people are motivated. It focuses on the direction or choice of behavioral patterns. The process theory to be discussed is Skinner's reinforcement theory.[2]

Skinner's Reinforcement Theory
The guiding principle of reinforcement theory is that human behavior is a function of its consequences. Or more formally stated, behaviors that result in desirable consequences will likely recur; those that result in undesirable consequences will be less likely to recur. This last statement is popularly known as Thorndike's law of effect.[3]

Although various revisions have appeared

in recent years, the basic concept behind behavior modification remains quite simple. Health behaviors that lead to desirable consequences are likely to be repeated. Health behaviors that lead to undesirable consequences are less likely to be repeated. This reasoning involves three components.

1. Stimulus: an event that leads to a response
2. Response: a unit of behavior that follows a stimulus
3. Reinforcement: a consequence of a response

The relationship is: a stimulus (event) leads to a response (behavior) that is reinforced (by a consequence). Note that none of these three components involves thinking. Behavior modification holds that current behavior is solely determined by a person's past history of reinforcement. Thus, according to behavior modification, if a particular stimulus–response pair is followed by a desirable consequence, it will be more likely that the stimulus involved will prompt the same response in the future. Conversely, if the consequence is undesirable, the response will be less likely to recur. In sum, the consequences of a person's behavior are made dependent upon his or her response to a stimulus.

Types of Reinforcement. From a nursing perspective, there are at least four types of reinforcement available for modifying patient behaviors as summarized in Table 6-2; two strengthen or increase behavior, whereas the other two weaken or decrease it.

POSITIVE REINFORCEMENT. A means of strengthening behavior, positive reinforcement provides

TABLE 6-2. TYPES OF REINFORCEMENT

1. *Positive reinforcement.* Strengthens behavior by providing a desirable consequence when a desirable behavior occurs.
2. *Avoidance learning.* Strengthens behavior by teaching individuals to respond in ways to avoid undesirable consequences.
3. *Extinction.* Weakens behavior by withholding a desirable consequence when an undesirable behavior occurs.
4. *Punishment.* Weakens behavior by providing an undesirable consequence when an undesirable behavior occurs.

a desirable consequence when a desirable behavior occurs. It thus increases the likelihood that a desired behavior will be repeated. For example, a nurse will praise an adolescent for consistently returning to the ward at the scheduled time. Positive reinforcers can include extra time off, bonus credits, etc.

AVOIDANCE LEARNING. A second means of strengthening behavior, avoidance learning, occurs when individuals respond in ways to avoid undesirable consequences. For the adolescent who returns to the ward at the scheduled time, the nurse avoids intense questioning of the patient, who in turn learns that being on time diminishes the likelihood of being interrogated as to his or her activities.

EXTINCTION. As a means of weakening behavior, extinction attempts to eliminate an undesirable behavior by withholding a desirable consequence when the behavior occurs. Under such conditions, the undesirable behavior will diminish and eventually become "extinct" as a result of not being positively reinforced. For example, withholding a ward pass may result in the adolescent's maintaining a consistent on-time schedule. Presumably the adolescent will eventually realize that chronic lateness is not producing a desired consequence.

PUNISHMENT. A second means for weakening behavior, punishment provides an undesirable consequence when an undesirable behavior occurs. For example, if the adolescent is late for a scheduled meeting, punishments could include withholding privileges, probation periods, or restriction in other life areas. According to Skinner, punishment has the effect of reducing the tendency to act in a given way, at least in the short run. Punishment is considered by many to be one of the least understood and most abused aspects of behavior modification.[4]

FACTOR THEORIES

The mathematical approach to personality, according to William W. Meissner, focuses on objective measures of personality and the application of such statistical techniques as analysis of variance and covariance and factor analysis to assess the role of personality factors in an individual's personality.[5] This approach involves the correlation and simultaneous measure of multiple factors, which are reduced to a defined set of functional units and then used to determine particular patterns of personality.

The factor analyst attempts to make a diagnosis similar to that of a clinician. The difference is that the factor analyst measures the variables according to a specific formula rather than assessing them on a relatively intuitive basis. For example, R. B. Cattell developed 16 factors to provide a profile of the functioning personality.[6]

LEARNING THEORIES

Learning theories provide a major contribution to nursing practice in offering a basis for health teaching and an understanding of a patient's health beliefs.

Building on the memory concept, it has been assumed in psychology that learned experiences form the basis of much of human and animal behavior. Experiences, stored as memory, determine much of current perception and performance.

The theories of learning that have accumulated over the years have followed a traditional research protocol that begins with a systematic set of observed events, develops a hypothesis and experimentation to confirm or refute hypotheses, and leads, ultimately, as the theory matures, to laws. A characteristic of a good theory is that it is modifiable and testable, able to accommodate new information and new challenges.

With the advances in the field of learning theory, it is still true that the fundamental bases of theory remain rooted, in large measure, in systematic theoretical formulations based on long experimental investigations by a relatively small group of scholar scientists: Hull, Skinner, Pavlov, and Thorndike.

Learning theorists differ over the definition of learning. One group relates learning to measurable, observable events in the physical world whereas a second group is concerned with describing basic processes that the theorist believes are necessary for learning to take place. However, regardless of the approach, there appears to be general agreement that learning is a change in behavior that results from practice, whether the practice reflects encoded neural pathways or a strengthening of certain responses. Moreover, learning is viewed as an intervening process that links organismic states before and after a change in behavior occurs. There is also a general assumption that learning represents a long-term change in behavior and is separate from changes induced by such factors as fatigue and maturation.

Learning then may be defined as a change in behavior potential resulting from reinforced practice. So considered, reinforcement becomes an example of an empirical law of effect that is basic to much of contemporary learning theory.

In 1931, Thorndike stated the law of effect:[7]

Acts followed by a state of affairs which the individual does not avoid, and which he often tries to preserve or attain, are selected and fixated, while acts followed by states of affairs which the individual avoids or attempts to change are eliminated.

In 1932, Thorndike modified his law and indicated that rewarded responses are always strengthened but that punished responses do not always diminish in strength, thus leading to an emphasis on reward as a primary determinant of behavior.

Conditioning

Conditioning is viewed as a case of learning. Hull, in many of his writings, described the classical Pavlovian conditioned reflex as a special case of law of effect, assuming reinforcement to be operative in such simple learning examples as well as in higher-order learning.[8] Many theorists accept a rough dichotomy between two types of conditioning: classical (Pavlovian) and instrumental (operant).

The pioneer in classical conditioning, the Russian physiologist Ivan Pavlov, observed in his work with gastric secretions in dogs that stimuli that were often present at the time the dogs were offered food came to evoke salivation, even though the dogs could not see or smell food. Pavlov assumed that the stimulus of footsteps came to be associated with food. His research was directed toward an analysis of this event, which he called the "conditional reflex"—the reflex that would occur, given certain conditions.

Hull's Learning Theory

Hull dealt with the complexity of consideration of the stimulus–response construct and the law of effect. He began to develop a mathematical model around the concepts of response potential as well as calling for mathematical consideration in measurement of the structure and intensity of the stimuli, all of which he believed influenced the ultimate learning that emerged in the human system.

Hull's approach to learning theory is strongly mathematical and neurophysiological. He sought to establish a theory of behavior, which he equated with learning, that could be quantified and tested in accordance with scientific method.

The cognitive aspects of personality are the focus in theories of learning. These theories have exerted considerable influence, specifically on Jean Piaget's work on child development.[9] One major contribution by Piaget is his description of the child's cognitive development. The sensorimotor period extends from birth to about 2 years, and the goal is for the child to gradually develop the capacity to evolve new sequences of behavior that increase in complexity. The preoperational period—from 2 to 7 years—is the beginning of the child's conceptual ability, although this ability still remains relatively unintegrated in this period. The period of concrete operations include the period from 7 to 11 years, and during this time the child's thought processes become more organized and function with greater stability, reasonability, and consistency. The period of formal operations ranges from age 11 on into adolescence. The child begins to understand the principles of causal thinking and scientific experimentation. He or she is also able to plan and carry through experiments and draw logical inferences from the results.

Piaget's work has been an important contribution to nursing care of children. Its delineation of cognitive development as a critical variable in planning care or teaching children helps nurses assist the young patient to a level of optimal health.

Critics of the learning theorists say that they all attempted to explain learning without the entanglement of meaning. The learning theorists who were most involved in behaviorism were trying to bypass the subjective experiences of the human organism and the role of those experiences in learning motivation, behavior, and social interactions.

COGNITIVE AND COMPUTER SCIENCES

The classical constructs of motivation, factor, and learning theories were not sufficient to provide understanding of the human brain and its impact on behavior. In the late 1940s, unrest was developing with the school of behaviorism. At a conference, Lashley realized that before new insights about the brain, or about computers, could be brought to bear in the psychological sciences, it would be necessary to confront behaviorism directly.[10] He raised the topic of serially ordered behavior, posing the research question of explaining complex organized behaviors such as playing tennis or speaking—phenomena not explained by traditional learning theory of associative chains between a stimulus and response. His thesis was that behavioral sequences have to be planned and organized in advance and originate within the individual as opposed to emanating from an external stimulus. This thesis also challenged two dogmas of neurobiological analysis: the belief that the nervous system is in a state of inactivity most of the time, and the belief that isolated reflexes are activated only when specific forms of stimulation make their appearance. Lashley, suggesting "every bit of evidence available indicate[s] a dynamic, constantly active system, or, rather, a composite of many interacting systems," advanced a new research agenda focusing on the complexity of human behavior and language.[11]

While the behavior sciences theorists were investigating human behavior, another group of scientists were investigating how machines could emulate the brain and provide faster computers.

With the advent of digital computers after World War II, interest in how the brain processed information emerged in engineering research in the fields of mathematics, computer science, cybernetics, and information theory. As the computer engineer pushed science technology to its limits using traditional computer architectures, scientists began to investigate how the brain processed data, recognizing this as a way of solving more complex problems and building more powerful computers.

This research has taken two directions: (1) biologic based on the neuronal model; and (2) the field of artificial intelligence.

There had to be some convergence of these fast-advancing contributions from the psychological and computer sciences in a model or framework to guide in the understanding and researching of basic fundamental human phenomena such as language, planning, decision making, problem solving, and creativity. Cognitive psychologist Howard Gardner traces the history of the interdisciplinary effort to solve the classic problems of Western thought: the nature of knowledge and how it is represented in the mind.[12] Contributing to this cognitive science research are the constituent cognitive sciences of philosophy, psychology, artificial intelligence, linguistics, and the border disciplines of anthropology and neuroscience. The key theoretical inputs to be focused on in this discussion include: mathematics and computer science, the neuronal model, cybernetic synthesis, information theory, and neurophysiological syndromes.

Mathematics and Computation

Since the earliest days of human history, people have aspired to free themselves from the drudgery of calculation. The abacus is believed to be one of the earliest calculating machines, having been used extensively in pre-Christian Rome and Greece as well as in Egypt and China. It was not, however, until the great rise of interest in natural philosophy in Western Europe in the 17th century that interest arose in the development of calculating instruments. With the predictive abilities of the new physical theories of Galileo, Descartes, and Newton, there came a real desire to use these theories, and this called for substantial calculating.

In the early part of the 17th century, John Napier invented the logarithm, which simplified the task of multiplying and led to the development of analog calculating machines. In 1642, Blaise Pascal built a simple machine whose arithmetic operations made it the first digital calculating machine. English mathematician Charles Babbage realized that if the entire process of a calculation could be automated a great speed-up could be achieved. Lady Ada Lovelace, an associate of Babbage's, worked with him on building his "difference" machine. It was a mechanical device used to calculate mathematical tables. In her letters to Lord Byron, the British poet laureate, Lady Lovelace described the basic command of today's digital computer, the traditional "conditional jump." Basically, the command tells the computer to do one thing if a certain condition exists and if it does not exist, do another thing. This major contribution by Lady Lovelace, rarely cited in computer history, was only discovered through patent litigation in the 1940s when von Neumann applied for patent rights on his computer. Lady Lovelace's letters, which proved her contribution, had come to light because of literary research, not computer research, and were cited in the litigation investigation. This shows how diverse research areas can overlap and assist each other and also demonstrates feminist contributions, which are not well recognized. Ada, a programming language, was named for Lady Lovelace in the 1980s.

In 1936 Allen Turing proposed the idea that a machine could carry out any possible, conceivable calculation. Briefly, the machine could execute any kind of program or plan that could be expressed in a binary code, for example a slash or a blank. One needed to be able to clearly express the steps needed to carry out the task (programming) and the Turing machine would scan the tape, regardless of length, and carry out instructions.[13] This Turing machine was the prototype for our modern-day computer.

In building upon Turing's ideas, John von Neumann explored the idea of devising a program to instruct the Turing machine and thus introduced the stored program that was kept within the computer's internal memory.

From the introduction of computers, scientists began to search for a machine to perform like the brain. The most difficult part of this research, thus far, has been developing the rules of human thought, that is, the discipline of artificial intelligence.

Artificial intelligence is the study of how the mind processes information and how it can be emulated by computer programs. Scientists became interested in how the mind processes because the computer, no matter how fast or powerful it is, cannot match the human mind in solving certain types of problems. A simple example is pattern recognition. Even a small child can see an automobile and immediately identify the make, model, etc., whereas the most powerful computer must search its memory or data base car by car to identify the car, which can take minutes.

The earliest applications in artificial intelligence are knowledge-based or expert systems. Knowledge-based systems are computer programs that emulate the deductive processes of experts in the field to solve specialized problems. For example, computers have been programmed to diagnose diseases using patient symptoms. The algorithms developed to do this processing were derived from working with doctors who were experts in the field. Law enforcement agencies are using expert systems to profile murders, and oil companies are using expert systems to process geological data to find oil.

In addition to programming the computer to emulate human thought other scientists are investigating how the brain processes data and if computers can be designed using logical elements connected together as neural elements are in the brain. The brain is considered to be a very powerful parallel processor, that is, it can process many facts simultaneously, whereas most of today's computers are serial processors. There are now emerging new parallel computers, but the ability to easily program these machines to solve problems in parallel needs to be developed.

The Neuronal Model

Warren McCulloch and Walter Pitts, in 1943, showed that the operation of a nerve cell and its connection with other nerve cells (a so-called neural network) could be modeled in terms of logic. Nerves could be thought of as logical statements, and the property of nerves firing (or not firing) could be compared to the operation of propositional calculus (in which a statement is either true or false). This led to the idea that the human brain could be thought to be operating according to the principles of logic and thus as a powerful computer; rather than trying to build machines that mimic the physiological level of the brain, analogies with the thinking that goes on in the human brain could be pursued at a higher level. This could lead to logical constructs for human problem solving that could be converted into logical and mathematical propositions to be embodied in a computer program.[14]

Mathematician Norbert Wiener was engaged in parallel pursuits at the Massachusetts Institute of Technology (MIT). He advanced beyond his contemporaries in his conviction that the issues of control engineering and communication engineering are inseparable. He put forth the then-radical notion that it is legitimate to describe machines that exhibit feedback as "striving toward goals," as calculating the difference between their goals and their actual performance, and as then working to reduce those differences. Machines were purposeful. Wiener's thinking was applied to the central nervous system as follows[15]:

The central nervous system no longer appears as a self-contained organ, receiving inputs from the senses and discharging into the muscles. On the contrary, some of its most characteristic activities are explicable only as circular processes, emerging from the nervous system into the muscles, and re-entering the nervous system through the sense organs, whether they be proprioceptors or organs of the special senses. This seemed to us to mark a new step in the study of that part of neurophysiology which concerns not solely the elementary processes of nerves and synapses but the performance of the nervous system as an integrated whole.

This critical contribution of the idea of the feedback loop led to a concept of mind as more than physiology and response. And in 1961, Wiener introduced his neologistic science as follows: "We have decided to call the entire field of control and communication theory, whether in the machine or in the animal, by the name Cybernetics."[16] In his book he set down an integrated vision—a linkage of developments in understanding the human nervous system, the electronic computer, and the operation of other machines. He underscored his belief, as well as that of von Neumann and MacCulloch and Pitts, that the functioning of the living organism and the operation of the new communication machines exhibited crucial parallels.[17]

Information Theory

Another key progenitor of cognitive science was Claude Shannon, an electrical engineer at MIT who is credited with devising information theory. He stated that all information can be represented with binary codes. His basic theory was that any analog signal, such as sound, can be encoded with a minimum number of codes. This made possible computer processing of natural phenomena such as voice and music. (For example, the new digital networks of the telephone companies are a result of his research.) This led to the notion that information can be

thought of in a way entirely divorced from the specific content or subject matter—that is, simply as a single decision between two equally plausible alternatives. Wiener explained the importance of this conceptualization as: information is information, not matter or energy. The basic unit of information is the bit (binary digit), that is, the amount of information required to select one message from two equally probable alternatives.

Neuropsychological Syndromes

Neuropsychological syndromes represent a convergence of disciplines (i.e., surgery, linguistics, psychology). It was discovered that there was much more regularity in the organization of cognitive capacities in the nervous system than was allowed for by wholly environmental accounts of mental processes. Furthermore, the patterns of breakdown could not be readily explained in terms of simple stimulus-response disruptions. Rather, in many cases, the hierarchy of behavioral responses was altered. For example, in certain forms of aphasia the general sentence structure was preserved (speaking in complete sentences) but the patient could not identify the verb and subject within that framework. In other aphasia the sentence structure broke down but words carried meaning. Thus it was learned that the human mind is layered and that cognitive operations are laid down in layers; injuries to the brain indicated that certain layers could be disrupted while others remained intact. For example, an individual can generate grammatically correct sentences but not be able to retrieve the meaning of specific words in sentences. Or the converse is true that a person can communicate meaning with individual words but cannot generate a grammatically intact sentence.

Only recently have cognitive scientists begun to question whether they can, in fact, afford to treat all information equivalently and to ignore issues of content. This information theory was constructed in terms of the use of the computer to process information concerned with physics and the hard sciences (e.g., engineering). In the human system, a unit of information is not equivalent to all other information. There must be a value orientation, or weighting. What is emerging is the information processing theory in human systems. It is another way of thinking about mind and behavior.

INFORMATION PROCESSING THEORIES

Information processing theories are based on studies of sensation, perceptions, and cognition. By sensation is meant simple (unembellished), immediate, conscious awareness by a person of both external and internal stimulation. It consists of a response to an amorphous energy stimulus with minimal signal and symbol information. Perception refers to the use of the senses to obtain information about the environment, its objects, events, and conditions. It consists of a response to a stimulus with signal and/or symbol informational value. Cognition refers to obtaining, organizing, and using sensory and perceptual information from the environment, from past experience, and from such mental activities as plays and strategies. Examples of cognitive activities are memory, problem solving, thinking, and language.[18]

Sensation, perception, and cognition have long been regarded as important factors in psychopathology because much of the phenomenology of psychopathology can be related to deviations in these areas. Until recently, the experimental work has lacked a systematic coherence, with findings often arising unexpectedly in the course of investigations aimed at other goals.[19]

The relationship among sensation, perception, and cognition offers a systematic way and a uniform framework for studying human behavior. This framework is an information processing approach. The goal of information processing investigations is to identify how incoming external stimuli or intentionally engendered stimuli enter the central nervous system (CNS) and result in some kind of final response. That is, information processing investigates how incoming stimuli are transduced, selected, coded, stored, and transmitted through the CNS. Information processing can be regarded as an organizing principle, a way of conceptualizing some of the dynamic complexities that are known to characterize human behavior.[20]

Information Processing

What exactly is meant by human information processing? Perhaps the best way to answer that question is to consider an example of a behavioral act, such as listening and retaining an hour's lecture by a professor for a future test. What terms or definitions are used to describe the hour transaction? First, the professor speaks from lecture notes. This is the auditory stimulus. The professor is beginning a chain of events and processes between the presentation of the auditory stimuli and the student's response to them, which in this case is to write key themes on paper. This act entails a large number of stages and controlling or modifying processes between the stimulus and the response.

What stages and processes are involved in the example of remembering key ideas from the lecture? The first stage has to do with sensation. This initial processing stage is called **sensory registration**; specifically, in the auditory case, it is called echoic memory. The physical energy of the professor's speech is translated (**transduced**) into electrical impulses in the nervous system of the student. Specifically, the auditory vibrations from the professor's words stimulate the listener's ear and thus generate electrical impulses in the acoustic nerve. These sensory impulses are transmitted to the cortical level, where they are perceived as a simple sensory message, namely, as a phonetic sound. In this sensory state, however, the sound is not necessarily categorized as a number; it simply remains as a sound without any informational signal or symbol value.[21]

If no further processing is to be done to the auditory stimulus, such as ascribing meaning to it by labeling it as a letter or number (pattern recognition) the sensory memory for the sound decays and the sound is not remembered. A large number of auditory sensations to which people are subjected are not processed beyond the stage of sensory registration. Persons are constantly bombarded by many more stimuli than they can or do respond to and these stimuli are ordinarily regarded as "noise."

If the words heard were not the ones the student expected to hear or was familiar with, the student would not pay much attention to them. This fact illustrates the importance of attentional factors in information processing. Attention is a major influence on what is or is not processed as well as how it is processed.

In the example, because the students are anticipating a test, they presumably would process the sensory memory. The next stage of processing is perceptual and is called **pattern recognition**. When the phonetic sounds are given meaning by the listeners, auditory pattern recognition has occurred. Pattern recognition is accomplished by a comparator-type process in which the stimulus patterns to be identified are compared with patterns previously stored by the listeners as part of their long-term and short-term memories.

The next stage of processing is **short-term memory**, which is a cognitive process that follows pattern recognition. This memory has to last long enough for the student to write key words on the paper. Therefore, to help students remember, the professor usually repeats key terms during a lecture. This **rehearsal** is one of several ways in which they can facilitate memorization. Without rehearsal, their sensory memory of the words following pattern recognition would decay rapidly.[22]

The Nature of Processing

A key concept in informational processing is the nature of processing. However, a process is not observable by itself. In any processing experiment, the only elements that can be directly observed and measured are the initiating stimulus and the resulting end-response. The intervening processes are hypothetical constructs; they cannot be directly measured but must, instead, be inferred. Processing can be analyzed in terms of several general questions.[23]

What Is Being Processed? The *what* question refers to whether the primary influence of the stimulus is due to its physical energy or to its formation, that is, energy processing or information processing.

Variations in the nature of the stimuli presented relate to the differences in what is being processed for the three domains of processing, sensory, perceptual, and cognitive.

Across the three domains of processing there are differences with respect to the relative importance given to energy and information. Sensory processing is concerned with measuring the effects on the response of precisely varied amounts of stimulus energy; in cognitive processing the major emphasis is on the information content of the stimuli; and perceptual processing falls in between sensory and cognitive processing. For example, the response to a visually presented word may be thought of as first entailing the sensory processing of contrast and color; next, the perceptual processing of lines, angles, and letter forms; and, finally, the cognitive processing of the meaning of the word.

Where Does Processing Take Place? The *where* of processing introduces questions about the underlying physiology and can be viewed in at least two ways. The first approach considers whether the processes occur relatively more peripherally or centrally in the nervous system. The second approach considers in which hemisphere of the brain the processing is most likely to be located.

When Does Processing Occur? Processing approaches assume that a sequence of stages takes place between the presentation of the stimulus and the subsequent response. Generally the stages can be described as (1) the input stage, at which the energy and information components of the stimuli are incorporated; (2) the classification of the components; (3) the organization of the classified components; (4) the interpretation of what has been processed; and (5) the output stage, which culminates in the response. The number and type of stages involved may differ for different types of stimuli, for different tasks, and for the person at different phases of practice or experience.

The Three Processing Domains

The three processing domains, sensory, perceptual, and cognitive, can be characterized in several ways.

1. They approximate a traditional division among psychological concepts.
2. Each domain relates to a different time period after the presentation of the stimuli. Sensory processing refers to the briefest, immediately poststimulation periods of time, usually for periods of up to a maximum of 1 second. Perceptual processing refers to slightly longer periods of time after the stimulus presentation, periods of up to about 5 seconds. Cognitive processing refers to even longer periods of time after the stimulus presentation, and the exact type of cognitive processing depends, in part, on the duration of the phenomenon under consideration. Such specific temporal distinctions are only approximations and are subject to modification with further research.

3. The three processing domains can be distinguished according to the nature of the stimulus material. The applied stimulus can be either of the energy type, in which case the response of the organism depends on the physical characteristics of the stimulus, such as its intensity, or of the signal type, in which case the response depends more on the accrued meaning or significance of the stimuli.

Application to Patient Care

Several researchers propose that information processing may be applied in psychiatric patients and that the process differs in mentally healthy individuals. For example, Kraeplin described schizophrenic patients as having difficulty in shifting attention, a kind of perseverative behavior influenced by the patient's rigid fixity of focus on some trivial portion of the environment. In general, both energy and information are processed in the three domains (sensory, perceptual, and cognitive), because energy is the carrier of information. Energy stimuli are those that can be defined completely with reference to their physical characteristics, e.g., wave frequency or intensity for light. The description of informational stimuli is more complicated because the term information is used loosely to mean stimulus complexity or the amount of stimulus patterning. Also, the quality of information depends on the individual.

A theory with an informational processing premise that has been proposed on depression suggests that depression is a defense reaction mounted to cope with anxiety arising from a defect in the patient's information-processing mechanisms. Because of increasing anxiety, the patient stops analyzing incoming sensory information and becomes lethargic and unresponsive to incoming stimuli.

Information processing theory has become an area of focus in investigation of learning deficits in children and organic conditions in the elderly. And in the 1980s, the application of the cognitive sciences has been advanced through the neuropsychological syndromes as related to post-traumatic events. Beginning work in this area has been by Horowitz, Figley, van der Kolk, and Hartman and Burgess.[24-27]

Summary

This chapter has reviewed recent contributions from the behavioral and cognitive sciences to understanding motivation, learning, and information processing. The relationship of the computer to the human brain has been a focus of intense study that has brought additional insights to clinicians working in the mental health field.

Questions

1. Describe an animal research project that contributed to learning theory.
2. How is Maslow's hierarchy of needs used in nursing?
3. Describe the information processing of a telephone conversation.
4. How has nursing research contributed through the cognitive sciences?

REFERENCES AND SUGGESTED READINGS

1. Maslow, A. H. *Motivation and Personality* (2nd ed.). New York: Harper & Row, 1970.
2. Skinner, B. F. *Science and Human Behavior*. New York: Free Press, 1953.
3. Bachrach, A. J. Learning theory. In H. I. Kaplan & B. J. Sadock, (Eds.), *Comprehensive Textbook of Psychiatry/IV*. Baltimore: Williams & Wilkins, 1985.

4. Skinner, op. cit.
5. Meissner, W. W. Theories of personality. In A. M. Nicholi, Jr. (Ed.), *The Harvard Guide to Modern Psychiatry*. Cambridge: Mass.: Harvard University Press, 1978, p. 135.
6. Cattell, R. B. *Personality: A Systematic, Theoretical, and Factual Study*. New York: McGraw Hill, 1950.
7. Bachrach, op. cit.
8. Hull, C. L. *Principles of Behavior: An Introduction to Behavior Theory*. New York: Appleton-Century-Crofts, 1943.
9. Piaget, J. *The Construction of Reality in the Child*. New York: Basic Books, 1954.
10. Lashley, K. S. In search of the engram. *Symposia of the Society for Experimental Biology*, 1950, 4, 454–482.
11. Jeffress, L. A. (Ed.). *Cerebral Mechanisms in Behavior: The Hixon Symposium*. New York: Wiley, 1951, p. 135.
12. Gardner, H. *The Mind's New Science*. New York: Basic Books, 1985.
13. Davis, M. *Computability and the Unsolvability*. New York: McGraw Hill, 1950.
14. Heimes, S. J. *John von Neuman and Norbert Wiener*. Cambridge, Mass.: MIT Press, 1980, p. 211.
15. Wiener, N. *Cybernetics, or Control and Communication in the Animal and the Machine* (2nd ed.). Cambridge, Mass.: MIT Press, 1961, p. 8. (Originally published, 1948.)
16. Ibid., p. 11.
17. Gardner, op. cit.
18. Kietzman, M., Spring, B. & Zubin, J. Perception, cognition, and information processing. In H. Kaplan & B. Sadock (Eds.), *Comprehensive Textbook of Psychiatry/IV*. Baltimore: Williams & Wilkins, 1985, p. 157.
19. Ibid.
20. Ibid.
21. Ibid.
22. Ibid., p. 158.
23. Ibid., pp. 160–161.
24. Horowitz, M. J. *Stress Response Syndromes*. New York: Jason Aronson, 1976.
25. Figley, C. R. (Ed.). *Stress Disorders Among Vietnam Veterans*. New York: Brunner/Mazel, 1978.
26. van der Kolk, B. A. (Ed.). *Post-traumatic Stress Disorder: Psychological and Biological Sequelae*. Washington, D.C.: American Psychiatric Press, Inc., 1984.
27. Hartman, C. R., & Burgess, A. W. Information processing of trauma: Case application of the model. *Journal of Interpersonal Violence*, 1988, 3(2), (in press).

Chapter 7

Theories of Personality

Ann Wolbert Burgess

Chapter Objectives

The students successfully attaining the goals of this chapter will be able to:

- Define and identify 10 personologists.
- Explain the core and periphery of personality.
- List the defining characteristics of the conflict model, the fulfillment model, and the consistency model.

Psychiatric nursing concerns itself with the mental health of people. Before studying the problems people have that might bring them to the attention of a psychiatric nurse or clinician, it is helpful to review what social scientists (i.e., the wide range of people who study aspects of human behavior) have to say about humans and human personality.

CONCEPTUAL FRAMEWORK

A useful framework for the study of theories of personality is set forth by Salvador R. Maddi and includes the following basic assumptions derived from a comparative analysis of various personality theories.[1]

1. People who are expert in the study and understanding of personality may be called "personologists."[2] Library shelves indicate that there are many people in the field of psychology and psychiatry who write on personality and can be called personologists. These are people who will be discussed in this chapter in terms of their contributions to understanding human beings.

Their work involves theorizing about personality through research, diagnosis, or psychotherapy. In personality research, the aim is usually to study the similarities and differences in observed behavior both within each person and across all people. In diagnosis, the personologist will use a number of tests of personality skills to determine a person's problems or capabilities. In research, groups of people generally will be studied, or if only a few individuals are studied, the concern will be with how representative they are of people in general.

2. Personologists generally restrict their attention to individual's behaviors that seem to have psychological importance in the expression of thoughts, feelings, and behaviors of humans.

3. They are concerned primarily with adult human beings because of the belief that personality does not congeal until sometime after childhood. The process of personality development is critical and many personologists attempt to explain their theory in terms of a historical orientation.

4. Personologists concentrate on the complexity and individuality of life. This individual focus is in contrast to sociologists, who concern themselves with similarities and differences of behaviors produced by membership of persons in the same socioeconomic class, e.g., voting behaviors or the social roles of new fathers; or to a neurophysiologist who might concern himself with the similarities of behavior of persons under the effects of marijuana; or to a geneticist who studies the structure of an individual from a genetic perspective.

5. Implied in personologists' theories is a reliance upon the idea that personality is a structured entity influencing behavior; the emphasis is on characteristics of behavior that show continuity over time and the assumption that personality, if it changes at all, changes slowly.

Definition of Personality

What is personality? Although various descriptions prevail, one definition set forward by Maddi is

a stable set of characteristics and tendencies that determine those commonalities and differences in the psychological behavior (thoughts, feelings, and actions) of people that have continuity in time and that may or may not be easily understood in terms of the social and biological pressures of the immediate situation alone.[3]

Core and Periphery of Personality

Two concepts important to personality are (1) core; and (2) periphery. Personologists tend to make two kinds of statements relevant to the core and periphery of personality.

Core Personality

The **core of a personality** describes the common factors or those inherent attributes of humans. These common attributes do not change much in the course of living and exert an extensive, pervasive influence on behavior.

Many theorists will describe one or two core tendencies; for example, all behavior constitutes an attempt of the individual to actualize his potential. Core theorizing also includes core characteristics of an individual.

Periphery Personality

The **peripheral aspects of a personality** delineate the differences in personality. These attributes of personality tend to be concrete and more readily observed. These attributes are generally learned, rather than inherent, and have a relatively circumscribed influence on behavior. They are mainly used to explain differences among people.

It is at the peripheral level that the theorist makes a major statement concerning the concrete styles of life that differ from person to person. The need for achievement or a compulsive trait are examples of concrete peripheral characteristics. The function of peripheral characteristics is to permit the understanding of differences between people.

Theorists differ as to how many concrete peripheral characteristics they describe; the greater the number, the greater the concern for individual differences. Sometimes the term *trait* is used. When traits are clustered into groups, the term *type* or *typology* may be proposed. The personologist states the different styles of life that are possible. Typically, one or more types are designated as ideal ways of life, whereas the others are considered nonideal or kinds of psychopathology.

The link between the core and periphery of personality is usually assumed to be development. Generally, the core tendency and characteristics are expressed in a particular environmental context. The resulting experience of reward, punishment, or knowledge congeals into concrete peripheral characteristics and types. The type of personality developed by a person is frequently understood to be a function of the family setting in which he or she matured. Those developmental conditions recognized to be favorable are regarded as leading to the personality type or types specified as ideal. The other, less adequate developmental conditions supposedly culminate in the less desirable personality types.

MODELS FOR PERSONALITY THEORIZING

Using a comparative analysis approach to the various theories of personality proposed, Maddi outlines three basic models for personality theorizing: the conflict model, the fullfillment model, and the consistency model.[4]

In the conflict model, the individual confronts two opposing forces. Life is necessarily a compromise, which at best involves a dynamic balance between the two forces and at worst, a foredoomed attempt to deny the existence of one of them. There are two versions of the conflict model. In the psychosocial version, the source of one force is in the person as an individual, but the source of the other force is in groups or societies. In the intrapsychic version, both great forces arise from within the person, regardless of whether he is regarded as an individual or as a social entity.

In contrast, the fulfillment model assumes only one great force and localizes it in the person. This model construes life as the increasingly great expression of this force. Although conflict is a possible occurrence in this model, it is neither necessary nor continuous. And when it occurs, it is considered an unfortunate failure in living. There are two versions of the fulfillment model. In the actualization version, the force is in the form of a genetic blueprint determining the person's special capabilities. Living fully is the process of realization of the capabilities. In the perfection version, the emphasis is on ideals of what is fine, excellent, and meaningful in life. The great force consists of striving toward these high ideals.

In the consistency model, there is little emphasis on great forces; rather, there is emphasis upon the formative influence of feedback from the external world. Life is to be understood as the extended attempt to maintain consistency. This model assumes no predetermined capabilities or ideals as the guides to living. This model has two versions. In the cognitive dissonance version, the relevant aspects of the person, in which there may or may not be consistency, are cognitive in nature. There may be inconsistency between two thoughts, or between an expectation and a perception of occurrences. In contrast, the activation version emphasizes consistency or inconsistency between the degree of bodily tension of activation that is customary for the person and that which actually exists at the time.[5]

CONFLICT MODEL: PSYCHOSOCIAL VERSION

Sigmund Freud

Classical psychoanalytic theory as described by Sigmund Freud and his followers is acknowledged as the cornerstone of the psychodynamic approach.[6] Alternate and supplementary points of view have been presented by Alfred Adler, Carl Jung, Karen Horney, and Harry Stack Sullivan, who have deemphasized the importance of instincts and (except for Jung) have emphasized social and cultural determinants of behavior. The psychodynamic approach is not without its limitations. At best, it presents an incomplete understanding of human behavior. Nevertheless, many of the concepts of the psychodynamic approach have proven invaluable in understanding mental health and mental illness and normal and abnormal human behavior.

Sigmund Freud (1856–1939) is described by Maddi as a man deeply serious about and committed to his work, his family, his colleagues and his friends.[7] His brilliance, tenacity, and independence was marked by social rejection that is a frequent concomitant of such accomplishments. Perhaps because of this rejection, Freud drew his circle of followers closely around him, insisting on loyalty.

Freud wrote a great deal and changed his mind often. He had a profound influence on personology. It is a tribute to him that as members of his inner circle left, they went on to develop influential theories of their own.

Freud viewed the basic tendency of living as maximizing instinctual gratification, while minimizing punishment and guilt. This view includes a position on (1) the basic drives or instincts; (2) the levels of awareness and agencies of the mind; (3) sources of punishment and guilt; and (4) the mechanisms of defense whereby instincts are satisfied while punishment and guilt are avoided.

Instincts

Freud proposed a number of instincts that are common to all people. These instincts form the core characteristics of personality. All instincts, according to Freud, have a source, a type of energy or driving force, an aim and an object. The source of an instinct is rooted in the biologic character of the individual in the process of metabolism. Freud makes it clear that psychic manifestations (thoughts, wishes, and emotions) are dependent on somatic activities and processes. For this assumption, Freud's theory is viewed as biologic rather psychological in nature.

Instincts have their sources in somatic processes and are characterized by the tension and pressure toward action of biologic deprivation states. The instinct says: "I want gratification now." The other agencies of the mind, as well as society, decide whether, when, how, and in what form these drives will be gratified. Such negotiations or compromises form the basis for conflict, which may ultimately result in psychopathology. The overall aim of instincts is satisfaction or the reduction of tension.

There are three kinds of instincts, all subsumed under the concept of the id. The id is a core characteristic of personality. Freud argued for a group of instincts that function to preserve biologic life, calling these self-preservation instincts such as the need to obtain food, air, and water. Although these life instincts are obviously basic, Freud paid less attention to them than the sexual instinct, the energy of which is called *libido*. In the latter part of his career, Freud began to theorize about a third instinct, the death instinct. His interest in this followed World War I and may well have been influenced by his own confrontation with death after he developed jaw cancer.[8]

The id is the core characteristic of personality that is comprised of the life, sexual, and death instincts. The wishes and emotions of the id are deeply self-centered and selfish in nature. It is this inherent selfishness that makes conflict inevitable. In addition, the parts of the personality called ego and superego are considered parts of the core.

Levels of Awareness

The levels of awareness approach divides the mind into three parts: the unconscious, the preconscious, and the conscious. The unconscious consists of repressed ideas and repressed feelings, which become partially apparent in dreams, slips of the tongue, and forgetting. The unconscious is not logical, it contains contradictory ideas and feelings, and it has no conception of time. For example, it may simultaneously love and hate, believe in irrational concepts, and feel that an event that occurred 20 years ago happened only yesterday. The unconscious is closely related to drives and instincts previously described. The sexual instincts in particular have their derivatives embedded in the unconscious process. The preconscious, which includes ideas and feelings easily made conscious, censors wishes and represses unpleasant ideas and feelings. In contrast to the unconscious, the preconscious supports the reality principle and respects logic. The conscious refers to all that is in awareness.

The above ideas were inferred from the observation that neurotic symptoms seemed to result from the repression of unacceptable wishes that were not in the conscious mind of the patient. When these unconscious wishes were made conscious again, the neurotic symptoms would often disappear.

Punishment and Guilt

The sources of punishment and guilt are in the communal requirements of society. When people transgress the rules and regulations of civilization, they are punished by other people acting as representatives of the society. All living has the aim of maximizing instinct gratification while minimizing punishment and guilt, and this is precisely what Freud meant when he said that all behavior is motivated.

The core theorizing not only involves a position on the nature of the instincts and the sources of punishment and guilt but also includes a position on the mechanism whereby instinct gratification is maximized while punishment and guilt are held to a minimum. This mechanism is contained in the concept of defense. If people express their instincts fully in action they will be punished by other people. If they fully recognize their instincts even without acting on them they will experience guilt. And yet the instincts are inexorable forces pushing for expression. This state of affairs is the major conflict of life, according to Freud, and is eased somewhat through the process of defense.

Defenses

Defenses are described as working as follows. When an instinct becomes strong enough to make a difference, an alarm reaction occurs in the form of anxiety. This anxiety reaction represents the anticipation of punishment and guilt and triggers the defensive process. Defenses operate unconsciously.

The concept of defense is preeminent in the achievement of a compromise of balance, which is the healthiest state. There are always defenses and thus the distinction is made in terms of whether the defenses promote the effective compromise of balance or the ineffective denial of one of the two opposing forces. Chapter 8 further discusses ego mechanisms.

Periphery of Personality

The Freudian position on the periphery of personality is contained in the classification of character types. A character type is a group of traits that is expressive of (1) particular underlying defenses; (2) a particular underlying conflict; (3) a particular response on the part of others to an underlying conflict; or (4) any combination of these. Traits are concrete peripheral characteristics. Character types reflect on development. The major stages of psychosexual development are the oral, anal, phallic, latency, and genital stages.

Harry Stack Sullivan

Harry Stack Sullivan (1892–1949) was an American physician who was greatly influenced by William Alanson White, a neuropsychiatrist. During his early career, Sullivan researched schizophrenia. Although considered a brilliant psychotherapist, he did not write in a formal manner; rather, his publications consist of papers originally given as talks.

Two core tendencies described by Sullivan are the pursuit of satisfaction and the pursuit of security. The tendency toward satisfaction has its source in the biologic survival requirements of the organism. The more the person is deprived of these biologic requirements, the stronger is the tendency toward satisfaction. The tendency toward security has a psychological, rather than biologic source, namely, the social arena of interaction between people. The insecurity of a person registers as tension or anxiety.[9]

The pursuit of satisfaction and security are core tendencies because they are the natural endowment of all humans. Sullivan also speaks of humans' need for power and physical closeness which propels humans into the world of interpersonal relations. The formation of a core tendency is almost identical to Freud's, namely, the maximization of satisfaction while simultaneously minimizing insecurity.

Sullivan distinguishes three classes of defense: dissociation, parataxic distortion, and sublimation. Dissociation involves the exclusion from awareness of experiences and impulses that would be anxiety provoking if conscious. Parataxic distortion is a defensive avoidance of reality, the function of which is to preserve the feeling of security. Sublimation occurs when the goals of impulses are incompatible with the self-system and are unwittingly exchanged for socially approved goals so that the impulses may achieve partial expression without threatening security.[10]

CONFLICT MODEL: INTRAPSYCHIC VERSION

In contrast to the psychosocial version of the conflict model in which the inevitable conflict is between the individual and the group, the intrapsychic version locates the conflict within the psyche. It is not dependent upon the difference between living alone and living in the company of others.

Otto Rank

Otto Rank (1884–1939) was a member of Freud's inner circle and considered a brilliant nonmedical contributor to the psychoanalytic movement. In fact, his training in philosophy, psychology, history, and art was viewed as a welcomed stimulus to the thinking of the group.

The core tendency in Rank's theory is that all functioning is expressive of the tendency to minimize the fear of life while at the same time minimizing the fear of death.[11,12] The terms life and death are specific to Rankians. Life is equivalent to the process of separation and individualization, whereas death is the opposite, namely union, fusion, and dependency. Early in his career, Rank considered the birth trauma the most significant event in life. He later developed his theory to consider it only the first in a long series of separation experiences that are as inevitable as death itself. To avoid separation and individuation is to deny life and death; thus, the person is caught between two poles of conflict that is as basic as being alive.

Periphery of Personality

Three personality types are described by Rank. The personality type called the artist is the Rankian ideal. This person has accepted both the fear of life and the fear of death, both the inevitable pressure toward individuation and the unavoidable longing for union, and achieved integration of the two. The neurotic personality type expresses the tendency toward separation to the exclusion of the tendency toward union. The neurotic seems fixated at the level of counterwill and the personality is weak on integrating principles. His sense of separateness is likely to be ridden by hostility and moralistic rather than ethical guilt. Characteristics of the neurotic would probably be hostile, negativistic, arrogant, isolationistic, critical of others, highly guilty, and so on. The final personality type, that of the average man, is someone who expresses the tendency toward union to the exclusion of the tendency toward individuation. The average man is inferior both to the artist and the neurotic man because he has never even seriously entertained the possibility of his own individuality. The average man's characteristics would include conformity, dependability, superficiality, suggestibility, and lack of dissatisfaction.

Carl G. Jung

Carl G. Jung (1875–1961) provides an extraordinarily complex theory. Perhaps because of the influence of his clergyman father, Jung first wanted to study philology and archaeology. However, he chose to study medicine and his early interest in psychiatry was spurred by Eugen Bleuler and Pierre Janet. The early relationship between Freud and Jung was mutual admiration, and Freud regarded Jung as his successor. However, the relationship became fraught with theoretical and personal disagreements, and in 1914 Jung resigned his membership, again emphasizing the competitiveness between strong and creative personalities.

The notable differences between Freudian and Jungian theory are Jung's deemphasis of sexuality and a greater emphasis on spirituality. The overall direction of Jungian theory is the tendency toward attainment of selfhood.[13] There are several core characteristics including the conscious mind that is comprised of conscious perceptions, thoughts, memories, and feelings. The ego directs the business of the day. The personal unconscious can become conscious with a shift in focus of attention and a relaxation of defenses. The collective unconscious, which does not reflect individual experience but rather the accumulated experience of the human species, is Jung's striking, unique, and controversial concept. According to the concept, all of the events that have happened to people for eons of human history make their contribution to the life of each contemporary person in the form of a sort of species memory. The accumulated culture of mankind is lodged in the infant's psyche at birth, in the form of a collective unconscious. All that is human, indeed everything in the universe, according to Jung, exists, changes, and thrives as a result of conflict and opposition.

Periphery of Personality

Jung's conceptualization of personality types is the distinction he makes between the attitudes of introversion and extroversion. The introverted person is concerned with the internal world or his own ruminations, whereas the extroverted person is concerned with the external world of things and people.

In summary, in the conflict model, life is viewed as a compromise, the purpose of which is to minimize the conflict.

FULFILLMENT MODEL: ACTUALIZATION VERSION

In the fulfillment model, life is not considered to be a compromise, but rather the process of unfolding of one force. In the actualization version of the fulfillment model, the perspective is humanistic.

Carl Rogers

Carl Rogers (1902–), a psychologist with background training in the biologic and physical sciences, studied at Union Theology Seminary and then transferred to Columbia University, where he was influenced by the humanistic philosophy of John Dewey. After practicing in a guidance center, Rogers became a university professor and researcher and was influenced by theorists who stressed the importance of an individual's self-view as a determinant of behavior.

Rogers views the core of personality as the tendency of humans to actualize their potentialities.[14] Maddi summarizes Rogers' view of the core tendencies of personality as: (1) the inherent attempt of the individual to actualize or develop all of his capacities in ways that serve to maintain and enhance life; and (2) the attempt to actualize the self-concept, which is a psychological manifestation of the first tendency.[15] The needs for positive regard and positive self-regard are secondary or learned offshoots of these core tendencies, explaining the motivational mechanism whereby the actualization of self-concept is attempted.

The characteristics of the core personality are (1) the inherent potentialities, which define the ways in which the actualization tendency will be expressed; and (2) the self-concept, which defines the ways in which the self-actualizing tendency will be expressed. These tendencies and characteristics are at the core of personality because they are common to all people and have a pervasive influence on living.

While the inherent potentialities are genetically determined, the self-concept is socially determined. This makes it possible to distinguish between the two sets of core characteristics; that is, a person's sense of who and what he or she is may deviate from what the inherent potentialities suit him for. Rogers calls the nature of society's influence conditional positive regard. It is assumed that he means that the situation in which only some but not all of the person's actions, thoughts, and feelings are approved and supported by the significant people in his life. Thus, a person develops a self-concept based on how and what others have regarded. An individual's self-concept is based on conditions of worth, i.e., standards for discerning what is valuable and what is not valuable about oneself. Conditions of worth as a concept serve much the same logical function as Freud's superego. The existence of conditions of worth in the self-concept bring into operation defensiveness that is similar to that suggested by Freud. However, for Freud, defensive operations lead to the most successful life, whereas for Rogers, defensive operations lead to a restriction on living.[16] Conditions of worth and defensive processes are considered crippling, a state called

incongruence. The only way for this condition not to cripple a person is for him to have had experience as a child of unconditional positive regard from a significant person. This, Rogers states, means an atmosphere of valuing and loving more than it means an absence of all constraints. Roger's definition of full functioning persons are those who (1) respect and value all manifestations of themselves; (2) are self-aware; and (3) are flexible and open to new experiences.

In terms of periphery of personality, Rogers outlines characteristics of the fully functioning person as follows: openness to experience, ability to show positive and negative emotion, reflectiveness, flexibility, adaptability, spontaneity, inductive thinking, and creativity.

Abraham Maslow

Abraham Maslow (1908–1970) researched and wrote about normal and creative people. Maslow developed his position slowly over his career and was responsive to and influenced by the work of other like-minded personologists such as Gordon Allport, Carl Rogers, and Kurt Goldstein.

Maslow agrees with Rogers and Goldstein in imputing to the person as a core tendency the push toward actualization of inherent potentialities.[17] For Maslow, the actualization of inherent potentialities includes development of a self-concept. In his core personality there is also the tendency to push to satisfy the needs ensuring physical and psychological survival. Both survival and actualization tendencies are part of the core personality. His position is not in the conflict tradition, in which survival and self-actualization are antagonistic to each other.

The casting of Maslow's survival and actualizing tendencies in motivational terms has been popular. According to Maslow, the actualization tendency is growth motivation, whereas the survival tendency is deprivation motivation.[18] Deprivation motivation refers to urges to strive for goal states, at present unachieved, in order to relieve the tension state, in order to recover homeostatic balance. Growth motivation does not involve the repairing of deficits so much as the expansion of horizons. Satisfaction has to do with the realization of capabilities or ideals through an increasingly complex process.

The core characteristics of personality are contained in Maslow's list of needs organized in terms of the degree to which satisfaction of each is a prerequisite to the search for satisfaction of the next. Maslow lists physiological needs, safety needs, needs for belongingness and love, and esteem needs. The needs are arranged in hierarchical order, moving from physiological needs through safety needs to the needs for belongingness and esteem.

Maslow describes the person achieving self-actualization in terms of what the person would be like. He uses such words as "creative living," "peak experience," "unselfish love," and "unbiased understanding."

Periphery of Personality

The only personality type that Maslow concerns himself with is that which attains complete psychological maturity. These are people who have fully actualized themselves, and common traits of these people' turn out to be: realistic orientation; acceptance of self, others, and natural world; and spontaneity.

In summary, in the actualization version of the fulfillment model, people are conceptualized as trying to become what their inherent potentialities actually suit them to be. For example, if the person is highly intelligent, fulfillment will involve a life in which intellectual endeavor is frequent.

FULFILLMENT MODEL: PERFECTION VERSION

Alfred Adler

Alfred Adler (1870–1937) began his medical career practicing general medicine. He then shifted to psychiatry and became a charter member of the Vienna Psychoanalytic Society. He resigned his office and membership after criticism of his ideas by the Society and went on to found his own group.

Individual Psychology

Adler's core tendency of personality is the striving toward superiority or perfection. Adler became convinced early in his career that aggressive urges were more important in life than sexual ones. He elaborated on this position by identifying as the basic drive in human beings the will to power.

Adler indicated that the striving toward superiority is innate and that it may evidence itself in a number of ways. Some of his thoughts on the precise sources of "the great upward drive" are organ inferiority, feelings of inferiority, and compensation.

After the break with Freud, Adler shifted the content of the core tendency from sexuality to aggressiveness. Adler's "will to power" clearly views social interaction as extraordinarily competitive in nature. In Adler's final position, both the individual and social sides of humankind are inherent and there is no antagonism between them.

The result of expressing the superiority tendency is the formation of a style of life. The style of life is a pattern of characteristics, determined both by the feeling of inferiority and the compensatory attempts the person engages in.[19]

Eric Fromm

Eric Fromm (1900–), trained in psychology and sociology and psychoanalysis in Europe and came to lecture at the Chicago Psychoanalytic Institute in 1933. Although Fromm's viewpoint includes elements of the conflict model and of both actualization and perfection versions of the fulfillment model, Maddi believes the perfection aspects of his position to be paramount.[20]

Fromm distinguishes between animal nature (biochemical and physiological bases and mechanisms for physical survival) and human nature (the ability to know itself and the things that are different from it).[21] True to the fulfillment model, Fromm does not assume a basic antagonism between humankind and society. He does stress humans' nature to achieve expression in ways that are effective and possible. As in other fulfillment positions, Fromm believes that when peoples' nature is pervertedly expressed, the blame is society's.

The core characteristics associated with the core tendency are the needs for relatedness, transcendence, rootedness, identity, and frame of reference.

Existential Psychology

Existential thought consists of a set of attitudes for living. Founders of the field all knew Freud and were heavily influenced by his thinking early in their careers.[22–24] But the major intellectual influences on them were Kierkegaard and Heidegger. Being-in-the-world is a basic core characteristics intended to emphasize the unity of person and environment.[25,26] Person and environment are essentially one and the same. For Rollo May and other existentialists, being is so essentially a matter of choice that a person can even choose against it by committing suicide, by precipitating nonbeing.[27] Achieving one's potential involves a painful and continual process of soul-searching and divisions, in the face of doubt and loneliness.

There are three broad modes of being-in-the-world. These are *Umwelt* (the biologic experience), *Mitwelt* (the social experience), and *Eigenwelt* (the personal experience). It is natural to consider the ideal to be a vigorous expression of all three. When this happens, there is a tendency for the three to merge, producing a unitary whole. This unitary quality of being-in-the-world is another criterion of an ideal personality according to existentialists.

To summarize, the consistency model emphasizes the importance of information or emotional experience the person gets out of interacting with the external world. The model assumes that there is a particular kind of information or emotional experience that is best for the person, and hence, that he will develop a personality that increases the likelihood that he will interact with the world in such a way as to get this kind of information or emotional experience. The personality is determined much more by the feedback from interaction with the world than it is by inherent attributes of a person.

CONSISTENCY MODEL: COGNITIVE DISSONANCE VERSION

The important elements in the determination of consistency are cognitions, that is, thoughts, expectations, attitudes, opinions, and perceptions. All cognitive dissonance versions of the consistency model assume that discrepancies between cognitive elements produce an emotional state that provides the energy and direction for behavior. Discrepancies produce anxiety, which in turn produces behavior—the aim of which is to reduce the discomfort.

George Kelly

George Kelly (1905–1966) is less well known than the other personologists described because he did not publish as much as others. The core tendency of personality in Kelly's view is the person's continued attempt to predict and control the events he experiences.[28] Kelly advocated taking as a model for humans, not the biologic organism or the frame of happiness and unhappiness, but rather, the scientific pursuit of truth. Truth is not necessarily what pleases or satisfies us in the straightforward terms of our desires but rather what convinces us of its inexorable reality. The scientific pursuit of truth is the empirical procedure of formulating hypotheses and testing them out in the tangible world of actual experience.

The first step in attempting to predict and control one's experience is to engage in the construing of events. The process of construing is the construct. A core characteristic of personality, the construct is an idea or abstraction that has a dichotomous nature, i.e., good–bad. Kelly's basic unit of personality is the personal construct. Personal constructs are organized into construction systems, which constitute the personality.

Less well defined are the common types of character derived from the cognitive dissonance of the consistency model.

CONSISTENCY MODEL: ACTIVATION VERSION

Fiske and Maddi

Donald Fiske (1916–) and Salvador Maddi (1933–) state as the core tendency of the activation version of the consistency model that the person attempts to maintain the level of activation to which he is accustomed and that is characteristic of him. According to Fiske and Maddi, activation is a neuropsychological concept, referring on the psychological side to the common core meaning in such terms as alertness, attentiveness, tension, and subjective excitement, and on the neural side to the state of excitation in a postulated center of the brain.[29] Three dimensions of stimulation include intensity (physical energy), meaningfulness (importance of a stimulus to the individual), and variation (change, novelty, and unexpectedness). The dimensions of stimulation that can influence activation are chemical, electrical, and cortical excitation. Everyone is assumed to have an activation level and a core characteristic of personality.

Maddi and his students, building on the core theorizing that he and Fiske offered, discuss the periphery of personality in terms of three basic kinds of similarity and difference among people.[30] The first consideration is the characteristic curve of activation. That is, everyone has a characteristic activation curve that begins upon waking, moves to a high point during the day, and then declines rapidly as sleep approaches. The second basic consideration of similarity and difference between people involves the average peak of a person's characteristic curve of activation. Some people have a high activation and some have a low activation point. The high-activation people spend the major part of their time and effort pursuing stimulus impact in order to keep their activation level from becoming too low whereas the low-activation people put their major time and effort into avoiding impact in order to keep their activation level from getting too high.

The third consideration involves the anticipatory and correctional techniques used for maintaining actual activation at the characteristic level for maximum impact. Impact implies intensity, meaningfulness, and variety of stimulation. Terms to distinguish people at this third level include approach motive as being high or avoidant. The approach motives are often called needs and the avoidance motives are often called fears. The activation theory continues to expand its periphery components with external and internal traits, expanding the possible number of personality types to 24. In defending this staggering number, the theorists argue that the personality theory is new and will be refined as it is used and tested.

Summary

This chapter conceptualizes the myriad theories of personality into three models based on the conflict theory, fulfillment theory, and consistency theory. In comparison with consistency theories, both fulfillment and conflict theories put much greater emphasis upon an inherent nature as a component of personality determining life's course. According to fulfillment theories, life is an unfolding of the human's inherent nature. And even when conflict theories stress society as an important force in living, they assume that personality is in large measure an expression of inherent characteristics. For both fulfillment and conflict theories, the content of personality is much more set by virtue of the attributes the individual brings into the world than is true of consistency positions.

Consistency positions concern themselves much more with the compatibility between aspects of content than with what the content actually is. For consistency theorists, the content of personality is largely learned and represents the history of feedback resulting from interacting with the world.

Questions

1. How is a comparative analysis helpful to understanding different theories?
2. Which of the three models do you favor and why?
3. Differentiate between core and periphery of personality and give examples.
4. Define personality.
5. Identify the defining characteristics of the conflict model, the fulfillment model, and the consistency model.

REFERENCES AND SUGGESTED READINGS

1. Maddi, S. R. *Personality Theories: A Comparative Approach*. Homewood, Ill.: Dorsey Press, 1972.
2. Murray, H. A. *Explorations in Personality: A Clinical and Experimental Study of Fifty Men of College Age*. New York: Oxford, 1938.
3. Maddi, op. cit., p. 9.
4. Maddi, op. cit.
5. Ibid.
6. Freud, S. *New Introductory Lectures to Psychoanalysis* (W. J. H. Sprott, trans.). New York: Norton, 1933.
7. Maddi, op. cit.
8. Freud, S. Instincts and their vicissitudes. In S. Freud, *Collected Papers* (Vol. 4). London: Institute for Psychoanalysis and Hogarth Press, 1925.
9. Sullivan, H. S. *Conceptions of Modern Psychiatry*. Washington, D.C.: William Alanson White Psychiatric Foundation, 1947.
10. Ibid.
11. Rank, O. *The Trauma of Birth*. New York: Harcourt, Brace, 1929.
12. Rank, O. *Will Therapy and Truth and Reality*. New York: Knopf, 1945.
13. Maddi, op. cit.
14. Rogers, C. *Client-Centered Therapy*. Boston: Houghton Mifflin, 1951.
15. Maddi, op. cit.
16. Ibid.
17. Maslow, A. H. *Motivation and Personality*. New York: Harper & Row, 1970.
18. Ibid.
19. Maddi, op. cit.
20. Ibid.
21. Ibid.
22. Fromm, E. *Man for Himself*. New York: Holt, Rinehart & Winston, 1947.
23. Binswanger, L. *Being-in-the-World: Selected Papers of Ludwig Binswanger*. New York: Basic Books, 1963.
24. Boss, M. *Psychoanalysis and Daseinanalysis*. New York: Basic Books, 1963.
25. Frankl, V. *The Doctor and the Soul*. New York: Knopf, 1960.
26. Binswanger, op. cit.
27. Boss, op. cit.
28. Kelly, G. A. *The Psychology of Personal Constructs* (Vol. 1). New York: Norton, 1955.
29. Fiske, D. W., & Maddi, S. R. (Eds.). *Functions of Varied Experience*. Homewood, Ill.: Dorsey, 1961.
30. Maddi, S. R., & Propst, B. Activation theory and personality. In S. R. Maddi (Ed.), *Perspectives on Personality: A Comparative Approach*. Boston: Little, Brown, 1971.

Chapter 8

Ego Functions, Self-Representation, and Mechanisms of Defense

Ann Wolbert Burgess

Chapter Objectives

The students successfully attaining the goals of this chapter will be able to:

- Name ten functions of the ego and how they are used in an assessment.
- Explain the role of ego defenses as a means for coping with psychological conflict and anxiety.
- Define the components of the self-representation system, specifically self-image and self-esteem.
- Name styles of personality defense based on research on ego development and ego mechanisms.

The term personality has many connotations, and knowledge of an individual's personality style is important for understanding that person's psychological strengths and vulnerabilities. The characteristic qualities of individuals are described by noting the prevailing nature of their character traits.

One way to understand personality styles is to study the development of the ego and the mechanisms of defense. Ego is used to denote that part of the personality that perceives, experiences, judges, and controls behavior. Ego is often equated with character or personality structure. This chapter discusses the development of the ego, ego functions, and the ego mechanisms of defense. This knowledge is essential for students of human behavior as they

begin to work with the defensive styles of people under stress, that is, stress from a physical and/or mental health problem.

During the past two decades, the attention of psychodynamic theorists has turned from studies of instincts and their vicissitudes to a careful and comprehensive study of the ego. The structural approach that set the ego apart as a distinct agency provided the stage for these later formulations. The major contributors to writings on ego psychology include Anna Freud, Erik Erikson, and contemporary theorists.[1-3] Studies of the ego have taken two major directions, each of which has considerable clinical importance. The first is the study of various ego functions that are primarily conflict-free and result from maturational aspects of intellectual functioning. The second is the study of the major mechanisms of defense of the ego.

THE AGENCIES OF THE MIND

Contemporary psychodynamic theory divides mental functioning into three major systems or agencies, each of which has different functions. These are the id, the ego, and the superego. Behavior may be understood as a result of the interaction among these three systems. It must be remembered, however, that the id, ego, and superego are theoretical constructs or ways of organizing our ideas about mental functioning. Therefore, it is meaningless to ask whether or not these agencies exist. But it is meaningful to ask to what degree these concepts are useful in making sense of the behaviors that we observe in health and illness.

The Id. The id represents the primitive instinctual drives that seek gratification. It is the major source of psychic energy and provides the power for the functions of the superego and ego. This instinctual energy, with which the infant is endowed at birth, knows no time or logic and is unconscious. It wants its wishful and irrational impulses to be immediately and totally discharged according to the pleasure principle.

The Ego. As the instinctual demands of the growing infant become incapable of reducing tension, the ego emerges. Wanting something is not enough. The ego then brings the reality principle to bear. It mediates the demands of the environment and the demands for instinctual satisfaction. It sees to it that the discharge of tension is appropriate. It decides how to act and when to act. Whereas the id originally comes into conflict with external reality, eventually conflict occurs within the mind, between the ego and the id. In this situation, the ego may prevent the id's instinctual discharge.

The Superego. The superego is the last of the three systems to develop. In contrast to the id, which strives for pleasure, the superego strives for perfection and morality. It is little wonder that these two systems (the superego and the id) are often in conflict. The standards of right and wrong adopted by the superego result from rewards and punishments and from approving and disapproving behaviors by the parents and

other important people in a person's early years. An important part of superego development arises from an attempt to please parents and not lose their affection. "I will do the right thing and they will love me." With superego formation, it might be said that the child has internalized the parent's belief as to what is right so that now there is an automatic signal inside. The ego must now deal with the superego, a force that is sometimes as irrational and unreasonable in its standard of right and wrong as the id is in its demands for pleasure. When these standards are not met, a person may experience terrible guilt, a fear of punishment, diminished self-esteem, and remorse. The superego may oppose both the id and the ego. The conceptual model of id, ego, and superego illustrates this system (Fig. 8-1).

The dimensions of the superego described above resemble the conscience. There is a less well-described subsystem of the superego, the ego-ideal, which is an incorporation of that which a person has been approved of and rewarded for. A person does what is right not only out of fear of punishment but also out of a desire to please and be rewarded.

Ego Functions

In common usage, the concept of the ego is grossly oversimplified, its meaning global and vague. The related concepts of ego strength and ego weakness suffer similar limitations in clinical practice.

However, as a result of the continuing efforts of psychodynamic theorists and ego psychologists, it is now possible to begin to define the ego by a finite number of functions that necessarily overlap and have a dynamic relationship with one another. Understanding these ego functions, at least from a descriptive and, hopefully, from a dynamic point of view, has the potential to increase nurses' abilities to help patients.

Research investigations continue to categorize ego functions. Ego functions have been described by Bellak and Sheehy in a comprehensive study of ego functioning (see Table 8-1). Nurses will benefit by being familiar with the ego functions as they are discussed in patient evaluations, especially in assessing the strengths and assets of the patient (see Chapter 29, Psychological Testing and Psychological Measurement). The assessment list of ego func-

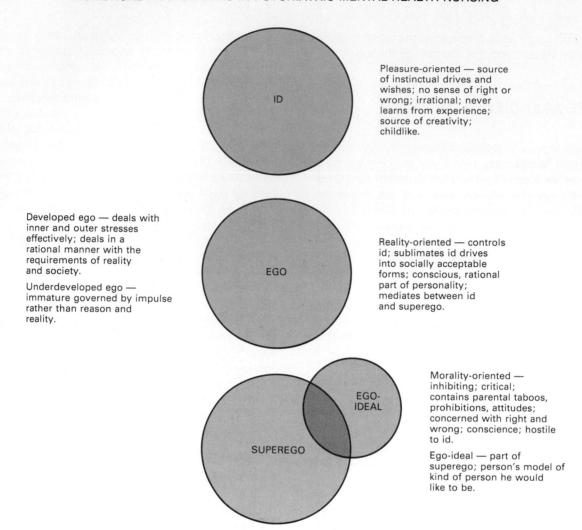

Pleasure-oriented — source of instinctual drives and wishes; no sense of right or wrong; irrational; never learns from experience; source of creativity; childlike.

Developed ego — deals with inner and outer stresses effectively; deals in a rational manner with the requirements of reality and society.

Underdeveloped ego — immature governed by impulse rather than reason and reality.

Reality-oriented — controls id; sublimates id drives into socially acceptable forms; conscious, rational part of personality; mediates between id and superego.

Morality-oriented — inhibiting; critical; contains parental taboos, prohibitions, attitudes; concerned with right and wrong; conscience; hostile to id.

Ego-ideal — part of superego; person's model of kind of person he would like to be.

Figure 8-1. Conceptual model of id, ego, and superego.

tions may be used as part of the mental status examination, and it also may be used as a checklist to focus on deficient areas of ego functioning that are troublesome for the patient. Since this type of ego assessment may prove useful to nurses in specific settings, additional readings on the subject are recommended, such as the text by Bellak, Hurvich, and Gediman.[4]

In summary, the ego regulates the self, maintains the balance between drives and values, and preserves the integrity of the individual. It serves as a monitoring device, constantly scanning the environment for possible threats, necessities, and opportunities. Concurrently, it remains in constant contact with the internal physiological state. However, because it has the capacity to perceive anxiety, the ego performs a signal function and in order to perform its adaptive function of discrimination, it also must per-

ceive and test reality. As stated by Wilson and Kneisl, "The ego or self-system is a controlling agency that recognizes messages, receives input, stores memories, discriminates perceptions, integrates life experiences, and acts to guard the vital balance."[5]

Ego Development

With such essential functions, the following questions arise: How does the ego develop? What are the key phases in the process? What implication is there for the nursing care of psychiatric patients?

In the psychodynamic framework, ego development refers either to the development of multiple processes, cognitive functions, defen-

TABLE 8-1. ASSESSMENT LIST OF EGO FUNCTIONS AND THEIR COMPONENTS

Perception of Reality

1. The ego tests reality in three major ways:
   A. Makes a distinction between stimuli perceived internally and externally.
   B. Maintains accurate perception of external events.
   C. Maintains accurate perception of internally experienced events.
2. The ego exhibits a sense of reality in four major ways:
   A. Maintains an accurate interpretation of self-identity and self-esteem.
   B. Establishes clear boundaries between self, others, and the world, in general.
   C. Sets boundaries on the extent of derealization between thoughts and reality.
   D. Sets boundaries on the extent of depersonalization between self and others.

Perception of Others

3. The ego achieves a balance in relationships between self and others in four major ways:
   A. Maintains a balance in degree and kind of relatedness between self and others that is neither narcissistic nor symbiotic in nature.
   B. Evidences maturity rather than primitivity in relationships with others.
   C. Maintains a balance to the degree to which others are perceived independently of self.
   D. Evidences consistency in relationships with others.

Judgment

4. The ego makes judgments and evaluations of internal and external conditions in terms of:
   A. Anticipating the consequences of intended behavior.
   B. Manifesting the anticipation of the intended behavior.
   C. Using social behaviors appropriate to the external events.

Control of Thoughts, Feelings, and Actions

5. The ego regulates and controls thoughts, feelings, and actions in the following ways:
   A. Directs the expression of the impulse.
   B. Employs delay mechanisms.
   C. Employs control over intrusive thoughts that seek impulsive action.

Thinking and Cognitions

6. The ego regulates cognitions in the following ways:
   A. Management of memory.
   B. Ability to conceptualize.
   C. Precision in language communication.
   D. Ability to cognitively regress acuity for relaxation purposes.
   E. Ability to allow new configurations to emerge in thinking.

Synthetic-Integrative Functioning

7. The ego evidences synthetic-integrative functioning in the following ways:
   A. Permits degrees of reconciliations of incongruities.
   B. Permits degrees of freedom from impairment of patterned thinking.

Prioritization of Human Needs

8. The ego makes selection of the needs to be gratified by the following:
   A. Separates primary from secondary needs.
   B. Manages excessive stimuli input.

Defensive Functioning

9. The ego evidences defensive functioning in the following ways:
   A. Manages weaknesses or obtrusiveness of defenses.
   B. Evaluates success or failure of defenses.

Mastery-Competence

10. The ego evidences achievement of mastery-competence in the following ways:
    A. Evaluates competence in terms of how well a person performs in relation to his or her capacity to actively master and affect his or her environment.
    B. Provides feeling of competence as measured by a person's expectations of success on actual performance.
    C. Notes discrepancy between actual competence and feelings of competence.

Source: Adapted from L. Bellak and M. Sheehy. "The Broad Role of Ego Functions Assessment," *American Journal of Psychiatry*, 133, no. 11 (1976) 1259–1264.

ses, and interpersonal skills or to early infancy, when ego processes are thought to first emerge. It is well known that nonclinical assessment of this patterning has been most difficult to achieve and has only occasionally been attempted.[6] Bellak, Hurvich, and Gediman and others have presented complex inventories for determining arrays of ego processes from interviews, behavioral observation, and test data.[7,8]

Loevinger's and Wessler's description of

ego development appears to be a promising approach best characterized as taking account of the individual's integrative processes and overall frame of reference. Their conception of ego development assumes that each person has a customary orientation to him and to the world and that there is a continuum (ego development) along which these frames of reference can be arrayed.[9] Ego development is involved with individual coping and adaptation—processes highly relevant for understanding impairments and gains in the maturational process.

The conceptualization of ego development is drawn from several theories dealing with the development of self, cognition, character, morals, and interpersonal traits. As noted by Candee, "Ego development is marked by a more differentiated perception of one's self, of the social world and of the relations of one's feelings and thoughts to those of others."[10]

Loevinger and Wessler have delineated stages of ego development sequentially ordered and independently defined by age.[11] Each of the ego development stages differs from the others along dimensions of impulse control, conscious concerns, and interpersonal and cognitive styles. The three major stages are outlined below.

Early Stage

Individuals at the earliest stages of ego development, termed **preconformists**, are impulsive and fearful and have stereotyped cognitive styles that are dependent or exploitative interpersonal styles. Persons at this level tend to be concerned with acceptance and status. Their interpersonal style varies from being dependent to manipulative to obedient. Their conscious concerns focus on self-serving dimensions, bodily feelings—especially sexual and aggressive, self-protection, wishes, things, advantages, and control. Inner stages are expressed in terms of clichés, stereotypes, and moral judgments (i.e., concrete aspects of traditional sex roles, that is, physical causation as opposed to psychological causation).

Middle Stage

Individuals at the middle stage of ego development, termed **conformists**, show evidence of conformity to external rules, shame and guilt for breaking rules, and dawning realization of standards, contingencies, and the ability for self-criticism. Their interpersonal style aims at being helpful, belonging to groups or conforming, and showing interest in interpersonal relationships. Conscious preoccupation includes appearance, social acceptability, social conformity, consciousness of the self as separate from the group, and increasing adherence to and recognition of psychological causation. Their cognitive style shows increasing sophistication in an awareness of individual differences (as opposed to stereotypical clichés), and their interests are expressed in broad terms and directed toward including other relationships.

Later Stage

In the later stage of ego development, termed **postconformist**, individuals show evidence of coping with inner conflict through a high degree of self-awareness; they also reveal much more cognitive complexity and have interpersonal styles that emphasize mutuality and respect for individual differences.

SELF-REPRESENTATION

A lively debate is going on about a related concept to ego development, that is, the development of a self-representation system, especially that of self-image and self-esteem. Much of the current discussion focuses on developmental deviations and the psychopathology originating from the self-representation system.

Self-experience dimensions have been discussed for years by social scientists, especially in the psychoanalytic areas. In the clinical realm, however, previous discussions most often characterized self-representations as relatively minor determinants, or by-products, of psychopathology. Major forces noted in clinical case discussions are more typically defensive styles, involving the management of unconscious impulses and inner conflicts stemming from past unresolved personal problems. The issue of whether self-image, self-esteem, and other "self-processes" are essential causes of psychopathology or of one subset of diagnoses (e.g., narcissistic personality disorders) has been brought forward in large part through Kohut's contributions.[12] Hauser and colleagues argue that a self-psychology model that gives such major weight to self-pathology has many ramifications, raising questions, for example, regarding the place of conflict in ego development;

the importance of impulses as motivating forces; the theoretical and clinical relevance of structural concepts of ego, id, and superego; and the interpretation of transference phenomena.[13]

Self-Image and Self-Symbolization

Self-images are those concepts, held at varying levels of awareness, through which a person characterizes himself. The notion of self-image is referred to in discussion of both ego and identity development. Within many nursing discussions about identity are predictions about and descriptions of self-image processes. Self-esteem is the self-evaluative aspect of self-images. The dimensions of self-image complexity range from full complexity to polarization or simplicity.

The concept of a unified self-experience has extended throughout the history of philosophical and psychological theories. Plato expressed the essence of personification with his idea of a unified, spiritual "soul." The literature on "self" is equally well established in the psychiatric nursing literature.

Self-symbolization phenomena are defined under various labels including self-image and self-representation. Self-image generally means conscious expression of self through a sensory mode, that is, visual, whereas the term self-representation is used to cover a wider gamut and includes behavior. For purposes of definition and clarification, Horowitz and Zilberg recommend the term *self-concept*, which may be expressed in any mode of representation.[14]

EXAMPLE: THE EXPERIENCE OF "I"

Because subjective experiences may be organized by multiple self-concepts, the "I" of one state of mind is not necessarily the same as the "I" of a person's next state of mind. In this respect, the "I" experience may be viewed as transitory. The phenomenon may be seen in the meditative experiences where a determined effort is made to erase boundaries of "I-ness" to achieve a state of mind without a sense of separateness.

On the other hand, the "I" experience, if it is organized to contain multiple self-concepts, can be relatively enduring. A person can remember different "I" experiences and can identify a continuity of self-development. In fact, one aspect of this has been called advanced ego development.[15]

One's self-organization may be noted in several ways. For example, one may observe how a new reality does not accord with one's inner symbolic structure. Recognition within oneself that one has acquired a new skill may evoke not only pleasurable affective responses but also a mild, transient depersonalization until the self-organization concepts modify into congruence with the change. This is reflected in such statements as, "Was that me?" and "I could not believe I was able to do that." Negative changes, as in the loss of a mental or bodily capacity, may evoke not only unpleasant effects, but they have the same kind of derealization or depersonalization.

EXAMPLE: SELF-ORGANIZATION

Let's take an experiment to note the impact of a major stressful event on self-organization. The example is a female college student who has achieved a reasonable level of development, perhaps with some residual obsessional traits, and evoke a threat to self-system. With a healthy level of adult development, this student organizes thought by the knowledge that she has derived from different states of mind, and she realizes that she may behave in ways that seem opposites as she cycles through these states. For example, she knows that she is stubborn in some states and warm and kind in others. And she knows that these character traits are complementary halves of a conflict in attitudes. She also knows that in different states of mind she will view others as attempting to dominate her, as submitting to her, or as cooperating with her. In a similar manner, she knows that others shift their own attitudes toward her as they also pass through varied states of mind.

Thus, this woman is able to tolerate her own ambivalence and that of valued companions. Concepts of estrangement and hostility will be known in relation to those of mutuality and tenderness. Because of the self-organization structure, the flow from one state to another state of mind is smooth and seamless rather than disjunctive. This person is able to view interpersonal situations unfolding in her environment according to various self and role relationship concepts, and she knows that various possible patterns of action can modulate them into adaptive combinations.

Now we will evoke a threat to her self-organization and observe what happens. We tell her she has failed her course work and must leave school. There is a retreat to a less advanced level of functioning and organization. In terms of thought processes, it could mean the simultaneous association of some negative self-concepts but also the inability to adapt to other self-concepts. That is, the woman in our experiment would not be sure that she is also kindly when she is in a stunned or angry state of mind and may have to undo her helplessness because she feels guilty by shifting into a flagrantly kind state of mind. Then, feeling anxious over submissiveness to the needs of others, she might have to shift back again.

Now let us presume that the subject of our experiment had had a more pathological developmental course and one that renders her vulnerable to more turbulent frustration when she is upset. When the stressful event occurs, she loses the capacity to associate different self-concepts within even a transiently active self-structure. We would observe clinically a person who was thinking and acting in one state of mind (that is, depression) as if she had only the self. She would not or could not acknowledge the attributes of her other states of mind.

This observation brings us to discuss what is termed **splitting**. Splitting can be described as simultaneous and parallel thinking without association between the organizational subsystems. The segregated processes concerning internal needs, events, and plans would be organized by different self, object, and relationship concepts rather than contained within a self-organization structure.

A regression in a vulnerable person may reach a point, according to Kernberg, in which self, object, and relationship concepts are compartmentalized into those that are all good or all bad.[16] Or it may progress further, as described by Rosenfeld, into a chaotic mixture of fragments of good and bad concepts.[17] The states of mind organized by these chaotic fragments are so anguished that the transitions between all-good and all-bad concepts, although stormy and deviant from reality, are preferable. Stabilization at the all-good, all-bad level is defensive against further regression of self-concept, and yet it is also the result of a deficiency, an inability to maintain a balance to the self-organization structure. All of these statements may support the concept of borderline personality structure, but they also argue in favor of the existence of the splitting process and question whether splitting is a defensive maneuver or the result of deficiencies in capacity for higher-level mental operations.

MECHANISMS OF DEFENSE OF THE EGO

As stated by Binstock, the hypothesis underlying the psychodynamic model of the human mind is that all human behavior makes sense; that is, whatever comes from the mind of a person is subject to rational explanation and the explanation is to be found through further information about that person.[18] Thus, the psychodynamic model places the psyche (ego, self, mind, soul) in the center as the active agency with the goal of making sense of the behavior. The absence of ego places the individual under the control of instinctual drives. The presence of ego gives personality its boundaries and its direction.

The psychodynamic investigation is a search for signs of conflict and for the missing link (i.e., why the person is under stress or upset), which is the intrapsychic fact (i.e., carried inside the mind). For example, a patient cried uncontrollably throughout an interview. Upon closer examination of dates and events, it was learned that the interview was a one-year anniversary of the death of a close friend. The patient had "forgotten" the date. To be aware of the anniversary may be too painful in her daily activities and work, yet she weeps in the presence of a caring person.

If the mind is in conflict with itself, it must have some way of defending itself. It does, and the mechanisms are called the ego defenses.

Defenses Against Knowing

One conflictual area for the ego has to do with cognition and knowing. To know something may produce mental conflict and pain. Thus, there are ego mechanisms for "not knowing." The most common defense is **suppression**. This is the effort "not to think about it," or "putting it out of mind." Suppression is the conscious focusing of the mind first on one topic and then on another. However, what is conscious is simply that which is receiving attention at the moment; what will receive attention next is still preconscious at that particular moment.

A second "not knowing" defense is **repression**, and this mechanism operates unconsciously. This unconscious phenomenon is demonstrated operationally by the fact that when the person is made aware that a defense mechanism is in action, it no longer works. Repression may be viewed as motivated forgetting. For example, once an interpretation is made regarding a fact that has been repressed, it is unlikely that the repression will continue to work ("You overslept and missed class because you didn't want to go.").

The distinction between suppression and repression can be clarified by noting that the person probably tried suppression first, willing himself not to think about the distressing affect welling up inside him, not to connect the feeling with anything. Once the connection has been made (the missing link), the person may be able to recall these efforts at suppression. In some individuals, the use of suppression is so excessive that it is difficult to know if repression is also being used. For example, the person may say, "How would I know what I am doing? You cannot expect someone like me to know why I am crying."

Just as the use of suppression is usually constructive (healthy and adaptive), so is the use of repression. It is a remarkably efficient measure when adaptively employed, constituting a decision that one has done as well as one can in resolving a conflict, so it is as well to forget about it. The remarkable degree of amnesia most people have about events in their childhood is normal, healthy, and adaptive. On the other hand, the state of mind that is called schizophrenia can be understood as the inability to use repression. Without repression, the mind is something worse than a confusion—it is a cauldron of chaos.

We learn nothing about the person's state of health from the fact that he is employing mechanisms of defense. However, we can learn a great deal about the person's personality style (character type) and his general health or illness by noting which mechanisms of defense are most prominently employed and how well they are working.

Although any mechanism of defense has its healthy, adaptive uses, this is less often true of the third way of "not knowing"—the mechanism of **denial**. Denial involves an assertion that something that is rather obviously true is not true—that, in fact, something else quite different is true. ("The fact that Jim died on this date is a mere coincidence—it could not have a connection with my crying.")

Denial is most common in early childhood, when it is most appropriate; that is, dangers seem mostly external and are best left to adults who know how to cope with them. The capacity to employ repression normally appears at about the age of five and is soon followed by the construing of dangers mostly from within the psyche and best dealt with by oneself. Heavy use of denial at a later age is most characteristically encountered in persons with substance abuse, psychosis, and with organic brain conditions. The mechanism of denial is, of course, used by all of us, especially when we are psychologically depleted or confronted with overwhelming news ("I can't believe it is true.").

Intervening in the "not knowing" defenses must be done carefully. For example, making an interpretation of a person's denial may result in the following:

NURSE: I don't like to disagree with your statement that you are perfectly calm, but why are you shouting and screaming and shaking your fist?

CLIENT: Oh, that's just my style when I'm trying to make a point.

The interpretation is met with active opposition, and the denial is mobilized more fully against the next repetition of that same interpretation. Denial is best approached when the nurse is confident of success of an interpretation and then should be made as though denial did not deserve the main thrust of the sentence. For example:

NURSE: Since it is perfectly clear to me that you are angry, I wonder if you did not deceive yourself that way in other situations?

Confrontation is a forceful demand that the patient face what he has been avoiding knowing. This can be a useful corrective to a situation in which the nurse has gone along with the denial for an exceedingly long time, but it should be done with caution as it is often a remedy to the nurse's frustration with the patient. Confrontation may be heard from observers saying, "He should snap out of it," or "This patient should be confronted."

These three defenses against knowing—suppression, repression, and denial—are straightforward ways of opposing cognition. The various interventions include **suggestion** (ideas verbally offered to the patient about the missing links), **clarification** (making a connection between something conscious and preconscious such as saying, "Did you ever cry before?"), and **interpretation** (making a connection between the conscious and unconscious).

In a related defense mechanism, **rationalization**, the person offers a good reason for his actions instead of a true (reality-true) reason. For example: "I didn't go to the library to study because of the weather." Once one is able to use repression, the technique of "alibiing" becomes the well-known mechanism of rationalization.

Reality-Distorting Defenses

Defenses may be classified according to their relationship to reality. Denial can be classified as one of the reality-distorting defenses. Two other reality-distorting defenses are projection and introjection, both having their origins in early infancy, even before denial. Their persistent use at later ages tends to be even less adaptive than does that of denial.

Projection consists of treating something inside oneself as being outside oneself, such as: "They look scared." **Introjection** is the reverse: "You're going to have an easy day, nurse—I've already solved everyone's problem on the ward." The very essence of what is defined as reality is the distinction of what is inside and what is outside onself. The blurring of this distinction for defensive purposes is called "not knowing about reality," "having poor reality testing," or "breaking with reality."

Denial is a denial of reality, not only in the sense of saying that which is not so, but also in often construing the problem as external.

Paranoia makes strong use of projection: "It is the other group who is so hostile." It also uses denial: "The world is not indifferent to me; it is preoccupied with me." Mania makes strong use of denial: "There are no dangers." And it also uses introjection: "Everything I need is inside." It may be useful to view mania as a defense against fear rather than as a defense against depression.

It is not the use of reality-distorting defenses per se that is maladaptive but the relative absence of reality-respecting defenses. The constant use of denial, projection, and introjection with the hard data of perception (reality) can be just as misleading as it can be creative.

Projection and introjection play a major part in the formation and connection of persons, relationships, and groups. Social organizations, for example, begin with sorting people into "ingroups" and "outgroups" by means of projecting stated characteristics onto others and their leaders while incorporating virtues and ideals shared from other respected groups.

Projection and introjection may also be combined, as in identification with the aggressor. For example, a young child is traumatized after being bitten by a large dog. Months later the child is observed crawling under tables and barking and biting peoples' legs. The child introjects the characteristic of the anxiety object and thus assimilates the anxiety experience. The child is transforming himself from the person threatened into the object that makes the threat. In identification with the aggressor, one observes a preliminary stage in the development of the superego. The mechanism is adaptive only so long as the ego employs this mechanism in its conflict with authority, i.e., in its efforts to deal with anxiety objects. When the mechanism is carried over into aggressive outbursts, the resulting behavior may be dangerous, as in the adolescent who identifies with the aggressor who has victimized him and begins to victimize younger children.

Other mechanisms that distort reality include dissociation and fantasy. **Dissociation** is a splitting off from awareness of some aspect of an experience. The repressed material continues to affect behavior. For example, a 39-year-old respected, married physician with two children admitted through his lawyer that he had raped 22 women and sexually assaulted at least 10 others, including a nun, over a 4-year period. The lawyer described his client as "two people"—one dutiful by day and one degenerate by night.[19]

Fantasy is a strategy used by an individual to escape temporarily from the demands of everyday life through nonrational mental activity. The thinking of children is heavily laden with fantasy; it is the process they use as they develop ego strength to assimilate and deal with the world of reality. Adults may revert to fantasy under stress because it offers temporary relief from pressures. The use of fantasy has also been advocated in the treatment of sexual dysfunction as a stimulus for sexual arousal. However, the unconscious use of fantasy can pull a person away from reality and can make him less amenable to any degree of adaptive functioning.

Reality-Respecting Defenses

One measure of adaptive functioning is the person's proclivity for reality-respecting defenses such as suppression and repression. Four other reality-respecting defenses that appear in the course of development between denial and repression are particularly characteristic of obsessive-compulsive phenomena. These are: (1) (doing and) undoing, (2) reaction formation, (3) intellectualization, and (4) isolation. These defenses are less efficient than repression itself: undoing is particularly inefficient; reaction formation is less so; and isolation and intellectualization are almost as efficient as repression.

Undoing involves alternatively expressing the different sides of a conflict. It encompasses balancing conflicting motives, something that all behavior embodies. Undoing is a compromise formation of multiple motives competing for access to action. In normal behavior, this compromise is generally effected so smoothly that the presence of competition or conflict is undetectable, such as after locking a car door, going back and turning the key in the lock to ensure that the lock is locked. The motive is conflicting: wanting both to lock and to unlock the door.

In usual behavior, conflict recurrently interrupts this smooth flow by condensing behavior into differently motivated parts. This is seen in everyday phenomena of "slips" of the tongue, ear, pen, or memory. For example, receiving communications with one's name misspelled may be taken as an understandable error, yet with some feeling about the sender's lack of attention to detail. A client forgetting an appointment points out the conflict in motive.

Reaction formation involves dealing with something that one does not want to know is on one's mind by emphasizing the opposite consciously and by focusing a great deal of attention on the opposite, for example, feeling compassion toward a rival for an advanced position and constantly checking on that person to make sure the person is not working too hard.

The defense of **intellectualization** is the use of verbal inquiry or explanation for an anxiety-provoking situation. Professional jargon may serve this purpose and is sometimes a method of writing difficult patient reports.

Isolation consists of the relative removal of emotion from the ideas with which it is associated. The mental contents seem as though they have had the color bleached out of them. In isolation, an empirical observation can be made; for example, a delay in telling about something serves isolation. Silence is a signal that the person is probably finding something too emotionally affect-laden and that he is waiting for the emotional immediacy to pass. There is a relatively constructive role for isolation, although there may be some extremes ("Do you suppose calling my wife 'Mom' was a manifestation of my repressed Oedipus complex?"). Talking or writing on difficult subjects calls for the use of isolation as well as professional jargon.

Ego-Supportive Defenses

There are several additional reality-respecting and ego-supportive defenses, including displacement of affect, sublimation, somatization, and altruism.

Displacement of affect assigns one idea or object to another and occurs at all levels of health and development. Most frequently, the nurse will listen to the client's concerns about himself, his life, and his relationships repeatedly expressed as concerns about other people: "I know a person who has this problem." Displacement is central to phobias and thus makes it easier for the client to talk about an issue.

Sublimation is the displacement of affect in conformity with higher social values. This mechanism is an asset and a sign of ego strength. Sublimations involve the capacity to work and pursue conflict-free interests.

Somatization is the expression of emotional discomfort and psychosocial stress in the physical language of bodily symptoms. Social, cultural, and ethnic forces modify the basic tendency to express psychological distress in somatic terms, and they influence the ways bodily complaints are expressed. Cultures differ in their beliefs about disease and health and in their attitudes toward different parts of the body and about the value or stigma attached to medical and psychological care. These cultural forces foster the expression of certain bodily complaints and discourage other symptoms. Thus, the most common somatic complaints differ in various cultures.

Altruism is the surrender of one's own wishes to another person's. The attempt to find wish fulfillment vicariously is comparable to the interest and pleasure with which one watches a game in which one has no stake oneself. The use of this mechanism is the displacement of one's wishes and dreams onto another person.

For example, a mother, inhibited from spending any money on herself, has no hesitation in spending lavishly on presents for her daughter. A secretary who would never venture to ask for a raise in salary for herself goes to a supervisor and demands that one of her coworkers should have her rights on a specific matter. Or it may be observed that parents delegate to their children their projects, hoping that their children will fulfill ambitions that they themselves have failed to realize.

What does an assessment of ego defenses mean for the nurse working with the individual client? In practice, it is important to note the predominant mechanisms that are characteristic of the person. When seeing the client at an initial interview and at a time when the client is experiencing heightened subjective distress, the manner in which he deals with intrapsychic conflicts will undoubtedly be obvious.

DEFENSIVE STYLES

The concept of coping and adaptation has received major attention in the health care literature. Methods of defense or coping have been well studied in the area of physiology and in response to invading organisms or physical trauma. In the psychological literature, coping has been discussed under the concept of defense mechanisms. However, there has been some confusion and debate over what defense mechanisms are and how they relate to coping, diagnosis, and care. As Laplanches and Pontalis note the problem:

It is generally agreed that the ego puts the defense mechanisms to use, but the theoretical question of whether their mobilization always presupposed the existence of an organized ego capable of sustaining them is an open one.[20]

Categorizing Defense Mechanisms

In her book, *Ego and the Mechanisms of Defense*, Anna Freud in 1937 advised that it was probably best to abandon the attempt to classify ego defenses and instead to study in detail the situation that called for the need for coping or defense.[21] This advice has been generally heeded until George Vaillant developed a hierarchy of ego functions. Vaillant's study of a sample of men selected for psychological health showed that these individuals tended to progress through the ego function levels over the course of their life-span and that each level was associated with a different level of adaptation to life.[22] His 12-year follow-up study of heroin addicts suggested that patients tended to recover sequentially through these levels.

Battista tested Vaillant's hierarchy of ego functions on a clinical population of 78 new patients admitted to a community mental health center. The results of this study provided empirical support for Vaillant's hierarchy of ego functions associated with distinct levels of health and illness and suggested the following modification:

level 1 (psychotic)—delusions, schizoid fantasy, denial of reality, hallucinations; level 2 (immature, or characterological)—acting out, projection, displacement; level 3 (neurotic)—somatization, repression, passive-aggression, reaction formation; level 4 (mature, or healthy)—altruism, suppression, sublimation, intellectualization, anticipation, humor.[23]

In a nursing study of coping and adaptation following traumatic crisis, Burgess and Holmstrom conducted a follow-up study of 81 rape victims years after the rape incident. This study found that victims recovering fastest used more adaptive strategies, including positive self-assessment, defense mechanisms of explanation, minimization, suppression and dramatization, and increased actions. Victims who had not yet recovered by 4 to 6 years had more maladaptive mechanisms such as negative self-assessment, inaction, substance abuse, and acting on suicidal thoughts.[24]

Defense Mechanism Styles

Bond and colleagues identified crucial questions relating to defense mechanisms and styles including the following: What phenomena can be labeled defense or coping mechanisms? Can these phenomena be measured? Do defense or coping mechanisms cluster into defensive styles? Can defense styles be measured? Along which function are defense styles organized? Can defense styles be related to the developmental stage reached or to other unique information about ego functioning?[25]

TABLE 8-2. CONTRIBUTORS OF DEFENSE MECHANISMS

Sigmund Freud	Anna Freud	Kernberg/Klein
Regression	Sublimation	Splitting
Repression	Displacement	Omnipotence with devaluation
Reaction formation	Denial in fantasy	Primitive idealization
Isolation	Denial in word and act	Projective identification
Undoing	Identification with the aggressor	Psychotic denial
Projection	Altruism	
Introjection		
Turning against the self		
Reversal		

Source: Adapted from Michael Bond, et al., "Empirical Study of Self-Rated Defense Styles," *Archives of General Psychiatry*, vol. 40, no. 3 (1983).

Bond and his colleagues suggest that defense mechanisms can be seen both as a conflicting influence that limits growth and as an adaptive technique that protects and enables the person to function psychologically.[26] This theme is noted in the writings of Sigmund Freud, Anna Freud, Otto Kernberg, George Vaillant, Haan et al., and Semrad et al.—all clinicians who have studied mechanisms of defense.[27-32]

To answer the question as to which phenomena can be labeled defense or coping mechanisms, Bond et al. summarized the published literature on defense mechanisms in terms of the definition of the mechanism by the contributor. (see Table 8-2). They used the term "defense mechanism" to describe not only an unconscious intrapsychic process but also behavior that is either consciously or unconsciously designed to reconcile internal drive with external demands.

To answer the questions relating to the measurement of defense styles, Bond and colleagues designed a study using a self-administered questionnaire that indicated a person's perception of his defensive style. This questionnaire was tested on a sample of 98 psychiatric patients and 111 nonpatients.[33] Table 8-3 outlines the four resultant defensive styles.

Examples of the test questions used to measure defenses are cited as follows:[34]

"If someone mugged me and stole my money, I'd rather he be helped than punished." (Reaction formation)

"There's no such thing as finding a little good in everyone. If you're bad, you're all bad." (Splitting)

"If my boss bugged me, I might make a mistake in my work or work more slowly so as to get back at him." (Passive–aggressive behavior)

"I always feel that someone I know is like a guardian angel." (Primitive idealization)

Description of Defense Styles

Defense Style 1. This style consists of apparent derivations of defense mechanisms usu-

TABLE 8-3. DEFENSIVE STYLES

Style 1 *Maladaptive Action Pattern*	Style 2 *Image Distortion*	Style 3 *Self-sacrificing Style*	Style 4 *Adaptive Defense Style*
Withdrawal	Omnipotence	Reaction formation	Suppression
Regression	Splitting	Pseudoaltruism	Sublimation
Acting out	Primitive idealization	Denial	Humor
Inhibition			
Passive aggression			
Projection			

Source: Adapted from Michael Bond, et al., "Empirical Study of Self-Related Defense Styles," *Archives of General Psychiatry*, vol. 40, no. 3 (1983).

ally viewed as immature, namely, withdrawal, regression, acting out, inhibition, passive aggression, and projection. The common feature determined for this style is that all behaviors indicate the person's inability to deal with his impulses by taking constructive action on his own behalf. The acting-out person requires controls. The withdrawn or inhibited person needs to be actively drawn out. The passive–aggressive person acts to provoke anger in the person with whom he is involved. The regressed person requires someone to take over and do something for him. The projecting person puts the blame and responsibility on others instead of accepting his own impulses. This style might then be labeled "maladaptive action patterns."

Defense Style 2. This style consists of apparent derivations of omnipotence, splitting, and primitive idealization. The essence of these defenses is to split the image of self and other into good and bad and strong and weak. This differs from the style 1 defenses in that it is image-oriented rather than action-oriented. This style could interfere with interpersonal relationships but not necessarily with achievement and accomplishment. These defenses could be invoked in the service of constructive adaptation in situations of stress by persons who do not use them habitually; e.g., one way of dealing with severe physical illness may be to trust in the omnipotence of the physician. These defenses may also be used nonadaptively by persons with chronic difficulty in forming mature relationships. In the literature, this style is associated with narcissistic and borderline personalities. Style 2 can then be described as the "image-distorting" defenses.

Defense Style 3. This style consists of apparent derivatives of two defenses: reaction formation and pseudoaltruism. The mechanism of denial is also included. The defenses of reaction formation and altruism reflect a need to perceive oneself as being good, kind, helpful to others, and never angry. Patients often come to the attention of clinicians when they suffer a loss and their characteristic pattern cannot synthesize their anger and anxiety. They then become depressed. Style 3 can be characterized as "self-sacrificing" defenses. It is speculated that other defenses could be identified with this style such as obsessive–compulsive, intellectualization, undoing, and isolation.

Defense Style 4. This style consists of apparent derivatives of suppression, sublimation, and humor. These defenses are clearly associated with good coping skills. Suppression allows for an anxiety-producing conflict to be put out of awareness until one is ready to deal with the issue. Humor reflects a capacity to accept the situation while taking the edge off the painful aspects of it. Sublimation uses the anxiety-provoking impulse in the service of a creative response. All three defenses are associated with a constructive type of mastery of the conflict— by putting it aside temporarily, by making a joke out of it, or by transforming it into a creative product. Style 4 can be labeled "adaptive" defense style.

The research data suggest there is a progression from the maladaptive action patterns, through the image-distorting defenses, to the self-sacrificing defenses, and finally to the adaptive defenses along the line of constructive dealing with the vicissitudes of life.

The least mature people have behavior problems. The image-distorting group have problems in realistically viewing themselves and others and thus have relationship problems. The self-sacrificing group have more stable relationships but cannot fulfill their creative potential. The adaptive group of defenses reflects a shift from a preoccupation with control of raw impulses, to a preoccupation with all important others, and finally to creative expression of one's self. Other studies have reflected this shift.

For example, Semrad, Grinspoon, and Feinberg have suggested that as patients improve, they go from using primitive to more mature defenses.[35] Vaillant in his studies found an increasing use of mature defenses over time.[36]

Understanding the style of defense that a person uses, as well as the degree of psychosocial maturity that style reflects, can be extremly useful in assessing the potential of a patient to recover from an illness and perhaps in predicting what type of treatment would be most appropriate when several models are available. For example, the recovery of a patient with acute paranoid schizophrenia whose habitual defenses are the self-sacrificing type may be facilitated by providing the individual with work that he or she views as helpful, while at the same time giving medication and psychotherapy. Conversely, someone who uses more adaptive defenses, i.e., humor, sublimation, and suppression, might recover best using creative arts as in occupational therapy as an adjunct to medication and supportive psychotherapy. In applying the theoretical concepts to clinical practice, O'Toole addresses the dynamics of shame;[37] Lego provides case illustrations to the development of the self;[38] and Welt discusses the role of envy in interpersonal relationships.[39]

Summary

Personality structure and style provide important data for nurses in the interview and treatment of patients. Major strides are being made in understanding ego development and the mechanisms of defense. This chapter presents current research findings in three major areas: (1) ego development in terms of ego functioning and stages of ego development; (2) the self-representation system, especially self-image and self-esteem; and (3) mechanisms of defense of the ego including reality-respecting and reality-distorting defenses and defensive styles.

Questions

1. How do ego functions differ from ego defenses?
2. How does anxiety relate to ego defenses?
3. Give examples from patient interaction of reality-respecting and reality-distorting defenses.
4. Give examples from patient interaction of the four styles of personality defense.

REFERENCES AND SUGGESTED READINGS

1. Freud, A. The Ego and Mechanisms of Defense (C. Baines, trans.) (Rev. ed.). New York: International Universities Press, 1966.
2. Erickson, E. H. Childhood and Society. New York: Norton, 1950.
3. Reiser, M. F. Are psychiatric educators "Losing the mind"? American Journal of Psychiatry, 1988, 145, 148–153..
4. Bellak, L., Hurvich, M., & Gediman, H. Ego Functions in Schizophrenics, Neurotics, and Normals. New York: Wiley, 1973.
5. Wilson, H. S., & Kneisl, C. R. Psychiatric Nursing. Reading, Mass.: Addison-Wesley, 1988, p. 289.
6. Hauser, S. T., Jacobson, A. M., & Noam, G. Ego development and self-image complexity in early adolescence. Archives of General Psychiatry, 1983, 40, 325–332.
7. Morris, M. M. & Myton, C. L. Ego function: Enhancement through Social Interaction. Journal of Psychosocial Nursing, 1986, 24, 17–22.
8. Prelinger, E., & Zimit, C. An Ego Psychological Approach to Character Assessment. Glencoe, Ill.: Free Press of Glencoe, 1964.
9. Loevinger, J., & Wessler, R. Measuring Ego Development (Vol. 1). San Francisco: Jossey-Bass, 1970.
10. Candee, D. Ego development aspects of new left ideology. Journal of Personal Social Psychology, 1974, 30, 621.
11. Loevinger & Wessler, op. cit.
12. Kohut, H. The Analysis of Self. New York: International Universities Press, 1971.
13. Hauser, et al., op. cit.
14. Horowitz, M. J., & Zilberg, N. Regressive alterations of the self-concept. American Journal of Psychiatry, 1983, 140, 284–289.
15. Loevinger & Wessler, op. cit.
16. Kernberg, O. Borderline Conditions. New York: Aronson, 1975.
17. Rosenfeld, H. Psychotic States. New York: International Universities Press, 1965.
18. Binstock, W. The psychodynamic approach. In A. Lazare (Ed.), Outpatient Psychiatry. Baltimore: Williams & Wilkins, 1979.
19. Dowd, M. Rape, the sexual weapon. Time, September 5, 1983, p. 28.

20. Laplanches, J., & Pontalis, J. B. *The Language of Psychoanalysis*. London: Hogarth Press, 1973, p. 109.
21. Freud, A., op. cit.
22. Vaillant, G. Natural history of male psychological health: The relation of choice of ego mechanism of defense to adult adjustment. *Archives of General Psychiatry*, 1976, *33*, 535–545.
23. Battista, J. P. Empirical test of Vaillant's hierarchy of ego functions. *American Journal of Psychiatry*, 1982, *139*, 356–357.
24. Burgess, A. W., & Holmstrom, L. L. Adaptive strategies and recovery from rape. *American Journal of Psychiatry*, 1979, *136*, 1278–1282.
25. Bond, M., Gardiner, S. T., & Christian, J. Empirical study of self-related defense styles. *Archives of General Psychiatry*, 1983, *40*, 333–338.
26. Ibid.
27. Freud, S. Inhibitions, symptoms and anxiety (1926), In *The Complete Psychological Works* Vol. 20, trans. by J. Strachey. London: Hogarth Press, 1964.
28. Freud, A., op. cit.
29. Kernberg, op. cit.
30. Vaillant, op. cit.
31. Haan, N. A., Stroud, J., & Holstein, C. Moral and ego stages in relationship to ego processes: A study of hippies. *Journal of Personality*, 1973, *41*.
32. Semrad, E. V., Grinspoon, L., & Feinberg, S. E. Development of an ego profile scale. *Archives of General Psychiatry*, 1963, *28*, 70–77.
33. Bond, Gardner, & Christian, op. cit.
34. Ibid, p. 334.
35. Semrad, Grinspoon, & Feinberg, op. cit.
36. Vaillant, op. cit.
37. O'Toole, A. W. The phenomenon of Shame, *Archives of Psychiatric Nursing*, 1987, *1*(5), 308–317.
38. Lego, S. The development of the self, *Archives of Psychiatric Nursing*, 1987, *1*(5), 318–321.
39. Welt, S. R. The psychodynamics of envy, *Archives of Psychiatric Nursing*, 1987, *1*(5), 322–333.

Chapter 9

Life-Span Developmental Theory

Ann Wolbert Burgess

Chapter Objectives

The student successfully attaining the goals of this chapter will be able to:

- Name three historical documents that discuss the concept of life cycle.
- Discuss the role that developmental tasks play in Erik Erikson's theory of personality.
- Compare and contrast the features of child and adolescent development with features of midlife crises.

The past several decades have witnessed a growing interest in life-span developmental theory. This interest has been documented in nursing curricula and research agendas as well as through the growth of the social security system, pensions, and medical insurance plans.

It is important to recognize that the course of a person's life is not a simple, continuous process; rather, there are qualitatively different phases. The view of the life course has been derived from the preadult years. The developmental perspective has been the main province of the field of human development. It is well accepted that there is a temporal order in the first 20 years or so of life. All human beings go through a sequence of periods—prenatal, infancy, early childhood, middle childhood, pubescence, and adolescence. Researchers are now distinguishing between early, middle, and late adolescence. Although everyone travels common developmental periods on the way to adulthood, this path is experienced in a variety of ways as a result of differences in biologic, psychological, and social conditions.

This chapter reviews the investigation of normal development processes throughout the life-span, building on the early efforts of Freud, Jung, Erickson, and Piaget and continuing to the contemporary clinicians who are raising the understanding of the second half of the life cycle to the sophisticated theoretical level that obtains for the understanding of childhood.

LIFE CYCLE PERSPECTIVE

There are three historical documents that reflect interest in the concept of the life cycle: the Talmud of the Hebrews, the writings of the Chinese philosopher Confucius, and the writings of the Greek lawmaker-poet Solon. Each of the writings present a male-oriented view of the ages of man that Levinson describes as major seasons of a man's life cycle as follows: (1) a formative preadult time lasting until age 15 to 20; (2) an early adult season until about age 40 in which the man establishes a marriage, family, and occupation; (2) a middle adult time between the years of 40 and 60 when the intellectual and moral powers of adults are most fully recognized; and (4) a late adult season beginning around age 60 until death.[1]

Carl G. Jung was one of the first contemporary voices in the mental health field to focus on the life cycle across the life-span.[2] He used a metaphor referring to age 40 as the "noon of life" and emphasized the need to understand the afternoon and evening in the individual's own terms.

Most theories of personality development suggest that individualization is normally completed by the end of adolescence. If one accepts this theory, the unresolved conflicts and problems of adulthood are seen as caused primarily by failures in childhood development. The therapy helps to modify the unconscious conflicts, defenses, and fixations formed in childhood in order to assist the individual to function better as an adult.

Jung took the position that the personality developed by adolescence assisted people to begin living as adults and assuming the responsibilities required of them by family, work, and community. He suggested that the next major opportunity for personal growth was around age 40, when individuals had the opportunity to embark on a mid-life phase.

Concurrently with Jung's work, Arnold van Gennep, a Dutch anthropologist, was studying the life cycle from a social perspective.[3] His book *Rites of Passage* (1908) dealt with major life events such as birth, death, marriage, and divorce. A society deals with such events by constructing rites of passage sanctioning the transition in and out of the life event. For society, rituals are thus a form of control, helping to ensure that its members become secure from generation to generation. Persons in passage or transition are psychologically vulnerable and a potential threat to society because they are poorly integrated into the groups they are leaving as well as the groups they are entering.

In 1933, José Ortega y Gasset, a Spanish his-torian–philosopher, wrote *Man and Crisis* in which he identified, on the basis of both individual and societal considerations, five generations, each representing a phase of the life cycle.[4] These phases were: (1) childhood, age 0 to 15; (2) youth, age 15 to 30; (3) initiation, age 30 to 45; (4) dominance, age 45 to 60; and (5) old age, age 60 plus.

The last figure in this historical review is Erik Erikson and his seminal book, *Childhood and Society*, published in 1950.[5] His use of the word *childhood* in the title reflects Erikson's early focus on children. The historic importance of the book is that it places childhood within an articulated framework of the life cycle and encourages the study of adult development. A limitation of Erikson's developmental stages of childhood is that his formulation reflects a unifocus on ego development. This singular focus is also noted in Freud's posited stages of psychosexual development and Kohlberg's posited stages in moral development.

ERIKSON'S DEVELOPMENTAL THEORY

Erikson, a student of Sigmund Freud, expanded the work of his teacher, who had described the psychosexual development of the child, and included developmental tasks from adolescence to old age. The eight basic life issues as defined by Erikson are outlined by task, conflict, and approximate age level (Table 9-1).

Erikson attributed a central or nuclear conflict to each of the eight developmental life issues. His theory further states that a relatively successful resolution of the basic conflicts, associated with each level of development, provides an important foundation for successful progression to the next stage. Whatever the resolution of these conflicts—mastery or failure—the result significantly influences personality development.[6]

Trust as a Basic Life Issue

The infant is truly a dependent individual in that his total existence depends on resources outside the self. The infant's behavior gradually becomes more discrete in terms of finding the food, discriminating what goes into the mouth, learning to delay immediate gratification, and putting other objects into the mouth.

TABLE 9-1. ERIKSON'S DEVELOPMENTAL THEORY

Task		Conflict	Approximate Age Level
Basic trust	vs.	Basic mistrust	Infancy (0–18 months)
Autonomy	vs.	Shame and doubt	Toddler (18–36 months)
Initiative	vs.	Guilt	Childhood (1½–3 years)
Industry	vs.	Inferiority	Latency (6–11 years)
Identity	vs.	Role confusion	Adolescence (12–19 years)
Intimacy	vs.	Isolation	Young adulthood
Generativity	vs.	Stagnation	Adulthood
Ego integrity	vs.	Despair	Elderhood

(Adapted from Erikson, E., 1963.)

As infants gain motor development (at the oral, biting phase), they progress to oral, visual, and manual grasping and to letting go and holding on to objects. One sees the beginning signs of self-stability and continuity through attention, focus, concentration, and discrimination of objects in depth and dimension.

The positive reinforcement of parents encourages infants in their development. Infants develop self-trust by relying on what they see and hear. The beginning feelings of confidence and faith develop from learning that they will receive or get done what is needed. Mastery of the task implies that as the infant achieves, he is weaned; that is, he loses as he gains. Erikson views this development crisis as the origin of optimism or pessimism. Erikson clearly states, "The firm establishment of enduring patterns for the solution of the nuclear conflict of basic trust versus basic mistrust in mere existence is the first task of the ego and thus first of all a task for maternal care."[7]

Parents or caretakers perform the life-propelling functions for the infant. In the second 6 months of life, out of this symbiotic relationship the ego is born with the original ego arising from identification with these primary caretakers. This is the first of many identifications that contribute to the development of the ego.

By 18 months, the infant is able to differentiate self from others, and the infant's ego separates from the maternal symbiosis. These first 18 months have been named the **oral phase** after the predominant zone of bodily contact with the environment.

Failure to master this first ego task leads to varying forms of dysfunctions and/or psychopathology. Behavior disorders of adults termed oral behaviors include: clinging and demanding behavior; impulsive greed; deep feelings of in-

ternal division; distrust (giving up) and reactive rage; and the need to bite, fight, and take rather than receive. Other problems include the failure of adequate self–other differentiation (resorting to reality-distorting defenses), the dread of abandonment, extreme anxiety, basic mistrust, feelings of helplessness, and a tendency to treat all relationships as though they were the same. Other dysfunctions include sociopaths, severe character styles, and persons with addictions, including sexual perversions. A lifelong underlying inability to trust is seen in adult personalities in whom withdrawal into schizoid and depressive states is frequent. Erikson comments on this behavior:

The re-establishment of a state of trust has been found to be the basic requirement for therapy in such cases. For no matter what conditions may have caused a psychotic break, the bizarreness and withdrawal in the behavior of many very sick individuals hide an attempt to recover social mutuality by a testing of the borderlines between senses and physical reality, between words and social meanings.[8]

Autonomy as a Basic Life Issue

The infant progresses from the earliest months of passive intake and dependent receptiveness through the end of the first year to active and aggressive oral behavior. In this second phase of the life cycle, Erikson describes muscular maturation as setting the scene for two simultaneous sets of social modalities: holding on and letting go. The resolution of these two conflicts may be hostile or benign. That is, to hold can become a destructive and cruel retaining or restraining, and it can be a pattern of care. To let go may also be destructive, or it may be a relaxed "to let pass."[9]

Continued verbal and motor development result in beginning communication by the child and upright walking. As children experiment with autonomy, they try to assess control through negativism, self-will, compliance, and dawdling. The developmental crisis of the two- to three-year-old is shame and doubt about control and loss of autonomy.

Erikson further discusses this phase:

What enduring qualities are rooted in this muscular and anal stage? From the sense of inner goodness emanates autonomy and pride; from the sense of bad-ness, shame and doubt. To develop autonomy a firmly developed and convincingly continued state of early trust is necessary. . . . Firmness must protect him against the potential anarchy of his yet untrained judgment, his inability to hold on and to let go with discrimination. His environment must back him up in his wish to "stand on his own two feet" lest he be overcome by that sense of having exposed himself prematurely and foolishly, which we call shame, or that secondary mistrust, that looking back which we call doubt. . . .[10]

The achievement of autonomy—the secure separateness that can bear loss and disappoint-ment—is the ego's task in the period of ego de-velopment that falls roughly between 1½ and 3½ years of age. It is the obsessive–compulsive phase of development. This achievement of au-tonomy corresponds roughly with the acquisi-tion of secure reality-testing and solid ego strength. But again, the reality upon which the ego is establishing a firmer grip is primarily a social reality. This time of socialization has been named the anal phase after the main social con-cern and the bodily zone of most interest to the child and to the people around him. It coincides with the mastery of language, beginning with the ability to say no.

Power is the issue in this phase of devel-opment: Who is big and who is small? Who is strong and who is weak? Who is active and who is passive? Because the child always loses this one, he learns devious ways of exercising power. The child is assisted in this process through developing mastery in speech and mo-bility, which begins to reassure him that he is at least becoming more powerful. Still, the weapons of the weak are used: withholding ("I can't go now."), and passive–aggressive mar-tyrdom ("I'm trying hard. I couldn't help it; it was an accident."), as well as alibis and lying ("I was playing so hard I forgot."). When the child's sense of autonomy falters, the resultant feeling is shame and doubt.

A reasonable level of ego strength involves a sense of autonomy customarily expressed by a basic comfort about the adaptive level of func-tioning expected for one's age. This comfort also permits individuals to find enjoyment in activ-ities, that is, to have fun in one's life. The ability to tolerate being a separate person (i.e., mas-tering separation anxiety) signifies the adapta-tion to loss.

Morality in this phase tends to be retribu-tion in kind: an eye for an eye. The dominant approach to impulse control is reaction forma-tion; that is, the sin is making a mess. The basic anxiety is the fear of loss of love, but "love" tends to mean approval. The person performs well in order to gain favorable attention. This behavior trait is seen in obsessional–compulsive persons. Less healthy characters engage in power struggles through passive–aggressive means. Those with paranoid characters become more concerned with power than with love as a means of seeking adaptive functioning.

Another method in which to make infer-ences about the relative strength or weakness of a person's ego is to assess the person's tolerance for frustration and his ability to accept delay in the gratification of wishes. If autonomy is lack-ing, there is dependence on the other person to arrange for the impulse to be gratified and to manage the dangers. Only the person who has mastered autonomy and expects to be adequate will eventually find a way to reach the desired goal.

The second nuclear conflict to be resolved is autonomy versus shame and doubt. Phase-related adult characteristics of this task are put-ting things into their place, being organized, meticulous, compliant, or rebellious. If feelings of shame and doubt are strong, adults may be characterized by stubbornness and overcom-pensatory control, jealous reform or compulsive cleanliness. Failure to resolve this basic conflict may result in adult traits of cleanliness or dir-tiness, orderliness or sloppiness, punctuality or disregard for time, rebellion or defeat and avoid-ance.

Initiative as a Basic Life Issue

The child now has a growing cognitive ability with the capacity to conceptualize and inter-nalize relationships. Children can express feelings, and they can anticipate, worry, grieve, and brood. Their ability to imagine and wish is increased. They frequently project all blame onto others, for example, onto their mother or a sibling. There is a heightened awareness and curiosity of the self. This interest or love for the self is called **narcissism** and is at its height between the ages of three and six.

In locating themselves in respect to their family, children focus specifically on the parents, and thus we have the development of the family triangle relationship. The major source of conflict in children from ages three to six evolves from what Freud describes as the Oedipus complex. Erikson comments on this phase:

. . . the increased locomotor mastery and the pride of being big now and almost as good as father and mother, receives its severest setback in the clear fact that in the genital sphere, one is vastly inferior; and furthermore that not even in the distant future is one ever going to be the father in sexual relationship to the mother or the mother in sexual relationship to the father. The very deep consequences of this insight make up what Freud has called the Oedipus complex.[11]

It is from this phase of development that the psychoanalytic theory of sexuality has its origin. Each of the previous two psychosexual phases of infantile sexuality (oral and anal) contributes to the infantile sexual development. Now in the Oedipal phase, the sexual orientation develops more fully. Infantile genitality, as Erikson says, is destined to remain rudimentary, a mere promise of things to come.[12]

The issue of sexuality overtly develops. Girls tend to seek out a new element in the relationship with the father, and boys with the mother. The Oedipal child becomes interested not only in his body but also in the bodies of those around him. The main focus of pleasurable feelings shifts to the genitals. The genital differences of people are particularly heightened.

Psychoanalysts write of the fears that the male child develops in his dread of losing his genital organ or being "castrated." The concept of castration anxiety comes from this developmental phase. Erikson states:

Infantile sexuality and incest taboo, castration complex and superego all unite here to bring about that specifically human crisis during which the child must turn from an exclusive, pre-genital attachment to his

parents to the slow process of becoming a parent, a carrier of tradition.[13]

The phase-specific crisis is between initiative and guilt. Mastery of the crisis implies identification with the parent of the same sex and subsequent internalization of values and sanctions in the form of conscience, superego, and ego-ideal.

Failure of task performance at this stage of development may produce serious consequences in adult life. Erikson states that the resolution of the basic conflict is a split between "potential human glory and potential human destruction." The child becomes divided within himself. When the superego becomes cruel and uncompromising, deep-rooted resentments and regressions may develop toward the parent who did not live up to the new conscience the child set up for himself. As Erikson points out, one of the "deepest conflicts in life is hate for a parent who served as a model . . . but who was found trying to get away with the very transgressions which the child can no longer tolerate in himself."[14] Other important results of task failure in this period of development result in hysterical behavior, intense anxiety or guilt, and antisocial personalities.

Industry as a Basic Life Issue

With the resolution of the Oedipus phase, the stages of infantile psychosexual development are completed, and the child now enters into the first major social system outside the family; this period of development is called latency. This phase usually lasts from age six through age eleven. The expression of infantile sexual energies into nonsexual energies is termed **sublimation**. This mechanism remains active throughout life as the ego rechannels drive energies into socially acceptable means of discharge. It is during latency that the resolution of the three previous phases of development results in increased ego control over instinctual drives.

One can see this process by observing in grammar-school children how personality traits and patterns reflect reactions against earlier infantile sexual and aggressive drives. For example, aggression and cruelty are replaced by sympathy and concern for others; messiness gradually eases into cleanliness; exhibitionistic tendencies give way to modesty; and selfishness and greediness are replaced by cooperation and willingness to share.[15]

Tasks in this developmental period are the acquisition of special skills, incorporating social values and patterns, and competition and interaction with peers and authority figures. The child looks beyond the family and begins to interact with another social system.

School presents a new challenge to children in that it puts to the test the preparation they have for learning. It has been found that neurotic, deprived, or abused children do not listen or use the kind of communication that teachers depend on for their work with children. This type of child may be poorly prepared to learn or may lack pleasure in learning. This problem may be complicated by attitudes of passivity and defiance, which may lead to underachievement. This, in turn, leads to inferiority and low self-esteem.[16] As Erikson describes the task of this phase:

The child's danger, at this stage, lies in a sense of inadequacy and inferiority. If he despairs of his tools and skills or of his status among his tool partners, he may become discouraged from identification with them and with a section of the tool world. To lose the hope of such "industrial" association may pull him back to the more isolated, less tool-conscious familial rivalry of the Oedipal time. . . . Many a child's development is disrupted when family life has failed to prepare him for school life, or when school life fails to sustain the promises of earlier stages.[17]

Identity as a Basic Life Issue

The major task in adolescence, as described by Erikson, is the development of a sense of identity. The phase-specific tasks for the adolescent may be identified as gaining independence from the family, integrating new-found sexual maturity, establishing meaningful and working relationships with peers of both sexes, and making decisions about life work and goals.[18]

Erikson defines this fifth stage of personality development as identity versus role confusion. He points out that the form of ego identity is more than the sum of the childhood identifications, that it is the accrued experience of the "ego's ability to integrate all identifications with the vicissitudes of the libido, with the aptitudes developed out of endowment and with the opportunities offered in social roles."[19] The danger of this stage is in role confusion.

Erikson states that when role identity is based on strong previous doubts as to one's sexual identity, delinquent and outright psychotic episodes may present themselves. He advises that if these incidents are diagnosed and treated correctly, they do not have the same pessimistic significance that they have at other ages.[20]

Intimacy as a Basic Life Issue

The personality development phase of adulthood is generally divided into two subcategories: young adulthood and middle adulthood. For each of these stages, Erikson has identified tasks to be mastered. The critical task for the young adult is to enter in an involved, reciprocal way with others sexually, occupationally, and socially.[21] The mastery of this phase results in intimacy and solidarity; the failure results in isolation. Essentially, the person completes the transition from the family of origin to the family of procreation. It is in this period that the young adult strives to achieve the first phase of sexual (genital) maturity, and he seeks a sense of intimacy with a partner of his choosing. Erikson further defines this stage: "Body and ego must now be masters of the organ modes and of the nuclear conflicts, in order to be able to face the fear of ego loss. . . ."[22] He also states, "It is integral to a culture's style of sexual selection, cooperation, and competition."[23]

Generativity as a Basic Life Issue

The second stage of adulthood is achieved during the middle years of adulthood, the years 30 to 60. It is during this period that a sense of generativity leads to productive and creative work. In past decades, this has meant child rearing for women. In contemporary times, both women and men are increasingly sharing parenting functions so that both may pursue meaningful careers outside the family structure.

This particular area of developmental crises is currently receiving major attention. Traditionally, greater emphasis has been placed on researching and understanding child, adolescent, and young adulthood issues of development in contrast to mid-life or older adulthood issues. There is a marked departure from this focus, specifically to the area of mid-life crises, and to a lesser degree to the problems of the older adult.

Two important points regarding mid-life crises are (1) that this area is an increasingly popular subject of study; and (2) that it is being studied on a gender basis; that is, researchers are studying issues for men and women independently of each other, being careful not to generalize one set of findings to another group.

The mid-life research on men has been led most recently by psychologist Daniel Levinson and his colleagues. Levinson and his colleagues interviewed 40 men—10 each of business executives, biologists, novelists, and blue-collar workers—who were between the ages of 35 and 45.[24] In addition, they studied a secondary sample of biographies, autobiographies, novels, poems, etc., portraying the lives of many other men in different countries and historical periods. Their findings propose a universal human life cycle consisting of specific eras and periods in a set sequence from birth to old age, that is, a psychosocial theory of adult development.

The era is the basic unit of the life cycle and lasts roughly 20 years. The eras are: preadulthood, 0 to 20; early adulthood, 20 to 40; middle adulthood, 40 to 60; late adulthood, 60 to 80; and late, late adulthood, 80 to death.

Each era has its own distinctive character. The character of living changes from one era to the next. The change is profound and requires a transitional period of some 4 to 5 years. The early adult transition is a bridge between preadulthood and early adulthood and is part of both eras; it usually starts at about 17 and ends at 22 (plus or minus about 2 years). The mid-life transition links early and middle adulthood and normally lasts from about 40 to 45. The late adult transition is from 60 to 65. There are additional periods within each era. The tasks of the transition periods are listed below.[25]

The basic developmental process in adulthood is the evolution of the individual life structure. The life structure is the underlying design of the person's life at a given time. It is a patterning of self-in-world and requires an accounting of both self and world. It provides a context in which to consider more specific matters of clinical importance, such as major life events and crises, as well as the entire range of psychiatric signs and symptoms.

TASKS OF THE TRANSITION PERIODS

1. Early adult transition (ages 17 to 22). The tasks of this period are to terminate preadulthood and initiate early adulthood. In it, the person is on the boundaries between two eras.

2. Building a first adult life structure (ages 22 to 28). In this period the tasks involve entering the adult world—forming an occupation and forming love relationships of a more enduring kind, often marriage and family.

3. The age 30 transition (ages 28 to 33). The central developmental task of this period is to question and modify the initial adult life structure. Developmental crises commonly occur here. The person finds his first life structure flawed, but considerable turmoil attends any attempts to change it.

4. Building a second life structure for culmination of early adulthood (ages 33 to 40). For men, this period has the character of settling down and becoming one's own person. Men who formed a seriously flawed life structure in their early 30s are thought to be at high risk for having a developmental crisis between ages 36 to 40 as the structure becomes unendurable. Data are not yet available regarding this period's specific characteristics for women.

5. The mid-life transition (ages 40 to 45). The developmental tasks in this period are to question the current life structure, terminate early adulthood, and create a basis for entering middle adulthood. The individual confronts various polarities such as young–old, masculine–feminine, destructiveness–creativity, and attachment–separateness. In this period, the individual may begin a process of individuation and genuine personality flowering or a process of spiritual and psychological decay.

6. Building an initial life structure for middle adulthood (ages 45 to 50). Levinson's research ended here, but there are reasons to believe that the series of transitional and stable periods continues.

Levinson and colleagues relate Erikson's seventh stage of generativity to their research as follows:

In every stage, developing is a process in which opposite extremes are to some degree reconciled and integrated. Both generativity and its opposite pole, stagnation, are vital to a man's development. To become generative, a man must know how it feels to stagnate—to have the sense of not growing, of being static, stuck, drying up, bogged down in a life full of obligation and devoid of self-fulfillment. He must know the experience of dying, of living in the shadow of death.[26]

The mid-life crisis research on women has been pioneered by B. Neugarten through a study of 100 men and women that stressed that certain characteristics of middle age were important for this group. The theme of reassessment of the self is most salient, and the concept of time is established in relation to the time left to live rather than the time since birth. One important finding from this study was that men and women use different criteria on which to base their sense of middle age. Married women in this study identified their age status in terms of launching their children into the adult world.[27]

Women psychologists and social scientists are studying the effects of work and motherhood on the life cycle of the family. Additional research is looking at the importance of biologic functioning for women and at such issues as the menopause, long stereotyped as dominating the mid-life phase for women. Malkah T. Notman, a psychiatrist, states that

however inappropriate it may be to consider women *defined* by their biological destinies, there is nevertheless, a considerable reality to biological concerns, and awareness of them is important. For women, life does take place within the limitations of a biological timetable which influences [their] options.[28]

Notman argues that it is important to distinguish a woman's concerns about reproductive potential separately from her concerns about individual fulfillment and self-realization as a woman because the traditional stereotype is that a woman's role is focused on motherhood rather than on a broader view of womanhood. In reality, Notman continues, many women have not found their children or their role as mothers predominantly gratifying, but rather have found the child-rearing process to be stressful, draining, and conflict-producing.[29] Thus, the traditional stereotype imposes stress if a woman finds conflict in her role as a mother and not necessarily in her role as a woman.

The period of mid-life for women is viewed by some women as a time for self-expression. The potential for autonomy; for changes in relationships; and for the development of their occupational skills, contacts, and self-image—all have the opportunity to start after childbearing is completed.[30] The life issues of separation and autonomy, however, need to be kept analytically distinct from the feeling states of aloneness and isolation.

Ego Integrity as a Basic Life Issue

The crisis of aging confronts the person with the finite boundary of the personal life cycle, which is death. The predominant theme in this stage of development is ego integrity versus despair. As Erikson states:

Only in him who in some way has taken care of things and people and has adapted himself to the triumphs and disappointments adherent to being the originator of others or the generator of products and ideas—only in him may gradually ripen the fruit of these seven stages. . . . It is the acceptance of one's one and only life cycle as something that had to be . . . and that for him all human integrity stands or falls with the one style of integrity of which he partakes.[31]

Failure to achieve ego integrity is identified by Erikson as despair.[32] The theme of this age period is loss, and thus without adequate emotional support to sustain and bear the losses, it is understandable why the older adult is vulnerable to despair.

In defining the full cycle of human life, Erikson cites the parallel of trust as the first of the ego values, with adult integrity as the last of the ego values, by saying, "Healthy children will not fear life if their elders have integrity enough not to fear death."[33]

CONTEMPORARY ADULT DEVELOPMENTAL THEORY

There is a history of pessimism in the clinical treatment of older patients. Freud wrote on the lack of elasticity of the mental process when people reach their fifties and believed that older people were no longer educable. Even if the elasticity were present, Freud wrote, "the mass of material to be dealt with would prolong the duration of the treatment indefinitely."[34] However, other analysts such as Abraham and Jelliffe had been conducting successful therapies with older patients and were optimistic about treating this age group.[35,36] The struggle between the two divergent views may be noted in the literature across the decades.[37]

The skepticism underlying the treatment of older people was addressed by Butler and Lewis, who related avoidance of older patients by therapists to the following six factors: (1) aged patients stimulation of therapists' fears about their own old age; (2) conflicts about parental relationships mirrored in work with patients of the same age as the therapist's parents; (3) anticipated therapeutic impotence stemming from a belief in the ubiquity of untreatable organic states in the elderly; (4) a wish to avoid "wasting" therapeutic time and skills on older individuals; (5) fears that the patient might die during treatment; and (6) a desire to avoid colleagues' negative comments about efforts directed toward the elderly.[38]

A belief that dynamic therapies were suitable, even preferred, forms of mental health treatment for older patients led psychiatrists Nemiroff and Colarusso to publish their clinical insights and recommendations for treatment, which follow.[39]

Adult Developmental Stages

Following Erikson's model, Colarusso and Nemiroff divide adulthood into four broad stages: early (ages 20 to 40), middle (ages 40 to 60), late (ages 60 to 80) and late-late (ages 80 and beyond).[40] However, because of the limited research on adult developmental process, the absence of biologic demarcators, and the tendency of major tasks to overlap (for example, becoming a parent), the authors find the stage framework less useful to understanding adulthood than childhood.

More salient, Colarusso and Nemiroff observe, are adult development tasks, which are outlined as the following: the aging process in the body; increased awareness of time limitation and death; illnesses or deaths of parents, friends, and relatives; changes in sexual drive and activity; markedly altered relationships with parents, young adult children, and a maturing spouse; the assessment of career accomplishments and the recognition that not all personal goals will be reached; and planning for retirement. Many of the symptoms presented by patients in this age group will either be expressed in terms of these tasks or be partially caused by a failure to have engaged them successfully.[41]

Adult Developmental Lines

Following Anna Freud's developmental lines for childhood, Colarusso and Nemiroff develop similar lines for adulthood as follows: (1) intimacy, love, and sex; (2) the body; (3) time and death; (4) relationship to children; (5) relationship to parents; (6) mentor relationship; (7) relationship to society; (8) work; (9) play; and (10) finances.[42]

Clinical Implications of Adult Developmental Theory

Some of the major clinical implications of adult developmental theory described by Colarusso and Nemiroff are summarized as follows.[43]

1. Older patients need not be treated superficially. Selected individuals are suitable for dynamic psychotherapy and psychoanalysis, regardless of chronological age.
2. An adult developmental orientation, as expressed through adult development lines and tasks, and a developmental history of the life cycle add new dimensions to the diagnostic process and therapeutic effort.
3. Symptoms are a condensation of experience from all phases of development, not a simple expression of infantile conflict in the adult present.
4. Thoughts about the aging body, time limitation, and the individual's own death—central issues in the psychic life of every adult patient—are often avoided by patient and therapist alike.
5. Sexual thoughts, feelings, and activity remain as powerful, dynamic issues until death.
6. In the second half of life, transference is a more complex phenomenon, taking a variety of forms. Special attention should be paid to the adult past as a source of transference.
7. Similarly, countertransference responses to the older patient are complicated, since they are reflections of the therapist's infantile and adult experience with his or her parents and other significant figures.

WOMEN'S MULTIPLE ROLES IN THE LIFE CYCLE

It is only recent scholarship that has identified sex bias in psychological theories and methods, documented the pervasive and destructive effects of gender inequality, and examined the stresses that differentially affect women by virtue of their subordinate social status.[44] Alan Stone in his 1980 presidential address to the American Psychiatric Association suggested the development of a new psychology for women, one that would make necessary "a new conception of all our human values and all the paradigms of psychiatry."[45] Carmen and colleagues argue for a multidimensional approach to patients' mental health problems when they say:

Traditional psychological theories have relied largely on intrapsychic explanations of how people think, feel, and behave . . . and have not always recognized the extent to which an individual's identity, psyche, and sense of self derive from the social context.[46]

Women have a tendency to become deeply involved in several different roles simultaneously. Contemporary theories of women's development take into account that women are more oriented than men to the needs of those around them, tend to define their sense of self and their life satisfaction in relation to a context of relationships, and traditionally use their power to increase the power of others.[47-49]

Women have traditionally been responsible for the health and well-being of their spouses, children, and parents. They have been considered to be the appropriate primary caregivers when anyone defined as a family member needs physical or emotional nurturing. Today, many women have added full-time paying jobs to their full-time jobs of homemaker, spouse, and mother, and frequently their employment also involves caregiving.

The competing and sometimes conflicting roles, as well as the stress of traditional and felt responsibility for important aspects of other people's lives, put considerable strain on women's resources. On the other hand, women may profit from multiple roles with increased social and financial resources, increased sense of self-worth, and greater life satisfaction.

Women are increasingly assuming new roles, without the relief of having their traditional roles reassigned. Some of these multiple roles include the following.

Employment

The entry of large numbers of women into the labor force is one of the most striking trends in this country. In 1984, some 54 percent of all women 16 years of age and older were working or looking for work. In the 25 to 54 age group, nearly 70 percent were in the labor force.[50] Overall, 66 percent of women with school-age children are in the labor force, including half the mothers of 1-year-olds. This represents a 200 percent increase in working women since World War II, compared to a 50 percent increase for men in the same period. Yet studies indicate that working women continue to maintain the major share of child care and housework responsibilities, primarily at the expense of their leisure activities and sleep.

Another contemporary social trend is reflected in the aging of the population. This has profound implications for middle-aged women, since they continue to be the major caregivers for the elderly. The National Center for Health Services Research in 1982 estimated that women constitute 72 percent of the approximately 2.2 million people caring without pay for the 1.2 million frail elderly persons living at home.

Today, the majority of women between 20 and 60 years of age are employed or in training, including increasing numbers of two potentially vulnerable groups: mothers of preschool children and women who were socialized to expect to be supported as housewives. Role stresses may well exist as part of the alternative life cycle pattern for the different subgroups of women employed at various organizational levels and in different types of occupations, e.g., professional or nonprofessional and occupations traditionally considered to be female or male.

Caregiver Role

Women have traditionally been the primary caregivers in our society, both in the home and on the job. Childhood afflictions impose a disproportionate burden on the mother in terms both of parental guilt and of the practical burdens of either caring for the seriously ill child at home or making the difficult decision for institutional care. With deinstitutionalization of the mentally disabled, mothers may have to care for chronically mentally ill or retarded children throughout their lives.

Studies have found consistently that families provide the vast majority (80 to 90 percent) of health and social services received by older people. The women—wives and daughters— were specifically identified as the major care-

Chapter 10

Communication Theory

Carol R. Hartman

Chapter Objectives

The students successfully attaining the goals of this chapter will be able to:

- Describe communication as a process of behavioral maintenance and behavioral change.
- Identify what influences communication.
- Describe the communication process.
- Define the relationship between spoken and nonspoken behavior.
- Identify the selected models and theories of communication, moving from simple to complex.
- Compare and contrast models and theories of human communication used in psychiatric mental health nursing practice for the individual and for the family group.
- Understand the important tenets of a model for observing the communication processes and its therapeutic effects—Neuro-Linguistic Programming.

Communication—what is it? Communication is a continuous activity of information generation, information exchange, and information processing.

For years, humankind has attempted to distinguish itself from lower forms of animals by distinguishing the communication experience as unique. However, investigation of animal life has demonstrated the existence of rather elaborate communication patterns among various species. More often than not the communication patterns of animals consist of gestures, smells, sounds, and postures. All of these "activities"

are frequently associated with status and power within a group or are related to reproductive acts or the claim of territory for food.

In detailed studies, particularly of animals that live in groups and have a considerable period of time for rearing their young, communication patterns have been discerned in regard to training the young in hunting, food preparation, nest building, and the expression of affection. The lack of recorded communications among animals such as writings has challenged researchers to investigate whether animals move beyond the level of sign communication

117

to that of symbol communication, in which symbol manipulation and abstract reasoning come into play. Inquiry into the communication patterns of dolphins and whales are examples of these efforts.

CONCEPT OF COMMUNICATION

Of what importance is this to a definition of communication and the practice of psychiatric nursing? As a concept, communication is essential for the maintenance and the evolution of all life forms. Life is a continuous process of information exchange and information processing. The concept of communication directs attention to the processes involved in the generating, exchanging, and interpreting of information. Since communication is essential to growth and development, delving into the intricacies of communication provides critical information as to how life is influenced and changed. Not only does the concept organize our thinking about patterns of maintenance and change; it also broadens our scope to recognize that, in human terms, communication goes beyond the spoken and written word.

Given these propositions, it is now understandable that when two people meet for the first time, such as a nurse meeting with a client in his home, there are at least 2000 bits of information exchanged between them within the first few seconds of meeting. The spoken and unspoken behaviors of both people and the arrangement of clothing and other inanimate objects in the environment all become part of the information exchange. In addition, the process of exchange engenders experiences for both parties, experiences that will increase the amount of new information. What is consciously attended to in the interchange is only a small part of all that has taken place.

WHAT INFLUENCES COMMUNICATION?

Culture

A discussion of the universality of gestures and expression has led to lively debates regarding the inherited characteristics of human language and expression. These studies have focused on congenitally blind and deaf children cross-culturally. Similarities in crying, coughing, and being surprised are examples of evidence offered for inborn traits.[1]

Anthropologists believe that culture determines language and gesture. Different cultures vary in the rules they apply to the expression of emotional behavior. Compare an American baseball player and a Japanese Samurai. There also are rules governing intimacy that vary from culture to culture and from class to class. And there are cultural rules for status, for example, who should speak to whom, rights of questioning, and order of speaking. Certain unspoken gestures take on cultural meaning and are emblems. For example, raising the middle finger and the index finger to form a *V* for victory has a special meaning in the United States. A circle made by joining the index finger and the thumb representing "A-OK" is another example of an American emblem. In Russia, the raising of your hands over your head and clasping them together is a means of graciously acknowledging the recognition of the group, whereas in the United States it is interpreted as a gesture of triumph and superiority. When one thinks of Italian movies or French movies, many of the gestures of the actors depict cultural variations in meaning and expression.[2]

Sexual Variations

In the United States there are many assumptions about gender differences in expressive behavior, for example, that women express more emotion than men in their verbal and facial expressions. Research has not always upheld the specified differences. However, research has demonstrated that there are certain response differences that usually include qualities of speakers that can be attributed to their sex. In a study of tonal breathing characteristics, more judgments were made about female speakers than about male speakers. Thinness of voice in women led to attributions of immaturity and sensitivity but had no effect on the judgments of male speakers. Males with throatier voices were described as mature, sophisticated, and well adjusted, whereas deep-voiced women were seen as boorish, ugly, lazy, and sickly.[3]

Again the discussion of the relative influence of gender on communication characteristics is debated as to whether differences arise out of cultural determinants or innate determinants. This has come about because the study of communication patterns of the very young and the very old does not necessarily indicate differences for sex. Some argue that this is because there are hormonal changes at these times. The important aspect of the influence of sex is that at least socially and culturally, patterns of expression do tend to vary between the sexes. It is worthwhile noting what these patterns are and how they do vary, particularly in terms of the attribution of personality characteristics.

Socioeconomic Background

"The rain in Spain is mainly on the plain . . . I think she's got it!" says Professor Henry Higgins in the musical *My Fair Lady*. This delightful musical, based on George Bernard Shaw's *Pygmalion*, underscores the class differences with regard to speech patterns and syntactical variations, as well as semantic differences, to say nothing of nonspoken behavior. Education, vocabulary, personal experiences, relative status positions—all become important factors in determining variations in patterns of communicating as well as providing an experiential basis for differences in the interpretation of spoken and nonspoken behavior. In addition, other implicit aspects of social structure generate rules of communicating and expectations, privileges not readily recognizable but clearly manifested in communication behavior.

Social Distance

Age, status, and, at times, gender, dictate the degree of familiarity and the amount of receptivity to the communications of another. For example, a worker on the assembly line is overheard stating, "Gee, I'm surprised the boss knew me and stopped and spoke." In hospital settings, patients are often reluctant to ask anything of the doctor because of a sense of social difference—therefore distance—and an expectation that they have nothing of value to say or that what they would say would not be understood by the doctor. In the mental health field, the concept of social distance and its relationship to a free flow of communication was recognized and the development of indigenous workers came about. The same principle of distance operates in the establishment of many types of self-help groups such as Alcoholics Anonymous.

At times there are very subtle factors that are criteria for one person and not another, and these can create social distance. Such criteria might reflect rules of privacy and intimacy.

Power Relationships

Ascribed and prescribed power in interpersonal relationships is most evident in the type, direction, frequency, and content communicated. Relative levels of power are ascribed by attention to tone of voice and body posture, as well as the phrasing of words. Power is ascribed in a specific manner to people regardless of social position. Strength and weakness are inferred from these communication behaviors.

For example, a patient may come on a ward believing he is a king and in fact attract a relatively higher degree of attention from staff and perhaps privilege by his bearing in relation to other patients. Or a physician who is unsure of himself may find that neither patients nor nursing personnel attend to his requests as they do to other physicians.

There are many ways the relative notions of power are expressed and played out in human interactions, and since social position alone does not establish power in a relationship, it is important to assess how it is interpreted.

Number of Receivers

The size of a group determines how often a person will speak and what he will say. Some people are shy in small groups and in one-to-one relationships, but they have little difficulty giving a lecture. For others the reverse is true. Small-group participation is often anxiety-provoking because of the personal processing required by an individual who does not want to compete or have himself compared with others.

Patterns of initiating, confirming, negating, and speaking freely can all be influenced by the number of people involved in the communication sphere.

Internal State

How one feels subjectively greatly influences patterns of communication. Here we come closer to recognizing our reliance on patterns of communication in the mental health field. How a person communicates becomes an integral dimension of inferring feeling states. Yet because of all the factors that influence communication and how one interprets the behavior of another, care must be taken that the observer indeed is correct in concluding what the internal state of another is by virtue of the other person's behavior. Nevertheless, it is valid to note that emotions such as fear, anxiety, sadness, and elation influence posture, gait, voice, and language. Part of knowing people is learning what their behavior is in relation to their statements of their internal state.

Drugs

The various forms of communication, including sending out information, receiving it, and processing it, are affected by drugs. Although people are familiar with some aspects of drug influence on sending messages, such as in cases of intoxication, there is need for continued research in this area. This is particularly true in the area of drugs used over a long period of time. The influence of drugs in learning, e.g., storing information, utilizing it, and communicating the information, needs considerable clarification.

Other Considerations

There are other considerations that influence communication behavior. For instance, loss of sensory acuity from specific diseases of special sensory organs as well as other forms of ill health can alter expectations regarding communicating behavior at all levels. Variations in communication behaviors may in fact signify that there are underlying disease processes occurring. For example, distraction, slurring of speech, and problems of recalling immediate events can indicate interference with brain functioning.

Another important factor already suggested but worthy of underscoring is that of age. Attending to the differences in communication processes of young children and adolescents can help facilitate better relationships between adults and children. The same is true of older people.

This does not cover all the many factors that influence communication. Rather it is a breakdown of aspects of human experience that make up the personal set of an individual and of groups of individuals and that ultimately regulate behavior and characterize communication patterns.

HOW DO WE COMMUNICATE?

Asking the question of how we communicate is a first step in discerning salient characteristics of human communication patterns. Two broad categories of how we communicate have been the subjects of research and theorizing. These two categories are spoken behavior and nonspoken behavior (often referred to as nonverbal behavior).

Spoken Behavior

Spoken behavior is basic to communication, and words and their use and emphasis are tools or symbols to express ideas and feelings.

Speech can be studied from a variety of perspectives, as outlined below:

Phonology. Phonology is the study of how sounds are put together to form words. Investigation of the developing speech of children is often focused on the evolution of sounds to words.

Syntax. Syntax refers to how sentences are formed from words. Implicit in the study of syntax is grammar. Syntactical patterns have been associated with different ages and different psychological states.[4]

Semantics. Sematics is concerned with the interpretation and meaning of words. Considerable emphasis has been placed on the thematic aspects of language in the practice of different types of psychotherapy and in the development of nursing practice. Investigations and analyses of verbatim transcripts of interviews have focused on theme development. This study has led to concepts regarding psychological conflict and motivation. Underscored in this area of study has been the distinction between private and shared meaning. **Denotation** refers to words that carry a general meaning. **Connotation** refers to the use of a word that has a particular meaning to that person. Confusion as to meaning can be seen in a small child who objects to having a woman introduce her own mother to him. He may object because the use of the word *mother* connotes for him his mother. As yet the denotative meaning of *mother*, a type of relationship, is not clear to him. The fact that words have this twofold potential for meaning (private and public) and that the choice of words is influenced by the context the person finds himself in, suggests that there is great room for misunderstanding.

Pragmatics. Pragmatics is the investigation of how we participate in conversations with one another. In the area of verbal communication, particular attention is paid to how the participation of those in conversation either confirms or disconfirms the experiences of another person. Consequently, the language that is used is assessed in the context of nonverbal or paralinguistic phenomena, such as intonation, pauses, rate, amplitude, and pitch.

Paralanguage. Paralanguage consists of those nonverbal aspects of speech, such as tone, tenor of voice, etc. Many researchers in paralinguistics believe that it is these aspects of speech that convey emotion. Consequently, it is felt that studies of paralanguage are important in personality research as well as in the study of psychopathology. Variables such as intonation, pitch, volume, rhythm, voice quality, frequency of pauses, etc., are all important paralanguage in conveying information regarding affective states.

Nonspoken Behavior

There is a wide variety of nonspoken behaviors to be observed such as body language, writing, spatial behavior, autonomic nervous system responses, and clothing and symbols. These behaviors are discussed below:

Body Language. Body language has become an interesting area of studying behavior and what one believes is being communicated about the personality and intentions of another. Unfortunately, it has taken on a parlor game quality of interpretation. That is, people have attempted to generalize from posture, gait, mannerisms, gestures, and facial expressions what is going on within another person. Although it is often true that stooped shoulders, slow gait, and

slowed speech have been associated with people who are depressed, it is not universally true that all depressed people appear this way nor that people who slouch, have a slow gait, and speak slowly experience depression. Utilization of information communicated in body language is most useful when the total context is taken into consideration.

Writing. Writing is an area in which little research has been done by professionals. Yet there is the area of graphology and handwriting analysis that has been the province of lay people for many years. Some graphologists claim they can interpret emotional distress and other personal problems by an analysis of people's handwriting. Their approach has been to develop categories of styles and then relate them to certain personality traits and characteristics. Limitations in these efforts always result from the fact that taking one particular behavior, albeit a complex one, and trying to draw definitive conclusions about that individual runs a high risk of error. In the area of semantics, there have been studies of suicide notes whereby attempts are made to relate content and themes to variables that might in fact predict suicidal behavior.

Another area of writing not explored in great depth, either for diagnostic purposes or treatment purposes, has been diaries, journals, and biographical sketches. The trials of assassins and persons who attempt to murder prominent people have sometimes disclosed the premeditated behavior as recorded in personal journals.

Spatial Behavior. Spatial behavior (proxemics) concentrates on the psychological implications of the use of space. When one walks on a psychiatric ward, it is interesting to observe who sits where and how close these positions are to people, activities, and strategic aspects of the ward such as the nursing station. Anthropologists pioneered in the study of space, noting how tribal living arrangements were set up and how space related to other aspects of tribal life, as well as how it influenced patterns of communication.

Sommer in 1965 studied the connection between spatial arrangements and group tasks. He found that competing pairs sat opposite one another, conversing pairs sat diagonally, and cooperating pairs sat side by side.[5]

Autonomic Nervous System Responses. Autonomic nervous system responses constitute a large area of study. Tearing, blushing, crying, pallor, gastrointestinal sounds, and breathing patterns have always been the province of expert clinicians. One such man, Dr. Milton Erikson, the father of hypnotherapy, used autonomic responses such as breathing to pace his use of language and induced hypnotic states.

Calibrating (visually measuring) tics and other nonspoken mannerisms to the topics under discussion often clues the clinician to the fact that the topic has more significance than might be consciously apparent to the client.

Of particular significance in this area are studies that correlate patterns of verbal behavior and thought with changes in physiological states. Gottschalk in 1975 found a correlation between outwardly manifested hostility and matching patterns of speech with increases in diastolic blood pressure in women with essential hypertension.[6]

Other important attempts at linking body movements (kinetics) to language have been done by Birdwhistell and Dittmann[7,8]; for example, the slightly downward motion of the head, eyelids, and hands at the end of a declarative statement and the slight upward tilt of the head at the end of a question.

A model linking language and movement is presented by the California group that coined Neuro-Linguistic Programming as the name for their model. This model links eye movements with certain linguistic patterns. The model will be discussed in more detail in the next section.[9]

Clothing and Symbols. Clothing and symbols are another area of nonspoken behavior that is integral to the process of communicating. In the area of clinical practice observing the care and the appropriateness of dress are part of the assessment. Inferences regarding psychological organization and social responsiveness are examples of information drawn from dress and clothing.

In addition, the wearing of jewelry, such as wedding rings or special amulets, also conveys information. Styles and customs tell us about group life, for example, the habit of a nun or the uniform of a policeman. The dress of adolescents can tell us about their social group and conformity. Also, certain aspects of grooming communicate information such as heavy makeup or no makeup, beards, and hairstyles.

The discussion thus far of how we communicate attempts to describe categories of salient dimensions of spoken and nonspoken communication. In addition, examples of research

and clinical implications were identified. The next question is why is it so important to link language and movement together.

The Relationship Between Spoken and Nonspoken Behavior

As recipients of communication, we readily recognize from the discussion thus far that we have an internal response to the total communication experience with another person. It is also clear that much of what the other is communicating may be well out of the consciousness of that person. By the same token, the same is true of us. Much of what we communicate is out of our awareness. Consequently, we are sending and receiving many "messages" at a time. Understanding is enhanced when we recognize the potential for confusion and make an effort to be sensitive to the feedback in order to adjust our communication patterns. This adjustment is facilitated when we realize that the tone of our voice and our facial expression and posture may present to the other person information that is experienced as not congruent with our words.

In addition to understanding how these two dimensions of communication (spoken and nonspoken) come together in interpersonal exchange, it is important to understand how they operate intrapersonally. What we are discovering is that there is an internal system of communication that has physiological consequences, and there are physiological experiences that have psychological consequences. Attending to speech as well as body movement in a more comprehensive manner opens a window as to how behavior is maintained and changed both by the individual and through interaction with others.

THEORETICAL MODELS OF HUMAN COMMUNICATION

A Gradation of Theoretical Complexity

Theories are statements of logical propositions designed to give some order to experience, to allow for prediction, and to focus on a specific area of study. Among other characteristics, theories contain suppositions regarding cause and effect. General theories of communication are closely related to theories of learning. This is

A ——————— B message

Figure 10-1. Diagram of Hullian theory of communication. *Hull, C. L., A Behavior System, New Haven: Yale University Press, 1952.*

quite natural since learning is concerned with the storage, intake, and utilization of experience. Consequently, theories regarding learning will have a measure of representation in theories of communication, since the communication process is essential for learning to take place. The summary of theories of communication will focus on the dyad, that is, communication between two entities.

The most simplistic theory of communication places emphasis on the sender and the receiver (Fig. 10-1). This is based on Hullian notions of drive reduction and stimulus–response phenomena.[10] Briefly: A is the initiator of a communication; the communication is designated the "message"; and B receives the "message." Understanding occurs if A selects the right message and if B accepts, without interference, the right message. Assumed in this theory are the following: (1) that there is a correct message; and (2) that sender and receiver are relatively independent of one another, having little influence on the meaning of the message but great responsibility for the sending and the skills involved in receiving the message. Emphasis is placed on the denotative aspects of words, syntax, and semantics; and skill is based on selection and appropriateness of words.

Belief in this model typifies many arguments between people that carry both an overt and a covert message that one or the other is to blame. For example, A says, "I told you not to put the car in the garage." B replies, "You told me that you weren't sure you were going to use the car."

The next level of theorizing regarding the communication process emphasizes reciprocity in interaction. Basically, this theory assumes that communication is an interactive process and effective communication comes about when reciprocity is achieved by utilizing the process of feedback to ensure there is agreement as to the meaning of the message. What is emphasized in this theory is: (1) that each person has a perspective; and (2) that it is important for each to step into the meaning framework of the other. What is left out of this theory is the complexity of the communications exchanged in the inter-

action and the lack of explanation as to how interpretation occurs and becomes part of the communication process. In this example, the whole area of pragmatics is not addressed nor is it explained how meaning is derived and how it influences communication behavior.

In clinical practice and in interpersonal relationships, this theory leads to the expectation that one person can know the experiences of another in a direct way, and it is assumed that words carry this directness of information. Difficulties arise when, from a simplistic position, one person assumes that his impression and response to what is being said by another person are exactly the same as the experience being sent by the other person. This assumption conveys the expectation that people can know the thoughts and experiences of another person if only they put themselves in the other person's position. Failure to "understand" continues to create a pattern of blame in miscommunication.

The next level of theory development takes into account the pragmatics of conversing and the complexity of meaning. This step moves communication from the levels of an action and interaction to the level of transaction.

An important aspect of the spiraling complexity of two people conversing has been presented by Laing, Phillipson, and Lee.[11] For them, behavior is the result of the personal perception of experience. Perceptions serve a decisive functional role in the behavior generated from experience. By way of demonstrating the complexity engendered in the communication process by perception, the following set of perceptions can be addressed in a dyadic exchange:[12]

1. How does B think of me?
2. How does B think I think of him?
3. How A thinks of himself or herself.

The same three perceptual considerations are operant for B. This means that at any point in time, six dominant perceptual dimensions can be in process when A and B interact. Consequently, the event, although shared between A and B, will have decidedly different experiential meaning for each of them as shown in the accompanying cartoon. Further, meaning will be a function of how each person answers the three questions in terms of the ongoing experiences of communicating.

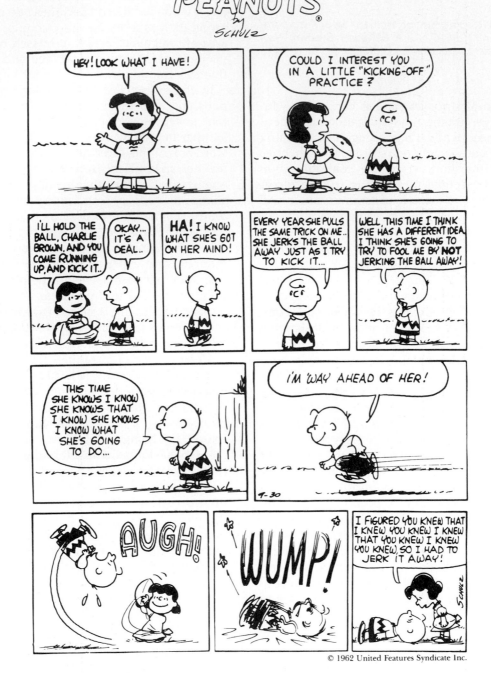

This cartoon illustrates a variety of communication messages. Differential experiential meanings are being expressed by Lucy and Charlie Brown; the final result is very clear.

The most complex theory to be presented is that meaning is derived from personal psychological constructs.[13] The theory has resulted in a model called Symbolic Interactionist Model of Communication (Fig. 10-2).

Basically, the model accounts for communication on an interpersonal level and an intra-personal level while also incorporating the tenets of the transactional model just set forth. The model was first proposed in 1966 by J. E. Hulett, Jr.[14] The structure of the model contains the following: (1) input, which refers to any stimulus, external or internal, that engages the individual in an interpersonal interaction for some specific

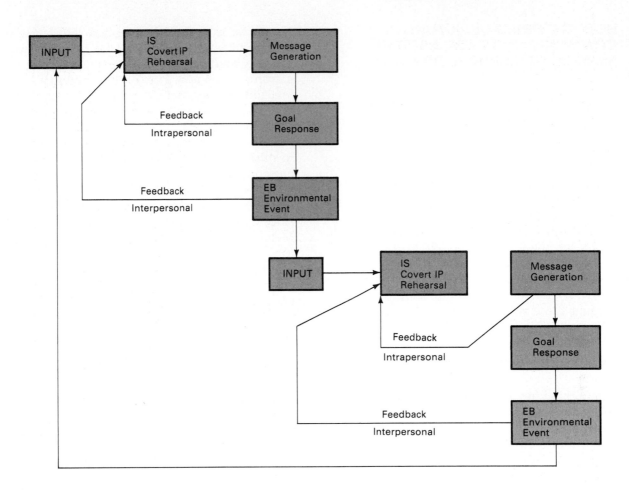

Figure 10-2. Symbolic interactionist model of human communication. IS = Internal State; IP = Internal Processes; EB = External Behavior.

goal; and (2) covert rehearsal. The first unit of covert rehearsal is the **cognitive map**, which is a structure of how meaning is derived for the person. This map is a source of information and contains the stored resources for filtering and interpreting messages from without and from within. The second unit of covert rehearsal includes the processes that generate behavior. These are: (1) the message generation, which is the actual act of delivering the message; (2) the environmental event, which in part refers to the new information generated by the delivered message; and (3) the goal response.

All of these structures are shown in Figure 10-2. They represent phases in the communication process. Communication can be examined from the unique functions of each phase and as a total process. Critical to this model are the phases of covert rehearsal and the recognition of the environmental event that emanates from the message generation. Interpersonal

feedback loops allow the individual to test out how well the message is formed and how it is received, thus working toward a goal response that has been negotiated between both parties.

Relevant assumptions regarding communication are generated by this model. Messages are organized by running internal processes that select behaviors arrived at in response to the perceptions of the individual. There is a trial run of these behaviors, and the individual selects those that he views as having the most success in conveying meaning. Success is a function of the person's cognitive map and the criteria and processes employed in generating the organized behavior as well as the two feedback loops and the environment. Whatever is communicated at a point in time can never be repeated. Communication is complex and ongoing. Meaning is not transferred; rather it is inferred and negotiated.

HOW THEORIES OF HUMAN COMMUNICATION ARE USED IN MODELS OF CLINICAL PRACTICE

The next major question to be asked is how are these theoretical considerations used for therapeutic results in the psychiatric–mental health field?

We will conclude this chapter with a review of models that have been used in an effort to alter disturbed behavior patterns. All of these models assume that disturbed behavior is in part, if not totally, mediated by dysfunctional communication. These models further assume that attention to communication behavior assists in diagnosing structures that maintain disturbed behavior and that therapeutic strategies aim at altering these structures.

Psychiatric Nursing Models

The nursing models of Mellow, Peplau, and Orlando have all emphasized the process of communication.[15–17] Each model states goals of communication within the therapeutic process. Yet none of the models focuses on the structure of the communication process itself. Rather, the models were developed through statements of belief and expectation regarding human beings, growth and development, and human relationships. Implicit principles guided and differentiated the relationships and therefore the type and focus of conscious communication efforts.

Generally, all of these models assumed that communication is dynamic and ongoing. Primary emphasis was on the spoken word, and great attention was paid to the development of semantics and themes from which motivational constructs were assumed operant and responsible for behavior. The centrality of motivation in developing the goal of behavior recognized the importance of personal experience. Consequently, style and techniques of communicating were aimed at facilitating the expression of personal meaning so that a more common meaning of events could be arrived at between two people. Each of the nursing models focused on different types of interpersonal experiences by which the latter could be accomplished.

Mellow espoused the use of an experiential model.[18] By this she meant that the nurse was to relate to the total behavior of the patient (her work was with severely psychotic individuals).

No matter how disturbed or bizarre or socially unacceptable the behavior, the behavior was basically assumed to be conveying meaning regarding the internal state of the individual. Mellow did not advocate condoning the patient's behavior; rather it was a matter of accepting the behavior as meaningful communication. The nurse would stop it if it was injurious to self or to others, or if it was totally disruptive to the environment.

The mayor objective of the nurse's behavior was to make contact with the patient through a sincere desire to communicate and understand. Meeting the patient at his individual level of functioning established rapport and created an internal state of trust for the patient.[19]

Peplau developed her conditions for therapeutic communication from many of the premises inherent in the Interpersonal Theory of Psychiatry outlined by Harry Stack Sullivan.[20,21] All behavior was developed through the context of interpersonal relationships. Disruptive behavior arose out of noxious interpersonal relationships that affected the dominant level of thinking and consequently the type of communications derived from the thinking patterns.

The relationship of the nurse to the client offered a corrective experience for the client, and this possibility was assured when the nurse paid attention to how she behaved with the client. The behavior of the nurse could detract or provoke anxiety in the client.

Style and approach emphasized talking with the client and attending to the process. The objective was to help the client to rely less on distorted patterns of thinking for solving interpersonal problems. Peplau outlined types of interviewing techniques that were designed to focus on the client and on an examination of the relationship of thinking and behaving. There was a major focus on themes and patterns associated with words and nonspoken behavior.[22]

Orlando believed that the deep levels of meaning and their relationship to disturbed behavior were in the province of psychotherapy and a treatment relegated more to psychiatrists than to psychiatric nurses. Use of the milieu and of the ongoing life experiences for confronting and altering disturbed behavior was the objective of Orlando's teaching of the nurse–patient relationship. Interaction, confrontation, and negotiation were the prime communicative skills to be developed by the nurse. Where a patient distorted reality, the nurse was to assume responsibility for supporting and guiding the patient in making contact and eventually negotiating reality more independently.[23]

Although Mellow, Peplau, and Orlando had different styles and a different focus of efforts, they all adhered to basic humanistic values, which pervaded their teaching and writing about the communication process. These values were that all behavior is purposeful, each person is unique, and the nurse must be aware of her own behavior and its impact when conversing and interacting with another. Implicit were the rights of another and that meaning was negotiated. Interpretation, on the other hand, was viewed as based on an understanding of deep structures of personality requiring a different and more extensive type of training.

These women set the value patterns inherent in concepts related to the therapeutic use of self. As psychiatric nursing practice continues to evolve, its commitment to the therapeutic use of self has led its practitioners to adopt, modify, and use increasingly more specific models of communication arrived at by a variety of clinicians from different backgrounds. These models have helped the nurse comprehend practices, which, while effective, appeared to emanate from intuitive capacities. In fact, nurses were early advocates of using communication and structured experiences in the care of emotionally disturbed people.

Clinical Models Derived by Other Disciplines and Influential in Psychiatric Mental Health Nursing Practice

Family Theories
During the late 1950s and through present time, a movement developed to understand the most severe mental disorders and to find ways to intervene. This movement directed therapeutic efforts toward the family unit. With a family perspective, clinical researchers became aware of the impact of the patterns of relationships and their role in both generating and maintaining deviant behavior. The works of many of these people have led to what is called the structuralist approach. Implied in this concept is that function is derived from structure. Roles in the family were defined by the structure of the communication patterns and the explicit and implicit rules each member was required to follow. Clinical writings in family work and research concentrate on the pragmatics of communication.

Intervention is viewed as being most successful when it is directed at altering noxious structures, thus changing the amount and frequency of deviant and misleading messages in the family unit.

A brief presentation of some key structural concepts will be given to demonstrate the clinical application of strategies based on family theories of communication.

Triangling. M. Bowen introduced the concept of triangling to the area of family work.[24] Triangling involves three people. At times a triangle involves two people against one. At other times it involves one person caught in the crossfire of two people. The object of the clinician recognizing this phenomenon is to stop the process and help the trio determine who is at odds with whom and to deal with the differences directly rather than scapegoating the third person. Where people are attempting to engage a third person to join sides, efforts are made to help the two opposing forces settle their differences without involving the third. Thinking of a child and parents getting a divorce and all that can happen helps clarify how assessing this process leads the clinician to more purposeful efforts in changing the dysfunctional communication system.

Double Bind. G. Bateson introduced the concept of the double bind from his studies of families with schizophrenic members.[25] Basically, the concept states than an individual is continually punished for his correct discrimination of the context of a message and the meaning directed toward him. The result is that the person gives up his accurate perception. An important aspect of the relationship in this pattern is that the person who is in the double bind cannot leave the relationship. This can occur because the person is a child or in some way through both internal and external factors experiences helplessness. The constant disqualification by another of one's perceptions as well as an adoption of this pattern by the individual involved leads to a distorted sense of reality as well as self. Imagine yourself in a situation with an important person who appears to be interested in what you think and what you see with regard to him and that person then tells you in many different ways that you are wrong. This is the experience of a double bind. Now imagine that you are completely dependent on this person!

Qualification/Disqualification. Qualification and disqualification are additional concepts proposed by Bateson.[26] Qualifying statements are clear, congruent statements of fact and motivation. Disqualifying statements lack congruence, increase paradoxical meaning (Does the person mean the opposite of what he is saying?), and lead to vagueness. For example, a couple have just fought over the household bills. She asks, "Do you love me?" (Tone is firm, declarative.) He answers, with his back to her, "Yeah, I think so." (Words are mumbled.) Patterns of speech reflect the frequency of use of qualifying and disqualifying statements. These patterns can vary with people and the context, or they can represent the characteristic style of an individual. Intervention is aimed at enhancing the person's ability to use qualification and to negotiate these patterns from others.

These are but a few examples of concepts derived from basic theoretical considerations regarding communication and applied to the area of family therapy. They have been presented to demonstrate the evolution of techniques for altering pathological states through addressing how people converse with one another rather than focusing on their motivations and personal meanings. For this group the symptom is the disease. Thus, there is absolute reliance on the process of communication for both cause and change.

Transactional Analysis

In 1964, Eric Berne presented his thesis that through the manner and the consistent style of people relating to one another, a paradigm could be developed indicating their internal state of psychological organization, referred to as "ego state."[27] Berne defined his ego states as adult, parent, and child. He hypothesized that at any point of transaction between people, they would be relating to one another from one of these ego states.

Complementary transactions are defined when each party is relating from the same, complementary ego state, i.e., adult to adult, child to child, parent to parent. For example, two people are in a heated discussion and each is yelling at the other, "This is not fair; you shouldn't do that. I want what is mine." A common response from an observer might be, "They're both acting like children." An adult-to-adult transaction would be identified by both parties qualifying the different experiences of one another and negotiating the difference.[28]

Cross transactions are defined by an exchange between two different ego states. For example, a college teacher assumes a parental state and the student assumes a child state. In this arrangement, the flow and the quality of the transactions will defer to the power position of the teacher. Differences between the two, rather than being negotiated, will be handled in an autocratic manner by the teacher and in a submissive and/or rebellious manner by the student.[29]

Ulterior transactions are defined by transactional acts that are not congruent. They are complex, implying one type of transaction on an overt level and a hidden motivational intent on another level. It is at this level that Berne coined the concept of games, i.e., games people play. These interpersonal games are many, and like games, they have rules. These rules are transmitted in the nonspoken and spoken behaviors of each party, and they are further negotiated from the respective ego states of those involved. Examples are adult sex games. On the surface a man and woman meet. While ostensibly acting as two adults, the woman begins to act demurely and defer to the man. She asks his advice, she doesn't argue with him, she follows his lead, she acts helpless. The game can be called Being Feminine; the ulterior motive can be Catch the Man.[30]

To avoid a pejorative use of the term *games*, people devoted to the further development and evaluation of the efficacy of this model advocate four broad areas of assessment as a means of confirming the ulterior transactions of an individual. These areas are:

Derive a behavioral diagnosis from the nonspoken and spoken communication patterns of the individual; that is, identify the behavioral patterns and their consistency and intensity.

Derive a social/operational diagnosis from the consistency, intensity, and frequency of patterns in social transactions.

Derive a historical diagnosis from an establishment of the behaviors in past relationships and in past transactions.

Derive a phenomenological diagnosis from the transactions that occur between you and the client.[31]

Cognitive Models of Therapy

As one can note from the foregoing discussion of the transactional analysis model, both semantic and pragmatic factors are considered in structuring therapeutic strategies from the assessment of a client's communication behavior.

Cognitive restructuring has been formalized as a treatment model by H. Ellis and Aaron Beck.[32,33] These authors and others have noted in their clinical practice that the linguistic structures people apply in using language to express themselves represent either facilitating or debilitating internal strategies for deriving meaning from their experiences. These strategies address an internal, intrapsychic, pragmatic process, one that is related to certain emotional states such as depression, anxiety, fear, and confusion. The brain is the regulative structure of behavior and is continually processing information. One aspect of this process is often an out-of-conscious dialogue with oneself. For example, the reader may be saying to himself, "I wish the author would get to the point so I can go on with this and make some sense of it." (Tension and irritation may be experienced.) "Some of this is interesting though." (Tension is reduced, interest is increased.)

The task of the therapist is to make the person aware of what he is saying to himself and the emotional state encountered, and where appropriate, to provide an examination of the person's beliefs and the unrealistic dimensions of beliefs such as cause–effect relationships and distortions of probability. For example, "I shouldn't make mistakes." This statement implies a proposition regarding perfection—an assumption that the person must be perfect, that perfect exists, and that all mistakes are a function of the individual. Many types of behavior and emotional states can emanate from this statement. Depression, anxiety, avoidance of activities, extreme focus on details, and criticism of others for being in error are examples of behaviors generated by such a statement.

This model has become rather important because it lends itself to more stringent research activities. In the treatment of depressive disorders, studies have demonstrated its effectiveness when compared to other interventions, including drug therapy.

Neuro-Linguistic Programming

The last clinical model that rests on basic theories of communication is that of Neuro-Linguistic Programming.[34] John Grinder and Richard Bandler were the first to coin the term Neuro-Linguistic Programming in 1975.[35] Joining them in the development of their model in its earlier phases of development were Leslie Cameron-Bandler, Judith DeLozier, Robert Diltz, and David Gordon.[36,37] There is an ever-increasing membership contributing to the development of the model. These contributions are being shared through extensive workshops. With the exception of Stephen Lankton, author of Practical Magic, the major publications on this subject have been produced by the original founders and developers of the model.[38]

The linking of the nonspoken and spoken dimensions of communication has moved both the clinician and researcher closer to eliminating the mind-body split. Recognition of the cybernetic relationship (internal communication) between physiological processes, emotional and thinking processes, and social transactions helps explain why it is possible for a variety of psychotherapies to have positive effects regardless of the particular theory about what is causing the disordered behavior or how it developed in the person. What research has demonstrated is that all types of therapy work when an expert clinician is involved in communicating with the client or clients.

It was this fact that spurred the Neuro-Linguistic Programming group to investigate just what did happen when an expert clinician worked with client(s). If theory did not make a difference, what did? That is, what went on in a therapeutic session when a client's behavior changed? Virginia Satir, a renowned family therapist, Fritz Perl, father of Gestalt psychotherapy, and Milton Erickson, the renowned developer of medical hypnosis, were key therapists who allowed Bandler and Grinder to investigate their therapeutic styles.*

The following observations were made by Bandler and Grinder of these three therapists:

1. Each therapist was intimately tuned in to the most minute details of how his or her client communicated, both verbally and in nonspoken behaviors.
2. Each therapist had sufficient behavioral flexibility to match and pace salient aspects of these behaviors. This was done frequently out of the conscious awareness of the client and often of the therapist. These therapists' abilities correlated with a demonstration of trust for them by the client.

---

* Historical background was given by Leslie Cameron-Bandler at the first Practitioner Workshop on NLP given in Boston, Mass., Fall/Spring 1980–81.

3. When clients were matched and paced for a period of time, they would change their behavior in accordance with the efforts of the therapist. These changes altered the transactional patterns of the individual with the therapist and/or the individual to him- or herself. These changes were most often in the direction of more behavioral flexibility, genuine emotional expression, and awareness of self and others with increasing tolerance for differences.

4. The therapist used both small and specific behaviors for change as well as large complex units of behavior.

5. The therapists did not use the thematic content so much for change as they did for the establishment and maintenance of rapport; rather, the content addressed was the structure of the communication experience. The manipulation through communication strategies on the part of the therapists forced clients to experience what they said and did in a different way. The therapists did not tell the client what to think, feel, etc.; rather, the strategies created new experiences that were basic to eventual change.

As already indicated, the group began to study in detail large and small units of therapist behavior and its impact on clients. The same was done for clients' impact on therapists. The many patterns that were observed were organized into the Neuro-Linguistic model. The model is not seen as incompatible with other theories of therapy, since all of the theories eventually guided the therapists in some critical aspect of the larger communication process.

Important guiding assumptions of NLP™ are as follows:

Meaning is dependent upon the personal set of an individual. Although meaning is negotiated through words, action gives the context to the message. Meaning is not transferable; rather it is inferred and is ultimately a personal psychological experience.

All behavior has a positive intention. The question about any behavior is whether it is effective and efficient, not hurtful, in achieving an objective.

There is a cybernetic relationship between physiological responses, psychological responses, and social transaction; therefore, change in any of these systems will cause change in the other systems.

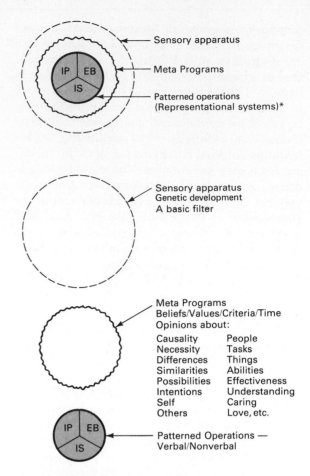

*Representational Systems: A = Auditory, V = Visual, K = Kinesthetic, Eye Movements, Body Posture. EB = External Behavior; IS = Internal States; IP = Internal Processes.

Figure 10-3. A schematization of the individual. *Adapted from Master Practitioner Program, Boston, Mass., 1981–82, Leslie Cameron-Bandler, Director.*

The model is schematized in two capacities, first the individual and second a dyad.*

Because all systems have a cybernetic relationship, homeostasis as well as change is facilitated by feedback loops within and between units conceptualized. See Figure 10-3.

Three Transacting Units. The individual is conceived of as consisting of three major transacting units. Unit 1 is the sensory apparatus. It

* The scheme can be generalized to groups and their subparts and to transactions between groups. Because of this, the model has been applied to business as well as to therapy and education. Source: Leslie Cameron-Bandler, "Schematic Representation of the Individual, Dyad," presented at the Master Practitioner Program, Boston, Mass., Fall 1981–82.

is a basic filter for all incoming and outgoing information. Genetic potential is realized through the transactions of the individual and the environment and through the processes of growth and development.

Unit 2 consists of major belief patterns. Major belief patterns are attitudes, beliefs, and values inferred in linguistic patterns. These patterns of belief are referred to as the Meta Program. Meta Program characteristics reflect patterns of belief, criteria, time such as past, present, and future orientations, patterns of causality, necessity, differences, similarities, intentions, self-orientation, and other-orientation. Meta programs can have specific relationships to particular contexts such as work versus home. Meta programs not only filter information but they contain important criteria for selective attention to experiences.

Unit 3 is patterned operations. Patterned operations are further broken down into categories of external behavior, internal states, and internal processes. Internal states and internal processes are inferred from external behavior. All we know of another person is what we observe from his or her outward behavior. Nonspoken behavior as well as verbal behavior gives us information about structure of internal states and internal processes. The following shows how the three major transacting units come into play when two people communicate:

Nurse Smith is new to an Eastern hospital. She is eager to know the staff she is working with and to perhaps make friends. She is from the West Coast and has been used to open and friendly encounters. She is walking down the hall when the physician in charge of the unit she is working on stops and says, "Hello, finding your way around?" [He makes eye contact and smiles and has stopped walking.] Nurse Smith stops, looks at the doctor, smiles and responds, "It's a bit confusing, but I'm learning . . . [pause] . . . I was wondering. . . ." [Interrupted by the doctor, now moving on] "That's fine, let me know if you need anything." He walks away.

Nurse Smith's meta program reveals critical beliefs about herself in relation to others. She believes herself friendly and that other people are friendly, and further she believes that it is possible to have friendships in the context of a work situation. She also has a desire to make friends and is looking for opportunities to so do. This mind-set is important as it becomes a basic filter by which she is going to selectively screen and interpret the behavior of another person, in this case the doctor.

The doctor considers himself friendly and consid-erate. He wishes to make contact with a new employee. He has the desire to convey that he is available for assistance in the work situation. These are the critical aspects of his meta program.

The nurse and doctor meet. The nurse takes in the doctor's behavior on the initial aspect of their meeting. His eye contact, smile, and direct question are interpreted by her as being friendly. He asks her a question; she flashes onto the many new things she has encountered. In a split second she makes a picture of herself sitting down and talking to the doctor. She makes a decision to ask if he has time to talk, perhaps have coffee; but before she can ask him, he is moving on.

When the doctor stops and says hello to the nurse, he sees her smile and hears her say something to him. He says to himself, "I'm glad I stopped, but I'd better get on to my next appointment." He moves on, giving a surface message that he is available to listen.

The next day while walking down the hall, Nurse Smith sees the doctor; she has a picture of him walking away the day before. She feels her face flush and she says to herself, "I'm not going to deal with that snob." She looks straight ahead and moves rapidly on with a short, "Hello."

The doctor coming down the hall sees Nurse Smith. He recalls her words the day before, and he reflects on their friendly tone. He has time for coffee and as he approaches her, he is perplexed by her downcast eyes and rapid walk. He nods in response to her "hello."

This example points out the units of behavior considered by both parties involved in relating self to others. Key aspects of verbal and nonverbal spoken behavior are taken into account, such as stopping, eye contact, smiling, and tone of voice. These become criteria that, through the filter of the meta program, proclaim oneself acceptable to another and vice versa. In addition, in the nurse's mind's eye, she actually envisions a future event that she has concluded as possible by virtue of her interpretation of the doctor's behavior. By the same token, the doctor's internal dialogue to himself draws conclusions regarding the nurse's interpretation of their encounter. The re-encounter is now coded in an entirely different way for Nurse Smith, and the doctor is confused as to what happened.

The interesting aspects of how information is stored and then represented in language moves to a discussion of eye movement patterns and language. Information is stored and interpreted kinesthetically (feelings, tastes, odors), visually (images, colors, hues), and auditorially (tones, pitch, amplitude, intensity). Language is an attempt to express these personal experiences. Words are a symbol for these experiences, not the experience.

According to research on eye movement and storage of information, when persons look to their left and then to their right, they are most apt to be attending to internal dialogue. If persons look up to their right, they are often responding to a remembered internal picture. To further establish the representational system being used by an individual, the predicates (verbs, adverbs, adjectives) used will correspond to the eye movements. See Figure 10-4 and accompanying exercises.

Representational Systems. The individual will usually have a dominant representational system that will bring the event to mind. However, the person is rarely aware of this process. This teaches us that a person does not respond to the direct sensory experience of an event; rather, a person responds to the experience out of his cognitive map and mapping procedures. What is stored and acts as a resource of information in the future is the consequence of these processes. The concept of representational systems and the ability to track them with careful observations should allow us to enter into a communication experience with another person

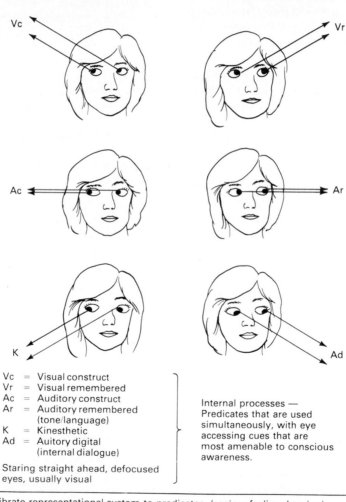

Vc = Visual construct
Vr = Visual remembered
Ac = Auditory construct
Ar = Auditory remembered
        (tone/language)
K   = Kinesthetic
Ad = Auitory digital
        (internal dialogue)

Staring straight ahead, defocused eyes, usually visual

Internal processes —
Predicates that are used simultaneously, with eye accessing cues that are most amenable to conscious awareness.

Questions to ask to calibrate representational system to predicates (seeing, feeling, hearing):

1. What did you *see* at the circus?

2. How do you *see* your garage and woodworking equipment?

3. What did your 3rd grade teacher look like?

Visual Remembered

1. Make a *picture* of a clown with donkey ears and red polka dots on his pants.

2. Imagine seeing yourself in an astronaut suit, walking to the elevator, going to the top of the launch missile.

Visual Construct

Figure 10-4. General patterns of eye accessing cues (right-handed person—based on U.S. citizens).

with increased flexibility. If we do not experience another as seeing our point, it may be traced to the fact that the person receiving our words hears them but cannot make logical sense out of them. Since a picture is worth ten thousand words, it is useful to return to our mind's eye picture and determine if we are putting into words the associations we have in mind, since our friend does not have direct access to the picture in our mind.

EXERCISES RELATING TO FIGURE 10-3

1. Make up a song about water and wind.
2. What would you say to a customer who said you cheated him? } Auditory construct

1. How do you *feel* when you are scolded?
2. How do you *feel* about sex? } Kinesthetic

1. Repeat what I *last said* to *you*.
2. What did your wife *last say* to *you*? } Auditory remembered

1. What did *you* last *say* to yourself?
2. When *you* are proud, what do *you* say to yourself? } Auditory digital

Add to these questions, being careful to state your question only in the terms of the representational system you are trying to elicit.

Do not be misled by initial eye movements because of overlapping systems. Remember, your input is auditory to other people. They may repeat your question, make a picture, and from the picture develop or recall auditory or kinesthetic information. By the same token, an individual may just take in questions and respond by *feelings*; and from feelings he moves on to visual or auditory experiences. The initial accessing eye movements are the lead system, informing you how information is initially taken in by a person. Predicates indicate the dominant system that gives more or less conscious meaning to the person of what was taken in and processed.

The developers of the Neuro-Linguistic NLP™ have made extensive use of their observation of language and eye movement patterns in developing and testing therapeutic interventions. Without going into further descriptions of the logic of these intervention strategies, it is apparent that knowing the impact of representational systems on the communication process

and the basic manner of identifying them can enhance conversing with another person or group by increasing rapport and providing a flexibility in self-expression that demonstrates an appreciation of the unique manner in which another person arrives at understanding. Rather than focusing on the intentions of another person regarding what we said, we can attend to how we said what we did, and whether it fits with the sensory mode of another person. If not, we can alter our patterns.

Meta Program. Intrinsically related to the awareness of kinesthetic, visual, and auditory representational systems is the concept of the meta programs. Meta program refers to the attitudes, beliefs, values, and opinions of a person. A basic assumption is that a written or spoken sentence leaves out information that is ultimately filled in by the receiver of the written or spoken word. It is further assumed that it is confusion over the surface structure and the deep structure that leads to communication problems. In a therapeutic transaction, it is considered valuable to elicit the deep structure of a sentence to establish experiential resources of an individual and to provide options for change. Bringing into awareness informational experiences basic to what is being said, such as the pictures, tones, feelings, and mannerisms, enriches the meaning.

NLP™ originators have identified what they call "meta program violations." Attention is directed to the syntax of speech patterns. The term *violation* is used because the surface structure of the language contains unspecified words and unclear denotation. For example, "The book is on the table." This sentence is correct grammatically, yet critical references are deleted and have to be filled in, such as which book, which table, and in what room. Deletions of this type are readily recognizable; but it is much more complex to recognize deletions manifested in generalizations and distortions. An example of this complexity can be found in the analysis of the statement. "Life without love is not worth living." When a person makes this statement, we have little information as to what is meant in general or specifically. First, this statement contains a presupposition, that is, a fundamental assumption that under certain circumstances, life is worth living. The assumption can be made more specific by clarifying what is worthwhile and not worthwhile. On the surface one may argue and say that love was specified.

Love is a nominalization, and it is derived from the verb "to love." Returning to the verb form would at least elicit from the person what behaviors are believed to be equivalent to the act of loving for that person.

With the expression of the underlying experiences that give meaning to the statement for the sender, there will be corresponding physiological states manifested in nonspoken behavior patterns. That is, by asking the person to detail how he knows he is loved can engender the physical components of the state. The observer can now know from the nonspoken behavior of the person what he or she means by the "state of being loved and that life is worthwhile." The nonspoken behavior changes, as well as the spoken behaviors, can now be used as an outcome indicator of behavior change. Thus, by attending to the communications on

all levels, it is possible for a therapist to elicit the desired outcome behavior a client is seeking, thereby establishing behavioral criteria for evaluation of therapeutic efforts. In fact, this is precisely how expert clinicians operate; they achieve critical behavior change during their therapeutic interviews. If a client is anxious, the therapist elicits a state when the client was not anxious but relaxed; now the therapist knows behaviorally how the client will be when not anxious—there is an outcome state.

The preceding discussion highlights the model of Neuro-Linguistic Programming. As a model it incorporates basic theories of communication and links them with neurophysiological patterns of behavior. As a model it becomes a powerful tool in developing and testing therapeutic strategies designed to operate on many levels of awareness.

Summary

The chapter has covered the following: definition of communication, parameters that influence the style of communication; culture, sex, socioeconomic background; social distance; power relationships; number of receivers, internal states; drugs and other factors. How we communicate addressed spoken behavior including phonology, syntax, semantics, pragmatics and paralanguage as well as nonspoken language. The relationship of spoken and nonspoken language was addressed in a presentation of various theoretical models of communication. The theories were presented from the simplest, based on a stimulus–response paradigm to the most complex, the symbolic interactionist model. A brief review of how psychiatric nursing theorists addressed communication was presented. Other clinical models which have influenced psychiatric nursing practices regarding communication and therapy were presented. These included family therapy models, transactional analysis, cognitive therapy and Neuro-Linguistic Programming.

Psychiatric nursing has put a primary emphasis on the process of communication. In addition, key beliefs and values regarding the individual have contributed to the success of the many nurse practitioners. Their practices have respected the uniqueness of the individual. Thus, when engaged in conversing and acting with clients, they have attempted to avoid forcing their interpretation of life onto the client. Recent multidisciplinary efforts at therapeutic interventions have cast more light on the communication process as the primary vehicle for change. From these efforts, models have been developed in clinical practice that facilitate creative ventures in using communication as the fulcrum for behavior change. As yet, clinicians continue to use a variety of models and blends of models in clinical practice.

Questions

1. Describe with examples eight factors that influence communication.
2. Identify five ways that spoken behavior can be studied.

3. Describe six ways in which nonspoken behavior may be observed.
4. Explain gradation of theoretical complexity as it relates to models of communication.
5. Identify with examples three psychiatric nurses who have emphasized the process of communication.
6. Identify the key concepts in the following treatment models:
   a. Family therapy
   b. Transactional analysis
   c. Cognitive restructuring
   d. Neuro-Linguistic Programming

REFERENCES AND SUGGESTED READINGS

1. Eibl-Eibesfeldt, I. Similarities and differences between cultures. In S. Weitz (Ed.), *Nonverbal Communication*. London: Cambridge University Press, 1974.
2. LaFrance, M., & Mayo, C. *Moving Bodies: Nonverbal Communication in Social Relationships*. Monterey, Calif.: Brooks Cole, 1978.
3. Addington, D. W. The relationship of selected vocal characteristics to personality perception. *Speech Monographs*, 1968, *35*, 492–503.
4. Weintraub, W. *Verbal Behavior: Adaption and Psychopathology*. New York: Springer, 1983.
5. Sommer, K. Further studies in small group ecology. *Sociometry*, 1965, *28*, 337–348.
6. Gottschalk, L. A. A computerized scoring system for use with content analysis scales. *Comprehensive Psychiatry*, 1975, *16*, 77–90.
7. Birdwhistell, R. L. *Kinetics and Context*. Philadelphia: University of Pennsylvania Press, 1970.
8. Dittmann, A. T. *Interpersonal Messages of Emotion*. New York: Springer, 1972.
9. Diltz, R., Grindler, J., Bandler, R., Bandler, L. C., & DeLozier, J. *Neuro-Linguistic Programming: The Study of the Subject of Subjective Experience*. Cupertino, Calif.: Meta Publications, 1980.
10. Hull, C. L. *A Behavior System*. New Haven: Yale University Press, 1952.
11. Laing, R. D., Phillipson, H., & Lee, A. R. *Interpersonal Perception*. London: Tavistock, 1966.
12. Ibid., p. 22.
13. Köhler, W. *Gestalt Psychology*. New York: Liverwright, 1947.
14. Hulett, J. G., Jr. A symbolic interactionist model for human communication. *A.V. Communication Review*, 1966, *14*, 14.
15. Mellow, J. The experiential order of nursing therapy in the treatment of acute schizophrenia. *Excerpta Medica*, International Congress Series, No. 187, Psychiatric Research in Our Changing World, Proceedings of an International Symposium, Montreal, October, 1968.
16. Peplau, H. *Interpersonal Relations in Nursing*. New York: Putnam's, 1952.
17. Orlando, I. J. *The Dynamic Nurse–Patient Relationship*. New York: Putnam's, 1961.
18. Mellow, op cit.
19. Ibid.
20. Peplau, op. cit.
21. Sullivan, H. S. *The Interpersonal Theory of Psychiatry*. New York: Norton, 1953.
22. Peplau, op. cit.
23. Orlando, op. cit.
24. Bowen, M. The use of family therapy in clinical practice. *Comprehensive Psychiatry*, 1966, 7.
25. Bateson, G. *Steps to an Ecology of Mind*. New York: Ballantine, 1972.
26. Ibid.
27. Berne, E. *Games People Play*. New York: Grove Press, 1964.
28. Ibid., p. 30.
29. Ibid., pp. 103–104.
30. Ibid., pp. 109–113.
31. Ibid., p. 75.
32. Ellis, H. C. *Fundamentals of Human Learning, Memory, and Cognition* (2nd ed.). Dubuque, Iowa: Wm. C. Brown, 1972.
33. Beck, A. *Cognitive Therapy and Emotional Disorders*. New York: International University Press, 1976.
34. Hartman, C. R. Neurolinguistic programming. In C. Beck, R. Rawlins, & S. Williams (Eds.), *Psychiatric Mental Health Nursing*. St. Louis: Mosby, 1984.
35. Bandler, R., & Grinder, J. *The Structure of Magic*. Palo Alto, Calif.: Science and Behavior Books, 1976.
36. Diltz, R., Grinder, J., Bandler, R., Bandler-Cameron, L., & DeLozier, J. op. cit.
37. Gordon, D. *Therapeutic Metaphors*. Cupertino, Calif.: Meta Publications, 1978.
38. Lankton, S. *Practical Magic*. Cupertino, Calif.: Meta Publications, 1980.

PART III

The Nursing Process in Psychiatric Mental Health Nursing

A major advance in nursing practice has been the development and acceptance of a framework for practice called the nursing process. The basic approaches and concepts that are part of the nurse's inventory of resources in caring for a troubled human being are discussed. Standards of nursing practice are highlighted in the sections in which they are most applicable.

CHAPTER 11: PSYCHIATRIC MENTAL HEALTH NURSING

Psychiatric nursing is viewed in terms of its past history, its current state of identity, and its future potential. Nursing research is emphasized.

CHAPTER 12: ASSESSMENT PROTOCOLS IN PSYCHIATRIC MENTAL HEALTH NURSING

A patient assessment is the first step in the nursing process, starting at the patient's point of entry into the health care system. Additional assessment protocols include functional health status and the mental status examination.

CHAPTER 13: NURSING DIAGNOSIS

The history and implementation of nursing diagnosis is presented within the framework of case examples and nursing care plans.

CHAPTER 14: SPIRITUAL DIMENSIONS OF PSYCHIATRIC MENTAL HEALTH NURSING

Religiosity is sometimes a major behavioral characteristic of a psychiatric patient. This chapter puts into perspective the spiritual and religious needs of people and looks at dysfunctional patterns and nursing care plans within this area.

CHAPTER 15: THE THERAPEUTIC ALLIANCE AND THE NURSE–PATIENT RELATIONSHIP

The therapeutic use of self, including attitudes and human qualities, is a key asset in establishing the therapeutic alliance and conducting a good interview. The various types of interviews as well as specific interview techniques are presented.

CHAPTER 16: COMMUNICATION AND THE THERAPEUTIC PROCESS

Understanding and observing the structure of rapport is a basic step in the development of the therapeutic process and communication strategies. This skill paves the way for promoting change in the interactional structure of the patient.

CHAPTER 17: STALLS IN THE THERAPEUTIC PROCESS

Practice is an essential component to conceptual understanding and to achieving competence in any specialty area. This chapter identifies the problem areas frequently encountered in the therapeutic process through the concept of the stall.

CHAPTER 18: LEGAL ASPECTS OF PSYCHIATRIC MENTAL HEALTH NURSING

The issue of patients' rights has been highly visible for the last two decades. This chapter describes, with case citations, the legal aspects of practice and implications for practice.

Chapter 11

Psychiatric Mental Health Nursing

Ann Wolbert Burgess

Chapter Objectives

The students successfully attaining the goals of this chapter will be able to:

- Trace the nursing care of the mentally ill from the 1800s to current times.
- Explain how the Mental Health Act of 1946, the establishment of NIMH, the Comprehensive Community Mental Health Act of 1963, the President's Commission on Mental Health in America 1978, and the 1981 Omnibus Reconciliation Act have all influenced the development of psychiatric nursing.
- Interpret Standard IX of the ANA Standards of Psychiatric Mental Health Nursing practice and describe the research process.
- Outline role options for psychiatric mental health nurses, especially the scientific-research role.

Psychiatric mental health nursing is in a state of exciting evolution and advancement. Communication is at an all-time high with the launching of a new refereed journal, *Archives of Psychiatric Nursing,* in 1986. In 1987 the inaugural convention of the American Psychiatric Nurses' Association was held October 15 to 17 in Baltimore. This new psychiatric nursing group brings together psychiatric and mental health nurses who are engaged in the direct care in a wide variety of practice settings throughout the United States.

Although its historical roots can be traced over a period of several centuries, psychiatric mental health nursing's current position as a specialty area in nursing and as a mental health profession really started in 1946. That year marked the passage of the Mental Health Act, which provided federal funds for the support of psychiatric nursing at both the undergraduate and graduate levels.

During the four decades following the passage of the Mental Health Act, psychiatric nurses have developed expertise in the roles of managers of the patients' hospital environment; psychotherapists for individuals, groups, and families; therapists and counselors for suicide prevention and crisis intervention; clinical specialists for special populations, supervision, consultation, and education; and researchers to study human responses to mental health problems.

As psychiatric nursing has moved from its historical custodial function to the widespread challenges described above, it has enjoyed the opportunity to improve the care of the psychiatrically ill and the emotionally distressed, while at the same time acting as advocate for the optimal level of mental health for people, strengthening the knowledge development in nursing, and enhancing the professional growth of the psychiatric nurse.

As a result of these challenges posed both to nursing and psychiatric nursing and as we enter the last decade of the twentieth century, we note that nursing has emerged with clear and distinct statements as to its domain, its scope of practice, its art and its science. The research and theory-development movement in nursing has had a powerful effect on advancing the profession. Effectively, over a four-decade period, nursing in general and psychiatric nursing in particular faced and resolved an identity crisis. Now the critical developmental task is to maintain nursing's productivity and the challenge is to expand and advance its knowledge base. Nursing, in many ways, has come of age.

This chapter reviews the development of psychiatric mental health nursing by describing early models of mental healing; reviewing nursing care of the mentally ill before 1946 and the major political and legislative developments; and outlining role options for the psychiatric mental health nurse. This chapter also presents a vision for nursing students, who often have a limited amount of time for the study and practice of psychiatric mental health nursing.

THE MYSTICAL MODEL OF MENTAL HEALING

The story of mental healing starts with the history of people. To early humans, mental life was something either supernatural or something to be ignored.

The concept of mystical or supernatural causes accounting for the destiny of a person is not uncommon today. Many superstitions lend credence to this concept. "Whatever will be will be" or "That was meant to be" are examples of such beliefs when tragedy strikes.

The historical origins of this mystical model

of viewing mental illness lie in ancient or even prehistoric times. Primitive man viewed disease as an evil spirit that took possession of the body as punishment for an offense against the spirit world. When man offended the demons of nature, he invited their revenge. This revenge might strike down an individual, his family, the village community, or an entire tribe. Therefore, the primitive art of mental healing was the art of driving hostile spirits away. The possibility of dying a natural death was unknown to primitive people. To them death was caused by the spirit world.

This view of illness is believed to have been in effect around 2500 B.C. and was dominated by attitudes of fear and superstition. It became evident that mental patients were turned out into the hills. Skulls with trepanations (drilled holes) were found far from the rest of the village. Restraints and actual physical rejection were the only types of care provided to these unhappy victims.

Undoubtedly, the primitive world had its share of psychiatric problems. Epileptics, eccentric individuals, and psychotics often were the witch doctors of the village. They were able to capitalize on the weakness or power, as it were, of their minds. The supernatural concept of illness was a major influence during this period.

THE CUSTODIAL MODEL OF MENTAL HEALING

The historical origins and treatment models of custodial care, the second evolutionary model of care, can be traced back to Greek and Roman times. Enlightened attitudes of humane treatment and concern prevailed in this period. The care included sedation with opiates, music therapy, good physical hygiene, and humane management of the patient's daily activities. This concept of care, however, was abandoned when the Roman Empire deteriorated, and the supernatural concept again prevailed until the eighteenth century.

In the nineteenth century, the mentally ill were collected together and someone was paid to watch over them. This particular model developed out of necessity because families could not bear the full responsibility of guarding or tending to the mentally ill person. Thus developed the model of custodial care, supported financially by private and community efforts. Mental difficulties at this time were considered irreversible, and therefore protecting society from these deranged individuals took precedence over treatment models.

These mental institutions operated on the concept of detention rather than treatment. State hospitals rapidly became too large and overcrowded. Such institutions were, and still are, the only source of psychiatric help for many citizens. The social-psychiatric problems inherent in this system and the organization of patient care are the concerns of mental health specialists today. Although patient care services have developed markedly in many state hospitals, severe problems still remain.

Thus the mental hospitals assumed a custodial role early in American psychiatric history. Their goal was to keep the patients safe, to guard them, and to manage them because they were incapable of managing their own lives.

Mental hospitals at this time functioned in an autocratic way, rendering patients helpless by their treatment. The patient was seen as defective, incompetent, and potentially dangerous. His rights were denied him, and he was considered an incapable citizen in our society. The patient was forced into an institutional mode of behavior. Families were not allowed to take an active role in the treatment process and, in many instances, were even discouraged from visiting. The stigma of being a mental patient was communicated to the patient. There was a continual increase in social isolation and an increasing pattern of conformity to the needs of the institution.

The institution did provide "custodial care." Shelter, rest, and food were supplied to the patient. Under the existing conditions, however, this was not the most effective treatment. Losing more and more of his options, interacting mainly with other psychotic patients, and dealing with a nontrained and frequently punitive staff, the mental patient became more institutionalized, more chronic, and less able to return to his family and community.

Where these conditions still exist, the possibility of change must be raised by the community. The attitudes and social consciousness of people are what make the difference in care models. Until a community feels concern and responsibility for the mental illness of its people, change cannot occur.

NURSING CARE OF THE MENTALLY ILL: 1860–1946

A history of psychiatric nursing would not be complete without a brief background on Florence Nightingale, who is well acclaimed as the founder of modern nursing.[1] Born to wealthy upper-class parents in 1820, Florence Nightingale resisted all pressures to stay within her social class and marry, preferring instead to follow her vocation of nursing the sick. At age 31, she obtained her first nursing experience with the Protestant deaconesses at Kaiserswerth in Germany and two years later traveled to London to reorganize a small hospital in Harley Street, the Institution for the Care of Sick Gentlewomen in Distressed Circumstances. The reorganization was a major success and led Sidney Herbert, secretary of war in the British cabinet, to invite her to undertake a mission to the Crimea. On October 21, 1854, Florence Nightingale sailed for the Crimea with 38 nurses, and within a month found that she had more than 5000 men in her charge.[2]

In July 1860, the Nightingale training school for nurses was opened at St. Thomas's Hospital in London. It is from this date that modern nursing is said to commence. This model of training nurses was brought to America in 1873. In May of that year the Bellevue Hospital School of Nursing began to train nurses in the Nightingale method of nursing; in October the Connecticut Training School opened; and in November the Boston Training School began. Linda Richards, one of America's first trained nurses, believed that the mentally sick person also needed nursing care. This belief led to her initiative in creating schools of nursing in state hospitals. In 1882, she worked with Edward Cowles, the medical director at the McLean Hospital in Belmont, Massachusetts, to begin the first psychiatric training school in the United States.[3] By 1890, this two-year program had graduated 90 nurses. The value of this school was so quickly appreciated that within 10 years there were 19 American institutions providing psychiatric training programs.

In 1886, McLean Hospital took another step forward by establishing an affiliation with the Massachusetts General Hospital whereby credit for a full nursing course was given upon completion of the senior year at the hospital. In England a similar program was in effect, and a certificate was given to the graduates from the Medico-Psychological Association.

Despite these promising beginnings, by the end of the nineteenth century the vast majority of professional nurses who worked in psychiatric hospitals had little or no training in psychiatry. For the most part, they adapted their training in the physical care of psychiatric patients—assisting in the administration of medications, hydrotherapy, and the maintenance of hygiene. Their effectiveness was certainly enhanced by their kindness and understanding, but there was no systematic program of psychiatric nursing care.

Many difficulties were encountered in the development of psychiatric nursing in America. The greatest problem was that there seemed to be little demand for the so-called "asylum-trained" nurse. By 1916, half of the mental hospitals in the United States still had no school for their nurses. These hospitals employed attendants at very low wages and provided them with very poor living conditions. However, there were about 40 mental institutions that were operating some sort of training school for their nurses, although the standards for admission and graduation, by comparison, were much lower than those for schools of nursing in general hospitals. During this time nurse educators were working toward establishing psychiatric nursing affiliations for students enrolled in schools of nursing in general hospitals, but the goal was never realized. It is no wonder that nursing of the mentally ill was so slow catching on.

By 1935, only half of the then existing diploma schools of nursing offered psychiatric nursing in their curriculum. Although the first textbook on psychiatric nursing—Harriet Bailey's *Nursing Mental Diseases*—was published in 1920 by the Macmillan Company (New York), its educational value was largely ignored. And psychiatric nursing was not a requirement for state registration until as late as 1952.

Up to 1946, nursing leaders pioneering in psychiatric care primarily worked with the long-hospitalized psychotic patient. This was the patient population left untreated or even unattended in some institutions. These nurses provided general nursing care for the mentally ill with minimal financial return. Wages were extremely low, and many nurses with advanced academic education had to settle for room, board, and uniforms. This is the heritage and backbone of the kind of nurse who aided in mental healing in the first half of the 20th century.

DEVELOPMENTS IN PSYCHIATRIC NURSING SINCE 1946

Political and Legislative Developments

In the 1940s and 1950s, there were a series of political and legislative developments that significantly influenced the advancement of the psychiatric field in general and psychiatric nursing in particular.

The Mental Health Act of 1946 provided training and research funds and grants-in-aid to all the states for clinic and service components. In 1949, the National Institute of Mental Health was established to begin to identify and promote goals and priorities for the mental health field. During the early 1950s, public concern for the mentally ill continued to grow as the conditions of state mental hospitals were exposed.

In 1955, President Eisenhower signed into law the Mental Health Study Act, thus establishing a Joint Commission on Mental Health and Illness. The charge to the commission was to analyze and reevaluate the human and economic problems of mental illness and to make recommendations for action. After extensive analysis and evaluation of the needs and resources available to the mentally ill, in 1961 the Joint Commission published *Action for Mental Health*, which laid out the groundwork for the further development of national mental health policy. This report placed strong emphasis on community-based services by calling for a reduction in patient population through the closing of large state hospitals; the development of mental health services in local communities; and the upgrading of quality of care in the remaining state hospitals so that patients could be returned as quickly as possible to their own communities. The recommendations set into motion a major change in the mental health field and resulted in an emphasis on the development of community-based services as opposed to large, inpatient facilities as the locus of treatment. The main thrust of treatment was prevention-oriented, and federal regulations mandated that services be provided to large-catchment-area, population-defined, geographic groups. A full range of services was offered, including psychiatric nursing. Within this clinical atmosphere, nurses had considerable opportunities to implement new roles.

In 1963, President Kennedy signed into law the Community Mental Health Centers Act, which authorized monies for construction of community mental health centers. However, financial assistance to communities for the development of services was not provided until 1965 when Congress amended the Community Mental Health Centers Act to include initial staff grants for professional and nonprofessional personnel. It was proposed that staffing grants would be funded for a relatively short period of time (51 months). Theoretically, community mental health centers would be self-sufficient by the end of the staffing grant period. However, by the late 1960s, it was clear that the majority of the nation's community mental health centers would not be self-sufficient within the 51-month time frame. Therefore, Public Law 91–211 was passed by Congress in 1970 to extend the staffing grants for another eight years. Then, in 1975, the Congress amended PL 91–211 with PL 94–63, which authorized funds to create new community mental health centers and to continue existing centers.

The next major mental health legislation grew out of the 1978 *Report to the President from the President's Commission on Mental Health*. The report recommended the following: (1) the development throughout the country of mental health services that would be responsive to changing circumstances and to diverse cultural and racial backgrounds; (2) adequate funding from the public and private sector to finance services; (3) assurances that appropriately trained personnel would be made available; (4) provision of services for populations with special needs such as children, adolescents, and the elderly; (5) establishment of a national priority to meet the needs of the chronic mentally ill; (6) coordination of mental health services with other health and human service agencies and with personal and community support systems; (7) extension of the knowledge base with respect to treatment; (8) focus on the prevention of mental illness; and (9) assurances that freedom of choice is guaranteed.

The recommendations of the report were implemented through the Community Mental Health Centers Extension Act, which was signed into law by President Carter in 1978. This law addressed the recommendations of the Commission on Mental Health. In the interim came the election of a new president (Ronald Reagan) whose attitudes and policies regarding the funding mechanisms for social programs, including mental health, were vastly different from those of his predecessor. The Reagan Administration was committed to decentralizing the dispersement of funds, moving from a federal to a state level, and to increasing the involvement and financial commitment of the private sector to social programs. Consequently, the Community Mental Health Centers Extension Act of 1978 was never fully implemented.

This was a bitterly contested issue that included extensive lobbying efforts by mental health professionals and organizations, and finally the act was replaced by the Omnibus Reconciliation Act, which was signed into law by President Reagan in 1981. The Omnibus Reconciliation Act created a block grant mechanism for direct funding to states for the provision of mental health services, with considerable discretion left to the states as to how the funds were to be spent. In addition, the amount of financial support provided by the government for mental health services was reduced. This clearly reversed the strong federal governmental role in the provision of mental health services for the people of the nation, with the intent of strengthening state- and community-level commitment to its people.

Of all these various political and legislative developments between 1946 and the 1980s, of importance to psychiatric nursing is one of the recommendations made in the 1978 Commission report regarding who shall provide mental health services. The report clearly identified psychiatric nurses as fully recognized members of the interdisciplinary mental health team and stated that they should be eligible for third-party reimbursement for services.

Education of Nurses in Psychiatric Nursing

World War II profoundly affected psychiatric nursing. Nurses returning from service were eligible under the GI Bill for advanced education. The three existing graduate programs leading to a masters degree were unable to meet the demand. The passage of the National Mental Health Act of 1946, enacted in response to the overwhelming numbers of psychiatric casualties encountered both in selection of men for service and in response to combat, provided funds for graduate education in nursing, psychiatry, psychology, and social work. This funding influenced the scope and direction of nursing and psychiatric nursing education.[4] Instrumental in shifting the physician-directed psychiatric nursing practice toward the emergence of theory-based nursing practice were Theresa G. Muller and Hildegard Peplau. Muller was influential in obtaining recognition of nursing as the fourth professional discipline in mental health. She established four of the early programs leading to a masters degree in psychiatric nursing at Catholic University, Boston University, Indiana University, and the University of Nebraska. Her emphasis was on the need for graduate education and on interdisciplinary preparation as a means of establishing collaborative interdisciplinary practice. Clinical practice, rather than functional specialization, was a clear emphasis in these programs.[5,6]

Another major impetus for psychiatric nursing resulted from a study by the National League for Nursing in 1950, which concluded that special training was required for psychiatric nursing. This report coincided with the renewed interest in psychiatric care precipitated by World War II. The new legislation encouraged the nurse to fill a wide variety of roles, especially because there was a shortage of staff in the care of the mentally ill.

Doctoral Nursing Education

Doctoral education in nursing gained momentum in 1955 when the United States Public Health Service (NIH) initiated the Special Predoctoral Research Fellowships, which could be used to finance doctoral education. Fellowships were awarded directly to students. A second program, the Nurse Scientist Training Program, provided grants to schools of nursing. These funds were used to finance doctoral (Ph.D.) education of nurses in disciplines related to nursing. One intent of the program was to help build a core of faculty who would be prepared to develop doctoral programs in nursing. In 1960 there were only four programs; opportunities for nurses wanting to pursue doctoral study were truly scarce. Teachers College at Columbia University offered an Ed.D. in Nursing; this was the oldest and best established, having been started in the 1920s. The University of Pittsburgh established a Ph.D. program in 1954. In 1960, Boston University established a program that awarded the D.N.Sc. in psychiatric mental

health nursing, and New York University began offering a Ph.D. in Nursing. As predicted, the Special Predoctoral Fellowships and the Nurse Scientist Training Program were successful—both provided opportunities for education and financial support that had not been available previously. It is estimated that over 500 nurses received support through these programs. Two indicators of the success of these training programs, observes Nicoll, is that many of the nurses who received support through these programs have continued to be very active in nursing, contributing through research, practice and publication.[7] Second, a core of scholars were prepared to take on the task of developing doctoral programs in nursing. The task of implementing these programs is well underway at over 25 universities.

ANA and Councils of Practice

The American Nurses' Association (ANA), as the official organization of nursing, has many areas of responsibility as well as many varieties of functions. Of importance to this discussion are the specialities of practice within the ANA. Each speciality council establishes committees to conduct the work of that division, such as preparing a statement relevant to the practice for that council.

Statement on Practice
In 1967, the Division on Psychiatric and Mental Health Nursing practice published its first *Statement* on psychiatric nursing practice. This *Statement* has contributed greatly to the historical development of nursing practice and education. Between 1967 and 1974 the Executive Committee of the Division on Psychiatric and Mental Health Nursing appointed an ad hoc committee to revise the *Statement* in keeping with the contemporary scope and rule of practice. In particular, the three contemporary advances that have had the most impact on the mental health sector and the nursing profession were as follows:

1. The strong trend toward community-based, short-term treatment models, with a concomitant emphasis on de-institutionalization.
2. Emphasis on the assurance of quality care.
3. Significant developments in the arena of litigation and mental health services.

The ad hoc committee began the task of revision in January 1975 and published the revised *Statement on Psychiatric and Mental Health Nursing Practice* in 1976. Sections of this *Statement* will be reprinted in various sections of this text. Of particular importance to this section on the interrelationship of general nursing and psychiatric nursing are the following assumptions and principles[8]:

MENTAL HEALTH CARE AND NURSING: COMPONENTS OF COMPREHENSIVE HEALTH CARE*

Comprehensive health care is an intricate complex of services to individuals, families, and society. Its purposes encompass promotion and maintenance of health; prevention, detection, and treatment of illnesses; and restoration to the highest levels of health. A high degree of interdependence is inherent to health care: among the elements of service, in the relations between the disciplines, and with the public. Nursing contributes to virtually all aspects of the health care delivery system, inclusive of those services identified as mental health.

Current controversy about the proper role of the mental health system and its linkages with other health and social systems reflects the pervasive changes in this sector in recent years. Nursing practice reflects the belief that mental health is a critical and necessary component to health and to the fullest possible utilization of human potential. Nursing has particular responsibility to speak out on behalf of the public's need for holistic and humane services. Nurses have participated and will continue to participate in the recent trends away from custodial, inequitable, and fragmented services. Continuing evidence of unresolved problems, especially in environmental conditions and discontinuities in service which violate human dignity, impel nurses to work more effectively as consumer advocates.

Accountability for professional practice recognizes the public's right of access to needed services and the freedom to choose among alternatives. That same principle requires that the mental health disciplines define the legitimate scope of their authority and expertise through discipline-specific and collaborative means.

Standards of Practice

The ANA Division on Psychiatric and Mental Health Nursing Practice, through its Executive Committee and the Standards Committee, revised the 1973 *Standards of Psychiatric-Mental*

---

* Reprinted with permission from American Nurses' Association, Kansas City, Mo.

Health Nursing Practice in 1982. Sixteen standards were formulated and will be reprinted in this text under the appropriate topic area. The purpose of the *Standards* is to fulfill the profession's obligation to provide a means of improving the quality of care. The *Standards* reflect the current state of knowledge in the field and are therefore subject to testing and subsequent change. Since *Standards* represent agreed-upon levels of practice, they have been developed to characterize, to measure, and to provide guidance in achieving excellence in care.

A rationale is provided for each standard, and criteria are developed to measure each standard. The criteria are divided into *structure, process*, and *outcome*. They are intended to provide a means by which attainment of the standard may be specifically measured. The criteria for each standard are not exhaustive.

THE EVOLUTION OF THE PSYCHIATRIC NURSE'S ROLE

The identity of psychiatric nurses, as viewed by themselves as well as by others, was clearest when it was most circumscribed. This role was the custodial nurse of earlier days, or the manager of the milieu, the 24-hour-a-day nurturant figure, and the executor of physicians' orders of recent days. Essentially the traditional role was that of a secondary, supportive service provider within the context of the administrative and status hierarchy of the mental hospital or inpatient service of a general hospital.[9]

As opportunities for diverse roles have multiplied, the professional identity of the psychiatric nurse has become blurred. In community mental health settings and programs, the psychiatric nurse has been required or allowed to assume many of the services of a primary service practitioner. As Ellen Davis and E. Mansell Pattison state:

The tasks and functions of psychiatric nurses in community mental health are often indistinguishable from those performed by the psychologist, social worker, and with few exceptions, the psychiatrist. Thus, role diffusion is quite outstanding in the case of the psychiatric nurse.[10]

Questions now before the profession, questions that nurses must ask themselves, are: (1) whether in some of their contemporary roles they are different from social workers, psychologists, or psychiatrists; (2) whether there is an "essence" to psychiatric nursing regardless of their role; and (3) whether psychiatric nursing should retreat to a unitary, more clearly defined role.

Shirley Smoyak, a family therapist and nurse-educator, effectively addressed the question of whether the psychiatric nurse should return to an older unitary role. She observed that when nurses were educated to be deferent, self-effacing subordinates who react rather than create or initiate, they contributed little to the psychiatric nursing literature. However, today one has only to review current journals and book reviews to see an increase in nursing contributions to the professional literature over the past decade.[11]

In a study conducted by Davis and Pattison on the roles of the regional mental health nurses in Orange County, California, it was learned that the nurses who were psychiatric mental health nurse specialists functioned with a high degree of independence. They provided the following activities: assessing the nature of the person's pathology and evaluating the need of the person for crisis intervention, outpatient treatment, or hospitalization; writing a psychiatric evaluation of the person's conditions; recommending court-ordered hospitalization when the individual would not voluntarily accept treatment; testifying in court; providing psychiatric nursing services to individuals at home; providing aftercare for patients discharged from state institutions; assisting individuals and families in carrying out physician's orders; conducting individual and group therapy; assisting with vocational and social rehabilitation; meeting with community organizations and workers in other agencies; and prompting an exchange of information about mental health.[12]

The problem of role differentiation among the four mental health professions of psychiatric nursing, social work, psychology, and psychiatry is a difficult one. All four groups are attempting to deal with their own professional identity crises by attempting to rediscover their historical roots, discover their natural expertise, and define their boundaries and areas of overlap. Before the community mental health movement, the professionals traditionally operated within narrowly defined roles. As Davis and Pattison state:

The physician diagnosed and treated the patient; the social worker worked with the client's relatives and social agencies; the psychologist "tested" and hopefully confirmed the doctor's diagnosis; and the nurse nursed, for example, provided custodial and maintenance services for the patient. In the closed system of the hospital, the stereotype of the nurse's role was most fixed.[13]

The *Statement on Psychiatric and Mental Health Nursing Practice* also speaks to the commonalities shared by the psychiatric disciplines.

Because by their nature comprehensive mental health services require the participation of more than one discipline, psychiatric and mental health nursing is practiced largely in collaboration and coordination with a variety of other professions working with and on behalf of the client. Some overlapping of roles and shared functions among the psychiatric disciplines are to be expected. This is attributable, in part, to mental health theory and methods currently available, and also to the increasing demands of a more sophisticated public for access to mental health services as a right. Nurses participate in planning and evaluation of interdisciplinary care so as to make the most effective use of and foster the expansion of health care team knowledge and skills.

An example of an activity shared among all disciplines occurs in the use of the guided verbal exchange in assisting patients to resolve their problems. This major intervention technique is represented by goal-directed conversations, group sessions, counseling, psychotherapy, and psychoanalysis. Effective use of this technique, or other modalities of treatment, is dependent upon the competence of the worker, her/his qualifications of education and experience, the established policies of the health care facility, and the availability of qualified personnel.

All disciplines in the mental health field have access to the same body of knowledge on which professional education and improvement of practice are based. Free, reciprocal exchange of knowledge among disciplines reflects a mature commitment and capacity for collaboration. The individual nurse's continued professional development through education and experience enhances the ability to contribute knowledge to patient care. Registered nurses qualified by education and experience for supervisory and administrative functions may well assume leadership in interdisciplinary patient care and in staff development programs. As new nursing knowledge and practice develop, nurses are responsible for keeping others informed, including professional colleagues, employers, and consumers.[14]

With the advent of role dysfunction in all mental health disciplines, each group is struggling with its own identity. Psychiatry, for example, in its rediscovery of its biologic/medical roots, is making considerable strides in developing reliable diagnostic criteria, in understanding the biologic mechanisms for the major mental disorders, in studying the interface between neurology and psychiatry, and in developing expertise in organic differential diagnosis of psychiatric symptoms.

Some elements of a nursing identity can be inferred from our previous discussion of nursing theory and nursing research. This identity has been made explicit in the *Statement on Psychiatric and Mental Health Nursing Practice* by the ANA Division on Psychiatric and Mental Health Nursing Practice:[15]

Psychiatric and mental health nursing, like all other specialties in nursing, has discrete as well as shared functions for which it is responsible to society. The major distinguishing characteristic of psychiatric and mental health nursing practice derives from the synthesis of knowledge and experience of both nursing and mental health. Chronologically, the professional nurse first acquires a generic base in the theory and practice of nursing which then provides the continuing substrate for the development and use of the more specialized competencies in mental health. Aspects of nursing which support the distinctive contributions of nurses to comprehensive mental health care include:

1. Nursing's commitment to holistic and continuous personal care of individuals, founded on theory and clinical practice, which utilizes content from the social, biological, and physical sciences;
2. Nursing's primary focus on helping persons attain their highest possible level of health, which includes but transcends traditional illness orientations;
3. Nursing's integration of content and experience related to both the medical and social systems models in the conduct of its clinical practice and research;
4. The use of the nursing process as the dominant modality, involving systematic and identifiable steps which must be accounted for, professionally, in terms of quality.

Contemporary Dimensions of Role

At various times nursing has been depicted as a series of tasks and technology (e.g., a subset of medicine); as a broad, compassionate, and supportive human service; and as a science of human health and behavior across the life-span. This last conceptualization includes understanding of the biologic, behavioral, social, and cultural factors in health and illness and the definition of health outcomes and indicators of health status.[16]

Psychiatric Nurse as Clinician

From the sensitivity and exploration of a one-to-one relationship, the psychiatric nurse of today has gained the ability to explore both in depth and scope the power of relationship and communication in the total healing and health maintenance process. Thus the psychiatric nurse is engaged not only in interesting and involving work with individuals and their problems, but also with individuals and larger groups who are concerned with maintaining and protecting positive mental health. Psychiatric nurses are actively involved in innovative efforts at the three levels of nursing practice: primary preventive intervention, secondary preventive intervention, and tertiary preventive intervention. In the area of primary intervention, we find for example psychiatric nurses involved in educational programs directed at helping children to protect themselves. The scope of psychiatric nursing involvement in the area of secondary preventive intervention is extensive, from nurses setting up crisis teams, to psychiatric nurses using home visits to help family members who are coping with illness or devastating tragedies such as natural disasters.

In tertiary intervention, nurses are active in the community in such projects as arranging for housing for the homeless, developing volunteer soup kitchens for the homeless, and working with self-help groups to pass active legislation to protect the interests of severely mentally ill and retarded people.

A major advancement has been the participation by psychiatric mental health nurses in the private practice model of health care delivery and entering the competitive arena for third-party reimbursement. In many states, psychiatric nurses are now reimbursed through the patient's insurance benefits.

Psychiatric Nurse as Researcher

Nursing research has long been considered an integral part of nursing practice. Nursing research is critical to all subspecialty areas in nursing. Of importance here is *Standard XI*, which specifically emphasizes the importance of research in nursing.[17]

As McBride observes, an era of intense research and theory development is unfolding.[18] The speciality of psychiatric mental health nursing has contributed significantly to the present maturity of the nursing profession and there is every reason to believe that we will continue to be on the cutting edge.

Practice-based research has been a dominant method of psychiatric nursing research. The 1950s witnessed dramatic progress in the field of psychiatric nursing. Gwen Tudor Will reported her study on psychosocial nursing in an inpatient hospital setting. The thesis of the Tudor article in 1952 was that the social milieu of a psychiatric ward operated to maintain deviant patient behavior. While working with sociologists over a six-month period exploring the social dimension of psychiatric care, Tudor observed that a discrete pattern of mutual avoidance emerged between the staff and a female patient. After making notes of her observation,

Tudor initiated her intervention. Gradually she began to disrupt the pattern of withdrawal in response to this woman by initiating conversation with her, moving closer to her, and eventually engaging her in activity. Not only did her pattern with the woman change, but so did the response of other staff members and patients. To test her concept of "mutuality" with regard to social withdrawal, Tudor supervised a nursing student's intervention with this patient, reversing the pattern of withdrawal. The study's importance was in challenging the notion that social withdrawal was a sign of mental illness. It now was seen as a behavior sensitive to the social context in its development and maintenance, which emphasized the critical role of the nurse in manager of the social milieu of the ward environment.[19]

STANDARD XI
Research

The nurse contributes to nursing and the mental health field through innovations in theory and practice and participation in research.

RATIONALE

Each professional has responsibility for the continuing development and refinement of knowledge in the mental health field through research and experimentation with new and creative approaches to practice.

STRUCTURE CRITERIA

1. Formal opportunities exist for nurses to conduct and/or participate in research at appropriate educational levels.
2. Mechanisms ensure protection of human rights.

PROCESS CRITERIA

The nurse—

1. approaches nursing practice with an inquiring and open mind.
2. utilizes research findings in practice.
3. develops, implements, and evaluates research studies as appropriate to level of education.
4. uses responsible standards of research in investigative endeavors.
5. ensures that a mechanism for the protection of human subjects exists.
6. obtains expert consultation and/or supervision as required.

OUTCOME CRITERION

The nurse has published contributions to theory, practice, and research.

Gertrude Schwing's *The Way to the Soul of the Mentally Ill* became available to nurses in the United States (after translation) in 1954. Schwing emphasized the mother surrogate role and corrective nurturing experience in the rehabilitation of severely disturbed patients. Sechehaye also addressed the symbolic meaning of language and nonverbal behavior with patients. Her work demonstrates the power of human communication in treating the mentally ill.

Reviewing psychiatric nursing's clinical contributions beginning with the one-to-one relationship, we discover how the nurses' presence took on meaning that helped people get themselves and their lives into focus. As Judith Krauss observes, psychiatric nursing's roots lie in the relationship of caring.[21] One milestone was Hildegard Peplau's work defining the importance of interpersonal relations in nursing. The work of Peplau emphasized how the nurse worked with a client to gain reasoned control and flexibility over unreasonable thoughts and experiences.[22] Other nurses continued to expand on these concepts; one such was Dorothy Gregg, who discussed reassurance and the role of the psychiatric nurse.[23]

In an excellent analysis and report on the development of a conceptual base for psychiatric nursing, clinician Suzanne Lego cites the three theoretical frameworks of Hildegard Peplau, June Mellow, and Ida Jean Orlando as being the most influential in the field.[24] Peplau's interpersonal relations framework has had the most far-reaching impact. This framework draws heavily from Harry Stack Sullivan's interpersonal theory and, to a lesser degree, from learning theory. In essence, the framework provides a system within which the nurse helps the patient to examine situational factors, with the focus on improving interpersonal competencies that have been lost or never learned. Peplau emphasizes the following steps: observing behavior, describing and analyzing the behavior with the nurse, formulating the connections noted, testing, and integrating new behavior. In addition Peplau describes the importance of the nurse assessing her own interpersonal behavior as it affects the therapeutic relationship, the work roles of the psychiatric nurse, and the phases of the nurse–patient relationship.[25]

June Mellow's theoretical framework, called nursing therapy, was derived from work with schizophrenic patients in an intensive one-to-one relationship.[26] Nursing therapy as a clinical specialty within psychiatric nursing was first introduced into the professional literature in 1953. This approach to psychiatric treatment involves intensive therapy by a graduate nurse working with a emotionally disturbed patient. The concern of nursing therapy is with giving the patient an opportunity to participate in a corrective emotional experience in order to facilitate the integration of his overwhelmed ego.

The work of nursing therapy is divided into two phases: the experiential phase and the clinically investigative phase. Initially, the work of nursing therapy took place in the experiential phase. This incorporated and emphasized the advantages of the traditional aspects of the role of the psychiatric nurse. Specifically, the concern was with such factors as living through highly charged emotional experiences with the patient, sharing everyday human interchange with him, setting limits, providing controls, satisfying regressive needs, providing an identification figure, and providing therapeutic punishments. The emphasis was on sharing experiences rather than hearing about them from the patient after they occurred. The goals were aimed at resolution of the acute phase of the illness as a preparation for long-term psychotherapy with the psychiatrist.

The work of nursing therapy then broadened to include the clinically investigative phase. In this phase, the needs of the patient shift to gaining insight into his personality structure and to developing mastery over his conflicts. The nurse needs to be prepared to cope with transference phenomena and to use skills similar to those needed for psychoanalytic psychotherapy. Mellow's work articulated the process in which the nurse participates and creates an experiential mode of restoring people lost to their internal processes, terrified and alone. The Mellow framework was used as the core clinical component of the Boston University Doctor of Nursing Science program in 1960 to 1966.

Ida Jean Orlando's theory of the dynamic nurse–patient relationship appeared in the literature in 1961. Orlando describes her theory in terms of the nurse observing the patient's need or distress and helping him to "express the specific meaning of his behavior in order to ascertain the help he requires so that his distress may be relieved."[27] Additionally, the nurse is encouraged to explore her observations or reactions with the patient.

It has been demonstrated in psychiatric mental health nursing that the quality of care will improve as the scientific base for practice is strengthened. One task of the research movement is to disseminate research findings to other nurses. Research reporting has shown improvement in two areas. First is the strengthening of writing itself. In a study comparing the scientific rigor of published psychiatric and mental health nursing research between 1970 and 1985, results suggest that research articles are more likely to be published in clinical rather than research journals, study is more likely to be conducted in fulfillment of an academic degree, the author is more likely than in earlier years to be a nurse with higher academic degrees, and the article is better written, with more sophistication in study design and execution.[28] The second area of improvement is the trend away from the publication of research results only in general research journals (e.g., *Nursing Research, Research in Nursing and Health, Western Journal of Nursing Research*) to its becoming an integral part of specialty journals (*Journal of Psychosocial Nursing, Issues in Mental Health, Perspectives on Psychiatric Care, Archives of Psychiatric Nursing*).

With the strengthening of the research process, McBride predicts a shift in focus over time from isolated pieces of research to a program of research.[29] The nurse researcher will be building on her own work and faculty will build on the strengths and resources of their institution. This notion has been encouraged and supported by the Division of Nursing, U.S. Department of Health and Human Services, through the concept of cluster grants.

McBride also recommends that the character of the research done by psychiatric mental health nurses be changed in certain ways.[30] First, there should be focusing on the development of large data bases; there needs to be concern with evaluation research; and there should be a connection between research and policy making. Also, according to McBride, there needs to be emphasis on the phenomena of concern, e.g., human response to mental health problems. With the implementation of programs of research, there will be needed state-of-the-art conferences where the findings of several researchers converge.[31]

A COALITION FOR PSYCHIATRIC NURSING ORGANIZATIONS

As we move into the last decade of the 20th century, there are efforts to make psychiatric nursing stronger within the total nursing arena. At the invitation of Patricia C. Pothier, chairperson of the ANA Council on Psychiatric and Mental Health Nursing (PMHN), the leadership of each of the four national psychiatric nursing organizations met at ANA headquarters on June 10, 1987.

The purpose of the meeting was to explore how the four organizations (ANA Council on PMHN, American Psychiatric Nursing Association [APNA], Society for Education and Research in Psychiatric Nursing [SERPN], and Advocates for Child Psychiatric Nursing [ACPN]) could work together for the advancement of psychiatric and mental health nursing. Specific goals were: (1) to identify common goals, areas of overlap, and specific differences in goals and interests; and (2) to explore mechanisms for continued collaboration with the National Institute on Mental Health.

Each of the groups affirmed the need and desire for cooperative efforts. Through discussion the groups were able to identify common, differing, and overlapping areas of concern.

The ANA was recognized as the major body responsible for regulation of nursing practice. ANA was also the organization identified with the resources to provide policy leadership for all nursing and support of the more specific goals of psychiatric nursing.

APNA was recognized for its focus on the provision of continuing education to its members. In addition, APNA regularly produces and distributes a comprehensive psychiatric nursing publication.

SERPN concentrates on activities related to the interface of education and research in psychiatric nursing and works in the area of political advocacy.

ACPN places emphasis on practice issues related to children, adolescents, and their families. ACPN also addresses advocacy concerns for professional education of child psychiatric nurses.

These major goals were viewed as separate, yet complementary to the needs of psychiatric nursing. It was also recognized that each group might engage in policy activity and political advocacy related to its unique goals. However, each group will apprise the others and seek their support in regard to policy activity so that psychiatric nursing can speak with "one voice" on issues of common concern and thereby gain strength from the support of collective numbers.

The leaders agreed to take to their executive

boards the following proposal for consideration: that an annual meeting of the four psychiatric nursing organizations' leaders (two representatives from each) be held in conjunction with a regularly scheduled annual meeting of one of the participating organizations, and that this collaborative mechanism be designated the Coalition of Psychiatric Nursing Organizations (COPNO).

The goal of COPNO meetings would be to explore issues of mutual concern and to plan jointly sponsored initiatives. The responsibility for these meetings would rotate among the organizations on an annual basis. In addition, ongoing communication between the groups would be implemented by telephone conference calls as issues arose during the year. The coalition would share informational materials such as newsletters, publications, and minutes on a regular and timely basis.

The openness of discussion by these leaders and the tentative agreement on future direction clearly indicated that the time had come for this type of collaboration. The coalition leaders agreed to strive to promote quality psychiatric nursing practice and to endeavor to keep psychiatric nursing on the cutting edge of the profession.[32]

In summary, psychiatric mental health nursing research is fast gaining momentum. There are new and innovative nursing issues to be studied: the concept of focused care; respite care; the chronically mentally ill; short-term hospitalizations; work with children, adolescents, and the elderly. There need to be testing of the psychiatric nursing taxonomy, confirmation of a comprehensive approach to patient care, and development of a nursing practice model that concurrently evaluates the efficacy of psychiatric nursing interventions.

Summary

This chapter has reviewed the historical roots of the nursing care of the mentally ill. Various external forces, including legislative and economic factors, have provided the necessary momentum for psychiatric nursing to continue to develop into its current profile. Two important documents for psychiatric-mental health nursing practice are described in this chapter, (1) *Statement on Psychiatric and Mental Health Nursing Practice* and (2) *Standards of Psychiatric and Mental Health Nursing Practice*, and will continue to be implemented throughout this text.

Questions

1. Who defines and regulates the standards and statement on psychiatric mental health nursing practice?
2. How do psychiatric nursing and general nursing relate to each other?
3. Compare and contrast the development of psychiatric nursing with the development of nursing research.
4. What are the similarities and differences between the four psychiatric disciplines of psychiatry, psychology, social work, and psychiatric nursing?
5. How do you view the current and future role of the psychiatric nurse?

REFERENCES AND
SUGGESTED READINGS

1. Nightingale, F. *Notes on Nursing: What It Is and What It Is Not*. Philadelphia: Lippincott, 1946. (Originally published, 1859.)
2. Cook, E. *Life of Florence Nightingale*. London: 1913.
3. Doona, M. E. *Travelbee's Intervention in Psychiatric Nursing* (2nd ed.). Philadelphia: Davis, 1978, p. 261.
4. Critchley, D. L. Evolution of the role. In D. L. Critchley & J. T. Maurin (Eds.), *The Clinical Specialist in Psychiatric Mental Health Nursing*. New York: Wiley, 1985, pp. 12–13.
5. Muller, T. G. *The Nature and Direction of Psychiatric Nursing: The Dynamics of Human Relationships*. Philadelphia: Lippincott, 1950.
6. Johnston, R. L., & Fitzpatrick, J. J. Relevance of psychiatric mental health nursing theories to nursing models. In J. Fitzpatrick, A. Whall, R. Johnston, & J. Floyd (Eds.), *Nursing Models and their Psychiatric Mental Health Applications*. Bowie, Md.: Brady, 1982, pp. 1–15.
7. Nicoll, L. H. Three landmark symposia. In L. H. Nicoll (Ed.), *Perspectives on Nursing Theory*. Boston: Little, Brown, 1986, pp. 91–92.
8. American Nurses' Association, Division on Psychiatric and Mental Health Nursing Practice. *Statement of Psychiatric and Mental Health Nursing Practice*. Kansas City, Mo.: American Nurses' Association, 1976. p. 1.
9. Davis, E. D., & Pattison, E. M. The psychiatric nurse's role identity. *American Journal of Nursing*, 1979, *79*, 298.
10. Ibid.
11. Smoyak, S. Family therapy. In F. L. Huey (Ed.), *Psychiatric Nursing: 1946–1974: A Report of the State of the Art*. New York: American Journal of Nursing Co., 1975.
12. Davis & Pattison, op. cit.
13. Ibid., p. 299.
14. American Nurses' Association, op. cit., pp. 3–4.
15. Ibid., p. 4.
16. Gortner, S. The history and philosophy of nursing science and research. *Advances in Nursing Science*, 1983, *5*(2), 289.
17. American Nurses' Association, Division on Psychiatric and Mental Health Nursing. *Standards of Psychiatric-Mental Health Nursing Practice*. Kansas City, Mo.: American Nurses' Association, 1982.
18. McBride, A. B. Theory and research: Present issues and future perspectives on psychosocial nursing. *Journal of Psychosocial Nursing and Mental Health Services*, 1986, *24*(9), 31.
19. Tudor, G. E. A sociopsychiatric nursing approach to intervention in a problem of mutual withdrawal on a mental hospital ward. *Psychiatry*, 1952, *15*, 190–195.
20. Schwing, G. [*A Way to the Soul of the Mentally Ill*] (R. Edstein & B. H. Hall, trans.). New York: International Universities Press, 1954.
21. Krauss, J. B. Nursing madness and mental health. *Archives of Psychiatric Nursing*, 1987, *1*(1), 3–15.
22. Peplau, H. *Interpersonal Relations in Nursing*. New York: Putnam's, 1952.
23. Gregg, D. Reassurance. *American Journal of Nursing*, 1955, *55*, 171.
24. Lego, S. Psychiatric nursing: Theory and practice of the one-to-one nurse–client relationship. In F. L. Huey (Ed.), *Psychiatric Nursing: 1946–1974: A Report of the State of the Art*. New York: American Journal of Nursing Co., 1975.
25. Peplau, op. cit.
26. Mellow, J. Nursing therapy as a treatment and clinical investigative approach to emotional illness. *Nursing Forum*, 1966 *5*(3), 64.
27. Orlando, I. J. *The Dynamic Nurse–Patient Relationship*. New York: Putnam's, 1961.
28. McBride, op. cit.
29. Ibid.
30. Ibid.
31. Ibid.
32. Pothier, P. C. Coalition of psychiatric nursing organizations proposed. *Pacesetter*, 1987, *14*(5), 1.

Chapter 12

Assessment Protocols in Psychiatric Mental Health Nursing Practice

Ann Wolbert Burgess and Carol R. Hartman

Chapter Objectives

The students successfully attaining the goals of this chapter will be able to:

- Identify three types of assessment in psychiatric mental health nursing practice.
- Employ the nursing assessment process in patient care situations.
- Describe the essential components of the patient's perspective.
- Identify the purpose of the three types of assessment.
- Assess a patient's family network through the use of a genogram.
- Interpret Standard IV of the ANA Standards of Psychiatric Mental Health Nursing Practice.

This chapter describes the entry of the patient into the mental health care system and the first stage of the nursing process, assessment of the patient. Three types of assessment are presented: (1) the patient's request; (2) the nursing assessment for functional status; and (3) the psychiatric assessment for mental status. The patient's request provides information about the circumstances that brought the individual to seek mental health attention. The nursing assessment for functional status provides a way for the nurse and the patient to become oriented to each other while eliciting information preliminary to arriving at nursing diagnoses supporting positive mental health. The psychiatric assessment provides information about the presence or absence of psychiatric symptomatology for consideration of a DSM-III-R diagnosis.

While we recognize that nursing students and beginning level nurses may not be conducting all three types of assessment of patients they care for, it is important to know the content, rationale, and outcome of each assessment protocol. A generalist-level nurse will use aspects of the formal psychiatric assessment for assessing side effects for symptoms, reality orientation, impulse control, defensive styles, and character traits that are relevant to ongoing behavior in the milieu environment. Nurses who are working as the primary psychotherapist in a clinical setting will combine the patient's request and the patient's functional and mental status into a complete report that will guide and direct therapy and provide input to the generalist nursing team for the 24-hour care of the client. The patient's request assessment is a useful technique to use periodically with patients to ensure that their needs are of first concern.

The process of assessing begins the nursing process as the systematic ordering of the steps that provide the organizational structure for nursing practice. These steps form the basis for the *Standards of Psychiatric Mental Health Nursing Practice* as described by the American Nurses' Association Division on Psychiatric and Mental Health Nursing Practice.[1] These steps include the conceptual framework for patient care, the assessment of the patient's status, the nursing diagnosis, the plan for nursing action, the implementation of the plan, and the evaluation of nursing care (Table 12-1). For optimal care, these sequential steps are used concurrently and recurrently in nursing practice.

ASSESSMENT AND DATA COLLECTION

The purpose of the first step of the nursing process, assessment, is to collect data on the functional health status of the patient in order to make a formulation and nursing diagnosis of the health concerns and problems. The nurse uses such skills as observing, encouraging the patient to talk, listening, and keeping the interview focused on collecting essential data.

Data are collected from the patient, the family, the physician, the psychologist, the social networks (which include extended family, neighbors, and significant people), and the

health care team. The format for collecting the necessary information on the person and his reason for seeking care may be decided on by the individual nurse or by the admission team. Data may be obtained from a formal interview, informal observation, medical records, or by talking with family and health team members.

The Individual Nurse

In many cases, the nurse is the first staff member a patient sees after admission to an inpatient unit. At this time the assessment and plans for initial care are made. In the community, a patient may present himself at a mental health clinic and the interview between the nurse and patient takes place there. Home visits by nurses often provide clinically rich data.

The Admission Team

In some mental health settings, the initial assessment interview(s) is conducted by a staff member, and then the admission team meets to discuss the data and plan the care. The team may consist of the nurse, psychiatrist, social worker, psychologist, mental health workers, occupational therapist, and students.

Some of the goals of the admission team are to prepare the family to work with social service, to communicate the agency's concern for family problems (financial, child-rearing), and to allow the patient to participate in decisions. The team also presents precisely what the hospital can do. This action minimizes the fear of the patient and family that the treatment is forever or indefinite. Other useful goals of the team conference

TABLE 12-1. SEQUENTIAL STEPS OF THE PSYCHIATRIC MENTAL HEALTH NURSING PROCESS

Conceptual Framework	Assessment	Nursing Diagnosis	Planning	Implementing	Evaluation
Patient request Functional health status Mental status	Data collection from: Patient Family Health team Social network	Analysis of assessment areas and prioritizing of health problems	Patient request Long-term goals Short-term goals Outcome criteria Nursing actions	Implementing planned nursing actions Observing patient response	Evaluating outcome Criteria

are to evaluate the suicidal, destructive, or regressive potential of the patient and to determine to what extent the family can exercise control or to what extent the family is unable to manage the deviant behavior.

ENTRY INTO THE MENTAL HEALTH SYSTEM

The act of bringing a mental health problem to the attention of clinicians sets into motion a series of procedures established either by the institution or by the professional. Entering into an authority system of any type, such as general health, mental health, or criminal or civil justice, is stressful for people because they are not familiar with the set procedures. People are very often (1) swept along by the day-to-day workings of the agency; (2) caught up in the protocol that is routine to the clinicians since it constitutes their daily work but new to the clients and thus not fully understood by them; and (3) questioned extensively about their reasons for coming into the system. These things may not be done exactly against a person's will, especially since consent forms are usually part of the agency policies, but more may be done than the patient ever bargained for. Thus, it becomes especially important to learn how people enter the mental health system and their perspective in terms of requests and goals in order to continually address patient care according to a humanistic view.

How the Person Comes for Help

How is the decision made for the person to come to the hospital or clinic? How does he finally come to the attention of the physician or nurse? People arriving for psychiatric care come by various ways. For example:

A 19-year-old boy arrived at the emergency room of a general hospital asking to be admitted to the psychiatric unit because he felt depressed and had suicidal thoughts. He had come to the hospital after asking the police for assistance. The police, believing that the young man might kill himself, drove him to the hospital. This person did not ask his parents to bring him, but he did not come alone. He felt the police would help. They did. The way in which this person

came for help is the significant point: he sought out the police, an authority figure, a symbol of limit-setting, perhaps even a symbol of punishment.

A 16-year-old male arrived at the psychiatric unit of a general hospital on a stretcher. Although he was visibly agitated and shaking, he kept saying, "I'm all right." His parents were with him. He needed both physical assistance and his parents to come with him to the hospital. The way in which this patient came for help is the significant point: he sought out a community service, the ambulance service, and his parents to bring him to the hospital. For some reason the parents were unable to manage their son themselves in order to bring him for help.

A 21-year-old arrived at a state hospital accompanied by her father, her boyfriend, and her parish priest. This young woman came for help with three males: one from her family network, one from her peer group, and one from a community group. The significant point is that this young woman sought out males rather than females, males with different roles and different symbolic meanings, when she was in distress and also included members from her total social network group.

The Patient's Perspective on the Problem

When people are asked why they came to the hospital or clinic, their first words often tell more about them than the several paragraphs that follow. For example, when the person says, "I am here because my father said I had to come," the person is saying that he is here because his problem was uncomfortable for his father, not because it was primarily distressful to himself.

As indicated in the above example, many people have been advised or convinced that they should come to a hospital. The family physician, a psychiatrist, or a community agency such as the police, school, or court may be responsible for advising the person to seek psychiatric help. The person may be relieved to be in the hospital; he may be indifferent; or he may be angry and resentful. Many acutely psychotic people who do not see the need for hospitalization are brought in. They say, "I don't need to be here. I'm not sick."

Other reasons for a person being advised to seek help are: "It was more my wife's request than anything else." "I'm here to appease my family." "I'm here because my brother beat me and took me to the cop station. They found tracks on my arms and took me to a doctor and the cops took me to the hospital.'' Or take the following example:

A 16-year-old male is admitted because his behavior is a problem to his foster parents. His problems revolve around his being truant from school and because he feels suppressed by his foster parents in regard to the friends he can choose and the outside activities he can participate in. He had a bad experience with marijuana in which he misinterpreted a water tank as a flying saucer. He resents baby-sitting for his foster brothers and sisters and says that they do not mind him. He says, ''I feel like killing them.''

Some patients seek hospitalization because of a control issue. In the above example, the 16-year-old was expressing a need for controls, although this was not his reason for coming to the hospital; his foster parents brought him to the hospital because they felt unable to control him and were advised by the family physician to do so. When people who have difficulty controlling their thoughts, feelings, and actions are admitted to the psychiatric unit, they might say: ''I lit a fire in the school trash can.'' ''I felt there was something wrong with me. Mostly I had the feeling of wanting to kill myself.'' ''I took an overdose of sleeping pills and my roommate found me.''

Some people seek hospitalization because they are looking for protection and comfort in exchange for the noxious environment in which they are currently living. On admission, these people might say: ''I was afraid of my husband. Because my fear was so great, I wanted to be safe for the night.'' ''I had to get away from the family bickering and my father's beating me. I couldn't stand it any longer. I was going out of my mind.'' ''I need a rest physically and mentally and wanted to survive without sleeping pills at night.''

Some people come to the hospital requesting help because they perceive the hospital as a place to obtain help for psychiatric symptoms. These people realize that they have psychic distress and will say: ''I was depressed; I was running in circles and had to stop.'' ''I felt sick and strange.'' ''I think people are watching me.'' ''I feel I am mentally ill.''

Some people perceive they are having emotional difficulties, but they state their reasons for being in the hospital in terms of a specific problem to be solved. These people might say: ''I have a drug problem.'' ''I need help in talking to people.'' ''I want to cut down on my medi-

cation to determine the cause of my stomach ailment and headaches.''

The Patient's Perspective on Mental Health Care

For many years such mental health professionals as Sigmund Freud, Kurt Lewin, and Herbert Maslow studied the concept of human need. These men were scientists investigating specific human problems; they did not necessarily attempt to meet the needs of people they were studying.

For the past several decades, however, meeting patients' needs has been a major goal of psychiatric nursing in planning patient care. Nurses have been putting the concepts and theories into practice. Ida Orlando Pellitier, a nurse-clinician, describes the development of treatment methods based on the hypothesis that satisfaction of needs leads to mental stability and that dissatisfaction of needs leads to mental instability.[2] For the most part, however, what the patient has ''needed'' has been determined by the professionals' clinical judgment rather than by direct verbal response from the patient. The *Standards of Psychiatric and Mental Health Nursing Practice* address this neglected area of planning patient care in Standard IV, which emphasizes the importance of client input in the assessment, planning, implementation, and evaluation of the nursing care program.[3]

The Patient's Request

Patients, in most situations, know how they would like to feel and how they hope the professional can help them to achieve this end. However, because patients may be afraid of being disappointed or being made to feel ridiculous, they seldom relate their expectations to the professional. Consequently, the professional often assumes that patients do not know what they want. For this reason it is important for nurses to demonstrate their concern for their patients and continually to ask questions to find out what the patients really want. This strategy is based on the assumption that patients know how they would like the nurse to help and that the nurse can be more effective by learning the patient's requests.

It is important to distinguish between patient request, patient complaint, and patient goal. Sometimes nurses think they know the request after hearing or reading in the chart the patient's chief complaint. The complaint is the patient's initial statement as to what is bothering him, for instance, "I am in pain." The goal is what the patient would like to accomplish or how he would like to feel, for instance, "I would like to feel well enough to be able to work." The request is how the patient would like the nurse to respond to help him achieve the desired goal. He might request medical intervention: "Give me some medicine for the pain." He might request clarification: "Help me understand why I am having this pain." He might make an administrative request: "Would you write a letter to my employer that I am ill?"

In the studies of how well clinicians elicit these three data points (request, complaint, goal), it has been found that the complaint is invariably elicited, the goal is usually elicited, but the request is often not elicited.[4] In such situations, the negotiation process will be seriously impaired if the nurse does not know the patient request.

Research on patient requests has been conceptualized from various population groups. One research project was led by Aaron Lazare, who with a clinical research team set out to learn from patients at the Massachusetts General Walk-In Psychiatric Clinic what they wanted from the professionals who were there to serve them. From the analysis of several hundred interviews, patients' requests were classified into fourteen categories as follows.[5]

Administrative Request

The patient is seeking administrative or legal assistance from the clinic to help him with his current dilemma. The specific request may be to provide a disability evaluation, a medical excuse to leave work, a medical permission to return to work, permission to drive, admission to a hospital, or testimony in court. The power to grant or deny these requests is delegated by society to particular professionals or institutions. The power may be subsequently rescinded, or, as in the case of therapeutic abortions, may no longer be necessary.

Advice

The patient wants guidance about what to do in personal or social matters. He may already have formed an opinion, but he now wants professional advice. He wants to know the "right" thing, the "best" thing, or the "wisest" thing to do. He may want the advice in order to have the clinician share the responsibility for a decision he is about to make.

Clarification

The patient wants help to put his feelings, thoughts, or behavior in perspective. He does not want to be told what to do but would rather take an active role in the therapeutic process. Often, the patient wants help so that he can make a decision himself. He wants to understand; he wants to see his choices. The patient usually sees his problem as being acute and not a part of an ongoing neurotic pattern.

Community Triage

The patient is requesting information on where in his community he can get the help he needs. He sees the clinic as an available resource that has the necessary information.

Confession

The patient feels guilty about what he has said, thought, or done. He hopes that by talking to the therapist he will feel better. Specifically, the patient wants to be forgiven. He hopes the clinician (authority figure) will see the misdeed as medical or psychological in origin and therefore not bad.

Control

The patient is feeling overwhelmed and out of control. He may fear hurting himself or someone else, or going crazy. He is saying, "Please take over. I can no longer manage."

Medical

The patient sees his problem as being physical in origin, like any other medical condition, as opposed to psychological or situational in origin. He often refers to his problem as "nerves" or as a "nervous condition." The patient, accordingly, hopes for medical treatment, for example, pills, ECT, hospitalization, or medical advice. He expects to take a passive role in the treatment.

Psychological Expertise

The patient believes that the source of his problem is psychological rather than physical or situational. He is asking the professional to explain to him why he thinks, feels, or acts the way he does. The patient anticipates playing a passive role in the interaction, contributing only that information that the expert requires.

Psychodynamic Insight

The patient perceives his problem as psychological in origin, as evolving from his early development, and as having a repetitive quality. As a result, he is left feeling unhappy, unfulfilled, but not overwhelmed or out of control. He expects to take an active, collaborative role in talking about the roots of his problem and hopes that a better understanding of his problem will enable him to change.

Reality Contact

The patient feels that he is losing hold of reality. He wants to talk to someone who is psychologically stable and "safe." He is requesting the clinician to help him "check out" or "keep in touch with" reality so that he will feel that he is thinking straight and not losing his mind.

Social Intervention

The patient sees the problem as residing primarily in the people or situations around him. Because he feels that he does not possess the resources to effect the necessary change, he is asking the clinic to intervene on his behalf. He is asking not for the legal powers of the clinic but for its social influence.

Succorance

The patient is feeling empty, alone, not cared for, deprived, or drained. He wants the clinician to care, to be involved, to be comforting, to be warm and giving so that he can feel replenished and warm inside. It is not so much the content of the interchange that is requested as its effective quality of warmth and caring.

Ventilation

The patient would like to tell the clinician about various feelings and affect-laden experiences. The patient anticipates that "getting it out" or "getting it off his chest" will be therapeutic. He feels that he is carrying around a burden, which he would like to leave with the clinician. In contrast to confession, the patient does not feel guilty and does not need or want forgiveness.

Nothing

Patients who make no request are a heterogeneous group. They may have been referred without proper preparation; they may be psychotic; they may have problems, but they are not seeking help at this time; they may want help, but they are reluctant to state the problem; they may not need help; or they may be in the wrong clinic.

Eliciting the Request

An important clinical technique is how to elicit the patient's request. Sometimes the patient will state the request spontaneously at the beginning of the interview. If this does not happen, the patient's request is best elicited after the nurse learns the patient's complaint and some background of the present concern. This early interaction establishes the rapport and alliance necessary for elicitation of the request and is described as follows.*

Eliciting the request too early in the interview and before the patient states his problem increases the probability of placing the patient in the position of adversary rather than collaborator in the assessment process. For example, "You asked me what I want. You do not even know what is wrong with me." On the other hand, eliciting the request at the end of the interview deprives the nurse of the opportunity to negotiate or work with the patient.

The most successful way of eliciting the request is by asking: "How do you hope (or wish) I (or the hospital or clinic) can help?" Try to avoid questions such as, "What do you want?" or, "What do you expect?" because they are apt to be perceived as a confrontation. The words *wish* or *hope*, in contrast, give the patient permission to state requests he does not necessarily expect will be granted.

Sometimes the patient's response to the question will be, "I don't know. You're the nurse." Or, "I just want to feel better." In this case, the patient may have had a rather specific request in mind that he is reluctant to state. Eliciting the request then requires persistence, persuasion, and compassion. The nurse might say, "You must have some idea when you decided

---

* The sections of this chapter on patient requests are reprinted with permission from Lazare, A., et al. The customer approach to patienthood.[4] Copyright 1975, American Medical Association.

to come to the clinic," or "It is important for me to know what your wishes are even if I may not be able to fulfill them."

It is not easy for patients to tell nurses what they want. Patients often perceive that it is their role to state their problem but not to evaluate how the help should be provided. The patient, however, does have the right to take his business elsewhere if he is not satisfied. Patients often perceive a health care person or agency as having the power to say "no." As a result, the patient must hint at his request rather than boldly state it. Or patients may find it difficult for a variety of personal reasons, for example: "A caring nurse would know what I wanted without my saying." Or, "Who am I to ask for anything?" Others feel a loss of pride in having to ask for something.

The difficulty in stating what one wants, wishes, or hopes for is not limited to the nurse–patient relationship. It is deeply rooted in our culture. For example, in seeking certain employment positions, a person does not always believe his best chances are when he asks for the job but rather if someone else submits his name for the position. The childhood ritual of blowing candles out after a wish or breaking a wishbone carries with it the pressure to keep the wish to oneself in order to have the best chance of its coming true. In academic settings, students are often reluctant to express their wishes regarding either lectures or clinical experiences for fear of influencing a grade.

The initial statement of the request may be incomplete or may be stated in such general terms that it requires elaboration to achieve more detail for clinical utility. The nurse could say, "You said you want me to help you to understand this situation better. What in particular did you want me to understand?" Or, "You thought you would feel better if I talked with your family. How do you hope I can talk to them?"

When the request has been finally stated and elaborated, it is important that the nurse acknowledge that she has heard and has understood the request. Otherwise, the patient may wonder whether the nurse heard the request, was offended by it, or didn't believe it worthy of a response.

The elicitation of the request undoubtedly depends on more than timing and phraseology. Certainly the nurse's attitude of interest and receptivity is crucial. One frequently observes a patient hinting or alluding to the request, apparently waiting for some response from the nurse that will indicate that it is acceptable to continue to be more specific.

As the interview progresses, the nurse should listen for elaborations of or changes in the request resulting from the developing relationship between the nurse and patient. The patient thinks to himself: "Now that I have more trust in you, let me tell you what I really want," or, "Now that you have responded to my initial request, it occurs to me that there is something more important that I need."

Negotiating the Request

The initial interview may be viewed as a process of negotiation between the nurse and the patient, taking the patient's request as a starting point. A basic assumption is that a patient's request for care is usually reasonable and always negotiable. This approach makes the patient more understandable and diminishes the nurse's sense of helplessness. It is the nurse's task to elicit the patient's request, collect the relevant clinical data, and enter into a negotiation. As a result, it is hoped that the patient will feel his perceived needs have been heard and responded to, while the nurse will feel that she has been not only comprehensive but responsive to the patient. The negotiation should facilitate a relationship of mutual influence between nurse and patient to the benefit of both parties.

There are many clinical situations in which the patient's statement of what he wants is exactly what he needs, for example: "I don't want to be woken up at midnight for my medication. I wish to sleep." Using the customer approach, the nurse has the chance to learn important information early in the interview and profit from the patient's ideas, a commonly ignored source of diagnostic data.

When the patient's request is clinically appropriate, making a careful diagnosis of the request can be very important in determining the precise clinical intervention. For example, the patient who needs "ventilation"—talking over fears and concerns about his mental health—requires the nurse to take the role of an interested listener. If the nurse breaks in to make interpretive comments and provides advice or some other intervention the patient has not requested, the clinical plan can fail.

In an ideal negotiation, the patient exerts

his influence in several ways. First, since the request has considerable diagnostic value, the patient is providing the nurse with valuable information. Second, the statement of the request itself obliges the nurse to consider the legitimacy of the perceived need and to explain why an alternative formulation might be more valid. Third, the patient has the right to evaluate and ultimately accept or reject any treatment proposal. In the process he may expect to receive from the nurse a further explanation, an alternative treatment plan, or a statement that the staff cannot meet the request.

The nurse is simultaneously exerting influence by the clarification and evaluation of each request in regard to whether it is clinically appropriate, clinically sufficient, and clinically feasible. If a request is clinically inappropriate, such as a request for medication where there is little chance that the medication will be effective, the nurse attempts to educate the patient so that he will change the request.

Impasses in negotiations are common, and remedial strategies are varied. It may be helpful to understand the patient's perception as to the nature of his health concern and to inquire what he has tried before. It may be helpful to know the patient's fears about his health and what he specifically does not want to happen. It may be helpful for the nurse to restate the formulation in the patient's words in order to facilitate communication.

The Patient's Goal

It is important to ask people who come for mental health services how they hope that they might feel and behave and how they hope that the facility might help with these goals. The patient may never be satisfied until the goal(s) is accomplished. For example, a person's problem may have been medically defined as schizophrenia. This person might say, "I am here because of my husband." When you ask her what she thinks the hospital can do for her, she says "You have to tell him to stop coming home and beating me because when he does, my hallucinations start up again." All the antipsychotic medicine will not change the problem because the husband keeps coming home and beating her. Somehow, the husband will have to stop beating his wife in order for the hallucinations to cease.

When people are asked, "What do you

want to accomplish while you are in treatment here?" they respond in a number of ways. Some responses are specific. For example, hospitalized patients have given the following responses.

SCHOOL-RELATED: "I want to get better so I can go back to school."

WORK-RELATED: "I need to be able to go home and go to work when I leave."

SOCIAL-RELATED: "I want to be able to speak up in groups."

FAMILY-RELATED: "I want to get on the right track with my husband, cooperating with him and to stop hurting myself and him."

"My husband and I have to get some marriage counseling and try to have a better marriage. If this does not work, I will have to cope with the situation the way it is."

SELF-RELATED: "I need to be as good as I was before I started taking drugs."

NURSING ASSESSMENT OF FUNCTIONAL HEALTH PATTERNS

The key elements in formulating a nursing diagnosis for people with emotional problems or distress are patterns of interaction, methods of coping, emotional status, and general life style. For psychiatric nurses to develop appropriate intervention, the careful collection of this information is critical. Throughout the assessment process, which may vary from one to five interviews, the main task of the nurse gathering the data is to remain in touch with how the patient is feeling. The therapeutic intent is to diminish the distress symptoms of the patient as well as to obtain the necessary information for a nursing diagnosis.

The goal of the collection of data is to assess for patterns defined as a sequence of behavior over time. Sequences of behavior, rather than isolated events, are the data used in clinical inference and judgment. This protocol will discuss the nursing assessment of functional patterns derived from Marjorie Gordon's eleven functional health patterns incorporated within the assessment form devised by University Hospitals of Cleveland, Hanna Pavilion Nursing Department (Fig. 12-1).[6]

The order of collecting data varies according to the presenting needs of the patient as well as

University Hospitals of Cleveland

Hanna Pavilion

Patient Assessment

DATE AND TIME OF ADMISSION _____

I. HEALTH PERCEPTION/HEALTH MANAGEMENT PATTERN
VITAL SIGNS   T: _____   P: _____   R: _____   BP: _____
STATE OF HEALTH   GOOD: _____   FAIR: _____   POOR: _____
DISTURBANCES IN PHYSICAL AND MENTAL HEALTH (DESCRIBE): _____

_____
_____
_____

PREVIOUS TREATMENT

YEAR	FACILITY	REASON	TREATMENT	EFFECT

MEDICATIONS

NAME	DOSE	FREQUENCY	EFFECT/ALLERGIES	REASON	LAST DOSE

SUBSTANCE USE HISTORY (ALCOHOL, DRUGS, TOBACCO)

SUBSTANCE	AMOUNT	FREQUENCY	LENGTH OF TIME	RECENT CHANGE IN USE

COMMENTS: _____
_____
_____
_____

II. NUTRITIONAL/METABOLIC PATTERN
HEIGHT FT/IN: _____   CM: _____   WEIGHT LBS: _____   KG: _____
APPETITE GOOD: _____   FAIR: _____   POOR: _____   RECENT CHANGE _____
FOODS AND FLUIDS CONSUMED IN AN AVERAGE DAY: _____

_____

ASSESSMENT	CLEAN	INTACT	UNKEMPT	DRY	CRACKED	ADDITIONAL COMMENTS
SKIN						
HAIR						
NAILS						
TEETH/GUMS						
MUCOUS MEMBRANES						

Figure 12-1. A sample assessment form. (From University Hospitals of Cleveland, Hanna Pavilion Nursing Department, Constance Harris, Leanne Sladewski, Bridget Thiel, and Julia Voss, with permission.)

II. NUTITIONAL/METABOLIC PATTERN

	YES	NO	DESCRIBE
FOOD ALLERGIES			
DIETARY RESTRICTIONS			
RECENT CHANGE IN DIET			
VITAMIN SUPPLEMENTS			
DISCOMFORT WITH EATING			
MECHANICAL DIFFICULTIES			
WOUND HEALING DIFFICULTIES			
DIFFICULTY OBTAINING FOOD			
DIFFICULTY PREPARING FOOD			

COMMENTS: _____
_____
_____
_____
_____

III. ELIMINATION PATTERN

	YES	NO	DESCRIBE
BOWEL DISTURBANCES			
BOWEL PREPARATIONS			
URINARY TRACT DISTURBANCES			
RECENT CHANGE IN ELIMINATION			

COMMENTS: _____
_____
_____
_____

IV. ACTIVITY/EXERCISE PATTERN

SELF CARE ABILITIES	INDEPENDENT	ASSISTED	UNABLE	DESCRIBE
EATING				
BATHING/GROOMING				
DRESSING				
TOILETING				
AMBULATING				
TRANSFERRING				
STAIRS				
LAUNDRY				
HOUSE CLEANING				

LEISURE TIME ACTIVITIES	YES	NO	DESCRIBE
HOBBIES			
REGULAR EXERCISE			

INTERFERENCES WITH ACTIVITY	YES	NO	SOMETIMES	DESCRIBE
DIZZINESS				
DYSPNEA				
CHEST DISCOMFORT				
PAIN/EDEMA OF:				
FEET				
LEGS				
HANDS				
JOINTS				

COMMENTS: _____
_____
_____
_____
_____
_____

2.

Figure 12-1. *(continued)*

V. SLEEP/REST PATTERN
AVERAGE HOURS OF SLEEP EACH NIGHT·   RECENT CHANGE:

	YES	NO	SOMETIMES	COMMENTS
DIFFICULTY FALLING ASLEEP				
DIFFICULTY REMAINING ASLEEP				
FEEL RESTED ON AWAKENING				
USE OF SLEEPING AIDS				
NAPS DURING THE DAY				
HIGH ENERGY LEVEL				
LOW ENERGY LEVEL				

COMMENTS: _____

_____

_____

_____

_____

VI. COGNITIVE, PERCEPTUAL PATTERN
MENTAL STATUS QUESTIONNAIRE (COMPLETE FOR PATIENT 60 YEARS OF AGE OR OLDER)
(THE FIRST 10) QUESTIONS ARE FROM R. L. KAHN, A. I. GOLDFARB, M. POLLACK,
AND A. BECK, "BRIEF OBJECTIVE MEASURES FOR THE DETERMINATION OF MENTAL
STATUS IN THE AGED" AMERICAN JOURNAL OF PSYCHIATRY, 117, (1960b): 326-328)
ARE THE FOLLOWING QUESTIONS ANSWERED CORRECTLY?

	YES	NO
1. WHERE ARE YOU NOW?		
2. WHERE IS THIS PLACE LOCATED?		
3. WHAT IS TODAY'S DATE? DAY OF THE WEEK?		
4. WHAT MONTH IS IT?		
5. WHAT YEAR IS IT?		
6. HOW OLD ARE YOU?		
7. WHEN IS YOUR BIRTHDAY?		
8. WHAT YEAR WERE YOU BORN?		
9. WHO IS THE PRESIDENT OF THE U.S.?		
10. WHO WAS PRESIDENT BEFORE HIM?		
11. SPELL THE WORD "WORLD" BACKWARDS?		

TOTAL THE NUMBER OF QUESTIONS ON THE MENTAL STATUS QUESTIONNAIRE ANSWERED INCORRECTLY
AND CHECK BELOW TO INDICATE THE DEGREE OF COGNITIVE IMPAIRMENT.

_____ 1-2 ABSENT TO MILD
_____ 3-5 MILD TO MODERATE
_____ 6-8 MODERATE TO SEVERE
_____ 8-11 SEVERE

ORIENTATION   PERSON: _____   PLACE: _____   TIME: _____
PAIN PERCEPTION/PAIN TOLERANCE
    HOW DO YOU MANAGE PAIN? _____
    WHAT CAUSES YOU TO HAVE PAIN?

SENSORY PERCEPTUAL ALTERATIONS	YES	NO	DESCRIBE
DELUSIONS			
PERSECUTORY			
GRANDIOSE			
RELIGIOUS			
SELF-ACCUSATORY			
SOMATIC			
HALLUCINATIONS			
AUDITORY			
VISUAL			

-3-

Figure 12-1. *(continued)*

SENSORY PERCEPTUAL ALTERATIONS (CONT'D)	YES	NO	DESCRIBE
HALLUCINATIONS (CONT'D)			
TACTILE			
OLFACTORY			
HOMOCIDAL IDEATION			
PAST THOUGHTS			
PAST ACTION			
CURRENT THOUGHTS			
CURRENT PLAN			
ACTION ON PLAN			
SUICIDE POTENTIAL			
CONTROL OVER YOUR LIFE			
FEEL LIKE GIVING UP			
FEEL GUILTY			
PAST THOUGHTS OF SUICIDE			
PAST SUICIDE ATTEMPT			
CURRENT THOUGHTS OF SUICIDE			
PLAN FOR SUICIDE			
RECENT SUICIDE ATTEMPT			
ATTEMPT IN THE HOSPITAL			
CURRENTLY AT RISK			
NURSING SUICIDE PRECAUTIONS			
FAMILY HISTORY			

RATIONALE FOR NURSING SUICIDE PRECAUTIONS _____

OBSESSIONS			
COMPULSIVE BEHAVIOR			
RITUALISTIC BEHAVIOR			
PHOBIAS			

EDUCATION: _____

EMPLOYMENT: _____

ASSESSMENT
SPEECH: _____
HEARING: _____
VISION: _____
GAIT: _____
PSYCHOMOTOR ACTIVITY: _____
ABILITY TO FOLLOW DIRECTIONS: _____
COMMENTS: _____

VII. SELF-PERCEPTION/SELF-CONCEPT PATTERN
DESCRIBE YOURSELF　PHYSICAL: _____
PERSONALITY: _____
INTELLIGENCE: _____
WHAT DO YOU LIKE THE MOST ABOUT YOURSELF? _____

4.

Figure 12-1. *(continued)*

VII. SELF-PERCEPTION/SELF-CONCEPT PATTERN (CONT'D)

WHAT DO YOU LIKE LEAST ABOUT YOURSELF? _____

WOULD YOU LIKE TO CHANGE ANYTHING ABOUT YOURSELF? _____

HAVE THERE BEEN ANY RECENT CHANGES IN YOUR BODY? _____

EFFECT OF ACTUAL OR PERCEIVED CHANGE. _____

ASSESSMENT

	NORMAL	UNKEMPT	MALODOROUS	BITTEN	DIRTY	OTHER (DESCRIBE
HAIR						
SKIN						
NAILS						
MOUTH						
CLOTHES						

COMMENTS: _____

VIII. ROLE-RELATIONSHIP PATTERN

FAMILY NAME	AGE	ROLE	QUALITY OF RELATIONSHIP GOOD	FAIR	POOR	SUPPORTIVE YES	NO
SIGNIFICANT OTHERS							

SATISFACTION WITH RELATIONSHIPS	YES	NO	COMMENTS
FAMILY MEMBERS			
FRIENDS			
SOCIAL ACQUAINTANCES			
CO-WORKERS			
CLASSMATES			
EMPLOYER			
TEACHERS			

HOW ARE PROBLEMS HANDLED IN YOUR FAMILY? _____

HOW DO FAMILY MEMBERS/SIGNIFICANT OTHERS FEEL ABOUT YOUR PROBLEMS? _____

WHO MAKES DECISIONS IN YOUR FAMILY? _____
MOST SUPPORTIVE? _____
LEAST SUPPORTIVE? _____

5.

Figure 12-1. *(continued)*

FAMILY ACTIVITIES _____

DO YOU EVER FEEL LONELY? _____ WHEN? _____
WHAT DO YOU DO WHEN YOU FEEL LONELY? _____

DESCRIBE:
  SPEECH _____
  EYE-CONTACT _____
  NON-VERBAL BEHAVIOR _____
  INTERACTIONS WITH FAMILY/SIGNIFICANT OTHERS IF OBSERVED _____
  _____
  _____

COMMENTS: _____
_____
_____
_____

IX. SEXUALITY/REPRODUCTIVE PATTERN

	YES	NO	COMMENTS
CHILDREN			
PREGNANCIES			
ABORTIONS			
MENSTRUAL HISTORY			
MENARCHE			
REGULAR MENSES			
MENOPAUSE			
TREATMENT FOR V.D.			
CONTRACEPTIVES			
SEXUAL RELATIONSHIP			
SEXUAL DYSFUNCTION			
SEXUAL ASSAULT			

COMMENTS: _____
_____
_____
_____

X. COPING/STRESS TOLERANCE PATTERN

RECENT CHANGES	YES	NO	COMMENTS
SCHOOL			
WORK			
FAMILY UNIT			
HEALTH			
FINANCES			
HOME			
OWN ILLNESS			
OTHER'S ILLNESS			
DEATH OF SIGNIFICANT OTHER			
MARITAL STATUS			

WHAT MAKES YOU FEEL TENSE (OR OTHER APPROPRIATE TERM)? _____

WHAT DO YOU DO WHEN YOU ARE FEELING TENSE (OR OTHER APPROPRIATE TERM)? _____

WHAT HELPS RELIEVE TENSION FOR YOU? _____

COMMENTS: _____

6.

Figure 12-1. *(continued)*

XI. VALUE/BELIEF PATTERN
WHAT IS IMPORTANT IN YOUR LIFE? _____

WHAT GOALS HAVE YOU SET FOR YOURSELF? _____

RELIGION: _____ DO YOU TURN TO YOUR RELIGIOUS BELIEFS WHEN YOU ARE
HAVING PROBLEMS? _____
WILL BEING HOSPITALIZED INTERFERE WITH YOUR PRACTICE OF YOUR RELIGIOUS BELIEFS?

HOW CAN WE HELP YOU TO PRACTICE YOUR RELIGIOUS BELIEFS? _____

COMMENTS: _____

II. CONTINUING CARE
DESCRIBE YOUR CURRENT LIVING SITUATION. _____

DOES YOUR CURRENT LIVING SITUATION MEET YOUR NEEDS? _____

WHAT HELP DO YOU THINK YOU WILL NEED AFTER DISCHARGE? _____

WHAT CHANGES WOULD YOU MAKE IN YOUR LIVING SITUATION? _____

WHO WILL BE AVAILABLE TO HELP YOU AFTER DISCHARGE? _____
DID YOU HAVE FOLLOW-UP CARE AFTER YOUR LAST HOSPITALIZATION? _____
    WHERE? _____
DO YOU EXPECT TO HAVE FOLLOW-UP CARE AFTER THIS HOSPITALIZATION? _____
    WHERE? _____
    HOW WILL YOU GET THERE? _____
    HOW WILL YOU REMEMBER APPOINTMENTS? _____

XIII. ADDITIONAL DATA
_____
_____
_____
All-- _____
_____
_____
_____
_____
_____

PRELIMINARY ASSESSMENT COMPLETED BY: _____ DATE: _____
                                      (SIGNATURE AND TITLE)   Time_____

PRIMARY NURSE ASSESSMENT COMPLETED BY: _____ DATE: _____
                                       (SIGNATURE AND TITLE) Time_____

10/85

7.

Figure 12-1. (continued)

the nurse's own set of clinical skills and competence. For example, if a patient is admitted via the emergency service talking in a confused manner and his vital signs are clear, a sociocultural history would be a secondary priority. Laboratory studies and cardiovascular monitoring would be the first priority.

The *Standards* cite two important rules of the assessment process. First, the nurse has a responsibility to inform the patient of their mutual roles and responsibilities in regard to the data-collecting interview. The nurse needs to inform the patient who she is, why she wishes to interview the patient, and what the goal of the meeting entails. Concurrently, the patient needs to inform the nurse regarding his intent to cooperate as well as discuss the meaning of the interview. Second, the nurse uses clinical judgments to determine what information is needed. As a nurse gains proficiency in conducting admission interviews, she reduces the amount of time needed to ask specific questions. However, if a student wishes the experience in conducting a full tri-level assessment (patient request, functional health status, and mental status), as is outlined in this chapter, the patient should give permission for such an assessment, since much of the questioning may well be repetitious and already recorded in the patient's chart.

Beginning the Interview

The beginning of the functional status interview is the sensitive gathering of present and past experiential and historical data primarily from the patient view. The style of gathering information is in contrast to the more structured psychiatric mental status assessment with an organized set of questions and dialogue.

The nurse introduces herself and orients the newly admitted patient to the unit. The nurse then sits down and says, "I would like to do a nursing assessment, the first part of which deals with your being here at the [hospital, clinic, etc.]. The second part of the interview deals with your understanding of how your past experiences have influenced your being here now."

This initial part of the interview includes observing the patient, how the patient makes initial contact with the therapist, and the gathering of essential identifying demographic information (name, address, type of work, names of family members, etc.).

Questions then may include some of the following:

- What [issue or problem] brings you here at this time?
- How long has this issue existed after first noting it?
- What do you believe is causing or contributing to it?
- What, if anything, alters or relieves the problem?
- What do you believe has to be done, and by whom?
- How will you know and how will it be that the problem has been adequately dealt with?
- How do you understand what might possibly be done?
- What are your expectations regarding what others might do to either alleviate or contribute to more stress?
- Who and what resources are available at this point in time?

The patient's ability to provide answers to the above questions rests on the skill of the nurse in establishing a therapeutic alliance, as described in Chapter 15, whereby the patient feels safe and that he or she can trust the nurse. The answers provide the nurse with an overall view of how the patient comes for assistance at this particular time. The assessment now turns to the eleven functional health areas.

Health Perception–Health Management Pattern

The first pattern to be assessed describes the perceived status of the health and well-being of the client and the manner in which his health is managed. The objective in assessing this pattern is to obtain data about general perceptions, general health management, and preventive practices. This means inquiry as to health habits and the patient's general level of health care behavior such as adherence to mental and physical preventive health practices, medical or nursing prescriptions, and follow-up care. Vital signs are taken during the admission process.

Questions that may be helpful in eliciting health status information include the following:

- How do you perceive your current health

(good, fair, poor) and past health? What previous treatment have you had?

- What medications are you currently on?
- In terms of health habits, what is your daily use of coffee, tobacco, alcohol, drugs?
- Are you concerned about any particular types of health issues?
- How much knowledge do you feel you have that is accurate and constructive regarding how your body functions and operates?
- To what, if anything, do you attribute your current difficulty?
- In growing up, were there periods of time that you were concerned or puzzled about yourself, your body or your development; how did you come to terms with those periods or are any of them still a puzzle?

Nutritional–Metabolic Pattern

The physical development of a person is important. Document height and weight. The eating and nutrition pattern of clients has long been a concern of nurses. The nutritional–metabolic assessment describes the food and fluid consumption pattern relative to metabolic need and indicators of local nutrient supply. The assessment objective is to collect data about the daily food and fluid consumption, daily eating times, the types and quantity of food and fluids consumed, particular food preferences, and the use of nutrient or vitamin supplements. The assessment should include observations of skin lesions and the general ability to heal, the condition of skin, hair, nails, teeth, gums, mucous membranes, and measures of body temperature.

Questions to ask the patient include the following:

- Is your appetite good, fair, poor? Have there been changes?
- What are your food and fluid preferences?
- What times of the day do you eat? How much?
- What are your usual habits for eating?
- Have you noted alterations in your eating patterns?
- Are you concerned about it or is anyone else concerned?
- Do you have any food allergies, dietary restrictions, recent changes in diet; use a diet supplement; have any discomfort in eating, any mechanical difficulties in eating, any

difficulty with wound healing, any difficulty in obtaining or preparing foods?

Elimination Pattern

The next pattern to be assessed is that of the excretory functional system (bowel, bladder, and skin). Information regarding the individual's regularity of excretory function as well as any changes or disturbances in time pattern, mode of excretion, or quantity is included. Questions to be asked include:

- Do you have any bowel or bladder changes or disturbances?
- What are your usual habits of elimination?
- Do you use laxatives or specific foods?
- Do certain foods or travel or activities interfere with regularity?

Activity–Exercise Pattern

Another important pattern to be assessed is that of exercise, type, quantity, quality of activity, leisure, and recreation. In addition this area includes activities of daily living that require energy expenditure, such as hygiene, cooking, shopping, eating, working, and home maintenance. Factors that interfere with the desired or expected pattern for the individual (such as neuromuscular deficits and compensations, dyspnea, angina, or muscle cramping on exertion, and cardiac/pulmonary classification, if appropriate) are noted, as are the activities the patient undertakes as recreation either with a group or as an individual. Emphasis is on the activities of high importance or significance to the individual. Questions to consider asking include:

- What are your self-care abilities: eating, bathing, grooming, dressing, toileting, ambulating, transferring, stairs, laundry, house cleaning?
- Leisure time activities: What is your usual day like; what are your hobbies and regular exercise?
- What are your favorite activities? Has there been an alteration in your sense of joy or pleasure in these patterns? What sports do you enjoy?
- What have your school and work patterns been? How have they been altered? Are

there any concerns you have as to how the hospitalization is going to impact on daily school and work patterns; general activity patterns?

- Has there been any of the following to interfere with activities: dizziness, dyspnea, chest discomfort, pain or edema of feet, legs, hands or joints?

Sleep–Rest Pattern

Preoccupation with sleep, or its lack, is a common psychological complaint. The objective in assessing a sleep–rest pattern is to describe the effectiveness of the pattern from the patient's perspective. The assessment covers patterns of sleep and rest–relaxation periods during a 24-hour day. It includes the individual's perception of the quality and quantity of sleep and rest and his perceptions of energy level. Also noted are aids to sleep as medications or nighttime routines that the individual employs.

Questions to ask patients include the following:

- How have you been sleeping?
- Are you sleeping too little or too much? What seems to assist you? In what environment do you sleep best?
- Do you have any of the following: difficulty falling asleep; difficulty remaining asleep; feeling tired upon awakening; napping during the day?
- How do you rank your energy level: high, medium, or low?

Cognitive–Perceptual Pattern

Assessment of the cognitive–perceptual areas includes the adequacy of sensory modes, such as vision, hearing, taste, touch, or smell, and the compensation of prosthetics used for physical impairments. Reports of pain perception and how pain is managed are noted when appropriate.

Cognitive functional abilities, such as language, memory, and decision making, are also assessed. The specific observations made by the nurse are discussed under the mental status assessment. Essentially, the nurse observes the client's language skills, grasp of ideas and abstractions, attention span, level of consciousness, reality testing, and any aids required for communication.

Role–Relationship Pattern

The interaction of humans is a major aspect of the work in psychiatric mental health nursing. People engage in many levels of relationship. The objective of role–relationship pattern assessment is to describe a patient's pattern of community, family, and social roles. The patient's perception about his or her relationship patterns is also a part of this assessment.

An important aspect of this assessment pattern includes gathering data about the patient's cultural and community background. An individual needs to be understood within the context of his own family and other social relationships. The assessment of these factors also includes some knowledge of the person's socioeconomic background. Data may be obtained from a direct interview with the client or family and from the client's history of education, employment, and financial stress.

The nurse assesses the influence of a patient's culture on his emotional difficulties by exploring the following areas of a patient's life: ethnic background, beliefs about the nature of illness, and attitudes toward life. The cultural functional health pattern in these areas shows how a patient's value and belief system affects his or her life.

In assessing the impact of ethnicity on the patient's current emotional difficulties, the following information is useful to obtain:

- What is the patient's nationality? Are both parents from the same ethnic group? How many generations have been born in the United States?
- What languages does the family speak?
- What customs/values does the patient think are special or unique to his/her group?
- How does this family or ethnic group view mental illness?
- What is the manner in which the ethnic group deals with feelings?

Family Communication Styles
What are the communication styles within the family? Every family has its own special rules, channels, and styles of communication. Various family constellations form the family structure.

In the sibling world, which brothers and sisters form an alliance? In the parent–child world, which child or children do the parents favor or differentiate between? In the grandparents–child world, which child do the grandparents single out? In the aunt–uncle world, which niece or nephew do they single out?

Which members of the family talk to whom and when? Often, communication between patient and family is neither very distinct nor clear, and it can be easily identified as a problem during the admission process. For example:

An 18-year-old female is brought to the clinic by her father who says, "I can't communicate with her at all. I'm not easy to get along with myself, let alone talk with her." The stepmother says, "I don't understand the girl either. Ever since she has been on drugs I know less what to talk to her about."

The father expressed his guilt about not being more involved with his daughter, but since his remarriage his interest in her activities has markedly declined. The history shows that the parents were divorced when the patient was nine years old and that she lived with her mother until her mother remarried. She then lived with various relatives until she became pregnant at age 16, at which time she went to live at a home for unwed mothers. After her daughter was born, she lived with the baby in an apartment and supported herself on money received from Aid to Dependent Children. She has been on drugs for the past year, receiving LSD, marijuana, speed, and mescaline from three Hells Angels men in the next apartment. She made three suicide attempts in the last year primarily because someone had rejected her. Her main symptom developed when she felt that the "neighbors were trying to get her." She then became frightened and called her father.

Much of this patient's difficulty centers around her feeling rejected—that no one cares. There is reality in both feelings because no one directly shows that he cares. She has no direct communication with anyone who is important to her. One of the main goals of hospitalization is to strengthen and repair ties with family and important people so that they can provide care and the succor that she vitally needs in order to stay alive.

The Family's Perspective on the Problem

The way the family perceives the patient's problem may be either similar to or dissimilar to the way in which the patient perceives his problem. For example, a father may say, "My daughter is so depressed. She lies around all day and cries." This may be exactly how the patient describes her problem.

In another example, a father and mother may say, "Joe is such a problem. He argues and fights with everyone, and if he is going to do that and keep us all upset, we don't want him at home." This family perceives the patient's problem as unacceptable behavior to them. They want the hospital to take their son and make him not a problem at home.

In still another instance, the parents may say, "Mary is so bad. She runs with a wild group and takes drugs." This family views the daughter's problem in moralistic terms. The members of the family may be divided on how they see the problem. The mother may say, "I cannot stand to even see my daughter. She told me she was a homosexual and I could never talk with her again." The father may say, "My daughter told me her problem and that she does not intend to change. That is her decision and what can I do about it? What she does in her personal life is not going to affect my talking with her as my daughter." In this example, it will be necessary to work with the parents in repairing any estrangement.

When there is a conflict between how the family and patient view the problem or a conflict between parents on how each views the child's problem, it indicates a need for negotiating goals in order not to stall the therapeutic process.

Differences in Patient and Family Goals

The assessment of the family's goals for the treatment of the patient is essential. It is important to ask the following questions:

- Are the goals for the patient and family different?
- If they are different, does this mean that the goals are couched in interpersonal terms rather than in intrapsychic terms?
- Does the family really want something different from what the patient wants?
- Is the family aware of this?
- Does the family want the patient to recover?
- If so, recover to what?

Some of these questions may not make sense until some case histories are considered, especially histories of alcoholics who have recovered from their addiction. For example, many times the wife who had complained bitterly during the course of the husband's long drinking history will leave or divorce the husband when he is in good health. For dynamic reasons, his being an alcoholic met some of her psychological needs, and when he returned to health, he presented new and intolerable difficulties and demands.

It is important to assess the family members who are important to the patient. Who comes with the patient to the hospital and who visits the patient? Who is present and who is not and why? Are there missing people important to the goals for treatment? The following example shows that the mother and daughter at the admission conference feel angry toward the missing father:

An 18-year-old young woman presents at the psychiatric clinic accompanied by her mother. She states, "My father is not here because he cares more about his teaching and his students than he does about me."

Later in the interview it becomes apparent that the triad relationship of mother, father, and daughter was significant in the daughter's problem:

The patient stated that after an injury to her neck 19 months previously, she had not been the same since. She dropped out of school and was then tutored. She changed tutors because the first one "told me I was dumb and he never gave me a chance."

After she dropped out of school, her somatic symptoms appeared concerning her neck and stomach. The symptoms pointed to appendicitis, but she was "too uptight" to have surgery.

The father doubts the daughter's somatic complaints. Both the mother and daughter blame the father for poor communication. The daughter's relationship with the mother is better, but she doubts her mother's ability to deal with the father.

The daughter is angry with the father and his treatment of her mother. She gets irritated with her mother's "crumbling to father's wishes." She gets depressed and speaks of suicide.

The daughter is in conflict because she feels disappointed that the father does not show care or concern for either her or her mother and because she feels frustrated in her own attempts to feel secure, to be able to attend school, and to be able to develop her own friends. Because conflict immobilizes her, she can see no alternative except suicide. Patient, family, and hospital goals have to be well negotiated in order for therapeutic progress to be made in this case.

The Genogram

The genogram (Fig. 12-2) is a shorthand technique used to identify the membership structure of a family as well as "mapping" some of the events and influences that have shaped the family's life.* The client will have learned first from the family: how to trust, how to deal with pain and loss, how to communicate, how to make decisions, and how to handle crises and changes. The individual will have been subjected to spoken and unspoken expectations as to what kind of person to be; what kind of knowledge and which relationships are valuable to acquire from the larger community; and in many families, how males and females should behave and experience the world differently. Whether or not the child was planned, whom she or he was named for (or thought to be like), and what else was happening in the family around the time of conception and birth can all be important shaping forces in the individual's development.

In order to fully understand the nature of a client's current problem and the request that brings him/her into the mental health care system, it is important to look at the entire family system in the present and over time. The nurse should collect data aimed at compiling a picture of the family—who its members are now and in the past, what events and crises have occurred in the life of the family, what the family's strengths and weaknesses are, who is close to whom, and who the outcasts are and why. As these questions and others are answered, it may become clearer what family factors might have played a part in bringing the client to the point of his present predicament. The family data will facilitate planning a focus for nursing intervention and can be a valuable part of the intervention itself.

The genogram is a structured technique and has many advantages. For example, the structure may often decrease the client's anxiety in the initial interview and can provide a relatively nonthreatening way to learn information that often takes a much longer time to emerge in the therapeutic relationship. The genogram also has the obvious advantage of building a context in

---

* This section on the genogram is written by Gloria Edelhauser Shapiro.

which to consider all future data. For these reasons it is often useful to work on the genogram with the client in the initial assessment interview. It can be introduced after the client gives a description of the problem that caused him to seek help. The client can be told that it is customary to take some time to learn who the people are in his family in order to better understand the current problem, and that the usual way of accomplishing this is to draw a family "map." However, if the client is too upset to focus on the genogram, it should be deferred.

Constructing the Genogram. Ages are put in the center of the symbols for people. Dates of events (day, month, and year if possible) appear next to the appropriate symbols. Other data can be noted at the discretion of the interviewer. Figure 12-2 illustrates the most common symbols and how they fit together.

Other information that can be noted on the genogram includes: chronic diseases (including alcoholism), causes of deaths, incidents of incest and other sexual trauma, ethnicity and religion of family members, dates of immigration (if pertinent), geographical location of various members, and occupations. Be sure to find out both formal names and "nicknames"—identify family members with the name they go by, but also include their formal name if they are named after someone else in the family.

Using the Genogram for Further Assessment. As you and your client build the genogram, encourage the client to talk about important members of the family. What does he know about the other members? What is his relationship like with them? Is it different now from when they were younger? Who is the family member the client is closest to? Whom does the client *not* get along with? Are there any family stories about various members? Any secrets? What do others in the family think about them? Are they esteemed or are they "black sheep,"

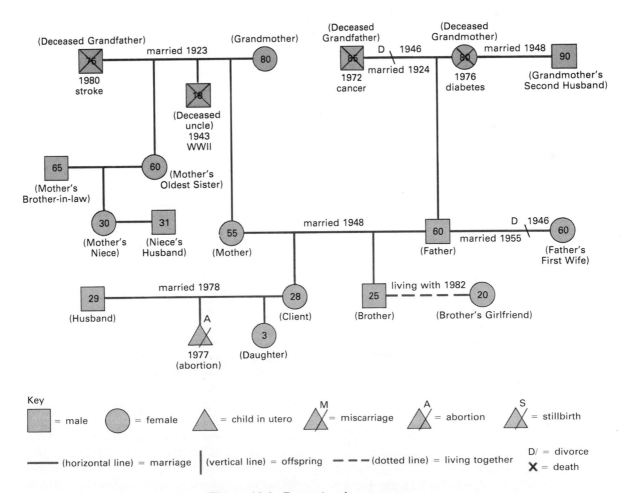

Figure 12-2. Example of a genogram.

etc.? You may ask the client to give a few adjectives for each person; then look for patterns.

Clients are often more comfortable revealing information about their family if the interviewing style is relaxed. It is essential to maintain an accepting and nonjudgmental demeanor. If the nurse does not act surprised or judgmental as the client describes things about other family members that he may consider embarrassing or shameful, it will begin to lay the groundwork for a trusting atmosphere in which the client can talk frankly.

The following example is a portion of an assessment interview with Sally, a young woman who came to a mental health center complaining of depression with no clear precipitating event. The beginning steps in constructing a genogram are shown in the four small diagrams.

NURSE: Let's start with you Sally. Where are you in your family—the oldest, the youngest?
SALLY: I'm the youngest.

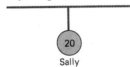

NURSE: Are your folks together?
SALLY: No, my father died when I was two; my mother got married again to my stepfather.
NURSE: What is your mom's name?
SALLY: Helen.
NURSE: How old is Helen?
SALLY: 52.

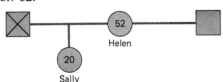

NURSE: Then she must have been 34 when your dad died.
SALLY: Yes. I guess she had a really hard time; she never talks about it though.
NURSE: Who told you about her hard times?
SALLY: My brother told me. He remembers her crying and then she had to go away and we stayed with my aunt for awhile. No one ever talks about it, but I think she went to a mental hospital.
NURSE: It sounds like a very difficult time for your family. I'd like to know more about that time, but let's put some of those folks down on the chart first, so I can see who's who in your family. What's your brother's name?
SALLY: Jack, he's the oldest—he's 30, and Joe is in the middle—he's 26.

NURSE: What was your dad's name?
SALLY: Jonathan.
NURSE: Is that what everybody called him?
SALLY: No, they called him Jack.
NURSE: What do you know about your dad?

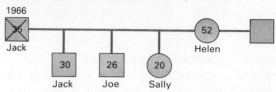

SALLY: Well, he was a carpenter; he was working on a job when he got killed; he fell off a roof. Some people say he was drinking, but he was a wonderful carpenter. He built our house all on his own. I used to walk around the house wondering what he must have been like. I thought maybe the house could tell me. Maybe that's why my stepfather wants to sell the house.
NURSE: How old was your dad when he died?
SALLY: 35—They say my brother will be dead by the time he's 35 too, the way he drinks.
NURSE: Which brother?
SALLY: Jack.
NURSE: What's your stepfather's name?
SALLY: Ron. He's 40. He's OK. He used to live next door with his mother until she died; that's when he married my mother.
NURSE: When was that?
SALLY: Five years ago.
NURSE: Oh, I forgot to ask earlier, do you know when your parents got married?
SALLY: I think they got married the year before my brother was born.

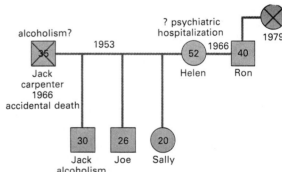

One can see even at this early phase of work on the genogram that some important issues are beginning to emerge that lend direction to the assessment of Sally's depression. The sudden death of her father at an early age, some apparent family secrets around which communication is closed down, Sally's longing to know more about her father, the importance of the family house to Sally and its connection to her father in her feelings, the mystery around how her mother dealt with her grief, and a possible family pattern of using alcohol as a solution to other problems—to name the most obvious issues. A likely hypothesis at this time would be that the threatened sale of the home her father built is a precipitant and the therapeutic issue is unresolved grief, perhaps for other family members as well.

The genogram can generate a sound framework of data on which to build a treatment strategy, and the same data can be used in many different treatment models as a basis for planning interventions.

It is useful to keep in mind that the emotional and mental functioning of a person never takes place in isolation. In order to assess the nature and meaning of a client's problem, the nurse needs to know about the people who make up the client's family system, about the events that have impacted on their lives, and about the coping mechanisms they have used to handle problems. The genogram can be a useful technique for collecting family information in the nursing assessment process.

Economic, Environmental, and Political Factors Affecting the Client's Health

Knowledge regarding the patient's economic level and environment is helpful for the nurse to obtain during the assessment process. People who have limited economic resources are often under a considerable amount of stress. Concern or worry about financial matters has been proven to have a negative effect on one's health status. The nurse may ask the patient the following questions:

- Are you employed? If so, is the work productive and satisfying?
- Do any political factors influence your work situation?
- Are you able to meet your financial obligations?
- Does your financial position cause you worry or concern?
- Are you anxious about losing your job in the near future?
- Do you have any outstanding debts that are of concern to you?

The environment may also affect one's mental health. Does the home environment provide the basic comfort needs? Do family members have enough space for privacy? Have there been any recent changes within the environment or changes in membership?

The political factors affecting health status can vary from sex-role stereotyping and discrimination in work conditions to feeling pressured and harrassed by situations affecting the individual's life-style.

Personally Significant Support Systems

An assessment area of importance regarding the hospitalized person is the visiting pattern. It is important for the nurse to observe who comes to visit the patient and what the visiting style is. Some families visit the patient singly; other families gather the entire clan for the visit. Often cultural mores determine visiting customs. Friends, peers, or community people may visit only when the family is not there, or they may prefer to come in their own group. The nurse can assess the significant support systems as well as inquire regarding other unutilized support systems.

It is important to assess the patient's mood and his reaction to visitors before, during, and after the visit. Occasionally it may be observed that the visits are so upsetting to the patient that they must be limited or possibly restricted to certain people. The nurse usually can determine this and may set limits on visitors.

The nurse should observe how the visitors physically act when they are with the patient, for this can indicate the patient's position in the group. Is there physical contact, for example, shaking hands, kissing, or embracing, when the visitors meet the patient or end the visit?

The following two examples show the patient's extreme dependence on parental figures. The issue of succor or needing to be cared about will undoubtedly come up in the nursing care plans. In these particular examples, healthier ways of dealing with dependent needs would be recommended and implemented.

During one admission conference, a 17-year-old daughter being admitted sat right next to her mother. The daughter cried and held her mother's hand during the entire conference.

A 20-year-old college sophomore presented in an extremely agitated and confused state at a general hospital emergency ward. He kept saying, "They will kill me if you leave." The father made arrangements to stay all night with the son. The mother, after her son's admission to the psychiatric unit, was observed sitting next to her son's bed, cradling his head in her lap, stroking his head, and saying, "Everything will be all right."

Demands can be placed on family members to make them feel guilty. An example is given below:

An 80-year-old woman is hospitalized with pneumonia. She holds her son's hand as he prepares to leave at the end of visiting hours and says, "Please don't leave me. I get so lonely at night and the nurses don't pay any attention to me at night."

The nurse's observations of this type of situation can be most helpful. For example, the patient may make increasing demands on the visitor and play upon his guilt feelings in order to make him stay. The nurse can then say to both family and patient, "It is time for the visit to end. I want to prepare Mrs. Smith for the evening and it is important for you to be home with your own family." The nurse should also talk with family members to ensure that they have the opportunity to express their feelings about how they feel the hospitalization is progressing.

Another important observation point is where and how visitors sit in relation to the patient. Does the patient sit alone? Is there any ally in the group? Is there an alliance against the patient? The nurse can observe if a patient is shut out of conversations by a domineering person.

Questions to include in an assessment for role–relationship patterns include the following:

- Do family and friends know you are in the hospital? Do you want particular people to know or to not know about your distress?
- What do you believe other people think or know or might think or know about being in the hospital?
- Do you have major concerns with regard to how people may think or feel or react?
- Do you have a best friend; within your family? With whom do you feel the closest?
- Who is in your social network and who is most problematic to you?
- On a scale of 1 to 10 how comfortable do you feel with people?
- What kinds of things annoy you the most?
- What do you believe you do that annoys people?
- How were you disciplined in growing up?

Who disciplined you? How frequently were you hit and where? Were all the children disciplined in such a manner?
- In reflecting on the discipline in your family, on a scale from 1 (normal) to 10 (abusive) how would you rate the behavior in your family? If siblings, how did you treat one another? Were the fights physical? How were they mediated? How aggressive were you and others?

Self-perception–Self-concept Pattern

A person's concept of himself is critical to mental health. Thus, the objective of this assessment is to describe the patient's pattern of beliefs and evaluations regarding general self-worth and feeling states. Problems the client or others identify and explanations or reasons they identify for the problem are also important.

Part of the assessment is the determination of the cause of the precipitating event that led to the patient's hospitalization or need for psychological assistance. By listening for the "last straw," one can assess the critical dynamic issue that is problematic to the person. The issue or reason is called *dynamic* because there is psychological meaning in why it has occurred.

There is a dynamic issue to every situation. For example, did the precipitating event mean a loss of love or a loss of people giving to the person in an emotional way? Or is the person one who needs to feel that he is a good person but now feels that he is a bad person? Or is the person one who needs to feel in control and now feels out of control? Or is the person one who needs to win and now feels that he is going to lose? Or is the person one who needs to be admired but no longer feels that anyone admires him?

The same precipitating event for two patients can have two different meanings. For example, a person dies. To one patient this means the loss of someone who cared and gave him something he needed. To another patient it means that because he had been so angry at the person he has contributed to that person's death, and now the patient feels that he is a bad person. He may feel that he could have done more to prevent the death.

The dynamic issues may be viewed as follows:

To be Cared About, Loved, and Protected

People who have strong needs for security, acceptance, and protection are prone to develop psychiatric symptoms when threats to these needs occur.

A person who has these needs predominating may become ill because of the loss of someone who provided them. The person may not return to normal health until the sources for succor are reestablished. These needs are often referred to as the *external supplies of life*. For example, it often happens that the death of one mate leads to the death of the surviving mate within a short period of time. This is frequently the case in elderly couples. It is felt that the emotional needs met by each mate are so great that no one else could substitute for the surviving mate.

An example of this dynamic issue is: A 45-year-old single teacher from the East Coast moved to the West Coast to accept an excellent teaching position. Her move required that she leave her mother, with whom she had lived all her life. This was a very difficult decision to make. Shortly after assuming her new role, she became severely depressed. She required hospitalization and electroconvulsive therapy before she was able to return to the community and her work. The loss of her mother's caring, coupled with a strange and unfamiliar environment, placed too great a strain on her emotionally. Until she was able to adjust to the new location, the new people, and the new interests, she needed support and succor from the hospital milieu and staff.

Patients suffering from schizophrenia are known to have reacted unfavorably to situations in which genuine caring and succor were lacking. When they are unable to take it upon themselves to find a substitute, someone else must provide this model of care. For example: A bright 18-year-old male student who had managed to achieve well academically in his small hometown high school became disorganized and lost under the pressures of a large and impersonal university in which competition was high. The student had been fifth in his high school class of 50, but now he must compete in college with the best graduates from all high schools. The pressure increased his feelings of inadequacy and social failure, and he became ill over the issue of needed security, comfort, and protection.

The resolution of this issue calls for return-ing the person to a situation in which he can depend on a caring person.

To Be in Control, To Be Good

People who place a high value on being good, conscientious, and in control may become symptomatic when there is a threat of the possibility of their being wrong or bad. Sometimes the "bad" is only in the form of thought or wishes, but even this is intolerable for them. For example: A 39-year-old woman became severely depressed after the birth of her fifth child. The baby was a great strain emotionally, physically, and financially. Although she said she was happy to have the baby, her inner thoughts were saying she wished she did not have the baby. She felt guilty because of these thoughts and became depressed.

Psychological assessment of this issue implies providing a model of care aimed at helping the person feel more secure in being a responsible and conscientious woman. The therapeutic task is to help her bear the painful feeling over which she feels guilty. The exploration of her thoughts and feelings is an attempt to free the "bad" thoughts. If she is encouraged to talk, she may be able to see the reality of the ambivalent feelings that mothers have from time to time toward their children. By listening, the nurse shows that she is not afraid to hear these thoughts and feelings. The human element is stressed with this mother so that she may understand the ideal and the real. No one can be good and perfect all the time. The mother has to make peace within herself about her ambivalent feelings.

Another example of this dynamic issue is a 23-year-old single female who is admitted for attempted suicide. When she is asked, "What do you hope to accomplish while you are here?" the patient responds, "To get better and be a good person again." The issue of being good and not bad is significant in planning treatment to help her to see her suicidal behavior in realistic terms rather than just in moralistic terms. People whose dynamic issue is to be in control tend to be logical and orderly in their approach to problems. They are conscientious and punctual. When there is a threat to the loss of control over their bodies or their abilities to function effectively, they may develop psychiatric symptoms.

To Be Strong, Secure, and to Achieve

The need for achievement and to be strong and secure is an important issue. People become upset when they are in situations in which they feel weak and insecure. For example, victims of rape whose dynamic issue is to be strong become upset when they believe they were not aggressive or strong enough to avert the rape. One victim with this dynamic issue would not talk to a nurse about her concerns as to whether people were helpful to her after the rape (as with the dynamic issue of being protected and loved) or about feeling bad in a moral sense (as the dynamic issue of to be good and in control) but instead would discuss feeling defeated and powerless.

The question to be asked regarding dynamic issue is, What is the dynamic meaning of the event that brings the patient for help?

A person's self-concept is usually derived from interactions within the family. Thus, the following questions are important to ask:

- In growing up, what type of statements were used to describe you, to praise you, to teach you, to criticize you, to scold you; by whom were these comments made?
- How useful were these comments in your life?
- What comments do you believe influenced you the most as to how you presently think about yourself?

Sexuality–Reproductive Pattern

Sexuality–reproduction is part of the total being of a client. The objective of assessment in the sexuality–reproductive pattern is to describe problems or potential problems.

To counsel patients about intimate concerns, the nurse must first be comfortable with his or her own sexuality. Nurses require self-esteem, a positive body image, and resolution of their own sexual identity. The patient should not be burdened by the nurse's sexuality. Nurses need to autognose their sexual reactions to patients to avoid behaving in ways that induce anxiety to the patient around issues of sexuality.

Nurses need to have an accurate perception of the social, cultural, and religious principles that guide the patient. They must also be aware of their own value system so that they may accept the sexual preferences of their patients without being threatened or judgmental. There must be genuine concern for the individual or

family and regard for any information shared as confidential.[7]

Once the nurses feel comfortable with sexual issues, they must also consider the patient's feelings. N. F. Woods states that numerous situations provoke anxiety in patients. They may regret divulging sexual data because of fear of reprisal or guilt. Invasion of privacy and embarrassment may be felt from physical examination of breasts and genitalia. Cultural taboos may prohibit sexual discussion or examination by professionals of the opposite sex. The patient's clothing may be removed, arousing fear of loss of control, or loss of sexual identity, privacy, attractiveness, and esteem.[8]

The nurse can facilitate the patient's comfort when taking a sexual history by utilizing several approaches:

1. While negotiating the patient contract, let the patient know you will be asking questions of a personal nature. Explain that this will facilitate uncovering problems requiring assistance.
2. Do not force the patient to talk about sex. If the patient seems hesitant or anxious about a question, ask whether he would prefer it to be brought up at another time. There is no need to dwell on the sexual portion of the assessment beyond eliciting the information necessary for therapeutic intervention.
3. Allow the client to talk by providing open leads: "After an operation (illness, accident) like yours, many men and women have concerns about sexual functioning. What are some of your concerns?" or, "Some of the questions they ask are . . . (give example). Do you have any of these questions?"
4. Be matter-of-fact in your approach with an emphasis on acceptable behavior. You might explain, for example, that sexual desire in old age is perfectly normal, or masturbation is often practiced in order to release sexual energy. Follow up this statement by asking the client's opinion.
5. When asking sexual questions, begin with the least sensitive and work up to the most sensitive. Information may often be elicited by asking about the ideal rather than the real. For example, ask how the relationship differs from the way the client had expected or would like it to be.
6. Do not use terminology that the client

won't understand. If the client uses unsophisticated language, don't express shock or disapproval, as that may end the discussion.

7. Finally, if you feel uncomfortable discussing sexual problems, you might state, "I feel that Mary Jones would be far more helpful in discussing that area with you. May I make an appointment for you to see her?"[9]

Taking the Sexual History

The extent of the sexual history should be proportionate to the patient's needs. The greater the potential for the patient's condition to affect his sexuality, the greater the need for sexual base-line data. Chapter 16 discusses the interview techniques that the nurse should use. It is again important to emphasize that the interview take place in a quiet, private location with the patient in a comfortable position. Because of the sensitivity of the subject, it is better addressed during the latter portion of the interview, after the nurse and patient have had a chance to speak for awhile. There is no one best place to introduce the topic, but it may seem more appropriate as part of the systems review related to reproduction or the genitourinary system or as part of the social and family history.

An excellent resource, *Assessment of Sexual Function: A Guide to Interviewing*, includes two guides for history taking and assessing performance, and covers each age group.[10] As a general tool for identifying sexual problems, this author has developed the acronym *caritas* as a reminder of the areas to be covered. (Note that the word *care* is derived from *caritas*.)

c Concern: What is the patient's definition of the real or potential concern? What is the patient's goal?

a Attitudes: What attitudes, beliefs, and values are operating? How does the patient feel toward himself, sexual expression, and practices?

r Relationship: What is the type and quality of the patient's relationship (marriage, homosexual, stable, . . .)? Who else needs to be involved and at what point?

i Illness: What effect does illness (physical, emotional, surgical, or drug treatment) have on the patient's sexuality?

t Trust: Trust is one of the most important aspects in resolving sexual problems. Does the patient have enough trust in the significant others (nurse, physician, mate) to be open for help?

a Awareness: How aware is the patient of the dynamics of sexuality? What is the patient's knowledge and what must the patient (and family) be taught?

s Sensuality: What techniques, environments, or experiences have improved or hindered sexual expression?

Another sexual assessment skill that nurses must have is the ability to identify cues. Patients whose sexual problems are unaddressed may send out verbal and nonverbal hidden messages. A person may complain of vague problems,[11] or say, "I'm not the man (or woman) I used to be." A teenager may begin a sentence with, "I have a friend who. . . ."

Unmet sexual needs may result in inappropriate patient behavior. Woods notes that flirting with members of the opposite sex may indicate the need to prove oneself sexually attractive. Sexual "acting out"—touching nurses' breasts and using sexual remarks—was seen in men whose sexual self-image was threatened. Exposing the genitals may be a means of gaining control or attention.[12]

M. Oberleder states that sexual "acting out" in the elderly is a cry for help. We all retain the need for warmth and touching, and holding a patient's hand is an acceptable way to prevent a sexual pass. A far greater problem resulting from sensory and sexual deprivation is sexual regression, "the pathological and unconscious sexualization of body functions, such as eating, urinating and defecating."[13] Institutionalized elderly are often deprived of the sensations of warmth, moisture, softness, and smoothness, and therefore may resort to "messing." Nursing intervention should be aimed at substitution, giving warm baths, back rubs, and soft items to the person, and reinforcing appropriate behavior. Regression may also be prevented by ensuring that the patient is adequately prepared and sensitively handled during genital–rectal examination.[14]

Questions to ask the patient include the following:

• Age of puberty (e.g., onset of secondary sex characteristics)?
• Menstrual history including menarche, regular menses, menopause?
• Autoerotic activities such as masturbation, nocturnal dreams?
• Age of sexual activities (e.g., what, when,

and how did you first learn and experience sex)?

- Any history of sexually transmitted diseases?
- In your own evaluation, as we have gone through this discussion, has there been any of these experiences that you would evaluate as being either unwanted, confusing, exploitative, or abusive?
- Have you ever felt frightened in a sexual situation?
- Were you ever told that you "asked" for it, that having sex was your fault?
- To what extent do you believe you were a knowledgeable and fully cooperating person in the sexual encounter?

Coping–Stress-tolerance Pattern

Stress is a part of living. Part of positive mental health is the ability to cope with and tolerate stresses. This functional pattern is critical to assess in the context of the current stressor in the patient's life that has resulted in his need to seek assistance and counseling.

A special technique to illustrate life events within the patient's life-span is the behavior–event lifeline. This visual aid is the construction of a behavior–event lifeline placed along a chronological axis (Fig. 12-3). This lifeline outlines past or current changes in the person's life

(e.g., school, work, family unit, health, finances, home, illness, other's illness, deaths, marital status) and can be constructed as the nurse listens to patients describe significant events in their lives. The data to be elicited for the lifeline include *both* the event and the behavior or symptom.

CASE EXAMPLE

A 45-year-old married mother of four seeks counseling because of feeling increasingly anxious after watching television accounts and reading newspaper stories on a highly publicized rape case in the local area. She reported having been raped by a stranger 2½ years previously. She received about six crisis counseling sessions for six months after the rape. She repeatedly stated how "embarrassed" she felt that she was still having trouble "coping" with the rape. The nurse–therapist saw the patient four times over a two-month period and the lifeline shown in Figure 12-3 was constructed.

This lifeline guide was very useful in the counseling of the patient to illustrate the linkages between the life event and the behavioral symptoms. The linkages were identified as follows:

1. Patient reveals her rape to a nurse while hospitalized a third time for asthma. The patient awakens during a nightmare of the rape and tells

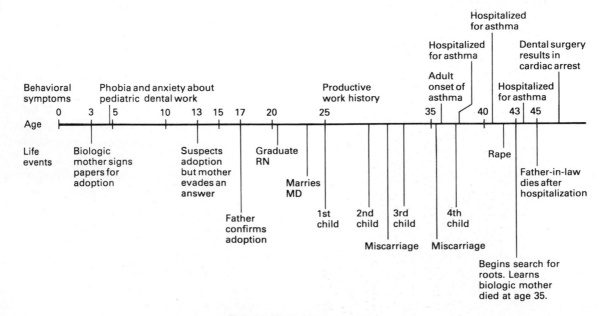

Figure 12-3. Lifeline guide.

the nurse in a "half-awake" state. This is her first disclosure to anyone three months following the rape.

2. In counseling, the patient describes another "half-awake state." She is 13 and recalls mother coming into her bedroom to check on her. The patient has been suspecting that she is adopted and asks mother. Mother says, "You must be dreaming; go back to sleep." When she is 17 father confirms that she was adopted.

3. Patient's first memory of an anxious state is at age 4 when she recalls needing extensive dental work. She is so resistive that she is medicated ("put to sleep") during the dental work.

4. At age 35, develops severe adult asthma and requires hospitalization.

5. After the rape, begins an adoptive search for her biologic family. Learns her biologic mother died at age 35 from pneumonia.

6. Experiences an anxiety attack during a visit to her father-in-law who was hospitalized for a stroke. She panicked seeing him restrained and unconscious (flashback to her rape).

7. Routine dental surgery results in a cardiac arrest; patient resuscitated. Had tried unsuccessfully to refuse general anesthesia. Only learned of the cardiac arrest by reading the nurse's notes.

In counseling, the patient was able to consciously link the symptoms of anxiety and panic to childhood events as well as adult events. This awareness helped reduce her anxiety.

Value–Belief Pattern

Personal constructs are values, expectations, self-perceptions, habits, and identification of critical events. The value–belief assessment is tapping into these constructs.

The terms "spirituality" and "religion," while differently defined, are often used synonymously or interchangeably. Spirituality is a universal phenomenon that has been defined by the conference on nursing diagnosis as the life principle that pervades the entire being of a person (i.e., emotional, moral-ethical, intellectual, and physical planes) and generates a capacity for developing higher values. Spirituality may include the recognition of an individual's ultimate dependence upon a Supreme Being, but it is not contingent upon or restricted to religious beliefs or values. The term "religious" is applied to delimit those spiritual beliefs that include the concept of a deity.

An individual whose spirituality does encompass the belief in a deity may belong to an organized system of worship, which is called a "religion." Religions are characterized by: (1) beliefs, to which those professing the particular religious preference are expected to adhere; (2) norms, which are used to regulate the behavior of the members of the particular religious system; and (3) rites and practices, which are used in the particular system of worship. Even when an individual does believe in a deity, he or she may not necessarily profess adherence to the tenets of a specific religious denomination.[15]

Shelly and Fish stress the universality of spiritual needs.[16] Thus, it is important that a major assessment area concern the spiritual beliefs of the client. A few questions that are useful in helping to elicit information relevant to spiritual or philosophical beliefs are as follows:

- Are you a member of an organized church group? If so, do you participate in church services? How often? Any change over the years?
- Does your religious practice differ from that of your family? If so, how?
- Does your philosophy of life affect your day-to-day living?
- Do you believe religion has an influence on health and illness?

Diagramming Religious Practices

Based on the concept of genogram, a religiogram is a map of the religious activities of a family. By completing such a diagram, the nurse can quickly visualize the continuity and tradition of religious values of the patient, his or her immediate family, as well as family members from several generations and components. If a patient has symptoms that could reflect unresolved conflicts in the area of religious or spiritual needs or has clear religious symptomatology (described in Chapter 14), the religiogram may open up important areas of discussion. A religiogram may be completed by the patient or jointly with the nurse. It also may be added to a genogram or completed separately.

The following example illustrates a religiogram completed by a nursing student and her patient (Figure 12-4).

Mrs. Jones, a 48-year-old married mother of three children was admitted with a diagnosis of depression. At the time of her marriage 25 years previously she stopped attending the church that she had attended through high school and

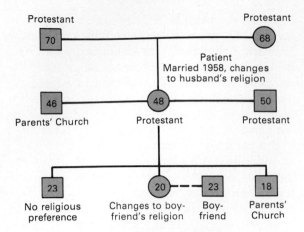

Figure 12-4. A religiogram.

joined the church that her husband and his family attended. This behavior and decision caused conflict between the women and her mother; the conflict had remained unresolved at the time of admission. The nurse learned the patient's 20-year-old daughter had joined the church of her boyfriend.

The religiogram can generate a sound framework of data on which to build a treatment strategy, and the same data can be used in treatment models as a basis for planning interventions.

Questions to ask include the following:

- Do you practice a religion?
- Is there anything that you want that would help or support in carrying out the religious activities while in the hospital?

Continuing Care

Although the nurse is assessing the patient for his current condition, the future is also a consideration, and thus the following questions will be useful for the patient's continuing care.

- Describe your current living condition.
- Does your current living situation meet your needs?
- What help do you think you will need after discharge?
- Who will be available to help?
- Have you ever had follow-up care after a hospitalization?

Concluding the Assessment Interview

As a conclusion to the functional health status assessment, a series of questions and discussion can bring closure to the interview and help the nurse in the formulation of current and continuing care for the patient. These questions elicit information that helps the nurse know something about the person in a straightforward manner and convey that she is interested in the whole sphere of experience.

- What are your expectations of being here?
- What is your expectation of the staff here?
- What have you noticed that helps you feel better, think better, behave better than you are at present?
- What do you believe to be your greatest assets both personally and interpersonally?
- What areas do you find are problematic for you personally, interpersonally, and in achieving?

The time orientation of a patient is important to assess. Questions related to time orientation include the following:

- Where do you find yourself thinking the most: things in the past, present, or future?
- When you think of the past, what kind of thoughts come to mind? When you think of the present what kind of thoughts? When you think of the future what kind of thoughts?
- When you think about time, where would you most like to be: the past, present, or future?
- Are there special things you regret? Are there special things that you are afraid of? Are there special things that you want to do or achieve in the future?

Other concluding questions to close the interview include:

- In comparing yourself to when you really felt the best about yourself and the world and today, what are the differences that you note in how you feel, how you think, how you behave?
- Of all of these things that we have talked about, what are some of the things you think are important in relation to what is now concerning you?

If the patient says none of these, the nurse then proceeds to the question:

• What is of most concern to you now?

Case Formulation From the Nursing Assessment

Nursing is a holistic science that treats the totality of the client. Primary prevention intervention is aimed at maintaining a state of wellness. Secondary prevention intervention aims at minimizing the client's negative response to an acute health state. Tertiary prevention assists the client to maintain optimal functioning despite the presence of a long-term illness or disability. With that backdrop, we ask now how the data that has been collected can be assembled into a formulation for a preliminary nursing diagnosis that can look to a primary, secondary, or tertiary level of prevention through the interpretation of the patient request, functional status assessment, and mental status examination.

Health Perception–Health Management

The health assessment is used to alert both the patient and the nurse to any past or ongoing patterns in health needing evaluation and attention. We also assess the individual's personal views about his own body integrity. This assessment is important for providing and planning resources and service activities necessary to sustain positive physical health. It also taps into any health knowledge deficits and indicates areas of health teaching. In addition, it is a screening mechanism that alerts the patient and the nurse to more extensive assessment.

Nutrition–Eating Pattern

In this area of assessment, patterns are examined in terms of extreme irregularity as opposed to regular practices and any variations in the recent occurrence. Attitudes, beliefs, and values regarding food and food behaviors and rituals are important and may later be cross-referenced with specific types of eating disorders. The assessment in this area is used to ultimately support healthy eating patterns that are congruent with major religious and personal preferences.

Elimination Pattern

This pattern is examined in terms of regularity. It may be cross-referenced with psychiatric symptomatology such as depression.

Activity Pattern

The activity pattern level gives us general information on preferred activities both physical and nonphysical as well as information about the individual's capacity for recreation. It is evaluated for changes in the present and for excess or deficiencies over time. This area becomes a potential base of evaluation for the support of existing preferred activities and of the introduction of new activities that tap potential positive resources in the individual.

School and Work Pattern

Of particular importance is the assessment in the area of school or work for initial information regarding past and ongoing performance. Again we are looking for any disruption in performance. In addition, this assessment alerts the nurse and the patient to further needs and evaluation of specific abilities that may be underdeveloped such as reading, math, as well as information about the individual's anxiety level regarding personal performance. This area is important for nursing activities that strengthen and build essential resources necessary for the person to solve problems.

Cognitive–Perceptual Pattern

The cognitive–perceptual pattern provides an understanding of the adequacy of sensory models, such as vision, hearing, taste, touch, and smell. Reports of pain perception and how pain is managed are noted when appropriate. The cognitive functional abilities, such as language, memory, and decision making, also provide data on the level of current functioning.

Sleep–Rest Pattern

What can be gathered from the personal construct assessment? In sleep and rest patterns we can find out if the person has had a reasonable healthy pattern of sleep and rest or whether it has been irregular or if the pattern has shifted or changed as of recently. This information is to be related to the biologic assessment of the client and it has implications for the negotiation with the client of instituting behaviors around sleep and rest that are aimed at establishing regularity and a reasonable and constructive rest and sleep.

Role–Relationship Pattern

This is a representation of the perceptions and values placed by the patient on interpersonal relationships. Initially, one is evaluating for alterations in prior constructive interpersonal relationships and existing social resources. A lack of connections either of a recent nature or a long-term standing provides data for other levels of assessment and diagnoses of disordered states but also gives a preliminary estimate of the patient's capacity for and tolerance of attachment to others.

The assessment for family relationships and discipline is meant to elicit from the client information that may substantiate a past history of family abuse. In addition it gives some information regarding the patient's model for the expression and control of aggression. It is a preliminary assessment of the patient's capacity for impulse control. It gives further information that may be relevant for assessing a person's self-esteem and, more specifically, related past factors that have significant influence in the present on a person's positive regard for self.

Self-perceptual Pattern

The pattern of self-concept and self-perception provides information as to the individual's attitude about himself, including perception of his abilities (cognitive, affective, or physical), body image, identity, general sense of worth, and general emotional pattern. Patterns of body posture and movement, eye contact, and voice and speech also provide an indicator of self-concept. The time assessment is important in its contribution to understanding states of depression and anxiety. Generally speaking, people who are past-oriented tend to have depressed moods. Those who are future-oriented in a negative way tend to be anxious. Of course, there are exceptions as there are persons who are future-oriented only to doom and this is subtly linked to the past (I have had bad luck and it is only going to carry through). By the same token there is the seeming exception in the person who looks back and is frightened or has been exposed to fear, and they think to the future and they think it will happen again. This awareness and the specific thought patterns associated with these two emotional states allow both the patient and nurse to work on present-orienting

activities that reduce either depression and anxiety for a short period of time, allowing more constructive reflection on past and future and altering fixed thought patterns that perpetuate either anxiety or depression.

The questions regarding what was said to the person, an attempt to elicit actual comments of praise and criticism, are asked in order to make an assessment of past psychological abuse. This information also gives us an idea of the person's perception of personal attributes through the eyes of others, in particular the primary early relationships. This information is useful in the assessment of the person's present sense of self-esteem.

Sexuality–Reproductive Pattern

This assessment again provides information on sexuality patterns as well as a preliminary basis for uncovering sexual abuse. In addition, it gives information about early modeling of sexual attitudes and beliefs.

Value–Belief Pattern

It is important to recognize and acknowledge the spiritual and religious beliefs of individuals to assess if they have been disrupted in any way and whether this disruption is extremely problematic to the patient and if the patient is perhaps in need of some spiritual counseling. It is important to differentiate a loss of faith that emanates from spiritual conflict and value conflict related to a person's primary spiritual and religious orientation from a lack of faith that is secondary to other disordered states.

Again, the assessment is used to establish whether there is a pattern of religious and spiritual activities that supports and sustains a person, whether there has been an interruption in this pattern, and whether the person ultimately needs to examine this area to resurrect important positive resources for his mental health.

In summary, the formulating of nursing diagnoses from functional health status data can also assist with dynamic formulations that are important in any kind of ongoing counseling session. The information is helpful in sensitizing the nurse to the patient's response to the social milieu in which the nursing care is going to be carried out. It can also be useful in helping the client identify and clarify issues of concern that relate to present problems.

THE MENTAL STATUS EXAMINATION

The purpose of the mental status examination is to determine objectively and record observable aspects of the patient's psychological functioning. This contrasts with the history, which is based not on observable behavior but on recollections. The performance and recording of a mental status examination have several major functions:

1. It is an agreed-upon method of organizing clinical observations.
2. It provides a clinical base line for a patient's psychological state.
3. It provides specific information that assists in establishing certain diagnoses, for example, organic brain disease.

The mental status examination is important for two reasons. First, nurses will hear discussion of the mental status examination and will be able to read the results in the patient's chart. Second, many nurses, specifically those who are seeing patients in the community, are beginning to perform formal mental status examinations with an eye toward referring possible cases of organic brain disease for thorough medical examination.

The mental status examination generally includes the following categories: general appearance, speech, motor behavior, mood and affect, thought process, thought content, intellectual functions, judgment, and attitude.

General Appearance

In assessing the general appearance of the patient, special attention needs to be paid to grooming, dress, facial expression, and posture and gait. A note should be made of any definitive features that would identify the individual immediately.

A. Grooming: Is the patient taking care of his appearance? What is the appearance of the teeth, hair, nails, body? If a woman patient uses cosmetic makeup, is it done appropriately for the situation?
Example: A 60-year-old patient enters the emergency room with her face made up in a clown-like manner.

B. Dress: Is the dress appropriate for the season and situation?
Example: A young college man arrives to be seen at the walk-in psychiatric service in mid-July in boots and a long winter coat.
C. Facial expression: What is the patient's facial expression? Impassive, expressionless, excited, sad, angry, startled, suspicious, grimacing? Does the patient avoid eye contact, stare at the examiner, look around the room, stare down or into space?
D. Posture and gait: How does the patient sit in the chair? Erect, slumped down, on the edge of the chair, leaning forward, backward, on his elbows? When the patient walks, does he move quickly, slowly, with hesitation, a limp, head erect or hung down?

Speech

The nurse can assess several aspects of the client's form of speech.

A. Volume: How loudly or softly does the patient speak? Does the examiner have to adjust her position to hear?
B. Rate: What is the speed of the patient's speech? Rapid with very few pauses? Or are there long pauses between words?
C. Tone: Is there a wide range in the pitch of the voice sounds? Is the sound of his voice boring, tedious, or monotonous?
D. Productivity: Are the questions answered in one-word responses—a yes or no? Are details offered? Are questions expanded? Do simple questions yield complex or overly detailed responses?
E. Goal direction: Do the answers follow a logical sequence? Do the answers make sense? Does the focus remain clear?

Motor Behavior

The nurse should assess for posture, gait, tics, tremors, posturing, grimaces, and other abnormal bodily movements. The speed of these movements is important to note. Is there a general slowness of movement? Does there appear to be much effort expended just to talk, walk, or gesture? Or do the movements appear to be intense and rapid? The behaviors that include nail biting, wringing of the hands, tapping of the foot, and chewing movements may be clues to the individual's anxiety, and an increase or decrease of these behaviors can be noted as the interview progresses and deals with emotionally charged material.

There are a number of abnormal motor behaviors that are frequently related to specific mental disorders. *Echopraxia* (the pathological repetition by imitation of the movements of another person) and *cerea flexibilitas* (waxy flexibility) are often seen in catatonic schizophrenia in which a person can hold his body in one position for a long period of time. *Catalepsy* (a generalized condition of diminished responsiveness) often is characterized by trance-like states and immobility and can occur in organic and psychological disorders. *Cataplexy* is temporary loss of muscle tone and may be precipitated by surprise, laughter, or anger and is seen in schizophrenics.

A *compulsion* is an insistent, repetitive, intrusive, and unwanted urge to act in a way contrary to one's usual wishes or standards. The suffix *mania* is used with Greek terms to indicate a preoccupation with certain kinds of activities or a compulsive need to behave abnormally. Examples are: *egomania* (the pathological preoccupation with self), *erotomania* (the pathological preoccupation with erotic fantasies or activities), *kleptomania* (the compulsion to steal), *megalomania* (the pathological preoccupation with delusions of power or wealth); *necromania* (the pathological preoccupation with dead bodies), and *pyromania* (the morbid compulsion to set fires).

Mood and Affect

The term *affect* refers to what the individual is feeling at the moment—the emotional state and the outward appearance. Several areas can be noted when assessing affect.

A. Range: Limited or narrow—only a few emotions are expressed.
Wide or labile—frequent shifts between very different emotions.
Example: A 39-year-old depressed woman vacillates between crying and laughing about her current experiences.
B. Intensity: The quality of emotion expressed—flat with little energy or exaggerated with great energy.
C. Types: Different categories of emotions—sad, fearful, happy, angry, elated, etc.

D. Appropriateness: Does the affect expressed fit the content being expressed?
Example: Appropriate affect—A young woman is crying and fearful as she describes an attempted rape.
Example: Inappropriate affect—A 40-year-old man smiles when describing how angry he is at his father.

The individual's subjective description of his feeling is his mood. Ask the patient to describe his mood. Have there been any mood changes noted? If so, were these changes in mood rapid, cyclic, or situational? Assess the patient's dominant mood during the interview, i.e., depressed, anxious, angry.

Anxiety Level of Patient

In the assessment picture it is helpful to identify the patient's level of anxiety and the defense mechanisms he employs to diminish and allay anxiety. Anxiety is an uneasiness, apprehension, or fearfulness stemming from anticipated danger. Anxiety occupies a focal position in the dynamics of all human adjustment and serves as the driving force for most of our adjustments in life.

Symptomatically, anxiety has both psychic and somatic components. The psychic manifestation is the sensation of apprehension and the critical perception of discomfort. It is perceived by the conscious aspect of the personality. The somatic manifestations are the result of physiological responses of the various bodily systems. For example:

1. Cardiovascular response—may be tachycardia or palpitation.
2. Gastrointestinal response—may be anorexia, nausea, vomiting, cramps, or diarrhea.
3. Respiratory response—may be rapid or slow respiration.
4. Genitourinary response—may be urgency or frequency of urination.
5. Musculoskeletal response—may be various muscular aches or joint symptoms.

In order for the nurse to formulate an accurate nursing diagnosis and an effective intervention, the patient's level of anxiety must be identified as well as the defense mechanism employed by the patient to allay or diminish these feelings. The level of anxiety experienced by a person may be determined by asking the patient for his subjective experience and by the nurse's observation of the patient's behavior.

Peplau's model of assessing anxiety levels according to the perceptual interference experienced by the patient is a useful assessment tool for the nurse to employ. She identifies four levels of anxiety: mild, moderate, severe, and panic—as outlined below.[17] Each stage of anxiety has its particular effect on the sensory perception of the individual. (Chapter 21 expands on the concept of anxiety.)

Mild Anxiety Levels. Mild anxiety levels can motivate learning and stimulate growth and creativity in the individual. During this stage a person's sensory field increases, and he is alert to the environment and able to sharply discern what he is experiencing, thus maximizing the options available for decision-making.

Moderate Anxiety Levels. Moderate anxiety levels tend to narrow the perceptual field and block out peripheral stimuli. The patient does not attend to all the factors operating in the environment, but is still able to focus if another person directs him to do so. The choices available to a person at this level are restricted.

Severe Anxiety Levels. Severe anxiety levels severely reduce a person's perceptual field. The primary goal of the individual is to obtain relief from the feeling. With much direction from another, he is able to attend to a specific area. At this stage, self-awareness is greatly diminished and choices are severely limited.

Panic Levels. Panic levels of anxiety result in the individual's loss of control. He becomes disorganized and is in need of help from another human being in order to function. The perceptual field is blocked and the level of self-awareness is almost absent. The feelings associated with this level are dread, terror, awe, and danger. If such a state continues over a long period of time, exhaustion and death may result because the human organism cannot withstand such an overwhelming experience for an extended period of time.

When assessing the patient's anxiety level, the nurse should ascertain if she fully comprehends the situation that the client is experiencing. Then she may assess whether the anxiety level seems appropriate to the situation. Are the defense mechanisms used by the patient effective in decreasing anxiety level? What is the price of this relief? Do the mechanisms interfere with perception of reality, isolate the patient from others, immobilize creative energies? Does the patient's anxiety level stimulate or facilitate personal growth, happiness, and satisfaction, or

does it inhibit and thwart attainment of these goals? All of these questions need to be addressed by the nurse prior to formulation of a diagnosis and development of an appropriate nursing intervention.

Defense Mechanisms

The defense mechanisms previously described in Chapter 8 are adaptive functions of the personality (the ego structure) and are specific intrapsychic processes, operating unconsciously. Defense mechanisms are employed to seek relief from emotional conflict and freedom from anxiety. Defenses are considered successful if they abolish the need for immediate gratification or if they find substitute gratification. Table 12-2 reviews the various types of defense mechanisms and gives examples of each.

Thought Process

As the nurse attends to the content of the patient's speech, observations may be made regarding disturbances in the thought processes, in the structure and rate of association, and in the flow of ideas. Among the areas to be considered are:

A. Form: Does the client's thinking and communication proceed in a relatively clear, understandable manner? The following examples describe thought disorder abnormalities:
  1. Circumstantiality—The person digresses into unnecessary detail and unusual thoughts before saying central idea (often seen in patients who are schizophrenic).
  2. Incoherence—Difficult to follow or understand the patient because of an impairment in the manner of speech.
  3. Blocking—Sudden stopping in middle of sentence with no understanding of why.
  4. Loose association—Lack of logical order in content.
  5. Neologisms—New words or condensations of words (often seen in psychotic disorders).
  6. Word salad—An incoherent mixture of words (often seen in schizophrenia).

TABLE 12–2. DEFENSE MECHANISMS AND EXAMPLES

Compensation—A conscious or unconscious attempt to overcome real or imagined inferiorities or inadequacies.
Example: An underweight, short 15-year-old boy joins the weight-lifting club at school.

Conversion—Elements of intrapsychic conflict are disguised and expressed symbolically through physical symptoms.
Example: A patient currently involved in a divorce situation cannot move her legs although no organic basis for her symptoms can be found.

Denial—The unconscious disavowal of thoughts, feelings, wishes, needs, or external reality factors that are consciously unacceptable.
Example: A 65-year-old male continues to plan for future projects within his work environment even though his retirement is imminent.

Dissociation—The detachment of emotional significance from an idea, situation, object, or relationship.
Example: A rape victim describes her rape experience with a bland, flat affect.

Displacement—The redirection of an emotion from one idea, object, or person to another.
Example: A 5-year-old girl who was angered by her teacher in school yells inappropriately at her mother.

Identification—The unconscious adoption or patterning of the personality characteristics of an admired other.
Example: A young soldier begins to socialize with his friends, just like his sergeant.

Introjection—The symbolic assimilation (of taking into self) of loved or hated attitudes, wishes, ideals, or persons.
Example: A 16-year-old girl decides not to participate in her friend's stealing expedition. (She has introjected her parents' values.)
Example: A 25-year-old man stands and walks just like his father.

Projection—The attributing to another person or object of thoughts, feelings, motives, or ideas that are unacceptable to self.
Example: A 30-year-old college professor accuses a colleague of wanting to be the chairperson of the department.
Example: A 50-year-old psychiatric patient is certain that the hospital food is poison and that the staff wants to kill her.

Rationalization—An attempt to modify unacceptable motives, feelings, needs, or impulses into ones that are acceptable.
Example: A 37-year-old man who was passed over for a job promotion says the new position was not challenging enough.
Example: A young college graduate who did not get accepted into graduate school says he did not really need more schooling.

Reaction formation—The direction of overt behavior or attitudes in the opposite direction to the individual's underlying motives, feelings, or wishes.
Example: A 35-year-old women has unconscious feelings of anger and hatred for her father; but when he visits, she is polite and sweet-mannered.

Example: A 13-year-old girl has a crush on her 17-year-old neighbor; but when she sees him, she talks about how much he annoys her with his mannerisms.

Regression—The return to an earlier and subjectively more comfortable level of emotional adjustment.
Example: A 5-year-old girl, the week before starting kindergarten, becomes clinging and fearful of leaving her mother.
Example: A 28-year-old career woman cries uncontrollably when confronted with negative feedback from her boss.

Repression—The involuntary banishment of unacceptable or painful thoughts, feelings, and impulses into the unconscious.
Example: A 17-year-old parent has no recollection of hitting his infant son.
Example: A 45-year-old European businesswoman has no memory of the frequent air raids she experienced as a young child.

Sublimation—The diversion of unacceptable instinctual drives into socially and personally acceptable channels.
Example: A 35-year-old lawyer whose early life was emotionally barren becomes a successful prosecuting attorney. His anger and rage are channeled into prosecuting criminals.
Example: A 13-year-old junior high school student has an intense crush on her science teacher. She does outstanding work in his class and receives an A+ in the course.

Substitution—The replacement of an unattainable or unacceptable need, emotion, drive, or goal by one that is attainable or acceptable.
Example: Instead of becoming a class office candidate, a young woman college student becomes a campaign manager.

Suppression—The voluntary relegation of unacceptable ideas or impulses from the conscious mind.
Example: A college student is angry at his friend for not calling. He goes to the library and puts it out of his mind.
Example: An accountant in a large business organization feels a strong sexual attraction to her boss. When at work she consciously puts the feelings out of her mind.

Symbolization—The mechanism by which an external object is used to represent an internal idea, belief, attitude, wish, or feeling.
Example: During the late 1960s, the hair and dress style of young people symbolized their feelings and attitudes toward authority and the prevailing values of the culture.

Undoing—An endeavor to actually or symbolically erase a previously consciously intolerable experience.
Example: A husband and wife have an intense emotional argument at breakfast. The husband brings her flowers when he comes home from work.
Example: Lady Macbeth's ritualistic hand washing was an attempt to undo the crimes she and her husband had committed.

7. Perseveration—Repetition of the same response to different questions (often indicates organic involvement).
8. Echolalia—The pathological repetition of words used by one person.
9. Condensation—One symbol stands for a number of others and results in the fusion of various ideas into one.
10. Flight of ideas—Describes a succession of thoughts without logical connections.
11. Retardation—The slowing down of thought process.

B. Disorders of perception: Perception is the capacity to be aware of objects and to discriminate between them. The nurse can assess the patient's perception of reality during the interview and determine if any of the three major perception disorders are present: illusion, hallucination, or depersonalization.
1. Illusion—The misinterpretation of some real external sensory experience.
Example: The patient looks out the window and sees the shadow of the tree as a real person and hears the wind calling his name.
2. Hallucination—Sensory perceptions without external sources. Hallucinations may have different origins such as psychosis, a brain tumor, drug reaction, drug overdose, alcohol overdose, sleep deprivation, and hepatic failure. They may be vague sounds, flashes of light, or recognizable voices, faces, insects, or odors. There may be one or more of the following types:
   a. Visual—Hallucinations of sight.
   b. Auditory—Hallucinations of sound.
   c. Olfactory—Hallucinations of smell.
   d. Tactile—Hallucinations of touch.
   e. Gustatory—Hallucinations of taste.
   f. Visceral—Hallucinations of sensation.

Note: Auditory hallucinations are the most common. In evaluating them one should ask the patient if he can identify the voice and sex of the person. Also is the voice friendly or threatening? What is the voice saying to the patient? (Important to assess the directive of the hallucination.)

3. Depersonalization—A feeling that one is outside of one's body. This often is accompanied by a derealization in which the person feels a kind of strangeness about his immediate surroundings, almost like being in a dream.

C. Delusions: Delusions are a process by which a person adheres to a false or unreasonable idea from which no logic or experience can dissuade him. The patient's views, opinions, or ideas differ greatly from those generally accepted. There are five types of delusions:
1. Persecutory—Person believes there is an organized conspiracy to hurt or harm him in some way.
2. Somatic—Person is certain that his body is deteriorating from within or that someone is in his brain.
3. Grandeur—Person believes that he is a famous or an important person, i.e., God, Clark Gable, Queen Elizabeth.
4. Guilt—Person believes that his "bad" thoughts have power to affect or influence others.
5. Influence—Person believes his thoughts are being controlled by objects or persons outside of himself.

D. Phobias: Phobias are a persistent unrealistic, obsessive fear or dread of an object or situation, held by a person. Four major phobias are:
1. Acrophobia—Fear of heights.
2. Agoraphobia—Fear of open places.
3. Claustrophobia—Fear of closed spaces.
4. Panphobia—Fear of everything.

Thought Content

The nurse can assess thought content by listening carefully to the patient's preoccupations, ambitions, and dreams. By assessing the major themes and issues discussed by the patient, the nurse can identify the dominant themes that the patient is expressing. For example, does the patient relate most of what he considers his difficulty to a sense of failure, fear of harm, loss of an important person, phobias, fear of losing impulse control, or certain ritualistic compulsive behaviors?

An important area for the nurse to assess is the suicidal and homicidal ideation. The patient should be asked if he has had any thoughts about hurting himself or hurting others. If the answer to either of these questions is yes, the following data must be obtained:

1. Does the thought only occur infrequently—or is there a serious plan?

2. When did the thought start and how often does it occur?

3. Does the patient have the means to implement the thought or plan?

4. Has the patient told anyone else about his thoughts or plans?

Intellectual Functions

The nurse can assess an individual's general intellectual capacity by listening to his history. The patient's level of knowledge can be measured against the years of formal education and family and cultural background. The following four sections are helpful in an evaluation of a person's intellectual function:

A. Sensorium:
1. Level of attention and consciousness—How alert is the patient?
2. Person—Does patient know who he is, i.e., name and age?
3. Time—Does the patient know the day of the week, month, and year?
4. Place—Does the patient know where he is, where he lives, and how he got to where he presently is?

B. Memory:
1. Recent—Can he remember the events of last week, what he had for breakfast, the name of the examiner?
   Anterograde amnesia is the absence of memory of recent events.
2. Remote—Simple facts, e.g., who was last governor of state? The current president and the president before him, etc.?
   Retrograde amnesia is the absence of memory for past events.
   (Test for recent memory: Name three objects and ask patient to recall in 5 minutes, 10 minutes, etc.)

C. Concentration:
1. Focus of responses—Does patient have difficulty in focusing his answers? Is the patient easily distracted?
2. Simple calculation—Can patient perform simple math additions, subtractions, etc.?

The following is a sample exercise to test a person's level of concentration.[18]

Stage 1:   Add any two small whole numbers.

Stage 2:   Multiply any two small whole numbers or spell the word *world* backward, or state the number of nickels in $1.35.

Stage 3:   Name the days of the week backward, or perform a "serial threes" test—that is, subtract 3 from 100, then an additional 3 from the result, and so on until he reaches zero. (Normal standard: Fewer than two errors in 120 seconds or less.)

Stage 4:   Name the months of the year backward, or perform a "serial sevens" test—that is, subtract 7 from 100, then an additional 7 from the result, and so on until he reaches zero. (Normal standard: Fewer than four errors in 90 seconds or less.)

Stage 5:   Repeat a random series of numbers forward, beginning with a series of three numbers, then increasing the series by one number at a time. (Normal standard: A forward series of from five to eight numbers.)

Stage 6:   Repeat a random series of numbers backward, beginning with a series of three numbers, then increasing the series by one number at a time. (Normal standard: A backward series of from four to six numbers.)

D. Ability to abstract:
Can the patient see any pattern to his life? Is the patient able to interpret a proverb in a less literal personal manner? Or is his interpretation very concrete and personal? An exercise to test a person's capacity of abstraction is given below.[19]

Ask the patient to state the meaning of each of two proverbs, describing their application to his own present circumstances. Some useful proverbs are listed below:

Don't cry over spilt milk.
People who live in glass houses shouldn't throw stones.
Birds of a feather flock together.
A stitch in time saves nine.
The tongue is the enemy of the neck.
Don't count your chickens before they hatch.
The proof of the pudding is in the eating.
A rolling stone gathers no moss.
The squeaky wheel gets the grease.

Also ask the patient to describe the similarity between the objects in each of the pairs below:

An apple and an orange
A chair and a table
A fly and a tree
A child and a dwarf

E. Insight:
Does the patient recognize that he is having emotional or mental problems? What is his level of motivation to work on his difficulties? Is he aware of how his difficulties affect his life in general?

Judgment

The nurse assesses the patient's judgment by observing his ability to make and carry out plans, to take the initiative, to discriminate accurately, and to behave according to accepted practice.

A person's judgment may be considered impaired if his thoughts and actions are inconsistent with reality. To test for such a process, the nurse can ask such questions as, "What would you do if you found a stamped envelope in the street?" "Explain why criminals are put in prison." "Describe what you would do if stopped for speeding."

Attitude

The attitude of the patient may be assessed by observing if he is cooperative, evasive, arrogant, ingratiating, spontaneous, assertive, or withdrawn. What is the client's attitude about coming to the clinic or hospital? Toward the interview? These observations provide clues regarding patterns of relating to people as well as clues to the client's defense mechanisms.

─── CASE STUDY* ───────────────────────────

Patient Request Assessment:
  Joan, a 34-year-old single female, was brought to the mental health unit of the community hospital by her parents. Her general appearance was disheveled, anxious, and worried. She was restless and occasionally paced during the admission interview. The stated complaint was: "I have heightened emotions." Her request for assistance was for control. She was feeling overwhelmed with what had been happening in the previous week. Her stated goal was "to get my life in control."
Nursing Assessment:
  Joan viewed her health as good until about one year ago when she was diagnosed as having bipolar illness. She viewed her physical health as good without significant contributing factors to this hospitalization. A systems review was done without significant findings.
Nutritional–Metabolic Pattern:
  Her eating patterns are erratic. She reported having poor appetite during the past week but says she either eats a lot or very little. She appears 30 to 40 pounds overweight. Mother stated during the initial interview that Joan's boyfriend had been putting too much pressure on her to lose weight and that this was the cause of her present illness. Joan denied this.
Elimination Pattern:
  Joan reports having daily bowel movements with occasional episodes of constipation. She attributes the constipation to the erratic eating habits, knows she should eat better.
Activity–Exercise Pattern:
  Joan's history reveals periods of hyperactivity alternating with periods of fatigue. Her level of activity has escalated over the past 2 to 3 weeks. She occasionally swims, knows that she should establish a more consistent exercise program.
Sleep Pattern:
  She normally sleeps 6 to 7 hours per night. During the past week she has had difficulty going to sleep and has been waking early. She has slept 3 to 4 hours in the past few nights.
Cognitive–Perceptual Pattern:
  Joan wears corrective glasses or contact lenses. On admission she could not remember if her contacts were in or not. There were no changes in her hearing, taste, or smell. Her

_____

* This case study was written by Ethel Stoltzfus Shank.

memory was impaired as she had difficulty remembering events of the previous week. She seemed troubled by this. Her thought pattern was delusional at time of admission.

Self-perception—Self-concept Pattern:

Joan sees self as weak and inadequate due to hospitalizations in the past year. She sees self as competent in professional work but is worried about repeated hospitalizations. She regrets having moved back with parents about one year ago.

Role—Relationship Pattern:

Joan describes family situation as being very conflictual and feeling controlled by parents. She has had few close friends in high school and college. She does not have any siblings and has had few close friends at work.

Sexual—Reproductive Pattern:

Her menstrual periods have been regular and normal. She has never been pregnant but noted that she someday hopes to have children. Joan has been on birth-control pills but does not want her mother to know this.

Coping—Stress-tolerance Pattern:

A big stressor was her home situation. She felt that her parents were putting a lot of stress on her and she was feeling overwhelmed and unable to cope. She had tried adaptation by taking more medication (under the direction of her physician) and was very frustrated that this had not been adequate to prevent hospitalization.

Value—Belief System:

Joan had developed a complicated system of deceit and lying to her parents in order to "sneak off" with her boyfriend. She had gone away on weekends with him while her parents thought she was with a girlfriend. She expressed regrets and guilt about the deceit.

Mental Status Assessment on Admission:

1. General appearance: disheveled and disorganized, appeared anxious and troubled.
2. Attitude: cooperative, agreed to voluntary hospitalization at urging of parents.
3. Speech: rapid, pressured, and sometimes incoherent.
4. Motor behavior: hyperactive, unable to sit still.
5. Affective state: fearful and irritated, disappointed about need for hospitalization, reports frequent crying.
6. Thought processes: flight of ideas.
7. Thought content: delusional, confused, denies suicidal ideation.
8. Perception: denies A/V hallucinations.
9. Intellectual functioning: impaired, insight poor.
10. Orientation: oriented to person but not to time or place.
11. Memory: recent memory more impaired than remote.
12. Judgment: poor, thoughts and actions inconsistent with reality.

Psychosocial History:

Joan lives with her parents and commutes daily $1\frac{1}{2}$ hours to a larger city where she works as vice-president of a bank. She has had a good work record in the 11 years since she graduated from college. At present she works with investments and securities. She is very bright and probably of above-average intelligence.

Her relationship with her parents is very enmeshed and fused. She began seeing her boyfriend about 18 months ago. Her parents have been very opposed to the friendship and have forbidden him to enter the house or to make phone calls to the house. They have offered excuses that he is not good enough for her. The boyfriend is in his early thirties, also an only child, and has never been married.

Joan owns the house in which her parents live. Economics of the family are fused and complicated. Both parents are retired and in their early seventies. About a year ago she moved to an apartment in an attempt to be independent. The parents continued to send her bills, which she felt obligated to pay. She soon became ill and that confirmed mother's notion that she was unable to care for herself.

Joan reports that extended family relationships have always been distant. Father had one sibling, a younger sister living in Texas whom he has not talked to for many years.

Mother had two siblings. None of the grandparents are living. Joan remembers visits to grandparents as having always been stressful.

NURSING CARE PLAN

DSM-III-R DIAGNOSIS

Bipolar disorder, manic with psychotic features.

PRIMARY NURSING DIAGNOSIS

Enmeshed family system with diffuse boundaries related to low levels of individuation of family and overinvolved emotional relationship between parents and daughter. Refer to long-term goals for intervention.

SECONDARY NURSING DIAGNOSIS

Disturbance in balance of rest, sleep, activity related to hyperactivity.

GOAL

The patient will demonstrate a decrease in restlessness within 10 to 14 days and will establish and maintain an adequate balance of rest, sleep, and activity.

INTERVENTIONS

1. Decrease environmental stimuli.
2. Limit group activities in terms of size of group and frequency of activities based on the patient's level of tolerance.
3. Provide a consistent structured environment.
4. Promote exercise and recreational activities as part of rest–activity balance.

SECONDARY NURSING DIAGNOSIS

Low self-esteem related to feelings of losing control of self.

GOALS

The patient will discuss feelings of anxiety and helplessness and will be able to identify the relationship between anxiety and responses.

INTERVENTIONS

1. Encourage her to use stress management techniques to reduce anxiety before approaching problems.
2. Support positive actions she might take in viewing her abilities realistically.
3. Provide positive feedback for improved hygiene and appearance.
4. Encourage participation in unit therapeutic activities.
5. Assist her in identifying strengths.

SECONDARY NURSING DIAGNOSIS

Inadequate skills for daily living related to dependency on parents.

GOALS

Patient will verbally express feelings.
Patient will identify present skills and level of functioning in relation to living situation.

INTERVENTIONS

1. Establish therapeutic nurse–patient relationship.
2. Meet with client at least 20 minutes every day and evening shift.
3. Encourage interaction with other clients.
4. Model care and concern and encourage expression of feelings.

EVALUATION OF OUTCOME

Joan responded well to the therapeutic interventions and was discharged in two weeks. Her hygiene and appearance began to improve within 3 to 4 days. She continued her medications of thiothixene (Navane) and lithium carbonmate (Lithium). Within one week she became involved in therapeutic activities of group therapy, assertiveness training, stress management, and relaxation training. Her interactions with other clients were minimal. She recognized that being in the hospital was a stopgap effort in working on the problems. She wanted her parents to be involved in the therapy sessions. As she improved she showed insight into the problems of the family.

Family work was applied by providing structure and reframing of the problem. During her hospitalization her parents were present for two family sessions. The first one was somewhat chaotic because the therapist attempted to alter the family's transactional patterns. The second session was prior to discharge and focused on reframing of the problem and discharge planning.

LONG-TERM GOALS

1. To improve the family's ability to deal with crisis and to help them develop appropriate role relationships.
2. To reduce conflict and anxiety in the family.
3. To increase awareness of each other's needs.
4. To assist family members to separate from each other while maintaining emotional connectedness.

STRATEGIES TO BE USED IN WEEKLY FAMILY OUTPATIENT SESSIONS FOR 30 TO 40 SESSIONS

1. Enforce, in various ways, rules of the session, which preclude any family member speaking for each other.
2. Address each person by name.
3. Decrease disengagement of parents by encouraging dialogue between them.
4. Reframe the problem to elicit the parents' support.
5. Negotiate agreements to allow increased independence of the daughter.

Summary

This chapter has outlined psychiatric nursing assessment protocols in conducting the nursing process. The nursing process is a systematic way of identifying problems and solutions in order to be of service to patients and their families. It is the basic vehicle by which the purposes of nursing care are fulfilled. A case example is provided to illustrate the components of the assessment of the health and mental function or dysfunction of a patient.

Questions

1. What areas are included in conducting a patient request assessment, a nursing assessment of functional health status and a mental status examination?
2. Prepare a genogram, including three generations, on a client.
3. Identify defense mechanisms used by patients in your care for the past week.

REFERENCES AND SUGGESTED READINGS

1. American Nurses' Association, Division of Psychiatric and Mental Health Nursing Practice. *Standards of Psychiatric—Mental Health Nursing Practice*. Kansas City, Mo.: American Nurses' Association, 1982, p. 9.
2. Orlando, I. J. *The Dynamic Nurse–Patient Relationship*. New York: Putnam's, 1961.
3. American Nurses' Association, op. cit., p. 6.
4. Lazare, A., Eisenthal, S., & Wasserman, L. The customer approach to patienthood. *Archives of General Psychiatry*, 1975, *32*, 553–558.
5. Lazare, A., Eisenthal, S., Wasserman, L., & Harford, T. C. Patient requests in a walk-in clinic. *Comprehensive Psychiatry*, 1975, *16*(5), 467–477.
6. Gordon, M. *Nursing Diagnosis: Process and Application* (2nd ed.). New York: McGraw-Hill, 1987.
7. Krozy, R. Becoming comfortable with sexual assessment. *American Journal of Nursing*, 1978, *78*, 1034–1038.
8. Woods, N. F. *Human Sexuality in Health and Illness*. St. Louis, Mo.: Mosby, 1975, pp. 111–119.
9. Krozy, op. cit., pp. 1037–1038.
10. The Group for the Advancement of Psychiatry, Committee on Medical Education. *Assessment of Sexual Function: A Guide to Interviewing* (Vol. 8, Report No. 88). New York: The Group for the Advancement of Psychiatry, 1973.
11. Glover, B. H. Sex counseling for the elderly. *Hospital Practice*, 1977, 101–113.
12. Woods, op. cit., pp. 115–117.
13. Oberleder, M. Managing problem behavior of elderly patients. *Hospital and Community Psychiatry*, 1976, *27*, 329.
14. Ibid.
15. Fish, S., & Shelly, J. A. *Spiritual Care: The Nurse's Role*. Downer's Grove, Ill.: Intervarsity Press, 1978, p. 38.
16. Ibid.
17. Peplau, H. *Interpersonal Relations in Nursing*. New York: Putnam's, 1952.
18. Cohen, S. Mental status assessment. *American Journal of Nursing*, 1981, *81*, 1509–1511.
19. Ibid., p. 1510.

Chapter 13

Nursing Diagnosis

Santa J. Kozak and Karla J. Hannibal

Chapter Objectives

The students successfully attaining the goals of this chapter will be able to:

- Define nursing diagnosis and describe its application in psychiatric mental health nursing.
- Explain the steps of the diagnostic process.
- Explain the advantages of using a conceptual framework when applying the nursing process.
- Develop a diagnostic statement based on assessment data.
- Develop a treatment plan after a diagnostic statement has been developed and confirmed.
- Compare the specific psychiatric nursing diagnoses accepted by NANDA, and apply these diagnoses to case studies.
- Identify the present and future trends in research in psychiatric nursing diagnoses.

HISTORICAL ASPECTS

The term *nursing diagnosis* began appearing in the nursing literature in the 1950s as nurse professionals were redefining nursing practice independent functions to extend beyond the practical skills and duties of following physicians' orders and providing medical treatment. Abdellah's definition, "the determination of the nature and extent of nursing problems presented by the individual patients or families receiving nursing care" points out this separate focus of nursing that goes beyond medical protocols and treatment.[1]

In 1966 Durand and Prince defined nursing diagnosis as "a statement of a conclusion resulting from a recognition of a pattern derived from a nursing investigation of the patient."[2]

The responsibility of the professional nurse to describe health problems of patients and subsequently to prescribe treatment was stressed in the 1970s. Marjorie Gordon placed emphasis on the legal and educational aspects that contribute to enabling a professional nurse to make a nursing diagnosis. "Nursing diagnoses made by professional nurses describe actual or potential health problems that nurses, by virtue of their education and experience, are capable and licensed to treat."[3] In 1980 the American Nurses' Association (ANA) published a Social Policy Statement defining nursing as "the diagnosis and treatment of human responses to actual or potential health problems."[4] This definition was based on language used in New York State's Nurse Practice Act of 1972 and was incorporated into other states' Nurse Practice Acts throughout the decade.[5]

Recently more attention is being given to the etiology of the patient's response or condition, which has been included in a definition by Shoemaker. "A nursing diagnosis is a clinical judgment about an individual, family, or community which is derived through a deliberate, systematic process of data collection and analysis. It provides the basis for prescriptions for definitive therapy for which the nurse is accountable. It is expressed concisely and it includes the etiology of the condition when known."[6]

NANDA: A Brief History and Statement of Purpose

Although the term *nursing diagnosis* was first used in 1953, there was little systematic use of the concept until twenty years later when the ANA's *Standards of Nursing Practice* established that nursing diagnoses were to be stated on the basis of health assessment data.[7] The need to identify nomenclature relevant to nursing but not included in medical classification systems prompted Gebbie and Lavin, faculty members of St. Louis University, to schedule the first National Conference on Classification of Nursing Diagnosis in 1973. The task of the conference was to begin to develop a comprehensive system for classifying those health problems diagnosed by nurses and treated by means of nursing interventions. The National Group for the Classification of Nursing Diagnosis developed from the first conference.[8]

Participants in the conference came from all specialties of nursing and represented all regions of the United States and Canada. The name of the national group was changed in 1982 to North American Nursing Diagnosis Association (NANDA) so as to include the Canadian participants. As of 1987, NANDA has met seven times and has identified 83 accepted nursing diagnostic labels (Table 13-1).

"Accepted Diagnoses" refers to health problems that, in the opinion of the national group, can be diagnosed and treated by nurses. At the biennial conferences, students, staff nurses, educators, administrators, and researchers review identified diagnoses. Majority vote, through a mailed ballot, decides which diagnoses are accepted and recommended for further testing in clinical practice. Diagnoses are then reevaluated, refined, or deleted at the next conference. Before 1982, changes were made on the basis of opinion. Since then it has become established policy that any additions, modifications, or deletions are to be based on scientific research.[9]

The Seventh Conference was held in 1986. Various papers and posters on research studies concerning economic issues, impact of fee-based reimbursement for nursing care, use of functional health patterns and conservation principles to organize data to facilitate the identification of nursing diagnoses and multiple diagnoses were presented. As a result of the conference, 21 new diagnoses, an expansion of previous diagnoses, and NANDA Taxonomy I have been accepted.[10]

The Mental Health Special Interest Group that met at the National Conference consisted of interested conference participants.

The group discussed such issues as implementation of nursing diagnosis in multidisciplinary settings and how nursing differs from the practice of other professionals in the mental health arena; choosing nursing diagnoses in the psychiatric setting; computerization of nursing diagnosis; prioritization of nursing diagnoses; assigning a sixth Axis to DSM-III revision to incorporate the nursing role, and the need for a taxonomy of assets. The group asks NANDA to address the need for positive language in the proposed taxonomy, to investigate and possibly represent the nursing standpoint in the proposed DSM-III revision, and to consider the addition of a mental health component to the category "exchanging."[11]

NANDA's goals include the development and promotion of a taxonomy of nursing diagnostic terminology, the promotion of scientific research, and the provision of consultation to regional or special interest groups desiring to conduct programs of interest to members. NANDA strives to promote relationships with nursing and other health professionals and provides a mechanism for bringing issues of regional concern to the Board and the association.

There is a liaison between NANDA and the ANA through the Cabinet for Practice and its

TABLE 13-1. NANDA—APPROVED NURSING DIAGNOSTIC LABELS

Activity intolerance
Activity intolerance: potential
Adjustment, impaired
Airway clearance, ineffective
Anxiety
Body temperature, altered: potential
Bowel elimination, altered: constipation
Bowel elimination, altered: diarrhea
Bowel elimination, altered: incontinence
Breathing pattern, ineffective
Cardiac output, altered: decreased
Comfort, altered: chronic pain
Comfort, altered: pain
Communication, impaired verbal
Coping, family: potential for growth
Coping, ineffective family: compromised
Coping, ineffective family: disabled
Coping, ineffective individual
Diversional activity, deficit
Family processes, altered
Fear
Fluid volume deficit: actual (1)
Fluid volume deficit: actual (2)
Fluid volume deficit: potential
Fluid volume excess
Gas exchange, impaired
Grieving, anticipatory
Grieving, dysfunctional
Growth and development, altered
Health maintenance, altered
Home maintenance management, impaired
Hopelessness
Hyperthermia
Hypothermia
Incontinence, functional
Incontinence, reflex
Incontinence, stress
Incontinence, total
Incontinence, urge
Infection, potential for
Injury, potential for
Injury, potential for: poisoning
Injury, potential for: suffocating

Injury, potential for: trauma
Knowledge deficit (specify)
Mobility, impaired physical
Noncompliance (specify)
Nutrition, altered: less than body requirements
Nutrition, altered: more than body requirements
Nutrition, altered: potential for more than body requirements
Parenting, altered: actual/potential
Post-trauma response
Powerlessness
Rape-trauma syndrome
Rape-trauma syndrome: compound reaction
Rape-trauma syndrome: silent reaction
Role performance, altered
Self-care deficit: bathing/hygiene
Self-care deficit: dressing/grooming
Self-care deficit: feeding
Self-care deficit: toileting
Self-concept, disturbance in: body-image
Self-concept, disturbance in: personal identity
Self-concept, disturbance in: self-esteem
Sensory-perceptual alterations: visual, auditory, kinesthetic, gustatory, tactile, olfactory
Sexual dysfunction
Sexuality, altered patterns
Skin integrity, impaired: actual
Sleep pattern disturbance
Social interaction, impaired
Social isolation
Spiritual distress (distress of the human spirit)
Swallowing, impaired
Thermoregulation, ineffective
Thought processes, altered
Tissue integrity, impaired
Tissue integrity, impaired: oral mucous membrane
Tissue perfusion, altered: renal, cerebral, cardiopulmonary, gastrointestinal, peripheral
Unilateral neglect
Urinary elimination, altered patterns
Urinary retention
Violence, potential for: self-directed or directed at others

NANDA = North American Nursing Diagnosis Association.

Task Force on Classification of Nursing Phenomena as well as with the Nursing Organization's Liaison Forum (NOLF). Nursing diagnoses have been translated into Japanese, Chinese, Spanish, Italian, and French. Thus, the association will need to provide liaisons to the nursing associations of other countries.[12]

ANA Standards

The American Nurses' Association's *Standards of Psychiatric and Mental Health Nursing Practice*

identify the steps of the nursing process, including nursing diagnosis, as standards of care (Tables 13-2 to 13-5). These standards have been developed to provide a means to improve the quality of care delivered by the nursing profession.[13]

ANA Classification System

There has been lively debate within the psychiatric and mental health nursing specialty re-

TABLE 13-2. STANDARD II

DATA COLLECTION

The nurse continuously collects data that are comprehensive, accurate, and systematic.

RATIONALE

Effective interviewing, behavioral observation, and physical and mental health assessment enable the nurse to reach sound conclusions and plan appropriate interventions with the client.

STRUCTURE CRITERION

A means by which data are gathered, recorded, and retrieved is available in the practice setting.

PROCESS CRITERIA

The nurse—

1. Informs the client of their mutual roles and responsibilities in the data-gathering process.
2. Uses clinical judgments to determine what information is needed. Health data undergirding the nursing process for psychiatric and mental health clients are obtained through assessing the following:
    a) Biophysical, developmental, mental, and emotional status.
    b) Spiritual or philosophical beliefs.
    c) Family, social, cultural, and community systems.
    d) Daily activities, interactions, and coping patterns.
    e) Economic, environmental, and political factors affecting the client's health.
    f) Personally significant support systems, as well as unutilized but available support systems.
    g) Knowledge, satisfaction, and change motivation regarding current health status.
    h) Strengths that can be used in reaching health goals.
    i) Knowledge of pertinent legal rights.
    j) Contributory data from the family, significant others, the health care team, and pertinent individuals in the community.

OUTCOME CRITERIA

1. The client participates in the data-gathering process.
2. The client affirms the value of the data-gathering process. If illness precludes this capacity in the client, affirmation of the quality and ethical handling of the data is sought from the client's significant others and/or the nurse's peers.
3. The data base is synthesized and recorded in a standardized format.

garding the method to classify patient conditions or responses. Advocates for the use of the DSM-III-R classification system point to its current use by other disciplines in the field, while others believe the NANDA taxonomy should be adhered to. The third standard identified by ANA, diagnosis, includes both types of systems (Table 13-3).

Following the revision of the *Standards of Psychiatric Mental Health Nursing* in 1982, it became increasingly evident to the nurses in this specialty that there was a need for them to identify their own domain. Neither the DSM-III-R nor the NANDA taxonomy was fulfilling this need. In their February 1984 meeting, the Executive Committee of the Division on Psychiatric and Mental Health Nursing Practice of the ANA

"authorized support for the identification of the phenomenon of concern for psychiatric mental health nursing practice."[14] The task force that was formed to work on this project consists of a panel of nurse specialists with expertise in various age and diagnostic specialties within the psychiatric mental health field. They have developed a working draft of a classification system that incorporates nursing diagnosis terminology with DSM-III-R descriptions. There is still much work to be done to complete the list of human responses being classified. The testing and validation of the classification system will continue as the system is developed and refined. Efforts continue to be made to ensure that NANDA's nursing diagnoses system is integrated into this classification system.

TABLE 13-3. STANDARD III

DIAGNOSIS

The nurse utilizes nursing diagnoses and/or standard classification of mental disorders to express conclusions supported by recorded assessment data and current scientific premises.

RATIONALE

Nursing's logical basis for providing care rests on the recognition and identification of those actual or potential health problems that are within the scope of nursing practice.

STRUCTURE CRITERION

In the practice setting, opportunities are provided for validation of diagnosis by peers and for exchange of information and research findings regarding the scientific premises underlying nursing diagnosis among peers.

PROCESS CRITERIA

The nurse—

1. Identifies actual or potential health problems in regard to:
    a) Self-care limitations or impaired functioning whose general etiology is mental and emotional distress, deficits in the ways significant systems are functioning, and internal psychic and/or developmental issues.
    b) Emotional stress or crisis components of illness, pain, self-concept changes, and life process changes.
    c) Emotional problems related to daily experiences, such as anxiety, aggression, loss, loneliness, and grief.
    d) Physical symptoms that occur simultaneously with altered psychic functioning, such as altered intestinal functioning and anorexia.
    e) Alterations in thinking, perceiving, symbolizing, communicating, and decision-making abilities.
    f) Impaired abilities to relate to others.
    g) Behaviors and mental states that indicate the client is a danger to self or others or is gravely disabled.
2. Analyzes available information according to accepted theoretical frameworks.
3. Collects sufficient data to verify a diagnosis.
4. Makes inferences regarding data from phenomena.
5. Formulates a nursing diagnosis subject to revision with subsequent data.

OUTCOME CRITERIA

1. Nursing diagnoses are validated with the client when validation has a therapeutic purpose and is not clearly impossible or contraindicated. If illness precludes this capacity in the client, affirmation of the nursing diagnosis is sought from the client's significant others and/or the nurse's peers.
2. Nursing diagnoses are recorded in a manner that facilitates nursing, planning, and research.

ADVANTAGES OF NURSING DIAGNOSIS

The advantages of using the nursing diagnosis classification system have been recognized by various professional nursing organizations including ANA and NANDA, who are endorsing and promoting its use. The nursing diagnosis taxonomy clarifies the abstract knowledge of patient conditions and situations into conceptually sound, concise, and understandable definitions. Nursing concepts and theories can be developed and refined more systematically when based on a consistent, definitive terminology. As this body of knowledge grows and the scientific foundation for nursing is strengthened, the profession is being recognized as a specialized and autonomous member of the health care system. Nurses can define their various roles, functions, and the patient conditions they treat, providing a basis for reimbursement by third-party payers for itemized services. Communication between colleagues and other health care professionals is facilitated using a standard

---

TABLE 13-4. STANDARD IV

PLANNING

The nurse develops a nursing care plan with specific goals and interventions delineating nursing actions unique to each client's needs.

RATIONALE

The nursing care plan is used to guide therapeutic intervention and effectively achieve the desired outcomes.

STRUCTURE CRITERIA

1. The practice setting is one in which the nurse has opportunities to collaborate with others in the development of nursing care plans compatible with overall treatment plans.
2. Within the practice setting, mechanisms exist for nursing care plans to be recorded, communicated to others, and revised as necessary.

PROCESS CRITERIA

1. The nurse collaborators with clients, their significant others, and team members in establishing nursing care plans.
2. In the care plan, the nurse:
   a) Identifies priorities of care.
   b) States realistic goals in measurable terms with an expected date of accomplishment.
   c) Uses identifiable psychotherapeutic principles.
   d) Indicates which client needs will be a primary responsibility of the psychiatric and mental health nurse and which will be referred to others with the appropriate expertise.
   e) Stresses mutual goal setting and shared responsibility for goal attainment at the level of the client's abilities.
   f) Provides guidance for the client care activities performed by others under the nurse's supervision.
3. The nurse revises the care plan as goals are achieved, changed, or updated.

OUTCOME CRITERIA

1. The nursing care plan is recorded and available for review.
2. The nursing care plan shows evidence of revision and deletion of prescribed nursing actions as goals are achieved, changed, or updated.

---

vocabulary, contributing to greater consistency and efficiency in patient care.

The diagnostic process requires an organized approach to collecting and recording data, which assists the nurse in applying the clinical reasoning skills needed to make the diagnostic judgment. The treatment approach that is determined by the nurse is goal-directed and individualized, focusing on the etiology of the patient's condition rather than on signs and symptoms. Nursing practice has moved away from the medical model to specific values, concepts, and standards exclusive to nursing, promoting professional enthusiasm and motivation for nurses.[15]

Nursing education programs now incorporate nursing diagnosis into the organization, structure, and content of their curricula. Iyer, Taptick, and Bernocchi-Losey cite a survey by Gaines and McFarland of 74 National League for Nursing accredited baccalaureate and higher degree programs. It was found that 81.5 percent of the programs taught students the concepts and use of nursing diagnosis based on the National Conference System (NANDA).[16] More professional nurses are entering the work force with the knowledge and skills required to apply the diagnostic process in clinical practice.

Nursing research has been facilitated through the computerization of clinical data. The testing, validation, and evaluation of present and proposed nursing diagnoses can be achieved more accurately and comprehensively via computerized data retrieval.

TABLE 13-5. STANDARD V

INTERVENTION

The nurse intervenes as guided by the nursing care plan to implement nursing actions that promote, maintain, or restore physical and mental health, prevent illness, and effect rehabilitation.

RATIONALE

Mental health is one aspect of general health and well-being. Nursing actions reflect an appreciation for the hierarchy of human needs and include interventions for all aspects of physical and mental health and illness.

STRUCTURE CRITERIA

1. Independent nursing interventions are promoted within the practice setting.
2. Professional staffing patterns in psychiatric and mental health care settings are determined by the documented health care needs of the population served.
3. A mechanism exists to review and revise nurse–client ratios on at least a biennial basis to assure implementation of the standards of psychiatric and mental health nursing practice.

PROCESS CRITERIA

The nurse—

1. Acts to ensure that health care needs are met either by using nursing skills or by obtaining assistance from other health care providers when indicated.
2. Acts as the client's advocate when necessary to facilitate the achievement of health.
3. Reviews and modifies interventions based on patient progress.

OUTCOME CRITERIA

1. A record of intervention is derived from the nursing care plan.
2. Interventions are validated with client and peers.
3. Peers corroborate that interventions are guided by the nursing care plan and are therapeutic.

DEFINITION

There are many definitions for nursing diagnosis found in the literature. These definitions vary in specificity and focus, as noted in the introduction to this chapter. Several authors of books and articles on the subject of nursing diagnosis have identified common features that highlight the basic principles of what the term means. The following seven statements specify and clarify these common features.[17-19]

1. The process of determining a nursing diagnosis is an independent function of a professional nurse.

   There are many skills and areas of theoretical knowledge that a nurse must possess in order to make the clinical judgments necessary when diagnosing. As the nurse gains experience in clinical situations, the identification of altered or dysfunctional health response patterns can be made with greater accuracy. The patient responses that are given a nursing diagnostic label are conditions that the nurse can independently identify and treat.

2. A nursing diagnosis is a short, concise summary statement about a patient's response to an actual or potential health problem or health state of the patient.

   The diagnoses for patients are arrived at from judgments and conclusions resulting from the nurse's analysis of patients' assessment data. The summary statement indicates how the patient is affected and includes the etiology of the health problem or health state when known. The majority of nursing diagnoses are statements describing a patient's response to actual or potential health problems; however, there are diagnoses that describe a patient's response to a health state that indicates an area for potential growth (i.e., wellness–prevention teaching need).

3. The health problem or health state that a patient responds to can be physiological, psychological, spiritual, or sociocultural in nature.

Nurses, in their attempt to provide holistic care to their patients, must assess these areas (whether it be individually, family, or community centered) to determine the specific strengths and limitations of the patient that indicate a need for nursing care. Nursing diagnoses can be associated with one specific aspect (e.g., psychological), but it is important to remember that effects of a health problem or health state may be seen in other areas.

4. The patient's response to the health problem or health state can be treated, maintained, or prevented by nursing care.

Nursing diagnoses are conditions primarily resolved by nursing care methods. The patient's problems or needs can be positively affected as a direct result of treatment provided by nurses.

5. A nursing diagnosis is a nursing judgment resulting from a conclusion that is based on subjective and objective patient data that can be confirmed.

Information for a patient data base may be obtained from a variety of sources including the nursing assessment. Documentation and organization of the data base assist in analyzing the information and formulating conclusions (inferences) based on the subjective and objective data (cues). These conclusions that indicate the problems, limitations, or potential areas for growth of a patient are then used to support the determination of the appropriate nursing diagnoses.

6. In order to arrive at an accurate conclusion and nursing diagnosis, the patient data should be organized to identify a pattern or cluster of signs and symptoms.

It is important to use a framework that enables the nurse to organize assessment data in human response patterns. This assists the nurse in determining which patterns are most affected and possibly dysfunctional. A nursing diagnosis is not made based on an isolated symptom or cue. The cluster of signs and symptoms

within a health pattern provides the supporting data for the nursing diagnosis.

7. A nursing diagnosis and its etiology, when known, is the basis for planning nursing care.

The nursing diagnosis defines the state of the patient by describing the effect a health problem or health state has on that patient. The etiology or risk factors contributing to the patient's response become the focus of nursing care, based on the rationale that the treatment of signs and symptoms is less effective and lasting than treatment that is directed at the underlying cause. Nursing diagnoses clearly identify the patient conditions that will be positively altered after nursing care is implemented.

CONCEPTUAL FRAMEWORKS

Conceptual frameworks refer interrelated concepts to a suggested theory.[20] Nurses use frameworks to understand phenomena of concern, providing guidance through each step of the nursing process. Frameworks can also provide a taxonomy for nursing diagnoses.

Nurses in psychiatric mental health nursing at this time build on traditional theories to guide their practice (e.g., psychoanalytic theory, developmental theory, systems theory). Conceptual frameworks enable nurses to collect data in a systematic and purposeful manner during the assessment phase of the nursing process. When interpreting the patient's health problems or state, the nurse uses a conceptual framework to provide a structure upon which to categorize the data, understand the factors that play a role in optimal health and disease, and interpret the data that will influence the choice of nursing diagnosis.

A conceptual framework is subsequently used in diagnosing to establish patient goals and prescribe nursing interventions to achieve the goals. A conceptual framework identifies health norms and describes rationale for nursing interventions. Establishing the rationale for a specific nursing intervention for a problem is a step toward promoting nursing to a science. Evaluation determines the level of achievement of the patient goals. If there is lack of progress toward the goal, the nurse can review each preceding phase of the nursing process using the concepts and interrelationships of the framework to determine the discrepancy.[21]

Use of Conceptual Frameworks in Nursing Diagnoses

Before the Seventh Conference, there was no common conceptual framework used when proposing or accepting nursing diagnoses. Gordon cited the advantage of the representation of the diversity in nursing but noted that the consequence has been that nursing diagnoses are different in levels of abstraction (Ineffective Individual Coping versus Rape Trauma Syndrome, Silent Reaction), ranging from the general to the specific. Each diagnosis serves as a separate framework to direct the organization of the data and account for empirical observations.[22]

FUNCTIONAL HEALTH PATTERNS

It has already been noted that the first phase of the nursing process, assessment, requires a systematic plan for collection and organization of information about the health status of a patient. Gordon's functional health patterns provide an assessment and organizational format. These guide the nurse in obtaining basic data, lead directly to nursing diagnoses, and permit a holistic approach to assessment. The functional health patterns also have the advantage of being usable with any conceptual framework.[23] Gordon's eleven functional health patterns (Table 13-6) are more practical when assessment data are being organized and analyzed since they describe the human functional patterns that are the focus of a nursing assessment.

Using the health patterns as an assessment tool provides data about all aspects of the patient's health status and health history, as well as relevant data about family, home, and community. The assessment data include patterns of health and illness, risk factors for physical and behavioral alterations, available adaptive resources, and present and past coping patterns.[24] Information is gathered from the assessment interview, observations, physical examination, previous records, and consultations from within the hospital and the community. The patterns demonstrate patient–environment interaction and include a developmental and a functional

TABLE 13-6. TYPOLOGY OF GORDON'S ELEVEN FUNCTIONAL HEALTH PATTERNS

Health perception–health management pattern: Describes client's perceived pattern of health and well-being and how health is managed.

Nutritional–metabolic pattern: Describes pattern of food and fluid consumption relative to metabolic need and pattern indicators of local nutrient supply.

Elimination pattern: Describes patterns of excretory function (bowel, bladder, and skin).

Activity–exercise pattern: Describes patterns of exercise, activity, leisure, and recreation.

Cognitive–perceptual pattern: Describes sensory-perceptual and cognitive pattern.

Sleep–rest pattern: Describes patterns of sleep, rest, and relaxation.

Self-perception–self-concept pattern: Describes self-concept pattern and perceptions of self (e.g., body comfort, body image feeling state).

Role–relationship pattern: Describes patterns of role-engagements and relationships.

Sexuality–reproductive pattern: Describes client's pattern of satisfaction and dissatisfaction with sexuality pattern; describes reproductive patterns.

Coping–stress-tolerance pattern: Describes general coping pattern and effectiveness of the pattern in terms of stress tolerance.

Value–belief pattern: Describes patterns of values, beliefs (including spiritual), or goals that guide choices or decisions.

(From Gordon, M., 1982, with permission.[13])

focus. Dowd and colleagues found that there was an increase in data supporting diagnoses when a focused assessment was used. Etiologies were identifiable from the data base.[25] Focused assessment tools facilitate a thorough and accurate data base rather than one influenced by the nurse's preconceptions or personal value system. (See Chapter 12 for a detailed assessment guide using the functional health patterns.)

How well do nursing students make diagnoses? In a study of 43 nursing students, subjects correctly accepted hypotheses of diagnoses if appropriate data were collected. They seldom made incorrect decisions if they had the necessary data. When there was insufficient data, subjects were more willing to accept incorrect diagnoses. This decreased the conflict of the felt need to solve the problem[26]

To ensure an accurate assessment, the nurse will find it beneficial to evaluate the following:

Accuracy Were cues correctly remembered and transcribed? Were cues misinterpreted because of preconceptions, language barriers, or misread nonverbals? Was the source reliable? Do any cues contradict each other?

Completeness Were all sources of data collection used? Were cues missed or not explored adequately? Was routine questioning stopped too soon in lieu of a more focused search (as a result of preconceived ideas)?

Validation If inferences were made, were they validated with the client and family?

Quality Was the quality of the assessment influenced by the nurse or client feeling "rushed"? (This could lead to false or incomplete data.) Were the patient's priority health concerns addressed promptly? (The patient may provide less than quality data if concerns weren't addressed. The patient will have little patience with the data collection process and will not understand its value.)[27] Was information sought to explain the presence of specific cues? (The nurse uses clinical knowledge to decide what additional information is to be collected.) Were a variety of assessment sources used?[28]

Description and evaluation of the patterns allow the nurse to identify functional strengths and dysfunctional patterns. Patterns, not isolated cues, are interpreted. During the assessment, a pattern that is based on the patient's description and the nurse's observations emerges. Patterns are identified through the nurse's cognitive abilities, although they may not be readily observable to the untrained eye.[29]

Use of the functional health patterns creates a holistic picture of the patient. The patterns are interrelated, interactive, and interdependent. Thus, a nursing diagnosis can be identified in one pattern while the etiology of the diagnosis is found in another pattern.

EXAMPLE OF ASSESSMENT DATA ORGANIZED INTO THE FUNCTIONAL HEALTH PATTERNS

Pre-encounter Data

A 32-year-old white single male admitted with diagnosis of Alcohol Abuse. Recent attempts at outpatient therapy were unsuccessful because of many cancellations by the patient. Health insurance is paid by parent.

Initial Observations

Slightly obese, clothes appeared expensive but soiled and wrinkled. Halitosis and body odor noted. Nails well manicured but dirty. Inappropriately smiling and laughing with personnel at nursing desk. Upon meeting the primary nurse, took her hand, squeezed it, winked, and told the nurse that he could tell she was well educated and that he was sure she would take good care of him and understand him unlike others he went to for help.

Admission Interview with the Patient

Stated he was admitted because of exhaustion, needed a rest, and that he had been unable to deal with the stresses of his job expectations and life, "because it's so crazy." The prime reason for admission was that his parents convinced him to be admitted to get some rest and deal with a drinking problem. He denied drinking is a problem for him, but was admitted to give in to their concerns, as he needed a rest anyways.

Mr. Thorne's affect became angry when discussing his relationship with his parents. Stated that they were "close," but that they constantly nagged him as if he were a child. They "nag" about his drinking and his inability to stay at a job. Has had five jobs in the past two years but explained they weren't right for him, he wasn't able to use his talents, or that they were too demanding. Visits parents every Sunday. Is an only child.

Described prior close relationships with two male friends, but after each of them married about two years ago, the friendships deteriorated. His friends no longer were interested in doing what he enjoyed (going to bars) and forgot about him as they became preoccupied with their wives. Denied sadness, rejection, or desire to look at possible ways to rekindle relationships. He identified being angry because they dropped him and showed that they didn't really care.

Dates occasionally. Usually sees the women two

to three times and drops them because they show by their actions that they don't care about him; they're not willing to give him help when he needs it. Describes self as being a loner until he can find the right woman who will take care of him.

Patient views himself as independent and in control of his life. Future plans and goals are to take a vacation in Europe per parents' promise as a gift for being willing to be admitted. Wants to get the "right" job, where he can use his talents and rapidly rise up the corporate ladder. Unable to be specific about talents or types of job positions he desires.

Stated that he has needed recent financial assistance from his family because his fatigue has prevented him from attending work on a regular basis. Feels that his parents are happy to give him the money because it makes them feel needed, so he doesn't feel guilty about it, and "they have more than enough money anyways."

Initially stated he only drinks socially. When pressed for specific details as to what, how much, when, and with whom, his voice became loud and angry and he began pacing in room. Prefaced his answer with denying that drinking is a problem for him, despite what others say. Admitted to stopping at a local tavern just about every night for a few vodkas to help him relax. Has had two accidents in the past year and was cited for driving while intoxicated but claims he was not drunk and knew what he was doing. Parents retained an attorney who was able to get the charges dropped. Admitted to blacking out once, but said he was very tired and hadn't eaten that day; it was not due to drinking. Stated he gets "a little tipsy a few times a week to have fun."

Smokes 2½ to 3 packs per day. Denied illicit or prescribed drug use. Takes aspirin about three to four times a week for headaches. Uses an antacid every day or two for a sensitive stomach.

Has difficulty falling asleep, uses an over-the-counter sleeping pill and a drink or two to relax. Usually falls asleep by 3:00 and frequently oversleeps for work.

Diet consists of coffee for breakfast, sometimes a doughnut; lunch and dinner are usually obtained from fast-food places—sandwiches, fried chicken, and pizza. Has never learned to cook for himself. Goes home for Sunday dinner once a week. Frequent snacking on candy bars for energy. No fresh fruit or vegetables in diet.

When asked about bowel and bladder elimination, immediately said "OK, every day, unless I'm under stress."

Oriented, good attention span, recent and remote memory intact. No delusions or hallucinations. No tremors noted. Stated he went on a retreat three months ago to try to relax. During the three-day period of the retreat, he had no alcohol, which only resulted in an increased feeling of nervousness and irritability. Used this example as "proof" that he does not have an alcohol problem.

Believes in God but emphasized he is "not a religious person."

Does not engage in any sports or athletic activities. Drives for even short distances.

Additional Observations

Had eye contact with nurse only when making jokes. When spoke of friends, self-concept, problems with jobs, and drinking behavior would fidget with hands, look at guidelines book, or attempt to change the subject.

Interview with Family

Father has arranged jobs for his son for the past several years, but the patient has either been fired because of poor attendance or left because the job wasn't right for him. Has never gotten a job on his own initiative. Has always used family or friends to find him a job. The boss of his present job has discussed with the father his concerns of the patient's chronic tardiness and absence. Within the past three months, interest in personal appearance has declined and the patient's boss has told the father that unless his personal hygiene and appearance improved, he would be fired. Parents explained that the problem of tardiness and absence is due to nightly drinking, frequently to the point of intoxication (per bartender's comments to father, who pays the bar bill).

The patient has never been completely financially independent. Parents routinely pay his health insurance. Dependence has increased the past two years. Frequently, when he visits on Sundays, he begins to cry, calls himself a failure and shows them letters from companies threatening to refer him to a collection agency and cut off his utilities. They have paid off all his financial debts several times to provide him with a "fresh start" but to no avail; the situation reoccurs.

Parents note a decrease in interest in his hygiene the past few months.

They expressed concern about their decision to relocate to Florida, which they shared with the patient three months ago. The patient has accused them of not wanting to be around him but has refused the offer from them to relocate with them.

Their goal for hospitalization is for their son to get the help he needs to stop drinking and to become more independent. "We want our son cured no matter what it costs!"

Physical Exam

Normal. Complains of frequent indigestion, relieved by antacids. No history of delirium tremens. Observable large cavities in teeth.

Old Records

Medical: Upper G.I. three years ago with a repeat one year ago; both normal.

FUNCTIONAL HEALTH PATTERNS WITH CORRESPONDING ALTERATIONS AND STRENGTHS

1. Health Perception–Health Management Pattern. Believes smoking decreases stress, e.g., smokes 2½ to 3 packs of cigarettes per day. Believes alcohol helps him relax, e.g., drinks alcohol every night, frequently to point of intoxication. Believes his smoking and drinking are within the norm. Believes his teeth are in adequate condition (but cavities noted during P.E.). Believes he has no time for sports.

2. Nutrition–Metabolic Pattern. Low daily intake of vitamins and minerals; does not meet daily requirements. Diet high in starch, fat, and sugar; lacks fiber. Height: 5 feet, 9 inches; weight 210 pounds. Slightly obese (recommended weight 175 pounds).

3. Elimination Pattern. Intermittent constipation; may be due to lack of fiber in diet.

4. Activity–Exercise. Sedentary life-style, no exercise program or active participation in sports. Leisure activity consists of going to bars and drinking. Decreased attention to personal hygiene past 3 months: body odor, halitosis, clothing dirty and wrinkled.

5. Sleep–Rest Pattern. Difficulty falling asleep. Uses over-the-counter sleeping pills. Oversleeps for work after falling asleep about 3:00 A.M. Complains of chronic fatigue.

6. Cognitive–Perceptual Pattern. Dependent on parents to make decisions and solve problems for him. Intelligent, has a B.A. degree. Recent and remote memory intact.

7. Self-Perception–Self-Concept Pattern. Verbal statements of positive self-concept were inconsistent with body language. Has frequent crying spells about the financial problems he gets involved in. Identifies experiencing anger but denies any sadness or feelings of rejection. Unrealistic expectations for job promotions. Demonstrates lack of pride or concern about his personal appearance. Continues to drink alcohol to excess, demonstrates poor job performance, and lives beyond his economic means in a destructive manner. Feels others are supposed to take care of him. Feels inadequate to care for self.

8. Role–Relationship Pattern. Expects others to be willing to take care of his needs. When others are unwilling or unable to "take care of" him, becomes angry. Describes relationship with parents as close, but he becomes angry when they nag him like a child. Dependent on parents for finances and to solve his problems (driving while intoxicated and procuring jobs for him). Angry because parents are relocating, believes they don't want to be around him. Unwilling to relocate with them, wants them to change their plans for him. (Manipulates friends and family; becomes angry when efforts are unsuccessful.) Hasn't made new friendships since he "lost [his] two friends." Parents support dependent relationship.

9. Sexuality–Reproductive Pattern. Attempted to manipulate nurse on first encounter. Avoidant regarding sexuality. Intimate relationships are of short duration.

10. Coping–Stress-Tolerance Pattern. Uses alcohol, denial, and rationalization to cope with feelings and stressors. Uses dependency or family's support for primarily financial and problem-solving situations. Has not availed self of other support systems, sabotaged previous attempts at outpatient therapy. Attempts to manipulate nursing staff to "take care of him." Unable to maintain a stable job performance and attendance.

11. Value–Belief Pattern. Believes in God, but does not attend church or appear to derive support from the belief.

COMPONENTS OF A NURSING DIAGNOSIS

There are three necessary components of a nursing diagnosis, which are described by Gordon's PES format.[30] The components include the problem or health state of the individual, family, or community (P), the etiology or related, risk, and contributing factors (E), and the cluster of signs and symptoms or defining characteristics (S).

The Problem

The first part of the nursing diagnosis is the problem described by the diagnostic title or category level. It is a concise description (two to three words) of the state of the person's health, either actual, possible, or potential (e.g., Ineffective Individual Coping). The diagnostic title reflects a cluster of signs and symptoms that has been researched and found to support a nursing diagnosis. Diagnostic titles that have been researched and accepted by NANDA can be found in Table 13-1.

If diagnostic titles are to convey a patient's problem, they need to be specific and they need to assist the nurse in planning goals. Indicating the focus of the problem also aids in the specificity (e.g., Knowledge Deficit: Side Effects of Medication). Modifiers are necessary for some diagnostic titles (e.g., Anxiety, Mild, Moderate, or Severe). The qualifiers, Actual, Potential, and Possible, describe the status of the patient problem and will be discussed in more depth in the following section.

The Etiology

The second part of the nursing diagnosis are the etiologic factors that are causing or maintaining the patient's problem. At present, the etiology is considered to refer to related, contributing, or risk factors. The etiology can be a pattern of behavior or of psychological, situational, or maturational factors in the environment. The etiology is an inference made by the nurse based on knowledge of theory and the ability to assess a dysfunctional pattern or state and risk factors that can be a causal link to the patient problem.

The specific etiology gives direction to the remainder of the nursing process. Nursing orders stem from the etiology and will alleviate the patient problem through modifying or eliminating the etiology (related, risk, or contributing factors). Two patients with the same diagnostic title but with different etiologies require two different forms of therapy (e.g., Actual Altered Parenting "related to lack of support between husband and wife" versus "related to interruption of the maternal bonding process").

An etiology is not listed in terms of a medical diagnosis; rather the nurse assesses the effect on the patient's life processes or life-style that can be amenable to independent nursing practice. For example, Potential for Injury related to organic brain syndrome is more appropriately stated Potential for Injury related to impaired judgment.

It is frequently difficult to assess the etiologic factors when a patient is first admitted. In these cases, "unknown etiology" may be used. Carpenito explains that "the use of 'unknown etiology' alerts nurses to the need to assess for contributing factors at the same time as they are treating the present manifestation of the problem."[31]

The diagnostic label and the etiologic factor(s) are linked together by the phrase "related to" to form the diagnostic statement. However, one needs to be cautioned against linking words that establish one cause and effect. There are usually a number of factors that contribute to a problem. The nurse identifies only those factors that are amenable to nursing care with complete certainty. Implications of blame could lead to professional or legal difficulties (e.g., Alteration in Health Maintenance "related to mother's use of cocaine" versus "related to mother's ineffective individual coping and inability to make thoughtful judgments").

The Signs

The third component of a nursing diagnosis is the cluster of signs and symptoms or defining characteristics. Each accepted diagnostic category has defining characteristics that permit discrimination among health problems. Although all the defining characteristics need not be identified, major characteristics, when listed, need to be present. A cluster of characteristics rather than isolated symptoms validates a diagnosis.

SAMPLE OF A DIAGNOSTIC STATEMENT SUPPORTED BY DEFINING CHARACTERISTICS

(Diagnosis was derived from assessment data provided in the example given in the preceding section.)

Ineffective Individual Coping related to personal vulnerability (dependent life-style)

- Inability to meet basic needs (not bathing or eating minimum daily requirements).

- Destructive behavior toward self (drinking to point of intoxication every night).
- Inability to meet role expectations (is chronically late or absent from work, financially dependent on parents).
- Inappropriate use of defense mechanisms (denies drinking is a problem despite loss of income caused by drinking).
- Verbalization of inability to cope.

Use of the Qualifiers: Actual, Potential, Possible

The qualifiers Actual, Potential, and Possible precede the diagnostic label to describe the stage of the diagnosis. The term Actual pertains to the diagnosis that has been validated by a cluster of accepted defining characteristics and an accepted etiology. When writing a diagnostic title, Actual is not used to preface the diagnostic title unless it is included in the diagnostic label (e.g., Actual Alteration in Parenting).

The qualifier Potential prefaces a diagnosis when describing an altered state that may occur if certain nursing interventions are not ordered and implemented. Defining characteristics are not present, but etiologic or risk factors are (exceptions: Potential for Violence; Potential for Injury; Family Coping Potential for Growth). A Potential diagnosis is preventive in nature or is used when health-promotion activities are indicated.[32] Gordon states that for the qualifier Potential to be used appropriately, the patient must be more likely than the general population to develop the problem. Thus, if Thorazine, which can induce sedation, is prescribed for a geriatric patient whose gait is already compromised, the nurse may assess for the diagnosis of Potential for Injury. There must be risk factors for the patient in order to merit the identification of a potential problem.

Carpenito explains that the qualifier Possible "describes problems [and areas of growth] that may be present but require additional data to be confirmed or ruled out . . . [and] serves to alert the nurse to the need for additional data."[33] Usually when Possible is used to describe a diagnosis, defining characteristics have not been identified but the presence of contributing factors is confirmed. Gordon warns that a danger of using the qualifier Possible is that the nurse may move toward premature closure rather than evaluating whether another diagnosis is more accurate.[34]

THE DIAGNOSTIC PROCESS

Diagnostic reasoning is "a process of determining a [patient's] . . . health state and evaluating the etiological factors influencing that state."[35] Carnevali describes the process as a complex observation and data gathering process in which the diagnostician is rarely applying the process to just one problem because multiple problems coexist.[36] The eight steps of the diagnostic process are interrelated and continuous and begin with assessment, which is ongoing.

1. Identify alterations in the patient's functional health patterns. The cues within each pattern are compared with the patient's previous base line and the developmental, standard health, and cultural norms. Dysfunctions (behaviors that are inconsistent with these norms) and potential dysfunctions (risk factors) are identified. When identifying a psychiatric diagnosis, subjective data are essential, but data from a neurological or physical examination are necessary to rule out organic pathology.
2. Identify significant relationships among cues within a pattern and from multiple patterns. The assumption that the etiology is found in multiple patterns is based on the interdependence and interaction of the functional health patterns and the belief that the patient responds as a whole person.[37] There can also be cues that may be in more than one relationship and indicators of more than one nursing diagnosis. The information collected may not match a textbook picture of a diagnosis; it is necessary to ascertain the meaning of concealed cues, to verify cues and to be able to put initial cues together so their relationship emerges.[38]
3. Identify cluster cues. Inferences (interpretations) are made and hypotheses are generated even when the nurse is performing the initial assessment. An advantage of clustering cues early in the process is that a focused search of related cues can be pursued, providing additional data. Inferences should be validated with the patient to help ensure accuracy.
4. Select functional health patterns that encompass cues and clusters. Since nursing diagnoses can be classified or grouped according to functional health patterns, selecting a dysfunctional health pattern can refer the nurse

to a number of possible nursing diagnoses. The definitions and critical and supporting defining characteristics can be reviewed to suggest further possible hypotheses.

5. Activation of hypotheses can occur in an initial assessment. However, these hypotheses must remain tentative, and the nurse needs to be seeking additional cues. Early activation and acceptance of a hypothesis can occur as an adaptive measure. An immediate hypothesis decreases cognitive stress by creating structure and direction for the nurse. Being able to label a problem brings a sense of closure and accomplishment. It has also been observed that once an opinion has been formed, a person tends to focus on data that is supportive of the opinion and to ignore nonsupportive cues.[39] However, if one employs clinical knowledge and theory, experience, and research to make a judgment regarding a hypothesis, it can again direct a focused search for cues to rule out or support the hypothesis.

Another factor that can influence activation of hypotheses is a nurse's lack of experience with specific client problems. Carnevali points out that "somatic diseases may tend to be recognized less quickly in a psychiatric setting."[40]

6. Testing of hypotheses is accomplished through three steps.
   a. Focus on critical characteristics to confirm or rule out hypotheses.
   b. As the range of hypotheses is narrowed, evaluate what led to favoring or disregarding hypotheses.
   c. Review the diagnosis to ensure that it describes the state of the patient. Match the cluster of cues and suspected etiologies of hypotheses with the nursing diagnosis profiles (lists of accepted defining characteristics and etiologies or related factors) for congruence. Assess which diagnoses have the strongest defining characteristics.
7. Label diagnosis with the "best fit" of defining characteristics and etiology.
8. Validate the nursing diagnosis (Table 13-7). If the diagnosis can not be validated, the nurse reevaluates the data collection and reshapes the data search or activates alternative hypotheses.

The results of a study that analyzed errors in diagnosis were presented at the Sev-

TABLE 13-7. DIAGNOSTIC VALIDATION

1. Does my synthesis of data demonstrate the existence of a pattern?
2. Are signs and symptoms that I used to determine the existence of a pattern characteristic of the health problem (or health state) that I identified?
3. Is the tentative nursing diagnosis amenable to independent nursing actions?
4. Have I clarified and verified information as necessary so that I understand the client's reports and have confidence in my observations?
5. Have I paid attention to diagnostic cues in the data?
6. Have I interpreted what the client reports mean or signify? Norms? In the context of other data?
7. Have I considered alternative explanations for the cues? Eliminated those not applicable in this client situation?
8. Have I recalled all the critical diagnostic characteristics for the hypotheses I am testing and assessed for these characteristics?
9. In my best (unbiased) judgment, do I have sufficient data to support the diagnostic hypothesis that I am about to formulate as a nursing diagnosis?

(Steps 1 through 3, from Price, M. R. Nursing diagnosis: Making a concept come alive. *American Journal of Nursing*, 1980, *80*, pp. 668–671, with permission. Steps 4 through 9, from Gordon, 1987, with permission.)

enth Conference, since errors occurred at major steps of the diagnostic process. During problem identification, information was not recalled accurately or the meaning of the data was not explored. At times data did not match the hypotheses that were generated, and priority areas of nursing concern were occasionally not focused on during the stage of hypothesis activation. Errors were made during the data gathering process for each hypothesis, which included the use of knowledge or experience that did not fit the data cluster. The stage of hypothesis evaluation was the source of errors made when premature conclusions were not tested or data were not confirmed or rejected when possible.[41]

Myers and Spies presented the results of a study which was to identify the terminology used by nurses in nursing diagnostic labels. The research showed no statistical differences between years of experience and type of diagnostic statement generated.[42]

PROCESS AND OUTCOME CRITERIA

Goals can be either process or outcome criteria, depending on whether they focus on nursing strategies to be used or on behaviors and status changes expected of the patient.

Process criteria are nursing goals that provide direction for the intervention. They guide the nurse in making the decision about what is to be accomplished with the patient and family (e.g., reduce patient's fatigue). Carpenito describes three major areas that process criteria strive to promote[43]:

1. Use of patient's resources to facilitate an optimal level of coping.
2. Identification of other resources to achieve an optimal level of coping.
3. Modification of the patient's activities of daily living and usual life-style when resources are compromised.

Process criteria assist the nurse in identifying the outcome of nursing care. However, process criteria are not the sole determinant of patient goals (outcome criteria). To guard against the nurse imposing her values, goals must be mutually set with the patient and family. If the patient is unable to identify goals, the nurse can make suggestions for the patient to choose. The patient's motivation will increase if the patient has an active role in the process and views the goals as valuable.[44]

Outcome criteria describe the anticipated change in the status or behavior of the patient or family after receiving nursing care. The criteria focus on eliminating or modifying the etiologic factor(s) of the nursing diagnosis, not merely the defining characteristics. Outcome criteria are determined before nursing care is planned. They are used to achieve two purposes: (1) to plan nursing care; and (2) to evaluate the effectiveness and validity of nursing care.[45] The goals that are listed on care plans are outcome criteria. They are written in terms of what the patient is to do, not of what the nurse is to do.

Components of Outcome Criteria

The components of outcome criteria are not entirely new to the nurse who has been writing behavioral goals or objectives. Outcome criteria have measurable verbs, are specific in content and time, and are realistic.

Measurable verbs describe the exact behavior or performance of the patient or family that the nurse expects to see or hear.

NOT MEASURABLE

accepts	appreciates
knows	understands

MEASURABLE VERBS

states	specifies
performs	administers
identifies	discusses
selects	assists
demonstrates	informs

Goals must be specific in content and time. Specificity pertains to speed and conditions under which the behavior is to be performed. Goals are dated. Frequently, under a long-term goal, there will be a sequential list of short-term goals. Specific conditions that may be included in the goal are accuracy, quality, and criterion-referenced conditions.[46]

Speed	Sets a time limit that is reasonable given the patient's health state and the patient's and nurse's capabilities and limitations.
Accuracy	Identifies a degree of performance quantitatively.
Quality	Indicates the standard that is expected in terms of a given acceptable procedure.
Criterion-referenced	Uses a book, pamphlet, or other resources as a guide. Criteria give direction to plans for meeting the objective. They also provide a measure to evaluate achievement of the objective.

Examples of conditions used in outcome criteria:

Accuracy	Will recite *3 out of 5* side effects of Thorazine that were taught by 1/5.

Quality   Will discuss how to resolve a
               conflict through *using the*
               problem-solving method by 3/7.
Criterion-   Will describe the steps of
referenced   Progressive Relaxation
               according to Bernstein and
               Berkovec by 2/8.[47]

Conditions may also include the experiences that the patient is expected to have before meeting the goal, e.g., "After two family meetings. . . ."

Outcome criteria must be realistic and include the patient's cognitive, psychomotor, and psychosocial abilities and limitations. Other important factors to consider are probable length of hospitalization and resources outside the hospital. Again, if outcome criteria are mutually set with the client and family, information can be obtained and shared so that realistic goals can be established.

A goal must always have a *measurable verb*, be *specific in time* and include at least one specific condition, all of which are *realistic*. A goal portrays an exact picture to others of what the patient is expected to do.

NURSING INTERVENTION

Nursing interventions include nursing actions that can apply to any number of individuals who share a similar problem. Standards of care (e.g., suicide precautions for a severely depressed patient) are examples of nursing interventions.[48] Nursing orders are used by some nurses to provide specific directions for nursing care and individualized care to clients. "Individualizing nursing orders increases treatment success rate."[49]

Translating a nursing intervention to a nursing order requires the nurse to think about the diagnosis, but also and more importantly, the etiology and the specific client and situation. Nursing orders assist the patient in meeting the outcome criteria that stem from the etiology. Gordon discusses the following areas, which the nurse must consider when writing nursing orders[50]:

1. Personal patient factors. The patient's unique characteristics—age, developmental stage, sex, culture, religion, family structures, and other personal characteristics—will influence interventions.

2. Patient's perception. The patient may believe certain causal factors are involved in the nursing diagnosis, despite their unrelatedness. Unless the interventions include methods to clarify perceptions, any intervention will fail because the patient will consider it meaningless and unrelated to the problem or area for growth.

3. Current level of compensation. The patient may be using resources, defenses, or strengths to compensate for the problem. Information about the compensation facilitates decision making about what kind of nursing assistance is needed and points out the strengths of the patient and family.

4. Problem magnitude and urgency. The severity of the problem must be considered when planning nursing orders. Some health problems may require immediate nursing action because of the risk that they pose to the patients or others. Potential for Violence and Potential for Injury require immediate interventions to reduce the risk factors.

5. Extended effects. Nursing actions may have effects on others (e.g., milieu in the hospital, or family or social group outside of the hospital). The possible effects of interventions on others must be considered before deciding on nursing orders. Interventions may also have positive or adverse effects on other nursing diagnoses or medical problems (e.g., the effects of seclusion for Potential for Violence on the nursing diagnosis of Social Isolation). Interactions among nursing orders and nursing diagnoses must be considered when planning care.

6. Cost–benefit factors. Each nursing order has a price and a consequence. The costs can be financial, psychological, or social. The consequences or benefits can be immediate or long-term changes in health and well-being or progress towards a long-range goal. The cost and benefits of nursing actions must be weighed against each other. If the benefit is long-term, can the patient and family wait or does the patient need an immediate "payoff"? The nurse must seek out the patient to determine what costs the patient is willing to pay for the benefit and whether the benefit is worthwhile to the patient. Cooperative

goal setting and planning of care is imperative.

To be successful, nursing interventions need to be individualized for the patient. Since the nurse will not have all the above information when writing the initial nursing orders, it is expected that nursing orders will be updated and modified as the nurse gathers more data about the patient and family.

Nursing orders are written sequentially to build toward the achievement of a specific outcome criteria. A withdrawn client is not usually expected to actively socialize with a group before being able to communicate on a one-to-one basis.

The sequential ordering of nursing orders will reflect the order of the outcome criteria.

Nursing orders (*patient-specific* nursing interventions) must contain the following[51]:

1. Date.
2. Directive verb.
3. Answers to the questions: What? When? How often? How long? Where?
4. Signature of the professional nurse.

EXAMPLE

Mrs. Thomas uses the defense mechanisms of rationalization and denial to avoid discussing the effects of her behavior.

Nursing Intervention

Encourage verbalization.

Nursing Order

3/9: Per contract, after breakfast, elicit from Mrs. Thomas a specific time period of 20 minutes to review and share perceptions regarding her entries in her notebook from the previous day.

Jane Doe, R.N.

NURSING DIAGNOSIS RESEARCH: PRESENT AND FUTURE TRENDS

Current Research

Many professional nurses throughout the country have demonstrated a commitment to using NANDA's accepted nursing diagnoses in clini-

cal practice. While some of the currently accepted diagnoses were based on clinical research and validation, the majority were based on expert opinion when they were accepted. Research in all areas pertaining to nursing diagnosis has been promoted to establish a strong scientific foundation. The development of the nursing diagnosis classification system has proceeded at a quicker pace than the research to support and refine the system. Areas that have been researched and that continue to need to be include the following[52–55]:

1. Diagnostic reasoning studies (including diagnostic skills, errors made in diagnosing).
2. Nursing process studies.
3. Utilization studies (including the implications and results of use of diagnoses in practice).
4. Education studies.
5. Identification studies (development of new categories).
6. Epidemiologic studies (rate of occurrence of a diagnosis in patient populations).
7. Validation studies (refinement of current diagnoses).
8. Treatment validity studies.

Much of the current research in nursing diagnosis is presented at the NANDA national conferences, and published in the proceedings of the conferences. Regional nursing diagnosis associations sponsor conferences periodically, providing an opportunity for researchers to present their studies.

Future Trends

The need for further research in all areas of nursing diagnosis is frequently stressed in the nursing literature on the subject. Research on the diagnostic categories must be pursued vigorously as each clinical specialty strives to identify the phenomena of concern within its practice. Much more research is required to improve the accuracy of diagnosing and the effectiveness of the use of nursing diagnosis in directing patient care.

Psychiatric Diagnosis: DSM-III-R

The revision of the third edition of the American Psychiatric Association's Diagnostic and Statistical Manual of Mental Disorders is known as

TABLE 13-8. PSYCHIATRIC–MENTAL HEALTH NURSING DIAGNOSTIC LABELS

Health Perception–Health Management
    Health maintenance, altered: Inability to identify, manage, or seek out help to maintain health.
    Injury, potential for: The state in which an individual is at increased risk for being invaded by pathogenic organisms.
    Noncompliance: A person's informed decision not to adhere to a therapeutic recommendation.
Activity–Exercise
    Diversional activity, deficit: The state in which an individual experiences a decreased stimulation from or interest or engagement in recreational or leisure activities.
    Growth and development, altered: The state in which an individual demonstrates deviations in norms from his or her age group.
    Home maintenance management, impaired: Inability to independently maintain a safe, growth-promoting immediate environment.
    Self-care deficit: A state in which the individual experiences an impaired ability to perform or complete bathing and hygiene, dressing and grooming, feeding, or toileting activities for himself.
Sleep–Rest
    Sleep pattern disturbance: Disruption of sleep time causes discomfort or interferes with desired lifestyle.
Cognitive–Perceptual
    Comfort, altered: chronic pain: A state in which the individual experiences pain that continues for more than 6 months in duration.
    Knowledge deficit: A state in which specific information is lacking.
    Sensory-perceptual alterations: A state in which an individual experiences a change in the amount or patterning of incoming stimuli accompanied by a diminished, exaggerated, distorted, or impaired response to such stimuli.
    Thought processes, altered: A state in which an individual experiences a disruption in cognitive operations and activities.
Self-perception
    Anxiety: A vague, uneasy feeling, the source of which is often nonspecific or unknown to the individual.
    Fear: Feeling of dread related to an identifiable source that the person validates.
    Hopelessness: A subjective state in which an individual sees limited or no alternatives or personal choices available and is unable to mobilize energy on own behalf.
    Powerlessness: Perception that one's own action will not significantly affect an outcome; a perceived lack of control over a current situation or immediate happening.
    Self-concept, disturbance in: body image: Disruption in the way one perceives one's body image.
    Self-concept, disturbance in: personal identity: Inability to distinguish between self and nonself.
    Self-concept, disturbance in: self-esteem: Disruption in the way one perceives one's self-esteem.
Role–Relationship
    Communication, impaired verbal: A state in which an individual experiences a decreased or absent ability to use or understand language in human interaction.
    Family processes, altered: The state in which a family that normally functions effectively experiences a dysfunction.
    Grieving, anticipatory: A state in which an individual grieves before an actual loss.
    Grieving, dysfunctional: A state in which actual or perceived object loss (object loss is used in the broadest sense) exists. Objects include people, possessions, a job, status, home, ideals, parts, and processes of the body, etc.
    Parenting, altered: actual/potential: The state in which the ability of nurturing figure(s) to create an environment that promotes the optimum growth and development of another human being is altered or at risk.
    Role performance, altered: Disruption in the way one perceives one's role performance.
    Social interaction, impaired: The state in which an individual participates in an insufficient or excessive quantity or ineffective quality of social exchange.
    Social isolation: Aloneness experienced by the individual and perceived as imposed by others and as a negative or threatened state.
    Violence, potential for: self-directed or directed at others: A state in which an individual experiences behaviors that can be physically harmful either to the self or others.
Sexuality–Reproductive
    Rape-trauma syndrome: Forced, violent sexual penetration against the victim's will and consent; the trauma syndrome that develops from this attack or attempted attack includes an acute phase or disorganization of the victim's life style and a long-term process of reorganization of life-style.
    Sexual dysfunction: The state in which an individual experiences a change in sexual function that is viewed as unsatisfying, unrewarding, or inadequate.
    Sexuality, altered patterns: The state in which an individual expresses concern regarding his or her sexuality.

TABLE 13-8. (*continued*)

Coping–Stress-tolerance
    Adjustment, impaired: The state in which the individual is unable to modify his or her life-style or behavior in a manner consistent with a change in health status.
    Coping, family: potential for growth: Effective managing of adaptive tasks by family member involved with the client's health challenge who now exhibits desire and readiness for enhanced health and growth in regard to self and in relation to the client.
    Coping, ineffective family: compromised: Insufficient, ineffective, or compromised support, comfort, assistance, or encouragement usually by a supportive primary person (family member or close friend); client may need it to manage or master adaptive tasks related to his or her health challenge.
    Coping, ineffective family: disabled: Behavior of significant person (family member or other primary person) that disables his or her own capacities and the client's capacities to effectively address tasks essential to either person's adaptation to the health challenge.
    Coping, ineffective individual: Impairment of adaptive behaviors and problem-solving abilities of a person in meeting life's demands and roles.
    Post-trauma response: The state of an individual experiencing a sustained painful response to (an) unexpected extraordinary life event(s).
Value–Belief
    Spiritual distress (distress of the human spirit): Disruption in the life principle that pervades a person's entire being and that integrates and transcends the individual's biologic and psychosocial nature.

DSM-III-R. All mental health clinicians use this classification in assigning a psychiatric diagnosis. These diagnoses are discussed in detail later in this text. They are used for each case study as part of the assessment data for the psychiatric nursing diagnoses.

Psychiatric–Mental Health Nursing Diagnoses

Following the Seventh National Conference on nursing diagnosis, 83 diagnostic labels were accepted for use in nursing practice (Table 13-1).

There are specific diagnostic categories that are frequently used by PMH nurses. These have been listed in Table 13-8 along with their definitions in order to clarify the use of nursing diagnosis in the PMH specialty. In the case studies that follow, the corresponding diagnostic statements and initial treatment plans are listed to assist in understanding the application of nursing diagnosis in PMH nursing practice. One diagnosis was identified for each case study. In practice, more than one diagnosis may be addressed in the care plan.

—— CASE STUDY #1 ——

Jerry is a 44-year-old white male who is seen bimonthly in the community mental health center for routine lithium blood level checks. He was diagnosed manic–depressive and prescribed lithium after six years of periodic psychiatric hospitalizations and trials on various medications. His wife died 18 months ago, leaving him to raise their four children, ages 6 to 17. Jerry reported during his last clinic visit that he had sold the family home and moved into a small three-bedroom apartment because of recurrent memories of his deceased wife that interfered with his concentration and often led to thoughts of his own death. His mood was relatively stable for several years prior to his wife's death; however, recently he has appeared more irritable and agitated and has been confronted at work because of "attitude" problems. Jerry acknowledged having problems juggling his work responsibilities and making sure his children are cared for. He described feeling worthless, that he is not able to succeed at his job, and that he is failing his family. He attributes this to a pervasive feeling of apathy about life in general since he no longer has his wife to share problems and successes with.

    Jerry missed his current appointment and the clinic nurse telephoned his home. Jerry was not at home but the eldest child talked with the nurse about some of the family's concerns. The children were aware of the mood swings and the decreased interest their father has shown in general. Jerry frequently complains of not being able to sleep, having little interest in eating, and feeling tired constantly. He does not talk to his children about their mother's death because he doesn't want to talk any more about "depressing" things as he is depressed enough. When Jerry showed up for his rescheduled appointment, he acknowledged that the children were probably having a rough time because they were on their own a lot. He did not mention that they might be having problems dealing with their mother's death and seemed surprised when this was mentioned by the clinic nurse. Jerry thought that there had been enough time since the death and that everyone "has gone on" with their lives. He explained his problems as stemming from his illness and wondered if the stress he felt could lead to a relapse. He appeared to be much more nervous than the previous appointment but did not exhibit any gross impairment necessitating a hospitalization at this time.

NURSING CARE PLAN

DSM-III-R DIAGNOSIS

Bipolar Disorder—Depressed

NURSING DIAGNOSIS

Dysfunctional Grieving related to lack of resolution of previous grieving response.

Defining Characteristics
- Verbal expression of distress at loss.
- Anger (irritability).
- Sadness.
- Difficulty in expressing loss.
- Alterations in eating habits, sleep patterns, activity level.
- Reliving of past experiences.
- Interference with life functioning.
- Labile effect.
- Alterations in concentration and pursuit of tasks.

GOALS (OUTCOME CRITERIA)

Long-Term
Jerry demonstrates minimal interference with work functioning and in family interactions within six months.

Short-Term

1. Jerry will acknowledge the unresolved grief issues he has and will work on a plan to resolve these issues within one month.
2. Jerry will acknowledge feeling in better control at work and with his family within two months.
3. Family will meet and discuss their feelings, problem areas, and plans to resolve problems (including each individual's responsibility) at least every two weeks.

NURSING INTERVENTIONS

1. Notify psychiatrist of father's emotional status and possible need for adjustment in medication based on lab results.
2. Discuss with father his feelings and perceptions surrounding his wife's death and the subsequent effects on him during weekly appointments.

3. Develop plan with father on how to resolve his grieving, focusing on working through the grief responses of anger, depression, and acceptance within first month of appointments.
4. Evaluate effectiveness of plan by questioning father on his feelings of control and level of functioning at work and at home.
5. Facilitate family meetings over the next several months to help members work on the loss of their mother, to identify current problems, and to develop plans to resolve these problems.

—— CASE STUDY #2 ——

Mary is a 37-year-old black female married for the last 12 years with two children from this marriage, ages 10 and 7. She was admitted to the hospital after ingesting 15 to 20 various pills she found in her medicine cabinet. Her husband found the opened bottles about 30 minutes after she reportedly took the pills and gave her syrup of ipecac and rushed her to the emergency room. She was unable to identify what she took specifically, but the pills included aspirin, cold tablets, and imiprimine hydrochloride, which had been prescribed for her but which she stopped taking several months earlier. She had overdosed on aspirin five years previous to this attempt after attending her only sister's funeral. She has sporadically seen a psychiatrist since then and had received a prescription for Tofranil one year ago. Her husband reported that although she had always been "high-strung" and nervous, lately she had been withdrawn and angry over minor problems. He stated that this change coincided with her discontinuation of the medication and the five-year anniversary of her sister's unexpected death (drowning). Mary works part-time as a clerk in a local grocery store and has no hobbies or other activities she participates in. She has cared for the children and kept the house clean but recently verbalized many complaints to her husband and the children about their lack of assistance with household tasks. She frequently misinterprets their concern for her as criticism and has told them to take care of themselves since they don't need her. She started drinking after her sister's death, to "calm her nerves." She used to drink several drinks every evening but has increased her intake of alcohol to five or six drinks a night over the last several months. Her husband voiced much concern over her recent comments that she's tired of feeling lousy and will do what she wants for once and doesn't care how it affects her. He has been unable to get her to return to her psychiatrist, or even open up to him about what is bothering her (other than the vague complaints).

NURSING CARE PLAN

DSM-III-R DIAGNOSIS

Depression

NURSING DIAGNOSIS

Potential for Violence: self-directed related to suicidal behavior.

Defining Characteristics

- Body language: wringing hands, tense posture.
- Increased motor activity: pacing, agitation.

- Self-destructive behavior: aggressive suicidal act—overdose.
- Substance abuse: increased daily alcohol consumption.
- Suspicion of others: states family doesn't want her around anymore.
- Increased anxiety level.
- Inability to verbalize feelings.
- Repetition of verbalizations: continuous complaints, demands.
- Anger.
- Vulnerable self-esteem.
- Depression.

GOALS (OUTCOME CRITERIA)

Long-Term
Identifies effective coping mechanisms to use when dealing with stress, by discharge.

Short-Term

1. Will not harm self throughout hospitalization.
2. Will identify sources of stress within first four days of hospitalization.
3. Will identify internal cues that correspond with heightened anxiety, anger, frustration within first week of hospitalization.

NURSING INTERVENTIONS

1. Verbally contract with patient every shift to:
   a. keep self safe;
   b. come to staff if patient has any thoughts of wanting to harm self.
2. Explore sources of stress with patient—assist patient in determining:
   a. what stressors are imposed externally (from others, environment);
   b. what stressors are self-imposed (expectations of self, misperceptions).
3. Teach patient to recognize internal cues (muscle tenseness, upset stomach, headache, jittery feeling) that indicate potential for loss of control.
4. Provide external control as needed initially (institution of suicide precautions, removal of any potentially harmful items) and encourage patient to assume responsibility for maintaining self control.

—— CASE STUDY #3 ——

John Mason is a 10-year-old white male living with his natural mother and two sisters (Jane, 4 years old; Julie, 2 years old). His parents divorced 2 years ago, shortly before Julie's birth, after being separated on and off since John was an infant. John has had numerous care-takers during the day since he was 4 months of age, when his mother began full time work. He cried easily and had temper tantrums throughout his preschool years when his mother was around, and behaved similarly for the baby-sitters, though less severely. John rarely asks about his father, whom he sees only several times a year. He is of average intelligence; however, his teachers have all expressed concern that he is far behind his peers socially. His teachers and his mother could not remember John ever having any close friends. They attribute this to his apparent inability to compromise and manage conflicts with others, becoming easily frustrated when he doesn't get his way, arguing, cheating, and quitting activities to continue play by himself. John spends much of his free time at home watching TV or playing with his toys. The neighborhood children used to ask him to play often, but as the arguments and episodes of cheating increased over the past several years, he has been excluded most of the time. He seeks out schoolmates and neighborhood peers to play but eventually quits playing with them if they don't exclude him first because of his diffi-culties in getting along with them. He engages in parallel play with his sister Jane occa-sionally but becomes easily frustrated and continuously attempts to tell her how he expects her to play. He does not spend much time with Julie because she is "such a baby." John denies belonging to or wanting to belong to any social organizations, including sports teams, though he spends much time watching basketball and football on TV. John claims he would have lots of friends, but everyone likes to argue with him and he gets tired of it. John was admitted to a child psychiatric evaluation unit because of the marked increase over the past 6 months in school truancy, cheating, lying and stealing, and verbal abuse directed at peers and adults indiscriminately.

NURSING CARE PLAN

DSM-III-R DIAGNOSIS

Conduct Disorder; undersocialized, nonaggressive

NURSING DIAGNOSIS

Impaired Social Interaction related to knowledge and skill deficit about ways to enhance mutuality.

DEFINING CHARACTERISTICS

- Observed discomfort in social situations (patient tenses up when with group of peers, usually remains on edge of groups).
- Observed inability to receive or communicate a satisfying sense of belonging, caring, interest.
- Observed use of unsuccessful social interaction behaviors (joins peers but becomes easily frustrated, angry, and quits).
- Dysfunctional interactions with peers and family (poor conflict management, controlling of others, cheats, lies).

GOALS (OUTCOME CRITERIA)

Long-Term
By the end of one month of hospitalization, will participate in social activities, exhibiting and verbalizing increased comfort and fulfillment with social relationships.

Short-Term

1. Will participate in group activities at least daily during first week of hospitalization.
2. Will follow staff's suggestions to solve conflicts at least twice by the end of the first week.

NURSING INTERVENTIONS

1. Each shift, review any scheduled group activities with patient and plan at least one group activity for patient if none scheduled.
2. Encourage patient to participate in group activities, provide positive reinforcement (praise, sticker) for patient's involvement.
3. Observe patient's interactions with others, noting when anxiety increases. Encourage patient to explore his perceptions and feelings at that time.
4. Teach problem-solving steps and use role play in different situations to help patient practice these skills every day.
5. Intervene during conflicts between patient and others when patient is not effectively managing situation:
   a. Encourage patient to identify the problem.
   b. Explore possible solutions (and consequences of solutions) with patient.
   c. Support patient in choosing helpful alternative and offer guidance to do so.
   d. After conflict is resolved, review with patient what occurred, and how it was more effective.

—— CASE STUDY #4 ——————————————————————————————————

Mrs. Mason (John's mother) is a 30-year-old white female with three children, divorced for 2 years from Mr. Mason (the children's father) after a chaotic marriage of 13 years. She married Mr. Mason shortly after they both graduated from high school and gave birth to John the next year. Mr. Mason worked for a long-distance moving company and was frequently gone from the home for extended periods of time. They live in the same city as Mrs. Mason's mother and father, who provided support to the family both emotionally and financially in the early years of her marriage. Mr. Mason would come home for several nights each month or two, with occasional separations lasting up to 10 months at a time. His arrival home caused much disruption because of his heavy drinking, refusal to assume any responsibility in maintaining the house, and eventual arguments with Mrs. Mason over financial matters. The money he gave Mrs. Mason to support her and John (and eventually the other children) was not sufficient, requiring Mrs. Mason to work full time. Mrs. Mason relied heavily on her family and friends to help out with caring for the children, especially John. Last year Mrs. Mason's parents moved south 1000 miles away because of her mother's failing health. Mrs. Mason has had much difficulty coping with this separation and source of support. She has become more easily frustrated with John's problems and acknowledged "being at the end of her rope" when John was suspended from school for truancy shortly before his admission. She has tried various forms of discipline to no avail—grounding, spanking, and chores. She feels capable of providing the needs for the girls but feels guilty that John's inability to get along with others may be a result of the arguments he's witnessed between her and Mr. Mason and the lack of attention she gave him when he was younger. She has attempted to compensate for this by allowing John much freedom with few responsibilities at home. She makes his bed and cleans his room, keeps snack food already prepared for him constantly, and only occasionally asks him to take out the garbage or rake leaves in the yard. At the time of John's admission, Mrs. Mason tearfully admitted that she was probably not helping John but did not know what he needed or how she should change.

NURSING CARE PLAN

DSM-III-R DIAGNOSIS

Adjustment Disorder

NURSING DIAGNOSIS

Ineffective Family Coping: compromised related to prolonged disability progression that exhausts the supportive capacity of significant people. (John's increasing problems contribute to mother's compromised ability to assist John in achieving more effective functioning.)

Defining Characteristics

- Significant person (mother) describes preoccupation with personal reactions (fear of John's losing control, grief over loss of support of parents, guilt over past problems and effects of these on John, fearful of own loss of control over John).
- Significant person (mother) confirms inadequate knowledge (of what is wrong with John and with her parental skills) that interfere with effective assistive or supportive behaviors.
- Significant person attempts assistive or supportive behaviors with less than satisfactory results (mother has tried various discipline practices and has attempted to get John to talk about what's bothering him but does not succeed in effecting a change in his behavior).

- Significant person displays protective behavior disproportionate (too much) to client's abilities or need for autonomy. (Mother usually does not delegate any responsibilities to John and assumes responsibility for tasks he can independently perform.)

GOALS (OUTCOME CRITERIA)

Long-Term
Mother will state that she feels more capable of helping and supporting John by time of his discharge.

Short-Term
1. Mother will identify how she has been affected by John's problems by the end of the first week of hospitalization.
2. Mother will identify other concerns or problems interfering with her ability to cope with John's problems by the end of the first week of hospitalization.
3. Mother will identify at least two sources of support she can turn to in the community when feeling overtaxed with responsibilities and worries, by the end of the second week of hospitalization.

NURSING INTERVENTIONS

1. Meet with mother twice weekly to discuss her perceptions and feelings of:
   a. how John's problems have impacted on her life;
   b. what other concerns, questions, or problems she has to deal with at present.
2. Assist mother in identifying what needs she has that are presently being unmet. Begin developing a plan with her for how she may get these needs met.
3. Encourage mother to identify present coping mechanisms she uses. Explore possible alternatives, especially in terms of support systems available to her (relatives, friends, community resources).

CASE STUDY #5

Rachel Lewin, a 66-year-old widowed female, was admitted to an acute inpatient unit after she was found wandering in the street with only her nightgown on at 3:00 AM She was disoriented to place and time. This has been the third time that Mrs. Lewin wandered out of the house during the night.

Mrs. Lewin moved in with her daughter and son-in-law, Mr. and Mrs. Braun, 6 months ago when she began having short periods of confusion. Mrs. Lewin gradually needed increasing amounts of supervision because of confusion, disorientation to place and time, forgetting where objects were, and difficulty with dressing (putting on her slip over her dress). She has been having difficulty carrying on conversations, loses track of what she's talking about, uses incorrect or nonsensical words, and changes the subject. Her daughter and son-in-law came home one time to find that she had turned on all the burners on the stove and had gone to bed. They then brought in a health aide to supervise Mrs. Lewin when they were not at home. Recently, Mrs. Lewin began feeling fearful that the aide was trying to kill her and consequently began striking out at the aide. She has also started to experience angry verbal outbursts in front of her young grandchildren.

Mr. and Mrs. Braun report that Mrs. Lewin has periods of lucidity when she appears to be depressed and talks of how she's ''not the same anymore'' and can't do the things that she enjoys (cooking and playing bridge). At times they find Mrs. Lewin sitting in a chair, staring at the floor and verbally unresponsive.

During the initial interview with Mrs. Lewin, she was oriented to place, but not time. She was preoccupied with finding a box of tissues that she misplaced. After two minutes she became angry that her mother (who is deceased) wasn't there to help her. She demonstrated a short attention span and was easily distracted by noise from the hall. Mrs. Lewin's long term memory was intact, but she was unable to remember the number of grandchildren she has (two). When given a choice of three nightgowns she deliberated several minutes, picking each one up and putting it down several times, then appeared frustrated. She soon became angry, yelling that she wanted to be in her own apartment.

NURSING CARE PLAN

DSM-III-R DIAGNOSIS

Primary Degenerative Dementia, Senile Onset: Alzeheimer's

NURSING DIAGNOSIS

Impaired Thought Processes related to sensory overload (inability to process excessive environmental stimuli).

Defining Characteristics

- Impaired attention span, distractibility (inability to keep conversation focused).
- Inappropriate behavior (wandering in streets when she's dressed in nightclothes, struck out at health aide).
- Impaired recall ability (short-term memory affected).
- Impaired ability to order ideas (puts on slip over dress).
- Impaired perception (believed aide was trying to hurt her).
- Impaired judgment (turned stove on and went to bed).
- Impaired decision making (becomes frustrated and angry when asked to choose among three options).

GOALS (OUTCOME CRITERIA)

Long-Term
Confusion and undesired behaviors will decrease in frequency within 3 weeks.

Short-Term

1. Will receive adequate rest and intake to promote optimal cognitive functioning within 5 days.
2. Through interpersonal contact and environmental cues, will make efforts to maintain contact with reality within 2 weeks (e.g., conversing, performing tasks, etc.).
3. Will accept assistance as needed to maintain activities of daily living.

NURSING INTERVENTIONS

1. Obtain information from family and patient as to patient's preferences and dislikes. Convey information to dietitian. Provide supplementary feedings of protein at 10:00 AM, 2:00 PM, and 8:00 PM, and encourage cranberry juice every 2 hours.
2. Encourage family members to visit during mealtime or be present with patient to help her focus on task of eating.
3. Monitor intake and output.
4. At bedtime and naptime (10:30 to 11:00 AM), keep door closed to decrease environmental noise. Use tapes of sedative music (chosen by patient and located in nightstand) to promote relaxation.

5. Keep a light on in room to decrease confusion.
6. Orient and reassure patient as needed when checking patient at least every half hour. Remain with patient when she is disoriented or agitated. Do not use restraints. Remind patient of events of prior day (e.g., daughter visiting, arranging flowers, etc.). Use tone and pace of speech to encourage her to focus on music and relax extremities and slow her breathing.
7. Encourage family to bring in familiar objects and pictures.
8. When interacting with the patient, refer to the date, pointing out the calendar with appropriate seasonal pictures.
9. Arrange for consistent staff from various disciplines to perform necessary tasks and procedures in room. Introduce any unfamiliar person to patient and explain task to be performed.
10. Control intercom so the patient is not disturbed by unfamiliar voices.
11. Tape a list of the whereabouts of possessions on her nightstand.
12. Use tapes of music (in nightstand) to help stimulate the patient and decrease the tendency to withdraw.
13. Use reminiscence therapy to promote active communication and to facilitate bridging the gap between past and present.
14. Involve Occupational Therapy to assess with the patient what hobbies she prefers and can learn. Have these readily available in her room to promote orientation to the present.
15. Involve in community group to promote increased interpersonal contact. Strongly encourage participation in group that meets after her midmorning nap when she tends to be most organized.

CASE STUDY #6

Mr. and Mrs. Braun invited Mrs. Braun's mother (Mrs. Lewin) to move in with them after she began experiencing periods of confusion. They discussed that although it altered their life-style, they both felt committed to care for Mrs. Lewin. They attended group support sessions for adult children who care for aged parents.

Mrs. Lewin's episodes of confusion became more frequent and severe. They came home one day to find that Mrs. Lewin had turned on the burners of the stove and gone to bed. They met with Mrs. Lewin's doctor and discussed the expected regressed behaviors resulting from the degenerative process of her disease. They contracted with an agency to provide a health aide to supervise Mrs. Lewin when they were at work or were out during the evening. Recently Mrs. Lewin has become very fearful of the aide, thinking that the aide was trying to kill her, and consequently began to strike out at the aide.

Mr. and Mrs. Braun have been candid with their 5-year-old and 7-year-old children about their grandmother's disease. They provided adequate reassurance as to their safety. However, they became concerned when Mrs. Lewin started to yell at them angrily and was unaware of who they were.

Mrs. Lewin wandered out of the house during the night, dressed in her nightclothes, and was found by local policemen, who know the family. Mrs. and Mrs. Braun requested hospitalization for evaluation after the last time she wandered out of the house. They have discussed their fears regarding the safety of Mrs. Lewin and their children. They have come to terms with the fact that placement in a nursing home is now necessary. They are asking for ideas of how they can continue to be involved with Mrs. Lewin's care while maintaining their jobs and taking care of their children.

NURSING CARE PLAN

DSM-III-R DIAGNOSIS:

Alzheimer's

NURSING DIAGNOSIS

Family Coping: Potential for growth related to readiness for seeking self-actualization.

Defining Characteristics

- Family members attempt to describe growth impact of crises on own values, priorities, goals, or relationships.
- Family member is moving in direction of health-promoting and enriching life-style that supports and monitors maturational processes and negotiates treatment programs.
- Family expresses interest in making contact on a mutual-aid group basis with another person who has experienced a similar situation.

GOALS (OUTCOME CRITERIA)

Long-Term

Family members will identify methods to facilitate their involvement and commitment with Mrs. Lewin's care while maintaining the functioning of their family unit.

Short-Term

1. Family will establish a realistic schedule that provides time to devote to their responsibilities (work, home, and leisure) and time to visit with Mrs. Lewin that will augment Mrs. Lewin's treatment within 3 days.
2. Will discuss the continuing impact of Mrs. Lewin's illness within 1 week.
3. Will identify support systems that can facilitate the promotion of health of their family within 10 days.

NURSING INTERVENTIONS

1. Provide verbal support to the family for their involvement and describe the positive impact on Mrs. Lewin's health. However, reinforce their need to take time to relax in order to be able to continue optimal support when they are with Mrs. Lewin.
2. Provide information to family when their presence is of special benefit to Mrs. Lewin's care (e.g., mealtime, bedtime). Again caution them against overextending themselves.
3. Review with them support systems in the community (e.g., clergy, friends, neighborhood associations, etc.). Suggest that they can be utilized to provide consistent volunteers to visit Mrs. Lewin when they are unable to visit. Encourage them to use them for emotional and spiritual support.
4. Refer family to the local chapter of Alzheimer's Disease and Related Disorders Association (ADRDA). Meetings are first and third Tuesday of the month. When they visit a day or two after a meeting was held, explore with them whether they attended, their comfort in the meeting, any questions or fears that surfaced, and whether they feel that they can use the organization as a support.

Summary

The ANA Standards of Practice established that nursing diagnoses are based on systematically collected assessment data. The nurse engaged in psychiatric–mental health practice can use nursing diagnosis to deliver individualistic care and to base future research in the area of nursing care for the psychiatric patient.

REFERENCES AND SUGGESTED READINGS

1. Abdellah, F. G. Method of identifying covert aspects of nursing problems. *Nursing Research*, 1957, 57(4), 4–23.
2. Durand, M., & Prince, R. Nursing diagnosis: Process and decision. *Nursing Forum*, 1966, 5(54), 51–64.
3. Gordon, M. Nursing diagnosis and the diagnostic process. *American Journal of Nursing*, 1976, 76, 1299.
4. American Nurses' Association. *A Social Policy Statement*. Kansas City, Mo.: American Nurses' Association, 1980, p. 9.
5. Ibid.
6. Shoemaker, J. K. Essential features of a nursing diagnosis. In M. J. Kim, G. K. McFarland, & A. M. McLane (Eds.), *Classification of Nursing Diagnosis: Proceedings of the Fifth National Conference*. St. Louis, Mo.: Mosby, 1984, p. 109.
7. Carpenito, L. J. *Nursing Diagnosis: Application to Clinical Practice*. Philadelphia: Lippincott, 1983, p. 3.
8. Gordon, M., Sweeney, M. A., & McKeehan, K. Development of nursing diagnosis. *American Journal of Nursing*, 1980, 80, 699.
9. Iyer, P. W., Taptich, B. J., & Bernocchi-Losey, D. *Nursing Process and Nursing Diagnosis*. Philadelphia: Saunders, 1986, pp. 83–84.
10. McLane, A. M. (Ed.). *Classification of Nursing Diagnoses: Proceedings of the Seventh Conference*. St. Louis, Mo.: Mosby, 1987, pp. xiii–xiv.
11. Ibid., p. 545.
12. Gordon, M. *Nursing Diagnosis: Process and Application* (2nd ed.). New York: McGraw-Hill, 1987, p. 405.
13. American Nurses' Association. *Standards of Psychiatric and Mental Health Nursing Practice*. Kansas City, Mo.: American Nurses' Association, 1982, p. 1.
14. Loomis, M. E., Toole, A. W., Brown, M. S., Pothier, P., West, P., & Willson, H. S. Development of a classification system for psychiatric/mental health nursing: Individual response class. *Archives of Psychiatric Nursing*, 1987, 1(1), 17.
15. Brooks, E. R. The starting point. *Nursing Management*, 1983, 14(6), 35–37.
16. Iyer, Taptich, & Bernocchi-Losey, op. cit., p. 82.
17. Lash, A. A. A re-examination of nursing diagnosis. *Nursing Forum*, 1978, 17, 334.
18. Shoemaker, J. K. Unpublished observation, letter to members of Delphi panel. April 4, 1983.
19. Shoemaker, op. cit. (1984), pp. 104–113.
20. Polit, D., & Hungler, B. *Nursing Research: Principles and Methods*, 3rd ed., Philadelphia: J. B. Lippincott, 1987.
21. Griffith, J. W., & Christensen, P. J. *Nursing Process: Application of Theories, Frameworks, and Models*. St. Louis, Mo.: Mosby, 1982, p. 39.
22. Gordon, op. cit. (1987), pp. 390–396.
23. Ibid., p. 9.
24. Carpenito, L. J. *Nursing Diagnosis: Application to Clinical Practice*. Philadelphia: Lippincott, 1983, p. 26.
25. Dowd, T. M., Grabau, A. M., Kolbe, M. R., Mann, D. W., McCabe, B. W., & Smith, D. R. A replication study evaluating the use of a focused data collection tool for the generation of nursing diagnoses. In A. M. McLane (Ed.), *Classification of Nursing Diagnoses: Proceedings of the Seventh Conference*. St. Louis, Mo.: Mosby, 1987, pp. 383–387.
26. Padrick, K. P. Tanner, C. A., Pulzier, D., & Westfall, U. E. (1987). Hypothesis evaluation: A component of diagnostic reasoning. In McLane, op cit., pp. 299–305.
27. Carlson, J. H., Craft, C. A., & McGuire, A. D. *Nursing Diagnosis*. St. Louis, Mo.: Mosby, 1982, p. 62.
28. Griffith & Christensen, op. cit., pp. 36–37.
29. Gordon, op. cit. (1987), p. 92.
30. Gordon, op. cit. (1976), pp. 1298–1300.
31. Carpenito, op. cit., p. 19.
32. Ibid., p. 20.
33. Ibid.
34. Gordon, op. cit. (1987), pp. 277–278.
35. Ibid., p. 19.
36. Carnevali, D. L., Mitchell, D. H. Woods, N. F., & Tanner, C. A. *Diagnostic Reasoning in Nursing*. Philadelphia: Lippincott, 1984, pp. 26–27.
37. Gordon, op. cit. (1987), p. 137.
38. Carnivali, op. cit., pp. 84–89.
39. Ibid., p. 41.
40. Ibid., p. 34.
41. Westfall, U. E., Tanner, C. A., Putzler, D., & Padrick, K. (1987). Errors committed by nurses and nursing students in the diagnostic reasoning process. In McLane, op. cit., pp. 341–342.
42. Myers, J. L., & Spies, M. A. Nursing diagnostic skills: A content analysis of spontaneously generated nursing diagnoses. In McLane, op. cit., pp. 324–331.
43. Carpenito, op. cit., p. 41.
44. Gordon, op. cit. (1987), p. 309.
45. Carpenito, op. cit., p. 41.
46. Griffith & Christensen, op. cit., p. 135.
47. Bulechek, G. M., & McCloskey, J. C. *Nursing Interventions: Treatment for Nursing Diagnoses*. Philadelphia: Saunders, 1985, pp. 36–39.
48. Carpenito, op. cit., p. 19.
49. Gordon, op. cit. (1987), p. 313.
50. Ibid., pp. 313–315.
51. Carnevali, D. L. *Nursing Care Planning: Diagnosis and Management* (3rd ed.). Philadelphia: Lippincott, 1983, p. 222.
52. Gordon, M. *Nursing Diagnosis, Process and Application*. New York: McGraw-Hill, 1982, pp. 318–321.
53. Gordon, op. cit. (1987), pp. 406–411.
54. Kim, McFarland, & McLane, op. cit.
55. McLane, op. cit.

Chapter 14

Spiritual Dimensions of Psychiatric–Mental Health Nursing

Eileen E. Rinear

Chapter Objectives

The students successfully attaining the goals of this chapter will be able to:

- Discuss the concept of spirituality and its relationship to coping and crisis theories.
- Describe the relationship between an individual's religious beliefs and the manifestations of his psychopathology.
- Discuss the use of nursing diagnoses related to spirituality and their application to a variety of client care settings.
- Describe appropriate nursing interventions for dealing with manifestations of spiritual awareness or distress within the context of the therapeutic relationship.

"Life is difficult," writes Peck in the opening line of his best-selling book, *The Road Less Traveled*.[1] Given the stark reality of his introductory remarks, one might wonder how it is that he managed to sell any copies of his work to a death-denying and pleasure-seeking society such as our own. Perhaps those who purchased his book simply failed to skim its contents before doing so; perhaps they were intrigued by his novel approach and assumed that he would lighten up in subsequent pages; perhaps they

were caught up in the seemingly endless stream of self-help books, all promising to hold the secrets to contentment and fulfillment within the confines of their covers; or perhaps, maybe just perhaps, Peck's candor sparked recognition of a truth locked deep within themselves, yet clamoring for expression, validation, and resolution. Regardless of the motivation of his readership, the tremendous success of Peck's book seems to suggest that the need for a personal spirituality, for a way of finding meaning and purpose in life, and for reconciling its injustices and incongruities is both universal and ongoing.[2]

Jourard has said:

Man needs reasons for living and if there are none, he begins to die . . . man is incurably religious. What

This chapter is adapted from Rinear, E. E., & Buys, A. M. Spiritual and religious dimensions of psychiatric–mental health nursing. In *Psychiatric Nursing in the Hospital and the Community* (4th ed.). Englewood Cliffs, N.J.: Prentice-Hall, 1985.

varies among men is what they are religious about. Whatever a person takes to be the highest value in life can be regarded as his God, the focus and purpose of his time and life.[3]

SPIRITUAL AND RELIGIOUS NEEDS

With Jourard's observations in mind, it seems easy to understand the common practice, among both laymen and professionals alike, of using the terms *religion* and *spirituality* interchangeably. Although it has been suggested that a more precise nomenclature might be developed by reserving the term *religion* to delimit those spiritual beliefs that encompass the concept of a deity, such semantic distinctions seem unnecessarily cumbersome, confusing, and restrictive in their practical application. Likewise, though it might be argued that a basic working knowledge of the religious beliefs of those population groups for whom nursing care is being planned is *essential* for the development of thoughtful and considered nursing interventions, it must also be recognized that not all nurses will view the acquisition of such background information to be either practical or essential, and that those who do have access to a wealth of related materials via the professional literature.

Peck's assertion that there is a tendency to define religion too narrowly and an assumption that religion must include a belief in God or some ritualistic practice or membership in a worshipping group has an inhibiting influence.[4] Thus, in an effort to avoid obscuring the more vital, central, and universal issues (e.g., those related to meaning and purpose, suffering, etc.) of concern to clients, a more global and generic approach to the topics of religion and spirituality will be used for this chapter. The terms will be used synonymously, and elements of coping and crisis theory will form the underlying conceptual framework.

HOMEOSTASIS, COPING, AND CRISIS

The concepts of homeostasis, coping, and crisis as related to psychological functioning suggest that there exists a reasonably constant balance between affective and cognitive functioning in people. Although this "homeostatic balance" may vary from individual to individual, its defining characteristic is the existence of a stability that is "normal" for each person and against which changes in psychological functioning can be evaluated. A healthy homeostatic balance requires: (1) stable psychological functioning with a minimum of dysphoric affect; (2) maintenance of a reasonable cognitive perspective on experience; and (3) retention of problem-solving skills.[5]

People are subjected to a variety of events and experiences that result in disruptions in the homeostatic state, the production of negative and uncomfortable affect, and a reduction in problem-solving skills. Such disruptive experiences, writes Caplan, are emotionally hazardous situations occurring when there is a shift or change in an individual's environment that alters relationships with others or expectations of self perceived to be negative.[6]

The concept of "threat" is inextricably bound to any discussion of stress, coping, and crisis. It has been suggested that "threat" offers a more unifying concept than "anxiety" because it takes into account the full range of affective responses (of which anxiety may be one) that individuals may experience in response to an emotionally hazardous situation. The awareness of threat invariably is followed by a process of cognitive appraisal in which individuals attempt through a series of continually changing judgments to evaluate the significance of the stimulus to their well-being.[7] Since the intensity of an individual's affective response to such stimuli may either heighten or diminish perceptual abilities, it seems reasonable to suggest that a feedback relationship between perceptual abilities and affective responses exists. Crisis theorists assert that it is the rise in stress (i.e., affective discomfort) accompanying an emotionally hazardous situation that summons an individual's coping behaviors and problem-solving skills to restore homeostatic balance and eliminate affective discomfort.[8]

Coping mechanisms thus are those psychological self-regulatory mechanisms that an individual uses to restore homeostatic balance and reduce affective discomfort following emotionally hazardous situations; as such, they are crucial not only to emotional well-being, but to stable psychological functioning as well.

Coping mechanisms may include a variety of cognitive processes and behaviors, which may operate at different levels of awareness (i.e., conscious, preconscious, unconscious, or a combination thereof) and exhibit varying degrees of adaptiveness, depending upon the characteristics of the individual and the situation involved.

While coping behaviors are best viewed as existing on a continuum manifesting varying degrees of adaptiveness, when an individual encounters a situation in which there is significant psychological threat, coping behaviors are more likely to be self-protective than oriented toward mastery.

In examining the relationship between coping and crisis, Burgess and Baldwin suggest that an emotional crisis may ensue if an individual experiences an emotionally hazardous situation and is unable to alleviate the stress generated by it through the use of previously learned coping behaviors or novel problem-solving skills.[9] Thus, an emotional crisis is characterized by an inability to effectively manage the stress associated with an emotionally hazardous situation.

Garland and Bush note that "the origin of coping behaviors remains an area of dispute," but that one hypothesis suggests that coping behaviors are learned through a process of trial and error, in which those behaviors that achieve favorable results (i.e., are reinforced) are repeated, refined, and eventually integrated into the individual's personal behavioral repertoire.[10] Since most people experience a diversity of life situations with which they must cope, skills in assessing as well as in flexibly reacting to various life situations typically are developed and expanded throughout the individual's lifetime.[11] Yet, it is believed that the process by which a person acquires a repertoire of coping behaviors is heavily influenced by his parents and siblings initially, and later, by members of his community.[12]

COPING AND RELIGION

Lovinger notes that most people maintain a relatively simple understanding of religion that has been erroneously assumed to be a function of the religion itself, when in actuality, it is a consequence of the discontinuation of religious education during the early teen (i.e., ages 13 to 14) years.[13] He states that, "most people stop learning in this area at the time when the stage of formal operations begins, and never acquire any abstract conceptual grasp of religion."[14]

Differentiation of Mature Versus Immature Religious Beliefs

Differentiating "mature" from "immature" religious beliefs, values, and expressions is obviously a difficult task and one that is often highly dependent upon the subjective orientation of the person making such determinations.[15] Although it has been suggested that "immature" religious beliefs might be differentiated from "mature" religious beliefs on the basis of their self-interest and self-justification, Field and Wilkerson note that at least within the context of psychiatry, by the time a person's religious preoccupations come to the attention of a professional, the immediate crisis has usually passed and the irrational nature of his religious preoccupations has already become obvious (e.g., the individual believes and tells everyone that he is Jesus Christ).[16]

Religious Symptomatology

Religious symptomatology has been defined as falling into two broad categories: personal crises and social crises. When religiosity is analyzed from the standpoint of personal crises, the relationship between an individual's religious beliefs and his psychopathology may be viewed as constituting either: (1) a direct causative factor; (2) an indirect precipitating factor; or (3) a factor that functions merely to supply the ideational form for the person's underlying illness.[17]

Direct Causative Factor
Factors that have been deemed important when viewing religion as a direct causative agent in the development of psychopathology have been: (1) a concept of God as extremely punitive and demanding; and (2) history of religious teachings that conflicted with biologic urges and thus gave rise to intense feelings of guilt and frustration. In the latter circumstances, the result may be the evolution of neurotic conflicts, which from an analytic standpoint can best be understood as representing the individual's inability to successfully resolve the conflict existent between his own unacceptable impulses and his own ego.[18]

Neurotic conflicts rooted in religious beliefs may express themselves in a variety of ways: for example, an individual who views God as being an all-powerful, protective, and sustaining parent figure may adopt a passive–dependent approach to the conduct of his life; an individual who seeks expiation of guilt or shame may involve himself in religious practices focused on achieving purity and cleanliness; or, an individual who believes that God requires pain and suffering may subject himself to humiliating or self-punitive practices as a consequence of his religious beliefs.

Indirect Precipitating Factor

Religion may be viewed as constituting an indirect precipitating factor in the development of psychopathology when it is used by an individual who is desperately seeking to avoid fragmentation of his personality. In such a situation, a person who feels that he is losing contact with his environment may seek an explanation for such feelings in religion because it has the capacity to explain unusual and unfamiliar occurrences. Such an individual may interpret his strong feelings as evidence of "conversion" or "salvation." In these instances, religious preoccupations are not the direct cause of the individual's psychopathology but rather an attempt on his part to cope with overwhelming stress and to avoid personality fragmentation. It has been noted that although people are generally not inclined to engage in intense thinking with regard to religion, crisis situations do arise that give impetus to such reflection.[19] Cavenar and Spaulding report that while religious "conversions" may serve to strengthen repression in depressed individuals, thereby aiding in conflict resolution for those with underlying hysterical personality traits, they do nothing to resolve the ambivalence or isolation of affect experienced by depressed individuals whose premorbid personalities were characterized largely by obsessive–compulsive traits.[20] Field and Wilkerson have further observed that when religiosity is motivated by an individual's need to ward off depression, his religious behavior will persist only as long as the need exists and the behavior is effective in combatting the dysphoric affect.[21]

Ideational Factor

The third relationship between religion and mental illness is that in which religiosity serves to supply the ideational form for the underlying pathology. In this situation, an individual may use religious beliefs to provide either a rationalization or verbal structure for his illness. It should be noted that this usage of religiosity is not confined to those who have had rigid religious upbringings. The schizophrenic patient may use religious beliefs not only to supply the ideational form for his illness but to correct two common processes associated with his psychopathology: namely, detachment from the world and alterations in affect. Thus the schizophrenic who is attempting to detach himself from reality may find support for such actions in religious teachings that suggest the world cannot be verified by reality testing. Similarly, the schizophrenic's altered affect may be justified by religious teachings that emphasize the importance of self-control and which, thereby, serve to reinforce his feelings of self-righteous anger. Finally, the prevalent use of symbolism in religion may be seen as having particular significance to the schizophrenic individual whose autistic thinking thrives upon the use of symbolic meanings.

Field and Wilkerson state that, "for the grossly ill, religiosity can be an obvious manifestation of the disease. But, religiosity as a psychiatric symptom may be much less evident and only observable to a professional."[22] These authors add, however, that since religion deals with an individual's spiritual development, it should in most cases serve to foster mental health by enriching the individual's personal and social life.

AUTOGNOSIS

A believer and a skeptic went for a walk. The skeptic said, "Look at all the trouble and misery in the world after thousands of years of religion. What good is religion?" His companion noticed a child, filthy with grime, playing in the gutter. He said, "We've had soap for generation after generation and yet look how dirty that child is. Of what value is soap?" "But soap cannot do any good unless it is used," protested the skeptic. "Exactly," replied the believer.[23]

When you consider your own spiritual and religious belief system, do you view yourself as a believer or a skeptic? If you are a believer, then what is it that you believe in? If you are a skeptic, what is it that you are skeptical about?

Importance of an Open and Investigative Approach

An open and investigative approach is essential for objectively assessing the maturity, or lack thereof, of an individual's spiritual beliefs and behaviors relative to his personality strengths, weaknesses, and general level of functioning.

One basic obstacle to effectively dealing with spiritual needs arising from within either the self or others is that the exploration and resolutions of such needs requires a person to confront his limitations, as well as to acknowledge his restricted sphere of control. Fish and Shelly observe that, "illness, suffering, and death serve to remind us that we are not very sufficient unto ourselves but are, indeed, very human and very helpless."[24] Bush stresses that anxiety most often is produced by some change, either internal or external, that we perceive to be threatening to our safety or well-being, and that "since our religious beliefs are very near the core of our being, any challenge to these beliefs will produce feelings of anxiety."[25] Gulko, in observing the behavior of chaplains at a large Veterans Administration facility, reported that clergy tended to adopt a "medical-model approach" to their clients and avoided any discussion of death, God, or religion, even though their clients were seen to engage in such conversations (in the presence of other staff members) among themselves.[26]

It seems obvious that a primary requisite for the effective management of spiritual needs involving either oneself or others is that of acknowledging the legitimacy and universality of these needs for all persons. Autognosis, that is, the process of "getting in touch" with one's own spiritual beliefs and values, is thus essential for the clarification and integration of such beliefs and values into one's own life, as well as for the resolution of underlying dormant conflicts that might otherwise become manifest within the context of the therapeutic relationship. Relling-Garskoff sums up the importance of autognosis to countertransference by noting that "countertransference is an unconscious process that takes conscious effort to recognize."[27]

ASSESSING SPIRITUAL AND RELIGIOUS NEEDS

The nature of a patient's spiritual and religious beliefs and needs, as well as the reciprocal relationship between these and his current illness or life situation, can be systematically assessed as part of the nursing admission history. Al-

though Stoll notes that in many instances such assessments are confined to inquiries regarding the patient's particular religious group affiliation, assessment of the following four key areas seems both practical and essential: (1) the patient's concept of God or of a deity; (2) the patient's sources of strength and hope; (3) the significance of specific religious rituals or practices to the patient; and (4) the patient's perception of the relationship of his spiritual or religious beliefs to his current illness or life situation.[28]

Field and Wilkerson emphasize the importance of evaluating the following three areas when dealing with patients who exhibit religious preoccupations as a manifestation of their psychopathology: (1) the patient's particular religious affiliation, if any (this is important because certain religious groups stress intense emotional experiences in which the client may have participated and also because a knowledge of the client's particular religious group affiliation may be useful in understanding his symbolic communications); (2) the date as well as the circumstances preceding the onset of the client's religious preoccupations; and (3) the manner in which the client has made use of his religious beliefs (i.e., as a direct causative factor, an indirect precipitating factor, or a factor that serves merely to supply the ideational form for his psychopathology).[29]

SPIRITUAL DIAGNOSES: MEDICAL AND NURSING

It seems evident from the information presented thus far in this chapter that none of the diagnostic categories contained within the American Psychiatric Association's *Diagnostic and Statistical Manual of Mental Disorders, 3rd Edition* Revised (DSM-III-R) have direct or universal applicability to the spiritual and religious dimension of a patient's psychopathology or life situation, although manifestations of spiritual distress may be expressed by any given number of behaviors or symptoms subsumed under a variety of diagnostic categories (e.g., schizophrenia, anxiety, and affective disorders).

In formulating nursing diagnoses that address a patient's spiritual and religious needs or concerns, the nurse may find it helpful to review the Spiritual/Religious Section of the Nursing

Assessment Protocol suggested in Chapter 12 in light of the following four key questions:

1. Does the patient give clues either verbally or behaviorally that suggest the presence of spiritual needs or concerns?
2. What is the patient's general affective response to the discussion of spiritual material?
3. Does the patient have access to those spiritual resources that he requires in order to successfully resolve spiritual concern or needs?
4. Does the patient show evidence of distorted spiritual beliefs or values that might require referral to other professional colleagues (e.g., clergy, other mental health professionals, etc.)?

Case Examples

Although it is beyond the scope of this chapter to present a detailed discussion of nursing interventions relevant to spiritual/religious needs, the following case examples are offered to assist the reader in this aspect of his/her nursing practice. See also Tables 14-1, 14-2, 14-3, and 14-4 that accompany the case examples and provide guidelines for each of the diagnosis.

CASE 1

PATIENT: Since John died I have no reason to go on. It's just no use.

NURSE: I hear how hopeless you feel now about your loss. What about John do you miss the most?

PATIENT: I guess the way that he made me feel important and special.

NURSE: I can see how you would miss such a feeling. What are some of the ways he did that?

PATIENT: He would tell me how much he enjoyed my cooking, and he would just look at me with such love in his eyes.

NURSE: It is hard to realize neither of these things will happen again and no one can exactly take his place.

PATIENT: It really is. We were married thirty years.

NURSE: I wonder what it would take for you to allow what he gave you to become part of you so you continue to feel that way.

PATIENT: I guess I would have to admit to myself that I really am important and special. Though I miss him a lot, I can go on.

NURSE: You and I can talk again about what you received from him that you will never lose, what you still need and will have to find other ways to get, and maybe what you need to let go of that only he could give.

PATIENT: I think John would have wanted me to do that. It won't be easy, but I am willing to try.

TABLE 14-1. GUIDE TO CHARACTERISTICS, GOALS, AND NURSING ACTIONS RELATED TO SPECIFIC DEFICITS IN MEETING SPIRITUAL/RELIGIOUS NEEDS
NURSING DIAGNOSIS: ALTERATION IN SPIRITUALITY (SPIRITUAL CONCERN OR DISTRESS) RELATED TO A LACK OF MEANING AND PURPOSE IN LIFE.

Characteristics	Goals	Nursing Actions
The patient verbalizes feelings of hopelessness. The patient questions the meaning of his/her own existence.	The patient will express a willingness to look for sources of hope and meaning in his/her life.	The nurse will acknowledge the patient's feelings and receive them in an atmosphere of acceptance. The nurse will provide the patient with his/her caring presence, but will not function

TABLE 14-1. (*continued*)

Characteristics	Goals	Nursing Actions
		in such a way as to increase the patient's conflicts or to impose on his/her world view (i.e., the nurse will lend the patient hope until he/she is able to mobilize this for him/herself).
The patient verbalizes the rejection of his/her former belief system or expresses ambivalence toward it.	The patient will be able to reaffirm his/her former belief system in light of a new understanding of what factors have interfered with this, or the patient will make clear revisions in his/her beliefs and values that are compatible with his/her current life situation.	The nurse will acknowledge the patient's current feelings in an atmosphere that is supportive and nonjudgmental. The nurse will assist the patient in describing his/her former belief system, and in reviewing factors that have threatened or weakened this (i.e., what happened and who was involved—including the patient's thoughts, feelings, and actions). Often the root of the threatening event can be traced to a problematic interpersonal relationship.
The patient expresses excessive or inappropriate humor or sarcasm about heaven, hell, or other religious topics.	The patient will be able to articulate the actual concern that is veiled in his/her use of humor.	The nurse will validate to the patient that he/she has observed a potential topic of concern. The nurse will pose questions useful in helping the patient to uncover any hidden concerns or message—if same exists.
The patient verbalizes anger toward God. The patient questions the meaning of his/her pain and suffering.	The patient will verbalize a chosen response to personal limitations.	The nurse will facilitate the expression of the patient's thoughts and feelings. The nurse will assist the patient in his/her search to find a personal meaning in what he/she is experiencing.

––––––– CASE 2 –––––––

PATIENT: Even God doesn't care anymore. I used to think I could count on Him.

NURSE: What happened to change your being able to count on God?

PATIENT: I feel so useless. Since my son left home and got married, I don't feel needed.

NURSE: You said God doesn't care anymore. I wonder if you also think your son doesn't care because he does not need you in the same way he did.

PATIENT: I guess so. My son used to tell me how he could not get along without me.

NURSE: I wonder if your feeling that God does not care could be related to your feeling useless and thinking your son does not count on you anymore.

PATIENT: Gosh, maybe. I don't really want my son to continue to need me. I want him to grow up, but it is hard to let him go.

NURSE: It is. Maybe it would help if you and I talk again about the changes that have taken place, what your beliefs are about them, and what you can do to get your needs met.

TABLE 14-2. GUIDE TO CHARACTERISTICS, GOALS, AND NURSING ACTIONS NURSING DIAGNOSIS: ALTERATION IN SPIRITUALITY (SPIRITUAL CONCERN OR DISTRESS) RELATED TO A LACK OF LOVE AND RELATEDNESS.

Characteristics	Goals	Nursing Actions
The patient states that God is remote or uncaring.	The patient will express a willingness to reevaluate the source(s) of his/her perceptions regarding God.	The nurse will assist the patient in exploring his/her thoughts and feelings relative to self, others, and God (i.e., the nurse will in a nonjudgmental manner facilitate a review of the area(s) from which the patient has reached this conclusion about God, and will assist the patient in recognizing his/her own use of projection and his/her beliefs about self that are rooted in the internalization of inputs that he/she has received from others).
The patient exhibits demanding behavior, or withdrawal, toward the nurse in his/her interactions with same.	The patient will demonstrate more assertive and goal-directed behavior.	The nurse will facilitate the patient's efforts to evaluate previously received inputs, to identify personal needs, and to articulate such needs once identified.
The patient verbalizes a loss of faith in the power or effectiveness of prayer. He/she expresses difficulty with, or the inability to pray; and/or he/she expresses anxiety that is related to the interruptions of his/her customary religious practices.	The patient will verbalize a sense of satisfaction with his/her current situation (i.e., prayer life and/or religious practices).	The nurse will investigate the meaning that prayer has (had) for the patient, as well as his/her previous experiences with prayer (i.e., including the patient's expectations of prayer and the outcomes experienced).
		The nurse will inquire about religious practices that the patient has considered as being important, as well as to the meaning ascribed to these by the patient. The nurse will assist the patient in resuming religious practices that have been constructive for him/her, or in determining acceptable alternatives to same when such practices are not possible.
		The nurse will assist the patient in increasing his/her awareness of his/her own inner religious experience—with or without its associated external practices.
The patient verbalizes loneliness due to the absence of his/her own system of spiritual support.	The patient verbalizes a greater degree of satisfaction with the supportive spiritual network that is available to him/her.	The nurse will inquire as to what person(s) comprised the patient's spiritual support system and to how this has changed. The nurse will assist the patient in recognizing his/her own needs in this area and in taking action to meet same.

TABLE 14-2. (*continued*)

Characteristics	Goals	Nursing Actions
The patient expresses anger directed toward clergy or other religious representatives.	The patient will be able to articulate expectations that were not met and to deal directly with the actual source of his/her anger.	The nurse will assist the patient in expressing his/her impressions of the situation—including his/her expectations, as well as what he/she perceives as having actually occurred. The nurse will assist the patient in determining where change might occur (i.e., either in the patient's expectations or in his/her response to the outcome), and in clarifying and resolving the precipitating situation ideally. The latter can be best accomplished if the persons directly involved can be included in the clarification and resolution of the situation.

——— CASE 3 ———

PATIENT: I really feel guilty for the way I treated my mother.

NURSE: What did you do?

PATIENT: She asked me to continue with the same church she went to and I didn't. When I married my husband, I changed to his church.

NURSE: Talk about how it happened.

PATIENT: I learned what his beliefs were and I found that they fit with my experience of God. I really feel this is where I belong.

NURSE: It sounds like you feel guilty because you did not meet your mother's expectations. However, you acted courageously on your own beliefs.

PATIENT: Yes, I do not feel guilty about that—only because my mother does not understand. So I just avoid the issue with her.

NURSE: What do you think you could do to relieve your guilt?

PATIENT: Now that I think about it, what I feel the most guilty about is that I now don't talk about religion to her at all, and that was important to both of us. I would feel better if I could talk over with her how I came to believe the way I do and how it feels right to me. Even if she still does not understand, I will feel relief.

NURSE: That sounds like a helpful plan. Let me know how it goes.

The nurse helped Jane to separate out her grieving over the loss of her boyfriend, and her quest for hope and meaning in her life. In relation to the grief, the nurse helped Jane to recognize it as the normal response it was, and she used some health teaching to help her proceed through it in a constructive way. In relation to the quest for hope and meaning, the nurse helped Jane to become aware of the inputs she had received, some of her related experience, of where she was currently, and of what she could do.

The following were among the interactions that took place:

NURSE: What messages did you receive as a child about hope and meaning in your life?

JANE: What I remember my mother saying is, "If you don't want anything, you won't be disappointed." I guess I thought the only thing that would give meaning to my life would be to have a husband and children like she did.

NURSE: What other inputs have you had since then?

JANE: Well, I have a teacher who really sets goals for herself, goes after them, and really seems to achieve them, so I have some doubts about what I learned from my mother about that. You know, too, this teacher seems to have meaning in her life and she is not even married.

NURSE: Those inputs are somewhat conflicting. How do they fit with what is going on with you right now?

JANE: Gee, I guess I'm really blaming myself for the disappointment about the breakup of the relationship with my boyfriend. If I had not wanted it to continue so badly, even though I know it was not good for me, it would not have happened. I looked at John as giving meaning to my life by becoming my husband. Maybe John isn't the right person for me, but the disappointment is due to the sense of loss right now. It does not mean that I don't want a relationship that will be constructive for me.

NURSE: You mentioned that your teacher seems to have meaning in her life. What do you think about taking the following statements, sitting with them for awhile, and see what answers come to you.

> What has given meaning and purpose to my life in the past was . . .
> What I have done so far to look for meaning and purpose is . . .
> Relationships that have helped me find meaning and purpose are . . .
> Relationships that have hindered me in finding meaning are . . .
> What helps me to make important decisions about my life is . . .
> I particularly enjoy . . .
> I know a belief is my own, rather than imposed upon me by . . .

In other sessions, the nurse carefully reviewed Jane's responses with her, accepted them, and then helped Jane see which of her beliefs were open to revision, which coping patterns had been destructive, and some alternatives that might be more useful. She also helped Jane recall previous helpful support systems, including a religious faith that had been helpful to her in the past. She suggested some potential new ones.

Interspersed with reviewing Jane's experience, the nurse did some spiritual health teaching. She reviewed signs of spiritual wellness, and as already noted, she helped Jane explore alternative beliefs, coping mechanisms, and support systems. The nurse stressed Jane's freedom and power to recognize and take action to meet her own needs. By making it clear to Jane that she had a right to accept her feelings, and to share them, Jane was able to eventually see that she was not the victim of the past but could make constructive choices for herself, regardless of what her previous boyfriend did or did not do.

Shortly before Jane's discharge from the hospital, the following interaction took place.

NURSE: What did you learn about yourself?

JANE: Well, one thing was that I have lots more to learn about myself! I realized I was looking to others for answers I can find only within myself.

NURSE: How are you going to use what you have learned?

JANE: I am going to continue to ask myself questions and keep some journal notes. When I feel stuck and unclear, I will look for someone to talk to—either you or another person that I can trust.

If Jane's inputs had included conflicting religious beliefs, it would have been useful to consult a clergy person of her faith orientation, particularly one with whom she had a good relationship in the past. This might have also provided an additional source of support for her.

Jane's own progress notes were a useful tool because they kept track of what might otherwise have been forgotten, and they provided a clear record of her progress in finding her own source of hope and meaning.

TABLE 14-4. GUIDE TO CHARACTERISTICS, GOALS, AND NURSING ACTIONS NURSING DIAGNOSIS: ALTERATION IN SPIRITUALITY RELATED TO MENTAL ILLNESS (PSYCHIATRIC DISORDER).

Characteristics	Goals	Nursing Actions
The patient expresses an obsession with religious thoughts; and/or the patient exhibits the use of compulsive and repetitious, ritualistic religious practices.	The patient will verbalize an increased personal awareness of his/her anxiety as it relates to these religious preoccupations. The patient will develop alternative behaviors to cope with his/her anxiety about religious issues.	The nurse will assist the patient in expressing his/her thoughts and feelings about religious issues, expectations, and inputs; as well as those behaviors used to cope with the anxiety generated by such issues. The nurse will encourage referral of the patient to a psychotherapist, so that he/she can be assisted in his/her acquisition of the skills necessary for use of the learning process (i.e., psychotherapeutic intervention should be focused on the underlying conflict, rather than on the symptomatic manifestation of the patient's distress).

SUMMARY OF NURSING INTERVENTIONS

As previously noted in this chapter, the first step in effectively managing the spiritual or religious needs of one's patient is acknowledging the relevancy, legitimacy, and universality of these beliefs for all persons, as well as their potential to provide a significant source of strength, hope, healing, and support for many people.

It is important that nurses who attempt to intervene in this aspect of a patient's care first achieve some personal degree of comfort with their own spiritual beliefs and values, as well as with "religious symptomatology" that may occur within the context of the therapeutic relationship. The nurse's approach must of necessity be one that is open, investigative, and nondirective (except when religiosity as a manifestation of psychopathology is operative) if the patient is to feel free to verbalize his own religious experiences, needs, and concerns; to question his own religious beliefs and values; and, when necessary, to identify and develop new and more adaptive strategies for managing his own personal spiritual needs.

The nurse must also recognize that in psychiatric–mental health settings, more than any other, the theoretical orientation of both the practitioner and the facility by whom she is employed will shape her conceptualization of and responses to spiritual and religious beliefs and needs. The use of a global, generic approach to religious needs enables the clinician to intervene effectively (e.g., to focus on dysfunctional thoughts if cognitively oriented; to focus on modification or extinction of ritualistic behaviors if a behaviorist) at the level of the patient's manifest symptomatology without entangling herself in a web of doctrinal, biblical, or traditional issues.

The nurse should further recognize that some religious needs and behaviors may fall outside her area of expertise—or even outside the domain of nursing—and as such will require referrals to other pastoral or mental health colleagues. Such referrals are usually indicated when a nurse views her own level of competence in this area to be insufficiently developed to deal with the: (1) recognition or reduction of a patient's affective discomfort relative to his spiritual needs; (2) effective management of a patient's religious preoccupations or ritualistic behaviors; or (3) correction of knowledge deficits specific to precise biblical or doctrinal interpretations, as well as a synthesis of a patient's previous personal religious experiences.

In stressful or crisis situations in which spiritual or religious needs and concerns seem to represent central or key issues, the following areas of inquiry and intervention may prove fruitful: (1) assessing the nature of the patient's spiritual belief system, the significance which these beliefs have had in his life, and the ways in which these beliefs have been affected by his current life situation; (2) identifying spiritual and religious resources that might serve as sources of support in the current situation; and (3) exploring those coping behaviors (both functional and dysfunctional) that the patient has used to deal with previous spiritual and religious needs and concerns, the reasons why such behaviors are no longer effective, and potential new strategies the patient may employ to deal with his present situation.

EVALUATION

It is important for the nurse to continue to assess and evaluate the patient's spiritual or religious needs, as well as the effectiveness of her nursing interventions in meeting such needs, and also, that such observations be recorded regularly on the patient's nursing care plan and chart.[30] Such documentation, to be meaningful, should include the patient's movement toward[31] or away from previously identified nursing goals, as well as any revisions in such goals or in the nursing interventions used to achieve them. It is ideal if the patient can be involved in the formulation of such goals and interventions initially as well as in the reevaluation and revision processes.

RESEARCH

Finally, the need for continued nursing research in this area is evident if nurses are to expand their knowledge and validate their interventions relative to the spiritual and religious needs of patients in all health care settings. Among the many potential areas of inquiry that might be examined are included: (1) common responses to spiritual needs and concerns, as well as manifestations of spiritual distress; (2) systematic data collection for the assessment of spiritual wellness or distress; (3) expansion of nursing diagnoses to include such categories as "mature" versus "immature" religious motivations, spiritual distress precipitated by "situational" versus "maturational" issues, or chronic spiritual distress related to developmental issues; (4) identification of psychiatric interventions based upon various theoretical orientations (e.g., cognitive, behavioral); and (5) mechanisms for evaluating the effectiveness of nursing interventions relative to identified goals for a client's spiritual care.

Summary

This chapter has provided a global, generic view of spirituality and wellness, drawing upon elements of coping and crisis theories to form its underlying conceptual framework. Manifestations of spiritual needs or distress in both psychiatric and nonpsychiatric settings have been presented, as have suggested nursing diagnoses, goals, and interventions. Finally, information regarding the documentation and evaluation of spiritual care has been included and potential areas for further nursing research identified.

Questions

1. What is the attitude of staff toward the spiritual/religious needs of patients in your clinical agency?
2. Describe a clinical situation in which you focused on the spiritual/religious needs of a patient.
3. What is the role of spirituality in relationship to crisis theory?

REFERENCES AND SUGGESTED READINGS

1. Peck, M. S. *The Road Less Traveled: A New Psychology of Love, Traditional Values, and Spiritual Growth.* New York: Simon & Schuster, 1978, p. 15.
2. Ibid.
3. Stoll, R. I. Guidelines for spiritual assessment. *American Journal of Nursing,* 1979, *79,* 1574–1577.
4. Peck, op. cit., p. 185.
5. Burgess, A. W., & Baldwin, B. A. *Crisis Intervention Theory and Practice: A Clinical Handbook.* Englewood Cliffs, N.J.: Prentice-Hall, 1981.
6. Caplan, G. *Principles of Preventive Psychiatry.* New York: Basic Books, 1964.
7. Garland, L. M., & Bush, C. T. *Coping Behaviors and Nursing.* Reston, Va.: Reston Publishing, 1982, p. 25.
8. Burgess & Baldwin, op. cit. p. 26.
9. Ibid.
10. Garland & Bush. *Coping Behaviors and Nursing,* p. 12.
11. Ibid.
12. Ibid.
13. Lovinger, R. J. Therapeutic strategies with "religious resistances." *Psychotherapy: Theory, Research and Practice,* 1979, *16,* 419–427.
14. Ibid., p. 420.
15. Field, W. E., & Wilkerson, S. Religiosity as a psychiatric symptom. *Perspectives in Psychiatric Care,* 1973, *11*(3), 100–105.
16. Ibid.
17. Ibid.
18. Ibid.
19. Ibid.
20. Cavenar, J. O., & Spaulding, J. G. Depressive disorders and religious conversions. *Journal of Nervous and Mental Disease,* 1977, *165*(3), 209–212.
21. Field and Wilkerson, op. cit.
22. Ibid., p. 104.
23. Christopher News Notes, April 1982, 12 East 48th Street, New York, N.Y. 10017.
24. Fish, S., & Shelly, J. A. *Spiritual Care: The Nurse's Role.* Downer's Grove, Ill.: Intervarsity Press, 1978, p. 22.
25. Bush, B. J. *Coping: Issues of Emotional Living in an Age of Stress for Clergy and Religious.* Whitinsville, Mass.: Affirmation Books, 1976, p. 71.
26. Gulko, J. Chaplain's medical approach to psychiatric patients. *Journal of Religion and Health,* 1983, *22*(4), 278–286.
27. Relling–Garskoff, K. Transferring the past to the present. *American Journal of Nursing,* 1987, *87,* 477–478.
28. Stoll, op. cit.
29. Field & Wilkerson, op. cit.
30. Peterson, E. A., & Nelson, K. How to meet your clients' spiritual needs, *Journal of Psychosocial Nursing,* 1987, *25*(5), 34–39.
31. Kennison, M. M. Faith: An untapped health resource, *Journal of Psychosocial Nursing,* 1987, *25*(10), 28–33.

Chapter 15

The Therapeutic Alliance and the Nurse–Patient Relationship

Ann Wolbert Burgess

Chapter Objectives

The students successfully attaining the goals of this chapter should be able to:

- Define therapeutic alliance and its relationship to the nurse–patient relationship.
- Discuss the relationship of human qualities and therapeutic use of self.
- Identify the opening, working, and terminating of a therapeutic interview.
- Give examples of eleven useful and facilitating verbal responses in interviewing.
- Identify questions that facilitate an interview and questions that stall an interview.
- Give examples of nine nonuseful or stalling interviewing responses.
- Record nurse–client interactions through the use of process recordings and nursing notes.
- Identify the goal in the supervisory process.

The process of establishing an alliance is a core component in implementing therapeutic communication strategies in psychiatric mental health nursing practice. It is a skill that is used in every nurse–patient transaction regardless of the amount of time for contact with the patient or the clinical setting. Its intent is a health-promoting impact. In the tradition of Hildegard Peplau, the alliance is that point of consensual validation and reality at which the patient and the nurse acknowledge that they are coming together to work toward a healthier state for the patient. It is a realistic acceptance that each person exists and is located in the present encounter.

The therapeutic alliance establishes certain ground rules. In an inpatient setting, the ground rules cover the following: where to go and from whom to request specific information; the space and territory of the individual and that of others; issues of conduct and personal hygiene; cooperative daily living arrangements such as recreation, eating, sleeping time, visiting times, passes to go on and off the unit, and rules of safety. In a community setting, in addition to the areas listed for an inpatient setting, the

241

ground rules cover the following: a consistent time to meet to review daily activities and agenda; agreeing to disagree; agreeing that if either one requests it, there can be outside consultation; and agreeing to keep communications open in the most positive and direct manner that each is able to. In addition to this agreement, each assumes responsibility for evaluating the work together to be sure it is achieving substantial objectives and goals that have primarily been negotiated and set by the patient.

An essential element of all psychotherapeutic transactions in psychiatric mental health nursing is the nature of the relationship between the patient and the nurse. Although this is a term that is frequently used, it is actually a very complicated matter. The patient enters into a therapeutic situation because of pain, suffering, maladjustment, or confusion and is seeking help from a care provider who is endowed, by virtue of her nursing education, with capacity to provide that help. Thus the patient brings to the professional relationship not only varying degrees of motivation but also some degree of expectancy and hope that the nurse will be able to help. The real attributes that patients bring to the therapeutic setting—their intelligence, their social and vocational competencies, their value systems, their resources, and their life transactions—all play a part in the therapeutic alliance and exchange, along with the nature of the patients' disorder and the quality and quantity of their defenses and resistances.

The art and science of conducting a good interview in terms of making pertinent clinical observations from useful information and establishing an alliance and a therapeutic relationship are psychiatric nursing's most basic and important tools. Neither nurse nor patient is passive in the process of the interaction; each reacts reciprocally. Thus, the therapeutic use of self becomes a key asset in helping people under stress, and all efforts to develop one's repertoire of skills are to be encouraged.

The Congress for Nursing Practice has defined psychiatric nursing as "a specialized area of nursing practice employing theories of human behavior as its scientific aspects and purposeful use of self as its art." This chapter will describe the attitudes and human qualities that are important in working therapeutically and effectively with people who are psychiatric patients as well as the specific dimensions of the relationship in which the work occurs.

ATTITUDES AND QUALITIES ESSENTIAL TO THE THERAPEUTIC RELATIONSHIP

The therapeutic relationship is an interpersonal process between a nurse and a patient. The purpose of the relationship is to facilitate the achievement of goals or objectives. These goals are established by the nurse and patient during the initial contact and are explicitly stated prior to the beginning of the relationship.

In general, the goals of a therapeutic relationship are directed toward producing behavior changes in the patient. These changes may be as basic as increasing personal hygiene activity or as complex as diminishing hallucinating or delusional experiences. The medium for the therapeutic relationship is the interview; the tool is the nurse. Therefore, a requirement for nurses involved in developing a therapeutic relationship is the ability to self-assess. Other qualities that are important for the nurse to develop are professional comfort, respect, optimism, a positive outlook about people, sensitivity, involvement, caring, patience, and persistence.

Self-Assessment

Examining one's attitudes and style is a very personal affair, for we are talking about our very self, our personality, and our unique identity. Self-assessing is, therefore, a difficult task. It involves being aware of the interpersonal assets and talents that the nurse brings to the situation. It further involves knowing what qualities and skills must be further developed within nurses in order for them to provide a more therapeutic interchange with patients.

From the very start it is essential to understand that this self-assessment process—the constant examination of feelings, attitudes, and actions—is essential in psychiatric nursing. It is as basic and fundamental as the stethoscope is to the medical nurse.

For some it may be more difficult to examine their attitudes than to analyze the expressions of their feelings or to view their behavior. Attitude is the statement of a person's position or stand on an issue. Ideally, each new situation should be started with a completely open mind. But how often is that the case? Take, for example, the student's original attitude toward the psychiatric nursing course. Some students have the attitude that psychiatry is the answer to the human dilemma, whereas others have the attitude that psychiatry is the reason for our dilemma.

It is essential that the student adopt the position that when examining feelings, attitudes, and actions or having them examined by an instructor or classmates, it is not to be a blaming or a breast-beating process. The nurse who is angry out of all proportion to the situation is not to be blamed. Rather there is something to be examined and understood. If a patient will not speak to a nurse, again there is something to be understood. Unless we adopt this attitude, we would be pretending that we are always loving, kind, and understanding in order to avoid criticism. Not only would this attitude be sheer pretense but it would also be hard to tolerate or justify.

Being Natural

Personality represents our unique identity. Those distinct personal character traits that distinguish us from every other human being establish us as individuals. During the years of personal growth, a stylistic pattern of communication and relating to people emerges as part of one's behavioral style.

Many people pass through life only dimly aware of their behavioral style and how it affects others. Yet people are aware of the principle that everyone is different and unique. Literature abounds in material on personality and behavioral styles, and colleges are well catalogued with courses on personality development and psychology. Understanding the human phenomenon of the uniqueness of a person is one step in the self-assessment process. The importance of understanding and developing one's natural behavioral style is to facilitate feeling secure and being therapeutic in nursing situations. Extracting the very best of humanness within oneself is to accent natural talents and to make use of one's special qualities.

Students should trust their natural behavioral style. Twenty years of living have taught interpersonal skills that others have perceived as therapeutic in the broadest sense. Unless you have absolutely no friends and unless all relatives completely avoid you, you do have natural talents.

Each of us has a natural style that in itself is so unique that it separates us from all other human beings. The student should ask "What are some of the characteristic and understanding ways that I have in dealing with people and what is it that people especially like about me and respond to?"

Students should start out by simply being natural and then seeing how much of their everyday interaction is therapeutic. They will find many aspects of their style that are perfectly acceptable in a social situation but may be inappropriate in a professional setting. It is these particular aspects of style that will be important to examine critically. However, unless one starts by being natural, one may lose valuable traits such as charm, softness, and warmth in the attempt to be "professional."

The professional style that a nurse finally adopts will be a special mixture of the natural self, together with some traits of several instructors and colleagues whose style and manner "feel right."

Professional Comfort

To be therapeutic, nurses should be comfortable in their professional role. Professional comfort comes most naturally from experience. Unfortunately, the discomfort of the inexperienced student is hard to conceal. This is illustrated by two nursing students during their first day on a ward:

A nursing student was in a four-bed unit, carefully checking her patient's name from her assignment list, when one of the patients said, "Hello, nurse." The student promptly said, "Just a minute, sir, and I will get you one."

The same day, another nursing student was taking the blood pressure of her patient when the patient, not knowing the status of the student, said, "How long have you been in nursing?" The student anxiously looked at her watch and said, "Exactly 10 minutes."

It may be helpful for you to think back to the time you first talked with a patient and remember your own degree of "professional comfort."

Students should be fully aware of the importance of professional comfort in the therapeutic process. At the same time they must be patient with themselves, for it takes time to acquire the experience.

Respect

Respect for the other person is crucial in all human interaction. It is of particular importance in the therapy of psychiatric patients. The term *respect* is used in the sense of paying attention to, observing carefully, and appreciating the worth and dignity of another person. The nurse communicates respect by taking the person seriously, by being honest, by listening well, and by regarding the patient as a person instead of an object. Failing to do the above by giving false reassurance or by infantilizing the patient is equal to saying, "I ignore your strength, I do not take you seriously, I am not interested in you, and I do not respect you."

Psychiatric patients commonly suffer from lowered self-esteem or even experience feelings of self-hate as part of their illness. Medical-surgical patients may share similar feelings because of their "lying around" and not being able to do an "honest day's work." Being able to communicate respect to the patient is therefore a powerful therapeutic tool.

Optimism (Every Patient Can Be Helped)

In order to be therapeutic, the nurse must believe that each patient can be helped. This may be hard to accept when a patient is seriously regressed, when he has been sick for a long time, or when he is grossly demanding and trying. Nevertheless, many regressed patients do make dramatic recoveries; patients who have been sick for a long time have been known to respond amazingly well, and demanding patients often become quite delightful when they recover.

Even in the most desperate of situations we must hold to our initial assumption that every human interaction has the potential for being therapeutic. Not everyone can be cured and not everyone can be rehabilitated, but some suffering can be relieved. The patient can be helped if he has hope; but he can only sustain a feeling of hope if the helper communicates that feeling to him.

There Are Positive Aspects to All People

Patients whom the students like and find interesting will usually respond to treatment more rapidly than patients whom they dislike. If this is true, students may face the seemingly impossible task of learning to like or at least finding something positive about an unpleasant, unattractive, hostile, uncooperative, or withdrawn patient. How can this be done? First, students must acknowledge to themselves how much they dislike the patient. You try to determine what it is about the patient that bothers you: his withdrawal, his hostility, or perhaps his personal grooming. Then you try to understand what it is about yourself that is bothered: possibly feelings of helplessness or anxiety about failing. If necessary you should discuss your feelings with a classmate or instructor. At this point you should more calmly take another look at the patient. You should attempt to understand the aspects of the patient's behavior that you dislike. You will find meaning. If the patient is trying to push you away, you will undoubtedly find a good reason for it if you review his past history. If he is withdrawn, you must feel this behavior is doing something for him. If the student enters into the world of the patient, his behavior will have meaning. At the same time you will find a real suffering human being, struggling in the best way he knows to survive. Using this approach, students are likely to find something about any patient to respect.

Sensitivity

Being sensitive is being acutely aware of the subtle changes in thought, mood, or behavior in another person. It is a feeling or a hunch that something is not right. It is listening, looking, and feeling more carefully and more intently than does the nonprofessional. In a sense, it is having one's own radar.

For example, the nurse enters the patient's room and senses that something is wrong. The atmosphere in the room feels different to the nurse. Perhaps the patient is more reserved and thoughtful. Instead of saying, "Good morning. How are you this morning?" the nurse might enter the room and just say, "Good morning." After a pause, if the patient does not respond, she might say, "I have the feeling there is something on your mind." Using the human quality of sensitivity, the nurse is able to communicate to the patient that she knows something is on his mind and that she is interested in listening to him. Almost all patients in this situation will respond favorably.

In another situation:

A patient group was gathering for an informal meeting and one patient remarked that Mary was missing. Other patients ignored the absence and the group started talking.

The nurse attending the meeting felt something was not right about Mary being missing. She went to the patient's room and saw that no one was there. Knocking on the bathroom door within the room brought Mary's response of "Leave me alone." The nurse heard a cracking noise and tried the door handle, telling Mary she was doing this because she was concerned about her. The door was locked. The nurse asked Mary to open the door, but there was no answer. The nurse then went to get the master key to unlock the door and when she did, she found Mary cutting her wrists with a piece of broken glass.

The nurse was paying attention to her own feelings of discomfort. This situation was picked up not only by the nurse but also by another patient who had first noticed Mary's absence at the group meeting. Because the nurse acted on her hunch that something was wrong, a problem situation was discovered that could be handled and resolved in time.

Involvement

One of the characteristics that distinguishes the nurse from other mental health professionals is the degree of involvement associated with patient care. The nurse has traditionally stood by the patient on a 24-hour basis through life-threatening situations and through chronic suffering. By continuing with this tradition, psychiatric nurses make their own unique contribution in the treatment of mental illness.

Involvement often takes the form of direct action. Listening and understanding may not be enough.

A nurse was helping patients wash and dress for the day. Two teen-age girls started fighting over a bottle of shampoo. In the struggle for the bottle, it fell and shattered. One of the girls grabbed the broken bottle and disappeared into the bathroom, closing the door behind her. The nurse opened the door in time to see the girl ingesting the contents of the bottle as well as the broken pieces of glass. The nurse forced the girl's mouth open and pulled out the pieces of broken glass. After the incident was reported and the patient was examined for any remaining glass in her mouth, the patient was X-rayed for any ingested glass.

The nurse's action was important to the therapeutic relationship with this particular patient as well as with the other patients who witnessed the event. The nurse was available at a critical time to intervene and resolve an upsetting situation with the patients. The emergency nature of the situation required immediate action. The nurse acted on the basis of her caring. She would not allow the patient to destroy herself. She involved herself by direct action in a way that instantly identified herself as a caring, protecting, significant therapeutic person. Discussing the incident immediately after it happened put the situation in perspective for all the patients involved.

Caring

A 17-year-old high-school girl on her admission to a psychiatric unit raised some questions about caring:

"I was walking down the street and I said 'hello' to a face I know. But no reply came. Probably in a hurry. Nobody has time anymore. Went to the beach. . . . The sun dominated the sky; it has a way of making you feel wanted. . . . As I left, I called 'good-bye' to the sun, but it didn't answer. I know it has other places to shine on. Now even my footsteps leave no traces; just as my 'hello' to a face and my 'good-bye' to the sun. Will I leave a trace? Will anybody care?"

The patient is describing her sense of insignificance: the feeling that she does not matter and that nobody cares. Her feelings of isolation and alienation are stated.

The quality of caring, as a genuine human concern, is important in the therapeutic alliance made with the patient. The patient must be made aware of the nurse's caring and must be convinced of the sincerity in order that progress may be made.

Feeling responsible for a person in terms of being involved with his well-being and by helping him to reach for mutually agreed-upon goals is in reality caring for the patient. As the patient works with the nurse on goals for recovery, he will use the nurse's humanness and strength to build back his own resources. In giving of herself, through her own uniqueness, coupled with an attitude of being genuinely interested in the patient and trying to understand and help him, the nurse will find the fundamentals of relating with the patient. Initially, the nurse should start by just listening and trying to understand the human process within the person, instead of trying to concentrate on specific interviewing techniques contained in some textbooks. Interest and caring about an individual are not technical skills; they are the basic arts of psychic healing.

Nurses do not need to tell the patient they care. They show concern for the patient by listening and by trying to understand the anguish or loneliness in the patient's heart. When nurses are comfortable enough to enable them not to worry about interview technique, posture, facial expression, and speech, their natural concern for people will begin to show. It is then that the patient will know that the nurse cares.

The patient must feel that the nurse is aware of the patient's goals, strivings, and wishes, and that the nurse is working hard in order to accomplish these goals.

Patience and Persistence

The importance of the patience that is required in the healing process of the mind is frequently underestimated in the psychiatric setting.

Working with severely depressed or regressed patients or patients with grave character disorders requires considerable (sometimes infinite) patience. This quality, coupled with the physical presence of the nurse, often achieves the first affirmative therapeutic results. There are frequently days and weeks when the nurse feels no progress is being made. The patient just sits or lies around and says, "Everything makes me depressed. I just want to be alone." A helpful approach in this situation is the patience that is demonstrated through the physical presence of the nurse. This approach can and often does set the stage for therapeutic success.

The ability to wait until the patient is ready to move may yield high dividends. As one patient put it, "I thought I could wait you out, but your patience won out and I decided to try it your way."

In another example involving a medical student:

The student was assigned to a depressed patient who was mute and said absolutely nothing. The student sat with him each day for two weeks. Technically, the student did not know the proper thing to say. He sometimes just sat with the patient. Sometimes he said things such as, "You must feel terribly low."

Mostly he just persisted. On the fifteenth day the patient turned to the bewildered student and uttered his first words: "You sure know what you are doing." Two weeks later the patient had recovered and was discharged.

It is important to remember that the therapeutic process must not be rushed and miracles should not be expected; the nurse must persist with the therapeutic attempts.

In summary, we want to reiterate the need for the nurse to be aware of her own behavior and how it affects the patient. Looking at her behavior is not always pleasant and is sometimes painful, but it is absolutely necessary if the nurse is to use herself to the fullest extent possible. As the nurse interviews a patient, it is imperative that she examine her responses and behavior. Does she feel repulsed when she's with a particular patient? Does she feel uncomfortable when the patient talks about certain subjects? Does she draw away when a patient expresses unacceptable thoughts? Does she have a feeling of compassion and empathy for the patient who seemingly has no support system outside himself? An awareness of your own feelings and of the resultant behaviors you exhibit is essential in the use of yourself with the patient.

Because so many psychiatric patients have fragmented and underdeveloped relationships with family and friends, they need the warmth of understanding, caring, and empathy. These feelings cannot be taught from a book. They are learned through experiences with other individuals. Nurses may continue to grow in their ability to care, understand, and empathize, but they must come to the patient with these basic assets already developed. The patients will sense through the nurses' behaviors and verbal exchanges whether they are giving of themselves in an unselfish manner, and will judge the nurses accordingly. Nurses get to know a great deal about patients and their problems from their interactions with them. Patients learn about nurses in the same manner. They know whether nurses respond to their needs for warmth, understanding, and respect. If they respond, patients will have found other human beings with whom they can discuss their feelings without fear. When this sharing occurs, nurses will know that they have been able to use their own strengths, weaknesses, and positive and negative behaviors to touch other individuals in a meaningful way.

TYPES OF NURSE–PATIENT INTERACTIONS

Nurse–patient interactions may be divided, generally, into two main categories: (1) social; and (2) therapeutic. In social exchanges both the nurse and patient are involved in discussing a situation, and both exchange their thoughts and feelings in a reciprocal fashion. For example, both nurse and patient may have a common interest in gardening. In a social discussion, the nurse would talk openly to the patient of her likes and dislikes in gardening. She would freely express her thoughts about types of plants, soil preparation, or whatever. It would be an experience of mutually sharing thoughts.

Therapeutic interaction, on the other hand, centers on the patient. Therapeutic interaction is seen as a verbal exchange between patient and nurse in which the patient's feelings and thoughts are the central focus of exploration. In a therapeutic discussion using the preceding example, the nurse would not share her likes and dislikes of gardening. Rather, she would make the patient's likes and dislikes the main topic of conversation. She would help the patient express what he liked or disliked about gardening, and her own ideas would not be discussed. Thus, in any given situation, e.g., medication time, mealtime, group social activities, etc., the nurse can use herself as a sounding board and a helper to allow the patient to discuss what is important to him. Her own ideas and interests need not be shared.

STRUCTURE AND USE OF INTERVIEWS

Interviews are one type of therapeutic interaction. The interview is a structured, goal-directed, time-limited encounter between nurse and patient. Two types of interviews are used in a psychiatric setting. The first type, which can be described as *fact-finding*, is conducted to help the nurse gain specific knowledge about an event. In this type of interview, the nurse has a goal to elicit specific data from the patient. There usually is a preset group of questions that are asked the patient. The patient request, functional status, and mental status examination, which are discussed in Chapter 12, are good examples of a fact-finding interview.

The second type of interview is referred to as the nurse–patient relationship or *one-to-one interaction*. This interview is useful in allowing the patient time to explore problems that have been unresolved up to that point. In this type of interview, the nurse and patient together identify and work on problems that, when resolved, will help the patient function in a more adaptive and effective manner.

The overall purpose of the interview is to provide a data base of information from which nurse and patient together can identify problems, set goals, and evaluate methods of achieving the goals that have been set. A review of nursing assessment, which was discussed in Chapter 12, would be helpful for the student who is interested in utilizing an interview to the fullest extent. If the student continues to see the patient on a regular basis, an opportunity exists for evaluation and modification of the goals that have been set. Thus the interview becomes a vehicle for helping the patient move toward emotional health.

The interview is also a valuable tool in helping students become comfortable in talking with patients. It provides students with a means of looking at their own behavior and how the patient is affected by it.

And finally, the interview is useful in providing an opportunity for the patient to establish a meaningful relationship with the student. It is through the formation of this relationship that the patient can experience becoming comfortable with another person. The patient, it is hoped, will use what he has learned from his talks with the nurse as he reestablishes relationships with his family and makes new acquaintances.

A word should be said about the length of the interview. Generally, the time should not exceed one hour. For patients who are acutely disturbed, severely regressed, or suffering from organic impairment, the interview should be informal (a therapeutic interaction) and brief (5 to 10 minutes) until the patient is well enough to tolerate regular meetings of increasing periods of time.

For the interview to be successful, the patient should be seen in a quiet place. It is distracting to try to talk on a busy ward where many patients are walking about and are likely to interrupt the interaction. Concern for privacy is vitally important. The more insistent one is upon uninterrupted interviewing, the greater the possibility of concentrating on the patient's thoughts and behavior. This holds true for the patient in both the general hospital or community setting. Find a quiet place to talk with the patient.

Your own comfort during an interview is essential in order to hear what the patient is saying and to be receptive to what the patient is having difficulty expressing. For example, it would be unwise to schedule an hour meeting during your lunch hour when you have already missed breakfast. When you are hungry, tired, or preoccupied, you are not going to be a good listener. By the same token, be sure that the time and place of the meeting are acceptable to the patient. He will be unable to respond effectively if he is hungry, sleepy, or unsure of the purpose of the interview.

PHASES OF THE THERAPEUTIC NURSE–PATIENT RELATIONSHIP

The Orientation Phase/First Phase

In the first phase of the therapeutic relationship, the primary goal is the establishment of the contract. The contract defines the purpose of the interviews and the meeting times and places, as well as the goals to be accomplished during the relationship.

If the nurse has not met the patient, an introduction is necessary. In the introduction, the nurse should include who she is, what the purpose of the interview is, and where and when she and the patient will meet, as well as the approximate length of each interview and the total number of anticipated meetings. For example, the nurse could say:

"Good morning, Mrs. Smith. I am Susan Jones, a student nurse from State University School of Nursing, and I will be coming here for the next five weeks as a part of my training. I am here to learn more about talking with patients. I would like to talk with you each Wednesday for about 10 minutes regarding any problems you are having. What would be a good time for you to meet with me?"

The process of becoming comfortable enough and establishing a talking arrangement between nurse and patient is not easy. The nurse and patient are two strangers, meeting together in a particular setting with the intent of getting acquainted. The following example describes some problems in beginning the interview:

STUDENT: Hello, Mrs. Smith [pause for recognition from the patient]. I am Susan Jones and will be here for the next five weeks to talk with you about anything that bothers you.

PATIENT: Where did you say you are from?

STUDENT: The State University.

PATIENT: Do you like the program?

STUDENT: Yes, very much. How long have you been in the hospital?

PATIENT: Two weeks.

STUDENT: What happened before you came to the hospital?

PATIENT: I wasn't doing too good. I was depressed and cried a lot. So my family sent me here.

STUDENT: Do you feel better now?

PATIENT: A little. I don't cry anymore. [pause] You want to go for a walk?

STUDENT: Sure—Where should we go?

Since the patient wants to know about this "stranger" who is talking with her, she asks about the student's nursing experience. The student was able to give brief answers to the patient's questions and then shifts the focus of the conversation back to the patient. The brief discussion of the patient's perceived problem, i.e., crying and depression, gives both the student and patient a sense of what the patient sees as her problem. Since the student may not feel comfortable enough to explore the problems related to the patient's depression, she quickly agrees to take a walk with the patient. The walk allows the nurse and patient to relieve tension and to further develop a relationship. As the student becomes more comfortable with the patient, she can provide the atmosphere that allows the patient to explore her feelings of depression.

For the relationship to develop and for the interview to proceed to the working phase, the patient has to respond positively to the feeling that there is something in it for her. She must sense that this relationship, although brief, will be meaningful. She must sense that this "stranger" will respect her, help her bear some of the pain that is in her heart, be trustworthy and honest, and be empathetic. If the patient senses these characteristics at the beginning of the interview, she will know that there is something in it for her. Students may erroneously feel that they must be brilliant, insightful, knowledgeable, and full of expert advice. The patient will expect none of these behaviors. She will expect neither a trained psychiatrist nor an experienced psychiatric nurse, but rather a responsive human being.

Many interviews begin with considerable stress and difficulty. The patient may vehemently refuse to talk, he may talk with much tension and anxiety, or he may be furious with the student. At this point, Chapters 1 and 2 might be reread to give you an idea of what feelings the neophyte psychiatric nurse and the patient experience. Examining your own and the patient's feelings should help you to become more empathetic to the patient's feelings and behaviors. Looking at your own feelings can also help you to remain objective. Chapters 1 and 2 should help you see and understand that the stress most often experienced is a natural part of the clinical situation and that it is not because of any unusual inadequacy within yourself.

In the introductory phase of the relationship, the patient and nurse are busy getting to know each other and are learning to be more comfortable together. At the initial interview, the nurse should help the patient be as relaxed and comfortable as possible. The nurse might say, "Sometimes it's difficult to talk with a person that you feel you hardly know." This statement could then be used to help the patient explore how he makes beginning relationships with other individuals.

The length of time involved in the introductory phase of the relationship varies from patient to patient. One patient may be reticent to discuss reasons for his hospitalization for several weeks. Another patient may start talking about his problems immediately after introduction. For this reason, the nurse must be able to "shift gears," so to speak, based on the verbal and nonverbal cues the patient gives. The pace of the interview is an individual matter, and it is imperative that the nurse let the patient set the pace.

Once the patient relaxes and begins to talk, the contract phase of the interview begins. Again, with some patients this transition occurs immediately, but with others it may take several meetings. For this reason, it is a good learning experience for the student nurse to have several patients so as to note individual differences in the evolution of the interview.

During this first phase, the nurse helps the client articulate his goals for the relationship. These goals will provide the direction and focus for the relationship. And the evaluation of these goals will be a consistent process during the next two phases.

Setting Goals

The task of setting goals in any therapeutic situation is essential to the anticipated gains for the individual. From the team standpoint, goals may be separated into the overall goal (long-term) and the subgoal (short-term). The overall goal tends to reflect the philosophy of the hospital or clinic, for example, determining when the patient may be out of treatment and returned to family and community. The subgoals are indicative of the intervening steps necessary to be taken in reaching the overall goal.

A necessary component in the task of setting goals is the inclusion of the goals the patient has for himself. It is hoped that the goals of the treatment team match the goals of the patient. When they do not, negotiation must take place.

The analogy may be made to the nursing student and the nursing education program. Generally, the overall goal for the student is to complete the program requirements of the school and to achieve the registered nurse's license. The various courses taken during the educational experience, such as liberal arts and science courses and the clinical nursing specialty courses represent the subgoals necessary to reach the overall goal of the registered nurse's license. The nursing students, however, also have personal subgoals related to personal fulfillment, family, and community that are necessary in order to complete the overall picture. A nursing program that fails to combine the goals of the student with the educational goals of the program will have as much difficulty in graduating students as the hospital will have in discharging patients when it fails to combine the psychosocial–economical–spiritual goals of the patient with the goals of the treatment team.

In the psychiatric setting, formulating goals begins with knowing exactly why the patient comes for treatment. For example, the patient may be hospitalized for an acute short-term crisis of possibly one or two months duration. It is important to know that the overall goal is to help the patient to return to the community and to prevent him from becoming a chronic patient. It is not necessary to announce this goal to the patient, but it should be uppermost in the mind of the nurse. Or if the patient is in a psychiatric hospital where the major treatment modality is long-term psychotherapy, the treatment goal might be confinement to the hospital for a year of intensive analysis.

Establishing a goal protects the nurse from trying to be everything to the patient. Goals are the reminders and limits to the reality within which one must work. The nurse does not have vague or unrealistic plans for the patient when the purpose or goal for being with the patient is clearly defined.

Some goals stated by patients may be misleading. Patients will say, "I want to establish meaningful relationships; I want to relate better to people; I want to understand myself better; I want to increase my socialization." Such statements tend to be psychiatric clichés, and the nurse should be alert to recognize them and to help the patient more clearly state what his expectations for therapy are.

Well-meaning as these goals may be, they are almost impossible to put into practice effectively. They are difficult to achieve and only serve to make both patient and therapist overwhelmed or confused. Well-thought-through, achievable short-term goals are more useful in a therapeutic program.

Goals may be stated in terms of activities of daily living.

What are realistic goals for the patient? What goals of psychiatric accomplishments can be established for a short-term setting? Depending on the behavior of the patient, some suggestions for short-term goals are listed below. The patient should be able to:

1. Talk about daily ward activities.
2. Perform a structured task, such as getting up for breakfast, or getting to school or work on time, or staying at school or work for the full time.
3. Discuss a particular incident that occurred at the unit that was upsetting or successful for the patient or others.
4. Look at the manner in which the patient's behavior leads to favorable or unfavorable reactions from other people.
5. Look at the patient's anxiety about specific situations and the reaction it has on him and others.
6. Determine whether the patient is suicidal.
7. Talk in order to clarify the patient's wishes and expectations in life and how the patient intends to obtain them.

The covert agenda of the patient is often overlooked. Although the nurse's goals are to help the patient, the patient may have totally different goals. It is necessary to keep this in mind because unless there is some merging of the goals, very little can develop. If the nurse's goal is to be a helpful listener and the patient feels like being helpfully listened to, the conversation usually goes well. If his goal, however, is to get the nurse to get him a glass of water because the other nurse has not been around to get him one, the nurse is going to have trouble. Or if the patient's primary goal is to leave the hospital and the nurse's goal is to merely help him understand his feelings, there will be little interchange.

The nurse might say, "What are you hoping or wishing for yourself? You look preoccupied." The patient might respond, "I'm being discharged in an hour and I am wondering if my husband is going to be his old self and start shouting and screaming at me." If the nurse's goal is only to listen, the approach will be irrelevant to the patient's goals. The patient will want and expect a more direct involvement on the nurse's part on how to deal with the potential situation that she dreads facing at home. Alternatives might be explored; for example, "Are you that fearful of your welcome at home?"

The role of the therapeutic person is to either convince the patient that staff goals are the right goals or to change staff goals to patient goals. If the staff is at an impasse with the patient, there must be a reevaluation of the situation with the staff team.

Find out what the patient wants. For example, "It seems as though many things are on your mind. What are the hopes and wishes you are experiencing and let's look at them." This will give a whole new area for discussion.

A final consideration of the task of setting goals is relevant to the teaching situation. This is identifying learning goals for the student. One learning goal may be learning to look for and to observe psychiatric symptoms, for example, schizophrenia, as part of the psychiatric nursing experience.

Learning goals such as these do not specifically aim at helping the patient. Nevertheless, it has been our experience that these learning goals do turn out to be therapeutic for the patient even though the primary aim is teaching. The teaching staff generally takes responsibility that the learning activity, such as teaching interview conferences, is not harmful to the patient.

In inpatient settings, helping the patient to be discharged from the hospital and to return to his family and community is usually the overall goal. This goal implies determining the patient's ability to cope and manage his life. The patient's wishes and expectations must be considered concurrently with the treatment team's goals. Otherwise, an impasse arises. Careful goal planning between staff and patient sets the stage for therapeutic progress.

A common reason for an unsuccessful interview is the failure of the nurse to define the goal and nature of the relationship at the start. For example, the nurse may never define what the limits of the relationship are. As a result, the patient may feel the need to form a social friendship from this newly developing relationship. At other times the nurse may not have made clear the number of visits to be expected and is upset when the patient responds with anger or annoyance when the relationship terminates. When a patient knows what to expect from the nurse and what the purpose of the relationship and interview is, he can make a valid judgment as to whether he wishes to become involved. The patient should always have the right to refuse an interview and to give his reason to the clinical team for further negotiation.

In the initial interview, the issue of confidentiality is addressed. The nurse's participation on the health team is stressed, and the patient is told that certain relevant information will be shared with the other team members in the form of verbal and written notes. The primary task of the nurse during this early phase of the relationship is to relate to the patient in a warm and caring manner. The goal is to decrease the patient's anxiety as well as the nurse's anxiety, and for the nurse to be open and emotionally available to the patient. The important qualities of accurate empathy, nonpossessive warmth, and genuineness, discussed in Chapter 16, are critical dimensions of the therapeutic relationship, and if felt by the client will greatly facilitate the movement of the relationship toward the working phase.

The Working Phase/Middle Phase

In the working phase of the therapeutic relationship, the nurse and client examine and explore data related to the stated goals identified in the orientation phase. Throughout this stage, these goals are addressed. Sometimes, as new information emerges, the client may decide to change the goals. The nurse helps the client formulate goals by validating, clarifying, and ordering the data. The nurse serves as an important reality agent for the client, supporting what is reasonable for the client to achieve during the limited time frame of their relationship.

The working phase of the relationship begins when the patient begins to feel comfortable with the nurse and starts discussing problems that have led to his hospitalization. Goals and objectives have been identified, and ways of meeting these established goals are now discussed. To accomplish this task, the nurse must continue to relate to the patient in a manner that is encouraging. The empathetic, understanding nurse will allow the patient to proceed to explore painful matters that he would otherwise keep "locked" within himself. During the working phase, the nurse observes; helps the patient talk; focuses the interview; and explores thoughts, feelings, and actions.

Observation

The unobtrusive observation of the patient is an ongoing activity throughout the interview. What is evident about the patient from his mannerisms and his style of communicating will contribute to a better understanding of him.

Generally, the nurse will focus on the patient's words, his mood, his emotions, and what he says or does not say. Observing the patient's appearance and the characteristics of his communication will also provide basic information. A keen power of observation is a much desired quality in nursing.

The initial observations of a patient's facial expression, manner of speaking, use of gestures, and general appearance tell us much about him. It will help us to perceive the thoughts and appraise the feelings that he has expressed about himself. We can then assess whether he is oriented or confused, sad or happy, or in contact with us or not. We can also, possibly, evaluate his social skills and determine whether or not he is regressed and withdrawn.

It is equally important to learn what the patient nonverbally implies as well as what he verbally describes. Almost all people have special ways of expressing anxiety that are as individualistic as fingerprints. Some will rub their eyes, tap their fingers, fidget, or light cigarettes a certain way. The pitch and tone of a person's voice can express emotions, as can the posture of his body and the movements and gestures of his limbs. Emotions affect the autonomic system as well as the central nervous system. Changes in breathing accompanied by flushing, signs of perspiration, and evidence of tears may be noted. When observing the patient, the nurse must be aware of the pitfall of becoming so intent on listening that the patient receives no response. If the nurse just sits with the patient and appears nonresponsive, the patient will feel unsupported and alone.

Being therapeutic is not just watching someone talk. One must be responsive in order to be therapeutic. If the nurse senses that a patient is experiencing anxiety when talking about his mother, for example, she should ask him if her perception of increased tension is correct. This question has at least two advantages. First, it allows the nurse to validate her perception, and second, it provides feedback to the patient about his nonverbal behavior.

A common misunderstanding on how much the therapist should say stems from confusion arising from being nondirective versus nonresponsive. To be *nondirective* allows the patient to choose the topic for discussion and to explore what is innermost in his mind without censorship from the therapist. This takes considerable skill and verbal exchange between patient and interviewer. In contrast, *nonresponsive* behavior on the therapist's part shows lack of concern and caring, or discomfort with the topic being discussed.

Helping the Patient Talk

Showing sincere interest in what the patient is saying will generally tell him that he is cared about as a human being. Showing this interest is one way the nurse can help the patient to talk freely. When she does not fully understand what a particular experience or situation means to a patient, she should inquire further and tactfully point out that what he is saying is not clear to her. Where he is able to clarify and explain, the situation becomes clearer and has more meaning to both the patient and the nurse.

In order to help the patient put some of his difficulties in perspective, the nurse must pay careful attention to details. For example, when the patient tells her that he cannot get along with his parents, she might reply, "Give me an example of a situation about which you disagree."

If the patient says that he can't think of one, then the nurse might suggest, "Talk about the last time you had a disagreement with your parents." It is more helpful to focus the patient on a recent problem than to delve into distant past experiences that are no longer real to the patient.

As a rule, when the patient continues to talk and new material appears, the nurse should be nondirective and should endeavor to let the patient maintain the initiative. When progress stalls, the nurse should try to learn why the patient is having difficulty in talking. When the block is discovered, she should emphasize it to the patient as something that should be discussed. With this technique the problem is dealt with directly. For example:

A 15-year-old patient had been talking well with his nursing student for a number of interviews. Suddenly he became withdrawn, just sat during the interview staring out the window, and responded with sarcasm to any remark of the student. She brought the problem to his attention by asking him what he was feeling that he could not say. He finally said that he thought that she was very pretty, that he liked her, but felt this was wrong and bad and so he had stopped talking to her. He felt this was the best way to handle his feelings.

As soon as the feelings were openly expressed, the nurse helped the patient see that these were human feelings and nothing to be ashamed of. The nurse could then go on to discuss what the patient would do when he felt he liked a girl in school and how he would handle his feelings of caring in general. Verbalizing his difficulties with the nurse gave the patient the opportunity to explore and resolve some of his problems with females in general.

In the nondirective approach, the patient takes the lead in the dialogue, and the nurse encourages the conversation without introducing new thoughts on the topic. She helps the patient to explain in more detail the situation that he is describing. Verbal methods that indicate a wish to hear more of what the patient is saying include using such phrases as, "I see," "Uh-huh," "Tell me more about . . . ," or simply nodding one's head. If the nurse is not comfortable with these methods, she can simply restate what the patient has said or use broad general cues such as, "And then what happened?" Tables 15-1 and 15-2 provide examples of useful and nonuseful responses.

Focusing the Interview

Once the goal has been identified, the nurse can guide the discussion toward that point. Patients may try to change to other topics or issues, especially if and when the subject matter makes them uncomfortable. Patients may also talk freely yet say nothing. Here the nurse's responsibility is to limit irrelevant talk. The patient's right to say what he wants to say does not mean that he can talk aimlessly and without some structure. Therefore, the nurse has a twofold job: She must keep the subject matter strictly to the point, and she must aid and support the patient in talking about what is either painful to him or what has made him want to change the subject. For example, the goal for this interview is to understand why Scott withdraws to his room when he is upset.

TABLE 15-1. USEFUL RESPONSES

Category	Example
Recognition	"I'm Jane Smith, a student nurse. What is your name?" "You have a new dress?"
Observation	"You look tense today." "I noticed that you haven't been sleeping. . . ."
General leads	"Tell me . . ." "Talk more about . . ." "Go on. . . ."
Broad openings	"Start at the beginning. . . ." "What is happening with you?"
Restating	"You are smoking more than usual."
Refocusing	"Go back and talk more about . . ." "You were talking about . . ."
Exploration	"Describe in detail . . ." "What happened first?"
Validation	"Are you saying . . . ?" "Did I understand you to say . . . ?"
Focusing	"Talk more about . . ." "Tell me about . . ."
Clarification	"You say you love your wife. What does love mean to you?" "Do you mean . . . ?"
Summarization	"You seem to have talked today about . . ." "You seem to be saying . . ."

TABLE 15-2. NONUSEFUL RESPONSES

Category	Example
Reassurance	"Don't worry." "Everything will be all right." "You look 100% better."
Rejection	"I don't like it when you . . ." "Don't talk about . . ."
Agreement	"You did the right thing." "I don't blame you at all."
Probing	"I want to hear more about . . ." "You should tell me about . . ."
Defensive	"We have good doctors here." "You are locked in for your own good."
Advice	"What you should do is . . ." "Why don't you . . . ?"
Clichés	"How are you today?" "Keeping busy makes you feel better." "Nice day today."
Belittling	"Everybody feels that way." "You shouldn't act that way."

NURSE: Tell me what happened yesterday morning, Scott.

SCOTT: I was playing table pool and things weren't going right and I broke the cue stick. I decided right then that the rest of the day was going to be bad so I went to my room and went to bed.

NURSE: Something bothers you about breaking the cue stick?

SCOTT: Sue said you can hammer on things in occupational therapy. Can you?

NURSE: I guess so. [Pause of a minute.]

SCOTT: I've been thinking of making a wallet for myself and—

NURSE: Scott, we were talking about yesterday morning.

SCOTT: Yeah. [Pause of a minute.] It made me feel destructive.

The patient had been troubled by his feelings of destructiveness. He subsequently tried to avoid thinking about them by changing the subject. He felt enough rapport with the nurse that when she brought him back to the subject, he was able to discuss what bothered him.

Listening

Just as the interviewer uses her eyes to observe, she uses her sense of hearing to keep the interview patient-centered. For example, what topics does the patient exclude from conversation? What does the patient sound like when he talks about his problems? Does the patient mumble when he discusses a threatening issue? And how does the patient see his problem? What part does he play in his present situation? Whom does he blame or praise? The nurse must listen for what is not said as well as what is said. It might be helpful, at this point, for you to review Chapter 10, which deals with various means of developing the communication process. In order to keep the interview patient-centered, the nurse needs to say little and listen carefully.

Thoughts, Feelings, Behavior

Another area that will be discussed in the working phase of the interview is the exploration of thoughts, feelings, and behavior. As the nurse interacts with the patient, she needs to first help him explore his thoughts about whatever situation he is discussing. The thoughts that the patient expresses gives good indications of what the patient feels about his situation. As a patient describes his thoughts, he will usually also discuss his feelings about what happened.

In order to understand the situation more completely, the nurse needs to know what the patient did, what he said, and what he thinks about both of these areas. An example may be helpful:

NURSE: Tell me more about your disagreement with your father.
PATIENT: Well, I wanted to go to the movies, and he said I couldn't go out, so I just blew up.
NURSE: What do you mean when you say "blew up"?
PATIENT: You know, I just started screaming at him and saying he never lets me do anything I want to do.
NURSE: It sounds as though you were pretty upset with him.
PATIENT: Oh, I was. I wanted to kill him.
NURSE: You felt you wanted to hurt him?
PATIENT: Yes, I guess that was it. I didn't want to kill him—just hurt him.
NURSE: What did you do when you had these thoughts?
PATIENT: I ran into my room and slammed the door. Then I threw a paperweight, and it went through the window.

NURSE: What happened then?
PATIENT: I started crying and crawled under the bed.
NURSE: What were you thinking about what happened?
PATIENT: I was afraid, and I knew my father would really be mad. He's really mean when he's mad . . . [pause] . . . and I was ashamed, I guess. I felt I should control myself better.

In this interaction the nurse has helped the patient to describe a painful incident and to explore his feelings about what happened. She would then need to follow the above discussion with identification of more appropriate ways to handle his disappointment, anger, and inability to interact effectively with his father. The depth of exploration would depend on the patient's anxiety level, the strength of the nurse–patient relationship, and the amount of time available for continued discussion. In a real sense, the nurse needs to convey to the patient that she understands his feelings of frustration and anger and believes that he can develop better ways to interact with his father.

Testing Behaviors

During the working phase of the relationship, the client may test the student nurse's commitment to the relationship. Does the nurse really mean what she says? Does she really accept the total person, including the inappropriate behaviors and feelings of the client? Some client behaviors that may be testing behaviors are:

1. Missing the interview appointment.
2. Coming late or leaving the interview early.
3. Displaying intense emotions.
4. Expressing dissatisfaction with the nurse's expertise as a counselor.
5. Asking the nurse to grant special privileges.
6. Asking for treats, food, cigarettes, etc.
7. Not talking during the interview.
8. Exhibiting unusual behavior.

The most effective strategy for surviving the testing stage is for the nurse to remain open, warm, congruent, and available to the client. It is important to understand the dynamics of such behavior so that the nurse does not personalize the experience and become angry and withdrawn. Testing behavior is often a clue to the nurse that she is getting emotionally close to her client. The client is testing the nurse to see if he can continue to trust her with himself. By reflecting to the client during this stage the possibility that he is experiencing feelings about the relationship may help him to understand the motivation for his behavior. When the nurse passes the client's test and continues to be available and warm and open, the testing behaviors diminish and the focus becomes the development of strategies to achieve the goals established in the initial phase.

Strategies for behavioral change are formulated during the working stage. During each session, the effectiveness of the strategy is evaluated. For example, the goal of the following interview is to help the client to cope more effectively with his anxiety:

NURSE: How do you want to feel?
CLIENT: I want to feel less nervous.
NURSE: What does nervous feel like?
CLIENT: Jumpy inside, stomach jittery.
NURSE: What helps you feel less jumpy and jittery inside?
CLIENT: Sometimes if I can stop and take some time out and deep-breathe.
NURSE: This will decrease the nervous feeling?
CLIENT: Yes, for a while.
NURSE: Could you try to stop and deep-breathe as soon as the first jittery feeling comes?
CLIENT: Yes, I think so.
NURSE: You do want to decrease your nervous feelings?
CLIENT: Yes, I do.
NURSE: And what you said is helpful?
CLIENT: Yes.
NURSE: So what would you do more often if you wanted to feel less nervous?
CLIENT: Guess I would take some time out and deep-breathe.

The strategy has been developed by both the nurse and the client. In the next meeting, the nurse will ask the patient about the strategy and will evaluate, with the patient, its effectiveness.

The intent of the evaluation of strategies is to help the client to understand the influence he has over his difficulties. The problem-solving abilities of the client are the main focus of the working phase, and the ultimate goal is for the client to be able to develop and change strategies for himself without the help of a professional. Thus the client learns how to develop his own corrective measures and is able to assess their effectiveness on his own.

In summary, during the working phase of the relationship, the nurse must be concerned with keen observation of the patient and with validation of her perceptions of the patient. She must help the patient talk freely about his problem, which can be accomplished by her use of appropriate questions and responses to the patient. Finally, she must listen to what the patient is expressing, help him focus on important details of what he discusses, and explore his thoughts, feelings, and behaviors. Strategies are developed during this stage and are evaluated for their effectiveness.

Termination/Ending Phase

Termination is the final phase of the therapeutic nurse–patient relationship. The nurse prepares the patient for this phase throughout the previous two stages. From the moment the contract is negotiated, the end date is known. This knowledge of the time frame for the relationship provides the structure upon which the relationship is built. During the working phase of the working relationship, the nurse reminds the patient of the number of weeks remaining. This information helps orient the patient to the reality that there is an end to their relationship.

There are common feelings of sadness, regret, and loss that are felt by both the nurse and the patient when they anticipate the end of their relationship. Saying good-bye may arouse memories of previous relationships that have ended and may touch feelings that are attached to past separation experiences. It is important that the nurse acknowledge her own feelings about saying good-bye to her client, and she should support her client's expression of emotions. Often the only clue to how a client is dealing with the termination phase is through his behavior. The behaviors that existed during the orientation phase of the relationship may reappear. Also, any behaviors that were testing behaviors during the working phase may reappear as well. Clients who have been able to change some of their coping behaviors may revert back to their old patterns. Usually these steps backward are only temporary.

Student nurses are encouraged to share their feelings about termination with their clinical peer group and instructor. It is important to the client and to the student nurse that both understand that their relationship has truly ended. There are no promises of continued involvement by the nurse via mail or telephone. The focus of this stage is on what has been accomplished during the relationship and what the client has learned.

If realistic goals were established in the orientation stage, then both the nurse and the patient will be able to see behavioral changes. For a patient to meet consistently with the nurse and be open to discussing his thoughts and feelings, a major accomplishment has occurred. Both the nurse and the patient are entitled to feel satisfied about their work together.

In the last meeting, the nurse supports the client's work and offers her belief that the client will continue to grow in the future. The ending note is one of hope and optimism of what the client will do and become.

THE SUPERVISORY EXPERIENCE

In psychiatric nursing the nurse's main tool for intervention is herself. The major learning experience that helps nurses increase their theoretical understanding of psychiatric principles and advance their clinical practice skills is clinical supervision. The focus of the supervisory meeting is on the nurse-supervisor's clinical practice. Supervision is recommended for all psychiatric nurses, regardless of their years in practice or level of competence. Both the supervisee and the supervisor agree to the goals and objectives of the supervisory relationship, and they contract for the educational objectives that are to be accomplished. The supervisee agrees to share her clinical interventions with the supervisor and to provide the supervisor with the data needed to meet the educational goals. The supervisor assumes the responsibility for helping the supervisee understand the dynamics of her clinical work and increase her clinical skills. The supervisee's feelings and behavior are discussed only as they relate to the supervisory relationship or the nurse–patient relationship. The supervisor's role is that of an educator, not a psychotherapist. The supervisee's problems are discussed only as they affect the learning process with the supervisor or impede clinical effectiveness with patients.

The most common form of supervision is the one-to-one meeting, in which the supervisor and supervisee meet weekly for a specific time.

The process of supervision requires that the supervisee bring to the meeting written nursing process recordings or audio recordings of her meetings with her patient.

The supervisee analyzes her data, extracts themes, formulates goals, and evaluates her nursing intervention. In the supervisory conference, she receives feedback from the supervisor regarding nursing process as well as suggestions and recommendations for the next meeting with her patient. The supervisor also reviews and makes suggestions on the record-keeping system for communications regarding nurse and patient.

Process Notes

The vehicle through which psychiatric nurses learn how to work effectively with psychiatric clients is the nursing process recording (Table 15-3). After each interview with her patient, the nurse writes down the actual dialogue and her thoughts and observations, as well as her theoretical understanding of what was happening in the interview. This process recording is shared with the psychiatric clinical nursing instructor, who provides constructive feedback for the next session with the patient. Sometimes student nurses have patients sign permission forms for the taping of the sessions. This happens only in accord with the policies of the unit and with permission from the clinical health team. Students should not decide to pursue the use of a tape recorder with clients until they have discussed the implications of taping with the clinical psychiatric nursing instructor. Initially, the writing of verbatim process recordings may be difficult, but with practice they become easier to write. Table 15-4 is an example of a student's process recording. The clinical supervisor writes comments on the process recording and usually a summary paragraph at the end. In this example, the instructor might write the following:

Jane, you were able to stay with Mary and not be put off by her defensive anger. Good work. Your hunches about what might have been going on were accurate and appropriate. Oftentimes, after clients have been verbal during one meeting, they have difficulty sharing in the next meeting. The content may have been painful or the process of sharing the content with you may have touched her emotionally. Do just as you did; stay with Mary and let her know that you are available for the time agreed and she can discuss

TABLE 15-3. NURSE–PATIENT INTERACTION FORM

Instructor's name _____
Student's name _____
Date of interaction _____
Patient's initials _____

Part I   *Introduction to the Interaction*
         (Physical description of setting and patient)
Part II *Goals*
         A. Long-term goals (behavioral measurements)
         B. Short-term goals (behavioral measurements)
Part III *Description of the Interaction:* Process Recording

Patient's behavior (Verbal/Nonverbal)	Nurse's reaction (Thoughts & feelings)	Nurse's behavior (Verbal/Nonverbal)	Analysis/Rationale

Part IV *Evaluation/Summary*
         A. Issues/Concerns.
         B. Themes.
         C. Effectiveness of interventions in relation to goals/met or not met.   10 page limit
         D. Plans for following interaction(s).   January 1989

(Sample of recording form used by Boston College School of Nursing, Secondary Preventive Intervention II B, Psychiatric Nursing form #NU204-02, with permission.)

whatever she chooses. Also, you might want to convey to her your understanding of how hard the last meeting was for her and your belief that she will be able to handle her feelings appropriately. In fact, you and she might discuss ways she could do this in your meetings. You might want to refer to your text for information on stalls in the therapeutic relationship as well as issues involved in the working phase.

NURSING INTERVIEWS AS DEFINED BY THE VARIOUS NURSING ROLES

The various roles of the nurse define the different kinds of nursing interviews. Roles must be defined for the patient too, and if role boundaries change, these boundaries must be restated.

TABLE 15-4. EXAMPLE OF PROCESS RECORDING

Nurse (Jane Smith)	Client (Mary Jones)	Observations	Theory
Hello Mary, it is our meeting time.	I am not talking to you today.	Mary appears angry. Her speech is rapid and her face is stern.	Could this be a form of resistance?
You seem upset about something.	I have nothing to say to you.	Mary's tone the same; face relaxing a bit. I am becoming anxious.	Is Mary displacing her anger on me?
You feel you have nothing to say?	Yes. Last time we talked it all out.	Mary's tone still tense; face and body less so.	Mary's possible need to protect herself from feelings aroused last time.
Last time we met you feel you said too much?	Yes. I felt bad when you left.	Mary seems less angry; more sadness. I felt less anxious.	Mary's anxiety about disclosing her sadness.
Tell me how you felt.	I began to cry, right after our meeting.		

For example, a role change occurs for the nurses when they make a home visit in order to assess the home and community adjustment of a patient previously treated in the hospital. The new role boundary must be defined for the patient, too.

Some of the various roles nurses assume are the following:

1. A nursing student on a psychiatric unit has a specific role and goal. It is a learning situation, and the final decisions are not made by the student alone. The patient should also know that the instructor is involved with the learning experience and that there is a dual goal of education and patient care. If a patient has further questions about the student role, he should have an opportunity to talk about the program. Specific questions could be directed to the instructor. The student uses the interview as a learning tool and receives supervision at all times.

2. Staff nurses on a psychiatric unit have defined and specific roles to which the patient is oriented when he is admitted. The patient knows what he can talk about to the nurses, what limits they will place on him, and how they will be therapeutic with him. He knows that they are part of the clinical team and that they work within the framework of the ward milieu. Staff nurses use the structured interview in planned meetings with the patient. They work out the goal for the interview as part of the ward treatment.

3. Nurse-therapists on a psychiatric unit usually take responsibility for the direct treatment of the patient and work closely with the psychiatrist who is the medical administrator of the case. They function as therapists and collaborate with the nursing staff in the total treatment of the patient. The nurse-therapist will define for both the patient and the staff the duration of the relationship, the goals of therapy, and the limits of the relationship.

4. The psychiatric nurse-clinician working within the general hospital defines her role to the ward in which she works with the nursing staff. The structured interview is used to provide the staff with more information for the psychotherapeutic handling of the patient. The nurse defines this role to the patient and then communicates her findings and recommendations to the staff.

5. The staff nurse working in the general hospital may do a structured interview in addition to regular nursing procedures, in an attempt to further clarify specific psychological concerns. The nurse works closely with the physician in order to maintain a consistent treatment plan.

6. The community mental health nurse is responsible not only for the patient and his present problem but also for understanding the family and community of the patient. In the interview the nurse must listen for the many facets of the problem in order to make a comprehensive assessment and evaluation of the situation.

7. The visiting nurse or public health nurse working in the community may talk with someone who has not yet defined himself as a patient. Often the interview is used to explore a social context for the problem. Sometimes the mother who is being seen for a medical problem begins to discuss her 15-year-old son who is frequently truant from school and who may be using drugs. The nurse uses the data from the interview to collaborate with other agencies in order to best handle the community problem, but at the same time is being helpful to the mother.

8. The clinic nurse in a psychiatric outpatient service is part of the clinic team that includes psychiatrist, social worker, psychologist, and rehabilitation counselor. Team members usually take turns conducting the initial interview with the patient, and later they discuss the patient at a team conference so that they can decide on treatment goals. The nurse conducts the initial interview in order to obtain the necessary information for the team meeting. How much time there is available for the interview determines how direct or open-ended the technique can be. For an indirect method of interview, for example, in the drop-in center or multiservice center, a data sheet to be filled in at the time of interview or immediately following is often provided. The role in this case is to remember the sequence and order of events as the patient talks to enable reconstruction of the interview later for presentation to the team for treatment plans.

9. School nurses who work in an elementary school or a high school use both the structured and unstructured interview. They see students who have physical and emotional problems, and they assess the need for follow-up care. The school nurse may collaborate with the family, teachers, administrators, and the community health center.
10. Nurses who work in an industrial organization are often the only health personnel in full-time attendance. Therefore, they have great responsibility for evaluating many presenting problems. They tend to know the employees who have been to the health office on other occasions. The industrial nurse may choose to use the structured interview when a new employee arrives. In an emergency, the interview is unstructured. The industrial nurse collaborates with the family, administration, and community.

Summary

The therapeutic use of self is a key asset in psychiatric nursing. Attitudes and human qualities that facilitate the therapeutic relationship include self-assessment, being natural, professional comfort, respect, optimism, positive outlook about people, sensitivity, involvement, caring, patience, and persistence. Also, the qualities of accurate empathy, nonpossessive warmth, and genuineness are key assets.

In addition to these skills, the verbal exchange between patient and nurse is an important part of the helping relationship. It is through these verbal exchanges that problems are explored, relationships developed, goals set, and nursing interventions carried out.

Therapeutic interactions between patient and nurse provide the framework for the development of the therapeutic nurse-patient relationship. There are three phases in the nurse-patient relationship. The *first phase* allows the two strangers to become acquainted. The *working phase* is the period in which the patient and nurse explore together the patient's felt problems and move toward goals that have been mutually set. The *final phase* or *termination* provides for the two individuals to evaluate their progress and the usefulness of the experience. The supervisory process is described in terms of nurse–patient interaction and record keeping.

Strategies described in this chapter that are useful in interviewing include verbal responses, use of questions, and nonverbal behavior. The process recording is described as a teaching method, and various clinical settings in which interviews are used are identified.

Questions

1. Through a process recording of a client interview, analyze the types of questions asked and the types of responses made by you.
2. Observe a client or patient group interaction and identify the types of silences that occurred during the meeting.
3. Through a process recording, identify (by autognosis) points where you used nonuseful responses during a client interview.
4. Give examples of ways you used an interview situation from past nursing experiences (other than psychiatric settings).
5. Give an example of a fact-finding interview and an example of a therapeutic interview.

REFERENCES AND SUGGESTED READINGS

American Nurses' Association Congress for Nursing Practice. *Standards for Psychiatric–Mental Health Nursing Practice*. Kansas City, Mo.: American Nurses' Association, 1982.

Blanck, P. D., Buck, R. & Rosenthal, R., eds. *Nonverbal Communication in the Clinical Context*, 1986, University Park, PA: Pennsylvania State University.

Bradley, J. C. & Edinberg, M. A. *Communication in the Nursing Context*. 2nd ed., 1986, Norwalk, CT: Appleton & Lange.

Davis, A. J. *Listening and Responding*, 1984, St. Louis: Mosby.

Dreher, B. B. *Communication Skills for Working with Elders*, 1987, New York: Springer Publishing Co.

Gruber, L. N. The no-demand, third person interview of the non-verbal patient. *Perspectives in Psychiatric Care*, 1977, *15*(1), 38–39.

Leininger, M. Caring: A central focus of nursing and health care services. *Nursing and Health Care*, 1980, *1*(3), 135–143.

Littlefield, N. T. Therapeutic relationship: A brief encounter. *American Journal of Nursing*, 1982, *82*, 1395–1400.

O'Sullivan, A. L. Privileged communication. *American Journal of Nursing*, 1980, *80*, 947–951.

Purtilo, R. B. *Health Professional/Patient Interaction*, 3rd ed., 1984, Philadelphia: Saunders.

Russell, B. V. Is the chief complaint really the problem? *Journal of Psychosocial Nursing and Mental Health Services*, 1983, *21*(12), 24–28.

Scully, R. Stress in the nurse. *American Journal of Nursing*, 1980, *80*, 911–914.

Smith, V. M., & Bass, T. A. *Communication for Health Professionals*. Philadelphia: Lippincott, 1979.

Chapter 16

Communication and the Therapeutic Process

Carol R. Hartman

Chapter Objectives

The student successfully attaining the goals of this chapter will be able to:

- Explain how key beliefs and behaviors can affect a nurse's capacity to be therapeutic.
- Identify factors that facilitate the therapeutic alliance.
- Determine how to set outcomes for therapeutic efforts.
- Describe how communication strategies alter a client's psychological structures and processes.
- Identify a client's major belief patterns and their relationship to personal resources.
- Identify direct and indirect communication strategies.

The initial steps in the overall therapeutic process are outlined in this chapter. The establishment of the therapeutic alliance precedes the working component of the nurse–patient relationship, the steps and dimensions of which are detailed in Chapter 15. This chapter will focus on the supportive component of the therapeutic relationship: establishing rapport, strengthening personal resources (coping), and setting outcomes for changing behavior.

The therapeutic relationship and the therapeutic process have underscored the conceptual context for therapeutic communication. To the novice in the area, there appears to be ready agreement to these concepts. However, to realize them is another matter. In Chapter 10, we covered various theoretical and clinical models that are being used to guide and investigate the efficacy of psychotherapeutic impact on the communication process. Although most interesting, how are they useful to a beginner?

STUDENT REACTIONS TO ENTERING THE MENTAL HEALTH SYSTEM

Most nurses find their first professional contact with the area of mental health practices in their role as students. Textbooks are aimed at students. A review of textbooks indicates that they introduce students to therapeutic communication strategies in subrole activities, such as the nurse's role in the one-to-one relationship and the family and group counseling roles. There is little focus on the therapeutic encounters within the nurse's general milieu, which, after all, represents the major province of the staff nurse. The limited duration of most clinical experiences in the student programs necessitates use of the one-to-one relationship for the purpose of teaching the student about therapeutic process. It is no wonder students are confused and unfocused when first attempting to define themselves within a specific mental health program, such as an inpatient unit, day hospital setting, or home follow-up visit. The following excerpts regarding the reactions of students to entering the mental health system in the first week of clinical practice have been taken from four student diaries. These excerpts demonstrate the personal mind-set of the students and its effect on their capacity to communicate.

EXAMPLE 1

My first day on the clinical area I felt a great deal of anxiety and apprehension. I did not know what to expect from the patients, the staff, or how to interact with the patients. I felt that I did not know enough about psychiatric nursing to qualify for patient interaction. I expected to start an uproar with my initial communication session with a patient. I thought that I would either say the wrong thing or not be able to think of anything to say at all. When I learned that I would be working on C-3 with all the "really crazy" patients, I was scared to death. However, after my first day, I realized that it wasn't going to be as bad as I had expected. The staff was very understanding and willing to help out in any way they could. They were very informative as to which patients to interact with. By the end of the day I felt comfortable in the clinical area. By the end of the week, all my fears and anxieties had abated. Communicating with the staff was going well, and I had picked a patient for my paper with whom I could communicate easily and who responded well to me. Interaction with all of the patients was much easier and I felt much more at ease in psychiatric nursing.

EXAMPLE 2

I was apprehensive about how I was going to initiate a conversation with a patient; but, I found, just as it is out of the hospital, I was able to strike up a conversation with some patients, and I was not able to do so with others. Many times this week it was the patient who spoke to me first and I listened.

EXAMPLE 3

I expected to find myself greeted by a bunch of so-called "crazy" people. I was afraid that I wouldn't act the right way or that I wouldn't be able to handle myself in a one-to-one situation. I found myself very anxious and uneasy for the first few hours at (the hospital), but I also noticed that the residents were just as uneasy. Later in the day the tension began to ease up, and I felt as though I was becoming accepted by the group and therefore owed them the same. I realized that (the hospital) is in its own little world and that I am an outsider.

EXAMPLE 4

It seemed less chaotic as the day went on. I approached and was approached by several patients. I found it difficult to pursue a lead, as with Mark: "It's safe here—the rats are outside and the mice are inside." I didn't know what to respond. Also, it was difficult to talk to Ray. I asked him what his hobby was and he said, "Discovering commies." I had no idea as to how to respond to that. I was more able to establish a relationship with Bob. I gave support to his expression of anger, but he reported that the staff felt it was inappropriate. I wonder what actually happened. Mark did something by moving away while talking about the Wizard of Oz uncovering what was already inside. Tom, who told me his name was Maxwell, said hello many times but moved away as conversations progressed. I had trouble with Cindy who was having difficulty staying in reality. She would try to talk but not hear me or tell me. She seemed unable to concentrate. I found it difficult to talk to someone whose senses are so distorted.

The outstanding revelation of these quotes is that a student coming into the psychiatric mental health environment has many preconceived ideas about what it will be like. These ideas have to be addressed because there is tremendous anxiety where the students alter expectations as to what is experienced and observed. The students recognize as a goal the ability to communicate with the clients, patients, and residents (notice the range of names applied to the people receiving professional care). However, there is something special about how, when, and where the students are to talk to these people. This "something special" is not clear except to note that these people have "problems," and somehow they and the nurses are to talk about these "problems." Problems become not only a focus but an expectation of how students will evaluate their effectiveness. If the patients on the unit talk with them about their "problems," the students expect to be on the road of therapeutic intervention. But what happens? The students discover that some people will talk to them and others will not. Therefore the students soon learn to approach people who tolerate their approach to them. The experience of the "other" (i.e., the patient) being comfortable in their presence makes them (the students) experience greater comfort with themselves.

To facilitate entry on the ward, the students rely heavily on their observations and interactions with the staff nurses. The students are greatly influenced by the staff and look to them for models of conduct. Their notes reveal that they first seek personal comfort, acceptance, guidance, and protection from the nursing staff. Next, the students move toward patients who are most receptive to them. It is further indicated that they are anxious to meet the expectations of the course.

There are always blessed mavericks in the student group. The last example (number 4) demonstrates a rather different report. The student documents interactions with people on the ward that are perplexing and confusing. This student puts down clear statements of experiences with various patients. When one patient seems to make "sense" to the student, the student dares to offer a specific statement of support for the patient's feelings of anger. When the student is done, the patient informs the student that the staff believe his anger to be "inappropriate." The student expresses the dilemma of who is to be believed: the patient, the staff nurses, or himself? One hopes that this does not curtail this student's ability to observe and risk talking with people who do not express themselves in typical ways. Let's hope this doesn't stop the student from considering what is meant by "appropriate" and "inappropriate" when applied to another person's personal experience.

FACTORS THAT GUIDE THERAPEUTIC STRATEGIES

The students' notes teach us much about the context in which a nurse is to implement the therapeutic alliance through therapeutic communication strategies. First and foremost, the system of interaction is a human social system. In this system, there are roles, rules, and power. These are not explicit; rather, they are implicit. The consequence of this structure is that a novice, the patient, and others hammer out by trial and error their personal construct of these critical factors. Rules are personal until they are tested and tried in human interaction. This learning is not easy for a beginner who has a limited time in the clinical setting.

Rules for interpreting behavior are often vague. What is considered therapeutic by one person may be viewed as irrational, superficial, or irrelevant by another person. What happens is that the criteria for effective communication are often based on what people *believe* should be happening rather than on what *is* happening. What can a student initially rely on?

THREE QUALITIES IMPORTANT TO THE INTERVIEWER

Three qualities that have been defined in the literature as important dimensions of the therapeutic nurse–patient relationship are: accurate empathy, nonpossessive warmth, and genuineness.[1]

Accurate Empathy

Accurate empathy involves more than just the ability of the therapist to sense the patient's "private world" as if it were the therapist's. It also involves more than just an ability to know what a patient means. Accurate empathy involves both the therapist's sensitivity to the patient's current feelings and the therapist's verbal facility in communicating this understanding in a language attuned to the patient's current feelings. At a high level of accurate empathy, the message "I am with you" is unmistakably clear, and the therapist's remarks fit perfectly with the patient's mood and content. At a low level of accurate empathy, the therapist may be off on a tangent or may misinterpret what the patient is feeling; the therapist may be evaluating, giving advice, sermonizing, or simply reflecting on his or her own thoughts and feelings rather than on those of the patient.

EXAMPLE 1: LOW LEVEL OF ACCURATE EMPATHY

PATIENT: [earnestly] Nurse, I need to know something.

NURSE: [sternly] Why are you wearing so much makeup?

PATIENT: [sadly] Is it normal for a woman to feel embarrassed, ashamed? Is it immature to want male attention and approval and feel so awful about getting it?

NURSE: [mechanically] Depends on what she is asking for.

PATIENT: [excitedly] Are you saying I am to blame?

In this example the nurse appears to be unaware of even the most conspicuous feelings; her responses are not appropriate to the mood or content of the patient's statements.

EXAMPLE 2: HIGH LEVEL OF ACCURATE EMPATHY

PATIENT: Nurse, I need to know something

NURSE: [warmly] What do you need to know?

PATIENT: [sadly] Is it normal for a woman to feel ashamed or embarrassed? Is it immature to want male attention and approval and feel badly about getting it?

NURSE: You seem to be feeling sad. Tell me more about what you are feeling.

In this case the nurse responds to the client's feelings and offers her an opportunity to explore her experience in depth.

Nonpossessive Warmth

The dimensions of nonpossessive warmth, or unconditional positive regard, range from a high level where the therapist warmly accepts the patient's experience as part of that person, without imposing conditions, to a low level where the therapist expresses dislike or disapproval or expresses warmth in a selective or evaluative way.

EXAMPLE 1: LOW LEVEL OF NONPOSSESSIVE WARMTH

PATIENT: [emphatically] Today, I am not going to work in the kitchen.

NURSE: [authoritatively] But you know that is your job.

PATIENT: There are mice there, and I do not like to work near them.

NURSE: If you do not go to work, you will not be able to participate in today's outing.

PATIENT: I do not want to go anywhere. [Storms out of the area.]

In this example the nurse is responding with negative regard and disapproval to what the client is expressing.

EXAMPLE 2: HIGH LEVEL OF NONPOSSESSIVE WARMTH

PATIENT: [loudly, emphatically] Today, I am not going to work in the kitchen.

NURSE: [warmly, concerned] You do not want to go to work today?

PATIENT: That's right. I hate those mice.

NURSE: There are mice in the kitchen?

PATIENT: Yes. Yesterday I saw one behind the stove.

NURSE: What was it about the mouse that upset you?

PATIENT: I think it will come and bite me.

NURSE: So you are afraid that the mouse will hurt you?

In this case the nurse communicates a deep interest and concern for the welfare of the patient and she helps the patient to clarify her fears.

Genuineness

Genuineness refers to the qualities of honesty and sincerity—when the therapist presents her true feelings; and it describes a high level of self-congruence whereby the therapist is freely and deeply herself. Thus, a therapist's response must be sincere rather than phony. It must express her real feelings and being, rather than her defensiveness.

EXAMPLE 1: LOW LEVEL OF GENUINENESS

PATIENT: I belong to the CIA and am on a very important mission here.

NURSE: [mechanically] Yes.

PATIENT: You don't believe me, do you?

NURSE: Sure I do. [yawns]

PATIENT: I worked on the Cuban invasion with President Kennedy.

NURSE: [indifferently] What year was that?

PATIENT: 1965 or 1963. Dates confuse me.

NURSE: That's not all that confuses you.

In this example there are striking discrepancies

between the nurse's statements and her non-verbal cues. There is also a lack of congruence between her feelings and responses.

EXAMPLE 2: HIGH LEVEL OF GENUINENESS

PATIENT: I belong to the CIA and am on a very important mission here.
NURSE: You are an important person.
PATIENT: You do not believe me, do you?
NURSE: I have difficulty in believing that you belong to the CIA.
PATIENT: I worked on the Cuban invasion with President Kennedy.
NURSE: Tell me about coming to the hospital.

In this case the nurse responds to the patient honestly and attempts to validate his need for importance. She then redirects the focus back to the reality.

PRINCIPLES OF PSYCHOLOGICAL LEVEL COMMUNICATION

Are there other factors that guide the development of therapeutic strategies? There are certain principles regarding therapy that become an important basis for effective communication efforts. These have been adopted from the teachings of Milton H. Erickson and Stephen and Carol Lankton.[2,3]

1. People operate out of their internal cognitive maps and not out of sensory experience. This has been said in many ways regarding the theories of communication, and it becomes a key principle in being therapeutic. A person's personal map is not the experience, and the experience is not the map. Therefore, when addressing therapeutic interventions, the impact is directed toward the *structure* of the person's map.

2. People try to make the best choice for themselves at any given moment. People do not want to set about to deliberately make mistakes or hurt themselves. People are trying to do something for themselves, and even suicide may be viewed as an attempt to do something positive. This principle changes the focus of intervention from a search for problems to a search for finding out what the person wants and what is an efficient, nonharmful way of reaching the goal. This principle challenges the strategy of blaming as a means of coping with ineffective consequences of behavior and invites open appraisal of behavior and choice.

3. What is said about the person is not the person. Language is the least representative of *experience*. It is only a guide, like a map of city streets. Knowing the map does not give you the *experience* of walking the streets and discovering the many important and uncharted characteristics. If the nurse places reliance on the word description of the person, conversing will be the interpretation of those words in the nurse's head and not based on the patient's nonspoken behavior.

4. Respect all messages from the patient. People cannot *not* communicate. Walking away, getting angry, and silence are all information from patients regarding their experiences. What the patients experience and interpret is the external behavior of the nurse. The nurse's basic worthwhileness is not being commented on; rather, it is her behavior.

5. Teach choice; never attempt to take choice away. This principle means that communication strategies are designed to keep the patients operating out of their own sense of power and choice. If the patients' behavior is unacceptable to the nurse, the objective of the communication from the nurse is to assist and encourage the patients to find a more acceptable manner of conveying their message.

6. Meet the patient at his model of the world. This principle does not mean that the nurse communicates that she agrees with the model, but rather that the nurse recognizes salient features of the patient's model and is able to match these features rather than superimposing her (the nurse's) model on the patient. A patient may believe that the world is unfriendly, hurtful, and dangerous. Certainly there are hurtful, unfriendly, and dangerous people, but the facts on how many, how much, where, when, and under what circumstances have been left out. There is no need to disagree with the patient; rather, explain how more choices can be made available.

7. The resources that patients need lie within their own personal history. A patient can only know that he is missing something if he has some idea of what it would be like to have it. This means that therapeutic communication strategies are aimed at recovering and uncovering personal resources within the patient. The nurse does not transmit nor can the nurse transmit her own resources. This guides communication processes toward how the person is solving a problem and what personal resources are needed for solution.

8. The person with the most flexibility will be the controlling element in the communicating process. This challenges the nurse to be free from personal bias and from concerns that interfere with responding to the patient's messages. Conversing with a patient is a creative process. The rules are set by the persons involved. These rules can be renegotiated and changed.

9. It is hard for the nurse and the patient to work on some type of change in behavior. It may be necessary to reduce the focus of the change. This negotiation guides the nurse in setting outcomes that can be achieved and realized. For example, if someone is distrustful of people, do not attempt to change this attitude to trusting most people. Rather, reduce the distrust slowly and recognize moments of trust with certain people and build up from that point.

10. The outcome of the nurse's intervention is determined at the psychological level of the patient; i.e., the structure of the internal map should be sufficiently changed so that the person behaves differently and experiences himself differently.

11. A person cannot *not* respond. This principle is meant to help the nurse recognize that there is always communication occurring. It is a matter of attending to the information and utilizing it.

MAJOR COMMUNICATION STRATEGIES

Major strategies of developing an alliance through therapeutic communication processes are those that assist in establishing rapport, ac-

cessing and establishing personal resources, assessing coping strengths, and setting outcomes for changing behavior. Skill in these strategies facilitates use of direct and indirect forms of communicating.

Establishing Rapport

Rapport is gained when the nurse *paces* the patient's world. Pacing is effected by mirroring, below the level of conscious awareness, the spoken and nonspoken behavior of the patient. Pacing is facilitated by an understanding of the eye scanning movements of a patient and the predicates used. In addition, this close attention to the total behavior of the patient allows the nurse to pick up incongruities in the patient that indicate mixed messages, such as a young woman who says she is not nervous talking with the nurse, but she begins to twist and turn a handkerchief in her hands.

Understanding the behavioral state of rapport and what reflective communications on the part of the nurse are necessary to establish rapport enables the nurse to regain rapport when the patient may have been led into experiences beyond his stress tolerance level. Rapport skills are essential in assessing and diagnosing a patient's issues and in using a variety of communication techniques in a therapeutic manner. Since the ultimate sense of whether intervention is effective is determined by the patient, it is important to know how to regain cooperative contact when negotiated efforts have gone awry.

Understanding the structure of rapport allows the nurse to address therapeutic messages in a style that is compatible with the style of the patient. Rapport is also essential in supporting the nurse's lead in moving a person from one perspective and source of personal information to another.

An important concept related to rapport building as well as all the other intervention strategies is that of *anchoring*.[4] An anchor is demonstrated when a particular pattern of behavior in one person elicits a consistent pattern of response in another person. For example, if a person smiles, wiggles his index finger, and mumbles something like, "I'm going to get you," while using a playful tone of voice, many infants and small children will giggle and curl their bodies to ward off a touch. Others may start to cry. In either case, the person has elicited an anchor in the child; that is, a total set of behaviors are set into motion that can be repeatedly elicited.

Anchoring is important in that it becomes a test of the extent of rapport established through pacing; when the patient begins to match the changes of behavior in the nurse, the nurse's behavior has become a positive anchor that can now be used to lead the patient into greater self-expression. Another component is anchoring for safety and is most essential in work with children.

Now, what does pacing mean in more specific terms? Pacing means the mirroring of spoken and nonspoken behavior of another in such a way that the other experiences a sense of being understood and possibly accepted. The matching of behavior creates familiarity and reduces initial differences that often become more of the focus of conversing than is useful for therapeutic outcomes.

Nonspoken behavior can be paced in various ways. For example, the rate of breathing can be paced by the observer nodding his head in rhythm with the breathing. Total body posture can be adopted, such as a person sitting back in a chair with his legs crossed. The concept of mirroring is used when the observer reflects back the same nonspoken behavior. Cross-mirroring occurs when the observer paces a nonspoken behavior with a different gesture, such as the breathing being paced by the head nodding.

Within the area of spoken behavior, the paralinguistic characteristics as well as the verbal patterns are reflected in the observer's behavior. Tone of voice, rhythm of speech, intensity, pauses, and tempo are all examples of paralinguistic patterns.

Verbal patterns that are most powerful in pacing and establishing rapport are predicates. Predicates are verbs, adverbs, and adjectives.

As discussed in Chapter 10, there are eye patterns that humans use when experiencing the different sensory modalities of visualization, kinesthetics, and audition. When most people make images in their mind, their eyes turn upward or point straight ahead with pupillary dilation. For example, if you recall asking someone when he last saw a friend, you may remember that his eyes moved upwards and to his left, and he said, "Let's see, when did I last see John?" The person is literally scanning his memory for a stored picture of the last time he saw John. Most often this is done unconsciously by the person.

Sometimes people will stare ahead and move their hands about, pointing to specific objects and people that are in their mind's eye. As an observer, we have the sense that the person is lost in his own thought rather than attending to what he can see in front of him. People deep in conversation can walk into doors because the external visual images are not being attended to. If one asks a person a question such as, "Can you see yourself skydiving?" the person can look up to his right and construct an image of himself skydiving. This is constructed imagery. The person may even step into the picture and imagine wind on his body, his eyes tearing, the sound of clothes flapping, and an excited knot in his stomach and mounting fear, at which point he can respond with, "No, I can't see myself skydiving. It would be frightening." Here the person is not only constructing images, but like the out-of-awareness sound track of a movie, the person is arousing feeling in his body (kinesthetic) and hearing imagined sounds (audition).

Eye scanning movements that correspond to a dominant recall or to the use of auditory experiences are eye movements to the lateral left and right positions. Eye movement laterally to the left indicates that the person is recalling words. When the person tilts his head to the left and looks down to the left, he is usually engaged in carrying on a conversation with himself. If you ask a person a question such as, "How might you decide to pay one bill before another?" he might posture with his head down, eyes to the left, and say, "Well, first I would ask myself, 'Do I have the money to pay for both bills?' I might say, 'No, pay a bit on both,' or I might say, 'Just pay one depending on how important the bill.'"

If one asks a person how he feels about abortion, the person is most likely to look down to his right before answering. This movement is associated with kinesthetic information, and since the question asked directed the person to a feeling state, he will move to where that information is stored in the brain, and for most people, the external movement of the eyes down and to the right indicates the kinesthetic representational system.

These patterns hold true for most people who are right-handed and are thought to be a function of hemispherical dominance in the brain. Rather than relying on these patterns being true for everyone, just pay attention to the client and the words he uses, his eye movements, and his eye scanning behavior when questions are asked such as, "How do you feel about that?" "What would you say?" "How do you see that point?"

The following examples demonstrate how important all aspects of pacing are to establish rapport:

NURSE: Your doctor feels that you will be able to leave the hospital by tomorrow or Saturday.

CLIENT: I can't see myself going. I just can't see myself returning to that household.

NURSE: I guess you feel scared of going home and picking up.

CLIENT: I can't see myself being able to do all of the work.

NURSE: I guess you feel alone and scared.

CLIENT: I don't know. I just know I can't imagine myself doing all that I did before.

NURSE: The doctor wouldn't let you go home if you weren't ready.

CLIENT: Can't you see . . . I'm not ready. . . . Isn't it clear to you . . . ? Can't you see my limited abilities. . . ? I haven't caught up.

This example demonstrates a mismatch of representational systems. This woman "sees" herself; she is not oriented to knowing how she feels. The nurse keeps making kinesthetic statements in an attempt to be empathetic. The client experiences this as not being understood. Each is talking a different language.

The following is an example of a student talking with a rather volatile adolescent on the ward.

JIM: I hate him, I hate him . . . damn it all . . . I hate the S.O.B. . . .
[Jim is yelling and pacing and hitting his fist on the table in the kitchen. The student is fixing coffee and observes Jim.]

STUDENT: [Remaining where she is standing, but looking at Jim, she matches his tone of voice and the tempo of his words.] I hear you, I hear you . . . who do you hate?

JIM: [stops pacing, his back to nurse as he stands at kitchen table, yells] You know who I hate . . . you know who I hate . . . dammit . . . you know. . . .

STUDENT: [Not changing position, in tone of voice matching Jim's, she says the following.] I should know who you hate . . . I should know who you hate . . . [changes voice tone, softer, slower rate] . . . but I don't Jim.

JIM: [turns and faces the student, tears in his eyes] I'm sorry . . . I . . . he isn't coming to the family meeting . . . he said . . . my father . . . [crying].

This brief example demonstrates the impact of cross-mirroring. The student, rather than matching Jim's words, matches the intensity and rate of his speech. This avoids escalation of Jim's physical banging behavior and gets his attention on the behavior of the student. In addition, the student refrains from interpreting or labeling the emotional reaction of Jim. She demonstrates its impact in imitating critical features of his communication. This allows Jim a chance to take charge and to relate to the nurse with more specific information, which is primarily useful to him. This example is at the heart of therapeutic intervention and demonstrates how rapport can be established by careful attention to the behavior of the client and the response of the nurse.

How can one learn how to put together all that has been outlined? Here are some exercises that the reader can do with interested colleagues that will assist in developing an awareness of the rapport skills, including addressing nonspoken behavior, eye scanning behavior, and representational systems, and using pacing and leading and anchoring skills. In addition to developing skill, these exercises can be fun.

EXERCISE ONE

Three people. Person A takes a most comfortable position while standing. Person B puts his or her body in the same posture as A. Person C checks A and B, making sure B simulates tension in the same muscle groups as A and the same weight shifts, in short has the same posture and facial expression as A. When the posture is as exact as possible, B is to relate how he or she feels, hears things, see things, and other experiences that come to mind. This is to be repeated by each participant until everyone has had a chance. Participants will increase their skill in observing posture and will have the unique experience of relating to the world in a very different manner.

EXERCISE TWO

Three people. A and B are to converse with one another. C is to observe when A and B begin to match nonverbal behavior and to attend to their match of predicates. Do this for 5 minutes. Next, A is to continue talking and B is to consciously make an effort to match A's predicates and nonspoken behavior. C is to observe and after 5 minutes, consult with B as to what is missing as well as responded to. Next, A is to continue to talk and B is to continue to mirror behavior; at some point B is to select a nonspoken behavior of A. This can be breathing rate, rate of speech, or head nodding. B is to institute a different behavior but one that follows the rhythmic intensity pattern of A's. This will be out of A's awareness. When B is ready, change the patterns of the complementary behavior and observe if the targeted behavior of A changes. If not, go back, pace the behavior again and try it over. Do this for 10 minutes. C is to observe and determine what pattern B is trying to alter. Repeat until everyone has had a chance. It is useful to take time to process the experiences with one another each step of the way. It is also useful if the observer (C) waits until B asks for feedback or is done.

EXERCISE THREE

Three people. A is the subject, B is the operator, and C is the observer. First A is to converse with B about anything of interest. B is to watch the eye scanning movements of A as well as the predicates and body posture. Do this for 5 minutes. B is then to consult with C as to what is observed. B and C then make up questions that will test the relationship of A's eye scanning patterns with predicates. For example, "Can you describe how your bedroom looks? Now go to the closet and tell me how your blouses and clothes are arranged." This will call upon visual memory. Next might be, "Can you hear a bird sing?" Check to find out if the person makes a picture of a bird, then hears the song, or if he hears the tones of the birds without making a picture in his mind's eye. Making a picture indicates that this person relies more on visual recall and then makes auditory associations. As another example, ask the person if he can remember the last thing his roommate said before he left in the morning. Or ask a person to make a picture of a monkey, then put the hindquarters of a donkey on the monkey, paint it blue, and put a top hat on it. This will draw upon visual constructive activities (usually to the person's upper right). It takes time to learn to observe these patterns in their more specific breakdown. What is important is that visual predicates and upward movement of the eyes occur. Lateral movements are associated with auditory experiences, and downward gazes (to the left) are associated with internal dialogue and kinesthetic states; also, movement of the mouth, smacking of the lips with taste, or flaring of the nostrils with olfactory experiences. You will also notice that the body posture of people accentuates representational systems. What is important is to observe a person and determine that person's unique patterns.

EXERCISE FOUR

Three people. A is to play the role of the client, B is to be the nurse, and C is the operator. In addition to the small cards with auditory, kinesthetic, and visual predicates, make out a card for each of the following: break rapport; be incongruent; develop a subtle mannerism; develop a subtle style of using language. A is to play the role of a client with typical concerns. As A is being a client, C is to flash instructions to change patterns. B is to establish rapport, maintain it, and accommodate pattern changes. C is to make sure that A establishes a pattern of sufficient character so that B has a chance to respond to it. C is to monitor B's capacity to adjust behavior to newly generated patterns. Take 20 minutes to do the exercise; change so all have a chance at the different activities. Process the experience with one another but limit time so each can participate.

These exercises are fun and challenging. Each role in the exercise is aimed at enhancing observational skill, recognition, and behavioral flexibility. Talking over the experiences of the exercise is useful but should be limited so that each person gets to participate. When giving feedback, each person gets to practice establishing and maintaining rapport.

The next important strategy to be considered is identifying personal resources.

Eliciting and Accessing Personal Resources

Eliciting resources is a major activity of the nurse. Accessing resources is the activity of the client.

What is a resource? For purposes of discussion, resources are patterns of experience that can be useful in a present situation but for some reason are not being used, or the patterns need to be developed more fully. Pattern development is at a critical stage in infancy. As the inherent potential of the infant interacts with the environment, inborn patterns become elaborated. In the first years of life, motor patterns, language patterns, and the rudiments of patterns basic to learning emerge and are developed. The infant and very young child are learning so much and at such a rapid rate that they are not conscious of learning but only of certain consequences. With an older child and then with an adolescent moving into adulthood, there is a complex history of experiences that have established patterns or that provide models for behavior.

When a client is stuck in his or her continued development, change occurs when the client is able to bring into awareness and use his own resources. Below is an example of a young woman trying to establish self-control.

The Technique of "Doing It": Accessing Coping Strengths

An example of accessing coping strengths through "doing it" was presented by an intelligent, attractive, 19-year-old woman who came to the nurse because of bulimia (a disorder of binge eating).

Sally's mother had called the nurse for an appointment. She was hysterical because she had just learned that for over a year, Sally had been binge eating. It was imperative for Sally to be seen right away. Sally was to return to college and the mother was most upset. There had been recent TV programs discussing the seriousness of the eating disorder.

Sally arrived with her mother. She was statuesque, nose a bit up in the air. Mother was attractive and terribly worried. The nurse, recognizing that the complaint was for a behavior that was reportedly out of control, decided that the first objective was to provide experience that would support personal control.

Sally noted pictures of the nurse's cats and remarked that she really enjoyed cats. The nurse used this opportunity to tell a little story about the cats. One was the mother cat, the others were the daughter cat and son cat, a convenient family, which in many ways was similar to Sally's family, including a missing father (in her case, a very busy business man). At any rate, the story reflected on the characteristics of the cat, emphasizing that the daughter cat, Claribell, was quite independent and would become most irritated with her mother's fussing and at other times went to her mother to be groomed and comforted. (This strategy will be discussed more under indirect methods of therapeutic communication.) Both Sally and her mother were interested and asked questions as well as sharing stories about the cat at their house. Mother was asked to remain in the waiting space and Sally was asked to go with the nurse to the private interview room. Thus, a phase of transition was provided for the separation of Sally and her mother as well as a concrete acknowledgment of Sally's independence.

In response to the nurse's opening question of what Sally's perspective was (Sally used visual predicates while talking about the cats. She looked straight ahead or slightly up rather than down, giving the appearance of her nose up in the air—so the nurse chose visual predicates.) on what happened to bring her to the visit.

SALLY: I really can't explain it. When I am at home,

I find myself sneaking around, gorging myself on food. [Tears come to her eyes, her face flushes.] I get frightened . . . I don't know . . . I really know myself pretty well . . . it's . . . I get so disappointed when I am at home. [At this point she is agitated, more tears, irritable tone.]

NURSE: I notice that you are struggling to maintain composure. How is it for you to show your feelings in front of me? [This was said in response to Sally's position that she knows herself pretty well.]

SALLY: [tears] It's all right . . .

NURSE: Your mother made the phone call. What are your thoughts about that?

SALLY: [Now crying more freely, head up.] At first I was upset, but secretly, I'm glad . . . I'm so frightened of what is happening. I don't feel I have control over my eating. [The nurse had not ignored Sally's statement of disappointment. Rather, the issue of control was still foremost and it was centered on the binge eating. Sally's statement of being out of control is the first issue to be addressed. This is in accordance with principles of working with people in crisis.]

NURSE: [Eating is a regular process. The reality is Sally sitting with the nurse and not running around looking for food. Furthermore, at this time, she is not interested in food. This is a fact and also demonstrates that she does have control and choice. What is apparent is that on a conscious level she does not believe she has choice. Because Sally is leaving the next day, the nurse is aiming at bringing into awareness the fact that Sally does exercise choice and has control, i.e., she *does it*.] You feel you do not have control over your eating. Has there ever been a time when you did have the feeling of control? [This is the beginning of eliciting the personal resource of self-control and choice.]

SALLY: [Sniffing, tears, straightens posture, looks at nurse.] Yes . . . I don't overeat at school, but that's because the food isn't too good . . . but . . . well, I like athletics and I like to keep my weight down. . . . I'm a gourmet cook. [Smiles with pride.] My brother and I ran a catering business when I was in high school. My mother is an excellent cook. The food is good at home.

NURSE: Sounds as if it would be . . . such high standards. . . . Well, when did you begin to sneak around, and binge?

SALLY: [Looks up to right, to her left, and then at the nurse.] Well, actually, it started in my senior year. I was on the soccer team and I discovered it . . . I mean, I had overeaten before a game. I felt full—this is a bit embarrassing—I put my finger down my throat and threw up. I was fine for the game. The next time I got full, I did the same thing . . . [tears] . . . now it's terrible. I sneak, overeat, throw up, it's exhausting. . . . [Looks at nurse with tears.]

NURSE: [nods slowly] This happens at home, but not at school?

SALLY: Yes. I get excited about coming home. I imagine how it's going to be. But when get home, it's never the way I imagine it. [Begins to cry, puts hands over face.]

NURSE: [Note "Never the way I imagine it" is not a clear statement. Also, Sally demonstrates how she sets herself up for severe disappointment. She sets expectations that are not realized at home. The first step is to clarify the reference. The nurse uses a matching tone of voice.] What is never the way you imagine?

SALLY: My parents. Oh, they are loving. They say they give us freedom to make choices . . . they are so careful not to force their point of view. I don't know what they think . . . it's just not the way I imagine it [sobs].

NURSE: On the bus you imagine things a certain way. How?

SALLY: That we can sit down and talk to one another. That we communicate . . . say something to one another rather than a bunch of words.

NURSE: We?

SALLY: My mother and my father. My father is never home; he has never been home. My mothers does all of the work. She is an interior decorator you know. She is busy . . . you don't sit and talk with her . . . she works all of the time, cooking, cleaning, never sits still and talks. I don't know what either one really feels. [Stares into space, tears coming down cheeks.]

NURSE: It's important to know how parents really feel. It's really important to make contact with parents as a young adult . . . it's important in preparing to leave and live your own life. Sometimes it can be perplexing figuring out how to do this.

SALLY: Talking to them is like talking to a wall. I guess, well, my family means a lot to me. We traveled and moved a lot, so I guess I expect a lot from them . . . from us.

NURSE: [Purposefully changing the subject.] Now, when you are on the bus, are you imagining yourself eating?

SALLY: [Looks at nurse, quizzical expression.] No. It's not a problem until I am at home. At home, I just find myself dreaming of the good bread my mother bakes, and I just don't let it go at one slice. I eat the bread with jam . . . it's good. It's not that I'm hungry . . . it's just good, tastes good. I say to myself, oh boy, this is good . . . be careful. You know you can't stop once you get started [looks at nurse]. I just don't have any control over it.

NURSE: I'm sure it seems that way . . . tastes so good and you can't stop . . . tastes so good . . . you don't want to stop at one or two pieces. Then you soon believe you have no control.

SALLY: That's right. I can't stop because I don't have control. [Looks at nurse, faint smile.]

NURSE: [Looking at Sally and maintaining the rate of speech and tone of voice.] That's right, I can't stop, I don't want to stop . . . because I don't have—

SALLY: [Interrupts with a surprised laugh.] I guess I do have control . . . [smiles] . . . I decide when I want to eat at school. I guess I decide when to eat at home . . . [pause] . . . but I'm so disappointed when I get home and it never works out.

NURSE: You don't feel you have much control over what happens to you with other people at home . . . your parents. [The nurse now reframes the experiences that create a sense of no control and disappointment.]

The interview went on from this point, linking patterns in growing up to what Sally wished to accomplish now. Time was spent in a joint interview with Sally and her mother at this same time. The joint meeting at the end of the interview was another coping or "doing it" experience, in which Sally's ability to express herself, to be in control, and now to ask for what she wanted with mother was a reality rather than something just talked about.

Eliciting resources by enjoining patients to demonstrate their capacity to behave in the way they desire to behave requires rapport, timing, and attention to not presuming from the surface structure of sentences that one knows the specific references and experiences a person is relating to. Also, getting up and directly demonstrating a behavior can be an anxious encounter with the nurse, both in doing it and in becoming aware of the control and choice factors involved. Care must be taken to structure the experience in a manner such that the patient does not draw negative judgments about himself. If this does occur, then the way the experience was put together must be dealt with to alter the negative propositions.

Certain questions help in eliciting resources such as, Has there been a time in the past when you behaved the way you want to behave now?

If a person cannot remember a time in the past or present, ask him if he knows someone who does behave the way he wants to. Then at least the person has a model to explore and emulate.

Another way of creating awareness of abilities necessary to achieve outcomes is to ask the client how he would go about helping you behave the way he wants to behave.

With specific symptoms such as self-control, anxiety, and depression, an individual's capacity to have some power over these states can be demonstrated by asking the person if the states get more intense and under what conditions. Have the person intensify the feeling state. This experience will assist in bringing into awareness internal psychological processes that are associated with the feeling states and over which the person has some control.

The psychological value of behaviors that at first appear symptomatic is to be watched for when engaging people in experiential activities. For example, a nurse was asked by a group of secretaries to have some activities to help them with the stress of their work. The nurse was teaching the group about relaxation techniques, one of which is thought stopping. The group was having success with stopping thoughts when one of the women said in a startled tone, "I can't give up worrying." The nurse realized that worrying served an important purpose for this woman. Originally, the woman thought she had no control over worrying. Now she discovered she did and was concerned because she had nothing to take its place for her. The nurse simply stated, "Worrying is important to some people. It could be a way of planning and making sure things of importance get done. However, being able to put the important process aside for a period of time for relaxation is important for effective worrying." The woman became visibly relaxed and nodded in agreement. The nurse went on with the program.

Eliciting resources by the direct method of accessing coping strengths through "doing it" is effective in the context of the nurse's ability to establish, maintain, and reestablish rapport. Spoken behavior and nonspoken behavior are considered together in evaluating when the resource has been fully accessed by the client.

Setting Outcomes for Changing Behavior

Although a great deal is written about the need to change dysfunctional behaviors, communi-

cation skills are needed to accomplish the task. Leslie Cameron-Bandler, in her Master Practitioner Program, outlined the following principles to assist in setting outcomes with the goal of changing behaviors*: First, using the schematicized outline of the person, outcomes can be evaluated by changes in the external behavior of the person, the internal state, and the internal processes. For example, role-play an internal process (talking to self differently), note the internal state, (feeling differently, e.g., relaxed).

Second, the impact of all therapeutic interventions either changes how the person sorts for positive or negative experiences, separates behaviors, combines behaviors, alters criteria, or forces the rehearsal of new behavior. These interventions, outlined by Leslie Cameron-Bandler, and implemented through the use of thoughtful questions, determine the efficacy of the therapeutic alliance.

Sorting Behaviors

Simply asking a person who feels anxious how he knows when he is relaxed begins to force a change in the personal sorting strategy being used by the person. Rather than concentrating on what causes anxiety and then feeling increased anxiety, he begins to recall relaxing experiences and his body relaxes. As the person focuses on being relaxed and how that is different, he has to begin to change muscle tension, breathing patterns, and ultimately mood and thoughts. The person has sorted out physical, perceptual, and cognitive experiences that are associated with relaxation. You have also made a change in behavior.

Separating Behaviors

Of particular importance in knowing when the patient needs to work on separating experiences is noting the causal links to certain characteristics of events that are made in the patient's mind. For example, a patient becomes very upset when mentioning his wife, who died 8 months ago. To help separate the painful memories and grieving over the wife, you might ask the patient about his wife when they were first married, using past tense; then select your language for past tense and move into when the wife was ill and how that was experienced, and then using present tense, ask the patient how

* L. Cameron-Bandler. Neuro-Linguistic Programming Master Practitioner Training Program. Boston, 1981, 1982.

he is feeling currently, e.g., what is that like for him? Then after her death what has it been like for him immediately after. The careful use of past, present, and future tense assists in separating thoughts, feelings, and behaviors regarding the event. Rather than continuing to be depressed over the death of a loved one, the person has to separate the event from the process of grieving.

To use the example of a woman having difficulty in relationships with men, rather than associating a bad feeling state with a particular situation or person, i.e., men, the female patient will separate the feelings held for her father from the feelings held for other men. For example, ask, "Has there ever been a man who was not angry with you like your father?"

To use a social example, instead of a community continually blaming the attractive woman who is raped, the community has to separate beauty and flirtatiousness from behavior that brutalizes and violates the rights of another person.

Combining Behaviors

In combining behaviors in a different manner, you seek to assist the person to transfer one positive behavior to another situation. Rather than relying on talking with people who know him, a person will also engage with new people in activities. Rather than paying attention only to how he looks as an adolescent, the youth will also pay attention to what he does and the impact it has on others. Rather than a city setting policies to reduce discrimination, it will fund projects aimed at increasing racial tolerance.

In a ward setting, the patient tells you she is comfortable with certain friends. You ask how she knows she is comfortable, what is being comfortable like with her friends. Then ask, "Taking that experience and feeling of comfort, imagine yourself talking to someone you know only slightly. How could you manage to increase your comfort with this less-known person?" This combining of behaviors will help move the person into being more comfortable with a stranger. You can have the person relate her feeling level of comfort with people on the ward.

Altering of Criteria

The altering of criteria for judging, setting priorities, and attending to specific experiences is a fourth way of setting outcomes and thereby changing behaviors. Rather than determining

the characteristics of someone by how he looks, the student now includes what that person does, and places this at a higher level for making a decision. The student can also take into consideration how the other person does, what he does, and how it impacts on others. A work group will change policies with regard to a new goal of building teams as opposed to supporting individual competition.

For example, a student draws the conclusion that the teacher cannot understand him because the teacher has gray hair. One would then ask the student what characteristics the teacher with gray hair would need so that the student knew he was being understood. Might there be other characteristics the student had not thought of? This helps move someone away from a stereotype.

Rehearsal of New Behaviors

Experiences provide structures that require the use of new, unfamiliar behaviors. For example, the isolate is placed in a church choir; the work group is sent on a retreat; or enemies join to help a group of people. In another example, a person rehearses a speech in preparation for giving it. The person is then asked: How was that for you?

Understanding how therapeutic communication works and where it works to effect change helps define how the nurse will set outcomes with a patient and how she can guide the patient by stating outcomes in behavior recognized as possible to achieve. Once the outcomes are set, then the nurse and patient work on implementing methods that give direction as to how to achieve them. Since the general outcome of communication interventions is aimed at changes in the "personal map" of another person, which is manifested in spoken and nonspoken behavior of the patient, the nurse and the patient now have tools to evaluate outcome.

Formulating the patient's outcome is the task of every therapeutic encounter. Unfortunately, it is the most frequently overlooked issue between the nurse and the patient. The outcome is usually assumed to be the resolution of the problem identified by the patient or assumed by the nurse. For example, a father feels compelled to have sex with his daughter and beat up his wife. The outcome is usually defined as stopping the behavior. The father may weep and express that he wants to stop this behavior. However, the desire to stop a behavior does not address what the person wants as an outcome.

The outcome is not stated as a problem, something not wanted; rather it is stated in the positive, that is, what the person wants. For example, the father may say he wants to be loving and accepting of the behavior of his wife, that he wants to enjoy sex with her, and that he wants to be with his daughter and be in charge of his behavior with her. People engage in change when they are motivated to change. When people experience change as restriction or deprivation, their motivation to institute and sustain change is lessened. People are more apt to change when they are trying to achieve something they want and when they become aware of their own resources and abilities to build on for that change.

THE PROCESS OF ASKING QUESTIONS

A primary communication tool in setting outcomes is the question. Questions are used to guide the patient in stating what he wants in positive terms, and they can facilitate the patient's awareness of resources and personal control. The following examples will demonstrate the process of asking questions and establishing outcomes.

Mr. Smith is lying on his bed when the nurse comes by.

NURSE: How are you today?
SMITH: Bad. [Puts left arm over face.]
NURSE: Bad?
SMITH: What's the use . . . not being here. . . . [Mr. Smith has a diagnosis of depression. His wife of 35 years is in the hospital undergoing radiation and chemotherapy. She is expected to go into remission; however, she will be weaker and it is not known how long the intervention will hold her.]
NURSE: [Moves toward the side of the bed and looks down at Mr. Smith who has not changed his posture.] Being where?
SMITH: On this earth. [Sighs deeply.]
NURSE: [matching rate of speech with Mr. Smith's breathing] How will not being on this earth help?
SMITH: [Long silence—chest is moving in convulsive spasms at times, then stops.] At least I won't feel the pain.
NURSE: Removing yourself from this earth will stop your personal pain?

SMITH: I know I sound like a coward . . . but. . . .
NURSE: [watching him, noting a change in his tone of voice, rate of speech] To whom?
SMITH: [Slowly removes his arm from his face—stares ahead] To myself . . . I don't know, maybe to you . . . to my wife, I don't know.
NURSE: Why not start with yourself? How do you sound like a coward to yourself? [Note that this comment separates self, nurse, wife. Also, the question focuses on the person, not on the general problem of feeling bad.]
SMITH: [Looks up at nurse's face for the first time.] I guess because I shouldn't be here . . . I should be with my wife. . . . [Tears course down his cheeks.]
NURSE: [looking at Mr. Smith] You should be with your wife . . . but something stops you . . . and you call yourself a coward.
SMITH: [now crying openly but maintaining eye contact with the nurse] It hurts so much . . . I . . . [sob] . . . her face, her arms . . . they have changed . . . [sob] . . . look at the way I'm behaving. . . .
NURSE: [measuring her tone] How do you want to behave?
SMITH: [with more intensity in his voice] Well . . . I don't want to be . . . slobbering all the time . . . depressed. . . .
NURSE: You cry, feel depressed, feel pain . . . looking at your wife. What has to be there to make a difference for you?
SMITH: [crying] That she's not sick.
NURSE: You don't want her to be sick and possibly dying.
SMITH: Oh, God [looks up, skyward, right arm on forehead] . . . I keep saying why . . . but that gets nowhere. . . .
NURSE: [Feeling a great temptation to put her arms around him, refrains, becomes aware of a sense of inner struggle and frustration.] Where do you want to get?
SMITH: I want to be in control [anger tone] . . . not useless . . . an emotional basket case.
NURSE: I'm confused. How does being emotional and useless go together?
SMITH: [tears subsiding, looks at the nurse in a more engaging, assertive manner] I . . . ah . . . well . . . I'm of no use to my wife if I get upset . . . I . . . she has enough without . . . uh . . . silence. [Eyes look down to his left, looks deep in thought.]
NURSE: Do I hear you right? Somehow you want to be with your wife, but believe your emotions get in the way. You have feelings. . . . What is it you want to feel when you are with your wife?
SMITH: I want to feel good . . . I don't want to just see her as sick. I want to see her well [tears]. She was so beautiful . . . now her eyes

[crying softly] show pain, fear . . . she is so thin. . . .

NURSE: [gentle tone of voice, Mr. Smith is again staring off into space, so her words are carefully matched so as not to jar his level of concentration.] Are your good feelings only in the past?

SMITH: [Looks at nurse, startled.] *No.* I love her very much.

NURSE: Have you told her that?

SMITH: No, I don't want to cry . . . in front of her. . . .

NURSE: You don't want to say you love her with tears in your eyes. In the past, did you ever tell her you loved her with tears in your eyes?

SMITH: [looking down toward his right, left, right, takes a deep sigh] Yes . . . several times. [looks at the nurse] I guess I want to be with my wife . . . you know . . . be with her now . . . not making comparisons with what was. . . .

NURSE: Let me see, you want to be with your wife now?

SMITH: Yes, I want to be able to enjoy our time together now. You know what I mean. . . .

NURSE: [Smiles] Not exactly . . . but you seem to be a bit clearer about what you mean. From an outsider's position, sounds worth working on.

This example is presented to demonstrate that setting outcomes is an ongoing function related to engaging a patient and meeting him in his struggle with existence. This is based on continually assessing and diagnosing the ongoing process of interaction with a patient. Therapeutic communication strategies are based on this level of diagnosing and outcome and not on the broader taxonomy of the disorders of affect. Further, it demonstrates that each encounter with a patient is eliciting from the patient what it is he wants. The process of elicitation has a therapeutic by-product to it and becomes a critical first step in further therapeutic efforts.

The next example demonstrates the process from an initial contact with a nurse. Jean is 27 years old. She had been drinking heavily over the weekend and had become uncontrollably upset and crying prior to hospitalization.

Jean is in shorts, attractive, tanned; facial expression is intense, bewildered; giggles as she responds to the following question.

NURSE: What brings you here?

JEAN: I don't know. Sally went to see Maggie and Maggie got on the phone and asked me when I was going to stop feeling pain and do something for myself . . . [leans forward, expectant expression].

NURSE: What is it you want to do for yourself?

JEAN: [Half laughs. The nurse smiles lightly. Jean resumes serious look and nods head in affirmative manner.] Well . . . I have been having a lot of stomachaches. I went to the emergency doctor. He did tests on me and told me there was nothing wrong. He gave me some pills and sent me home. One was Donnatal and one was Librax, like Valium. . . . When I found out what he gave me . . . I freaked out. . . .

NURSE: [looking at client] These pills meant something to you?

JEAN: Yes, I didn't want to be taking dope. . . . [Looks down quickly, then makes intense eye contact with nurse.]

NURSE: Dope's an issue?

JEAN: Yes . . . [tears]. My life is a mess . . . I don't know where to go. . . . [Looks expectantly at nurse.]

NURSE: You want to put some order in your life. You want direction?

JEAN: Yes . . . I don't know what to do. [Looks down at hands.]

NURSE: [The nurse notes that on repeated efforts to open up subject area, letting Jean take the lead, Jean has not responded. This is an important clue to Jean's present state. Several hypotheses are: she is very depressed; she is unable to contact her own sense of control over identifying what she has and what she wants; she relies heavily on other people to act in her own behalf, consequently reinforcing her sense of not being able to take charge and define for herself what it is she wants. She gets things from people, like medicine from the doctor, but she rejects it because it isn't what she wants.] Well, let me ask you this, how long have you felt this way?

JEAN: [tears in eyes] All my life. [Looks intently at the nurse.]

NURSE: Well, has it been worse lately?

JEAN: I don't know . . . I think so. . . . In the past when I have felt this way, I ran . . . went to Florida. [Smiles.] I felt better for a while. Then I ran back here I guess. [Face reddens, frowns, keeps gaze on nurse.]

NURSE: Seems hard to know where to begin . . . everything is in a jumble. Take a deep breath. [Jean does.] Let it out slowly. [Jean begins to relax, leans back.] Let's start at the beginning and I will ask you some questions about you, your life, your family [pauses, watching Jean, who smiles gently]. Tell me about your mom. . . .

JEAN: [Starts to talk, bursts into tears, pulls her legs up, bending over as if in severe abdominal pain.]

NURSE: [gently] You really meant at the beginning. . . .

JEAN: [trying to gain composure] She was never there . . . [sobs].

NURSE: Never there to do what?

JEAN: She was never there to talk to . . . [crying, looking at nurse, struggling for composure].

NURSE: Never there to talk about what? [This is getting closer to a statement of what Jean wants from seeing someone.]

JEAN: [Looks up at nurse.] About things . . . anything.

NURSE: Name one important thing.

JEAN: About being a woman. [Looks a bit surprised.]

NURSE: So, is it as if all your life you have felt confused, in a mess, because you don't know about growing up to be a woman . . . kinda run around, tried but not sure you have found out what you want to know . . . confused. . . .

JEAN: Yeah, something like that. . . .

NURSE: Then is that something you want out of coming here?

JEAN: [wiping tears] Yeah, something like that.

The interview went on. Jean had become enough aware of her running behavior to try and address her confusion when her search for who she was became too overwhelming. She readily answered questions regarding her extensive drug abuse, which she thought she had given up. Upon reviewing her present behavior, it became apparent that she was severely addicted to alcohol, although until detailing the amount she was drinking every day, she had not realized the fact that she was moving from drugs to alcohol to deal with her internal state. Much of this part of the evaluation was facilitated by the time taken to elicit, even though it is still global, Jean's outcome, to get into a relationship that would help her grow into a woman. During the interview Jean realized she had done much to help herself. Now there was this big piece of how she felt and acted when she was confused. Because she was on a daily drinking schedule of a quart and a half of wine, she agreed to an initial program of reducing her alcohol consumption.

As time progresses with Jean, setting outcomes will be a process she herself will carry out with far more independence than she displayed

in the interview. Jean is also instructive in demonstrating how a powerful internal state cut her off from her own resources and how restricted she was in constructive self-appraisal.

An exercise that can help develop skill in eliciting an outcome follows:

EXERCISE

Get into pairs. Person A focuses on something he doesn't want to do, a behavior such as procrastinating before doing homework or writing a paper. Person B is to keep asking A to search out what the behavior does for him. B is to continue until A comes up with a statement that convinces B of the most positive aspect of doing the behavior A doesn't want to do. B is to facilitate this process, maintaining rapport. When B believes it has been stated positively, B asks A what it is he wants instead and how he will know when he has it. B is to observe and note all of the postural changes, voice changes, and language changes. A is to report on any changes in feeling or thinking and to indicate if he believes the change can be achieved. If the answer is negative, B is to ask A what he thinks he needs to make the change possible and where and how he will get it.

This exercise will help the reader appreciate that all behavior serves some positive function. Maintaining rapport and using focused questions such as how, when, where, and what will help guide the patient. Notice that the question why has not been mentioned. A why question elicits a particular type of information. The next section will cover the particular use of why questions with regard to accessing and eliciting personal resources.

BELIEF PATTERN VIOLATIONS IN ELICITING AND ACCESSING PERSONAL RESOURCES

The concept of major belief patterns must be understood as an imaginary construct designed to consider those broad, holistic groupings of behaviors that are directed by central, key, personal beliefs—beliefs high on the scale of personal importance.* Beliefs not only give focus to behavior, but they provide patterned consistency. As such, they are usually arrived at with-

* This section is based on Practitioner and Advanced Master Practitioner Neuro-Linguistic Programming Workshops led by L. Cameron-Bandler, M. Lebeau, L. Conwell, and D. Gordon, Boston, 1982, 1983.

out the personal awareness of the individual. In addition, there is an efficiency to the beliefs because they play a big role in what is attended to and what is ignored. Consequently, they are a resource to a person as well as a limitation.

Interest in this human phenomenon occurred in the study of human potential because it was often observed that people who were set in their ways changed dramatically from just one experience. This experience could be a statement from a stranger or a complex personal experience, or reading a particular piece of work. In clinical practice, patients sometimes have identified a single experience in their therapy that had a profound effect and changed their entire lives.

Leslie Cameron-Bandler realized that in some manner the major values of a person were addressed in the single type of experience that resulted in profound change. Observing the work of very effective therapists, such as Satir, she discovered that the therapists demonstrated an ability to utilize the important value structure of a patient in such a manner as to change the direction of the person's life in a profound and critical way. She became interested in trying to observe those holistic patterns of people that so directed them and to identify salient features of the structure of the beliefs expressed by a person's behavior. She discovered that there were broad patterns of preference in attending to the world of experience. Some people focus on the world in terms of people; some look to their world for information. Others are seeking experiences of activity, and still others relate to the world in terms of things, i.e., machines, buildings, artifacts. In addition to attending to how people sort for their experiences in the world and how different situations may alter this sorting priority, other broad structural characteristics may be defined. Characteristics such as moving toward experiences or moving away can reveal inner patterns of thought. Another factor is the pattern of time preferred by the person. Is it past, present, or future? Characteristics of experiences also explain why people act in a certain way. For example, do they act out of what they personally think, feel, experience (self), or do they act most frequently out of what they think others think, feel, experience (other)?

The object of this section is not to go into the evolving aspects of therapeutic change through intervening at the belief pattern level because that is beyond the scope of this chapter. Rather, the above discussion is offered as an in-troduction to a useful aspect of the impact of language structure on the discovery and use of resources. What is proposed is that the semantic and syntactical aspects of language block awareness of personal experience necessary for behavior change. Use of the person's language by the nurse allows the person to change in a manner that is congruent and useful to that person. Thus the focus will be on how to identify and respond to belief pattern violations. These violations refer to patterns of language that exclude from awareness personal experiences that give special, out-of-awareness meaning to the message of the sender. When the message is not made explicit, it finds the receiver filling in the meaning from his own personal map of experience. The consequence of this experience is that the sender remains out of touch with important personal information that could be useful in considering change.

It is important to realize that working at this level of patterns of belief and thought can have a profound impact. Maintaining rapport, pacing the patient, and attending to the degree of personal tension aroused in increasing a patient's awareness is a responsibility of the nurse. Nothing is gained by rushing.

To underscore and demonstrate how powerful intervention at this level can be, a rich example is provided in a recorded excerpt of Dr. Margaret Newman's comments made to a group of nurse theoreticians and investigators of nursing diagnosis. In this excerpt she presents a clinical encounter that she argues needs some type of diagnostic scheme that addresses the whole person. Our answer is to explore the concept of belief patterns.

. . . I think, as we look at our definition and try to look at the specifics we have been dealing with, that we had to have a person, a whole person, in order to have a diagnosis.

The person whose life we examined was a university professor who had a medical diagnosis of hyperthyroidism, with all the classical symptoms of hyperthyroidism. She had been diagnosed and was on medication treatment for over a year, but her symptoms were not being controlled and surgery was imminent. She was dissatisfied with, or concerned about, having surgery and decided to seek another opinion, so to speak. She sought the advice of a practitioner who could look at her in a holistic way. These are some of the empirical indicators that this practitioner came up with.

The client was a person who took on an extraordinarily heavy teaching load. She was the type of person who could never say no when she was asked to do something, and therefore was involved in more committee work than most people would be in that particular situation. Not only that, she would end up being the chairman. In addition to her work responsibilities in her profession, she was involved with many organizations and again could never say no and so took on additional responsibilities in terms of committees. She had a strong commitment to her church. She also had a large family who were spread across the country and who called on her frequently for help; therefore, she was continuously in the process of supporting family members one way or another. She had a lot of friends and often did not have time even to eat. . . . These are sufficient empirical indicators about this person . . . which fit into the dimensions of the scheme: wakefulness, activity, relationships, material exchange, valuing . . . these represent guidelines for assessment. Now the practitioner involved said to the client, "I can see that your energy is being directed in many different directions and that this is your way of life, and I know I cannot tell you to change your way of life because that is you. The only thing I can say to you is, 'increase your energy intake.' In other words, sleep more and eat more in order to maintain the energy demands of your system." It seems too simple, doesn't it? Yet for this particular person it seemed to work, because after a period of time she could be maintained on minimal to no drug therapy.[5]

The impact of the clinician's intervention is understood when it is realized that what was in fact done was twofold. First, the clinician accurately recognized the patient's hierarchy of values: service, activity, and others. All of these factors were utilized in the message and in the manner in which the message was delivered. The patient was placed in a double bind. In addition, a paradox was invoked, that is, to do all that you are doing, you must do more. You must rest more and you must eat more. The patient could not *not* respond to the command. To not respond would go against her highest held beliefs about herself and about others and her responsibilities. In short, she had to change her ways to do what she believed she must be doing. She had to take time out for herself. Simply telling her to change her life, taking time out for herself, would be so incongruent with her major beliefs and patterns of behavior she would experience defeat before she began. Matching her model of the self and the world resulted in a structured message and command that she could follow. As indicated earlier, a first step in appreciating how we can intervene at the belief

pattern level is to learn how to identify and address some of the restrictive aspects of belief pattern characteristics realized in patterns of language use.

Characteristics that Reveal Belief Pattern Violations

Distortions, generalizations, and deletions are broad categories of characteristics of sentence structures that reveal belief pattern violations. (Table 16-1).* These three categories act upon one another. Specific violations will be discussed under each of the categories.[6]

Distortions
Distortions are a general class of belief pattern violations composed of broad categories of beliefs and values. They tend to limit a person's view of reality because of the structure of underlying assumptions. The belief pattern violations have been specified as follows: presuppositions, cause–effect, complex equivalents, and mind reading.

Presuppositions. Presuppositions are implicit assumptions in a patients communication that may, if taken for granted, cause limitations of a patient's choice about an experience. For example, "I'm afraid my life is going to be just like my mother's." This statement has the following presuppositions: (1) Daughters become their mothers; (2) life of one person can be repeated by another; and (3) the mother's life is to be feared. This belief holds great potential in limiting the patient's own choice of experience. She may limit how she interprets her successes and failures according to her notions of her mother's life.

Some strategies for challenging and prompting the examination of such underlying assumptions would be: How can your life be exactly the same as your mother's? What in your life is different from your mother's? Is there anything about your mother's life that is worthwhile? Name three positive things you have learned from your mother's life. What would

---

* For a comprehensive discussion of the structure of language, read R. Bandler and J. Grinder, *The Structure of Magic*, Palo Alto, Calif.: Science and Behavior Books, 1975.

TABLE 16-1. SUMMARY OF AN INTRODUCTION TO META PROGRAMS

Pattern	Example	Response	Recovery
Presupposition	If I had not made a mistake.	How does focusing on making mistakes help you now?	Separates event from process.
Cause-effect (how that stimulus makes that)	Make, force, cause, A ↔ B. He makes me dumb.	How do you know that?	Counter example.
Complex equivalent	Indicators as opposed to cause-effect: A = B. A is like B. If you loved me, you wouldn't do that. Love = that.	Has there ever been a time when I did that and you thought I loved you?	Counter example.
Mind reading	I understand. I know you're upset (tired, happy). You're insensitive.	How do you know that?	Complex equivalent or counter example.
Universal qualifier (provides a limitation for the person)	All, every, only, never.	Exaggerate. Has there been a time when it did? Didn't?	Counter example.
Lost performance (judgments)	Bad, crazy, wonderful, different, stupid, brilliant.	According to whom? What criteria? (How do you know?)	Performance criteria.
Modal operator	Should, must, have to, can't, impossible, as if.	What would happen if you did? Didn't? What stops you if you could?	Projected effect (expectation). Subsequential identified cause.
Deletion	I'm scared. I'm angry.	Who? What? When? Where?	Missing information.
Unspecified referential index	They, it, those people, things.	Which? What specifically? Which?	Specific reference.
Unspecified verbs	Learn, understand, profit, frustrate, dominate.	How specifically? In what way?	Specified verb.
Nominalization	Freedom, communication, learnings, problem, tension, depression.	Which specifically? Return to verb form. Recover deletion. How is it to be free?	More specific verb. Missing information.

(Adapted from Gordon, D. Meta Programs Introduction, The Practitioner Program in Neuro-Linguistic Programming, Fall 1980–Spring 1981, Boston, Mass.)

assure you that your life would be different? How do you come to believe that your life must be like your mother's?

Other examples of presuppositions are given below:

Presupposition: I always say, haste makes waste. This statement presupposes that: (1) speed of action is not desirable; and (2) nothing else is considered by me.
Challenge: Has there ever been a time it paid to hurry?
Response: Yes, when I put out the fire in the house. I'm capable of acting with dispatch. (Recovers a resource.)
Presupposition: My problem is not important. This statement presupposes that: (1) there are important

problems; and (2) my problem is of little concern to others.
Challenge: How do you know it is of no concern? Specifically, how is your problem not important?
Response: Well, it is important to me. I guess I'm making a judgment about someone else. (Opens up choice.)
Presupposition: John is a liar. This statement presupposes that: (1) John lies; and (2) John never tells the truth.
Challenge: What has John lied about? Does John ever tell the truth?
Response: In the beginning of our relationship he didn't lie, but now it's all the time. (Opens up an examination of change in behavior of another.)

Cause–Effect. Cause–effect statements express causal linkage between the patient's experience or response to some outside stimulus that is not necessarily directly connected, or where the connection is not clear. Examples are given below:

Cause–effect statement: I would have a happy life if it weren't for the way my parents raised me.
Challenge: How specifically did they raise you to make sure you had an unhappy life? How did your parents raise you to be unhappy? In what way did their raising you make for your unhappiness?
Response: I don't think they intentionally wanted me to be unhappy. Certain things weren't there for me to use today—like how to take responsibility. (Opens up determining more specifically what the person wants. Opens choice rather than blaming.)
Cause–effect statement: I stole the car because my buddy wanted it.
Challenge: Do you always steal because your buddy wants something?
Response: No, I can make my own decisions . . . it just seems that way. (Opens up choice by providing recognition of self-control.)
Cause–effect statement: My mother makes me feel guilty and depressed.
Challenge: Does your mother always make you feel guilty and depressed?
Response: Well, no it's mainly when I want to go out—and she wants me to stay with her.

Note that the presuppositions contained in all these examples of cause–effect infer that others are responsible for one's internal state and behavior. This is a most limiting belief and contributes to stalling personal change.

Complex Equivalents. Complex equivalents are revealed in statements where two experiences or events come to stand for each other but may not necessarily be synonymous. These statements reveal the personal criteria applied to experiences and events without conscious realization that they are not known or are not necessarily the same for other people. There is a presumption of similarity and agreement, which limits experience of learning from differences.

Complex–equivalent statement: If my boss liked me he would comment on my work.
Challenge: Do his comments always indicate he doesn't think much of you? What specifically about his comments leads you to believe he doesn't think much of you? What kind of comments lets you know he thinks positively of your work?
Response: Well, it's only when he gives me a correc-

tion—I guess you would call it a suggestion, that I don't think he thinks much of me . . . hmm. (Opens up choice, allows for consideration of assumptions regarding learning and being perfect.)
Complex–equivalent statement: When she raises her voice, it's proof she hates me.
Challenge: Has there ever been a time she yelled at you and you knew she didn't hate you?
Response: Yes. (Forces sort for positive yelling. Gives choice for interpreting the yelling.)
Complex–equivalent statement: I know he doesn't love me. He never kisses me good-bye.
Challenge: Is a kiss good-bye the only way you know he loves you?
Response: No; he does a lot around the house for me. It is something I would like though. (Opens up choice, points to asking more specifically for what she wants.)
Complex–equivalent statement: They don't think much of me, sending a student in to talk with me.
Challenge: Who would they send in to talk with you that would let you know they think something of you?
Response: I haven't seen my doctor since the first evening I got here. I guess I'm upset . . . taking it out on you. (Gives important information. Opens up opportunity to talk with student.)
Complex–equivalent statement: I know he is going to say no. He has the same look on his face as my father.
Challenge: Did your father ever look that way and say yes? Has anyone looked like that before and said yes?
Response: Well, not everybody is my father . . . but I bet he does say no. (Brings generalization into awareness; opens up choice.)

Mind Reading. Mind reading is a statement that claims that the person knows what is in the mind of another person without receiving specific information from the other person.

Mind-reading statement: The teacher doesn't care whether I pass or not.
Challenge: How do you know that the teacher thinks that?
Response: She didn't answer my questions in class. (Reveals complex equivalent for caring. It does not establish the motivation of the teacher, but it does begin to open up options for the person to find out what it takes to get the teacher to answer questions.)
Mind-reading statement: I'm sure John is sorry for what he said.
Challenge: How do you know John is sorry?
Response: I guess I really don't know. What I want to say is I am sorry you and John are having difficulty. (Opens up more direct expression of personal feelings.)
Mind-reading statement: You think I'm weak.
Challenge: What am I doing or saying that makes you think I think you are weak? (Note: Challenges to mind

reading often reveal the complex equivalents held by a person, thus indicating the selected types of cues from others used to draw conclusions. Challenges open up choice for people.)

Response: It's . . . it's . . . the look in your eyes, the tone of voice. (Information and important feedback.) It's like my father. (Opens up generalization from complex equivalents. Opens up opportunity for different experiences with someone.)

Generalizations

Generalizations represent the next category of belief pattern violations and are also influenced by the category of distortions. Generalizations represent the next highest representation of values and beliefs. They are characterized by references to time, amount, possibility, judgment, and opinion.

Universal Quantifiers.

Universal quantifiers are words that generalize a few experiences to be a whole class of experience. Words like *every, all, always, never,* etc., characterize these expressions.

Universal-quantifier statement: My father never listens to me.
Challenge: (Most often just requires an emphasized repetition of the word.) Your father *NEVER* listens to you?
Response: Well, hardly ever. (Opens up experience of being listened to. Opens up choice of behaviors.)

Lost Performatives.

Lost performatives are words that are basic to statements and judgments that an individual makes about the world that are primarily based on the individual's own experience. Certain words characterize these judgments and statements: *good, bad, crazy, sick, wrong, right, true, false,* etc. These statements and judgments contain criteria information regarding the individual making the statement. As well as generalizing, the individual is unaware of the criteria upon which the judgment is being made.

Lost-performative statement: I am too stupid to be a physician.
Challenge: By whose standards?
Response: My father . . . hmm . . . he always said I couldn't do things. Now I guess I have believed him all these years. (Opens up opportunity to stop generalization. Has own beliefs.)
Lost-performative statement: Look what you have done; now it's all crazy.
Challenge: How is it crazy?
Response: It wasn't supposed to go that way . . . let

me see, I guess it will work . . . didn't think of this way before. (Opens up opportunity.)

Modal Operators of Possibility and Necessity.

Modal operators of possibility and necessity are statements that refer to rules and limits for an individual's behavior. They are characterized by the following terms: *possible/impossible, can/cannot, should/should not, will/won't, may/may not, must/must not, need to, have to,* etc.

Modal-operator-of-necessity statement: I must not show my feelings.
Challenge: What will happen if you do?
Response: I think I will fall apart. (Information that allows person to explore further what falling apart means; opens up chance to recall experience where emotions were expressed and nothing bad happened. Opens up to take chance now.)
Modal-operator-of-possibility statement: I can't say I'll lead the group.
Challenge: What stops you?
Response: I need to feel more confident. (Opens up exploration of what is needed for confidence. Explores moments of confidence.)
Modal-operator-of-necessity statement: I want my way with him.
Challenge: What will happen if you don't get it?
Response: I'll feel terrible, but I know I will survive. (Separates negative feeling state from sense of competency. Opens up choice.)

Deletions

Deletions represent our last general category of belief pattern violations. Deletions are those pieces of information that tell us who, what, when, where. They specify actions and directions, and relate special information on how something is or does. Simple deletions occur when an object, person, or event has been left out of the surface structure (noun phrases, noun arguments).

Simple-deletion statement: I feel miserable.
Challenge: Miserable about what?
Response: My toothache. (Specifies conditions; points to action to relieve state.)
Simple-deletion statement: I received the call and then it fell apart.
Challenge: Received the call from whom? Specifically what fell apart?
Response: Jim, about Art's accident. I just became overwhelmed with fear. It reminded me of my accident when climbing. (Reveals connection of specific feelings with associated events. Opens up exploration of traumatic personal event.)

Lack of Referential Index. Lack-of-referential-index statements focus specifically on the person, subject, or object being left out of the surface structure.

Lack-of-referential-index statement: Life isn't worth living.
Challenge: Whose life?
Response: My life. (Opens up exploration of decision process. Provides specific information.)
Lack-of-referential-index statement: They always accuse me of something.
Challenge: Who always accuses you?
Response: The voices. (Information of private experience. Opens up opportunity for exploration.)

Comparative Deletions. Comparative deletions are statements that make a comparison but leave out what is being compared to what. Terms used are *good-best-better, more-less, most-least.*

Comparative-deletion statement: You are doing better.
Challenge: Better compared to what? Better for whom?
Response: To yourself at the beginning of the semester. (Information. Allows person to make his own comparisons and determine whether he agrees. Opens up choice.)
Comparative-deletion statement: You have the most potential for this work.
Challenge: I have the most potential compared to whom, what?
Response: To all the applicants thus far. (Information for making a decision. Opens up choice.)

Unspecified Verbs. Unspecified verbs are verbs that are not specific in the actions they are meant to depict.

Unspecified-verb statement: John bugs me.
Challenge: Specifically how does John bug you?
Response: He doesn't pick up the tools in the garage and this makes me angry. (Specifies emotional reaction to specific behaviors of another. Opens up choice of how to act.)
Unspecified-verb statement: Mary loves me very much.
Challenge: How does Mary show her love?
Response: She supports me when I have problems at work. She puts up with my bad habits and many more things. (Brings forth positive experiences with Mary. Useful in doing couples work. Builds on positive experiences.)
Unspecified-verb statement: This exercise frustrates me.
Challenge: How does the exercise frustrate you?
Response: When I'm frustrated, I get tense inside. I begin to think, this is happening and it shouldn't happen, and then I blow. (Information regarding internal state, internal processes. Opens up areas for change to reduce intensity of response. Opens up choice.)

Contrast the more specific verbs of *run, jump, kiss* with nonspecific verbs such as *learn, profit, dominate, understanding.* The nonspecific verbs require particular criteria that have to be made clear by the client.

Nominalizations. Nominalizations, as referred to in NLP terms,[7,8] are words that are derived from verbs describing complex processes. These are often treated as static concepts by turning them into noun forms. Nominalizations, unlike nouns, are not a person, place, thing, or object. Rather, they refer to actions that are erroneously treated as things or objects. Examples are *tensions, depression, freedom, communication, loving.* Compare with the nouns *thumb, neck, wagon, shoe.*

Nominalization statement: I want freedom from my depression.
Challenge: What is it to be free for you? What is it to be depressed? Not depressed? (Note the return to the verb form.)
Response: I can return to work, feel good with the kids, my wife, make decisions instead of crying and feeling sorry for myself or mad at everybody else. (Accesses times of feeling in charge. Gives comparisons. Indicates what is wanted and states the thoughts that get in the way.)

Nominalizations are at first difficult to recognize because people have a habit of treating abstract concepts as something real like a table or a chair. Labeling is an example of the improper use of nominalizations; i.e., he is schizophrenic; she is borderline; etc. These labels are developed supposedly to facilitate communication among particular groups of people. They do, somewhat, but because each person develops his own criteria, it cannot be assumed each is talking about the same thing, nor do the labels in these cases truly represent the person.

DIRECT AND INDIRECT THERAPEUTIC COMMUNICATION STRATEGIES

Direct Therapeutic Communication Strategies

The forms of direct communication to be discussed in this section include the following:

thinking that the intentions of others have some positive objective; reframing negative experiences to positive; the use of directives, identification, changed tense, stimulating curiosity, and giving parallel examples.

Avoiding Negative Forms of Communication

As has been stressed throughout the discussion thus far, there are patterns of expression from the nurse that can either facilitate or diminish patient expression and interaction. If the nurse has her own ideas as to how her questions should be answered, this will either stop or frustrate a patient's response. Talking too much about oneself, interrupting, being opinionated, and frequently using negatives are all examples of patterns of communication that have a direct bearing on restricting interaction by the patient and thus act as stalls. Because these behaviors are patterns, recognition is usually facilitated by the comments of another person, such as a nursing supervisor. Exploration of the patterns, i.e., how frequently they are used or what time they come up, becomes an important process in changing. Frequently, the nurse's concerns about what is expected, about the need to succeed rather than taking the time to learn, about experiencing self-control, about sustaining or gaining recognition, etc., are factors that operate to reduce the nurse's effective use of the communication process. The important point here is that ineffective communication may be due to the need for the nurse's personal survival rather than caused by any malicious intention on her part toward another. Respecting the positive intentions of oneself as well as patients reduces the use of negation. Rather, the behavior is addressed rather than suspected negative motivations which, when suspected, often arouse defensive behavior.

The nurse should also avoid self-fulfilling prophecies like the following: "This is going to hurt." "You are going to need to work hard if you want to change." The reader will note that these comments emphasize more or less painful negative experiences. Contrast these to the following statements: "I don't know how this will feel to you." "Let me know, I'll be curious as to your impression." "Change is a challenge, an adventure with ups and downs, but exciting."

We communicate to patients in causal statements in a very matter-of-fact way. It is important to acknowledge these statements, and where they are negative, restate them in the positive, enhancing terms. All behavior has a positive goal; pain is a signal. This is true of psychic pain as well as physical pain. Attempts to avoid pain, or to make it into something to be dreaded, only intensify tension and consequently the negative dimensions of an experience.

Reframing a Negative Experience to Make It a Positive Experience

Simply stated, reframing is the process by which information is exchanged with a patient that facilitates the patient's ability to take a negatively identified situation and put it in terms that increase his sense of mastery and control through choice and options. This is done by identification of the positive dimensions of behavior.

For example, the concepts upon which natural childbirth are built focus on recognition of the tension associated with competing muscle groups, so that the relaxation can be induced and control gained, thus reducing the intensity of pain. The mother, often with the aid of her husband, approaches the process of childbirth equipped with experiential tools and a sense of curiosity as well as of challenge in using them in their adventure into life. This is an example of reframing the idea that childbirth is a dreadful, painful, fearful event.

The nurse is in a critical position to reframe a client's negative interpretation of personal experience, as shown in the following example:

EXAMPLE

A depressed mother has been admitted to a psychiatric unit. She is having her initial evaluation with the staff nurse.

CLIENT: [crying] I shouldn't be here . . . just shouldn't. My husband has to work . . . take care of the kids. I just can't help it . . . I'm terrible, no good to anyone.

NURSE: You shouldn't be here . . . it's hard on your kids and husband. Yet, you made a decision to come into the hospital. How did you do that?

CLIENT: [crying] I just couldn't go on. . . . Every day in bed . . . things not changing. . . . That's not good for the kids [crying] . . . me . . . John.

NURSE: [slow tone of voice] So, you are saying you decided to come here to protect your kids, husband. . . . [Silence. Client is crying, head is down.] Sometimes the only way a person can help those she loves is to take time for herself. . . .

The client dried her tears. There was a slight affirmative nod of her head. The client went on with the interview. Later that day, the nurse overheard the client talking to a student nurse in the day room. She told the student that it was important for her to come into the hospital to help her with her depression so she could return to her family.

No doubt much of the high recovery reported of people who come into clinics, have an initial interview, and then are placed on a waiting list is in fact related to the reframing of their dilemma that brought them to the clinic in the first place. That is, the person's difficulties are not minimized, but they are stated in such a manner that the person feels positive about identifying his problem and taking action.

Directives

Directives are another form of positive communication intervention. Directives are tasks for patients to carry out when the nurse is not there. Such a directive may be designed to increase the patient's awareness of a behavior and the conditions under which it occurs. For example, the patient may be asked to keep a notebook for the next two days on the times he experienced disappointment. In the case of a patient who tends to be explosive, not attending to what he says or does when piqued, the nurse may ask him to pay attention to a factor leading to the explosion. This is aimed at getting the patient to respond to what annoys him prior to the buildup.

Directives are useful when the nurse does not see the patient every day. They emphasize that the patient has the ability to take charge of change and growth beyond the time of talking with the nurse.

Identification

Identification with another person is a strategy to use with people when they do not feel they have particular abilities. The nurse actively encourages the patient to identify someone he thinks does have the ability.

A dramatic story of how this works was told by an elderly woman who had fallen on the back steps during a snowstorm and had broken her leg. When asked how she had gotten up the stairs, into the house, and pulled herself to the telephone for help, she said she had watched a movie the night before. In the movie, a man in the Klondike had broken his leg in a blizzard. She watched him hold his broken leg together and pull himself backwards through the snow to protection. For this dramatic moment, this woman had emulated the man.

During certain stressful moments, people are seemingly cut off from their resources. Asking them to think of someone who could do the thing they believe they cannot do allows them to get in touch with their own resources, albeit in an indirect manner. The above example also underscores the fact that direct methods are often useful with people who are experiencing the confusing aspects of a crisis. Taking on the role of another is also a useful first step in having a person rehearse new behaviors.

Other Positive Forms of Direct Communication

Changing tense is a powerful direct method of instituting change. Mothers often use this technique with their children. A small child complains of a hurt finger and shows it to Mommy. Mother looks at the finger and states, "That hurt didn't it?" When a person has suffered a traumatic event in the past but is carrying it over into the present, the change of tense helps separate the past event from the present, so that the person can forget the hurt and look forward to the future.

Stimulating questions and curiosity in the patient is another useful form of direct communication when the nurse knows there is something the patient wants to do, or when the patient needs to explore other things for himself. The goal is to get the patient to seek information instead of the nurse telling him. This is more effective when there are three parties present—the patient, the nurse, and another colleague. The nurse and colleague can carry on a conversation about a particularly relevant issue but don't relate it to the patient. For example, a patient may be having a great deal of trouble with anxiety and tension. The nurse turns to her colleague and asks, "Have you heard from Jim yet and his experiences with the new relaxation program? He was most curious about carrying it out at work." The coworker goes into a discussion about Jim's success with the plan. This provokes curiosity in the patient, who begins to ask questions about the specifics of the new program.

Giving parallel examples, like the last concept, moves us a bit closer to indirect communication strategies, but it is considered direct because the parallel example is not disguised. The nurse selects an example of a state of affairs very similar to the patient's involving another person. This is often the key beneficial aspect of support groups where people come together because of similar shared issues. For example, a young woman who has just been raped and is in the emergency room, unable to talk, responded to the nurse who told her of a similar young woman and how the young woman revealed that her reluctance to talk was based on fear of judgment by the nurse and staff and fear that the rapist would retaliate since it was someone she knew. The example closely matched the presenting experience of the rape victim. The nurse filled in what she had learned from another patient. One might ask, what happens if the patient claims it isn't that way for her? It's still helpful because she is beginning to talk and recount her personal experience.

Indirect Communication Strategies

Indirect strategies are used in a purposeful way in advanced nursing clinical practice. They are presented here by way of introduction so that a beginning nurse can become aware of their use and can begin to use them spontaneously.

Illusion of Choice

Illusion is a most obvious form of indirect communication. It is a basic structure for many of the next examples. Its most common appearance is in child rearing where parents are attempting to motivate children to behave in certain ways. For example, the question to the young toddler, "Do you want your teddy bear in bed with you, or your dolly?" bypasses the issue of whether the child will go to bed. The issue is nonnegotiable; however, the child is given the choice of what to bring to bed with him.

Another example was presented by a student nurse.[9] She was on an accident floor. A man in his 60s was refusing to move and get around after his leg was broken. This was of great concern to his physician. The student knew the man was interested in gambling and playing poker. Therefore she went to him after taking care of him in the morning and said the following: "You know, the guys on this ward like me. As a matter of fact, I have noticed that by Friday, they are all getting better . . . walking, using their crutches. Now, I bet you that by next Friday, on that day, you are going to be feeling like taking on the world and walking. I'll put my money on Friday. Now, you may do it on Saturday, or Sunday. Or you might do it on Tuesday or Wednesday, but I bet on Friday."

In this example the patient is given the illusion of choice on several levels. He can choose when he will walk, and he can choose whether to cooperate with the student or not. Notice also how the example utilizes key important factors in the make-up and behavior of the patient.

Junko Logic

The phenomenon of junko logic occurs more often than we realize. It is the putting together of statements that appear to have a relationship to one another but in fact do not, or stating two or more facts and then linking them to a third as if they are related when they are not.

In one instance a nurse was seeing a patient who was recently home from being hospitalized after a heart attack. He was most anxious about his condition, so the doctor had given him an order for Valium and told him to do his walking. However, he just sat in a chair all day and did not do the prescribed walking. His fear attached him to the drug, and he was most skeptical about giving it up. The nurse said the following: "Well, after all, the important thing about drugs is the chemicals they put in your body. Therefore the way to get chemicals in your body that make you feel good is to begin to walk and exercise." Two weeks later the client was off the Valium and was enjoying himself on his walks outside.

Chemicals in the body were the focus (a truism), and the nurse told the patient to put them in his body by walking. He followed the command. There was a relabeling of what was important to the patient, i.e., having chemicals in his body; instructions were given as to how to achieve getting the important experience, chemicals, without taking drugs.

Embedded Commands

Without being aware of it, nurses often given commands. For example, "Most people stop before they get angry and report that they discover what provokes them and therefore feel in control and better." This statement appears rather straightforward. However, there are three embedded commands. By understanding how we can mark out what is important by tonal changes, we have the use of a communication strategy to effect change. Upper-case letters will be used here to indicate how the nurse delivered this last comment to give direction to behavior change. "Most people STOP BEFORE THEY GET ANGRY and report that they DISCOVER WHAT PROVOKES them and therefore FEEL in control and BETTER."[10]

Paradoxical Commands

A paradoxical command is used with people who are vacillating between two extremes; for example, where persons feel so anxious they believe they cannot relax; or where a parent insists that a child eat, and the child refuses to eat. Skilled clinicians such as family therapists have developed the use of paradoxical command in many life-threatening situations, such as that of the adolescent with anorexia nervosa. Such an example is the clinician who had lunch with a young patient who would not eat. As they sat together and began lunch, the girl picked up her fork but did not eat. The therapist ate his food with gusto and periodically reached over to the girl's plate and ate her food. The girl looked perplexed and then a bit annoyed. She didn't like the doctor, yet he insisted on eating lunch with her for the next week. She got so annoyed with his behavior that she began to eat the food on her plate while she was with him. The paradox was that rather than respond in opposition to her behavior, he intensified it by making sure she was not going to eat unless she really wanted to.

Therapeutic Double Binds

Therapeutic double binds are another example of indirect therapeutic communication strategies. The difference between therapeutic and nontherapeutic double binds is that the therapeutic double bind is used to help the person move on and broaden his options rather than lock them in a negative relationship. Good parental strategies use positive double binds. For example, "Would you like your teddy bear or Mr. Rabbit with you when you go to sleep?" People who tend to be polarized in their beliefs about their behavior and their ability to change respond well to double binds. For example, a woman insisted she could not say no to people. She was asked by the nurse to spend the next three days saying no to people on the ward who asked her to do something she didn't want to do. The patient was now in a double bind. That is, if she said she wouldn't do the exercise, she was saying *no* to the nurse. If she did the exercise, she has the experience of saying *no* to other people. She cannot not say *no* to someone.

Summary

In this chapter, the student is introduced to the use of theoretical models in the development of therapeutic strategies. First, the anxiety of the student is addressed, then characteristics and beliefs important to working therapeutically with clients is provided. Rapport-building strategies are presented. Other sections include guidelines for setting and evaluating outcomes of communication methods; eliciting and accessing personal resources: Meta program violations are explored in the context of challenges. The chapter ends with a discussion of direct and indirect communication strategies.

When the student understands the structure of rapport and how to observe its manifestation in relationships, a first step is taken in exploring more advanced techniques of therapeutic intervention. This exploration is further enhanced when the student realizes the areas of an individual's behavior and how change is manifested in them as a result of the structure of the interaction.

Questions

1. Give examples from your clinical work of three dimensions of behavior needed by a therapist: non-possessive warmth, congruence, and accurate empathy.

2. Give a clinical example in which you paced the client's world. What happened?
3. Give examples of the following: sorting behavior, separating behavior, combining behavior, altering criteria for judging, and rehearsing new behavior.
4. Give an example in which you elicited the resources of a client.
5. Give a clinical example of belief pattern violations: presupposition, cause–effect, complex equivalents, and mind reading.

REFERENCES AND SUGGESTED READINGS

1. Carkhoff, R., & Truax, C. *Toward Effective Counseling and Psychotherapy.* Chicago: Aldine, 1967.
2. Erickson, M. H. General introduction to hypnotherapy. In M. H. Erickson & E. Ross (Eds.) *The Collected Papers of M. Erickson* (Vol. 4). New York: Irving, 1980, pp. 1–13.
3. Lankton, S., & Lankton, C. *The Answer Within: A Clinical Framework of Ericksonian Hypnotherapy.* New York: Brunner/Mazel, 1983.
4. Dilz, R., Grinder, J., Bandler, R. & Bandler-Cameron, L. *Neuro-Linguistic Programming* (Vol. 1). Cupertino, Calif.: Meta Publications, 1980.
5. Newman, M. Nursing diagnosis and nursing theory. In M. Kim & D. Moritz (Eds.), *Classification of Nursing Diagnoses, Fourth National Conference.* New York: McGraw-Hill, 1982, pp. 225–226.
6. Lankton, S. *Practical Magic.* Cupertino, Calif.: Meta Publications, 1980.
7. Brockopp, D. Y. What is NLP? *American Journal of Nursing,* 1983, *83,* 1012–1014.
8. Knowles, R. D. Building rapport through Neuro-Linguistic Programming. *American Journal of Nursing,* 1983, *83,* 1010–1011.
9. King, L., & Novik, L. *Irresistible Communication: Creative Skills for Health Management.* Philadelphia: Saunders, 1983, p. 82.

Chapter 17

Stalls in the Therapeutic Process

Ann Wolbert Burgess

Chapter Objectives

The students successfully attaining the goals of this chapter will be able to:

- Define the stall concept as it applies to clinical practice.
- Describe stalls in terms of:
  behavioral style.
  judgmental feeings.
  ambivalent feelings.
  rescue feelings.
  feelings of pessimism.
  feelings of omnipotence and omniscience.
  setting goals.
  being reassuring.
  confrontation and misuse of the analytical approach.
  misjudging the patient's independence.
  labeling the patient.
  overidentification with the patient.
  nontherapeutic involvement.
  bearing painful feelings.
  being dishonest.
  listening.
  eliciting the patient's request.
- Describe stalls in the interview process.

An analogy may be made here to aerodynamics and a student pilot learning to fly an airplane right side up and safely. In Chapter 15 the prac- tice of being therapeutic was discussed as a guide to effective interaction with people. Stu- dent pilots also identify their assets and reactions and learn the dynamics and mechanics of flying. With this knowledge they then get into the cockpit of the plane and put theory into practice.

THE STALL CONCEPT

It is not until the student starts flying the plane that an actual stall is experienced. A stall means that the airplane has lost the lift that it needs to stay in the air. A variety of conditions can cause a stall. Although a stall will not necessarily put the plane out of control, it does mean that a corrective measure is necessary to help the plane resume its path of flight. A red light or buzzer in the plane alerts the pilot of a potential stall position in case he has not "felt" that the lift is gone. At this point the pilot must then consider his alternatives if he wants to stay aloft.

The psychiatric nursing student is now at the point where she has some concepts of therapeutic meetings with patients. The next step is to test what has been learned in the psychiatric setting. Here it is helpful to know the common stalls that impede the therapeutic process.

There are many situations that lead to a stall, and we will attempt to describe some of them. In addition, we will attempt to describe the warnings that signal a stall is imminent.

The stall warning occurs when you feel that something is wrong before the patient reacts unfavorably to the situation and you are into the stall. Ideally, you try to remedy the situation before the stall occurs. You will, however, feel that the stall is imminent because you will receive warnings such as a vague feeling of discomfort within yourself, the realization that the therapy is getting nowhere, the patient's sudden change in attitude toward you, his expression of hostility, your autognosis of your own withdrawal, or a feedback from the staff of the patient's reactions.

In this chapter we will mention some specific stalls and the general warnings of other potential stall situations. The corrective mechanism to "right the flight" or remedy the stall will also be given.

STALLS IN HUMAN QUALITIES

Behavioral Style

People beginning their training in the psychiatric mental health field often seem to have a pseudoprofessional approach, characterized by their looking and acting stilted and rigid. This may result from their trying too hard to follow the book and the prescribed rules. By the time their training has ended, however, they act far more natural, for they have learned to be themselves and are thus able to reveal their humanness and genuine concern for their patients.

When a nurse behaves in a pseudoprofessional way, the patient feels uncomfortable and wonders what is happening to this person who is supposed to know what she is doing. When the patient feels no confidence in the helping person, there is a stall. In this situation, the stall warning occurs when you notice yourself becoming tense, rigid, and stilted and wishing that you felt more professional.

In order to correct the stall, you should try to worry less about the rules concerning methods of listening and talking with people. Strict adherence to rules can prove burdensome and may hinder the development of the naturalness of one's skills. It is important not to abandon one's common-sense approach for the pretense of the professional approach. Being natural can impart the feeling of security and competence as a therapeutic person.

STALLS IN FEELINGS

Judgmental Feelings

Judgmental feelings surface when the nurse arrives at a clinical situation with an already formed judgment or prejudice. The word *prejudice* has a similar root to the word *judgment*. Prejudice is prejudging without having any actual data or experience. It is often opinion based on cultural values or upbringing.

The patient generally can tell when a person has negative feelings toward him. The patient feels isolated, ignored, or dealt with in an abrupt manner. The therapeutic progress stalls because the helping person unconsciously rejects him because of strong negative feelings.

The stall warning occurs when nurses realize that they have strong negative opinions of the person before even meeting him. In the staff report you may hear the patient described in highly negative judgmental terms, or perhaps the history of the patient may give you an uncomfortable feeling. You have a strong negative visceral reaction and you know that it comes from a previous unpleasant experience in your life.

A negative feeling triggers a strong reaction through the sensory system and adversely reflects the way one person looks, sounds, smells, or responds physically to another person.

In order to remedy this stall, nurses must realize the scope of their judgmental feelings and must be able to keep them in check so that they do not interfere with the therapeutic process. For example, if the nurses cannot stand a geriatric patient, they should be aware of it so that they can be therapeutic and polite. If they acknowledge this, they will not have to say at nursing report, "That old lady in 356—I wonder what she is ringing her bell for this time?"

The nurse brings all her feelings to any new situation and everything proceeds smoothly as long as the feelings are positive. For example, if the nurse says, "That patient reminds me of my grandmother. I really like her and want to help her," she probably will be therapeutic because of her positive feelings.

Judgmental feelings can help or stall the therapeutic process. What we are concerned about in this section are those judgmental feelings that hinder and stall.

The stall in the judgmental situation may be more easily detected by impartial staff members than by the nurse herself. The objective person may hear the stall as a labeling of the patient, such as, "The lady is just an alcoholic," or "We had another drug-abuse patient admitted last night."

For example, a student says, "I really dread going to the psychiatric nursing experience." The student probably has formed an opinion of the experience from past remarks made by relatives and friends regarding psychiatric patients or even from hearing other professionals talking about the clinical specialty areas. This is a judgmental feeling because the student has never experienced the situation personally, and thus the entire discipline is condemned beforehand.

The judgmental attitudes we all develop because of our upbringing become a pattern for searching inquiry when working with people with emotional illness. The ideal is to proceed above and beyond the judgmental attitude. This helps to understand the patient as a human being in his own right, rather than to see him as someone with unacceptable behavior. When two people talk together, what they say depends not only on what they want to tell each other but also on what they think of each other. Patients will be reluctant to reveal themselves to people who they feel will judge them critically.

There is no doubt that even nurses with considerable experience will at times find themselves automatically judging a patient. When they realize how nontherapeutic this is, they will then reassess their attitude. For example, nurses may find themselves reacting unfavorably to girls hospitalized for abortions, venereal disease, and illegitimate babies. This is not just a problem for beginning nurses; it is also a problem for the entire medical and nursing professions. Behavior that deviates from society's norms is difficult for people to accept. Two cases that illustrate this are drug abuse and alcohol consumption. These problems of society are compounded greatly when the medical-clinical professions tend to use judgmental terms in prescribing treatment. For example, the physician may say, "It's all in his head—just give him a tranquilizer. He is always complaining." Nurses also may assume judgmental attitudes from what the physician has to say about a patient. This approach, in itself, is far from helpful in dealing with or attempting to understand the problem.

No one is without bias and no one is without judgmental feelings. Our feelings and opinions about people and situations derive from our experiences and interactions in life. The question is how to facilitate the process of becoming more objective and less judgmental. How is one able to step back and look at the situation objectively and thereby prevent a stall in the therapeutic process?

The process of becoming objective is twofold and involves (1) autognosis of feelings; and (2) accepting the feelings and realizing it is not excessively harmful to have negative feelings about someone. However, it is harmful if the judgmental feelings are suppressed and then unconsciously acted upon. The patient will be rejected, ignored, and relegated to a powerless position.

The nurse has the right to be human, which implies the right to have judgmental feelings. There is, however, the ideal to which one should aspire. Even when the nurse cannot give up her judgmental feelings, she can recognize them as such. She can rise above the feelings and not let them interfere with the therapeutic process.

Ambivalent Feelings

The term *ambivalence* implies having both positive and negative feelings toward an object, a person, or an action. We have all experienced feelings of ambivalence.

The stall in the therapeutic process comes from denying ambivalent feelings, especially the negative aspects of the ambivalence. As a result the staff can become overly solicitous. It may be the nurse acting as "Suzy Goodshoes." Alternatively, the staff may handle the negative ambivalence by displaced anger.

The stall occurs when nurses simultaneously like and do not like the patient. They then feel guilty for their negative feelings. The anger does not come through because they are unwilling to be open and honest with their feelings. They may not dare be angry because nurses are supposed to like and relate to all their patients. If they cannot deal with their ambivalence, the anger comes through in covert ways, and the patient then senses something is wrong. A stall results.

The stall warning occurs when nurses notice themselves being overly nice to a patient or when they have either all positive or all negative feelings toward the patient.

Ambivalence is part of all human relationships. People who are in the health fields generally are there because they sincerely like people and wish to help them in stressful times. Too often it is assumed that one must have positive feelings for the patient at all times. Assumptions like this will only put a student or practitioner in direct conflict because ambivalence is a natural feeling in any relationship.

The nurse must realize that ambivalence is a normal feeling. If the nurse dislikes the patient a great deal, chances are there are positive feelings too, and she can still work with the patient even though she has negative feelings.

If you look closely at your own personal relationships, you will find that even with those you love, you can also be furious at times. For example, if you are shopping in a store and a child begins to fuss and cry, all attempts to pacify him only distract and upset you further. If you have not had such an experience, we suggest you spend an hour observing mothers shopping in the supermarket with their children. The ambivalent feelings are most evident when one is tired, upset, under pressure, or generally unhappy.

Despite the pain of ambivalent feelings, however, it is still better than having no feelings at all. Ambivalence shows that the nurse is real, and by acknowledging and dealing with her positive as well as negative feelings, a stall will not occur, and the therapeutic process will be facilitated.

A well-established psychiatric nursing principle states that patients need to be accepted exactly as they are. This means that the patient is seen as a person, but it does not mean that the nurse necessarily approves of his behavior. It may be that the nurse does not like the person or what he has done. If the patient has committed a crime, such as robbery or murder, this behavior will produce a negative bias or will induce prejudiced feelings in the nurse. It is difficult to acknowledge these feelings and still remain therapeutic in dealing with the patient. The following clinical example shows a staff reaction to a patient who had trouble staying within the limits of the laws of society:

A 17-year-old girl was referred to a halfway house residence by her social worker. Her presenting behavior pattern showed frequent environmental moves since age 11 when the total family was broken up because of the mother's psychiatric hospitalizations and the father's desertion of the family. In the previous six years, Susan had lived in 14 different foster homes. Her typical pattern was to become increasingly unmanageable after a three- or four-month period. She would refuse to meet the expectations of the home by coming in at odd hours, being truant from school, and ignoring her household duties. She would become verbally aggressive with the mother in the home, and this would inevitably lead to her referral back to the social worker. Her life-style made her a target for the drug culture, because her boyfriend was a pusher, and her promiscuity made her vulnerable to pregnancy and venereal disease.

In the new situation at the halfway house, Susan was pleasant, attractive, and bluntly honest regarding her pseudoinvolvement with people and her negative regard for the "establishment."

Susan first induced the staff to help her by appealing to their rescue feelings and by making them feel guilty. The staff felt that they could help Susan by being supportive and understanding. She responded by making the staff feel helpless and by behaving in her natural style. She did not abide by the house rules but instead brought drugs and alcohol into the house. She initiated some younger and more inexperienced patients to the world of drugs. This behavior provoked guilt feelings in the staff. When the staff finally said that they could not tolerate this deviant behavior, she burst forth with positive behaviors of cooking, cleaning, being pleasant, going to school, and promising to avoid all drugs. The staff again felt guilty after talking with the social worker and learning that Susan had no place to go because everyone had "kicked" her out.

The staff was ambivalent over discharging Susan because she was appealing as a human being in distress, but her behavior was not appropriate for the house. Ambivalence creates and perpetuates uncomfortable feelings that people find hard to compromise with. Here the staff needed repeated conferences to talk out their feelings and to recognize that their treatment model was not therapeutic for Susan with her manipulative abilities.

To be able to accept and possibly understand Susan's behavioral style helped them to avoid the conflict in feelings resulting from expecting behavior that Susan simply could not manage. The staff had to realize and to expect that this patient would lie, cheat, and manipulate because this was her life-style and she was accustomed to behaving in that manner. Expecting people to behave as society dictates when it is not their style sets the stage for judgmental and ambivalent feelings. It is comparable to expecting the alcoholic to give up alcohol because he is told it is harmful to his body.

The problem with ambivalence is that some people find it difficult to accept ambivalence in themselves. They suppress unpleasant feelings and try to counteract the negative feelings by being generous and altruistic, which only displaces their negative feelings. Therapy thereby stalls rather than progressing.

Rescue Feelings

Rescue feelings occur when the helping professional believes that he can do for the patient what no one else can do. The feeling is that one possesses the magic cure and can help the patient get better when everyone else has failed. Even though this is unrealistic, it can be helpful in small doses; this is the therapeutic side of the double-edged sword of rescue feelings.

Rescue feelings lead people to believe that there is some magical quality about them that can change a secluded, regressed psychotic person into an outpatient neurotic person. During the painful descent into reality, the nurse often becomes preoccupied with what can or cannot be done for the patient. This frequently prevents the nurse from seeing the patient as he really is.

The therapeutic process stalls when nurses ally themselves against the family or when they promise the patient more than they can reasonably deliver. The patient's hopes are raised sky-high; and when the nurse does not deliver, the patient feels hopelessly let down. The stall warning is there when you feel that you are clinically better than anyone else or when you feel the family has done everything wrong.

For example, a psychiatric resident physician allied himself with his patient against the family during the therapy. He advised the patient to get an apartment of his own, continue going to school, and everything would be fine. The patient agreed that this sounded like a fine idea and a family conference was arranged to tell the parents of this decision. At the conference the patient said to his parents, "I want to move out and get my own apartment. What do you think?" The parents replied, "Fine. Go ahead." The patient then said, "I think I am going to commit suicide."

This example shows that the patient was not prepared for such a major decision in his life, and he had to be hospitalized for a short period to help him recover and learn to deal with his feelings about this situation. This situation illustrates the potential for a permanent stall to the therapeutic situation. One must avoid making secret alliances with the patient. The patient often contributes to this by saying, "You are the only one who understands me." This statement should be a warning signal, and the nurse should then realize that she may be in for a problematic and difficult situation.

The stall warning occurs when the patient plays up to the nurse's omnipotence and she thinks that perhaps what he is saying is true. Possibly she feels that she is the only one who understands him.

In order to remedy the stall, the nurse will have to consider what is going to happen to the patient when he is discharged and she is not going to be there. This will help her put other relationships into proper perspective.

Sharing the responsibility with other staff members in order to accomplish treatment goals will usually be more rewarding and successful than thinking that the nurse and patient can solve the problem alone.

Feelings of Pessimism

At times, beginning nurses will have a difficult time understanding why the patient cannot comprehend his problem and why he cannot seem to be helped. This leads to feelings of pessimism about the patient's recovery. The nurses have listened to people say, "You can't teach an old dog new tricks. He has always behaved that way; he will never change." With this negative expectation about the potential of people to change and to be helped, any dialogue with the patient is likely to be antitherapeutic.

The stall here occurs when the patient realizes that the nurse feels that his situation is hopeless. The warning sounds when the nurse is feeling desperate and helpless in dealings with the patient.

The remedy for this stall is for the nurse to talk over such feelings with a staff member, supervisor, or instructor to try to get a therapeutic approach to the situation.

It is difficult for beginning nurses to grasp a person's potential for change, especially in psychiatric situations. Often the person is seen in terms of what he has achieved rather than in terms of what he could achieve. The positive adage, "Today is the first day of the rest of my life," should be reexamined in terms of individual potential.

If one looks for the negative side, the therapeutic leverage loses its reason for being. We all know people who have made slighting remarks about prominent people as if they were comparing them with the ideal. The human element of a person is lost in these remarks. What does stand out, however, is the unforgiving quality of the remark. In that context, who can be expected to change or grow and who can be helped?

Feelings about an individual's ability to change may be evaluated by looking at one's own capacity to change. Frequently, a low achiever in high school will do an about-face and become a high achiever in college once he identifies with what it is he wants.

In American politics there are examples of senators, governors, and presidents who were known to suffer from specific behavior disorders. Chronic alcoholics have withdrawn from alcohol and achieved much in public office. People do recover and go on to other important aspects of living.

People who know themselves well say that when teachers or parents had confidence in their ability to develop and grow, they did grow. Those who were unfortunate in having teachers or parents who thought they would not make it usually were the ones who failed. The expectation and positive attitude of the senior helping person determine in large part what the child or patient will do. Supportive encouragement by a person important to the patient, coupled with an optimistic expectation for the individual, will be effective in helping the patient develop and grow.

Feelings of Omnipotence and Omniscience

Nurses and others in the helping professions sometimes feel that they are all-powerful and all-knowing. The patient's ideas and feelings tend to be regarded as irrelevant because the professional thinks she or he can be a better judge of the situation.

The stall occurs when the patient becomes furious with the nurse for not listening to him and for thinking that she knows all the answers. The patient may respond by withdrawing and saying, "Everything is fine with me. I need nothing." Nurses sometimes misinterpret this as "the good patient who has no complaints." The nurse may have the feelings of omniscience, that the nursing care is excellent and all the patient's needs have been met.

The correction of the stall requires that the nurse take the time to listen to the patient's requests and to his perceptions of the situation. This information is essential in planning the patient care. If the patient's request is unreasonable or if the nurse feels that she cannot meet it, this information should be conveyed to the patient so that he knows it was considered. For example, if the patient asks whether or not he may telephone his family, and the staff feels that it would not be helpful to the patient at that time, the patient should be told why he cannot do as he requested. Then this request may be negotiated, thus giving the patient a part in the planning of his care.

Two examples, involving a doctor and nurse who were hospitalized medical and surgical patients themselves, are cited in order to illustrate feelings of omniscience displayed by nurses regarding the administration of pain medication.

SITUATION ONE

A doctor required emergency surgery when he was visiting in a strange town. He did not initially tell the nurse he was a doctor because he felt that it was irrelevant to the situation. Less than 24 hours after his appendectomy he was requesting pain medication every three hours, although he was not wearing a watch and did not know this. A nursing supervisor appeared at his bedside and asked him whether he knew he could become a drug addict the way he was requesting pain medication. He finally could not tolerate this and had to tell the supervisor that drug addiction usually needed a three-week period to develop and not a 24-hour period, and that the pain following surgery does justify medication around the clock.

SITUATION TWO

A nurse was hospitalized for back surgery. The pain was considerable and she requested her medication as frequently as she could but within the "proper" limits. The nurses showed such a suspicious attitude that she found herself going through "games" so that the nurses wouldn't think she was a drug addict. In desperation she told her physician, who finally decided to handle the situation by allowing her to keep her medication at her bedside.

Part of the problem in these two situations is that nurses somehow feel that they are in a position to judge how much pain a patient is having. Nurses are usually the first ones informed of the patient's pain and are instrumental in determining what and how much medication a patient receives. The nurse will say such things as, "He is getting too much medicine," or "He is not getting enough," or "He needs a weaker dose," or "He needs a sleeping medication."

Nurses should not be placed in the position of judging whether or not the patient is having pain. That is where the problem lies. The only real indicator as to whether or not the patient has pain is to listen to the patient. If he says he has pain, he has pain. All pain hurts. There is no all-embracing and infallible measure of pain. You simply cannot prove your pain threshold to someone else; you can only tell them. Nurses somehow feel that they should be able to sense or measure pain as indicated by how much the patient fidgets, is restless, or is contorted and doubled over. If the patient asks in a normal or even offhand manner for pain medication, the nurse may feel the patient

should justify this request. She may become annoyed with the patient if she does not feel that he is having enough pain. The annoyance may be reflected onto the patient by making him wait for the medication or by the nurse saying that the doctor must be consulted first.

When a patient says he has pain, the nurse should first determine what measures are available to relieve the pain. Trying to relieve the pain is being therapeutic; trying to prove whether he does or does not have pain is psychonoxious. The nurse might assess: Has the patient complained recently of pain? Does he complain after he has had visitors or when he does not have visitors? Does he have more pain at night than during the day? What circumstances surround the pain?

In contrast to feelings of omnipotence and omniscience are the feelings of humility and respect—humility in that perhaps the nurse does not have all the answers, and respect in that possibly patients can help out by stating requests and needs.

No human being knows all the answers, and certainly no nurse has all the answers to patient situations. There are times when no one is able to provide the answers to a given situation. Very often consultation with colleagues and supervisors is necessary to deal with clinical situations. The important point in correcting this stall is to realize that humility and respect go a long way in facilitating the therapeutic process.

STALLS IN THERAPEUTIC TASKS

Failure to Set Goals

The failure to set goals leads to confusion in the treatment triad of patient, physician, and nurse. The stall occurs when one member of the triad does not know all the facts. For example, the physician or the nurse may say, "What is the patient here for?" or "I wonder why the patient has not been discharged?" The therapy is not progressing satisfactorily when these questions are asked. It means that goals have not been clearly defined and communicated. The treatment is then stalled.

The remedy to be used in correcting this stall is for each person to begin communicating with the others to know what is occurring. The negotiation of goals implies that everyone is aware of what is going on in the therapeutic process.

For example, when the overall goal is interfered with, the patient may say, "I don't want to go home." This means that the patient has not cognitively agreed to the overall goal that he is to return to family and community when he has recovered.

When the physician and nurse know what the treatment goal is and the patient does not, the patient may say, "I don't know what I am doing here. Nothing gets done. No one tells me anything. The nurse says to ask the doctor, and the doctor is in and out so fast that he won't give me a straight answer anyway. I might as well leave and go somewhere else if I want an answer."

The patient feels ignored. This behavior disregards the needs of the patient. The patient can share remotely in the therapeutic goal by being verbally passive and doing what he is told, or he can be pleasant and uncomplaining—for example, asking only for such minor things as a washcloth in order to help himself. On the other hand, the patient may absolutely refuse to cooperate. The patient who is uncooperative may receive the label of a rebellious patient and may discharge himself against medical advice. This kind of stall in the therapeutic process tends to be irrevocable.

In order to avoid such a stall situation, it is necessary that interdependent relationships be established. For the whole to function smoothly, the parts must be synchronized and all must relate to the direction of the goal. The overall goal should include all team members. Each member may then have contributing aims or goals specific to his role.

When the treatment goals are not stated to the patient either before admission to the hospital or within the diagnostic and assessment period, this approach shows inconsiderateness for the needs of the patient. This method could imply that treatment may be forever and that the patient may never leave.

Beginning staff, not yet aware of what is therapeutic, may tend to compensate for this lack of setting goals by giving the patient that which he can either manage for himself or do without: a pat on the back, several different medications, extra appointment times, or a lecture to the patient's family. As the psychiatric staff member becomes more comfortable with the role and learns the therapeutic tasks, the patient is then seen as a distinct individual with requests and needs of his own.

False Reassurance

Reassurance may be therapeutic when it is based on fact. The surgeon says, "I am reassuring you that you do not have cancer. I have done a biopsy." He has the proof. This is also a supportive statement. If the reassurance is based on truth and concrete evidence, it is supportive. If the reassurance is not based on truth, the patient senses that it is insincere and this is false reassurance.

The stall occurs when nurses reassure a patient and the patient is smart enough to know that they are unable to really predict or prove the truth of the statement. For example, the patient has had a kidney transplant and the nurse says, "Don't worry, you have the best surgeon and you will be fine in a few weeks." The patient knows that the nurse does not have a solid basis for that information and thus sees her as one who no longer has anything of value to offer. The patient will not find this nurse a useful, supportive, or helpful person. He will probably withdraw and get angry.

Other stall situations that can be called false reassurance are as follows:

Reassurance is sometimes used under the guise of protecting the patient. A patient who has a diagnosis of a terminal illness and has not been told is often the recipient of this kind of reassurance. The patient may say, "I am feeling worse today. I wonder why I still have that pain?" The nurse with good intentions may say, "It should go away. Don't think about it; put your mind on other things." What actually happens is that the response protects the nurse's feelings. This answer to the patient avoids any further discussion. A better response might be, "The pain is making you uncomfortable and is worrying you. What are you thinking?"

False reassurance is commonly observed in dealing with children in pediatric nursing. The goal tends to be to complete the nursing procedure as quickly as possible regardless of the patient's feelings, for example, when giving an injection or changing a dressing. In this service, statements are made such as, "Just a little medicine to make you feel better." The child's concept is here-and-now, not future-oriented. Feeling better later does not make sense to him when at present the medicine feels painful. It is best to tell the patient that it will hurt or it will taste bad and that it is perfectly all right to cry. It is cruel to expect stoic behavior from children or adults. It is therapeutic to encourage genuine feelings.

In another case the nurse says to the patient preoperatively, "Don't worry, a herniorrhaphy is a very ordinary operation today and you will be up and about within a few days." The nurse's goal is to be supportive to the patient preoperatively. She feels that her statement is reassuring to the patient. Undoubtedly, the patient will have an uneventful postoperative course. The statistics are heavily in his favor. Nevertheless, the statement is actually denying the patient's concerned feelings regarding surgery. All the patient's real fears and anxieties are allowed to remain untold. Further exploration of the patient's concern is abruptly denied. Verbal reassurance is not supportive when it does not allow the patient to first express feelings of concern.

The nurse in the community talks with a patient who says, "I think I am going crazy." The nurse may then say, "But you don't have any of the symptoms and I don't think you are going crazy." This is nonsupportive reassurance. It is more useful to ask what "crazy" means to the person or what factors are leading him to feel as he does. Nurses should seek out and explore the anxious thoughts if they want to be helpful. This action shows the patient that he is being taken seriously and that the nurse can stand to hear what is going on in his mind. By allowing the patient to express himself, the powerful aspect of the anxiety is reduced to more tolerable limits.

Sometimes well-meaning reassurance can inhibit the patient. For example, if the patient says, "I need love and I can't get it," one response might be, "That is a basic human need and you are not alone in that feeling." This is going from a specific issue (the patient and his feeling) to a general issue (the feeling and everyone's need). This response will put the conversation in more general terms and will inhibit the patient from further talking about himself. A more useful remark would be, "What seems to prevent you from getting love?" The second response still supports the patient because he needs to be cared for, and it allows him to talk further about his feelings.

Another false reassurance situation occurs when the nurse tells the patient he can trust her. This is not particularly effective or reassuring to the patient. The nurse must demonstrate trust

and be prepared to have the patient test this before he will accept and agree that she is sincere about him as a human being and in helping him. The patient may ask, "Can I trust you?" The best response in this situation is to tell the patient that he will have to decide that for himself. That response is honest and allows the patient the option to make his own decision.

The stall warning is sounded when the nurse thinks that she is giving reassurance, and the patient does not respond. The lack of response may be one sign that the reassurance is felt to be false. Some examples of false reassurances are as follows:

"Don't worry about your illness. Think about going home."
"You will feel better tomorrow."
"Don't worry about it; everything will be fine."
"Your doctor is very good."
"Lots of people lead productive lives after such an operation."

Other warning lights flash on when you feel a strong urge to leave the room when talking with the patient, or when you hear your own words echoing as you talk, or when you hear yourself saying something that you would not want said to you.

It is normal to attempt to reduce human suffering. When a patient expresses his anxiety, the nurse will often automatically think of reassuring him. The nurse feels uncomfortable in helping the patient bear his anxieties and fears. For example, the patient says, "I am depressed. I don't want to live." At such a time it seems easier to say, "But you shouldn't feel that way. You have much to live for." These statements are false reassurances and can cause a stall. The stall is corrected by being supportive rather than reassuring. The nurse rectifies the situation by trying to understand the concept of support rather than by giving a reassuring statement.

Confrontation and Misuse of the Analytical Approach

To attempt to treat all dialogue as containing significant psychological messages having deep interpretations is not being therapeutic. People resent this intrusion and sometimes freely say, "Don't psych me out."

One reason why confronting the patient with a psychological interpretation of his behavior will lead to a stall is because it is inappropriate. For example, a patient is late for an appointment with the nurse and says, "I overslept and I am sorry I am late." The nurse then says, "You must be angry with me and not want to see me or you would have been here on time." The feeling the patient is left with is either total bewilderment or intimidation. Such a statement is not appropriate or germane to the situation. It is an interpretation of the patient's behavior that may or may not be correct. The correctness of the interpretation, however, is not the issue. These interpretations can stall the therapeutic process.

The interpretation of the patient's behavior depends on the role assumed by the helping person. In a role assumed by a staff nurse there are helpful ways of ensuring that the situation does not stall and yet the patient can begin to understand what his behavior means. For example, in the above situation a more exploratory approach to the details of the "oversleep" behavior might bring about the patient's understanding that his behavior was based on feelings about the appointment. The nurse might have responded, "Maybe it was easier to sleep through the alarm than to have to get up and come all the way over here for an appointment?" This might lead the patient in a less psychologically exposed way to be able to say that it is indeed difficult to talk to someone about painful issues.

Interpretations of behavior often are given for the shock value they impart. The manner in which they are offered may be and usually is nontherapeutic. For example, a patient is hallucinating and responding to the voices he hears by running up and down the corridor. To confront the patient with an interpretation such as, "That is crazy behavior. We don't want you to act crazy. You must stop," offers no support, understanding, or alternatives for the patient. A more helpful response might be, "I do not understand why you are running up and down. Something must be happening inside you that we do not know about. I will walk with you and see if it helps you feel better so that you can tell me what is upsetting you."

The analytical approach and use of interpretations are very important to seminar and class or staff discussion of patient behavior in trying to understand the patient. The interpretation technique is used mainly for teaching purposes and for understanding behavior—it is not to be conveyed back in an unsettling way to the patient. If interpretation technique is used during a therapy interview, it is done only after careful supervision and is generally not required as an initial nursing approach.

Currently, a large percentage of the people seeking psychotherapy are trying to understand and correlate their current day-to-day style of either relating adaptively to people or keeping people at a distance by using defense mechanisms. These ways of adapting may have less to do with early trauma than with ongoing styles of interacting. In therapy, styles have to be worked through in order to help the patient change and become more adaptive.

Often therapists will think that if the patient has an insight into his problem, he will be able to change. The insight concept, however, often works in reverse with the therapist saying, "Now I understand why the patient does such and such," but the patient does not understand. Therefore, there is no change in the way the patient behaves.

The nursing student is more helpful to the patient by staying with the here-and-now issues rather than trying to explore past history and attempting to make profound interpretations. There is no one simple reason for the illness. The patient's difficulty in living within his present existence is the issue.

Misjudging the Patient's Independence

The nurse needs to assess and evaluate how much to do for the patient and how much he should do for himself. The stall developing from infantilizing a patient occurs when he tries to exert his freedom and prove to you he can do something. He says, "See, I can go to the bathroom by myself. I don't need the bedpan." Then he gets out of bed when he is supposed to remain on bed rest. This behavior is a stall in the therapeutic process.

The patient may try to prove his point by leaving the hospital without permission simply because he was not allowed to go home for the weekend and is angry about the restriction because he felt he could handle the visit. It may be antitherapeutic to punish the patient for this behavior, and a better solution would be to reconsider the patient's request and reevaluate his independence.

The corrective measure is to try not to be oppressive in dealing with the patient when he has overridden the restriction placed on him.

The nurse may have to acknowledge that the situation was misjudged and asks the patient what he can do for himself. Or it may be the reverse. The patient tries to go beyond his limits and finds he still needs help from the nurse. For example, a patient may try walking after surgery, feeling he does not need the nurse, but may find after ten steps that he has to sit down. He has overestimated his capacities.

The stall warning is present when the nurse fails to ask the patient what he can do for himself and she assumes that she knows his limitations. This kind of clinical judgment is not helpful to the patient.

Similarly, as the nurse assesses what the patient can do, the issue of assessing how the family can deal with its own problems is important. For example, the patient may ask to have a phone call made for him or request the staff to tell his wife something. A member of the family may call the nurse's station to say that an uncle has died and will someone please tell the patient. The nurse must remember that these are family matters and that it is the family's and the patient's responsibility, not hers. The family should tell the patient unless it has been decided that the family is unable to handle that responsibility.

Doing anything more for the patient than he could do for himself is infantilizing, and anything less is withholding. For example, if a child wants to walk and he is carried, he will resent it. If the child has walked some distance and he is forced to keep walking, that is cruel and negative to his development. A good rule to follow is to do for the patient and family only what they cannot do for themselves. This protects against infantilizing.

Labeling the Patient

Labeling the patient instead of describing the patient's behavior dehumanizes the person. It is a singular way of not wanting to see the patient as a real, suffering person. To label a patient usually implies that the patient bothers the nurse and she has not autognosed her own feelings.

Labeling may be a result of patient requests, for example, "That cranky old man in room 407 who is always complaining now wants another cup of coffee." Or the labeling may refer to the patient's illness, for example, "The appendectomy wants to get out of bed today."

In psychiatric nursing the problem of labeling may be a troublesome area even for seasoned staff. This involves talking about people in terms of their ego control, their delusions, or their schizophrenia. The staff may say, "He is just a manipulator," or "He is just acting out," or "She is just a hysteric." Almost all labeling is preceded by the cliché "He is just a. . . ." This does not describe the patient as an individual who happens to be dealing with an episode of mental illness in his life.

Another stall involving labeling occurs when the statement is made, "The patient is not motivated for therapy." This may often be a way for the therapist to justify his failure to elicit a therapeutic response in the patient. Instead of admitting that he is partly responsible for the failure, the therapist blames the patient for not "being motivated."

Labeling may be a defense mechanism for the nurse. The labeling may occur when it is too difficult to see the person as a human being because his suffering is so great. For example, the nurse may think, "I don't want to think of Mrs. Jones as a person because she is about to die. It is easier to call her the cancer patient in room 389."

The corrective measure to the stall would be for the nurse to acknowledge her feelings and be painfully honest in her reaction. If the nurse does not like a patient, she should admit it to herself, and she should not call the patient a name. She must admit to herself, at least, that the patient makes her uneasy.

Labeling is sometimes done in the service of diagnosis. However, it is important to remember that a psychiatric diagnosis accounts for only a small percentage of the patient's behavior. Labeling sometimes seems to convince people that they know more about the patient than they really do. Labeling seems to make the professional feel better, as though he understands the situation better. If nurses do not have to label a patient, they are then free to see the patient as a real human being in distress. This view facilitates the therapeutic process.

Overidentification with the Problem

Overidentification with the patient and his problems is another human reaction of staff and beginning students that brings about a stall. For example, the patient will tell about his belligerent wife and the student agrees with him and says, "I know how mean she can be." The student then continues to see the patient as the victim of his unsatisfactory marriage. The student fails to see that the patient chose the wife in the first place and that the cruelty displayed in the marriage may be equally shared. One often hears a similar story when listening to a family complain about an alcoholic father. The family says, "Everything is his fault and is his problem. If he didn't drink, things would be just fine." They fail to realize the importance of their role in the situation. A patient simply does not live in a vacuum.

Overidentification with the patient's problem leads to a stall when the therapist says, "I understand your problem," or "That's not really a problem," or "I know what it is like." When you say, or even imply, these things, the nurse then becomes a sympathetic person and stops being a nurse. The patient feels that although it is nice to have someone sympathetic, he also needs someone who can provide a different perspective to the problem. If you cannot give him a new perspective, you have nothing to offer. Once you tell the patient that you agree with him, he may like you, but he is then convinced that there is nothing new to be learned and there is no more therapy taking place. Here there will be a stall.

The warning light is on when nurses cannot understand why a patient is in the hospital, or when they do not see that the patient has any problems, or when they feel too sympathetic to what the patient is describing.

To remedy the stall, the nurse must talk over the patient's vital part of his problem. The nurse can be therapeutic only by helping the patient look at the problem from all sides.

Nontherapeutic Involvement

Negative involvement means becoming involved with the patient in a non-nurse way. To feel that one can be the patient's mother, father, sister, brother, lover, or friend is nontherapeutic. Beginning students often face this dilemma when they say to the patient that they want to be a friend. This statement presents multitudinous problems.

It is often easier to assume a role one already knows than to work at learning a new one. The beginners in psychiatric nursing may not be convinced that they can be therapeutic. They feel that at least they can offer friendship. However, it is one thing to be friendly and another to be a friend. Nurses may want to be friends because they feel they cannot be therapeutic in any other way. As nurses develop therapeutic skills and more expertise, they learn how to put limits on friendships in order to be therapeutic.

The stall occurs when the nurse is the friend or buddy of the patient and she is no longer the nurse. If the patient does not have a nurse, he no longer has anyone to help him. By definition, the nurse ceases to be the professional. The patient may need a friend and he may ask the nurse to be his friend. He can, however, find a friend more easily than he can find someone who can offer professional help, which is why he is in the hospital or has come to the clinic.

A friend is someone with whom you maintain contact and to whom you may turn at any given time. The feeling of mutual reliance and comradeship is usually present and evident. However, to talk with the patient about one's personal life and its vicissitudes is not therapeutic for the patient and is strictly within the realm of social conversation. This limit to the relationship does not mean that the patient should know nothing about the nurse, for this would be equally unreal to the relationship. The same phenomenon may occur in the parent–child relationship in which the mother feels that it is modern and beneficial to be a friend as well as a parent to her child. Almost all children find it difficult to listen to parents' problems or to know how to relate to them. Children want parents to be parents. Patients want professionals to be professionals.

An example of nontherapeutic involvement was evident at one mental health clinic where many hippies came for help. The doctor felt that he should be like them in order to relate to them better. He removed his tie, grew long hair, and used the language of this group. The hippies became angry because they wanted the professional to be professional, and they did not want someone resembling their own group. That is why they came to the clinic.

Once the helping person abdicates the therapeutic role, the therapy stalls. Correcting the stall means developing therapeutic skills so that the nurse realizes the actual power she has as a nurse and as a therapeutic person.

A good rule of thumb to follow is to discuss with the patient only those facts regarding one's personal life that are public knowledge. Nurses who tell a patient they want to be a friend promise many things that they will be unable to fulfill. Do not try to provide something that the person can find elsewhere.

There are other examples of nontherapeutic involvements. For instance, to call the patient at home about something that is not concerned with a goal-oriented issue or to accept a patient's invitation for a social evening is to develop a personal social relationship that is nontherapeutic. Or, patients will deny the reality of the hospital setting and will blurt out this feeling during their interaction with the staff. To go along with this denial is not therapeutic.

Being honest and telling it straight are important therapeutic techniques, especially concerning role-appropriate attitudes and behavior. For example, it is natural for some patients to want to relate to the nurse in a non-role-appropriate manner, and they will ask such questions as, "Would you date me?" or "Could I have your phone number?" This frequently happens with young people and should be dealt with as a therapeutic issue, not as a social request.

It is important to make it clear that the relationship is a nurse–patient one and to define the limits of the relationship. When the patient makes such requests as wanting to see the nurse on off-duty time or after the psychiatric nursing experience ends, the nurse sometimes has to say that there are some difficult feelings to bear when relationships end.

Dealing with the patient's wishes to have a nonprofessional relationship by saying to the patient, "If you weren't a patient, I would give you my phone number," is another stall to avoid, for a week later the patient may be discharged from the hospital and he may then phone for a date. By not dealing with the reality initially, a more complicated scene may develop. The question becomes, What can the nurse now deliver to the patient and what has she promised? A better solution to that original situation would have been to have autognosed one's reaction initially and to have brought it up for discussion with staff members, the instructor, or supervisor. If one is unable to step back to view the situation clearly, others may be able to help.

The patient is in the hospital because he is genuinely ill. His illness is serious, and the nurse must be serious about therapeutic involvement. As long as her actions and words make clinical sense, the involvement is therapeutic.

Inability to Help Bear Painful Feelings

The inability to help bear the painful feelings of another person can lead to a stall. Nurses may feel so helpless or angry or incompetent that they wonder if they can be of help. They feel drained, as though they have nothing more to give, and consequently they withdraw. The warning of the potential stall comes when they feel that they want to withdraw.

The corrective approach to this stall is for the nurse to autognose the feelings of anger and helplessness and then to look calmly at how the patient's pathology fits into the situation.

In the general hospital setting, this stall in patient care is often seen when a nurse is nursing the dying patient. The staff feel so uncomfortable and inadequate in helping the patient with the dying process that they isolate the patient and withdraw to allow him to die alone.

An example in the psychiatric setting illustrates how difficult it is to tolerate the feelings of anger that a patient expresses as she yells and screams at a nursing student:

A nursing student was assigned to talk with April, a 29-year-old airline hostess who had been hospitalized for a three-month history of drug abuse and depression. The student entered her room and immediately had the impression of being backstage in an actress's dressing room. Perfume hung in the air; clothes and makeup were strewn everywhere. The student introduced herself and asked to talk with April about her hospitalization. April carefully looked the student over, threw her head back, and laughing loudly said, "Now I've heard everything. I'm assigned to a little student nurse who looks twelve years old and wet behind the ears. I'm supposed to tell you my problems. That is ridiculous. Get out of here, little Miss Nightingale." With that, April started to yell, grabbed a book, and threw it at the student.

Needless to say, this patient's behavior is not the kind that produces a cordial therapeutic nurse–patient relationship. The important step to be taken here is to learn how to accept and adjust one's own feelings when the patient's behavior is so upsetting and obnoxious.

One suggestion is to talk out these feelings with other people. This particular situation would be handled best at a staff or nursing report meeting to see what reaction other staff members were receiving. This collaboration will indicate how much of a pattern there is to this woman's behavior.

Bearing painful feelings is a difficult task,

but it can be one of the strongest aspects of facilitating the therapeutic process.

Being Dishonest

Being dishonest with the patient is a subtle and often unintentional act by the staff. Insufficient regard for this concept of honesty in a relationship may stall the therapeutic process.

If the patient feels that the nurse is not being honest with him, he simply will not trust her, and without trust there is no therapy. This is a stall. In order to correct the stall, the nurse may have to discuss the situation with the patient again and admit that she was wrong. If the nurse knows that she has done something dishonest to the patient and the patient withdraws, she should then assume that she has stalled.

Situations having stall potential of this kind are the following:

Failure to Keep a Promise
The nurse promises something to the patient and then fails to meet the promise. For example, setting an appointment hour and not being punctual or saying that she will get a certain medication and then not coming back with it may imply to the patient that the nurse is untrustworthy. A response such as telling the patient that everything will be all right when it won't be or telling him that he will be better in a certain length of time is dishonest.

Not Answering Truthfully
The nurse does not answer a simple, direct question truthfully. The patient may ask if the nurse is angry or upset. He is asking directly and openly about a feeling he thinks she has. If she immediately denies this when she is really angry, this may tell the patient that she is not always truthful. This may confuse him and increase his anxiety about his judgment of people's emotions. Do not forget that facial expression, tone of voice, and gestures may say more than words, and they can be interpreted by the patient as accurately as by anyone else.

If the patient asks the nurse if she is bored, she may feel she does not want to answer directly that she is. She might say, "Sometimes I feel you are trying to bore me." There are subtle yet effective ways of dealing with the honest answers to patients.

The various responses that can be made are more thoroughly discussed in Chapter 15. If students are to be at all adept in human relationships, they must treat patients with as much respect as family and friends are treated. In other words, one simply does not blurt out to friends such immediate responses as, "I don't like you when you stay in your room all day," or "You make me angry when you pout like that." Children are prone to tell friends they are "stupid" or "dumb" when the friends have hurt them or made them angry. This is a defensive mechanism with the child. It is neither kind nor respectful. If negative comments are felt appropriate, they are usually best stated in terms of the behavior that is annoying. Here, tact, common sense, and diplomacy are needed, and bluntness and dishonesty should be avoided. Treat your patient as you would want to be treated at all times.

Omission
The nurse is dishonest by omission. If the nurse neglects to tell a patient of conversation that she had with his family, it may prove difficult to handle when the patient finds out about it. And the patient inevitably does. This situation may be compared to the academic situation in which a previous instructor talks with a current instructor about a student's performance. The student usually finds out and inevitably has feelings about it.

Pitfalls in Listening

After one has attempted to listen, it should be helpful to review the following pitfalls involved in listening that may lead to a stall situation:

Being Too Verbal
The nurse becomes so verbal during the interview that she forgets to listen. The patient begins to think that the nurse is thinking ahead about what should be said next, rather than listening to his present thoughts. He thinks that the nurse would rather hear herself talk, and thus the therapy stalls. In psychiatric nursing, one needs to understand and distinguish between being therapeutically active and being therapeutically passive. The nursing student often has difficulty in developing the skill of becoming therapeutically passive in the interview situation. "Passive" in this case does not mean to imply "doing nothing," but rather denotes

being mentally alert and active. This process implies having an open mind and being able to absorb verbal meaning by listening attentively and with eager understanding.

Giving Advice

A second pitfall to avoid in listening is that the nurse may become involved in making decisions or giving advice to the patient. Not all advice leads to making decisions for patients, but some does. The stall in the therapeutic process is that once the nurse gives advice or makes a decision for a patient, she is taking away the patient's opportunity to do something for himself. She is taking away the therapeutic process. The potential for the stall to lead to a permanent block in the therapy is there if the nurse gives the advice or makes the decision. There isn't much that she can do to correct the stall at this point except to hope that the patient is similar to most people and will not take her advice. For example, a nursing student wonders about her decision to become a nurse and says to a friend, "I don't know if I want to continue studying to be a nurse." It would be defeating to have her friend respond with, "Of course you do. It is helping people. You should not change your mind." This does not at all agree with the student's feelings at the time. She is seeking help in thinking through her own thoughts in order to work out the problem. She does not want someone else to tell her what she should do.

Another situation illustrates how giving advice can be antitherapeutic. Almost all people have felt troubled or upset at times and have tried to seek out a friend for solace and understanding. When the friend interrupts what he is being told and prematurely gives advice, the person probably becomes annoyed, for what he really means is, "Be quiet and listen to me. I have something to tell you and please be a good listener." This wanting to be listened to is what the person in distress is attempting to tell the friend. Dominating the conversation rather than encouraging the dialogue is not helpful. Sometimes people will say, "Give us some advice," but what they really want to hear is what the other person thinks about the situation. Too often people get caught saying, "Why don't you do this and this?" or "Shouldn't you have tried such and such?"

For example, a student fails a test and thinks that she may not pass the course because of this. She seeks out a friend with whom to express her distress. When the student says, "I feel like I'll never get my R.N.," the friend may respond, "You shouldn't feel that way." The student may feel angry because she wanted to be listened to and not told what to feel. She really does not want advice because people do not generally take advice. The helping person may make some suggestions, but the student will make the decision and feel that it was a positive step for her, rather than feeling that it was someone's advice.

Giving advice may be used as a maneuver by the nurse in order to control the patient. The patient may feel that he has to please the nurse and will act out of compliance, but, of course, almost all people react negatively to this type of control.

Indifference

The nurse can stall the interview by responding in an indifferent manner and by presenting a bored appearance—faking attention, avoiding eye-to-eye contact, interrupting, and frequently requesting the patient to repeat what he has said. The stall warning occurs when the nurse finds herself becoming bored, at which point she must stop to autognose in order to determine who is producing the apathetic response—herself or the patient. One possible correction of this stall is for her to listen carefully to the patient in order to determine whether or not he is deliberately trying to bore her.

Emotionally Charged Words

The use of emotionally charged words in the course of the dialogue may stall the interview. Introducing a word that the patient cannot tolerate can quickly induce the stall. For example:

PATIENT: My mother is always complaining and picking at me for not getting up in time or for not cleaning my room.

NURSE: Your mother makes you pretty angry.

PATIENT: She is a wonderful person and she always tells me how she loves me. Oh, I have to finish that letter I was writing when you came in. . . .

This example points out the sensitivity of the patient to the word *angry*. If the nurse had chosen a less emotionally charged word, the patient might have continued expressing his feeling.

Some patients can talk about feeling uncomfortable about or displeased with their negative feelings, but others find the use of the words *anger* and *guilt* upsetting if they are used before they have said them themselves. Part of the skill in listening to the patient is in using low-keyed words such as *upsetting* or *uncomfortable* or to simply ask, "How did you feel about what she did?" When the patient feels comfortable and more familiar with his own feelings, he will choose his own words to illustrate his feelings. Once the patient has used a word, it is helpful to use that word back to him.

Another example in which the patient became verbally angry occurred when a psychiatric resident physician was interviewing a male patient. The man said, "My wife is hallucinating and she even managed to get herself admitted to a hospital." The resident said, "How long has she been acting crazy?" The patient yelled back, "My family isn't crazy. What do you mean?"

Sometimes the stall can actually be seen developing when the patient cringes or blanches when a particular word is used. The corrective remedy is to become adept at only using words that the patient first uses.

Changing the Subject

If the nurse changes the subject during the interview, the patient will think that the nurse really cannot stand to hear what he wants to say. If she cannot stand to hear what he wants to say, then the therapy is in a stall because she is not talking about what is important to the patient. The stall warning appears as the nurse observes the patient disengaging from the conversation. This phenomenon may also be observed through reviewing process recording notes or in supervision. To correct the stall the nurse might try to find out why she cannot bear to hear what the patient is saying. She might ask herself what unbearable feelings she has that prompt her to change the subject. It is therapeutic to stay with the issue that the patient introduces.

Repetition

When the patient feels he is not being understood, he will keep repeating the same complaint or request. Repetition means that he is not being understood, and this creates a stall. Correcting the stall means paying strict attention and listening carefully to what the patient is saying. There are three kinds of understanding: First, there is the distinct understanding of what

a person is really talking about. The person is clear about the issue, his feelings, and actions. What he says can be clearly understood.

Second, there is the understanding that requires discussion until there is satisfaction with the explanation. For example, a patient complained of a headache and kept requesting medication for this symptom. Repeatedly aspirin medication was used by the patient until the nurse finally decided to explore further the nature of the headache in order to determine why there was no relief. It turned out that the headaches were voices talking to the patient in a disparaging manner, and they were causing her great distress. The medication was not effective in relieving this kind of headache.

Third, there is the understanding that requires listening between the lines for the indirectly expressed messages. The listener must try to get a clear picture from the message. For example:

A woman called her doctor at 5 A.M. and said to him, "I have nothing to do today." The doctor was angry at her for calling at that hour and quickly terminated the conversation. Since she had never done this before nor spoken like that before, it became clear to him that another message was being given. The doctor checked into the situation and found out that her father had just died. She had devoted her days to taking care of him. She was trying to tell the doctor that her father had just died, but what came out was that she had nothing to do that day.

The point to be made here is that when a message does not seem clear, it may be helpful to keep working on what one thinks the person is really trying to say. When you feel something is not right, you are prompted to investigate further. The clearer the message from the sender, the greater the therapeutic stance that can be taken.

Stalls in Eliciting the Patient's Request

There is apt to be a great deal of wasted time and energy during an interview in which the patient request is verbalized either late in the interview or not at all. Instead of speaking freely about the problem, the patient may be preoccupied, wondering whether the nurse is kind enough, respectful enough, wise enough, understanding enough, and flexible enough to hear the request. "When will the nurse be ready to hear? When will I have the guts to come right out with it?'' The nurse, meanwhile, often unaware of these concerns, goes about the business of establishing nursing care plans, not understanding why the patient participates only reluctantly during the interview. On the other hand, when the patient has stated the request early in the interview and feels it has been supportively heard, he is apt to participate more freely and feel more satisfied at the end of the interview.

Listed below are two situations in which the nurse may stall the process of eliciting the request.

1. Changing the subject. The nurse may unwittingly discourage the patient from stating his request by changing the subject after the patient has hinted at the request.

2. The request elicited too late in the interview. The patient may feel there is no opening till the end of the interview: "By the way, would you . . . ?" Or the patient comes to a medical clinic for a general examination, and, as he is ready to leave the office, states the real request: "Please tell me if I have cancer." Had the patient made the request earlier and had the nurse perceived the request as legitimate and important, the nurse might have explored the reasons for the patient's concern and learned what kind of explanation would be most appropriate.

In many clinical situations, acknowledging the request or giving the patient what he asks for satisfies needs that must be met before a second request can be made. In cases of sexual assault, for example, the victim very often has a medical request upon entry to the emergency ward. Once reassured of her medical condition in terms of treatment of physical trauma, wounds, and prevention of venereal disease or pregnancy, the victim then makes a request for psychological assistance: "I keep thinking about the attack. Help me get rid of these thoughts." This statement illustrates the progressive aspect to the patient's request: that is, as a request is met, the patient progresses in her attempt to regain psychological equilibrium.

It is not uncommon for the request to be appropriate but not sufficient. For example, the patient who wants to talk out his fears and concerns about a chronic medical illness may also need referral for diagnostic tests. Or there are situations where the request is clinically appropriate but not clinically feasible because of the treatment facility. This dilemma should be stated directly and honestly to the patient. At least the patient has received clinical confirmation of what he wishes and can be referred elsewhere if necessary.

INTERVIEWING TECHNIQUES THAT AID AND ONES THAT STALL

Helping a person to talk freely depends on how clearly questions are phrased, what kinds of verbal responses are given, and how silences are used. The nurse's therapeutic use of self and patient-centered interactions enhance the individual's ability to explore his problems. These areas will be discussed in greater detail in order to help nurses improve their interviewing skills.

Use of Questions

As we have already discussed, questions are an important part of the interview. How they are phrased is crucial. One must be aware that questions can at times be inappropriate and irritating, and can, in fact, close or block the discussion. Therefore, the nurse should be familiar with the use of questions and should know when it is appropriate to refrain from asking them.

The questions that are most useful in an interview involve the use of *who, what, when*, and *where*. Such questions allow both patient and nurse to further explore what has been said. When questions are used appropriately, the patient will feel that the nurse is interested in him and will be less likely to have the threatened feeling of being given the "third degree."

An example might be useful at this time. A patient is explaining that his mother sent him to the hospital. The nurse needs further information before she can assess the situation:

NURSE: What happened just before you came to the hospital?
PATIENT: My mother got real mad and called the police.
NURSE: What happened between the two of you just before she called the police?
PATIENT: We were fighting about my girl friend.
NURSE: Tell me more about the fight.
PATIENT: Jane was standing there and my mother screamed at her to leave me alone.
NURSE: Who is Jane?
PATIENT: My girl friend.

NURSE: Who else was present?
PATIENT: No one.
NURSE: Where were you when the argument started?
PATIENT: At my mother's. Jane came to pick me up to go for a ride.

In this situation, the nurse effectively uses questions to explore exactly what happened before the patient's mother called the police. She would follow with other questions that would give her more data about the incident. It would be helpful to know what the patient did when his mother demanded that Jane leave, and also what Jane did.

Closed versus Open Questions
Asking a question that can be answered by *yes* or *no* is undesirable because it elicits very little information and blocks the flow of conversation. Questions that start with *do, would, could, can, were, was,* and *are* will often limit the patient to a nod of the head or a monosyllable. Some examples follow:

STUDENT: Do you like it here?
PATIENT: Yes.
STUDENT: Are you ready to talk today?
PATIENT: No.
STUDENT: Would you like a weekend pass?
PATIENT: Yes.

Compare these questions to those that follow: "What do you think about being here?" "It's time for our talk. Where shall we sit?" "What would you like to do on a weekend pass?" These questions invite discussion of thoughts about what was asked.

Double-Edged and Double-Barreled Questions
The double-edged and double-barreled questions are often used when the interviewer's anxiety level increases, or when she is expecting or wanting a specific answer to a question. A double-edged question is one that invites a predetermined answer. For example, "You don't mind if I sit by you, do you?" or, "You didn't spill these ashes, did you?" These questions are blocks in communication because they have a "built-in" response that the patient is hard pressed to ignore.

The double-barreled question is the asking of two questions at once. The patient will be confused about which question he should an-

swer. Examples of this type of question are: "Do you want to stay here or go home?" "Are you living with your mother or alone?" It is better to ask one question at a time in order to reduce confusion for the patient and for yourself.

Bombardment
Bombarding the patient with questions occurs usually when the nurse's anxiety level increases because of a silent or very quiet patient. The patient usually responds with even less verbal content when he is bombarded with questions. Here is an example:

NURSE: I notice you are rather quiet today.
PATIENT: [Shakes head in affirmative.]
NURSE: Is something bothering you?
PATIENT: [No response.]
NURSE: Why are you not answering me?
PATIENT: [Pulls back in his chair.]
NURSE: It's always better to talk about your problems. Now, tell me what's bothering you?
PATIENT: [Gets up and leaves room.]

In this situation as the patient shows less and less verbal response, the nurse becomes more demanding. As a result of her demanding verbal responses, the patient removes himself from the interaction. The nurse would have been more effective to sit silently following her question, "Is something bothering you?" The silence would have allowed the patient time to collect his thoughts and share those feelings that were important to him.

Probing Questions
Questions that begin with *how* or *why* are very seldom useful in a therapeutic interaction. These questions are often viewed by the patient as threatening, and he will be unlikely to give adequate answers. "How do you feel about your wife?" "Your family?" "Your job?" are difficult questions to answer. Students would do well to incorporate early in their interviewing the question, "What do you think about . . . ?" to replace, "How do you feel?" The patient will be more likely to tell you what he thinks in response to the former question than the latter, and will often incorporate how he feels in his answer.

Why questions are usually questions that put the patient on the defensive. "Why were you late for the interview?" immediately tells the patient that he's in trouble. Better to say,

"What has been happening with you?" This gives the patient a chance to discuss the reasons for his being late.

Some answers to questions will tend to incriminate or embarrass the patient. For example, the patient may think that his answers to such questions as, "Do you love your mother?" or, "Do you beat your wife?" may be damaging to himself. The interviewer can learn much more by asking, "What is it like between you and your wife?" and, "What do you think about your mother?"

Other Considerations

Along with bombardment of the patient with questions, one should consider *irrelevant* questions. Irrelevant questions are those questions asked a patient that either change the subject abruptly or seek information that is unimportant in the context of the patient interaction. Some examples may be helpful:

> PATIENT: I'm worried about going home.
> NURSE: How many children do you have?

Although the part of having children at home may be somewhat relevant, the number of children is immaterial. The patient is expressing a general concern of worry, and the nurse needs more information about his discomfort. The nurse would have been more in tune with the patient to ask, "What worries you about going home?" Take another example:

> PATIENT: Sometimes I feel very depressed and think about just giving up.
> NURSE: Tell me about your mother.

Here the nurse abruptly changes the subject to a "safer" topic for herself. It would be more helpful to the patient to find out what he means by saying "just giving up."

The *timing* of questions is important. The more positive the relationship, the wider the range of questions one may ask. Talking with the patient about a painful or sensitive issue (for example, previous failures) is more likely to be fruitful during the fourth interview than during the second. The patient should have the opportunity to move at his own pace, and the nurse should not bring up an issue prematurely by asking probing questions, even though they seem important at the time.

A *direct approach* is useful when there is se-rious concern over the patient's ability to control his behavior. The patient may have to be asked directly whether or not he is having suicidal thoughts. The psychotic patient may have to be asked how troublesome the voices are or what the voices are saying. The impulsive patient may have to be asked how much control he has and how much freedom he can handle without getting into difficulties with drugs or with the police.

In conclusion, how questions are phrased can add considerable mileage to the freedom the patient feels as he expresses himself. The nurse should think about what important issues there are to discuss with the patient and try to have the questions phrased as clearly and as simply as possible.

Verbal Responses

Certain responses to patients will elicit the therapeutic gains at which the nurse aims. Highest priority should be given to responses that bring about understanding. We have already discussed the positive benefits that are derived when one feels understood.

In addition to questioning, certain types of verbal responses can be used to help the patient talk more freely. These verbal responses give the patient a sense of being accepted and listened to. As nurses become more proficient in interviewing, they develop the ability to use these responses at the appropriate time and are able to evaluate the effectiveness of their response.

Useful Responses

Since there is often some difficulty in determining what response should be made in a given situation, the nurse must continually evaluate what the patient is trying to convey. Clarification of any parts of the conversation that puzzle her is essential. Listed in Table 17-1 are some types of verbal responses that may be useful. Although these are not the only appropriate types of responses to use, they will give the beginning interviewer a sense of accomplishment once they are mastered.

A word should be said about *reflection* as a strategy in interviewing. Instead of the nurse simply repeating a phrase or expression the patient has just used, it is usually more helpful to restate in slightly different words what has been said if clarification is necessary. Using

TABLE 17-1. USEFUL RESPONSES

Category	Example
Recognition	"I'm Jane Smith, a student nurse. What is your name?" "You have a new dress?"
Observation	"You look tense today." "I noticed that you haven't been sleeping. . . ."
General leads	"Tell me . . ." "Talk more about . . ." "Go on . . ."
Broad openings	"Start at the beginning. . . ." "What is happening with you?"
Restating	"You are smoking more than usual."
Refocusing	"Go back and talk more about . . ." "You were talking about . . ."
Exploration	"Describe in detail . . ." "What happened first?"
Validation	"Are you saying . . . ?" "Did I understand you to say . . . ?"
Focusing	"Talk more about . . ." "Tell me about . . ."
Clarification	"You say you love your wife. What does love mean to you?" "Do you mean . . . ?"
Summarization	"You seem to have talked today about . . ." "You seem to be saying . . ."

other words that approximate what was said by the patient helps the nurse validate that she has understood what has been said. For example, if the patient says, "I hate to go to work," and the nurse replies, "You hate to go to work," no new information has been requested. The nurse has no more understanding of the statement made, and the patient is likely to give no new information. It would be more helpful in this situation to reply, "What is it that you hate about your work?"

Responding to Patient Questions

There will be times when the patient attempts to turn the discussion into a nurse-centered interaction. The patient will try to change the focus of the discussion by asking the nurse a question. When the patient asks the nurse a question, the nurse is likely to become uncomfortable. After all, the nurse thinks she should be asking the questions. Often the nursing student has difficulty deciding on an appropriate reply.

The type of questions that the patient asks will vary from patient to patient. Some patients will ask about the nurse's personal life. For example, he might ask, "Do you ever fight with your husband?" "Where do you live?" "Have you ever taken drugs?" It is a good plan to turn the question back to the patient. "You wonder how I get along with my family? I'm wondering what prompted that question." It is more helpful to suggest talking about the issue than to give an answer. It is doubtful that patients really want an answer. Their curiosity about the nurse as an individual may just be uppermost in their mind at the moment, or the question to the nurse may be an attempt to avoid the issue. Answering personal questions, or treating the content of the questions rather than seeing these as part of the developing relationship, would be turning the nursing and therapeutic situation into a social exchange. Patients can talk this way with friends and acquaintances. Remember that the patient needs the nurse primarily as a nurse, not a friend.

When a patient asks a direct question about his condition, it is important to start by knowing how much information the patient has and what prompted the question in the first place. The nurse could respond with, "That was an abrupt question to ask. Tell me what you have been thinking of to cause you to ask that?" Telling the patient that it would help to look at and explore his thoughts and feelings about the issues defines the therapeutic role and does not place the nurse in an uncomfortable role.

Nurses need not feel guilty over not answering specific questions that the patient asks, any more than the nurse should feel she is expected to give advice. The patient will benefit greatly if he has to make his own decisions and resolve his own questions that relate to his life. The questions that nurses should answer are those questions that apply to them directly; for example, "Are you angry?" or, "Are you busy?" The nurse should answer questions about her own behavior simply and honestly.

Nonuseful Responses

Just as there are helpful responses that provide the opportunity for greater verbal exchange,

TABLE 17-2. NONUSEFUL RESPONSES

Category	Example
Reassurance	"Don't worry." "Everything will be all right." "You look 100% better."
Rejection	"I don't like it when you . . ." "Don't talk about . . ."
Agreement	"You did the right thing." "I don't blame you at all."
Probing	"I want to hear more about . . ." "You should tell me about . . ."
Defensive	"We have good doctors here." "You are locked in for your own good."
Advice	"What you should do is . . ." "Why don't you . . . ?"
Clichés	"How are you today?" "Keeping busy makes you feel better." "Nice day today."
Belittling	"Everybody feels that way." "You shouldn't act that way."

there are some responses that stall the communication process. These nonuseful responses frequently occur as a spontaneous reaction to our own increased anxiety or because we simply don't know what to say. When the student nurse feels the need to reassure, advise, defend, etc., she should quickly look at what is happening within herself. These responses are usually used to meet one's own needs. They are not helpful in a therapeutic situation. Table 17-2 gives some of the commonly used nonuseful responses.

Although these groups of responses are not by any means complete, they should give the beginning student some idea about ways to respond either appropriately or inappropriately. Rather than using reassurances or advice, it is more important to discuss with the patient the details surrounding a given problem. For example, a patient might say, "I hate this hospital." The student's first inclination is to defend by responding, "People here are trying to help you." A more useful response for the patient would be, "What do you dislike most about being here?" The first response closes communication, whereas the second allows the patient to explore what he dislikes about the hospital.

Nonverbal Behavior

It should be remembered that while the nurse and patient are exchanging verbal responses, they are also looking and listening for nonverbal cues about what is being said. For example, the patient may say, "I see I've made you angry." The nurse may reply, "No, I'm not angry," but her tone of voice, flushed face, and the whirl of her body as she moves away from the patient say a great deal more than her words. Her denial only confuses the patient and provides incorrect feedback for his perception of her feelings. A much more truthful response might have been, "Yes, you did make me angry, but there are other reasons for my being angry that aren't part of this conversation." Here, the patient gets a sense that, yes, he did correctly perceive the nurse's anger, but that he is not the sole cause of her disgruntled feelings.

The tone of voice used tells the patient or nurse a great deal about what the feeling is below the surface. The nurse may say, "You cannot touch me," in many ways. A high-pitched voice tone with rapid discharge of words shows the patient that the nurse is anxious, angry, or feeling threatened. But a calm voice with an evenly spoken sentence simply sets a limit. The patient is more likely to ignore the first statement than the last. If the nurse shows nonverbally that she is in control, the patient will be more likely to gain control of his impulse to touch.

The expression on an individual's face, his body movement, and his posture give important clues about what is being felt. For example, does the patient smile when he says he is feeling sad? Does he twist his hands and yet say he's feeling quite relaxed? Does he sit slumped in a chair and ignore the activity going on around him? These behaviors tell a great deal about what the patient is experiencing and needing to deny.

As the nurse looks at nonverbal behavior, she begins to sense what the patient's true feelings are. When the patient uses denial, the incongruency of what is said and what is observed should be gently pointed out to the patient. An example may be helpful:

PATIENT: I really don't feel anything for my husband anymore. He just doesn't mean much to me. [Tears in eyes and sad expression as she is saying this.]

NURSE: [pause] I notice you look sad when you say you don't feel anything for your husband. It must be a little difficult to sort out all the feelings you have about him.

PATIENT: [thoughtful] Yes, I guess your're right. Sometimes I hate him, sometimes I love him, and sometimes I think I really couldn't care less.

In this situation, the nurse points out to the patient the incongruity of her words and facial expression. She then helps the patient explore her true feelings about her husband. The nurse's response indicates to the patient that she is aware of the painful aspects of the situation the patient explores. By her softened tone of voice, her slight movement toward the patient, and the expression of concern on her face, the nurse tells the patient nonverbally that she does understand her pain. Of course, this type of interaction would usually take place after the individuals have come to know each other, and mutual trust and respect have been established.

In summary, the nonverbal responses of the patient and the nurse play an important role in the one-to-one relationship. By looking at her own as well as the patient's voice tone, body movement, and posture, the nurse can gain another dimension of understanding of what the two of them convey to each other.

Using Silences

Silences may be awkward to handle for the beginning student. There are generally four types of silence that develop in interviews. They are: the reflective silence, the silence of confusion, the disturbed silence, and the resistive silence.

Reflective Silence. The reflective or thoughtful silence is useful to collect thoughts and determine what should be said next. This type of silence can be used as an ally and a positive reinforcement for your work with the patient. Let the patient break this type of silence. It is wise to allow at least one or two silences to develop during an interview. Usually after a reflective silence the patient will share some significant information. In the beginning the student will feel that a minute silence is very long. However, the more comfortable the student becomes with reflective silence, the more productive her work

with the patient will be. Both the patient and student can use the silence to assess what has been said and decide what should be discussed further.

Confused Silence. Occasionally, there will be a silence that indicates confusion. The student may have inadvertently made a statement or asked a question that the patient does not understand. Or sometimes the student will be confused about what the patient has said. These silences should not be prolonged. As soon as the student understands that either she or the patient is confused, she should intervene with a statement to clarify the issue. For example, she might say, "I think I didn't follow what you just said," or, "You look puzzled. What questions do you have?" This type of silence usually becomes more confused and uncomfortable the longer it lasts.

Disturbed Silence. A third type of silence that occurs in interviews is the disturbed silence. In this silence, the patient or student senses that the silence is neither a comfortable nor thoughtful one. When the patient has grown silent and looks uncomfortable, the student could say, "You seem to be having trouble talking about what's on your mind," or, "What are your thoughts now?" These statements will give the patient a means of continuing the discussion. When the silence indicates unexpressed feelings such as anger or distrust, the nurse could say, "I sense that what I said has upset you." As soon as the student ascertains that the silence is not a comfortable one for the patient, she should help him talk about the reasons for the silence.

Resistive Silence. The final type of silence to be discussed here is the resistive silence. This type of silence almost always occurs sometime during the working phase of a relationship, but it may occur at other points in the relationship as well. This silence results when the patient for some reason decides that he will no longer talk with the student. Usually this type of silence is the result of anger on the patient's part or his need to control the interviewer.

When this silence occurs, it frequently evokes anger from the interviewer, and, in a sense, allows the patient to gain the control he wants. Angry thoughts the student may have include, "If he doesn't want to talk to me, I'll just leave now," or, "I don't have time to sit here doing nothing." It would be better for the student to gain control of her own feelings and then say, "I wonder what the silence is all about?" or, "We need to figure out why it is hard for us to talk together." After these statements, there will probably be more silence until the patient decides to discuss the problem. In the meantime, the student can effectively use the silence to gain control of her own feelings so that when the patient does begin to talk, she will be able to listen to him in an effective manner.

Summary

The analogy of an airplane stall to the practice of being therapeutic was made. A stall does not mean that the airplane is going to crash or that the therapeutic process is going to be irrevocably impaired. A stall means that corrective measures are needed in order to remedy the situation so that the plane may continue its path of flight or so that the therapeutic process may continue to be a helpful experience to the patient.

Specific and general stall situations were described. Stall warnings, as well as the corrective maneuvers applicable to the situation, were identified. In this chapter we discussed stall situations that are relevant to behavioral style, judgmental feelings, ambivalent feelings, rescue feelings, feelings of pessimism, feelings of omnipotence and omniscience, setting goals, being reassuring, confrontation and misuses of the analytical approach, misjudging the patient's overidentification with the problem, nontherapeutic involvement, bearing painful feelings, being dishonest, pitfalls in listening, and eliciting the patient's request.

Questions

1. Give an example of a stall in a general nursing situation.
2. What stall situations have you encountered in the academic setting?
3. Record a nurse–patient interaction and underline areas where there was a potential stall.
4. How do the technique of autognosis and the stall concept relate?
5. Describe a situation in which you stalled the interview and a situation in which the interview "crashed."

REFERENCES AND SUGGESTED READINGS

Bradley, J. C., & Edinberg, M. A. *Communication in The Nursing Context*, 2nd ed., 1986, Norwalk, CT: Appleton & Lange.

Davis, A. J. *Listening and responding*, 1984, St. Louis: Mosby.

Garant, C. Stalls in the therapeutic process. *American Journal of Nursing*, 1980, *80*, 2166–2169.

Purtilo, R. B. *Health professional/patient interaction*, 3rd ed., 1984, Philadelphia: Saunders.

Chapter 18

Legal Aspects of Psychiatric Mental Health Nursing

Joyce Kemp Laben and Colleen Powell MacLean

Chapter Objectives

The students successfully attaining the goals of this chapter will be able to:

- Discuss the concept of competency versus issues related to commitment.
- Define *voluntary, emergency involuntary*, and *indefinite involuntary admission* to inpatient psychiatric hospitals.
- Discuss the legal rights of psychiatric patients.
- Define *informed consent* and *aversive therapies*.
- Discuss the general legal issues in mental health care including clinical assessment and documentation, medication, malpractice, confidentiality and privilege, maintenance of potentially dangerous clients in the community, and forensic services.

There are special legal issues involved with the provision of care for individuals who manifest symptoms that are indicative of mental illness. Nurses who provide care for the mentally ill should be conversant with current legal problems and trends in order to ensure adequate care for patients. There has been a dramatic increase in the number of mental-health-related lawsuits in the last 15 years, which makes it imperative for mental health professionals to keep current with the law. Only those legal areas specific to the treatment of the mentally ill will be discussed in this chapter.

One of the major differences in admitting a patient to a mental hospital or a psychiatric unit rather than a medical–surgical facility is that of voluntariness. Ordinarily, an individual is allowed to choose the type and extent of physical care that may be available. However, society has permitted the "involuntary" treatment for the mentally ill in a variety of circumstances.

Deprivation of liberty occurs when involuntary inpatient treatment is required. Such deprivation of liberty is usually tolerated only when an individual is charged with a crime because of safeguards established by the Constitution. Involuntary inpatient treatment, therefore, must be viewed as an extreme treatment recommendation. Since legal issues vary according to whether mental health care is provided on an outpatient or inpatient basis, the legal issues will be analyzed according to this distinction.

HISTORICAL PERSPECTIVE

The public mental institution as a method of caring for the mentally ill is a relatively recent development in organized society's approach to mental illness. There was no reason for the common law in England, from which we derive most of our law today, to provide for adequate procedures for the involuntary commitment of the mentally ill because public institutions for the mentally ill were virtually nonexistent.[1]

The king of England had the authority to act as the general guardian of all infants, "idiots," and "lunatics." In acting in this role as *parens patriae*, the king or his representative was required to promote the interests and welfare of wards, but he was not empowered to sacrifice the ward's welfare for the benefit of others. During "lucid moments," the lunatic was permitted to manage his own property and to generally exercise his civil rights. This practice provided the basis for the *parens patriae* doctrine used by many states today in involuntarily committing patients to mental hospitals.[2]

If a person exhibited dangerous behavior, however, English common law and the early colonies in America allowed his removal from society. These individuals were generally placed in jails along with the criminals. This authority to remove dangerous people from society was based on the state's police power, which embraces all authority used by the states for the protection of health, safety, and the general welfare of citizens.[3] It is important to remember the concepts of *parens patriae* and *police power* because the justification for involuntary hospitalization today rests upon these doctrines.[4]

The treatment of the mentally ill and societal attitudes toward mental illness have ranged from the tortures of the Middle Ages, designed to exorcise the demons that were thought to be possessing the mentally deviant, to the humanistic view that is reflected in contemporary treatment circles. Perhaps the only common element in the history of formal governmental policies toward mental illness has been fear of the violence and destructiveness that have been thought inherent in the "madman."[5]

In the United States, there were few institutions for the mentally ill until the middle of the nineteenth century. Because of lack of resources, those confined were generally only those who were clearly "deranged" and violent. Therefore, until 1860, there was a dearth of statutory provisions relative to conditions for and limitations upon admission to mental institutions. The decision to admit to a facility was wholly within the discretion of the hospital administrator, who would often be under great pressure to admit indigent or dangerous persons in view of the lack of alternatives for support and care in the community.[6]

The movement toward the creation of state mental health institutions was stimulated by the crusading of individuals such as Dorothea Lynde Dix. From 1840 to 1880, Miss Dix conducted a personal crusade to expose the conditions existing in poorhouses and local jails where many mentally ill persons were ultimately placed. She effectively lobbied in many states for the creation of public institutions.[7] The increase in the availability of institutions focused attention on the need for rational and fair admission procedures, particularly for persons who refused to voluntarily admit themselves to hospitals.

The efforts of Dorothea Dix and other activists also brought reforms in the admission process, principally in the form of statutes requiring that no one could be involuntarily committed without a jury trial by peers. However, because of the increased interest in mental illness and the expansion in institutions, the common law requirement for "dangerousness" was changed. The result was that by the end of the nineteenth century, many states permitted commitment based upon a wide range of showings of mental illness and did not require dangerous behavior. Forms of these statutes remain in effect in most states.[8]

In *Addington v. Texas* (1979), the U.S. Supreme Court has reviewed the constitutionality of a state statute governing involuntary commitment. Previously, many state and lower federal courts had analyzed both the standards and procedures used in commitment statutes that allow the placement of persons in mental institutions involuntarily. This decision will be discussed later to demonstrate the current legal restrictions for involuntary hospitalization. In addition to the legal restrictions on the commitment to mental institutions, the development of new treatments, such as medication, facilitated the creation and expansion of community mental health services in the 1960s and 1970s, which resulted in the emphasis on the use of community care for the mentally ill.

Major issues of the 1980s include the right of patients to refuse antipsychotic medications and the passing of legislation by several states for mandatory outpatient treatment of individuals who have a prior history of dangerousness or noncompliance with treatment. An additional development has been the perceived failure of the deinstitutionalization movement in providing adequate mental health services in the community.

As reflected in newspaper articles across the country, the public has expressed concern for the homeless mentally ill, who cannot find the social support, housing, and other necessary services available upon release from a mental institution. The New York City policy to allow for commitment of persons who might face "serious harm within the foreseeable future" has been questioned because of the possible violation of civil liberties.[9]

Competency

There is a popular misconception that anyone admitted to an inpatient psychiatric facility loses his civil rights and is incompetent to handle his own affairs. Under current law this is inaccurate as it applies to voluntary as well as involuntary patients. Unless an individual has been found incompetent to manage himself or his affairs by a court and a guardian has been appointed, the person does not lose the right to make decisions relating to personal or business matters when he is admitted to a hospital.

It was only in the 1960s that most states separated the issue of competency from commitment in the commitment statutes. Until that time an individual was generally found incompetent at the time of commitment to the hospital. Unfortunately, when these issues were separated, the existing guardianship laws were not amended to provide the appropriate standards or procedures that would apply to the mentally ill incompetent person.

A person who is 18 or older is permitted to manage his own property and health in any way he chooses. If a person appears to be "incompetent," he is still legally competent until a court declares him to be incompetent and appoints a guardian or conservator to act on his behalf. Currently, most states have laws that authorize the court to find a person to be totally competent or incompetent. However, there is a trend to amend state laws to authorize the court to declare individuals disabled only in those areas of their life in which they are in fact unable to manage and to appoint limited guardians.[10] This would also provide for persons who may be incompetent but who may not require inpatient care.

Whether a nurse is providing care to inpatients or outpatients, there should be an assessment as to whether the person being treated has been declared incompetent. If this is the case, a copy of the court order for the record should be obtained and documentation as to who has authority to consent to treatment or authorize release of records should be established.

Types of Admissions to Inpatient Psychiatric Facilities

Generally, there are three types of admission to inpatient psychiatric hospitals: (1) voluntary; (2) emergency involuntary; and (3) indefinite involuntary (judicial commitment).[11] Any person can be admitted to a psychiatric hospital as a voluntary patient if he is mentally ill, in need of inpatient care, and is willing to seek admission. A voluntary patient must consent to all treatment and must be released upon request within a reasonable period of time, which will be specified by state law and may be from eight hours to two or three days after receipt of the request for release. If an individual refuses treatment or requests release at a time when he is a danger to himself or to others, the staff must look to state law to determine whether the person must be released or if a petition for judicial commitment should be initiated.

Historically, parents have been allowed to authorize the "voluntary" admission of juveniles under the age of 18. This practice, however, has been challenged in court in a number of states such as Georgia and Pennsylvania, and attorneys for juveniles have requested that no juveniles be admitted to a psychiatric facility without court approval.[12]

Other states, both through court decisions and amendments in state law, have recognized that at a certain age minors are "mature" enough to determine their own admission.[13]

This would still allow parents under certain circumstances to authorize the admission of younger juveniles. The Supreme Court authorized this practice in *Parham v. J. R. et al.* (1978) and stated that it was not a requirement that court approval be given on all juveniles admitted to psychiatric facilities.[14] However, it did find that some kind of inquiry should be made by a "neutral fact finder" to determine whether statutory requirements for admission are satisfied. The Court clarified that a formal or quasi-formal hearing is not required nor does it have to be conducted by a law-trained or judicial or administrative officer.

Most states provide for emergency involuntary admission to a psychiatric facility when an individual is thought to pose an immediate threat of serious harm to himself or others as a result of mental illness and is willing to seek treatment. This type of involuntary commitment differs from indefinite judicial commitment because it usually permits commitment without a court hearing for a short period of time.

State statutes have been narrowed in the past few years to require threat of actual physical harm before an emergency involuntary admission can take place. When this occurs, a law enforcement official or usually a licensed physician is authorized to take the person into custody for the purpose of an initial evaluation and eventual transportation to a psychiatric facility if this is determined to be appropriate. The person can then be detained for a brief period before a court hearing is held in order to determine whether emergency admission standards have been met and to authorize short-term hospitalization. Normally, aversive therapy such as electroshock treatment is not allowed during the initial detention. When the time period authorized for the emergency commitment ends, the person must be released; a petition must be initiated for an indefinite judicial commitment; or the person must agree to voluntarily remain.

The only instance in which a person may be detained in a psychiatric facility against his will for an indefinite period of time is through the judicial commitment process. Most state statutes allow this process to be initiated when an authorized official, physician, or family member files a petition for such commitment along with certification by two physicians or other mental health professionals that the individual is mentally ill, poses a likelihood of serious harm because of the mental illness, and suitable community resources are unavailable. Generally,

the standard for "likelihood of serious harm" is broader for indefinite judicial commitment than for emergency commitment and includes both immediate danger to self or others as well as more passive types of danger that can result from a person's inability to avoid or protect himself from harm because of mental illness.

Numerous court decisions in the past two decades reflect the severe attack that has been made on the judicial commitment process. Many people believe that since commitment results in deprivation of liberty, the procedures should parallel those provided in a criminal trial. While a few courts have agreed with this, most courts have demanded that procedures be used that provide due process without requiring total adherence to procedures used for criminal trials. The United States Supreme Court has now clarified that a commitment procedure does not have to duplicate the criminal process.

In addition to the attack on the procedures used in this process some authorities feel that involuntary commitment should be totally abolished, while some courts have said that only persons who pose an immediate threat of harm to self or others can be involuntarily committed.[15,16] The Supreme Court of the United States reviewed the indefinite commitment statute from the state of Texas and reviewed a variety of procedural issues. The Court ruled that the proof for involuntary commitment must be greater than a preponderance of evidence and that "clear, unequivocal and convincing" evidence is constitutionally adequate. The Court determined that the standard of beyond a reasonable doubt is not required, indicating that the Court selected a standard greater than that required for civil cases but less than that required for criminal prosecution.[17]

The Court also stated that the substantive standards and procedures for civil commitment may vary from state to state, as long as they meet the constitutional minimum. The opinion further held that the state has a legitimate interest under its *parens patriae* powers to provide care for its citizens who are unable to care for themselves as the result of mental illness and that the state also has authority under its police power to protect the community from dangerous tendencies of those who are mentally ill. Since this decision relies on the theory that the purpose of the commitment law is to "help" the person rather than punish him, *Addington* leaves unstated whether a person who is committed only because of dangerousness should be treated any differently than a person who is committed solely because of his need for care.

Legal Rights

When an individual is admitted to a psychiatric hospital, he maintains certain legal rights although he may be deprived of the freedom to leave the hospital. These rights are sometimes defined by state law so that mental health professionals should be familiar with patients' rights as defined by statute in the jurisdiction where they practice. As stated earlier, unless the person has been declared incompetent, the individual maintains the rights of any citizen such as the right to vote, to manage financial affairs, and to execute legal documents.

Because of the nature of confinement of a patient in an inpatient psychiatric facility, certain rights are given special focus. These include the right to communicate with his attorney in person, by letter, and by telephone. The patient has a right to receive mail without interference or censorship, the right to receive visitors, and the right to not be denied the basic necessities of life in the name of treatment. While these rights may be temporarily restricted (under certain circumstances), a mere claim by the staff that interference with these rights is necessary for treatment purposes is not sufficient to deny a patient these rights.[18]

A patient right that emerged in the late 1960s and early 1970s was a right to treatment once hospitalized. A landmark case for the right to treatment doctrine was *Rouse v. Cameron* (1967),[19] which involved a person found not guilty by reason of insanity and committed to a federal mental health facility. This case was the first to hold that society has a legal duty to provide adequate treatment and to ensure that confinement for purposes of treatment does not degenerate into punishment. The court did not characterize the right to treatment as a constitutional right, but instead it relied upon a District of Columbia statute that specifically cited this right. The court stated that the right to treatment would be satisfied by bona fide efforts of the staff consistent with present medical knowledge.

The most publicized case in the area of right to treatment is *Wyatt v. Stickney* (1971).[20] This Alabama case involved a district federal judge who threatened to sell state property in order to ensure that the state would have enough money to provide adequate treatment to its mental patients. The importance of this decision is that it establishes a constitutional basis for right to treatment for the involuntarily committed patients by analyzing the nature of the commitment process itself. The basis of this theory is that in order to justify the involuntary commitment of an individual and restriction of his freedom, treatment must be provided once he is hospitalized.

Wyatt states that treatment must provide realistic opportunities to be cured and established three categories necessary for treatment: (1) humane psychological and physical environment; (2) qualified staff personnel in sufficient numbers; and (3) individualized treatment plans. The court came to this conclusion after extensive expert testimony was provided. The facilities in Alabama have improved but the Wyatt standards never have been fully realized. Active court supervision has been relinquished and progress is measured by the "plaintiff's counsel, internal advocacy of quality assurance mechanisms, and accreditation by Joint Commission on the Accreditation of Hospitals."[21]

One case that has received widespread publicity is *O'Connor v. Donaldson* (1975), decided by the United States Supreme Court. It involved a Florida patient who was not considered dangerous but had been hospitalized against his will for over 15 years without treatment.[22] The findings of this decision have been greatly misrepresented. It does not state that there is a constitutional right to treatment; it does not require that all patients who are not receiving treatments be released from psychiatric facilities; and it does not require that all nondangerous patients be released. It is important to remember what *O'Connor* does state because it was the first United States Supreme Court case to discuss the issue of treatment for committed patients.

O'Connor does stipulate that a state cannot constitutionally confine without treatment a nondangerous individual who is capable of surviving safely in the community by himself or with the help of willing and responsible family members or friends. To do so, the court held, would be a deprivation of liberty.

A subsequent United States Supreme Court decision, *Youngberg v. Romeo* (1982), further reviewed the issue of "right to treatment."[23] This case concerned a person involuntarily committed to an institution for the mentally retarded. In the concurring opinion by Justice Burger, who also wrote the *O'Connor* opinion, he specifically states that there is no constitutional right to "habilitation."[24] The concept of "habilitation" for the mentally retarded individual is parallel to the concept of "treatment" for a mentally ill individual; therefore, this case is pertinent to the issue of "right to treatment." However, the majority opinion held that a committed mentally retarded person has a right to minimally adequate or reasonable training to ensure safety and freedom from undue restraints. Ultimately, the Court again declined to rule on whether an individual involuntarily committed to a state institution has some general constitutional right to training per se.

Interestingly enough, the right to treatment concept as espoused by *Wyatt v. Stickney* (1971) has lost popularity in some legal circles. There is a fear that to connect the right to treatment issue to the commitment process in order to justify deprivation of liberty only diverts attention from the more fundamental problems of permitting involuntary commitment. Many see this connection as using right to treatment as a justification of postcommitment deprivation of civil rights.[25] In addition, this is often applied by the courts only to those persons who have been involuntarily committed, thus raising the question whether voluntary patients have a right to treatment.

Informed Consent

It has long been an established axiom that adults who are of sound mind, that is, mentally competent, have the right to determine what will be done to their own bodies.[26] It has more recently been established that a person must not only give consent but must have enough information or knowledge of an anticipated procedure to be performed by health professionals to give an informed consent.

When a person enters a hospital for a mental illness, he does not abdicate his right to consent to treatment. A *voluntary* patient should have the right to refuse any kind of treatment.[27] An attempt should, however, be made to explain to the individual the various kinds of treatments and alternatives that might be available. Once the possible treatments and alternatives with relevant facts are presented to the patient, it is up to him to make the decision. Once that decision is made, even though it might differ from the mental health professionals' preferred choice, the patient should be allowed to pursue

the course he has chosen without repercussions from the staff. For example, if a patient chooses not to have electroshock therapy, other alternatives should be explored, and the staff should not withdraw their support from the individual even though the treatment choice differs from a recommended decision by a therapeutic team.

The real difficulty seems to arise when a procedure is recommended for an involuntarily committed patient and he refuses the treatment. In many instances, the patient is involuntarily committed, but he has not been found incompetent to manage his affairs. According to Roth, even committed patients must be given adequate information on which to base informed consent to intrusive procedures such as electroconvulsive treatments.[28] If they are not thought competent to make this decision, then a court should make the finding of incompetency, and an appropriate consent should be obtained from a formally appointed substitute such as a guardian.

In the past few years there have been several lawsuits pertaining to a patient's right to refuse psychotropic medication. The two major cases are *Rogers v. Okin* (1979), later entitled *Mills v. Rogers*, which originated in the State of Massachusetts, and *Rennie v. Klein* (1978) which originated in New Jersey.[29] Both of these cases were appealed to the United States Supreme Court, which sent them back to lower courts for resolution.

Both cases concerned the rights of involuntary hospitalized patients to refuse to take psychotropic medication. Because of the potential of incurable side effects such as tardive dyskinesia, patients were motivated to file suit to protect the right to refuse medication.

Currently the question of the right to refuse medication has not been finally resolved; however, it is clear that a voluntary patient does have the right to informed consent and the right to refuse medication unless the individual is manifesting behavior that is clearly dangerous to himself or others.

The guidelines for how to manage an incompetent involuntary patient seem to follow several courses: appointment of a court-ordered guardian who will make a decision using one of two guidelines or a combination of both. The first is "What treatment is in the best interests of the patient?" The second is a "substituted judgment" decision. What would the patient want if he or she were competent?

Some states use administrative procedures

such as calling in an outside psychiatrist consultant to examine a drug-refusing patient or establishing a specially appointed treatment team to evaluate the necessity of giving forced medications to an incompetent mentally ill person.[30]

There are certain steps that state systems or individual facilities can currently take. Procedures for how to manage a drug-refusing patient should be established. Guidelines for how to manage the involuntary patient refusing medication should incorporate state law, case decisions, rules and regulations, and consent decrees of the particular jurisdiction where the facility is located.

There is, however, no substitute for a therapeutic relationship between a patient and a mental health professional to resolve issues about medication. An ongoing dialogue over several days can assist in assessment of the patient's reason for refusing medication. Continuing inservice education about medication and its side effects is an important mechanism for keeping professionals informed about the current literature on the subject.[31]

Aversive Therapies

It is especially important to be careful and thorough in obtaining valid consent for particular intrusive procedures. Although the use of psychosurgery has substantially diminished, it is still occasionally performed. Since the effects of such a procedure are profound and can alter the personality, it is imperative that the person be competent to give consent, or if incompetent, that a court hearing occur to determine the validity of performing such a procedure.

Electroshock treatments (ECT) are still given throughout the country. The competent patient should be fully informed of all the facts about the treatment, including side effects. The patient can refuse the treatment. In at least one jurisdiction, only a court can consent to ECT treatments on a minor.[32] The parents cannot give such an authorization. According to Ennis and Emery, all jurisdictions allow substituted consent for incompetents.[33] The nurse should know what the law is concerning ECT in the state in which she practices. The hospital should have policies and procedures for obtaining consent.

In a recent study it was reported that ECT use is decreasing. More women than men receive ECT, but age and diagnosis are the most important factors in selecting to undergo the treatment. It is primarily used by white voluntary patients in private psychiatric facilities.[34]

There has been controversy about conducting research on hospitalized patients. The National Commission on the Protection of Human Subjects has compiled guidelines for research on the mentally infirm.[35] All research conducted on mentally ill patients in an institutional setting should be reviewed by an institutional review board, which is convened to protect the rights of human subjects. If there is a professional review board in a facility, all professional disciplines and consumer members from the community should be on the committee.

Least Restrictive Alternative Environment

One of the concepts in the delivery of mental health care is that of the least restrictive alternative. In planning mental health care, professional care givers should plan a treatment program that can be implemented in the least restrictive environment. If a person can be treated in a halfway house, or in his own home, it is a preferable alternative to that of involuntary commitment on a locked ward in a psychiatric hospital. A case that discussed this issue extensively is *Dixon v. Weinberger* (1975).[36]

This doctrine is based on the principle that the state may have a legitimate reason for wanting to treat an individual, but treatment must be provided in the least restrictive manner that can provide sufficient care for the patient's needs. Some states have enacted statutes that explicitly state this requirement. It is an important point to consider when planning care. Each person's specific needs at a particular time should be assessed. These needs should be reevaluated at frequent intervals to determine if the client might need a more or a less restrictive environment.

Right to Aftercare

As a result of the reduction of the inpatient population in mental hospitals during the last 20 years, large groups of people have been discharged into the community. Many of these individuals are placed in foster homes, nursing homes, and boardinghouses. Too frequently, there is no adequate follow-up of patients after discharge, either by personnel from state hospitals or community mental health centers. Nursing homes employ people who are not familiar with caring for persons with mental problems, especially those individuals who have remained in state hospitals for long periods of time. Fortunately, a growing number of personnel in nursing homes have been making an effort to upgrade the expertise of employees in this area.[37]

In regions of the country where large groups of patients have been placed in boardinghouses, there has been a public outcry about the lack of care for these people. There have been many reports of inadequate care and deplorable living conditions of former mental patients. One such report stated that one-half of the patients discharged from long-term facilities in New York City have been returned to the hospitals.[38]

During 1977, when the President's Commission on Mental Health held public hearings in communities across the country, reports of lack of aftercare for individuals in the community were repeatedly made. Based upon this testimony, a Task Force Panel was selected to study the problem and to make recommendations. This report, released in the spring of 1978, states that due process must be ensured for those individuals who are being considered for placement into the community, especially if it is against their wishes.[39] The concept that a patient has a right to due process upon being discharged from a hospital as well as upon admission is a relatively new concept.

Saphire has raised the question not only about the right to aftercare, but about the issue of retaining patients in the hospital because the individual does not have the personal resources to maintain himself in the community.[40] It is his opinion that aftercare should be viewed as being "constitutionally and morally mandated."[41] Because of the growing concern about aftercare in general, nurses should be aware that there is a possible constitutional issue that could mandate a right to aftercare. All patients, regardless of the setting of care, should have adequate aftercare planning by a professional staff that will ensure stabilization within the community for as long as possible. It is probable that if a patient is discharged with no aftercare planning, the professional health care givers could be held responsible for falling below a minimal standard of care.

The issue of the mentally ill homeless has generated much attention by the media nationally. A major issue in the city of New York is whether the definition of "danger of serious harm" can be expanded to include within the foreseeable future. Can individuals be removed from the street if they will suffer serious harm in the foreseeable future? The New York Civil Liberties Union asserts that Mayor Koch is attempting to rewrite state law without the requisite legal authority.[42]

GENERAL ISSUES IN MENTAL HEALTH CARE

Overview

In today's world of sophisticated, complex mental health care, many health professionals still have a simplistic view of the potential legal issues. Many so-called legal concerns are overstated, whereas others are not properly emphasized. As a result, critical issues such as confidentiality, privilege, informed consent, and documentation are often ignored in everyday practice.

There are several important points to remember when practicing psychiatric nursing in a community mental health setting: (1) know and provide the basic clinical care that is the responsibility of any nurse or mental health professional; (2) carefully document all recommendations and the basis for such recommendations; (3) document appropriate attempts at following through on the recommendations; and (4) be familiar with the mental health law in your state.

Clinical Assessment and Documentation

One of the most important aspects of delivering care to a mental health client is to accurately record the treatment that is being given and note why the decision was made to provide a specific kind of care. An overall psychosocial assessment should be made for each client and a treatment plan should be developed and updated as needed.

There should be an accurate recording of the treatment process. It is better to describe an event in detail than to label the behavior. For example, it is more delineative to record that the patient was visited at home and refused to come out of the bedroom for the 30 minutes while the nurse was there, than simply noting that the patient was withdrawn.

Another important issue to document is the crisis episode of a patient and the therapeutic intervention provided. The nurse's assessment of the crisis and the intervention should be recorded not only for the protection of the client, but also for the protection of the nurse, especially if the client later responds to the crisis situation with self-inflicted injury or follows through on other threats that were made. Although only a small percentage of patient records will be subject to public scrutiny as a result of a subpoena by a court or review by the patient, it is good practice to always document as though the record were going to be reviewed by a third party.

Medication

With the introduction of phenothiazines for treatment of persons with schizophrenia in the 1950s, the population of mental hospitals continued to decline, and many people are now treated in the community through the use of medication. All medications that are prescribed must be documented, including the continued use of the medication throughout the treatment.

There has been much concern recently about the long-term effects of medication on individuals who are mentally ill. Nurses delivering care to patients in the community should be particularly sensitive to individuals who are on drug therapy and complain of difficulties. It is imperative that any complaints of side effects from medication be immediately and accurately recorded and reported to the prescribing physician.

The sudden death of patients on large doses of psychotropic medications has been described in the literature. Nurses should be knowledgeable about the side effects of drugs and consult with the prescribing physician when toxic effects are noted. This is particularly urgent when there is an administration of phenothiazine therapy at high doses over a short period of time.[43] As evidence is accumulated on the toxic effects of psychotropic medication, nurses should review the most recent information published in the literature.

Malpractice

A matter about which all nurses and mental health professionals should be educated is that of malpractice. The term malpractice is often used interchangeably with negligence to define those acts of a professional person that are called into question because of lack of due care. Negligence is a legal dispute that comes within the field of tort law. A person who feels that he has possibly been injured as the result of the actions of a nurse would bring suit in a civil court for money damages for negligence.

There are certain elements that must be proven in order to win a case for negligence. The court will analyze all of the elements of negligence in relationship to the facts of the case before determining whether malpractice in fact exists.

Standards of Care
There is a legal fiction called the reasonably prudent man. Courts over a period of many years have relied on this concept to require nurses to function at a minimum standard that is equivalent to that of a reasonably prudent nurse delivering care in the same circumstances.

Legal Duty
Once a nurse initiates a professional relationship with a patient, a nurse–patient relationship is established, and the nurse is obligated to give care in an appropriate manner. In addition, if the nurse observes an action by another professional that she thinks breaches the standard of care and can predict or foresee possible harm to the patient, she has a responsibility to intervene and prevent the injury.

Causation
In order for a nurse to be found liable for negligence, the person bringing the lawsuit must show that there is a causal relationship between the professional's acts and the alleged injury. This is often difficult to prove, but the causal link must be established.

Injury
It must be established that an injury resulted to the plaintiff from the acts of the professional that can be recompensed by money damages.

An example of a potential malpractice issue

that is frequently raised regarding mental health professionals relates to the suicide of a patient after discharge from a facility or during off-the-ward activities. Courts generally have ruled in the following manner: If the staff has carefully observed the patient and he has not exhibited any suicidal behavior, verbally or nonverbally, the mental health team will not be held liable; however, if the individual has exhibited current suicidal tendencies and is discharged or given a pass, it is conceivable the ruling would not be in favor of the mental health staff.[44] It is imperative that communication about a patient's condition be reported verbally and also be written in the record.

Confidentiality and Privilege

Two concepts that are often misunderstood and are vitally important to a relationship with the client are confidentiality and privilege. Confidentiality relates to the responsibility of the agency and professional to keep all information, records, and correspondence confidential and private and to allow access by third parties to these records only under specifically defined circumstances. On the other hand, privilege specifically refers to the relationship of a particular professional to a client and provides protection of the information obtained from the client as a result of this relationship. Each state defines by law which professionals have privilege and whether this privilege is absolute. The professionals who most often are given privilege are ministers, psychiatrists, psychologists, and lawyers. Privilege can be asserted only by the client and does not exist unless there is a client–therapist relationship. When someone other than the client and the therapist was present when the information was conveyed, privilege would probably not attach.

A mental health professional should investigate in the state where he or she is practicing to determine (1) which professionals are granted privilege; and (2) under what circumstances information about the patient and records should be released. Usually records may be released only with the written permission of the client or by court order. In addition, there may be specific statutory exceptions to confidentiality, such as mandatory child-abuse-reporting laws or emergency situations.

MAINTENANCE OF POTENTIALLY DANGEROUS CLIENTS IN THE COMMUNITY

Although there has been an increasing amount of litigation in the mental health field, the majority of this litigation has been directed at state mental health inpatient facilities and has focused on such issues as appropriate standards and procedures for involuntary hospitalization, provisions for treatment in the least restrictive alternative, and right to treatment and to refuse treatment. However, the results of this litigation have directly influenced the practice of community mental health. Most states have now amended commitment laws to allow only the most dangerous persons to be hospitalized against their will, to limit time of hospitalization, and to mandate that services be provided in the least restrictive setting whenever possible.

This has resulted in an expansion of the range of clients that are now served at the community level. Fewer persons can be referred to hospitals when problems arise. More *potentially* dangerous clients must continue to be served at the community level and more chronic patients must be supported in the community. It is important for all mental health professionals to have a working knowledge of the mental health laws in the state in which they are practicing. This is particularly important when they determine that a client must be referred for inpatient care.

It is at this point that the concept of voluntariness becomes critical. The appropriate treatment should be discussed with the client so that he can make an informed decision concerning hospitalization, if possible. However, if the individual is unwilling to either seek inpatient care or is posing immediate threat of harm to himself or others, a decision must be made concerning involuntary commitment to a psychiatric facility.

If the individual does not pose a threat of serious harm based on his mental illness, it may not be possible or desirable to force the person to be hospitalized against his will. The professional should always determine whether all alternatives have been exhausted so that the individual can be treated in the community.

Another issue involving the care of individuals in the community is the potential danger to the third parties and the responsibility of the therapist to warn of the potential danger. *Tarasoff v. Regents of the University of California* (1974) is a case in California that has generated anxiety on the part of mental health professionals.[45] In this particular decision, an individual was in treatment with a psychologist, and in the course of therapy confided that he intended to kill a young woman whom he knew. The university police were notified by the psychologist and they briefly detained the client but made the decision to release him. The psychologist did not see the client again, and he made no attempt to warn the victim or her family.

The individual subsequently killed the young woman as he had threatened to do, and the family filed a lawsuit. The Supreme Court of California held that a duty to warn third parties existed when a therapist determines, or pursuant to the standards of his profession should determine, that his patient presents a serious physical danger to another person. The Court stated that this situation created an exception to the confidential relationship with the patient and that a potential victim can be warned since "the protection of privilege ends where the public peril begins."[46] Other states have adopted the Tarasoff concept to require notifying third parties about dangerous individuals. Kjervik maintains that although nurses have not been defendants in a lawsuit of this kind, when serving in a therapeutic capacity, they have the duty to warn.[47]

Several states have recently passed legislation known as mandatory outpatient treatment. These statutes were passed to allow mental health personnel to require individuals with a history of noncompliance in taking medication and a history of dangerousness to be subject to possible involuntary commitment or forcible examination if they refused to take medication once they were returned to the community. The due process protections vary from state to state but "all states fall short of granting outpatients the same procedural protections provided to inpatients."[48] The practice has been, however, to subject few individuals to preventive commitment orders."[49]

Forensic Services

Mental health professionals can be asked by the courts to evaluate individuals who have emotional problems and have been charged with crimes. In the past, there has been confusion about the information that mental health professionals should provide and the issues that they should address.

The first point that must be addressed is the competency of the individual to stand trial. This is a limited concept that relates to the mental condition of the defendant at the time of the trial. Competency can be defined as a defendant's ability to advise counsel, understand the charges against him, and understand the nature and object and consequences of the proceedings.[50]

The second point the courts usually request the mental health professional to address is an evaluation that relates to the insanity defense (criminal responsibility). An insanity defense plea relates back to the defendant's mental status at the time of the alleged crime.

Competency to stand trial is raised more often than the insanity defense and is an important concept, since the court and prosecuting attorney, as well as the defense attorney, have an obligation to ensure that the defendant is competent so that he can receive a fair trial. Most evaluations for competency to stand trial can be done on an outpatient basis. If a patient needs to be hospitalized, every effort should be made to enable him to become competent to stand trial as quickly as possible so that he may proceed through the criminal justice system expeditiously.

Until the 1970s, pretrial defendants could be institutionalized for years without being brought to trial or committed under the same standards as civil patients. The United States Supreme Court, in the decision of *Jackson v. Indiana* (1972) mandated a change in this process.[51]

In this particular case, a retarded deaf-mute resident of a maximum security unit was awaiting trial on criminal charges. Because of his disabilities, it was impossible for him to ever become competent to stand trial. Therefore, he was essentially given a life sentence without trial. The court held that Mr. Jackson was denied equal protection of the law because he was subjected to a "more lenient commitment standard and to a more stringent standard of release" than other patients in psychiatric hospitals.[52] The court also commented that persons under criminal charges who are hospitalized because of their incapacity to stand trial cannot be "detained more than a reasonable period of time necessary to determine whether there is a substantial probability that they will attain competency in the foreseeable future."[53]

As a result of this decision, patients cannot be kept for a long period of time in a mental institution on the issue of competency to stand trial unless they are committed according to the same standards that are applied to all civil patients. In order for a pretrial defendant to be detained in a mental hospital for more than a reasonable amount of time, the person must conform to the civil commitment standards of that state. It is still possible that an individual may be confined in a mental hospital with charges pending for a long period of time, but only if he meets the standards of commitment for any patient. The treatment goal is to assist the individual to become competent to stand trial.

New proposals have been suggested in the area of forensics as a result of the legally mandated changes. For example, several states have adopted a Guilty But Mentally Ill Statute (GBMI). This statute does not abolish the insanity defense but provides an alternative plan for those defendants who were mentally ill, but not insane at the time of the crime.[54]

Since most states are already required to provide services to persons who are convicted of crimes and become mentally ill, it would appear that the main purpose of this statute is to reduce the successful use of the insanity defense and to label the "mentally ill offenders."

In Tennessee, a psychiatric mental health nurse clinical specialist is considered qualified, after a training course, to testify to the issue of competency to stand trial. Qualified nurses in the future may be involved in this aspect of care in increasing numbers. In most jurisdictions, it is still considered necessary to have a psychologist with a doctoral degree or a psychiatrist testify on the issue of insanity or criminal responsibility.

Summary

There are a variety of legal issues related to the provision of mental health care. This chapter attempts to pinpoint and summarize the basic legal issues. In order to provide comprehensive mental health nursing care within the appropriate legal framework, it is imperative that a nurse educate herself about her state's mental health law and learn how to identify legal questions so that an attorney can be consulted when necessary.

Questions

1. How may a person be detained in a psychiatric facility against his will and for an indefinite period of time in your state?
2. How does the issue of informed consent relate to patients in psychiatric hospitals compared to patients in a general hospital?
3. Why is it important to record accurately patient care information?
4. Differentiate between the concepts of confidentiality and privilege and give examples of each.
5. A patient tells you during an interview of his wish to kill his wife. Discuss how you would handle this information and cite a legal case that had to deal with a similar situation.

REFERENCES AND SUGGESTED READINGS

1. Saphire, R. B. The civilly committed public mental patient and the right to aftercare. *Florida State University Law Review*, 1976, 4, 232.

2. Ibid.
3. Ennis, B. J., & Emery, R. D. *The Rights of Mental Patients; The Revised ACLU Guide to a Mental Patient's Rights.* New York: Avon, 1978, pp. 43–48.
4. Saphire, op. cit., p. 255.
5. Ibid., p. 232.

6. Ibid., pp. 229–242.

7. Ibid.

8. Ibid.

9. Wylie, M. Reinstitutionalization in New York. *The Family Therapy Networker*, 1987, 38–39.

10. Legal issues in state mental health care: Proponent for change. *Mental Disability Law Reporter*, p. 68.

11. Hemelt, M. D., Mackert, M. E. *Dynamics of Law in Nursing and Health Care*. Reston, Va.: Reston, 1978, pp. 101–102 and; Tennessee Code Annotated 33-601–33-604.

12. Bartley v. Kremens, 402 F. Supp. 1034 (E.D. Pa. 1975), vacated and remanded 97 S.Ct. 1709 (1977); J. L. and J. R. v. Parham, 412 F.Supp. 112 (M.D. Ga. 1975).

13. Tennessee Code Annotated 33-601; In re Rogers, Crim. 19558 Cal., (July 18, 1977).

14. Parham v. J. L. and J. R. 442 U.S. 584 (1978).

15. Szasz, T. S. *Law, Liberty and Psychiatry*. New York: Macmillan, 1963.

16. (Lessard v. Schmidt, 349 F.Supp. 1078 (E.D. Wis. 1974), vacated on procedural grounds 421 U.S. 957 (1975), reinstated 413 F.Supp. 1318 (E.D. Wis. 1976); Ennis & Emery, op. cit., p. 52.

17. Addington v. Texas, 441 U.S. 418 (1979).

18. Ennis & Emery, op. cit., p. 154.

19. Rouse v. Cameron, 373 F.2d 451 (D.C. Circuit, 1967).

20. Wyatt v. Stickney, 325 F.Supp. 781 (M.D. Ala. 1971), on submission of proposed standards by defendants 334 F.Supp. 1341, enforced 344 F.Supp. 373 (1972), affirmed in part, remanded on other grounds sub nom; Wyatt v. Aderholt, 503 F.2d 1305 (Fifth Circuit, 1974).

21. Parry, J. 1987 in review. *Mental and Physical Disability Law Reporter*, 12(1), at 8.

22. O'Connor v. Donaldson, 422 U.S. 563 (1975).

23. Youngberg v. Romeo, 102 Sup. Ct. 2452 (1982).

24. Ibid.

25. Saphire, op. cit., pp. 234–238, 268–274.

26. *Schloendorff v. Society of New York Hospital*, 211 N.Y. 128–129, 105 N.E. 92–93 (1914).

27. Report of the task force panel on legal and ethical issues. *Task Force Panel, Reports Submitted to the President's Commission on Mental Health* (Vol. 4, Appendix), p. 1434, Washington, D.C. 1978.

28. Roth, L. Involuntary civil commitment: The right to treatment and the right to refuse treatment. *Psychiatric Annals* 1977, 7(5) 50–244.

29. Rogers v. Okin, 478 F.Supp. 1342 (D. Mass. 1979), Rogers v. Okin, 634 F.2d 650 (1st Cir. 1980), Rennie v. Klein, 462 F.Supp. 1131 (N.J. 1978) at 1135, Rennie v. Klein, 476 F.Supp. 1294 (D.N.S. 1979).

30. Parry, J. A unified theory of substitute consent: Incompetent patients right to individualized health care decision-making. *Mental and Physical Disability Law Reporter*, 1987, 11(6), 378–385.

31. Laben, J. K., & MacLean, C. P. *Legal Issues and Guidelines for Nurses Who Care for the Mentally Ill.* Thorofare, N.J.: Slack, 1983.

32. Tennessee Code Annotated 33-320.

33. Ennis & Emery, op. cit., p. 139.

34. Thompson, J. W., & Blaine, J. D. Use of ECT in the United States in 1975 and 1980. *American Journal of Psychiatry*, 1987, *144*, 557–562.

35. Protection of Human Subjects, Research Involving Those Institutionalized as Mentally Infirm; Report and Recommendations for Public Comment. 43 *Federal Register*, 50–87.

36. Dixon v. Weinberger, 405 F.Supp. 974. (D.C. CIR. 1975)

37. Rowland, H. *The Nurses Almanac*. (Germantown, Md.: Aspen Systems Corp., 1978, pp. 458, 459.

38. Santiestevan, H. *Deinstitutionalization: Out of Their Beds and Into the Streets*. Washington, D.C.: American Federation of State and County and Municipal Employees, December, 1976, p. 15.

39. Report of the task force panel on deinstitutionalization, rehabilitation, and long-term care. *Task Force Panel Reports*, Submitted to the President's Commission on Mental Health, (Vol. 2, Appendix). Washington, D.C.: U.S. Gov't Printing Office 1978, p. 359.

40. Saphire, op. cit., p. 288.

41. Ibid., p. 295.

42. Wylie, M. op. cit.

43. Kremberg, R. Sudden death of a patient taking Phenothiazine. *Psychiatric Annals*, 1978, 8(7), p. 90.

44. Cohen v. State of New York, 382 N.Y. 2d 128, (1976); Torres v. State of New York, 373 N.Y.S. 696 (1975).

45. Tarasoff v. Regents of the University of California, 592 p. 2d 553, (1974).

46. California court reaffirms Tarasoff ruling, finds duty to warn third parties. *Mental Disability Law Reporter*, 1976, 129.

47. Kjervik, D. The psychiatric nurse's duty to warn potential victim of homicidal psychotherapy outpatients. *Law Medicine and Health Care*, 1981, 9(6), 11–16.

48. Stefan, S. Preventive commitment: The concept and its pitfalls. *Mental and Physical Disability Law Reporter*, 1987, *11*(4), 288–302 at 292.

49. Ibid., 296.

50. National Institute of Mental Health. *Competency to Stand Trial and Mental Illness*, (Crime and Delinquency Issues Monograph Series, DHEW Publication No. HSM 730-9105). Washington, D.C.: U.S. Government Printing Office, 1973, p. 20.

51. Jackson v. Indiana, 406 U.S. 715 (1972).

52. Ibid., p. 716.

53. Ibid.

54. Laben and MacLean, op cit.

PART IV

Clinical Modalities in Psychiatric Mental Health Nursing

There are a wide variety of clinical modalities in practice in the mental health field. These include pharmacotherapy, milieu management, individual psychotherapies, trauma therapy, crisis intervention, family and group work, consultative liaison, and community mental health work, as well as psychological testing and measurement. Each specific modality is addressed in this part of the book with accompanying history, theory, and description of practice. The first two chapters review the evolution of nursing thought and conceptual models of care in psychiatric nursing practice. The aim of these chapters is to help nurses understand the theoretical basis for the clinical modality in order to be able to practice the therapy, talk to patients about their progress, and to be able to refer or consider such modalities for referral.

CHAPTER 19: THE EVOLUTION OF NURSING KNOWLEDGE: CONVERGENCE OF PRACTICE AND RESEARCH

This chapter traces the development of nursing and its convergence with an articulated framework for practice. Contemporary nursing knowledge has moved into the twenty-first century with a major focus on research.

CHAPTER 20: CONCEPTUAL MODELS OF PSYCHIATRIC NURSING CARE

Four models that are currently being used in the understanding and treatment of mental illness are identified as the cognitive–behavioral, psychological, social, and biologic models of care. The psychiatric nursing activities prescribed by the ANA Council of Psychiatric Mental Health

Nursing Practice are discussed within the context of the models of care.

CHAPTER 21: PHARMACOTHERAPY

Psychopharmacology has had a major impact on the treatment of a wide range of emotional disorders. The nurse's role in the administration of medications has significantly increased, and thus this chapter addresses psychiatric intervention by use of medication.

CHAPTER 22: MILIEU THERAPY

An early identified role of the nurse was manager of the milieu or therapeutic environment of the patient. This chapter reviews the history of the concept of milieu and describes the current role of the psychiatric nurse in milieu management.

CHAPTER 23: INDIVIDUAL PSYCHOTHERAPIES

A major modality of patient intervention is individual psychotherapy. This chapter reviews some of the current types of psychotherapy used by all mental health professionals.

CHAPTER 24: CRISIS THEORY AND INTERVENTION

Crises or highly stressful life events are characteristic of the human life cycle. A model for assessment, diagnosis, and intervention is presented with case illustrations.

CHAPTER 25: TRAUMA THERAPY

Using a conceptual framework drawn from the cognitive sciences of information theory and cybernetics, the stress response syndromes, and psychodynamic formulations, a trauma learning model describes how child victims think and process information about sexual abuse. A case involving a three-year-old girl victim and five-year-old male schoolmate illustrate intervention principles that address the three information storage domains: sensations, perceptions, and cognitions.

CHAPTER 26: FAMILY WORK IN NURSING PRACTICE

Families are the most basic and essential subsystem in our society. Working with families is an important aspect of a holistic approach to nursing care. This chapter addresses family structure, functions, dynamics, and communication factors.

CHAPTER 27: WORKING WITH GROUPS

Groups maintain an important position in the structure of our society's organization. The nurse's role in group process and group therapy is discussed.

CHAPTER 28: LIAISON AND CONSULTATIVE ISSUES IN PSYCHIATRIC MENTAL HEALTH NURSING

The role dimensions of the psychiatric nurse have greatly expanded in the general hospital. This chapter discusses the psychological reactions of the medically ill patient and the therapeutic approaches to help this patient deal with anxieties about his physical illness. The chapter also discusses the role of the psychiatric nurse in the emergency room and in rural community mental health settings.

CHAPTER 29: PSYCHOLOGICAL TESTING AND PSYCHOLOGICAL ASSESSMENT

The tradition of measuring behaviors in a standardized and objective manner is presented along with a description of the reasons for referral and the types of tests and analyses. The aim of the chapter is to assist nurses to understand and to interpret psychological test reports included in the records of patients.

Chapter 19

The Evolution of Nursing Knowledge: Convergence of Practice and Research

Ann Wolbert Burgess

Chapter Objectives

The students successfully attaining the goals of this chapter will be able to:

- Trace the evolution of nursing knowledge from prescientific times through to the current research era.
- Identify the role of Florence Nightingale and nursing thought.
- Describe the importance of nursing's social policy statement to the professionalization of nursing.

Nursing has derived its practice from a multidimensional perspective. A review of the evolution of nursing knowledge relevant to research and practice addresses the different levels of human responses to health and illness. The determinants for the theories include sociocultural, neurobiological, cognitive or behavioral, developmental, interpersonal, general systems, and existential concepts and the resulting convergence has generated a wide range of conceptual models for practice. Nursing's commitment to holism and multiple models of practice suggest that the complexity of human responses to health and illness are determined by multiple pathways.

Although nursing practice does not have a long history of documented research on which to affirm its theoretical base, Ellis observes that

thinking nurses always must have used concepts, working hypotheses, assumptions, and presuppositions in their understandings of the world of nursing and nursing care.[1] Through the technique of historical analysis, we have good reason to believe that, indeed, many of the ideas first proposed by the early nurse leaders persist as themes in modern theory and practice. Historical analysis, according to nurse-historian Ellen D. Baer, attempts to interpret and explain events using particular world views or conceptual schemes. One such conceptual scheme, social history, is used by Baer to analyze the organization of nursing that developed during the last third of the nineteenth century.[2] This chapter reviews the development of nursing knowledge from the prescientific era through to the current research and scientific era, with atten-

tion to the social forces of the times as preparation to this section's discussion of clinical models for psychiatric nursing practice.

PRESCIENTIFIC ERA: THE ENVIRONMENT MODEL

The prescientific era in nursing includes the centuries before the emergence of modern American nursing in the 1870s. The earliest models of care of the sick derive from ancient history when nursing was recognized as one of the works of mercy of the Christian church. With the rise of monasticism, the care of the sick became a function of many religious orders. It was one of the services performed by communities organized under the rule laid down by St. Benedict in the sixth century.

The principles practiced by the sisters were provided by the religious rulers; for example, the principles outlined by St. Vincent de Paul provided the guidance for the Sisters of Charity. Pastor Theodor Fliedner and his wife, whose work influenced the later development of European nursing, laid the foundation of the deaconess movement at Kaiserswerth, Germany, in 1836. The focus and intuitive thinking during this period of nursing history were the gathering of religious women and men to care for the sick.

Florence Nightingale is considered a forerunner of nursing theory because her laws of health or nature provided the bases for health nursing and are reflective of a rational mode of thought or knowing.[3] Nightingale's nursing emphasized activities designed to alter a person's environment for restoration or promotion of health. She believed that the analysis and application of the "laws of nursing" would promote well-being and relieve suffering.[4-6] She early demonstrated her concern and commitment to the sick and indigent through her visits with them. Convinced of the need for reform in nursing, she had just opened an institution for the care of the sick in London when, in 1854, England's secretary of war asked her to undertake the nursing of soldiers in the Crimea.

Nursing, at this time period, was defined as an art and a science requiring an organized, scientific, and formal education. The scientific dimension derived from Nightingale's understanding of statistics, sanitation, logistics, ad-

ministration, and public health as well as the laws of health and symptoms of disease. Nightingale's emphasis on the patient's environment emerged, in part, out of her early Crimean war experiences with the sickness and death that occurred as a result of unsanitary environmental conditions of the wounded and sick soldiers at Scutari. The environmental D's of health were to be managed: dirt, damp, draughts, drains, drink, and diet. The significance of environment is reflected in Torres' reference to Nightingale's model as an "Environmental Therapy of Nursing."[7]

Nightingale differentiated nursing from medicine by delineating nursing's concern with the patient who was ill rather than the illness of the patient. Although nurses were to carry out physician orders, they were to do so only with an independent sense of responsibility for their actions. All women, advised Nightingale, were to practice health nursing, which required some practical teaching, and the goal of which was prevention of disease.[8] A nurse was, to Nightingale, any woman who had the "charge of the personal health of somebody," whether sick or well.[9]

Returning to the social context of this environmental era, the formalizing of nursing outside the home represented the invention of a whole new work arrangement that had broad economic, gender, and social class implications. The intimate nature of the work of nurses, once performed within families and now practiced in public arenas among strangers, further confounded attempts to categorize and organize the effort. Not surprisingly, several methods of organization developed. Each embodied ideal characteristics of its leading advocate and each concerned itself with the contextual issues in a manner that each leader hoped would gain acceptance for nursing.[10]

The first formal effort to organize the work of nursing occurred at the Nightingale Training School for Nurses at St. Thomas Hospital in London. Opened in 1860, the Nightingale School constituted a reform effort stimulated by the revelation of the scandalous care received by British soldiers during the Crimean War.[11] Grateful to the dogmatic, charismatic, complex Florence Nightingale for her legendary efforts on behalf of the soldiers in the war, British citizens contributed £44,000 with which ". . . to establish an institution for the training, sustenance, and protection of nurses and hospital attendants."[12]

NURSING AND KNOWLEDGE IN AMERICA: HISTORICAL OVERVIEW*

The Early Years

The relationship between nursing and knowledge is an oddly self-conscious one. Organized as a system of woman's work in the last half of the nineteenth century, nursing provoked prevailing fears that women who used their mental energies diverted and depleted their reproductive energies, especially at certain times. That exhausting physical work was not only permitted but necessary in nursing seems not to have disturbed the sensibilities of that generation's guardians of women's health. From the 1873 organization of nursing in training schools in America, women traded their physical labor as pupil–nurses for sparse and hurried instruction at the bedside in their attempt to become "trained" nurses and make themselves self-sufficient in a vastly changing society.

The accumulation of knowledge by self-identified nurses began almost covertly with Nightingale's nighttime studies of mathematics, science, and hospital reports in the 1840s.[13] Convinced that the absence of knowledgeable nurses caused the sick harm, Nightingale wrote to her cousin: "I saw a poor woman die before my eyes this summer because there was nothing but fools to sit up with her, who poisoned her as much as if they had given her arsenic."[14] Prevented by custom and her mother from direct learning activities, Nightingale, aided by her father, chose indirect methods by candlelight.[15]

Her American successors described similar situations in less than privileged circumstances. America's "first trained nurse," Linda Richards, wrote about her one-year (1872–1873) course during which the trainees worked 16-hour days, slept in rooms between the wards, received no pay, had only one free afternoon every second week, had no books or examinations and only a limited bedside instruction—yet, "if complaint was made that we did not do well, we were called to account."[16–18] Referring to the common practice whereby pupil–nurses donated their services to patients in the community while the hospitals collected the fees for that service, Hopkins' nursing superintendent Isabel Hampton chided her medical colleagues at the 1893

World's Fair that pupils had not entered hospital work to be "philanthropists."[19] Having attracted women to nursing work with promises of training, was it "not then a most serious responsibility on the part of such hospitals or training schools to see that the education is made as complete as possible?"[20]

The specific goals articulated by Hampton, a former teacher, at the 1893 Fair included a uniform curriculum in all schools, a three-year course of eight-hour days, specified entry periods, unified standards for applicants, a divided academic year as in colleges, and normal school courses for the nurses who would be the teachers.[21] A full decade passed before some of the best schools achieved even a few of these goals.

The awkward and ambivalent relationship between nursing and knowledge that began out of necessity and social custom became entwined in the developing nursing culture. The extensive fusion of preparation, even to sharing residence, with the work itself made nursing different from every other occupation for which knowledge was considered important. It reinforced the notion that nursing was "natural" to women and that its "higher" rewards were adequate. It strengthened the menial aspects of the nurse training, making them predominate, for without systematic inquiry into the nature of nursing and its application in varied situations to different individuals, thinking action could not replace rote doing. Nursing's only relationship with legitimate education came through courses for the teachers, who also administered the agencies. Special preparation for teaching and administrative tasks was accepted and the new Teachers' College welcomed the nursing teachers as students. Not surprisingly, the teachers and administrators who attended such courses chose areas of study relevant to their function, teaching and managing, and did not advance knowledge regarding nursing practice.[22]

By the late 1920s, small numbers of nurses engaged in and reported a more formal, though still rudimentary, kind of research that they called "studies" and that could be applied in practice. "[K]nowledge, interest and ideals are never an end in themselves; their function is to influence action. It is how we act, how we respond to this situation or how we conduct ourselves under one circumstance or another, that is the final test of knowledge."[23] Some of these studies compared cases of treating illness, oth-

---

* This section, through page 331, was written by Ellen D. Baer.

ers compared methods of problem solving in teaching students.[24] Even so, an unsigned editorial, presumed to be by Isabel Stewart, in Teachers' College *Nursing Education Bulletin* regretted that "It is not much exaggeration to say that the scientific content of nursing is little more than a thin veneer covering a large body of traditional materials and experience."[25] The nurses' concern about "the scientific content of nursing" echoed the entire medical community's post-Flexner (1910) preoccupation with meeting standards accorded to "professions": those occupations characterized by intellectual function with individual responsibility that are based on science and are learned over a long period of study, having specialized skills and knowledges, altruistic motives and a "tendency to self-government."[27]

Once again a war precipitated progress in nursing's search for sound educational and scientific foundations. Born at the Crimea with Nightingale, modern nursing grew with each American national catastrophe as well. World War II proved no exception. Aware that events in Europe and the Pacific might require an American nursing effort, the 1940 Biennial Convention of the American Nurses' Association (ANA) sent a message to President Roosevelt, offering its service.[28] Anticipating some response, representatives from the five major nursing organizations formed the Nursing Council on National Defense in July, 1940, with ANA President Julia Stimson as Council president.[29] In the 18 months available to them before the United States entered the war, the Council (renamed the National Nursing Council for War Service in 1942) assessed America's nurse power through a National Survey of Nurses, established an optimal ratio of nurse to military (1:154) and, most importantly, persuaded the government "that federal aid for nursing education was a legitimate and imperative defense measure."[30–32]

Professional Nursing

To continue the historical analysis, in the twentieth century, scientific advances and medical technology gave sick-care institutions the opportunity to do more than care for and protect people. Certain diseases could be cured, and institutional agendas shifted accordingly. Dependence no longer assured someone a place in an institution.[33] Illnesses susceptible to manipulation by new science and its technology became the preferred admitting criteria and nurses' caretaking role had to share its central position with the instrumentality of medicine. Further, the promise of cure dramatically altered institutions' potential benefits to society because cure returned sick people to health and to work. Society profited from the regained productivity and economic independence of recovered citizens.

By the mid-twentieth century, insurance had become the passport for hospital entry. Insurers who would not pay for diagnostic tests done on an outpatient basis but would pay for those done in a hospital guaranteed full or near-full occupancies, and nurses became traffic cops, directing the flow of patients to and from their multiple appointments in congested and increasingly specialized institutions. More than ever before, managing the bureaucratic mayhem occupied nurses' time and defined their success. Efficiency models, time and motion studies, and even assembly-line management methods inspired nurses' activities; caretaking became a by-product delegated to less-prepared, inexpensive armies of aides and technicians hired during World War II.

During the civil rights movement of the 1960s, ethnic, racial, gender, and consumer groups mobilized with zeal to reclaim their alleged abrogated rights. As members of these groups, individual nurses developed political agendas, sought advanced degrees, and resumed their caretaking roles with new interest in nurses' rights to practice autonomously. At the same time, nurses and physicians began extolling the virtues of comprehensive care, total care, holistic care, and primary care.[34] Specialist roles allowed nurses to advance in status and pay without having to move into administrative or teaching positions. Some specialists chose inpatient, acute-care clinical roles that focused on specific patient populations: oncology, clinical nurse specialists, and so on. Others, such as nurse practitioners, chose outpatient, generalist roles that involved providing primary care to broad segments of the population. Nurse anesthetists and nurse–midwives, pioneers in the two major nursing specialty areas, continued to practice in their established niches. But these were nursing pro-active agendas, and it is unclear whether they fit as well with institutional agendas as had nursing's earlier reactive modes of practice. Like the movements that spawned it, nursing's more assertive posturing upset the institutional social order.

Specific economic arrangements for nursing practice did not exist until the 1977 Rural Health Clinics Act (PL95–210) authorized reimbursement for nurse practitioner services in rural districts, dependent on individual state approval.[35] For the preceding century, although making up 40 percent of most health care institution budgets, the costs of nursing practice were subsumed into and reimbursed to hospital bed and board of clinical agency operating expenses.[36] Rendered economically invisible by such accounting practices, nursing was seen by administrators as a cost center and not as a revenue producing center.

Teachers and administrators in hospital schools of nursing did not encourage students to question the practices of their parent organizations. By the war's end, 70,000 nurses were eligible for GI benefits and nurses entered higher education in droves. The GI Bill gave many nurses financial access to higher education and, by 1972, more nurses obtained their basic nursing education in academic institutions rather than in hospitals.[37] Better equipped intellectually to question old practices and enlightened by 1960s activism, especially the women's movement, nurses began to assert themselves. At the same time, the health care system was getting into a bind. The rights movement combined with the enactment of Medicare and Medicaid legislation to create a demand for services that physicians could not meet, and the nurse practitioner movement began. More than 60 studies have proved the efficacy and cost-effectiveness of nurse practitioners as substitutes for more expensive physician care givers in outpatient settings.[38] Nurse–practitioners took advantage of a social need, staked a claim to good patient outcomes, documented that they achieved such outcomes, and now seek broader economic recognition of their work.

Although few researchers have assessed the direct impact of the advanced preparation of nurses on inpatient care, one major study showed that the institutions that employ advanced practice nurse specialists become "magnet" hospitals, attracting patients and staff with the greatest success.[39] The study points to the presence of clinical nurse specialists as a major factor in those institutions' "magnet" status.

Nursing's Social Policy

The professionalization of nursing was a move to secure nursing's position within society as a profession. The evolution of its professional status can most readily be traced by following the history of its national nursing organization. To understand its position today, nursing's meaning, identity, and social purpose, best described by nurse historians and philosophers, has also been codified by the profession into a social policy statement.[40] This statement, drafted by a seven-member task force appointed by the ANA Congress for Nursing Practice, outlined the nature and scope of nursing practice and a description of the characteristics of specialization in nursing. It ultimately answers the repeatedly asked question, "What is nursing?" and was drafted with the intent to facilitate decisions through which nursing can consolidate achievements of the past and move with wisdom and courage into its future of service to society.

Nursing is an essential part of the society out of which it developed and with which it has been evolving. In one sense, nursing can be said to be owned by society because nursing's professional interests serve the interests of the larger whole of which it is a part.[41] This mutually beneficial relationship between society and its profession is described in the ANA social policy statement as follows:

A profession acquires recognition, relevance, and even meaning in terms of its relationship to that society, its culture and institutions, and its other members. Professions acquire recognition and relevance primarily in terms of needs, conditions, and traditions of particular societies and their members. It is societies (and often their vested interests within them) that determine, in accord with their different technological and economic levels of development and their socio-economic, political and cultural conditions, and values, what professional skills and knowledge they most need and desire. By various financial means, institutions will then emerge to train interested individuals to supply those needs.

Logically, then, the professions open to individuals in any particular society are the property not of the individual but of society. What individuals acquire through training is professional knowledge and skill, not a profession or even part ownership of one.[42]

Authority for Nursing Practice

The authority for nursing, as for other professions, is based on a social contract, which in turn derives from a complex social base. Under the terms of the contract, society grants the professions authority over functions vital to itself and permits them considerable autonomy in the conduct of their activities. In return, professions are expected to act responsibly, always mindful of the public trust. Self-regulation to assure quality in performance is at basis of this relationship and is the hallmark of a mature profession.[43]

The Nature and Scope of Nursing Practice

Nursing is the diagnosis and treatment of human responses to actual or potential health problems. This definition points to four defining characteristics of nursing: phenomena, theory application, nursing action, and evaluation of effects of action in relation to phenomena.

The *phenomena of concern* to nurses are human responses to actual or potential health problems. Such responses include, but are not limited to, the following: self-care limitations, impaired functioning in areas such as rest, sleep, ventilation, circulation, activity, nutrition, elimination, skin, sexuality; pain and discomfort; emotional problems related to illness and treatment, life-threatening events, or daily experiences such as anxiety, loss, loneliness, and grief; distortions of symbolic functions, reflected in interpersonal and intellectual processes, such as hallucinations; deficiencies in decision making and ability to make personal choices; self-image changes required by health status; dysfunctional perceptual orientations to health; strains related to life processes; and problematic affiliative relationships.

Nurses use *theory* in the form of concepts, principles, and processes to understand the phenomena within the domain of nursing practice. The theoretical base for nursing is partially self-generated and partially drawn from other fields. The range of theories used by nurses varies through interpersonal, intrapersonal, and systems theories, with the latter providing explanations of complex networks or organizations, the dynamics of their parts and processes in interaction.

The aims of nursing *actions*, ideally based on theoretical formulations, are directed toward promoting health and preventing illness. Nursing actions are intended to produce beneficial *effects* in relation to identified responses.

Nursing is part of the total health care system. The term health care, not synonymous with nursing or medical care, refers to a composite of planned care provided by interdependent collaborative professionals. The scope of nursing practice, therefore, must be defined in concert with other health care professions.

Thus, the contents of the nursing segment of health care, has four defining characteristics: boundary, intersections, dimensions, and core.

Nursing's *boundary* expands outward in response to changing needs, demands, and capacities of society. As new needs and demands arise, and as a consequence of nursing research, the other three defining characteristics of scope begin to change, resulting in expansion of the boundary.

The nursing components of health care *intersect with other* professions in the health care arena. The intersections are not hard and fast lines separating nursing from another profession; the relations between nursing and medicine at these interfacings are especially fluid in situations where collegial, collaborative joint practice obtains.[44]

The *core* of nursing practice is the basis for nursing care, e.g., the phenomena of concern. Diagnosis of phenomena (e.g., human response) leads to the application of theory to explain the condition and to determine actions to be taken. The range of diagnostic categories within the scope of nursing practice is constantly undergoing expansion.

The *dimensions* of nursing practice include but are not limited to the philosophy and ethics that guide nurses. One of the most distinguishing characteristics of nursing is that it involves practices that are nurturative, generative, or protective in nature.[45] Nurses are also guided by a humanistic philosophy having caring coupled with understanding and purpose as its central features. Values include regard for self-determination, independence and choice in decision making in matters of health, respect for the individual unaltered by the social, educational, economic, cultural, racial, or religious attributes of the patient.

Nursing care is provided with an interpersonal relationship process to a patient, a family, or a group. It involves privileged intimacy—physical and interpersonal. Nursing is a laying-on-of-hands practice in which nurses have access to the body of another person in carrying out assessments, comfort care, and definitive treatments. Nursing includes an array of functions, including physical care, anticipatory guidance, health teaching, counseling, and the like.

Nursing practice demands professional intention and commitment carried out in accordance with the ANA Standards of Practice and the ethical code for nurses. Nursing is practiced at the generalist and specialist level. Each nurse remains accountable for the quality of her or his practice within the full scope of nursing practice. Variations within nursing practice result from differences in level of education, extent of experience, and competence in regard to the following: assessment and data collection, analysis of data, application of theory, breadth and depth of knowledge base, range of nursing techniques, need for supervision, evaluation of effects of practice, and identification of relationships among phenomena, nursing actions, and effects on patients.

All nurses are responsible for the inclusion of preventive nursing as part of generalized and specialized practice. Prevention in nursing is directed to promotion of health and disease prevention; securing prompt attention for medical diagnosis and treatment of disease, or as necessary when predisposition to a given disease is apparent from the nursing diagnosis; and early recognition and management of complications and other consequences arising from disease or therapy.

Nurses provide care to people in various states of their life-span, from birth through death. Nurses are ethically and legally accountable for actions taken in the course of nursing practice as well as for actions delegated by the nurse to others assisting in the delivery of nursing care. Such accountability may be accomplished through the regulatory mechanism of licensure, through criminal and civil laws, through the code of ethics of the profession, and through peer evaluation.

Nursing Process: An Organizing Framework for Practice

The ANA Social Policy Statement outlines the value that nursing places on an approach to practice in which investigation and action are interrelated. This approach, noted in the four characteristics of nursing that are reflected in the use of the nursing process, serves as an organizing framework for practice and is described in the Social Policy Statement as follows:

The nursing process encompasses all significant steps taken in the care of the patients, with attention to their rationale, their sequence, and related importance to helping the patient reach specified and attainable health goals. The nursing process requires a systematic approach to the patient's situation, which includes reconciliation of patient/family and nurse perceptions of the situation; a plan for nursing ac-

tions, which include patient/family participation in goal setting; joint implementation of the plan; and evaluation which includes patient/family participation. The steps in the process are not necessarily taken in strict sequence beginning with assessment and ending with evaluation. The steps may be taken concurrently and should be taken recurrently, as in the evaluation of the assessment or the plan of action.[46]

Recognition of the nursing process is reflected in the ANA Standards of Nursing Practice, which apply to all nursing practice. The standards describe a "therapeutic alliance" of the nurse and the person for whom he or she provides care through the use of the nursing process.[47]

The relationship between the characteristics of nursing, the nursing process, and the standards that reflect it are shown in Figure 19-1. The characteristics of phenomena and theory application are implicit in the standards involving data collection, diagnosis, and planning; that of action is referred to in the standards involving planning and treatment; and the characteristics of effects are related to the standards involving evaluation and revision.

The Discipline of Nursing

As nursing approaches the twenty-first century, a repeated theme in the literature is the quest for defining nursing knowledge.[48-50] In the interim, much has been written about nursing knowledge. A review of research problems, questions, and studies notes a *global* approach to the task. Donaldson and Crowley urge nurses to be clear about nursing as a profession and as a discipline.[51] By definition, these researchers write, a discipline is not global; it is characterized by a unique perspective, a distinct way of viewing all phenomena, which ultimately defines the limits and nature of its inquiry. They appeal for an identification of the essence of nursing research and of the common elements and threads that give coherence to a precise body of knowledge. Rather than continuing the use of energy in defining the nature of nursing, Donaldson and Crowley suggest focusing on the following themes: (1) Principles and laws that govern life processes, well-being, and optimum functioning of human beings—sick or well; (2) the patterning of human behavior in interaction with the environment in critical life situations; and (3) the processes by which positive changes

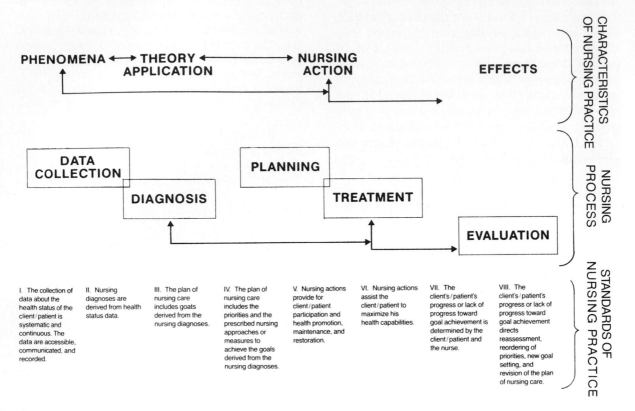

Figure 19-1. Defining characteristics of nursing practice: relationship to the nursing process and the standards of nursing practice. ANA Standards of Nursing Practice, Kansas City, MO: American Nurses Association, 1974. Reprinted with permission.

in health status are effected.[52] These themes may be considered boundaries of an area for systematic inquiry and theory development for making the nature of the discipline of nursing more explicit than it is at present.

What then is the discipline of nursing? Reminding us that, traditionally, human knowledge and inquiry have been considered in the context of disciplines, and that the two major types of disciplines are sciences and humanities, Donaldson and Crowley emphasize that nursing has both scientific aspects and aspects akin to the humanities, e.g. the arts.[53] They cite, for example, that human health is considered within nursing in terms of political issues, history, and laws of health. Therefore, they conclude, nursing as a discipline is broader than nursing science and its uniqueness stems from its perspective rather than its object of inquiry or methodology.

Disciplines can also be typed as academic or professional. The academic disciplines include sciences such as physiology, sociology, physics, and liberal arts disciplines such as mathematics, philosophy, and history. The aim of academic disciplines is knowledge development, and their theories are descriptive in nature. Professional disciplines, in contrast, are directed toward practical aims, generate prescriptive as well as descriptive theories and include basic, applied and clinical studies.[54]

Part of the reason for nursing's struggle in evolving, observe Donaldson and Crowley, is derived from the slow emergence of the recognition of its social relevance.[55] Because nurses give service related to the quality of human life, its value fluctuates often, depending upon the current social value of service.

Patterns of Knowing

The body of knowledge that serves as the rationale for nursing practice, observes Carper, include patterns, forms and structure that provide an understanding characteristic way of thinking about phenomena.[56] Carper identified four patterns of knowing from an analysis of the conceptual and syntactical structure of nursing knowledge.[57] The four patterns are distinguished according to logical type of meaning and designated as: (1) empirics, the science of nursing; (2) esthetics, the art of nursing; (3) the component of a self-knowledge in nursing; and (4) ethics, the component of moral knowledge in nursing.

Empirics and the Science of Nursing

The 1950s saw the emergence of the term *nursing science* in the literature. Since that time, as already described, there has been an intensity to the press for developing nursing knowledge. Some of the advance in nursing science is the representation of health as more than the absence of disease, rather viewing health as a dynamic state or process that changes over time. This conceptualization permits a classification for variations in health or levels of wellness as expressions of a human being's relationship to the internal and external environment.[58]

Science is the consensus of informed opinion obtained usually through research.[59] Science seeks to describe, explain, and predict events as it develops a body of understanding about the universe. Nursing science, as a form of human science, has as its object of analysis, the human organism, with particular reference to the human response states in illness and health across the life-span. Its aim is to generate a body of knowledge that can define patterns of behavior associated with normal and crucial life events such as catastrophic illness; depict changes in health status and predict how these are brought about; and along with other scientific fields, determine the principles and laws governing life states and processes.[60,61] Ultimately the aim of nursing science is prediction of the human response state.

Esthetics and the Art of Nursing

The "art" of nursing, once a dominant component (e.g., teaching of the nursing arts), has been relegated to a lesser position in the description of nursing. Carper suggests two reasons for the reluctance of nursing to acknowledge the esthetic component as a fundamental pattern of knowing in nursing.[62] The first was the effort to exorcise the image of the apprentice-type educational system of nursing. Within this system, the art of nursing was closely associated with an imitative learning style and the acquisition of knowledge by accumulation of unra-

tionalized experiences. The second reason is the restricted definition of the term *art*.

Several nursing authors discuss art and nursing. Wiedenbach speaks of the art of nursing made visible through the action taken to provide whatever the patient requires to restore or extend his ability to cope with the demands of his situation.[63] Orem writes of the art of nursing as being "expressed by the individual nurse through her creativity and style in designing and providing nursing that is effective and satisfying."[64]

Carper's study suggests that one esthetic pattern of knowing is empathy, that is, the capacity for participating in or vicariously experiencing another's feelings.[65] Empathy is controlled or moderated by psychic distance or objectivity in order to abstract what is being attended to. The esthetic pattern of knowing involves the perception of particulars as distinguished from universals; that is, understanding the uniqueness of an individual as separate from a class or group.

The Component of Personal or Self-knowledge

This component relates to the therapeutic use of self and the literature on self-knowledge. Difficult to teach, it is an integral aspect of psychiatric mental health nursing. It is concerned with the kind of knowing that promotes wholeness and integrity in the personal encounter.

Ethics as the Moral Component

This pattern of knowing focuses on matters of obligation or what ought to be done. Knowledge of morality goes beyond simply knowing moral codes and rules. Nursing's goals and actions involve choices to be made. Berthold writes that "goals are, of course, value judgments not amenable to scientific inquiry and validation."[66] Much of nursing's value orientation is related to the goal of patient independence and nursing actions to assist the patient in assuming full responsibility for himself at the earliest possible moment or to enable him to retain responsibility to the last possible moment. However, continues Carper, valuing independence and attempting to maintain it may be at the expense of the patient's learning how to live with physical or social dependence when necessary.[67] Differences in normative judgments may have more to do with agreements as to what constitutes a "healthy" state of being than lack of empirical evidence in the application of the term.

Ethical and moral values inherent in clinical practice have significantly influenced the perspective and value orientation of the discipline. A goal of nursing service is to foster self-caring behavior; thus, nursing interventions aim to foster individual independence rather than control and directly manipulate the person into a socially determined state of health.[68]

THEORY DEVELOPMENT

While the past 30 years have seen a particular emphasis on nursing theory development, the need for knowledge that is specific to nursing has been acknowledged since the writings of Florence Nightingale. This pioneer nursing leader focused on the environment, nourishment, and observation of the patient and on the interaction between patient and nurse. Nightingale was clear in her perception of nursing and its relationship to medicine and the patient[69]:

Pathology teaches the harm that disease has done. But it teaches nothing more. We know nothing of the principle of health, the positive of which pathology is the negative. . . . It is often thought that medicine is the curative process. It is no such thing; medicine is the surgery of functions. . . . Surgery removes the bullet out of the limb, which is an obstruction to cure, but nature heals the wound. . . . Medicine . . . assists nature to remove the obstruction. . . . And what nursing has to do, in either case, is to put the patient in the best condition for nature to act. . . .

Although the charge to nursing was clear over 130 years ago, it is only within the past several decades, observes Newman, that we have begun to discover the kinds of information that will assist us in establishing optimal health for people, in sickness and in health.[70]

Background

Since the late 1950s and early 1960s, nurse scholars and scientists have been involved in a theory-development movement in nursing. This movement has evolved, in part, from the development of research in nursing and a concomitant evolutionary shift in nursing to conceptual language. As nursing became autonomous from physician authority, there was increasing pressure to answer such question as: What is nurs-

ing? What is nursing research? What is nursing theory? What do nurses do?

Nurses quickly learned of the reciprocal relationship between theory development and research. As nurses became involved in research for nursing, observed Ellis, they became involved in theory development in nursing.[71]

The primary goal of nursing theory is the generation of knowledge specific to nursing. In the early days, the literature focused on the definitions inherent in the theory domain. A theory is formally defined as "a set of interrelated constructs [concepts], definitions, and propositions that present a systematic view of a phenomena by specifying relations among variables."[72]

Theory postulates specific relations among concepts and takes the form of a description, an explanation, a prediction, or a prescription for action. Any theory presupposes a more general abstract conceptual system; the concepts, definitions, and propositions of the theory are derived from the concepts and assumptions of the model.[73] Scientific theories are those that can be communicated and can be used and evaluated by others. They are produced by processes that are public, explicated, and open to evaluation against agreed-upon criteria. Scientifically tested theories are one important form of knowledge essential to effective professional practice of nursing.[74]

Theory development in nursing is old enough to have a past. As with many pioneering issues, isolated articles began appearing first. Gunter's 1962 article titled, "Notes on a Theoretical Framework for Nursing Research," was published by *Nursing Research* and eventually followed by variations on the theme, e.g., Brown's 1964 article on the importance of a theoretical framework in nursing research and the 1964 Wald and Leonard article on development of nursing practice theory. By 1971 the interest in the issue had created a forum for debate. Walker's understanding of the concept of nursing theory was criticized and Walker published a rejoinder.[75]

As interest was gaining momentum, three conferences on theory development in nursing, termed Landmark Symposia, were held in 1967 and 1968, with the purpose to bring together nurse scientists to discuss nursing theory and nursing science. These conferences provided a forum for established as well as emerging nurse scholars to come together to discuss the issues related to the development of the discipline of nursing. The result of the conferences was the publication of papers presented, the topics of which ranged from a theory of theories, research's role in theory development, borrowed and unique features of theory in nursing, a theory of clinical nursing, the nature of science and nursing, science and the helping professions, the pure and applied scientist and theories, and models and systems for nursing.

SCIENTIFIC ERA

With theory development well established, nurse scholars began refining and expanding the literature relevant to the science of nursing, the development, analysis, and evaluation of theory building, and the relationship between nursing theory, nursing research, and nursing practice.

Nursing science has been defined as the body of codified understanding of human biology and behavior in health and illness, with particular attention to response states.[76,77] In 1969, Abdullah discussed the nature of nursing science, stating that terms must be operationally defined and preferably observable and quantifiable.[78] Postulates are validated by testing deductions, which either helps to confirm the theory or leads to modifications of the postulates. The criterion for the assessment of scientific progress is an increase in scientific truths.

The emergence of conceptual frameworks in nursing in the early 1970s heralded another review of the relationship of theory development and philosophy of science. The early frameworks made no explicit linkage to philosophy of science; however, in the 1980s there is noted a shift in nurse theorist's thinking. For example, when Newman introduced a new theory of health, the viewpoint was of logical empiricism.[79] In 1983, one notes a shift in her thinking, where the emphasis is on process (not product) and revolution (not logic), from logical empiricism to historicism.

Every scientific theory is tied to some philosophical framework as the basis for understanding and assessing theory. Silva and Rothbart suggest there is the beginning of a metatheoretical shift away from a strongly empirical and logical empiricism and toward a more holistic and humanist approach more in line with historicism.[80]

Nursing Research

Research is the systematic process of scientific inquiry that is involved in the generation and testing of knowledge.[81,82] In nursing, research is a tool that both professional nurses and nurse scholars use to obtain the knowledge and information needed to make daily practice and administrative decisions.[83,84]

The ultimate goal of the nursing profession, writes Duffy, is to provide the highest quality services to the individual whom it serves.[85] All disciplines, in order to advance, must develop a scientific body of knowledge.

History

Harriett Werley, founder and first chairperson of the Council on Computer Applications in Nursing, was an early advocate of nursing research. To help place the *early* history of nursing research into perspective, we cite one of the 1976 presentations.[86]

It is generally recognized that advancement in an area or field comes about as a result of research; this should be no less true for nursing than for other fields.* Some would have us believe that research is new in nursing, and, therefore, that we should be patient about the slowness with which the research dimension is being developed. Some of us, however, do not see it as a recent development and are impatient with the fact that nursing leadership through the years has not viewed research as important, has not *expected* research to be developed and conducted, and has not seen to it that the criterion of research performance loomed large in nursing's reward system. In 1966 Virginia Henderson raised the question, "Do we not deny our function when we fail to investigate it?" She was, of course, concerned about the dearth of research in the practice of nursing.[87]

In my estimation, nursing research is not as new as some would have you believe when they mention its beginnings in the 1950s. Why, even I was actively encouraging research at that time! As I view it, research in nursing is as old as our heritage in nursing itself, which is generally

* This section, through page 339, is reprinted with permission from H. H. Werley, "Nursing Research in Perspective," in *Nursing in Illinois: A Bicentennial Glimpse*, College of Nursing Round Table Discussion, Chicago: University of Illinois, 1976.

thought to derive from Florence Nightingale. I think it is important for us to understand that, if we are interested in the "whence" and the "whither" of nursing research.

Florence Nightingale was, in fact, a great researcher, and if you doubt that, you should read some biographies on her, and more importantly you should examine some of the old documents that she developed to make her case about needing to clean up and systematize the health delivery system of her day. She produced well-documented data-based materials to justify her stance. I remember when in 1959 we were conducting a two-week nursing research conference at the Walter Reed Army Institute of Research, Dr. Bernard G. Greenberg made the point so well about her research contributions:

She was the person who kept prodding, you might say, all the English government officials about many of the things they were doing, not only in nursing, but in education, in social welfare, in hospital work, in penology, and many others. As a matter of fact, she gave a paper about a hundred years ago, before the Royal Statistical Society, on hospital statistics and the value of interpreting hospital statistics. That paper had a lot more insight as to the value of hospital statistics and their limitations than some of the papers I read today in . . . periodicals where they try to misuse or overuse the data available from hospitals. Florence Nightingale was more aware of the limitations in hospital data than some of our current research workers. . . . If anybody was a critical thinker, it was Florence Nightingale.

These remarks, in essence, will help us to put into perspective the older beginnings of nursing's research movement.

Unfortunately, there does not seem to have been much persistence to these older beginnings. In the late 1920s, Mary Marvin read a paper on "Research in Nursing" at the annual reunion of the Teachers College Alumnae in which she told her audience that "research and experimentation are universally recognized instruments or methods for finding out new facts and principles and for applying known facts and principles to the problems of everyday life."[88] She outlined six phases of experimentation that would help in developing nursing along safer, sounder lines. She commented on nursing instructors being impressed with the variety of methods of doing the same procedures and the lack of understanding of the principles involved, not only implying the need for research, but asking, "Is it too much to hope that some day every nursing procedure will be scientifically tested with the results measured, so far as it is possible to measure them?"[89] She saw scientific research as the means of developing nursing in a shorter time than could possibly be done by slow accumulation of knowledge gained through casual experiences, and she outlined some of the fundamental needs for undertaking research, including a journal in which to publish results and funds for projects.

It seems that eventually the research emphasis petered out, and it was a British physician, Margaret Jackson, who wondered about nursing's lack of research emphasis. Writing in *Nursing Times* in 1955, she said, "Research into nursing methods and appliances possibly began with Eve. Miss Nightingale and the generation of nurses trained under her aegis took it, of course, immeasurably further; but since their day it seems to have come to a dead end of evolution, like the frog."[90] She commented on aspects of nursing that had changed and that few nurses seemed to pause and ask themselves questions pertinent to their methods and equipment for purposes of improvement. She felt it was time that nursing research be revived.

Since nursing has generally looked to Florence Nightingale as a model, why was the model not followed for the more research-oriented aspects of nursing? Why was nursing so eager to follow only the nursing course work and not also the investigative aspects that should have provided the bases for that course work? We might, however, ask the same question about the present-day situation and wonder why research receives so little emphasis by comparison, even today. R. L. McManus shed some light on how the early emphasis on developing the work of the nursing organization may, in earlier years, have sidetracked the few universities concerned with nursing education from developing scholarly work in the art and science of nursing.[91] This, however, does not explain the persistent relative lack of emphasis on research, despite the fact that through the years, nursing has struggled long and hard to move its educational programs into universities where one of the functions of faculties is to conduct research to expand knowledge.

Most nurses think of nursing research as having had its beginning in the 1950s, for many nurses remember that the ANA started a series of studies to examine nursing functions around that time; and then in 1955, the American Nurses' Foundation (ANF) was established by the ANA. Less well known to nurses, unfortunately, are the earlier efforts that were exerted in the interest of research development that go back to the early 1940s, which were highlighted by World War II when it was clearly shown that more research generally was needed. The culmination of many individuals' efforts was the Public Health Service Act of 1944, which authorized the Surgeon General to encourage and support research through grants to various health institutions and to individuals.[92] Further legislation in the 1940s brought into existence the National Institutes of Health (NIH), which today we take for granted. Over time, Public Health Service reorganization to meet needs brought about the establishment of the Division of Nursing Resources in 1948 with its *intra*mural research program and in 1960 the creation of the Division of Nursing (as it is known today) when the Division of Public Health Nursing and the Division of Nursing Resources were combined.

In the early 1950s, increasing interest was shown by nurses and others in the research and consultation services of staffs of the Public Health Service; and thus in 1954, the Division of Nursing Resources was given the responsibility for developing an *extra*mural research program to encourage and support research and research training in all areas of nursing. Consequently, in 1955, a Research Grants and Fellowship Branch was established within the Division of Nursing Resources comparable to similar branches in the various institutes of NIH. Evllwynne Vreeland was its first chief; Fay Abdellah, whom many associate with this activity, headed the branch later. The application for grants and the review procedures to be followed were the same as for all extramural research programs of NIH, and in the fall of 1955 the first applications for nursing research grants were processed. This led to the establishment of the Nursing Research Study Section, and I was privileged to be one of its initial members.

There were also other developments that must be considered in placing nursing research in proper perspective. I will mention only a few of these: (a) the establishment in 1953 of the Institute for Research and Service in Nursing Education at Teachers College, Columbia University, which through the years has provided learning experiences in research for doctoral students; (b) the establishment in 1957 of a Department of Nursing Research in the Walter Reed Army Institute of Research—the first nursing unit in a research institution and the em-

phasis was on research pertinent to the care and health of people rather than on education; (c) in 1969, the establishment of the Center for Nursing Research (later called the Center for Health Research) in the Wayne State University College of Nursing—this was the first research center in a college of nursing; (d) the WICHE effort to regionalize the interinstitutional nursing research efforts; and (e) the efforts on the part of personnel in the Southern Regional Education Board (SREB) to bolster nursing's research efforts. Each of these developments has had a bearing on the general research movement.

ANA and Nursing Research

In 1958, at the ANA's 41st Annual Convention, members of the ANA Committee on Current and Long-Term Goals stated that "the future of nursing should increasingly be dependent upon the results of research in nursing undertaken by nurses themselves." In fact, Goal One read as follows:

Stimulate efforts by nurses and other specialists to identify and enlarge the scientific principles upon which nursing rests, and to encourage research by them in the application of these principles to nursing practice. Thus, historically, the impetus to stimulate nursing research came from ANA goal statements on research and the development of new knowledge.

ANA Blueprint for Research in Nursing
Although the ANA Committee on Research and Studies had been in existence since "the 1954–1956 biennium to plan, promote, and guide research and studies relating to the functions of the Association," it was the 1960–1962 ANA Committee that developed the ANA Blueprint for Research in Nursing, stating it was "not a complete statement of what is needed in the way of a research program in nursing, but is a guide for the shaping of a research program." The language of the Blueprint was careful to permit individual nurse scientists creativity and latitude in the selection of research topics. The six broad subject areas, with 78 identified study areas suggested for research in the 1962 document, were: (1) Nursing and Its Practice; (2) Nursing in the Social Milieu; (3) Communication and Decision Making in Nursing; (4) Organization and Operation of Nursing Services; (5) Education for Nursing; and (6) Structure, Functions, and Program of the American Nurses' Association.

In 1970, the ANA Committee on Research and Studies recommended dissolving the Committee and establishing a Commission on Nursing Research to parallel the Commissions on Nursing Education and on Nurse Services. As one of its publication tasks, in 1976, the ANA Commission on Nursing Research published the statement on *Priorities for Research in Nursing*. Two broad areas of priorities for research in nursing were identified: the practice of nursing, in which 12 study areas were included, and the profession of nursing, which included 6 study areas. The predominant focus was on clinical research, reflecting the increased emphasis that the profession was placing on the need for such research to expand nursing's scientific knowledge base and, concurrently, improving the quality of nursing care. The priorities identify that this impetus for the clinical emphasis was the profession's response to a changing social climate in which (1) the elderly population was increasing; (2) the focus of health care was shifting from acute to chronic illness; (3) the impact of life-style behaviors on health was being recognized increasingly; and (4) health promotion and self-care activities were emerging as cultural values. In addition there were increasing numbers of clinical nursing majors in graduate programs as opposed to the earlier majors of education and administration, making available doctorally prepared nurses to conduct such clinical research.

In 1981, the ANA Commission on Nursing Research published *Research Priorities for the 1980s: Generating a Scientific Basis for Nursing Practice*. Six "directions for research" were identified as priorities in generating knowledge to guide practice:

1. Promoting health, well-being, and competency for personal care among all age groups;
2. Preventing health problems throughout the life-span that have the potential to reduce productivity and satisfaction;
3. Decreasing the negative impact of health problems on coping abilities, productivity, and life satisfaction of individuals and families;
4. Ensuring that the care needs of particularly vulnerable groups are met through appropriate strategies;
5. Designing and developing health care systems that are cost-effective in meeting the nursing needs of the population; and

6. Promoting health, well-being, and competency for personal health in all age groups.

This ANA statement focused on clinical practice research, emphasizing health promotion, self-care, cost-effectiveness, care of cultural minorities and the underserved poor and rural clients.

Nursing Comes of Age: The National Center for Nursing Research

In 1987, the NIH celebrated 100 years of biomedical research. The NIH was founded in 1887 when, during a cholera epidemic, a Hygienic Laboratory was established at the Marine Health Service Hospital in Staten Island, New York, for the study of infectious diseases. That facility was moved to its current Bethesda location in 1935 and renamed the National Institutes of Health in 1948.

On April 18, 1986, Secretary Bowen of the Department of Health and Human Services (DHHS) announced the establishment of the National Center for Nursing Research (NCNR), authorized under the Health Research Extension Act of 1985, Public Law 99-158. The purpose of the Nursing Center is to conduct a program of grants and awards supporting nursing research and research training related to patient care, the promotion of health, the prevention of disease, and the mitigation of the effects of acute and chronic illnesses and disabilities. In support of studies on nursing interventions, procedures, delivery methods, and ethics of patient care, the NCNR programs are expected to complement other biomedical research programs that are primarily concerned with the causes and treatment of disease.

In January 1987, the first meeting of a National Advisory Council to the NCNR was held and in May 1987, nurse-researcher Ada Sue Henshaw, former chair of the ANA Cabinet on Nursing Research, was appointed Director of the NCNR. With a first-year budget of approximately $16,200,000 in support of research and research training, the NCNR is the newest addition to the NIH family. The NCNR is expected to thrive as it carries out its mission to augment the nursing science base that underlies effective patient care and the efficient delivery of nursing services, which benefit all individuals in the United States at some time in their lives.

Summary

Nursing depends on the specific knowledge of human behavior in health and illness, the esthetic perception of significant human experiences, a personal understanding of the unique individuality of the self, and the capacity to make choices within concrete situations involving particular moral judgments. Each of these patterns of knowing have meaning for nursing according to its distinctive logic.

Questions

1. Describe the evolution of nursing thought.
2. What contributions have been made to nursing thought in the 20th century?
3. When did nursing research begin?
4. What role does the NCNR play in nursing thought?
5. Identify three future directions for nursing thought in the 21st century.

REFERENCES AND SUGGESTED READINGS

1. Ellis, R. Foreword. In L. H. Nicoll (Ed.) *Perspectives on Nursing Theory*, Boston: Little, Brown, 1986, p. ix.
2. Baer, E. D. Nursing's divided house: An historical view, *Nursing Research*, 1985, 34(1), 32–33.
3. Reed, P. G., & Zurakowski, T. L. Nightingale: A visionary model for nursing. In J. J. Fitzpatrick & A. L. Whall (Eds.), *Conceptual Models of Nursing: Analysis and Application*. East Norwalk, Conn.: Appleton-Century-Crofts, 1983, p. 11.
4. Cook, E. *The Life of Florence Nightingale* (Vols. 1 & 2), New York: Macmillan, 1942.
5. Murphy, J. Toward a philosophy of nursing. In N. L. Chaska (Ed.), *The Nursing Profession*, New York: McGraw Hill, 1978, pp. 3–9.
6. Schlodfeldt, R. M. Nursing research: Reflection of values, *Nursing Research*, 1977, 26(1), 4–9.
7. Torres, G. Florence Nightingale. In *Nursing theories: The Base for Professional Nursing Practice*, East Norwalk, Conn.: Appleton-Century-Crofts, 1980.
8. Nightingale, *Notes on Nursing*, op. cit.
9. Nightingale, *Notes on Nursing*, op. cit.
10. Baer, op. cit., p. 34.
11. Seymer, L. R. B. *Florence Nightingale's Nurses: The Nightingale Training School 1860–1960*. London: Pittman, 1960.
12. Seymer in Baer, Nursing's divided house, op. cit., p. 34.
13. Baer, E. D. Nursing. In R. Apple (Ed.), *Women and Health Care*, New York: Garland Publishing Co., in press.
14. Woodham-Smith, C. *Florence Nightingale 1820–1910* (London: The Reprint Society 1952) pp. 44–50.
15. Ibid, p. 43 in an uncited quote, and 44–50.
16. Richards, L. *Reminiscences of Linda Richards: America's First Trained Nurse*, Boston: Whitcomb and Barrows, 1911, pp. 6–12 and 114.
17. Ibid, p. 12.
18. Ibid.
19. Hampton, I. A., et al. *Nursing of the Sick 1893*. Nursing papers published separately under the sponsorship of the National League for Nursing Education, New York: McGraw Hill, 1949, p. 6. Original source: *Hospitals, Dispensaries and Nursing*, Papers and Discussions in the International Congress of Charities, Correction and Philanthropy, Section III, Chicago, June 12th to 17th, 1893, under the auspices of the World's Congress Auxiliary of the World's Columbian Exposition. John S. Billings, M.D. and Henry M. Hurd, M.D. (Eds.), Baltimore: The Johns Hopkins Press, 1894.
20. Ibid, p. 7.
21. Ibid, pp. 8–10.
22. Baer, E. D. A cooperative venture in pursuit of professional status: a research journal for nursing, *Nursing Research*, 1987, 36(1), 18–25.
23. Schmidt, E. Correlation of theoretical and practice work, extracts from a paper read at the annual meeting of the NYSLNE, Nov. 1919, *American Journal of Nursing*, 1920, 21(3), 164.
24. Domitilla, Sister. An experiment in the Project Method of Teaching, Department of Nursing Education Section, *American Journal of Nursing*, 1920, 21(1), 30–37.

25. *Nursing Education Bulletin 1928–1943* 1(1), p. 2. The Bulletin's editor, Isabel Stewart, is the presumed author.
26. Flexner, A. Is social work a profession? *Studies in Social Work*, 1915, (4), The New School of Philanthropy, 5–10.
27. Newell, H. *The History of the National Nursing Council*, an undated, bound pamphlet located in the open stacks at Mugar Library, Boston University, p. 1.
28. Goosetray, S. Pres. represented the National League for Nursing Education (NLNE), Julia Stimson, Pres. represented the American Nurses Association (ANA), National Organization of Public Health Nurses (NOPHN), Association of Collegiate Schools of Nursing (ACSN), and National Association of Colored Graduate Nurses (NACGN). Newell credits Isabel Stewart as the instigator in forming an official committee to review nursing's preparedness for war.
29. *New Horizons in Nursing*, Josephine Nelson (comp.), New York: Macmillan, 1950, p. 71.
30. Newell, op. cit., pp. 2–7 and 10–11.
31. Baer, A cooperative venture, op. cit., p. 19.
32. Baer, E. D. Making the most of today's economic climate, *Nursing and Health Care*, 1987, 8(3), 143–145 provides the basis for most of this section.
33. Rosenberg, C. E. The aged in a structural social context: Medicine as a case study. In D. Van Tassel & P. Stears (Eds.), *Old Age in a Bureaucratic Society. Contribution to the Study of Aging No. 4*. New York: Greenwood Press, 1985, pp. 236–239. The author added the interpretations about nursing.
34. McGivern, D. O. The evolution of primary care nursing. In M. D. Mezey & D. O. McGivern (Eds.), *Nurses, Nurse Practitioners: The Evolution of Primary Care*. Boston: Little, Brown, 1986, pp. 3–14.
35. Maraldo, P. J. Politics and policy in primary care. In M. D. Meezy & D. O. McGivern (Eds.), *Nurses, Nurse Practitioners: The Evolution of Primary Care*. Boston: Little, Brown, 1986, 438–439.
36. Lauver, E. B. Where will the money go? Economic forecasting and nursing's future. *Nursing & Health Care*, 1985, 6(3), 135.
37. Bullough, B. The state nurse practice acts. In M. D. Meezey & D. O. McGivern (Eds.), *Nurses, Nurse Practitioners: The Evolution of Primary Care*, Boston: Little, Brown, 1986.
38. Freund, C. M. Nurse practitioners in primary care. In M. D. Meezy & D. O. McGivern (Eds.), *Nurses, Nurse Practitioners: The Evolution of Primary Care*. Boston: Little, Brown, 1986, pp. 305–333.
39. McClure, M. L., Poulin, M. A., Sovie, M. D., & Wandelt, M. A. *Magnet Hospitals Attraction and Retention of Professional Nurses*, Kansas City, Mo.: American Nurses Association, 1983.
40. American Nurses Association Congress for Nursing Practice. Nursing: A social policy statement, Kansas City, Mo.: American Nurses Association, 1980.
41. Page, B. B. Who owns the professions? *Hastings Center Report*, 1975, 5(5), 7–8.
42. Nursing: A social policy statement, op. cit.
43. Donabedian, A. Foreward. In M. Phaneuf, *The Nursing Audit and Self Recognition in Nursing Practice*, 2 ed., New York: Appleton-Century-Crofts, 1976.
44. The National Joint Practice Commission. *Statement on the Definition of Joint or Collaborative Practice in Hospitals*. Chicago: The National Joint Practice Commission, 1977.
45. Bevis, E. O. *Curriculum Building in Nursing: A Process*. St. Louis: C. V. Mosby, 1975, p. 171.
46. Nursing: A social policy statement, op. cit.
47. American Nurses' Association Congress for Nursing Practice, *A Plan for Implementation of the Standards of Nursing Practice*. Kansas City, Mo.: The American Nurses Association, 1975, pp. 4–5.
48. Schlotfeldt, R. M. The need for a conceptual framework. In P. J. Verhonick (Ed.), *Nursing Research, Vol. 1*, Boston: Little, Brown, 1975, pp. 3–24.
49. Fawcett, J. The relationship between theory and research: A double helix, *Advances in Nursing Science*, 1978, 1(1), 49–62.
50. Donaldson, S. K., & Crowley, D. M. The disciplines of nursing, *Nursing Outlook*, 1978, 26, 113–120.
51. Ibid.
52. Ibid.
53. Ibid.
54. Ibid.
55. Ibid.
56. Carper, B. A. Fundamental patterns of knowing in nursing. *Advances in Nursing Science*, 1978, 1(1), 13–23.
57. Ibid.
58. Ibid.
59. Gortner, S. R. Knowledge in a practice discipline: Philosophy and pragmatics, *Nursing Research and Policy Formation: The Case of Prospective Payment*, Kansas City, Mo.: American Nurses Association, 1984, pp. 5–16.
60. Gortner, S. R. Nursing science in transition, *Nursing Research*, 1980, 29(3), 180–183.
61. Donaldson and Crowley, op. cit. 1978.
62. Carper, op. cit.
63. Wiedenbach, E. *Clinical Nursing: A Helping Art*, New York: Springer, 1964.
64. Orem, D. E. *Nursing: Concepts of practice*, New York: McGraw Hill, 1971.
65. Carper, op. cit.
66. J. S. Berthold: Symposium on theory development in nursing: Prologue, *Nursing Research 17*, 1968, pp. 196–197.
67. Carper, op. cit.
68. Donaldson and Crowley, op. cit.

69. Nightingale Notes, op. cit.
70. Newman, M. A. Nursing's theoretical evolution, *Nursing Outlook*, 1972, *20*(7), 449–453.
71. Ellis, R. op. cit.
72. Kerlinger, F. *Foundations of Behavioral Research*, 2nd ed., New York: Holt, Rineholt and Winston, 1973, p. 9.
73. Fawcett, J. A framework for analysis and evaluation of conceptual models of nursing, *Nurse Educator*, 1980, *5*(6), 10–14.
74. Ellis, op. cit.
75. Walker, L. Toward a clearer understanding of the concept of nursing theory, *Nursing Research*, 1971, *20*, 428–435.
76. Gortner, S. R. Nursing science in transition, 1980.
77. Ibid.
78. Abdullah, F. The nature of nursing science, *Nursing Research*, 1969, *18*, 390–393.
79. Newman, op. cit.
80. Silva, M. C., & Rothbart, D: An analysis of changing trends in philosophies of science on nursing theory development and testing, *Advances in Nursing Science*, 1984, *6*(2), 1–13.
81. Kerlinger, 1973.
82. Brink, P., & Wood, M. *Basic Steps in Planning Nursing Research: From Question to Proposal* 1980, 2nd ed., North Scituate, Mass.: Duxbury Press.
83. Lindeman, C. A. Priorities in clinical nursing research, *Nursing Outlook*, 1975, *23*, 693–698.
84. Horsley, J. A., Crane, J., Crabtree, M. K., & Wood, D. J. *Using Research to Improve Nursing Practice: A Guide*, Orlando: Grune & Stratton, 1983.
85. Duffy, M. E. The research process in baccalaureate nursing education: A ten-year review, *Image*, 1987, *19*(2), 87–91.
86. Werley, H. H. Nursing research in perspective, *Nursing in Illinois: A Bicentennial Glimpse*, College of Nursing Roundtable Discussion, Chicago: University of Illinois, 1976.
87. Henderson, V. The nature of nursing. *American Journal of Nursing*, 1964, *64*, 67.
88. Marvin, M. M. Research in nursing: The place of research in improving the nursing care of the patient, *American Journal of Nursing*, 1927, *27*, 331.
89. Ibid., 334.
90. Jackson, M. Where should the nurse be trained? *Nursing Times*, 1955, *51*, 560.
91. McManus, R. L. Research—Its evolution, *American Journal of Nursing*, 1961, *61*(4), 76.
92. Vreeland, E. M. Nursing research programs in the public health service, *Nursing Research*, 1964, *13*, 148.

Chapter 20

Conceptual Models of Psychiatric Nursing Care

Ann Wolbert Burgess

Chapter Objectives

The students successfully attaining the goals of this chapter will be able to:

- Define the historical and contemporary origins of the four models of patient care: cognitive–behavioral, psychological, social, and biologic.
- Explain the nine therapeutic nursing activities as identified by the ANA Division on Psychiatric and Mental Health Nursing Practice.
- Explain how the nursing activities are used in the models of care.
- Discuss the benefits of occupational therapy and art therapy to encourage social competencies in patients.
- Describe how the models of care are determined for each patient.
- Interpret the *ANA Standards of Psychiatric–Mental Health Nursing Practice* specific to interventions.

A central issue facing psychiatric mental health nursing is theory development, a conceptualization of the patient care process that would facilitate and enhance patient care, teaching, and the development of research hypotheses. This chapter will review the importance of a conceptual framework for nursing and current models of care in the specialty area of psychiatric mental health nursing.

CONCEPTUAL MODELS OF NURSING

Conceptual models, observes Fawcett are important in guiding the development of the discipline of nursing.[1] Conceptual models of nursing have had a major impact on nursing education. Since 1972, schools of nursing have been required to identify their conceptual frameworks as an accreditation requirement of the National League for Nursing.[2] It is reported that between 1964 and 1981 at least 22 conceptual models, or theories, of nursing were published.[3] From a national survey of 691 graduate students and nursing faculty, Jacobson reports the best-known models to be Orem's Self-Care Model (1971), M. E. Roger's Life Process Model (1970), the Roy Adaptation Model (1976), King's Social Systems Model (1971), Newman's Nursing Theory of Health (1979), the Johnson Behavioral Systems Model (Grubbs, 1974), and Peplau's Interpersonal Theory of Psychiatric Nursing (1952).[4]

The term conceptual model as defined by Fawcett refers to ideas about the individuals, groups, events, and situations of interest to a science.[5] These phenomena are classified into concepts that are words bringing forth mental images of the properties of things. Concepts are abstract ideas that are linked to form propositions stating their interrelationships. These statements constitute the basic assumptions of the science (e.g., "People and their environments are open systems"). Thus, according to Nye and Berardo, a conceptual model may be defined as a set of concepts and those assumptions that integrate them into a meaningful configuration.[6]

Conceptual models specify the phenomena of interest to nursing science, encompassed by four essential concepts: person, environment, health, and nursing.[7] Existing nursing models define and describe person and environment and their interrelations. Essentially, the majority of conceptualizations view the person as a biopsychosocial being who interacts with family members, the community, and other groups, as well as with the physical environment. However, the schemes are presented in various ways such as adaptive systems, behavioral subsystems, or complementary four-dimensional energy fields. The models further include a definition of health, often describing both the well and ill person and environments conducive or detrimental to health. They also identify the goals of nursing, which usually derive directly from the definition of health.[8]

Initial efforts in psychiatric nursing have been implemented by Fitzpatrick, Whall, Johnston, and Floyd in their book, *Nursing Models and Their Psychiatric Mental Health Applications.* To quote from Whall's Preface, "These nursing models are currently developed to a level where concepts are at times defined operationally but the relationships between concepts have not

been explicitly developed. What is available to guide the practice of psychiatric mental health nursing has, for the most part, been 'borrowed' from other disciplines. . . . What is needed now is a merging of prevailing nursing views, a merger of the nursing models with existing psychiatric mental health theories. We believe the nursing models should be used to reformulate or change the existing theories for the purposes of nursing."[9]

Responding to the question of the ethics and methods involved in reformulation of borrowed theory, the authors continue, "We agree with those philosophers of science, such as Abraham Kaplan, who posit that concepts and theories are not 'owned' by any one discipline, but rather, that each discipline has a right and a responsibility to select from the available knowledge, and to modify and reformulate those theoretical positions to its own purposes."[10]

Even though psychiatric nurses may be comfortable with their attitudes, feelings, and style, they still need to know the specific activities and tasks that facilitate recovery for the patient. In the same way, the nurse may be comfortable with the tension and drama of the operating room, but this does not make her an effective operating room nurse.

The specific tasks and activities used in psychiatric nursing are best described within the different conceptual models of psychiatric mental health care. Many people may be puzzled in trying to understand how a psychiatric nurse selects relevant clinical data, formulates or makes a diagnosis of the patient's problems, and decides on a treatment program. In the psychiatrically ill person, is it the symptom complex, the "unconscious conflict," or particular undesirable behaviors that contain the key to clinical decision making? And why does one nurse emphasize individual therapy; another, family therapy; a third, a biofeedback therapy; and a fourth, tricyclic antidepressants—for apparently similar patients?

DIFFERENT MODELS OF CONCEPTUAL CARE AND THE NINE THERAPEUTIC NURSING TASKS

One major reason for the difficulty in understanding the thinking regarding psychiatric care is that several different conceptual models are implicitly used in the clinical formulation. The four most common models are the psychological, the social, the cognitive–behavioral, and the biologic (medical). When a patient is being treated, the kind of assessment obtained, the meaning assigned to certain historical facts, and the treatment modalities most often chosen depend on which model or combination of models is employed.

This chapter will discuss the nine therapeutic tasks as identified by the ANA Division on Psychiatric and Mental Health Nursing and will explain how these nursing activities are used in the four models of care.[11] The nine tasks are as follows: providing a therapeutic milieu; addressing the here-and-now living problems of clients; the use of the surrogate parent role; addressing the somatic aspects of clients' health; client teaching; providing for social competencies in client care; conducting psychotherapy; assuming a leadership role; and assuming a community action role within the context of the four conceptual models of care. The therapeutic activities are illustrated by four case histories of *one* patient, each formulated in terms of one of the four models.[12] *

CASE HISTORY OF MRS. JANIS: COGNITIVE–BEHAVIORAL VIEW

Mrs. Janis is a 53-year-old widow who has a history of depressive behaviors of anorexia, insomnia, feelings of hopelessness, helplessness, and worthlessness. These behaviors began shortly after the death of her husband, who had been the major figure in her life. Throughout the marriage he had been a continuous source of reinforcement to the patient. This quality of the husband's interaction with his wife had been evident since the marriage, at which time the patient was still depressed after her mother's death. The family stated that the husband had always ignored the patient's demands and pleas of helplessness while responding actively to the more positive aspects of her personality. After his death the patient began to complain to her children about her loss of appetite and her sense of helplessness and worthlessness. They responded to these complaints with frequent visits and phone calls, but the depressive behavior only worsened.

CASE HISTORY OF MRS. JANIS: PSYCHOLOGICAL VIEW

Mrs. Janis is a 53-year-old widow who became depressed a few months ago after the death of her hus-

---

* Lazare, A., 1973, pp. 345–351.[12] Copyright 1973 by the *New England Journal of Medicine*. Sections used with permission.

band. Although the marriage seemed happy at times, it is known that there were many stormy periods in their relationship. There have been no visible signs of grief since his death. Since the funeral, the patient has been depressed and has lost interest in her surroundings. For no apparent reason she now blames herself for apparently minor events of the past. Sometimes she criticizes herself for traits that characterized her husband more than herself. She had a similar reaction after the death of her mother 23 years ago. At that time, the patient and mother lived together. From the family history, it could be inferred that the relationship was characterized by hostile dependency. Six months after her mother's death the patient married. The patient seems intelligent, motivated for treatment, and had considered psychotherapy in the past in order to gain a better understanding of herself.

CASE HISTORY OF MRS. JANIS: SOCIAL VIEW

Mrs. Janis is a 53-year-old widow who has been depressed during the past few months after the death of her husband. He had been the major figure in her life, and his loss has left her feeling lonely and isolated. After his death she moved to a small apartment some distance from her old neighborhood. Although she is satisfied with her new quarters, she finds the community strange. Furthermore, she does not have access to public transportation, which would enable her to visit her old friends, children, and grandchildren. Since her husband's death, old strains between the patient and her children have been aggravated.

CASE HISTORY OF MRS. JANIS: BIOLOGIC VIEW

Mrs. Janis is a 53-year-old widow with a history of a depressive syndrome. During the past few months she has lost 20 pounds, has early morning awakening, and has a diurnal variation in mood manifested by feeling better as the day goes on. She describes herself as feeling hopeless, helpless, and worthless. There is some retardation of speech. She denies suicidal intent and presents no evidence of delusions or paranoid ideation. There are obsessional trends. Twenty-three years ago there was a similar episode of depression that remitted spontaneously. The patient has a sister who was hospitalized for a depressive illness that responded positively to electro-convulsive treatments.

These four histories could have been elicited from the same patient by four different nurses, each employing a different conceptual model of care to understand the patient. It can be seen from the case material above how the nurse, using one model to the exclusion of the others, unnecessarily limits the data base and nursing intervention options.

This chapter will describe these four models of care, which are the ones most frequently employed in mental health practice, by reference to the case histories above. It will then attempt to show the use of psychiatric mental health interventions helpful to the perspective of each model. It will also discuss the integration of these models into an eclectic approach for nursing practice.

COGNITIVE–BEHAVIORAL MODEL OF CARE

The cognitive–behavioral model of care can be classified as a learning model. The assumption is that both thinking and behavior are learned. This model looks at cognitive sets (thoughts) as well as at motor behaviors.

The notion that cognitions are the basis for behavior is part of the cognitive theory. Cognitive therapy as a system of psychotherapy has been best advanced by psychiatrist Aaron Beck at the Center for Cognitive Therapy at the University of Pennsylvania. In the early 1960s, Beck became increasingly aware that the conventional associations and productions verbalized by patients in therapy failed to yield the most clinical useful material. He noticed that parallel to the verbalized thought there was a "stream" of other thoughts that usually were not expressed. In order for the patient to become aware of this stream, active coaching to focus on it was required.[13]

An example was given by Beck of a woman who felt continuous unexplained anxiety while describing sensitive sexual conflicts. The patient was able to verbalize freely about these conflicts but continued to feel anxiety. Beck directed her attention to her thoughts *about what* she had been saying. Upon his inquiry, she noticed she had been ignoring this stream of thoughts and was able to report that she did not believe she was expressing herself, that the therapist was not able to follow her talk, that he was bored, and that he might try to get rid of her.[14] Beck concluded that the patient's anxiety had less to do with her sexual conflicts than with this second stream of thoughts dealing with the patient's self-evaluations and anticipations of his reactions.

Beck increasingly trained his patients to observe the stream of previously unreported thoughts by having them recall the thoughts they had prior to the unpleasant feeling.[15]

Because these thoughts emerged automatically and extremely rapidly, he labeled them "autonomic thoughts." The autonomic thoughts have several characteristics: prior to focusing they are vague and unformulated, but after focusing, they are discrete and specific; they do not result from reasoning or deliberation but arise autonomously and by reflex, without the patient's voluntary initiation; they are difficult to stop; they are completely believed no matter how illogical; and they are associated with or induce a variety of painful effects. Indeed, a cardinal principle of cognitive theory is that automatic thoughts, generally referred to as *cognitions*, are important etiologic factors in the production of dysphoric moods, maladaptive behaviors, and psychiatric syndromes.[16]

Many theories have identified cognitions as the mediator of behavior. Ellis, for example, theorizes that an event experienced at A does not determine how we react at C, but rather it is the thoughts that we experience at B that do so.[17]

The studies of Beck, Ellis, and Harper, Rehm, and Seligman all center upon an individual's control of his or her cognitive processes.[18-21] The work of Bandler and Grinder, Cameron-Bandler, and Diltz and colleagues on Neuro-Linguistic Programming provides us with a technology for examining the cognitive and behavioral aspects of a patient.[22-24]

Cognitive theory states that belief systems may reflect a sense that an event should not have happened to an individual. In such a case, the belief may well reveal a presupposition about the event based on the belief system. Behavior coming about as a result of such a presupposition may have little bearing upon reality, but it is logically derived from the belief system. Beck has identified patterns associated with such cognitive errors in depressives, for example, sorting for the negative, demanding perfection, arbitrary interpretation of events, and distortion of time. The dominant feature of cognition in depression is a negative view of oneself, the world, and the future.[25]

A critical component of cognitive–behavioral therapy is the belief that an individual may control his or her behavior and thereby his or her mental health. Thus Neuro-Linguistic Programming examines the structures of communication rather than its content. And Diltz et al., view behavior patterns as a result of cybernetic interaction between response, mind, and body.[26] Change can come about only when the pattern is disrupted. The result of such changes is an increase in flexibility in choosing ways of attaining life goals.

The behavioral model rests on the conceptualizations of Ivan Pavlov (conditioned learning theory).[27] To the behavioral therapist, both neurosis and psychosis are examples of abnormal behavior, behavior that has been learned as a result of aversive events and is maintained because it either leads to positive results or because it avoids deleterious ones. The overt symptoms (the learned behavior), not the secondary manifestations of disease or unconscious conflict, are to be treated because they themselves are the problem. The typical therapeutic course includes: (1) determining the behavior to be modified; (2) establishing the conditions under which the behavior occurs; (3) determining the factors responsible for the persistence of behavior; (4) selecting a set of treatment conditions; and (5) arranging a schedule of retraining. The conditions that precede the behavior may be modified by such techniques as desensitization, reciprocal inhibition, and conditioned avoidance. The conditions resulting from the behavior may be modified by positive reinforcement, negative reinforcement, aversive conditioning, and extinction.[28]

The behavioral model, resting on theoretical foundations from the early twentieth century, began its rapid growth in the late 1950s. Its derivative, behavior therapy, has enjoyed considerable interest in the clinical field during the relatively brief period of its existence. Behavior therapy offers several possible advantages over other forms of treatment, including shorter duration of treatment and applicability to a wider range of patients.

Considering the case history of Mrs. Janis according to the behavioral model, the nurse first identifies the behavior—anorexia, insomnia, feelings of hopelessness, helplessness, and worthlessness—which are regarded as pathological. Then the empirical relationship between the depressive behaviors and the antecedent and consequent environmental events that precipitate and maintain the depression is determined.[29] The death of the husband is interpreted as a sudden withholding of positive reinforcement of adaptive behavior. The attention received from family members inadvertently reinforces the depressive behavior.

In considering the case of Mrs. Janis, the nurse would begin to explore the premises of her sense of hopelessness. For example, is it her belief that the future only holds disappoint-

ment? If this is the case, one would begin to challenge this belief pattern by asking: Was there ever a time when something positive happened that you did not expect? Might this happen again, in the future?

The implication of the cognitive–behavioral model for nursing assessment and intervention is that attention must be paid to the structure of cognitive and behavioral experiences that are associated with negative states, such as depression. In the case of Mrs. Janis, we find that paying attention to her orientation to the future gives insight to a belief about the future that can only be associated with a state of negative feeling. If she truly believes that only bad things will happen in the future, she will not feel very happy when thinking of the future. Furthermore, that belief and feeling state will impact on present behavior.

The cognitive–behavioral approach underscores how the mind operates to regulate mood, affect, and behavior through the processing of information. Mrs. Janis's thinking demonstrates how the personal meaning construct of future is being processed within the client and the relationship of this processing to the client's present state of depression and her stated sense of hopelessness. Further elaboration on the information processing model appears in Chapter 25.

Treatment consists of reinforcing adaptive behaviors incompatible with depression and extinguishing depressive behaviors. These therapeutic goals may be accomplished by teaching the family to respond positively to the adaptive behavior instead of to the depressive behavior,[30] by purposefully encouraging the patient to express feelings incompatible with depression,[31] or by establishing a period of sensory deprivation that makes the depressed patient more susceptible to positive reinforcement.[32]

Nursing Activities and the Behavioral Model—Client Teaching

One of the nine psychiatric nursing activities identified by the ANA Division on Psychiatric and Mental Health Nursing practice applies to the behavioral model of care, as follows:

Teaching with specific reference to emotional health as evidenced by various behavioral patterns.

The nursing activity of client teaching is emphasized throughout all nursing curricula, and teaching in the psychiatric mental health field implies paying special attention to emotional health. Standard V-B describes this skill.[33]

PSYCHOLOGICAL MODEL OF CARE

Although there are many theories of personality and many psychotherapies, the psychological model in American psychiatry began with the work of Sigmund Freud and was modified by the subsequent work of Harry Stack Sullivan, Frieda Fromm-Reichmann, Erik Erikson, the ex-

istentialists, and many others.[34] Freud's revolution depended on the "conviction that psychological events, however obscure, were understandable."[35] Through the newly developed method of free association, he was able to reconstruct childhood experiences that he believed determined adult neuroses.

According to the current use of the psychological model, the developmental impasse, the early deprivation, the distortions in early relationships, and the confused communications between parent and child lead to the adult neuroses and vulnerabilities to certain stresses. As a result of these psychological determinants, we see patients who distort reality, who are prone

STANDARD V-B.
Intervention: Health Teaching

The nurse assists clients, families, and groups to achieve satisfying and productive patterns of living through health teaching.

RATIONALE

Health teaching is an essential part of the nurse's role with those who have mental health problems. Every interaction can be utilized as a teaching–learning situation. Formal and informal teaching methods can be used in working with individuals, families, groups, and the community. Emphasis is on understanding principles of mental health as well as on developing ways of coping with mental health problems. Client adherence to treatment regimens increases when health teaching is an integral part of the client's care.

STRUCTURE CRITERIA

1. Opportunities to use varied and appropriate teaching methodologies are available.
2. Appropriate teaching facilities and resources are provided within the practice setting.
3. Health teaching by nurses is specified in job descriptions.

PROCESS CRITERIA

The nurse—

1. identifies health education needs of clients.
2. employs principles of learning and appropriate teaching methods.
3. teaches the basic principles of physical and mental health.
4. teaches communication, interpersonal, and social skills.
5. provides opportunities for clients to learn experientially.

OUTCOME CRITERIA

1. Health teaching activities are recorded.
2. The client or family demonstrates acquisition of knowledge as a result of health teaching.

to depression, who avoid heterosexuality, and who fear success. The social setting may be changed, or psychotropic drugs may be given, but the pathology remains because the personality is pathological.

Therapy consists of clarifying the psychological meaning of events, feelings, and behaviors. The patient is taught how to experience appropriate affects and how to tolerate intolerable affects.[36] Forgotten events may be remembered, reexperienced, and then put into perspective so that the patient can be freed to see current situations as they really are. As a result, growth and maturity are enhanced.

Most important to the therapeutic situation is the nurse–patient relationship. It is the therapeutic alliance between the two that will enable the patient to remember what she has not wanted to remember and to abandon familiar but pathological ways of dealing with anxiety. It is through the vehicle of the therapeutic relationship—by experiencing these feelings toward the therapist—that the patient will relive pathological ties to important people and will have the opportunity for a "corrective emotional experience."[37]

The psychological model has exerted a great influence not only on American psychiatry but also on everyday thinking. Its derivative, psychotherapy, has become a commonly accepted treatment of choice, especially for the neuroses and personality disorders. Advocates of the psychological model, especially since World War II, have been able to translate the clinical insights derived from classical psychoanalysis and more recent developments of ego psychology into concepts that residents in nearly all training centers in the United States can utilize in the understanding of most psychiatric patients.

Returning to the case history of Mrs. Janis, the nurse, using the psychological model, first takes note of the problems in the marital relationship. She pays special attention to the absence of grief, which has psychological meaning and is related to the patient's ambivalent feelings toward her husband.[38] A similar reaction after the patient's mother's death suggests the possibility of a psychological connection between Mrs. Janis's feelings toward both her husband and mother. This is reinforced by the history that Mrs. Janis married only six months after the death of her mother. The patient's criticism of herself in terms that she had used to criticize her husband suggests Freud's concept

of introjection of the lost object.[39] Because the primary modality of treatment is psychotherapy, it is a favorable sign that she is motivated to gain a better understanding of herself.

Nursing Activities and the Psychological Model

Standard V-A of the *Standards of Psychiatric-Mental Health Nursing Practice* further delineates the importance of nursing interventions as psychotherapeutic activities.[40]

Three of the nine psychiatric nursing activities identified by the ANA Division on Psychiatric and Mental Health Nursing Practice apply to the psychological model of care:

- Working with clients concerning the here-and-now living problems they confront.
- Accepting and using the surrogate parent role.
- Conducting psychotherapy.

Here-and-Now Living Problems
In Chapter 3, a conceptual way of viewing mental distress was described through observing a person's thoughts, feelings, and behavior. Nurses can address patient's here-and-now living problems through the nursing management of thought, feelings, and behaviors.

Nursing Management of Feelings States.
The first task of the nurse dealing with a patient and a here-and-now living problem is to assess the feeling. Identifying the feeling and the degree of anxiety accompanying it is important. The following questions may serve as a guide in this process:

- What is causing the feeling? What is the precipitant?
- Is it anxiety or a specific feeling?
- Can the person talk about the feeling?
- What is the current life situation for the person?
- Is the person taking any drugs or medication?
- Does talking with the person increase or decrease the feeling?

After observing and identifying the feeling state, the nurse may try to decide whether the

STANDARD V-A.
Intervention: Psychotherapeutic Interventions

The nurse uses psychotherapeutic interventions to assist clients in regaining or improving their previous coping abilities and to prevent further disability.

RATIONALE

Individuals with and without mental health problems often respond to health problems in a dysfunctional manner. During counseling, interviewing, crisis or emergency intervention, or daily interaction, nurses diagnose dysfunctional behaviors, engage clients in noting such behaviors, and assist the client in modifying or eliminating those behaviors.

STRUCTURE CRITERION

The nurse who engages in psychotherapeutic interventions is minimally prepared as a generalist in psychiatric and mental health nursing.

PROCESS CRITERIA

The nurse—

1. identifies the client's responses to health problems.
2. reinforces those responses to health problems that are functional and helps the client modify or eliminate those that are dysfunctional.
3. employs principles of communication, interviewing techniques, problem solving, and crisis intervention when performing psychotherapeutic interventions.
4. uses knowledge of behavioral concepts such as anxiety, loss, conflict, grief, and anger to assist the client in coping, adapting, and dealing constructively with feelings.
5. demonstrates knowledge about and skill in the use of psychotherapeutic interventions specifically useful in the modification of thought, perception, affect, behavior, and motivation.
6. utilizes health team members to help evaluate the outcome of interventions and to formulate modification of psychotherapeutic techniques.
7. reinforces useful patterns and themes in the client's interactions with others.
8. uses crisis intervention to promote growth and to aid the personal and social integration of clients in developmental, situational, or suicidal crisis.

OUTCOME CRITERION

Clients state that they have been assisted in regaining or improving their previous coping abilities.

feeling is genuine or a defense against another unexpressed or unbearable feeling. Nurses do not uncover or point out the feeling; instead, they make it possible, by their support, for the patient to talk about the feeling.

Nurses deal with the feelings of patients by helping them put the feelings into words. This may lead to the patient's discovering feelings of which he was not previously aware. This technique helps him to be in touch with his feeling.

For example, the patient talks of his extreme anger with his wife. As the nurse sits and listens to him and his description of real situations, she helps him to bear the pain he has been avoiding. As he expresses his feelings to a therapeutic person, he may not have to be so angry with his wife, and he may be able to look at other feelings he has, perhaps the positive feelings. The anger has prevented him from feeling close to his wife.

Sexual feelings are another area in which people are hesitant to express themselves. The therapeutic person helps the patient to bear these feelings—to tolerate them and to talk about them. The goal is to help the person learn how not to push the feelings from consciousness or defend against them or act inappropriately on them.

Boredom and apathy are also subjective feelings common to many people. They are evoked by situations that one would rather not be in. For example, a person would like to prolong the weekend, but he must go to work on Monday. This presents the person with transitory feelings of apathy.

The nurse helps the patient to bear feelings that he thought were unbearable. Putting the feelings into perspective helps the patient understand how the feelings originated and what brings them out. The more a person can gain control of the feeling with words and understanding, the easier it is to bear.

Nursing Management of Defensive Thinking Techniques. In normal dialogue with a person who is not using grossly pathological defensive thinking techniques, the nurse can sit and listen to the person and can feel involved; and the patient can feel that the nurse understands and she can have a sense of progression in the nature of the discussion. But when a patient uses neurotic or psychotic thinking, it is common for nurses to get a feeling that they really do not understand. They feel bored, their minds wander, and they do not feel engaged. Moreover, they feel that the patient really does not say what is bothering him. They feel that something superficial is happening. In fact, this is true because something superficial is happening. The patient is avoiding the real issues of concern to him. These are some of the clues that indicate a patient is using defensive thinking techniques. By using these techniques the person avoids saying what counts, what is painful, and what is meaningful.

Another example of a defensive technique is when the nurse is lectured to by the patient. After the patient has been intellectualizing for an hour, the nurse really feels she has not learned anything. She feels that she has heard a lecture rather than a meaningful discussion. Or after sitting with a patient who is sad but who in fact has been telling jokes for the whole hour, the nurse feels like saying, "I don't know where that person is or where I am." The patient has managed to put her off. The jokes are avoidance techniques for avoiding dealing with her. The nurse knows it even though it may be difficult for her to describe the avoidance technique accurately.

As soon as the nurse is able to notice the avoidance during the interview, she may be able to say, "It sounds to me as though there are a lot of painful things you want to say that are difficult to talk about." Somehow she communicates to the patient that it is acceptable for him to tell her the feelings and that she is prepared to hear them. An alternative to helping the patient is knowing what the here-and-now issues are and how the person must really feel. For example, if someone has lost a spouse before coming to the clinic, the nurse can assume that the person is experiencing sadness. And if the person shows no sadness at all, then she can help the person deal with the lack of sadness and what feelings the person does express. We use this approach because clinical knowledge shows us the kind of feelings that usually occur with grief. The goal of the nurse is to translate the patient's defensive thinking into nondefensive, direct thinking.

Nursing Management of Behavior. Some people deal with anxiety or overwhelming feelings by behavior rather than by thinking out the problem or putting it into the proper perspective. For example, the acting-out patient may become suicidal when hospitalized and when prevented from acting on his feelings. In this case, the nurse should help the patient to understand and verbalize his feelings to keep him from defending against them with acting-up behavior.

The patient needs to be taught how to allow some time to elapse between the overwhelming feeling and his action. For example, if the patient were to say, "My brother said something rotten and I felt so angry I smashed him," the nurse would intervene by saying, "Your brother said something rotten; you felt angry. Tell me what that feeling was like."

The nurse tries to teach the patient to put into words that which he normally acts on immediately. She tries to teach him to delay the action by increasing his verbal skill and his understanding of the feeling. When he is about to act in a destructive manner, she sets limits on the behavior.

Surrogate Parent Role

There are specific skills that are part of a surrogate parent role. These skills include: encouraging the client to talk, listening, understanding, bearing painful feelings, setting limits, providing support, providing a corrective emotional experience, and aiding in the healing process of the mind.

Encouraging the Client to Talk.
Talking helps people feel better. The free expression of emotions is encouraged in psychiatry because emotions give importance to an experience and communicate this to other people. If a nursing student does not talk about her academic and clinical experiences to family and friends, the importance of her education is not transmitted to others; but if she does tell them of her nursing encounters, she finds that they will react favorably or unfavorably to what she says. Thus their behavior adds a definite dimension to the meaning of the experience for herself.

Talking brings emotions to the surface, often displaying to the patient what he has not realized before. By identifying his feelings, he has better control over them. For example, a patient fears a job interview after a hospitalization for a depression. Brooding over the problem by himself magnifies the fear. Talking about it to a therapeutic person puts the problem into proper perspective and helps the patient view the pending interview more realistically.

People are often frightened by intense feelings and emotions, their own as well as those of others. This accounts for the statement by some that it is better not to express how one feels. Part of this reasoning results from the fear that the other person will not be able to tolerate or be receptive to the feelings. This may occur especially if the other person suffers from the same anxiety. An example of this is the nursing student who fears failing her state board examinations. When this is discussed among nursing classmates, anxiety can run high, and some

students prefer to avoid this trauma altogether. When the fear is expressed to a truly supportive person who understands the situation, the anxiety can be more realistically viewed, and the feelings can then be expressed, shared, and resolved.

It is also important to consider cultural influences and the individual's upbringing as to how people feel free to express feelings. For some people who have difficulty talking, this may be a totally new experience. They may never be spontaneously verbal, but the difference evident in previous verbal behavior and current verbal behavior can be quite dramatic.

Listening.
Encouraging a person to talk and to express himself will not be helpful if the person feels that he is not being listened to.

Listening is a highly valued art that requires understanding, patience, skill, and perseverance. It is a grossly underrated art. It is often much easier not to listen than to listen. Although the discussion on the mechanics of listening may take only a few paragraphs, the pitfalls to be encountered and overcome in listening can fill many pages.

The concept of listening has major implications in the talking therapy of patient care. *Listening* implies a voluntary effort to understand what is being said. *Hearing*, as distinguished from listening, is the audible reception of the spoken word or noise.

Listening is most successful when there is a definite goal. Being in a crowd with many people who are talking at the same time shows the difficulty in knowing to what or to whom to direct attention. If there is no purpose, your attention will wander when someone is talking, or your mind will wander when you read a textbook.

Perhaps you have had the experience of being with a person who is talking, yet you are trying to hear the conversation of the person behind you. Or you have been in a class and found to your discomfort that you were not listening when a question was specifically directed toward you. By having the purpose of listening in mind as you listen, what is heard captures your attention. If this happens, you will start to actively think about the subject. The dialogue then becomes meaningful and important. When the speaker engages your interest, your voice and manner reflect enthusiasm and you respond to the speaker. The conversation then takes on meaning.

In talking face to face, the response the nurse gives, such as leaning forward when the patient says something important or nodding her head in agreement, is the nonverbal message to continue. In telephone conversations the tone and pitch of the voice are clues that you are listening.

If the nurse's listening behavior has been successful, the feeling of satisfaction is inherent in the dialogue. To feel that one has been successfully listened to is a therapeutic gain for anyone. It makes people feel important and respected.

Understanding. Although nurses may be successful in encouraging the patient to talk, and although they may be successful with their listening behavior and in their ability to show the patient that they are interested and care about his welfare, the entire purpose of the interchange will be missing unless they understand the patient and unless the patient realizes that they understand.

How do you show that you understand? If in talking, the patient expresses sadness, to listen is therapeutic, but to acknowledge your understanding of his distress in your own words indicates understanding. For example, to say to the patient, "Everything I hear you talk about speaks of sadness. Your heart must be aching today," is to communicate that you do indeed understand. It is therapeutic to offer statements expressing understanding with such remarks as, "I can see how hard that was for you to say," or "That must have made you feel better." Statements of this kind should indicate understanding of what the patient has endeavored to express.

Be precise with a message. Try to say exactly what you mean and be certain that the patient understands completely. If a goal is stated to the patient as, "It is important to work through problems in order to develop meaningful relationships," the patient may not understand what is expected of him. This expression may be far over his head and entirely incomprehensible to him.

When one is understood, one is no longer alone. When a person can verbalize what is on his mind, he feels more in control of the situation. He preserves his dignity and quality as a human being. The display of understanding and interest takes a person out of loneliness and isolation. To listen is therapeutic, but to understand goes far above and beyond listening.

Bearing Painful Feelings. A special dimension of listening and understanding is to help bear the feelings that the patient is trying to express. Nurses may find this a difficult skill to master. It is extremely difficult for some nurses to sit with a depressed or sobbing patient. Experience helps condition you to be able to sit for long periods of time with someone in psychic pain. The nurse should try to be able to help bear the sadness with the patient during stressful times.

If patients cannot bear painful feelings, they will deal with them in unhealthy ways. Some patients will develop psychotic thoughts; others will develop depressions or antisocial behaviors in response to the feelings. These reactions can be warded off or lessened by helping the patient to cope and bear the feelings.

It takes practice to be helpful; and even having had considerable experience, the therapeutic person often feels uncomfortable when helping the patient bear painful feelings. It is a learning process that requires many and varied encounters of these situations. For example, being able to sit with a crying patient in the general hospital is a skill that is learned and developed over a period of time. Let us use an example from child rearing: When a child wants something immediately, you attempt to help the child bear the tension. You do not give the child a pacifier or piece of candy every time he cries.

A clinical example of a situation in which grief feelings were not adequately resolved follows:

A 55-year-old woman was referred from the medical unit of a hospital to the psychiatric unit because she "refused to have a myelogram" to determine the cause of her back pain of 15 months duration. The symptom went back to her hospitalization following a car accident. The patient related the following: "We were returning from my son's home after a weekend. I was in the backseat of the car with my two grandchildren; my son-in-law was driving. He said I interfered too much and complained too much about his drinking. I wanted to drive because he was intoxicated but decided to say nothing. The car was swerving back and forth and suddenly missed a curve in the road. We went over the embankment. My daughter was killed in the accident."

The question was asked during the interview what other deaths the patient had experienced in her life and with considerable crying and sadness she said, "When I was 11 years old, we were all summoned into my mother's room as she was dying giving birth to my sister. . . . When I was 30 years old, I had three children; the boys were seven and five and one daughter was three weeks old. I went in to get her up from a nap and she was dead in her crib. . . . Eighteen months ago my husband was getting into his car and dropped over dead with a CVA."

Death and human loss are predominant issues with this woman. The main therapeutic task in the psychiatric setting is to sit and listen to her as she recounts her feelings of grief. This demands much from the nurse, but until the patient can make peace with the agonizing tragedies in her past, she will be unable to be free to live in the present.

Setting Limits. If emphasis is placed on the open expression of thoughts and feelings, it may seem surprising that setting limits on a patient's behavior can be an important part of the therapy.

It may be easier to understand if we begin with the normal child. A child left to himself may frequently behave in ways that are self-destructive. He might eat paint, walk in the middle of a busy street, or destroy the possessions of others. The child possesses neither the intelligence nor the inner controls to cope with the complexities of the outer world or the tensions of his inner world. The adult does this for him in order that the child may remain alive. The child can thus be free to gradually learn inner controls, and then he can learn to channel his drives into constructive outlets.

The medical–surgical patient has limits set on him by the nursing plan that the nurse implements. Limits are usually placed on his physical activities (getting out of bed, going to the bathroom), his diet, or even his visitors. Some patients, like young children, are often reluctant to accept these limits, even when their very survival is at stake. The patient may want so badly to deny being weak, sick, or dependent that he insists on behaving as if he were healthy.

In psychiatric units, where behavior is the very basic material one works with from moment to moment, limit setting takes on special importance. Nurses must decide if a hyperactive patient (mania, for example) is being overstimulated and needs to be controlled. They must decide whether or not suicidal patients must be restricted for their own protection. They must also decide when the adolescent patient needs to have someone say no in order for him to know someone cares. For example:

A 16-year-old female patient asked an aide if she would intercede for her and ask the physician to let her stay out until midnight. The aide asked the patient how she would feel if the response was yes. She replied, "Scared! If he let me out, it would mean he really doesn't understand me."

The nurse learns when limits are necessary from several cues: (1) if the patient's behavior is disturbing to everyone else; (2) if the patient seems to be upsetting himself by his own behavior; (3) if the nurse worries excessively about a suicidal patient; (4) if the nurse feels the patient is saying, "Please take over." When the nurse discusses concerns about setting limits with the patient, frequently the patient will give a clue that helps the nurse to make a decision. For example, the nurse says to a suicidal patient, "I am especially worried about you today and I am trying to decide whether you should stay on the ward." The patient may respond with relief, "You should be worried about me. I intended to walk right in front of a car."

The nurse first tries to set limits with a supportive verbal interchange. For example:

A patient was loudly banging on the piano much to the annoyance of other patients and visitors. The nurse went over and asked the patient to please stop or to play softly as it was disturbing to other people. The patient said, "You're not big enough to make me stop. Want to try?" The nurse said, "I'd be a fool to try that. I can't make you do anything, but I can talk with you for a while."

In this situation the nurse avoids a physical confrontation. She gently offers an alternative behavior that will be socially appropriate. There are times, however, when setting limits by using medication or by actual physical restraint may be necessary.

Setting limits on a medical or psychiatric ward is always necessary. The need for limits will be kept at a minimum when all the members of the team agree on a plan of care and keep the channels of communication open. When the staff disagrees—just as when mother and father disagree on the rules for their children—the patient will become anxious and will then begin to test the limits.

Providing Support. The nurse encourages the patient to talk. She also listens, understands, helps bear painful feelings, and sets limits. All these tasks are embodied in the truly supportive person. Providing support is the strength one person gives to another, and anyone in a therapeutic situation must be supportive.

Support helps people grow and become independent themselves. In the process of psychic development, support is necessary in order to sustain the individual through the pain of learning. Support provides trust and strength in the event of faltering during the experience.

Providing a Corrective Emotional Experience. The therapeutic process may be perceived as a corrective emotional experience. When the nurse responds to the patient in a healthy, direct, accepting, yet limit-setting fashion, the patient may be experiencing something quite new in his life. The patient, not convinced that the nurse "means business," may withdraw or express hostility toward her. The nurse persists, however, in her therapeutic attempts.

After a period of time the patient may alter his behavior, possibly because of his corrective experience with the nurse, and if the nurse respects and accepts him, he then begins to believe he is worthy of respect and acceptance. He may reciprocate these feelings to the nurse, and if the therapy succeeds, he may begin to generalize the healthy behavior to others.

For example, a 17-year-old male related the following:

A year ago things really started getting bad. I'd get so depressed I thought a great deal about killing myself. I seriously wanted to die. I began drinking a lot at that time. When my parents would go out, I'd drink all my father's liquor. He was pretty disgusted I guess and my mother was angry too, but they never said anything.

The point here is the parents' indifference to the boy's behavior. In order to provide a corrective experience, the nurse must show she is not indifferent to him, and by seeing him daily to talk over his experiences of the day, she can then set limits on him when his behavior is not appropriate to the situation. This physical intervention action shows that she cares about his well-being, and her presence each day indicates her concern and interest in him as an individual.

Aiding the Healing Process of the Mind. Nurses and physicians do not cure. The mind and body cure themselves, while the professionals help the normal healing process. We find this perspective a useful one, as we will attempt to illustrate with the following example:

A patient comes to the emergency ward with a knife wound. The surgeon cleans the incision, sterilizes the area, and stitches the skin. The wound then heals. Without the surgeon the would would still heal, but there would be considerable scarring.

In an acute psychiatric illness, the mind has suffered a wound that may be called *schizophrenia* or *depression*. It is a wound nevertheless. The mind will heal, for it will not remain in its tormented state for long; but *how* the mind will heal remains uncertain. If the healing process is not assisted and protected, scarring may occur. In psychiatry, scarring is chronicity. The patient, no longer acutely pained, is resigned, apathetic, and withdrawn. Many chronic schizophrenic patients who have been hospitalized for years have made this "peace" for themselves.

When the healing process is assisted, the mind is less likely to be subjected to scarring. In other words, with proper treatment, chronicity can be avoided. For example:

A patient who is overwhelmed by his insignificance and impotence develops the delusion that he is king of the universe. If he is neglected and treated as if he were insignificant, he might "decide" that his delusion is worth keeping. If he feels respected, supported, and important to someone, the patient will be more willing to give up the delusion of being king and will return to being a normal human being.

The hospital provides a nutrient environment for the patient who is psychologically depleted. He can rest from the stress and strain of his home environment and have his inner resources replenished.

Listen well when the patient says that he has come to the psychiatric hospital because his "nerves are shot" and he needs a good rest, or when the housewife says that the children are "driving her crazy and she just had to get away from them." There is a great deal of truth in what they say. The people expect the hospital to be the nutrient climate to enable the mind to heal properly.

Conducting Psychotherapy

The ANA Division on Psychiatric and Mental Health Nursing Practice identifies as one of the direct nursing care functions, the activity of psychotherapy. The nurse's actions and reflections in this activity are focused on a particular client or family, and the nurse assumes personal responsibility and accountability to the client for the outcomes of such actions. Standard V-F discusses psychotherapeutic interventions.

STANDARD V-F.
Intervention: Psychotherapy

The nurse utilizes advanced clinical expertise in individual, group, and family psychotherapy, child psychotherapy, and other treatment modalities to function as a psychotherapist and recognizes professional accountability for nursing practice.

RATIONALE

Acceptance of the role of psychotherapist entails primary responsibility for the treatment of clients and entrance into a contractual agreement. This contract includes a commitment to see a client through the problem presented or to assist the client in finding other appropriate assistance. It also includes an explicit definition of the relationship, the respective role of each person in the relationship, and what can be realistically expected of each person.

STRUCTURE CRITERIA

1. The nurse who engages in psychotherapy shall be qualified as a psychiatric and mental health nurse specialist.
2. An agency policy specifies the educational and experiential qualifications required of the nurse who functions as a psychotherapist.
3. Job descriptions of nurses expected to function as psychotherapists and to use specific treatment modalities shall include educational and experiential qualifications.
4. Work assignment and staffing patterns provide adequate time for conducting psychotherapy when that responsibility is included in the job description.
5. A mechanism for peer review exists within the agency or is established by the nurse in solo or group practice.
6. The psychiatric and mental health nurse specialist who conducts psychotherapy in private practice maintains an ongoing, regular, formal consultative relationship with a professional colleague.
7. The psychiatric and mental health nurse specialist in private practice utilizes physician services when needed.

PROCESS CRITERIA

The nurse—

1. structures the therapeutic contract with the client in the beginning phase of the relationship, including such elements as purpose, time, place, fees, participants, confidentiality, available means of contact, and responsibilities of both client and therapist.
2. engages in interdisciplinary and intradisciplinary collaboration to achieve treatment goals.
3. engages the client in the process of determining the appropriate form of psychotherapy.
4. identifies the goals of psychotherapy.
5. uses knowledge of growth and development, psychopathology, psychosocial systems, small group and family dynamics, and knowledge of selected treatment modalities as indicated.
6. articulates a rationale for the goals chosen and interventions utilized.
7. fosters increasing personal and therapeutic responsibility on the part of the client.
8. provides for continuity of care for the client in the therapist's absence.
9. determines, with the client when possible, that goals have been achieved and facilitates the termination process.
10. refers clients to other professionals when indicated.
11. respects and protects the client's legal rights.

12. avails self of appropriate opportunities to increase knowledge and skill in the therapies utilized in nursing practice.
13. obtains recognized educational preparation and ongoing supervision for types of psychotherapy utilized, e.g., individual psychotherapy, group and family psychotherapy, child psychotherapy, and psychoanalysis.
14. uses clinical judgment in determining whether providing physical care (especially procedures prone to misinterpretation, e.g., injections, enemas) will enhance or impair the therapist–client relationship and delegates such care as needed.

OUTCOME CRITERIA

1. The client articulates the elements of the therapeutic contract.
2. The client demonstrates responsibility for the therapeutic work.
3. The client demonstrates movement toward therapeutic goals or objectives.

SOCIAL MODEL OF CARE

A social model of treatment was practiced in psychiatric hospitals in the United States from the latter part of the eighteenth century to approximately 1860. It was introduced under the name of "moral therapy" first by William Tuke, a Quaker layman (1732–1822) in England, and later practiced by his great-grandson Daniel Hack Tuke (1827–1895), a leader of British psychiatry. During that time, social and environmental causes of mental illness were given serious consideration as moral treatment attempted to relieve the patient by "friendly association, discussion of his difficulties, and the daily pursuit of purposeful activity."[41] Treatment results compared favorably with those for patients hospitalized today. The social model received further impetus from Adolph Meyer and Harry Stack Sullivan in the first half of this century.[42,43]

The social view of psychiatric illness focuses on the way the individual functions in the social system. Symptoms are traced not to conflicts within the mind, not to manifestations of psychiatric disease, but to the "relationship of the individual to his manner of functioning in social situations, i.e., in the type and quality of his 'connectedness' to the groups which make up his life space."[44] Symptoms may thereafter be regarded as an index of social disorder.[45] Accordingly, when a socially disruptive event occurs, for example, a daughter's leaving home, a wife's dying, a geographic displacement by urban renewal, a war, or an economic depression, the resultant symptoms are seen as stemming from the social disorder.

The social model like the biologic, psychological, and cognitive–behavioral models, was revived in the 1950s. Since then the psychiatric ward has been viewed as a social system, the relationship between social class and mental illness has been established, federal legislation to provide psychiatric care for catchment areas in the community has been enacted, and epidemiologic studies have been carried out.[46–49] During these years, group and family therapy, day hospitals, and walk-in clinics provided new ways of treating the mentally ill patient without separating him from his social milieu.

In referring to the case history of Mrs. Janis, treatment consists of either reorganizing the patient's relationship to the social system or reorganizing the social system, because the personality is neither "diseased" nor in need of fundamental restructuring. Using the social model, the therapist may help the patient better understand how she relates to the social system and how better to satisfy her needs. If others do not seem to care, how can she get them to care? If her job is not stimulating, how can she find the right one? If her behavior is irrational, how can she learn to stop acting irrationally or how can her family better tolerate the behavior? If the therapist wants to restructure the "nuclear" social system, the patient may be seen with her family. The therapist who wants to impact the broader social system may also attempt to influence major social issues such as housing or education.

The nurse, using the social model to study the case, notices that the patient's social matrix has been altered in two ways. First, the patient has permanently lost the one person to whom she has been closest. She now feels empty and isolated. Second, by moving, she has placed herself in a situation in which she has lost access to those with whom she had previously related. In individual and group therapy, one could temporarily substitute a transitional social system. Simultaneously, the therapist would attempt to reestablish a social field in which the patient could be comfortable after discharge. To do this, the patient might be encouraged to move to a home where she could have better access to family and old friends. Work with the family might repair any estrangement. The patient might return to work, either paid or volunteer. Continued individual or group therapy might help her acquire social skills that she may never have needed to develop in the marital situation.

Nursing Activities and the Social Model

Four of the nine psychiatric nursing activities identified by the ANA Division of Psychiatric and Mental Health Nursing Practice apply to the social model of care.[50]

- Providing a therapeutic milieu, concerned largely with the sociopsychological aspects of clients' environments.
- Assuming the role of social agent concerned with improvement of recreational, occupational, and social competencies.
- Providing leadership and clinical assistance to other nursing personnel and generic health care workers.
- Engaging in social and community action roles related to mental health.

Providing a Therapeutic Milieu

There are several aspects to the nurse's increasing responsibility for patient care that have implications for the nursing management of the milieu. The nursing staff sets the ward tone and climate—whether it is to be a permissive or strict atmosphere, a cooperative or competitive atmosphere, or a caring or rigid atmosphere.

The nurse also is the one who sets the pace and adjusts the climate of the hospital unit. This responsibility involves judging with whom to spend time and in what capacity, with whom to sit in silence, whom to scold, whom to support, and whom to avoid a harmful dependent relationship with. In the hospital discipline, the responsibilities of the nurse have steadily in-

creased to the point where she usually makes the final decisions on the ward milieu.

This broadened responsibility has moved the psychiatric nurse from the subordinated position of asking that the doctor do something for the patient, to sitting with the patient and later collaborating with the treatment team to determine what the patient's problem is and helping decide what the patient care plan should be. In other words, when Mrs. Smith comes to the nursing station and says that she is feeling anxious and needs medication, the nurse does not immediately call the doctor for the medication order. Instead, the nurse takes the time to sit and talk with Mrs. Smith to find out why she is anxious. It may be learned that the patient is overly concerned because her husband is coming to visit that evening. Defining the issue as the patient's ambivalence toward the anticipated visit of her husband gives the team considerably more information, so it can consider what therapeutic plan should be used.

Standard V-E specifically deals with the milieu concept.[51]

Assuming the Role of Social Agent

The adjunct therapies such as occupational and art therapy are very important to this overall activity of attending to the social competencies in client care.*

Occupational Therapy. The goal of occupational therapy is the socializing of patients by countering the regressive aspects of the psychiatric illness. The aim is to increase self-esteem and to teach new occupational skills. A basic principle of occupational therapy is that people learn through activities.

Occupational therapy is an essential part of the total treatment program for a patient. Similar issues may be explored as in talking (psycho) therapy but in different ways. For example, the patient may say, "I want to gain more confidence." The occupational therapist then engages the patient in an activity and continues to talk about the issue of gaining confidence, but the patient is learning through his actions. This is in contrast to psychotherapy in which the patient has to verbally recall previous situations of success or failure.

---

* This section was prepared in consultation with Dawn Huber Warrington, O.T.R. Newton-Wellesley Hospital, Newton Lower Falls, Mass.

ENTRY PROCESS IN THE OCCUPATIONAL THERAPY SETTING. Assessment of the patient begins the moment he walks toward the occupational therapy room. Is the patient hesitant about coming into the room? How does he walk in? Does he seem fearful to be in the room? Once the patient is in the room, his reaction to the room as well as to the therapy should be observed. Occupational therapy rooms tend to be very colorful and perceptually stimulating with artwork and materials displayed in the room.

If this is the first time that the patient goes to the occupational therapy department, the therapist orients him to the room and explains the purpose of the therapy. Then the patient is asked to select an activity. Some patients say, "I don't know what I want to do. You pick one." Other patients may say that they do not like activities or that the activities are too hard. These responses are very meaningful. Is the person trying to say that he has trouble making decisions, or that he is dependent, or that perhaps he has had so many failures in his life that he does not even want to take a chance on making an occupational therapy item? The therapist then collects more data to confirm or reject possible interpretations.

If the therapist decides that a patient needs help with decision-making, she might take two items and ask the person to pick one. This action narrows the choice, and most people can select one item. The patient is also asked if there is someone he would like to make an item for. This question provides data on who is important to the person at that particular time.

The therapist might ask the person to look around the room and select an item he would like to try to make. After selecting one, the person is asked to talk about why he selected it. Some people say they have never tried such an item, or maybe they just like the looks of the activity. Or the therapist asks the patient which color or which material he wishes to use. These data help to evaluate the patient's ability to make a decision.

Projects are ranked from easy to complex. A project such as painting-by-number is usually considered a no-fail project, unless the person cannot concentrate well enough to stay within the lines. A complex project would include several phases.

SETTING GOALS. Ideally, patients set their own goals. However, the therapist may have to ne-

gotiate a goal. Also, because the person may have to change his goal, the therapist should determine if the activity is realistic. For example, one patient wanted to build an electric organ—an unrealistic goal because of the occupational therapy room facilities. The patient was helped to select a smaller project that could be finished within a certain time period and with the tools and room space at hand. The important part of the goal was that the person chose to do something he had always wanted to do, and the therapist helped negotiate the goal so that the person was successful in some aspect of his overall request.

Different patients have different goals. For example, the adolescent with impulse control difficulties may want a project that he can finish quickly—in one day. After the patient completes the project, the therapist may try to negotiate an activity that would take longer in order to increase the patient's attention span. A good project for this goal would be an item that required cutting, staining, and then glazing, for example, a multiphase project. The adolescent is then supported as he tolerates the time delay in finishing the project.

Some patients select projects that are not therapeutic to their problems. For example, a depressed patient who selects knitting becomes involved in a project that is repetitious and has no interactional stimulus. Knitting is better for someone with impulse control problems because it helps set internal limits on the patient. The depressed person needs interpersonal stimulus and an activity that requires that the therapist come back frequently for reinforcement or a project that requires that the person ask many questions.

There are many occupational therapy projects that are goal-directed in terms of the patient's therapeutic progress with life problems. Three major goals include: (1) establishing interpersonal relationships; (2) expressing feelings; and (3) freeing people emotionally.

Activities aid in establishing interpersonal relationships and reality testing. If a project is a success (growing a plant, for example), the socialization aspect in the occupational therapy room is important. In one case, a patient had a difficult time sitting in a group and sat outside the circle that had gathered around the worktable. The therapist talked with the patient and found out that she was fearful of sitting in the group. The therapist suggested to the patient

STANDARD V-E.
Intervention: Therapeutic Environment

The nurse provides, structures, and maintains a therapeutic environment in collaboration with the client and other health care providers.

RATIONALE

The nurse works with clients in a variety of environmental settings such as inpatient, residential, day care, and home. The environment contributes in positive and negative ways to the state of health or illness of the client. When it serves the interest of the client as an inherent part of the overall care plan, the setting is structured and/or altered.

STRUCTURE CRITERIA

1. Mechanisms exist within the practice setting that govern the establishment and maintenance of settings that are clean, safe, humane, and attractive.
2. Written policies and procedures that govern the safe use of seclusion, restraint, or aversive meassures are utilized when staff institute such activity.
3. The environment is characterized by features that facilitate therapeutic gains on the part of clients.

PROCESS CRITERIA

The nurse—

1. assures that clients are adequately oriented to the milieu and are familiar with scheduled activities and rules that govern behavior and daily living.
2. observes, analyzes, interprets, and records the effects of environmental forces upon the client.
3. assesses and develops the therapeutic potential of the practice setting on behalf of clients through consideration of the physical environment, the social structure, and the culture of the setting.
4. fosters communications in the environment that are congruent with therapeutic goals.
5. collaborates with others in the development and institution of milieu activities specific to the client's physical and mental health needs.
6. articulates to the client and staff the justification for use of limit setting, restraint, or seclusion and the conditions necessary for release from restriction.
7. participates in ongoing evaluation of the effectiveness of the therapeutic milieu.
8. assists clients living at home to achieve and maintain an environment that supports and maintains health.

OUTCOME CRITERIA

1. Within 24 hours after admission to a psychiatric setting, the client has been oriented to the milieu, including scheduled activities and rules governing behavior, unless unusual client circumstances interfere with the orientation process.
2. If restrained or secluded, the client can state the reason for such action and the conditions necessary for release, unless unusual client circumstances prevail.
3. The client demonstrates an awareness of the effects of environment on his health and incorporates that knowledge into self-care.

that when she felt comfortable, she should try to sit at the end of the table instead of outside the circle and that she should try to work her way gradually into the circle. The activity the patient was working on helped to provide entry into the circle, and this was an important step for the patient. Also, sitting around a table encourages patients to ask each other for input to their activities. It helps patients reach out to others and to find out that others, and not just the staff, care and can be helpful. Usually, the therapist does not know how to do all the activities that are available. When there is one activity that the therapist does not know, she and the patient can learn together. This encourages cooperative effort and decreases the omnipotence of the therapist. Other patients may know how to do an activity better, and their expertise is welcomed.

Another goal in occupational therapy is encouraging patients to express their feelings. In one case, an angry patient was unable to talk about her feelings in her psychotherapy. She came into occupational therapy, took a hammer and piece of wood, and pounded on the wood. During the second week of her hospitalization, the occupational therapist asked her to label each indented area in the wood. She did and identified anger at having to be in the hospital, and anger at her husband, her therapist, and her child. Identifying the anger was the first step in being able to express and talk about her feelings. Many patients find it helpful and therapeutic to pound something in a constructive way, such as leather or an ashtray.

Working on projects is one way to free people emotionally. Occupational therapy tries to bring into therapy what is occurring in the patients' outside environment. For example, one patient lost four jobs in one year, recently divorced his wife, and left his family. These data imply that this man starts something and then stops before it is finished. If, during occupational therapy, the therapist observes that he starts a project and then leaves it before it is finished, she might say, "I see you have started three different projects here and are having difficulty finishing them. Does this happen in your personal life?" In another example, a patient had an impulse control problem and the therapist observed that he started many different projects. This lack of following through can be confronted as he works on the project. If the patient is a dependent person, he may be encouraged to move into more independence. The therapist can also encourage him to help another person with a project that he himself has already completed.

EVALUATION OF ACTIVITIES. In evaluating a patient's progress it is necessary to look at the whole process from beginning to end in all areas. What feelings is the person struggling with—depression, anxiety, lack of confidence—and how does he move from that position? How does he deal with feelings and with other people? What can occupational therapy teach him?

When the therapist evaluates the activity, she must find out the goal of the person. Were the goals too low or too high? For example, evaluate two different people who worked on making ashtrays. One ashtray has good color and is neatly done and structured. The other ashtray is bizarre with contrasting colors and strange arrangements. The first ashtray may be considered good, but it may mean that the person is too controlled and rigid. The second ashtray may be good because the person was depressed and restricted and was able to loosen up and do something very abstract. The kind of activity and what it means in terms of the goal of the patient must be carefully evaluated.

In evaluating the progress of the person, the therapist may test the thought process. When she instructs a patient on an activity, she may omit one step in order to see if the patient is able to figure out the missing step. At the end of the project, the therapist evaluates how the person compensated for the missing step. If he managed well, that is a success and he is told this in the evaluation process.

Art Therapy. Art therapy may be part of the occupational therapy department or activities therapy department, or it may be a technique the nurse wishes to use in working with a patient. People who cannot express themselves verbally can often put their thoughts on paper. The use of art therapy encourages a person to reach a part of his potential not realized before. Art therapy helps people express what they feel in terms of color and design. For example, in one case, a patient drew a picture of a house, but she did not sign the picture. When asked about this, she expressed ambivalence about going home for the weekend. This information was helpful in the planning session for her visit home in terms of what she anticipated and how she might cope with certain situations.

After the patient has completed a painting or picture, the therapist asks the patient to explain the picture. The therapist may ask what the colors mean or what a certain shape or object is. It is very important to let the patient explain. The therapist cannot interpret what it means, but she can help clarify what the patient is trying to say. For example, one patient drew a multicolored picture in which there was a tree. The patient's interpretation of this was that she felt like the tree—lonely with the sun all around, but she could not feel the sun.

In another case, the patient drew a picture of her previous weekend at home during which she had had anxieties and fears. Many conflicts had developed, and she became angry at her husband and returned to the hospital feeling very depressed. She drew a picture of a rainbow with many colors and talked about each color in relation to her weekend. She said that whenever she is pushed, she gets angry and depressed and nothing comes out. The rainbow color of gray showed this feeling.

Another therapeutic technique is to take pictures drawn previously by the person and show them to him to see whether or not progress is being made. Pictures may be compared as to how the choice of colors changed and what certain objects mean within the picture. Color usually means feelings. Often, as anger and hostility decrease, there is an increase of feelings, typified by yellow or bright colors.

Art therapists can see change over time. For example, instead of many colors being run together, subsequent pictures will show definite boundaries. In exploring this with the patient, it may be learned that issues were clearing in her life and that the patient was able to talk about this in art therapy. In one case, a patient said that the brown color used in the painting were the pills she took and they helped her not to lose control. In every picture she used the color brown. This patient used to lose control and throw plates and furniture, a behavior that frightened her. Her goal was to have control and one way to have control was to take pills or to put the color brown in her paintings. Through talking about her paintings in art therapy, it came out that her father had deserted the family when she was in the second grade. As an adult, she sees her children starting grammar school and she fears that her husband will divorce her

and desert her. The color showed this in her work. Her talking about these issues and her painting showed definite evidence of her gaining control over this fear.

Providing Leadership

The nursing activity of providing leadership and clinical assistance to other nursing personnel and generic health care workers is further addressed in the ANA Division on Psychiatric and Mental Health Nursing Practice as follows[52]:

Psychiatric and mental health nursing embodies responsibilities for collaboration and coordination with those who may be working concomitantly with the client and with others whose expertise can enhance the quality of service. Most organized mental health settings employ an interdisciplinary team approach, which requires highly coordinated and frequently interdependent planning. Cooperative and collaborative efforts with other professional health care providers are an essential part of nursing service. Thus, a high degree of interdependence with colleagues in nursing and other professions is inherent, whether by formal or informal means.

In acknowledgment of this trend in the profession, Standards IX and X cite the need for the nurse to provide learning experiences for other nursing care personnel and for the professional growth of others.[53]

Engaging in Social and Community Action Roles

An important indirect psychiatric nursing activity is engaging in social and community action roles related to mental health. This activity is an indirect nursing action; that is, the activity is not directly related to patient care, but rather is nursing behavior in the service of a larger societal goal. Psychiatric nurses assuming this role are activists for various causes they believe important to the profession. One example of this role is a nursing group in Massachusetts that uses the acronym of NURS or Nurses United for Responsible Services, formerly Nurses United for Reimbursement of Services, is a grass roots nursing group founded in 1975. The group was organized by Boston area psychiatric nurses to promote independent nursing practice as per the passage of the Additional Acts Amendment to the Nurse Practice Act. Third Party Reimbursement, the initial goal of NURS, was achieved in November 1986. In 1987, a bill was filed to authorize health care facilities to accept for evaluation the credentials of Certified Clinical Specialists in Psychiatric and Mental Health Nursing, for clinical privileges and staff membership. This bill was enacted on September 1, 1987. The goal for legislative year 1988 is obtaining Medicaid Reimbursement and future goals include prescription writing and commitment privileges.

BIOLOGIC MODEL OF CARE

The modern origins of the biologic model can be traced to Emil D. Kraepelin, German psychiatrist, born the same year (1856) as Sigmund Freud.[54] Kraepelin's contribution was his application of the medical approach, or the *nosological conception*. By carefully observing groups of patients who exhibited similar symptom clusters through time, he was able to provide the classification of psychiatric illness, which, with some modification, is still in use.

The biologic model views psychiatric illnesses as diseases like any others. For each disease, it is supposed that there eventually will be found a specific etiology related to the functional anatomy of the brain. The clinician using the biologic model is primarily concerned with etiology, pathogenesis, signs and symptoms, differential diagnosis, treatment, and prognosis. Knowing the syndrome or disease determines the treatment. Although addressing patients with proper medical respect, the clinician keeps a distance in order to maintain objectivity. This contrasts with the psychological model in which the therapeutic relationship itself is both diagnostic and therapeutic.

The biologic model, after giving psychiatry its classification of mental illness in the late nineteenth century, has provided the conceptual foundations for (1) the development and use of the antipsychotic and antidepressant medications; (2) the development of mathematical techniques such as factor analysis, which facilitates the validation of clinical syndromes and predicts the response to drugs; (3) studies of the genetic transmission of mental illness; and (4) metabolic studies of psychiatric illness, especially the depressions. The most significant progress in the above four areas has occurred since 1950.

When the nurse applies the biologic model to the case history of Mrs. Janis, she elicits the history of the symptom picture and observes a group of symptoms and historical data consistent with the cluster of a unipolar depression. The patient's relationship with her family, her ambivalence toward her husband, and her motivation to understand her illness are interesting, and perhaps even relevant, but they are not central to the recognition of the illness. Antidepressant medications or electroconvulsive treatments would be the treatments of choice. The patient will be told that she is suffering from a depression, a psychiatric illness not uncommon in her age group. The illness is time-limited and, with proper treatment, has a favorable prognosis.

The important aspect of the nursing role in the biologic model is obtaining a base-line assessment of the key symptoms of Mrs. Janis that respond to drug intervention and secondary symptoms. This gives the nurse a comparison point for evaluating Mrs. Janis's response to drug therapy. If this woman were to receive electroconvulsive therapy (ECT), the nurse would assume an important function in orienting the client and family to ECT, preparing the patient for the treatment, assuring her that she will be present after the treatment to help the client regain her orientation to person, place, and time. In addition, the same principles of base-line information and evaluation and monitoring used in drug therapy would be applied here.

Nursing Activities and the Biologic Model

One of the nine psychiatric nursing activities identified by the ANA Division on Psychiatric and Mental Health Nursing Practice applies to the biologic model of care[55]:

Detecting and caring for somatic aspects of clients' health problems, including responses to drugs and other treatments.

Somatic Treatments

One of the major somatic treatments used in caring for the mentally disturbed client is pharmacotherapy. This type of intervention is discussed in Chapter 21. Standard V–D of the ANA *Standards* emphasizes the knowledge of somatic therapies and related clinical skills are used in working with clients.[56]

STANDARD V-D.
Intervention: Somatic Therapies

The nurse uses knowledge of somatic therapies and applies related clinical skills in working with clients.

RATIONALE

Various treatment modalities may be needed by clients during the course of illness. Pertinent clinical observations and judgments are made concerning the effect of drugs and other somatic treatments used in the therapeutic program.

STRUCTURE CRITERIA

1. There are policies and guidelines for provision of nursing care in somatic therapies.
2. Organizational policies regarding the client's rights for treatment or refusal of treatment are congruent with applicable laws.

PROCESS CRITERIA—

The nurse—

1. utilizes knowledge of current psychopharmacology to guide nursing actions.
2. observes and interprets pertinent responses to somatic therapies in terms of the underlying principles of each therapy.
3. evaluates effectiveness of somatic therapies and recommends changes in the treatment plan as appropriate.
4. collaborates with other team members to provide for safe administration of therapies.
5. supervises the client's chemotherapeutic regimen in collaboration with the physician.
6. provides opportunities for clients and families to discuss, question, and explore their feelings and concerns about past, current, or projected use of somatic therapies.
7. reviews expected actions and side effects of somatic therapies with clients and their families.
8. uses prescribing authority for medications as congruent with the state nursing practice act.

OUTCOME CRITERIA

1. Client responses to drugs and other somatic therapies are recorded.
2. The client incorporates knowledge of somatic therapies into self-care activities.

The convulsive therapies, insulin treatment, psychosurgery, and hydrotherapy are somatic therapies used in varying degrees within institutions. The nurse generally assumes a dependent functional role in working with the physician who has ordered the procedure.

Electroconvulsive Therapy (ECT). Electroconvulsive therapy was first introduced by two Italian psychiatrists, Ugo Cerletti and Lucio Bini, in 1937. The treatment consists of inducing a generalized grand mal convulsion by applying an electrical current to the head.

The treatment originated from the mistaken observation that epilepsy and schizophrenia were not likely to occur in the same patient. It was concluded that convulsions might serve as a treatment for schizophrenia. It was then learned that ECT was even more effective in treating some of the depressions.

ECT is used for both inpatients and outpatients. Because the apparatus needed for the entire treatment consists of a portable ECT box that can easily be carried and only needs a 110 AC voltage, therapy can be administered in any setting if necessary.

The patient usually receives three treatments per week. A minimum of six treatments, an average of nine treatments, and a maximum of 25 treatments are considered within a normal range for a single course of treatment.

ECT is primarily indicated in the treatment of a serious depression where drug therapy has failed or has produced untoward side effects, or where treatment cannot wait for the onset of action of drugs. ECT may be used in the treatment of acute mania, catatonic excitement, or catatonic stupor. The patient is always told of the treatment. The physician generally discusses this treatment with the patient. The term *electric shock* may upset some patients, and a more technical term to use is *convulsive therapy* or *treatments*.

The patient is told that a transient period of memory loss will occur after the treatment and possibly longer for recent events. If the patient is told that he will be asleep, will receive a treatment, and will wake up before an hour has passed with no memory of what happened, he is likely to cooperate. It is customary to have permission forms filled out prior to the first treatment.

The steps involved in the treatment are as follows:

1. Thirty minutes prior to treatment the temperature, pulse, respiration, and blood pressure are taken and any unusual findings reported to the physician. At this time the patient is reminded of the treatment and should be toileted to prevent incontinence during the treatment. Dentures and eyeglasses or contact lenses should be removed and food withheld or instructions given that nothing should be taken by mouth for at least four hours before the treatment. This will prevent any complications arising from aspiration during the treatment.
2. Then 0.8 mg of atropine sulphate is administered subcutaneously 30 minutes prior to treatment to decrease bronchial and tracheal secretions. This reduces the chance of respiratory embarrassment secondary to excessive secretions.
3. At the treatment table the anesthetist administers a quick-acting anesthetic such as intravenous sodium pentathol. The administration of an intravenous muscle relaxant such as succinylcholine chloride (Anectine 10–30 mg IV at 0.5–5 mg/min) is combined with the anesthetic. Positive pressure oxygen is administered for 2 to 3 minutes until the muscular paralysis caused by the succinylcholine disappears and the patient breathes spontaneously.
4. Nursing care during the convulsion is aimed at controlling the patient's body by holding the patient firmly in order to reduce the chance of dislocation and fractures. The convulsion itself starts with a tonic spasm of the entire body, followed by a series of clonic, jerking motions, markedly in the extremities. An airway is inserted after the anesthesia is administered in order to prevent the patient from biting his tongue or lips during the treatment. The patient usually sleeps for 20 to 30 minutes after the treatment and remains confused for 30 minutes more.
5. During the recovery stage the respirations and blood pressure are taken. The nurse stays with the patient until he is awake and able to answer simple questions and can care for himself. Since the patient will be in a confused, hazy state after the treatment, it will be necessary to have someone accompany him back to the ward if he's an inpatient; or to have someone drive him home if he's an outpatient. Emotional support is needed to help the patient feel more secure and relaxed as the confusion and anxiety decrease.

Modifications of ECT produce effects other than the classic convulsions. The electrical current can be regulated so that it merely stimulates the brain (this can be useful in the treatment of severe drug intoxications). The current can also be regulated to produce a loss of consciousness and sustain a minimum of quivering muscles. This kind of treatment is called *electronarcosis* and usually lasts from 3 to 5 minutes.

Another technique of convulsive therapy is the use of a drug such as Indoklon to induce the convulsion. In this method the patient is given the medication intravenously or by inhalation.

Insulin Treatment. In 1933 in Austria, Manfred Sakel (1900–1957) developed a method of insulin shock in treating psychosis. The purpose of insulin coma therapy is to induce a coma by the administration of increasing doses of regular insulin to a fasting patient. Hypoglycemic shock is affected this way.

The procedure involves the patient's receiving an initial dose of 15 units of insulin with daily increases until the coma is reached, about 2 to 3 hours after injection. Insulin doses needed to reach the coma vary from about 60 units to several hundred units. The coma usually occurs in 7 to 10 days. The dangerous stage of insulin coma therapy is during the early coma stage. The coma periods are gradually extended to an hour. The coma is terminated by awakening the patient through tube feedings of sugar solution. High carbohydrate feedings are given as soon as the patient is awake. The average treatment includes 5 to 6 comas per week for 6 to 10 weeks.

This method of treatment requires a well-trained physician and nurse team. The treatment team is necessary because of the precarious and time-consuming aspects of each stage of coma. The shortage of professionals and expense during World War II made this method less practical. After the 1950s, the increased knowledge and use of psychotherapy, psychopharmacology, and convulsive therapies have caused insulin therapy to lose much of its practical importance. The complications of this method, for example, the patient's failing to awake from coma or the development of acute and lasting symptoms of cerebral and cardiovascular damage, are not found in the more contemporary somatic therapies.

Psychosurgery. The modern method of psychosurgery was described by a Portuguese physician, Ega Moniz, in the 1930s. For this he earned a Nobel prize.

Neurosurgeons have since attempted several variations of various surgical techniques from the original method. The objective of almost all lobotomies is the cutting of tracts between the cortex, subcortex, and basal ganglia. If cortical tissue is removed, the procedure is called a *lobotomy*. If only white fibers are severed, the procedure is called a *leucotomy*.

Although lobotomy has lost its clinical importance, there is some resurgence in interest in psychosurgery by using surgical techniques producing less brain damage.

Hydrotherapy. The use of water as a relaxant has long been documented. Spas and baths are still popular in Europe, and other cultures and resorts advertise regimens of exercise, swimming, and massage. Water is equated with pleasure and relaxation.

The water bath as a somatic therapy for disturbed behavior was popular prior to the 1950s and the advent of drug therapies. The patient was placed in a large tub filled with carefully maintained warm water. Then he was covered with a sheet of canvas so that only his head protruded. Close supervision of patients by the nursing staff was essential to maintain their safety. The interpersonal aspect of this type of supervision undoubtedly was as effective as the soothing water bath.

DETERMINATION OF THE CONCEPTUAL MODEL

The nurse implicitly uses one or a combination of conceptual models to assess and plan patient care by the process referred to as *clinical judgment*. The selection may be made according to the results of outcome studies. Or it may be made on practical grounds: "This is the only available plan; let's make the best of it." Sometimes the decision rests on clinical bias. In this section we will attempt to describe some of the variables that determine the choice of conceptual models in patient care.

Clinical Bias

There are physicians, nurses, psychologists, and social workers who because of training, temperament, or clinical bias see a patient predominantly from one conceptual point of view. They may acknowledge the validity of other points of view, but they themselves prefer to use one model.

Sometimes there is a relationship between clinical bias and the geographic location of the psychiatric center. An association with a prominent psychiatric center leads one to identify with that point of view. This identification is also true in medicine. For example, in the insulin treatment of diabetes mellitus there are various viewpoints on how much the blood-sugar level should be controlled in the patient.

Diagnosis

Any functional psychiatric syndrome may be viewed predominantly from any one of the four major models. Certain syndromes, however, are more likely to be viewed by the biologic model than others. These are the schizophrenias, the involutional depressions, and the manic-depressive depressions. Consequently, it is from these clinical syndromes that more is known about genetics, epidemiology, symptom picture, course of illness, somatic treatment, and prognosis.

The neuroses, however, are more inclined to be viewed by the psychological model. It follows then that more is written about the psychodynamics of these syndromes than of the schizophrenias and the depressions.

Treatment

When there is an effective somatic treatment for a psychiatric illness, the biologic model is more likely to be used. Of all the syndromes, those most amenable to somatic treatment are some of the depressions and the schizophrenias. The depressions often respond to antidepressant medication and electroconvulsive therapy. Lithium carbonate has shown great promise in the treatment of the manic phase of manic-depressive syndromes. The phenothiazines, electroconvulsive treatments, and insulin coma treatments have been used with varying degrees of success in the treatment of schizophrenia.

Social Class and Other Attributes of the Patient

A number of studies have demonstrated the importance of the patient's social class in the application of the psychotherapeutic model.[57] Patients from the middle and upper social classes are more likely to be accepted for, and to continue in, psychotherapy. In contrast, patients from the lower class and the lower middle class have a poorer chance of being accepted for therapy, and they drop out of treatment at higher rates.[58] Other patient characteristics that determine the use of the psychotherapeutic model include responsibility, verbal intelligence, psychological mindedness, the capacity to form a close personal relationship, young adult age, history of effective adaptation prior to the current difficulty, likability, and attractiveness.[59]

Available Services

The available treatment resources are an important determinant of the choice of model. Psychotherapy clinics, especially when they are not overcrowded, attempt to apply the psychotherapeutic model in understanding patients. Walk-in emergency clinics, in responding to large numbers of patients, approach the patient with social and biologic perspectives that usually require less time from staff but are effective for many clinical conditions.

There are many small, private psychiatric hospitals that specialize in electroconvulsive treatment. Many patients who have unipolar depressions receive quick, safe, and effective treatment. Some of these hospitals, however, in their persistent use of the biologic model, determined in part by the service that is available to them, may overlook other treatment modalities based on intrapsychic and social models.

There are some psychiatric hospitals that specialize in social techniques (family therapies, therapeutic communities) or intrapsychic techniques (intensive long-term therapy). These institutions will usually use electroconvulsive therapy infrequently or not at all.

Clinics staffed with physicians, nurses, and social workers that treat large numbers of patients may have little opportunity for the long-term psychotherapy that is so often necessary for personality change. Therefore, they make use of the medical and social models that require less staff but are, nevertheless, effective in many clinical situations.

The Immediacy of the Social Situation

When the social cause is obvious, pressing, and immediate, the first consideration is rightly given to the social model. For example:

A 30-year-old married mother of three was referred for psychiatric care following an 8-month depression. Although the depression did not fit the endogenous picture, she was given electroconvulsive treatments without success (the medical model failed). It was then learned that her husband had become severely depressed just prior to the onset of the patient's depression. He arose at 4:00 A.M. each day appearing very morose. He had estranged himself from his mother and sister and spoke little with his wife. The children in their fear of him would cling to their mother. The patient complained of feeling unsupported and overwhelmed, and she developed a fear of being alone.

In this case the social model was used. The major task was to attempt to restore the relationship between the patient and husband. The social management would consist of helping the patient with a substitute social matrix (speaking to her priest, friends, family, or therapist), engaging the couple together, and helping the husband obtain psychiatric treatment. Intensive long-term psychiatric therapy for the wife at this time could have the negative effect of pulling her emotionally away from her husband and toward the therapist.

In general, a social situation in crisis can make intensive psychotherapy a near impossibility. A successful resolution of the social crisis, however, can produce such a dramatic clinical change that the patient often does not want psychotherapy. Indications for somatic treatment may likewise disappear.

It has been noted in a number of outpatient psychiatric clinics that many patients who are called to begin intensive psychotherapy after waiting several months for their turn decline to come. One of the reasons for this phenomenon may be that they had applied for treatment because of social crises, but during the waiting period the social crises were resolved, and the patient no longer felt the need for help.

Failure of a Model

Sometimes one model will prove effective when another fails. For example, a patient who has not responded to electroconvulsive therapy may well respond to individual therapy, and in reverse, a patient suffering a depression who has not responded to the treatment with the group experience may well respond to antidepressants.

Mixed Models

The therapist frequently uses two models simultaneously. An adolescent patient may be treated within a hospital setting by the nurse who maintains a supportive, sustaining relationship (social model) and at the same time by the psychiatrist who uses the intrapsychic model of individual psychotherapy. Without the

social model provided by the nursing staff, the patient may become suicidal, need longer hospitalization, and manifest behavioral disturbances.

Social and Biologic Models

A chronic schizophrenic patient (biologic model) is unmistakably identified as such in the psychiatrist's office. Yet he has lived with his family, served a useful social function, and has never been identified as a patient (social model). Because of a change in his environment (his brother left for the army), he has developed an increase in his delusional thinking. He begins to feel that people are against him and therefore starts to break windows. This behavior is intolerable to his family, who then bring him to the psychiatrist's office. Now he becomes a patient both socially and medically. He is given medication, becomes less delusional, and stops breaking windows. Given the original assessment of his social function, he is cured. Medically, his symptoms have been ameliorated, but he is still considered to be suffering from schizophrenia.

How the Use of One Model May Diminish the Use of Another Model

Clinicians who rigidly hold that one model is useful in understanding psychiatric phenomena will obviously find little use in alternative models. Even when a clinician may be equally skilled in all four approaches, the election to use one model may diminish the use of another.

For example, a certain psychiatric unit relies only on the principles of a therapeutic community (social model). The patient is encouraged to discuss painful issues in a group setting. Symptoms are treated with social controls and medications. Families are actively involved in the treatment program. In this situation it becomes difficult to use individual psychotherapy because the therapist–patient relationship might interfere with the group process. The discussion of painful feelings in individual therapy might communicate to the patient that the group and community are less important. Similarly, a hospital ward that encourages individual psychotherapy implicitly discourages maximal use of a therapeutic community.

Almost all psychiatric units, especially those connected with teaching hospitals, tend to claim that they utilize individual therapy as well as the social techniques of the therapeutic community. In practice, however, teaching, research, and clinical, economic, and other reasons determine which model predominates. This decision automatically determines that another will not predominate.

The phenomenon of the decision to use one model, thereby diminishing the use of another, may also apply in outpatient settings. An example may be the question of whether to treat a patient individually, together with his wife, or to combine the two. Seeing the patient as a couple may diminish the use of the psychological model by altering the therapeutic relationship.

Special Clinical Situations

There are special clinical situations in which a therapist who is knowledgeable and facile in all four conceptual models will favor a particular model:

1. In order to further the Army's goal of maintaining a fighting force in a combat situation, the therapist will find the social model extremely useful. Whenever possible, he will treat the soldier near the combat area, he will avoid defining him as sick or even as a patient, and he will return him to his military unit as soon as possible. Either defining the patient as medically ill or entering into an intensive therapeutic relationship is likely to keep him from returning to combat.

2. In treating a child, the parents are almost certain to receive some attention. It is clear that the patient's social milieu, the family, is having and will continue to have a major effect on the patient's problems.

3. A therapist knowledgeable in all four conceptual models is likely to use the social model if it is his job to treat a community. Economic and manpower reasons alone will justify this decision. He will become closely involved with the social agencies of the community; he will become acquainted with the problems of the school; he will do a large volume of consultation and teaching; and he will see only a few patients on an individual basis.

IMPLICATIONS FOR THE NURSE'S ROLE IN THE MODELS OF CARE

The Eclectic Approach

According to the eclectic approach, clinical psychiatric nursing uses information derived from all models of care. There are, however, two potential stall situations in eclecticism. First, many clinical teams may use data and methods derived from all models without knowing the models well enough to choose what is best for the patient.

Second, there is reason to believe that psychiatric nurses either become adherents to one particular model or they use bits of data from each model in an unsystematic way. At this stage of development, eclectic psychiatry and psychiatric nursing can best be learned and used by making the available models already in use explicit rather than implicit. This will prevent a stall situation and will help clinicians to consciously search for data relevant to successful treatment. It will also allow clinical judgments to be better understood by mental health practitioners instead of appearing as mystical conclusions.

Identifying the Therapeutic Leverage

In order to make a meaningful referral, it is important to know the therapist's area of expertise. The question to ask in evaluating the patient and his need is, "What model of care will give the greatest therapeutic leverage?" This leverage is essential in producing positive results. For example:

A 64-year-old alcoholic woman was referred to a psychiatrist by an internist. Her history stated, "She always drank too much." But her drinking had become extraordinarily excessive over the past 4 years, even though she had been a heavy drinker prior to this. She was frequently intoxicated, would defecate in her underwear, lose consciousness, be socially maladaptive, and she had a liver dysfunction.

To view this problem from the biologic model, that is, having the disease of alcoholism, there would be no treatment except to stop drinking, order vitamins, or administer disulfiram (Antabuse) therapy. To view this problem as a psychological process would prove extremely difficult. It would be difficult to treat a 64-year-old woman from a cultivated, Yankee background with a treatment that concentrates on the expression of feelings because she denies feelings and insists that everything is all right.

The problem could be defined socially. Four years previously, the patient's last daughter married and left her hometown. The patient then was alone with her husband, who also missed the daughter. In the past, the children provided emotional support for both parents.

The therapy was designed to meet with the husband and wife as a couple in order to try to help them give to each other what in reality they were not giving. Since there was so much embarrassment about the patient's having an alcoholic problem, it was more bearable for the patient to have the problem defined as a couples problem rather than as an individual problem. The therapist, being very interested and committed to the patient, partially took the place of her daughter. The social model was used because it provided the best therapeutic leverage. The process involved introducing a new person in the patient's life and changing her social milieu. Since the personality structure of the patient could not be altered and the alcoholism could not be adequately treated, the social model was the effective model.

Identifying the Nursing Approach

The nurse is an important link in the implementation of the social model of care. In this model the nurse becomes a transitional milieu for the patient in a special way that allows the patient to heal.

It is the nurse's role in the biologic model to administer medications, observe the symptom picture through time, and watch for resolution of the mental distress.

From an intrapsychic or psychological point of view, the nurse listens carefully to the patient for the dynamic issue, even when she is not the primary therapist to the patient. The nurse's understanding and interpretation of the patient's thoughts, feelings, and actions yield valuable data for the total team planning of care. If the nurse is in a primary therapist role, this model of care takes on specific dimensions.

For the nurse's understanding of colleagues in the mental health field, these four major models of care should be familiar ones. They will enable the nurse to know which questions to ask the patient. Questions may be asked from a biologic, social, psychological, and behavioral assessment standpoint.

In summary, if the nurses see themselves as eclectic in their conceptual frame of reference in psychiatric nursing, they then know what to listen for and how to interpret most effectively in the best interests of the patient.

Summary

This chapter focused on the therapeutic process and how the decision to use a certain model or models of care is made in the psychiatric mental health field. The health team's variability in thinking was discussed. The decision-making process of clinical judgment was presented; this included the various conditions of clinical bias, diagnosis, treatment, demographic data, available services, the immediacy of the social situation, failure of a model, mixed models, social and medical models, how the use of one model may diminish the use of another model, and special clinical situations.

The nine therapeutic activities identified by the ANA Division on Psychiatric and Mental Health Nursing Practice include: providing a therapeutic milieu, addressing the here-and-now living problems of patients, surrogate parent role, somatic care, client teaching, social competencies in client care, and conducting psychotherapy, leadership, and social activist roles. Also, Standards of Psychiatric Mental Health Nursing are included in the designated model of care.

Questions

1. How do you see the models of care being used in the clinical setting?
2. Do certain disciplines in the mental health field favor certain models? Give examples from your own clinical setting.
3. What implications do the models of care have for the nine therapeutic nursing activities?
4. Use the models of care to describe one client example, as was done in the text example.
5. Describe an eclectic approach to client care.

REFERENCES AND SUGGESTED READINGS

1. Fawcett, J. A framework for analysis and evaluation of conceptual models of nursing. *Nurse Educator*, 1980, *5*(6), 10–14.
2. National League for Nursing. Criteria for the appraisal of baccalaureate and higher degree programs in nursing. New York: National League for Nursing, 1977.
3. Jacobson, S. F. Studying and using conceptual models of nursing. *Image*, 1987, *19*(2), 78–82.
4. Ibid.
5. Fawcett, op. cit.
6. Nye, F. I., & Berardo, F. M. *Emerging Conceptual Frameworks in Family Analysis*. New York: Macmillan, 1966.
7. Yura, H., & Torres, G. Today's conceptual framework within baccalaureate nursing programs. New York: National League for Nursing, 1975, pp. 17–25.
8. Fawcett, op. cit.
9. Fitzpatrick, J., Whall, S., Johnston, R., & Floyd, J. *Nursing Models and their Psychiatric Mental Health Applications*. Bowie, Md.: Brady, 1982, p. *v*.
10. Ibid.
11. American Nurses' Association Division on Psychiatric and Mental Health Nursing Practice. *Statement on Psychiatric-Mental Health Nursing Practice*. Kansas City, Mo.: American Nurses' Association, 1976, pp. 5–6.
12. Lazare, A. Hidden conceptual models in clinical psychiatry. *New England Journal of Medicine*, 1973, *288*, 345–351.
13. Beck, A. *Cognitive Therapy and Emotional Disorders*. New York: International Universities Press, 1976.
14. Ibid.
15. Ibid.
16. Ibid.
17. Ellis, A. *Reason and Emotion in Psychotherapy*. Secaucus, N.J.: Lyle Stuart, 1962; paperback ed. New York: Citadel, 1977.
18. Beck, op. cit.

19. Ellis, A., & Harper, R. A. *A New Guide to Rational Living*. Englewood Cliffs, N.J.: Prentice-Hall, 1975.
20. Rehm, L. P. A self-control model of depression. *Behavior Therapy*, 1977, *8*, 707–804.
21. Seligman, M. *Helplessness: On Depression, Development and Death*. San Francisco: Freeman, 1975.
22. Bandler, R., & Grinder, L. *The Structure of Magic* (Vol. 1). Palo Alto, Calif.: Science and Behavior Books, 1976.
23. Cameron-Bandler, L. *They Lived Happily Ever After*. Cupertino, Calif.: Meta Publications, 1980.
24. Diltz, R., Grinder, J., Bandler, R., & Bandler-Cameron, L. *Neuro-Linguistic Programming: The Study of the Structure of Experience* (Vol. 1). Cupertino, Calif.: Meta Publications, 1980.
25. Beck, A. T. *Depression*. New York: Hoeber, 1967. Republished as *Depression: Causes and Treatment*. Philadelphia: University of Pennsylvania Press, 1972.
26. Diltz, R., Grinder, J., Bandler, R., & Bandler-Cameron, L., op. cit.
27. Pavlov, I. [*Lectures on Conditioned Reflexes*] (2 vols.) (W. H. Grand, Ed.). New York: International Publishing, 1941.
28. Urban, H., & Ford, D. H. Behavior therapy. In A. M. Freedman & H. I. Kaplan (Eds.), *Comprehensive Textbook of Psychiatry*. Baltimore: Williams & Wilkins, 1967, pp. 1217–1225.
29. Liberman, R. P., & Raskin, D. E. Depression: A behavioral formulation. *Archives of General Psychiatry*, 1971, *24*, 515–523.
30. Liberman, R. P. A behavioral approach to family and couple therapy. *American Journal of Orthopsychiatry*, 1970, *40*, 106–118.
31. Lazarus, A. A. Learning theory and treatment of depression. *Behavior Research and Therapy*, 1968, *6*, 83–89.
32. Kish, G. B. Studies of sensory reinforcement. In W. K. Honig (Ed.), *Operant Behavior*. Englewood Cliffs, N.J.: Prentice-Hall, 1966.
33. American Nurses' Association. *Standards of Psychiatric-Mental Health Nursing Practice*. Kansas City, Mo.: American Nurses' Association, 1982, p. 7.

34. Monroe, R. *Schools of Psychoanalytic Thought.* New York: Dryden, 1955.

35. Havens, L. L. Emil Kraepelin. *Journal of Nervous and Mental Disorders,* 1965, *141,* 20.

36. Semrad, E. V. *Teaching Psychotherapy of Psychotic Patients: Supervision of Beginning Residents in the Clinical Approach.* New York: Grune & Stratton, 1969.

37. Alexander, F., & French, T. M. *Psychoanalytic Therapy.* New York: Ronald, 1946.

38. Deutsch, H. Absence of grief. *Psychoanalytic Quarterly,* 1947, *6,* 12–22.

39. Freud, S. [Mourning and melancholia]. In *Collected Papers* (Vol. 4). New York: Basic Books, 1959, pp. 152–170. (First published in 1917.)

40. American Nurses' Association, *Standards,* p. 8.

41. Rees, T. P. Back to moral treatment and community care. *Journal of Mental Science,* 1957, *103,* 303–313.

42. Meyer, A. *Collected Papers of Adolph Meyer* (E. E. Winters, Ed.) (Vols. 1–3). Baltimore: Johns Hopkins Press, 1951.

43. Sullivan, H. S. *The Interpersonal Theory of Psychiatry.* New York: Norton, 1953.

44. Thomas, C. S., & Bergen, B. J. Social psychiatric view of psychological misfunction and role of psychiatry in social change. *Archives of General Psychiatry,* 1965, *12,* 541.

45. Coleman, J. V. Social factors influencing the development and containment of psychiatric symptoms. In T. J. Scheff (Ed.), *Mental Illness and Social Processes.* New York: Harper & Row, 1967, pp. 158–168.

46. Stanton, A. H., & Schwartz, M. S. *The Mental Hospital.* New York: Basic Books, 1954.

47. Hollingshead, A. B., & Redlich, F. C. *Social Class and Mental Illness.* New York: Wiley, 1958.

48. Caplan, G., & Caplan, R. B. Development of community science concepts. In A. M. Freedman and H. I. Kaplan (Eds.), *Comprehensive Textbook of Psychiatry.* Baltimore: Williams & Wilkins, 1967, pp. 1499–1516.

49. Leighton, D. C., & Leighton, A. H. Mental health and social factors. In A. M. Freedman and H. I. Kaplan (Eds.), *Comprehensive Textbook of Psychiatry.* Baltimore: Williams & Wilkins, 1967, pp. 1520–1533.

50. American Nurses' Association, *Statement,* pp. 5–6.

51. American Nurses' Association, *Standards,* p. 5.

52. American Nurses' Association, *Statement,* p. 9.

53. American Nurses' Association, *Standards,* p. 10.

54. Kraepelin, E. [*Clinical Psychiatry: A Textbook for Students and Physicians*] (A. R. Diefendorf, Ed. and trans.). New York: Macmillan, 1921.

55. American Nurses' Association, *Statement,* p. 5.

56. American Nurses' Association, *Standards,* p. 6.

57. Schaeffer, L., & Myers, J. K. Psychotherapy and social stratification. *Psychiatry,* 1954, *17,* 83–93.

58. Overall, B., & Aronson, H. Expectations of psychotherapy in patients. *American Journal of Orthopsychiatry,* 1963, *33,* 421–430.

59. Heine, R. W., & Trosman, H. Initial expectations of doctor–patient interaction as a factor in continuance in psychotherapy. *Psychiatry,* 1960, *23,* 275–278.

Chapter 21

Pharmacotherapy

Carol R. Hartman
Margaret Knight

Chapter Objectives

The students successfully attaining the goals of this chapter will be able to:

- Describe the history of psychotropic drugs.
- Describe the rationale for the current classification system for psychopharmacologic agents.
- List the drugs and their dosages currently used for the major diagnostic categories.
- Describe the linkages between drug action on the brain and human behavior.
- Associate major behavioral changes to drug toxicity and drug side effect.
- Carry out psychiatric–mental health nursing regarding pharmacotherapy intervention.

The use of somatic or biologic interventions is an important aspect of the nurse's work with the patient. Although the responsibility for prescribing drugs resides with the physician, the nurse's role is most essential and goes beyond the dispensing of drugs. In the mental health field, nurses are often the primary evaluator of behavior and have great influence over patients who receive drugs.

Since the heart of psychopharmacotherapeutics relates in general to the regulatory functions of the brain and in particular to neuroregulation, the nurse must be knowledgeable about the actions and side effects of drugs. This knowledge is particularly important because it is the nurse who will have the most frequent contact with the individual receiving the drug. Teaching individuals and their families about drugs is an extremely important responsibility of the nurse. In settings where the nurse will work with other professionals and paraprofessionals (nonmedical), the nurse's knowledge of drugs is essential in helping these professionals carry out their work with patients.

In addition to the very helpful aspects of drugs, there are serious issues in their use. Informed consent is imperative. Drug therapy carries with it a degree of risk, as do other therapies. These risks must be known by nurses and must be conveyed to patients and their families in an appropriate manner, i.e., by the physician, or by protocols. The nurse is in an important position to contribute to clinical information that confirms or refutes the efficacy of certain drugs. This may be done through direct observation and reporting, or through systematic study. Although somatic interventions place the nurse in close collaboration with the physician, the nurse is not relieved of independent responsibility regarding drug therapy. Assessment and reassessment of patient behavior are key tasks.

OVERVIEW OF NURSE'S ROLE

Pharmacotherapy, as a biologic intervention that blends the specifics of medical diagnosis with nursing diagnoses, demands a critical assessment of the patient. This appraisal needs to include the sociocultural and psychological as well as the physiological context in which the behavior is manifested. The nurse has three tasks at this level of assessment: (1) obtaining a base line of patient behavior; (2) monitoring the response pattern within the context of the drug regimen; and (3) teaching the patient and family about the medications.

Base-line Assessment

It is essential that the nurse have a base line of patient behavior before drug treatment is instituted. The functional status assessment protocol and the mental status examination (see Chapter 12) assist the nurse to assess with the patient his past response to drug therapy as well as the total drug history for the patient.

The functional health history includes the patient's beliefs and expectations regarding drugs, his willingness to participate in their use, myths and fears about taking drugs, and understanding of the risks and potential side effects in the use of psychotropic drugs. Direct questions as well as probing questions encourage elaboration of these themes. Behavior and thought patterns that interfere or limit these understandings must be fully noted by the nurse. Often, this part of the assessment strengthens the therapeutic alliance because of the thoughts and decisions by the patient. This empowerment of the patient can prevent regression. Personal commitment of taking drugs through knowledge and negotiation counteracts fears of

dependency, control by drugs and other concerns of the patient.

The mental status examination provides information about behavioral movement patterns such as spasms, flexibility, myoclonic movements, tremors, states of restlessness, rates and patterns of speech, and states of excitement. The examination assesses psychological processes such as perception, memory, thought content and organization, sense of self, distorted perceptions such as hallucinations (visual or auditory) and illusions as well as self-care domains such as grooming, appropriateness of dress and interpersonal patterns.

Monitoring of Behavior

The patient's behavior while on a drug regimen needs careful monitoring. The information obtained incorporates observations of patient behavior as well as self-appraisal by the patient and assists in eliminating or reducing the untoward effects of drug intervention.

Initial nursing evaluation schemes are enhanced if they include questions and criteria that allow for observation and interview data for a patient status report. When this information is included with basic physiological assessment indices such as weight, blood pressure, temperature, and a present history of the patient's health state and health habits, nursing conclusions can be made regarding the patient's response to an instituted drug regimen.

Drug Education

The psychoeducational needs of patients make clear the nurse's role in the variety of drug regimens used in psychiatric nursing practice. The nurse's knowledge of drugs becomes important not only for the monitoring of intervention programs but for the ultimate enhancement of the patient's independence and self-reliance.

An educational paradigm for drug taking which emphasizes that the chemical imbalances which when left uncorrected, influence thinking, perceptions and interpretation of information, counteract negative assumptions by the patient. Most negative assumptions by patients focus on drugs being a sign of total incompetancy, out of control, "crazy." The use of drugs aims at restoring balance to the body's chemical information-transmitting system when it is out of balance. The patient has to do the work to improve problem-solving skills but the drugs will assist in that thinking process. Parallels can be drawn with other physiological conditions, such as the use of insulin to process sugar in the body or medication that "thins" the blood by reducing blood clots. Nurses need to be prepared for reluctance and challenges by the patient who feels compromised by the need to take a drug.

For patients who have been on drug therapy for some time, the converse is true. They often need to understand that they can take the risk to reduce their need for drugs. This process is complicated by the fact that oftentimes patients have not felt they had any say in their drug intervention program. They have not learned self-monitoring procedures and consequently they lack confidence in their ability to communicate and negotiate either increases or reductions in their drugs.

Drug Regimens

Drug regimens can be divided into four major phases. Phase I is the initiation of drug treatment to control the acute period of a disorder. Phase II is the maintenance period when the lowest effective dose of drug is achieved. Phase III is the period of time when there is a cessation of drug therapy, and Phase IV is the drug-free period.

Given this overview of the nurse's role in the use and management of psychotropic drugs, the remainder of the chapter will focus on three major units of antipsychotic drugs, antidepressant drugs, and antianxiety drugs. The chapter focus will be on general principles of these drugs, their specific actions, and the nursing management of the patient and drug.

GENERAL CLASSIFICATION OF PSYCHOTROPIC DRUGS

Early in the discovery of antipsychotic drugs, they were referred to as *tranquilizers*. This term has not proven useful in distinguishing the drugs and their actions. Therefore an attempt to increase specificity has resulted in the present terminology: *antipsychotic* or *neuroleptic agents*; *antidepressant agents*; *mood-stabilizing agents*; and *antianxiety agents*. In addition, anti-Parkinsonian agents used in the treatment of certain side effects and amphetamine-like stimulants used in the treatment of hyperkinetic syndrome are part of drug treatment.

The classification of drugs to a great extent has a logic based on chemical structure and drug action. As discussed earlier, many psychotropic drugs were discovered by making slight molecular changes and studying the effect of these changes on behavior. These initial changes were made at the R_{10}, S, and R_2 areas of the phenothiazine triple ring. Figure 21-1 demonstrates the chemical derivation of antidepressants from the phenothiazine triple ring. In addition, Figure 21-1, reading across the top, shows major chemical chains added to at the R_{10} position. These changes—aliphatics, piperidines, and piperazines—were made to alter side effects and potency. The variations of effects of these manipulations are graphically represented at the bottom of Figure 21-1. Not all psychotropic drugs follow from these chemical structures; however, those that do can be expected to generally manifest similar clinical characteristics based on their structural grouping. Milligram potency, dosage range, sedative actions, psychomotor inhibition, autonomic reactions, stimulating actions, and extrapyramidal reactions can be related to structure not only for antipsychotic drugs but also for antidepressant drugs.

In the past decade drugs have been placed into groupings depending on the symptoms that they treat. The term *antipsychotic* has replaced the term *major tranquilizer* and *antianxiety agent* has replaced *minor tranquilizer*. *Antidepressants* remain, as they are specific to depressions, and *mood-stabilizing agents* have been added to refer to drugs such as lithium carbonate and certain anticonvulsant drugs that have proven effective in the treatment of affective disorders.

ANTIPSYCHOTIC DRUGS

Identifying Symptoms of Psychosis

It is necessary to identify what is being treated when antipsychotic drugs are being used. An important aspect of using drugs is a clear assessment of the target symptoms and a differential assessment of the possible etiology of the symptoms.[1] Anxiety in and of itself ought not to be treated with antipsychotic drugs, and psychotic states ought not to be treated with an-

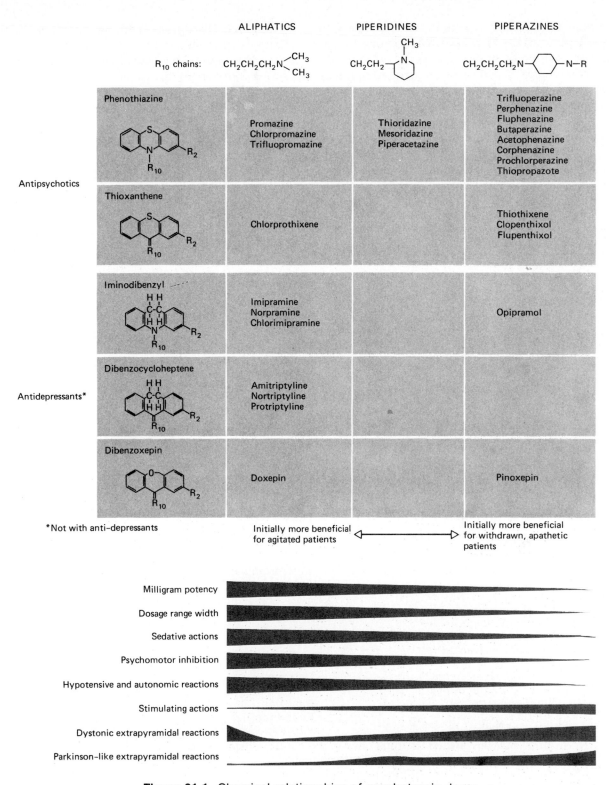

Figure 21-1. Chemical relationships of psychotropic drugs.

tianxiety agents. For the most up-to-date considerations of the classification of behavioral symptoms, physical status, personality structure, life stressors, and coping behaviors, the reader is referred to the *DSM-III-R*.[2]

Target symptoms most affected by antipsychotic drugs are negativism, combativeness, psychotic tension, hostility, hallucinations, acute delusions, and paranoia. Improvements in memory, judgment, self-care, seclusiveness, anorexia, insomnia and insight are only likely to occur secondarily to use of these drugs.[3] Confusion is to be carefully observed in using antipsychotic and antidepressant drugs. A target symptom approach clarifies what areas of behavior modification can be expected; and, as one can see, these areas of symptom control do not necessarily address all the behaviors that are disturbed in various diagnostic states, nor do they address other sociopsychological areas of interpersonal relationship that may contribute to or

perpetuate disruption in higher cognitive functions.[4]

A current listing of antipsychotic drugs and anti-Parkinsonian drugs is provided in Table 21-1.

Antipsychotic Drug Action

Research has indicated that antipsychotic drugs are most useful in the treatment of acute psy-

TABLE 21-1. ANTIPSYCHOTIC DRUGS AND ANTI-PARKINSONIAN DRUGS

Brand	Generic Name	Dialy Dose Range (mg)
I. *ANTIPSYCHOTIC AGENTS*		
A. *Phenothiazine derivatives:*		
1. *Aliphatics*		
a. Thorazine	Chlorpromazine	100–1000
b. Vesprin[a]	Triflupromazine	20–150
c. Sparine[a]	Promazine	25–1000
2. *Piperidines*		
a. Mellaril	Thioridazine	30–800
b. Serentil	Mesoridazine	50–400
c. Quide[a]	Piperacetazine	20–160
3. *Piperazines*		
a. Stelazine	Trifluoperazine	2–30
b. Trilafon	Perphenazine	2–64
c. Proketazine[a]	Carphenazine	25–400
d. Tindal[a]	Acetophenazine	40–80
e. Repoise[a]	Butaperazine	30–50
f. Prolixin, Permitil	Fluphenazine	0.5–20
g. Prolixin enanthate or decanoate	(long-acting injectable)	$\frac{1}{2}$–4 cc ($\frac{1}{2}$–4 cc every 2 or 3 wk)
B. *Thioxanthene derivatives:*		
1. Taractan (aliphatic)	Chlorprothixene	10–600
2. Navane (piperazine)	Thiothixene	6–60
C. *Butyrophenone derivative:*		
1. Haldol	Haloperidol	1–100
D. *Dihydroindolone derivative:*		
1. Moban	Molindone	20–225
E. *Dibenzoazepine derivative:*		
1. Loxitane, Daxolin	Loxapine	20–250
2. Leponex (experimental)[a]	Clozapine	60
F. *Diphenylbutylpiperidines:*		
1. Orap (experimental)[a]	Pimozide	0.3–0.5
2. Experimental[a]	Penfluridol	25–100 mg every 1–4 wk
3. Experimental[a]	Fluspiridcne	—
II. *ANTI-PARKINSONIAN AGENTS* (Drugs used in the control of side effects. They also have anticholinergic properties that can lead to toxic reaction.)		
Akineton[a]	Biperiden	2–6
Artane	Trihexyphenidyl	1–10
Benadryl	Diphenhydramine	25–200
Cogentin	Benztropine mesylate	1–6
Kemadrin[a]	Procyclidine	6–20
Symmetrel	Amantadine	100–300
Parsidol[a]	Ethopropazine	50–600
Disipal, Norflex[a]	Orphenadrine	50–300

[a] Infrequently used.

chotic states, both in people with good premorbid history and in chronically ill patients having an acute exacerbation of symptoms. The drugs target the symptoms of negativism, combativeness, psychotic tension, hostility, hallucinations, acute delusions, and paranoia.[5] Not all chronically psychotic patients require large doses of medication for maintenance, and many have responded to treatment without drugs. The risk of the prolonged use of antipsychotic drugs must be evaluated against the benefits, and every patient deserves opportunities to be medication-free. The major serious consequence of prolonged use of antipsychotic drugs is tardive dyskinesia, for which there is no known corrective treatment. However, research is being conducted with various drugs to try to reverse the tardive dyskinesia symptoms although none have been successful to date. In addition to those with a history of chronic and prolonged use of antipsychotic agents, elderly people are at high risk to this condition because of the drug's seeming impairment of higher cortical functions and psychomotor skills.[6]

The dosage schedules vary according to the potency of the drug and the individual differences. There are drugs available to minimize the unwanted pharmacologic effects of sedation, adrenergic blocking activity, and extra-pyramidal effects (see Table 21-1). Since the antipsychotic drugs are long-acting once a dose level to control symptoms has been achieved, a single dose can be given at bedtime. This permits the unwanted short-term side effects to occur during sleep. Also, sleep seems to ameliorate manifestations of extra-pyramidal side effects.[7]

In acute psychotic episodes, treatment with antipsychotic drugs may be brief, but in newly treated chronic patients, it might require three to six months of treatment before a change in medication is warranted. In schizophrenia, maintenance doses should be as low as possible while retaining therapeutic gains. Some forms of postpsychotic regression or depression may be related to the drugs rather than to the course of the illness. As behavior becomes more normal, the drugs become more noxious. The realization that people can be on low maintenance doses and still retain the needed effect came from patients themselves who took their own drug "holidays," reducing the amount of drug that was prescribed.[8]

Antipsychotic agents may impair physical and mental abilities, especially during the first few days of therapy.

These agents are metabolized in the liver and may cause hepatic toxicity. There is also excretion of these drugs via the kidney. Side effects and toxicity are not infrequent with antipsychotic drugs, yet as a group of drugs they are relatively safe.[9] Adults respond within a wide therapeutic margin. Most fatalities from overdoses have occurred with children or when these drugs are mixed with other drugs, which result in dangerous interaction effects.

To understand side effects, it is important to consider the anatomic location where it is thought that the antipsychotic drugs act. Four anatomic sites of action are[10]:

1. The reticular activating system of the midbrain where sensory input is monitored.
2. The amygdala and hippocampus, which are structures of the limbic system that provide emotional coloring attached to incoming signals, i.e., fear, fight, flight.
3. The hypothalamus, which governs the peripheral responses to meaningful sensory information through both the pituitary endocrine system and the autonomic nervous system.
4. The globus pallidus and corpus striatum, where extrapyramidal syndromes are elicited, perhaps coincidentally.

As one can see, antipsychotic drugs, although acting in certain areas to effect control over certain aspects of psychotic behavior, have the dubious distinction of affecting systems of the brain that are involved in many regulatory functions—particularly in motor and fine motor coordination. Side effects most frequently noted are those involving the extrapyramidal system.

Because antipsychotic drugs often produce signs of neurological dysfunction, the term *neuroleptic* was created. There is an effort on the part of clinicians in the United States to try and avoid the emergence of CNS side effects. An example of two drugs with a low incidence of CNS side effects are mellaril-thioridazine and closapine in dibenzoxazepine compound.[11] Common extrapyramidal symptoms are dystonia, dyskinesia, akathesia, Parkinson's syndrome, tardive dyskinesia, and choreathetoid movements. With the exception of tardive dyskinesia, the other symptoms occur and disappear within the first three to four months of drug treatment. Tardive dyskinesia, when it occurs, does so after three months. A detailed presentation of special problems follows, they are: tardive dyskinesia; extrapyramidal symptoms; rare side effects and common side effects. This will be followed by special nursing management considerations.

Special Problems

Tardive Dyskinesia

Tardive dyskinesia is a syndrome that usually occurs later in the use of antipsychotic drugs. It is more often associated with the higher-potency neuroleptics or antipsychotics. It is marked by repetitive, involuntary movements involving the mouth, lips, tongue, trunk, and extremities. It is usually preceded by the Parkinson syndrome. Anti-Parkinsonian drugs make the condition worse because of their anticholinergic actions. Decreasing the antipsychotic drug may temporarily reduce the symptoms of tardive dyskinesia, but the dosage would soon need to be increased to control the symptoms. This is true even if another antipsychotic drug is substituted. Sudden withdrawal of an antipsychotic drug may reveal the latent syndrome. Prominent features of the syndrome are face and neck movements including chewing, smacking and licking of the lips, sucking, tongue protrusions, tongue tremor with open mouth, wormlike movements on the surface of the tongue, blinking, and facial distortions. Neck and trunk movements include spasmodic torticollis, retrocollis, torsion movements of the trunk, hip rocking, and finally the choreoathetoid movements of the extremities (these are a combination of jerky, incomplete involuntary movements of the upper extremity combined with constant recurring series of slow vermicular [undulating] movements of the extremities). Sometimes this movement may be restricted to a finger (thumb) or a big toe. The movement is constant.[12]

Early detection of the disorder is most important to reduce the seriousness of the condition. For example, movements of the big toe can be so constant that the shoe top is worn through. In extreme conditions and with some young clients, despair has been so great they have committed suicide. All patients on prolonged use of antipsychotic drugs must be evaluated for some of the subtle signs. These signs are the wormlike movements of the tongue surface and the subtle spasmodic signs, particularly those of the arms. Although many drugs have been studied as a potential treatment for tardive dyskinesia, none have proved efficacious. The only known treatment at this time is discontinuance of the drug.

Extrapyramidal Symptoms

Dystonia is involuntary, irregular clonic contortions of the muscles of the trunk and extremities. Initially, patients often complain of a thick tongue, and inability to hold their neck straight. Other early symptoms include cog-wheeling[11] and difficulty speaking and swallowing. (Symptoms appear chiefly on walking, at which time the contortions twist the body forward and sideways [tortipelvis] in a grotesque fashion.) Sometimes the dystonia can be quite dramatic, resulting in oculogyric crises (rolling back of the eyes in the head) and opisthotonos (extreme arching of the back with the head thrown back). This extreme reaction occurs mostly in young males and early in treatment. Higher-potency drugs are more often associated with acute dystonias. This is easily treated, as are all of the extrapyramidal side effects with the exception of tardive dyskinesia, with anti-Parkinsonian drugs such as benzotropine mesylate (Cogentin) or with diphenhydramine hydrochloride (Benadryl). Dystonia requires immediate treatment. Problems arise when severe dystonia is not recognized as a side effect of an antipsychotic drug. Emergency measures such as tracheotomies have been performed unnecessarily and with danger to the patient.

Dyskinesia is impairment of the power of voluntary movement, resulting in fragmentary or incomplete movements.

Akathisia is an extreme inability to sit still. The body is in constant movement. There is pacing and constant movement of the feet. If you stop movement in the trunk, the person's pelvis and feet will move. This side effect is frequently mislabeled as agitation or severe anxiety, often resulting in an increase of problems. Patients describe feeling as though they are "jumping out of their skin" or that their extremities won't stay still.

Parkinson's syndrome is marked by muscular rigidity, immobile face, involuntary movement of the head, tremors, and pill-rolling movements of the forefinger and thumb. There can be salivation and drooling. In some ways the person appears rigid, not free to move, yet agitated.

Rare Side Effects

NEUROLEPTIC MALIGNANT SYNDROME (NMS). This is a rare side effect that has been referred to as extrapyramidal crisis. The symptoms of this condition include labile blood pressure, elevated pulse and temperature, anxiety, dyspnea, profuse perspiration, cyanosis, and seizures. The best treatment is discontinuance of the neuroleptic agent. Often, clients must be admitted to the general hospital setting for a symptomatic treatment of this disorder such as ice blankets, hydration, and control of blood pressure. Some literature suggests that bromocriptine mesylate and dantrolene sodium alone or together are useful in the treatment of NMS.[13,14]

AGRANULOCYTOSIS. Another rare complication is agranulocytosis, marked by sore throat, fever, severe itching, increased bruising, and bleeding. Medication must be stopped and the patient isolated from sources of infection; antibiotics may be given and the patient should be hospitalized. Periodic blood counts and other laboratory data can help to detect this problem before it reaches crisis proportions.

PROGRESSIVE OBSTRUCTIVE JAUNDICE. Progressive obstructive jaundice is another rare and serious reaction. Increased yellowing of the skin and sclera of the eyes are the most notable signs. The drug must be stopped. The patient can be changed to another drug because cross-sensitivity is rare.[15] The usual intervention for the liver disruption is bed rest and a high-protein, high-carbohydrate, low-fat diet.

Common Side Effects
Milder and more common side effects of antipsychotic drugs are listed as follows:

PSYCHIATRIC SYMPTOMS. Depression, anxiety, increased drowsiness, increased hallucinations, and aggravation of schizophrenic symptoms in borderline patients can occur. Usually decreasing the dose of drug or changing to another neuroleptic drug results in a decrease of these symptoms.

ANTICHOLINERGIC EFFECTS. These include blurred vision, flushing, pallor, and dry mouth. Reassurance usually helps. Urologic symptoms are less common, but there may be retention of urine, particularly with thioridazine (Mellaril). Also, there may be retarded ejaculation and painful urination. These symptoms can be handled by reducing the dosage if possible, and if not, a cholinergic drug (bethanechol chloride [Urecholine]) may be used.

CENTRAL NERVOUS SYSTEM SYMPTOMS. CNS symptoms include drowsiness and seizures

from a lowered convulsive threshold. In cases of seizures, drugs should be stopped or decreased and anticonvulsant therapy initiated. Mild forms of dystonia, dyskinesia, and akathisia may all be treated by anti-Parkinsonian drugs. Severe reactions have already been discussed. Impaired motor function must be dealt with by warning the patient and having him not involve himself in dangerous activities. Fatigue, lethargy, and weakness are mild and usually subside when the patient becomes active and moves around. Any problems in breathing are best handled by stopping the drug or reducing the dose.

CARDIOVASCULAR SYSTEM SYMPTOMS (IN MILD FORM). These include syncope and electrocardiogram changes. Not as common are ventricular tachycardia (usually with thioridazine) and coronary thrombosis (which has been suspected with imipramine hydrochloride), peripheral edema, and hypotensive crises. The heart rate changes may be handled by reducing the dose if possible, and other cardiovascular complications must be weighed clinically against the benefits with consideration of stopping the drug.

DERMATOLOGIC SIDE EFFECTS. The most common dermatologic side effect is photosensitivity, usually with chlorpromazine (Thorazine) and thioridazine (Mellaril). Staying out of the sun and wearing protective clothing are the best methods of dealing with this problem. Less common effects are skin rashes with edema on face, feet, or hands. Diphenhydramine chloride (Benadryl) may be used. A rarer effect is a deep pigmentation of the skin. This may occur with Thorazine.

ENDOCRINE SYSTEM SYMPTOMS. Common symptoms are obesity, menstrual irregularity, edema, abnormal lactation, and decreased sex drive for men and increased sex drive for women. These symptoms are usually handled by reassurance or trying another class of drugs.

METABOLIC SYSTEM SYMPTOMS. The symptom of cholestatic jaundice may be noted; another rare and dangerous side effect is hepatic necrosis.

OPHTHALMOLOGIC SYSTEM SYMPTOMS. Patients may manifest a mild disturbance in accommodation, in which the eye is not able to focus on an object, and miosis (small pupil). An ophthalmologist should assess the eye's ability to accommodate. Rare and serious side effects are glaucoma or aggravation of glaucoma, ulceration of the cornea, pigmentation of the retina (tissue darkening or discoloration in the eye ground), and fine reticular corneal opacities. The important treatment for eye involvement is early detection and consultation with an ophthalmologist.

GASTROINTESTINAL SYSTEM SYMPTOMS. These are uncommon and include fecal impaction (use mechanical aid to reduce the impaction and to prevent its reoccurrence), constipation, and diarrhea. More severe symptoms requiring cessation of the drug are paralytic ileus and perforating ulcer, for which hospitalization is necessary.

HEMATOLOGIC SYSTEM SYMPTOMS. As noted before, side effects in this system are rare and when they occur in the form of leukopenia, agranulocytosis, or purpura, the drug must be stopped and supportive measures instituted.

Nursing Management of Extrapyramidal Side Effects and Other Symptoms

The nurse is in an important position to help the patient withstand the side effects that will soon pass as well as those that need to be sorted out from the symptoms. Often patients have been placed on excessive amounts of drugs because nurses have confused reactions to the drug therapy with symptoms of the disordered state being treated. Therefore, a review of the nursing parameters of extrapyramidal side effects will be helpful here. These side effects fall into four general classes: (1) Parkinsonism; (2) dyskinesias and dystonias; (3) akathisia; and (4) tardive dyskinesia.

Parkinsonism Syndrome

Parkinsonism syndrome usually occurs after the first week of treatment but before the second month of treatment. The symptoms resemble Parkinson's disease, which has the following symptoms: akinesia (lack of interest, fatigue, slowness, heaviness, lack of drive or ambition, vague bodily discomforts), muscular rigidity, mask-like facies, shuffling gait, loss of associated movements, hypersalivation, drooling, alterations in posture, tremor, and pill-rolling movements.

The akinesia is often misinterpreted as depression or negativism. The weakness and lack of interest should be evaluated from the standpoint of muscle weakness. Usually, there is a lack of muscle strength in the individual's grip. In addition, increased muteness or any comments about feeling slowed down, heavy, in slow motion, or under water are further subjective signs of akinesia.

The lack of facial expression or "flatness" of the face is often mistaken for signs of chronic schizophrenia or depression. The difference is that despite the facial expression, the person uses language to express variations of emotional reactions in contrast to schizophrenic or depressed patients.

Body rigidity is often mistaken for anxiety, again a misdiagnosis that can lead to more medication rather than treating this as the Parkinsonism syndrome. Rigidity is tested for by holding the patient's elbow in the palm of your hand with your thumb positioned over the flexor tendons, extending and flexing the patient's arm, asking him to relax. If there is a consistent resistance—"lead-pipe rigidity," or a ratchet-like phenomenon known as "cog-wheel rigidity," this is evidence of drug-induced rigidity. It usually starts two to three days or two weeks after drug therapy is begun.

The stooped posture and the lack of associative movements such as the moving of arms while walking are often mistaken for depression. If the person was not like this prior to drug treatment, the chances are that such changes in posture and movement are connected with the drug.

Tremor, particularly in the hands, will be noted. The amount of tremor is usually more than in Parkinson's disease. The hand tremor interferes with fine motor coordination. Patients may try and hide the tremor, feeling embarrassed or attributing it to their emotional state.

The muteness and alterations in posture are often mistaken for worsening schizophrenic syndrome. Unfortunately, any increase in medication increases the symptoms. If left unchecked, incontinence, fever, and coma can ensue.

Improvement of these symptoms usually occurs slowly with the reduction of the dose of the drug and by the addition of an anticholinergic drug. Sometimes switching a patient to a different antipsychotic drug removes the symptoms. After two to three months the symptoms will usually disappear. It is important to recognize this since anti-Parkinsononian drugs have powerful anticholinergic effects, and it is important to get the patient off them as soon as possible.

Dyskinesias and Dystonias

Dystonic reactions and acute dyskinesias (i.e., involuntary, abnormal movements of various types) and oculogyric crises typically occur during the early hours or days following an increase in the dosage of antipsychotic drugs. The symptoms are episodic and recurrent, lasting from minutes to hours. Involuntary contractions are common, particularly around the jaw, mouth, face, and neck. These may be trismus (lockjaw), dystonia or dyskinesias of the tongue, opisthotonos (spasms of the neck that arch the back and pull the head backward), or eye closure.[16] These symptoms are seen more commonly in males. The importance in recognizing these rather frightening symptoms as being drug-related is that they can often be misdiagnosed in an emergency situation. Consider the following example:

A mental health worker reported that her daughter was about to have a tracheotomy performed in an emergency room when she came in with oculogyric crisis, torticollis, protrusion of her tongue, and opisthotonos. Fortunately, the mother informed the physician that her daughter was on an antipsychotic drug and he administered diphenhydramine (Benadryl) intravenously, and the tracheotomy was avoided.

The symptoms of dystonias are painful and frightening. They can be acute, or they can be milder. Once these occur, the dosage of the medication should be lowered to avoid further episodes. Because the patient may complain of his eyes rolling up in his head or suspect peculiar things going on with his jaw, a nurse might wrongly assume the patient is delusional rather than having a drug-related response.

Akathisia

Akathisia, with the most common effects of feeling restless and agitated, the "walkies and the talkies," can be mistaken for anxiety and agitation. These symptoms are most uncomfortable, and patients often refuse to take medications because of them. It is difficult to concentrate and read and do simple tasks. The way of differentiating akathisia from anxiety is to note whether it gets worse when the drug is increased or if the subjective experience of the patient is different. The patient usually experiences the restlessness as something different. He also will report feeling better walking around and will identify an internal sense of restlessness that was not experienced before. The incidence peaks within 6 to 10 weeks with a decline in 12 to 16 weeks. Anti-Parkinsonian drugs and the shorter-acting benzodiazapines will reduce the symptoms as well as encourage the patient by demonstrating that the effects of akathisia are time-limited.

Tardive Dyskinesia

The most serious extrapyramidal syndrome is that of tardive dyskinesia. If detected early, it can be reversed by stopping the drug therapy. Clients on antipsychotic drug therapy, and in particular on long-term therapy, must be screened every 3 months for the disorder. The earliest signs are excessive blinking and fine, vermiform movements of the tongue. The symptoms then progress with a fluctuating course until, finally, they interfere with activities of daily living, such as bathing, dressing, or even eating. The symptoms can be suppressed only by intense, voluntary effort. During sleep they are absent. They are very embarrassing to clients, and some people have committed suicide because of them.

There is active research attempting to find a cure for tardive dyskinesia and to find drugs that will not cause the syndrome. For years it was thought that children, who appear to have fewer side effect reactions to antipsychotic drugs, were relatively free from this disorder. Unfortunately, this is not the case.

At present, the rule is to place people on antipsychotic drugs for the shortest time possible and for people who are on long-term maintenance to use the least amount of drug and to institute "drug holidays." Drug holidays refers to the practice of allowing clients to be off drugs for two or three days at a time. This is possible with some of the antipsychotic drugs because they have a residual effect over several days because of the manner in which they are stored and metabolized by the body.

When tardive dyskinesia is identified, drugs used to treat extrapyramidal reactions should not be used, as these may exacerbate the condition. Increasing the antipsychotic drugs is contraindicated because it masks the symptoms and can lead to toxicity.

TABLE 21-2. ABNORMAL INVOLUNTARY MOVEMENT SCALE (AIMS) EXAMINATION PROCEDURE

Either before or after completing the examination procedure, observe the patient unobtrusively, at rest (e.g., in waiting room).

The chair to be used in this examination should be hard, firm one without arms.

1. Ask patient whether there is anything in his mouth (i.e., gum, candy, etc.) and if there is, to remove it.
2. Ask patient about the *current* condition of his teeth. Ask patient if he wears dentures. Do teeth or dentures bother patient *now*?
3. Ask patient whether he notices any movements in mouth, face, hands, or feet. If yes, ask to describe and to what extent they *currently* bother patient or interfere with his activities.
4. Have patient sit in chair with hands on knees, legs slightly apart, and feet flat on floor. (Look at entire body for movements while in this position.)
5. Ask patient to sit with hands hanging unsupported. If male, between legs; if female and wearing a dress, hanging over knees. (Observe hands and other body areas.)
6. Ask patient to open mouth. (Observe tongue at rest within mouth.) Do this twice.
7. Ask patient to protrude tongue. (Observe abnormalities of tongue movement.) Do this twice.
8. Ask patient to tap thumb, with each finger, as rapidly as possible for 10 to 15 seconds, separately with right hand, then with left hand. (Observe facial and leg movements.)
9. Ask patient if he/she is incapacitated from any abnormal movements (observe activities avoided).
10. Ask patient to stand up. (Observe in profile. Observe all body areas again, hips included.)
11. Ask patient to extend both arms outstretched in front with palms down. (Observe trunk, legs, and mouth. Note any extra movements.)
12. Have patient walk a few paces, turn, and walk back to chair. (Observe hands and gait.) Do this twice. (Observe for block movement—moves as unit, rigid, as opposed to flexible.)

INSTRUCTIONS: Complete examination procedure before making ratings. MOVEMENT RATINGS: Rate highest severity observed. Rate movements that occur upon activation one *less* than those observed spontaneously.	CODE: 0 = None 1 = Minimal, may be extreme normal 2 = Mild 3 = Moderate 4 = Severe

		(Circle one)
FACIAL AND ORAL MOVEMENTS	1. Muscles of facial expression, e.g., movements of forehead, eyebrows, periorbital area, cheeks; include frowning, blinking, smiling, grimacing.	0 1 2 3 4
	2. Lips and perioral area, e.g., puckering, pouting, smacking.	0 1 2 3 4
	3. Jaw, e.g., biting, clenching, chewing, mouth opening, lateral movements.	0 1 2 3 4
	4. Tongue. Rate only increase in movement both in and out of mouth, *not* inability to sustain movement.	0 1 2 3 4
EXTREMITY MOVEMENTS	5. Upper (arms, wrists, hands, fingers). Include choreic movements (i.e., rapid, objectively purposeless, irregular, spontaneous), athetoid movements (i.e., slow irregular, complex, serpentine). Do *not* include tremor (i.e., repetitive, regular, rhythmic).	0 1 2 3 4
	6. Lower (legs, knees, ankles, toes), e.g., lateral knee movement, foot tapping, heel dropping, foot squirming, inversion and eversion of foot.	0 1 2 3 4
TRUNK MOVEMENTS	7. Neck, shoulders, hips, e.g., rocking, twisting, squirming, pelvic gyrations.	0 1 2 3 4

TABLE 21-2. (continued)

GLOBAL JUDGMENTS	8. Severity of abnormal movements.	None, normal Minimal Mild Moderate Severe	0 1 2 3 4
	9. Incapacitation by abnormal movements.	None, normal Minimal Mild Moderate Severe	0 1 2 3 4
	10. Patient's awareness of abnormal movements. Rate only patient's report.	No awareness Awareness, no distress Aware, mild distress Aware, moderate distress Aware, severe distress	0 1 2 3 4
DENTAL STATUS	11. Current problems with teeth or dentures.	No Yes	0 1
	12. Does patient usually wear dentures?	No Yes	0 1

From Department of Health, Education and Welfare, Public Health Service. Washington, D.C.: U.S. Government Printing Office, 1980.

In prolonged treatment, evaluation should be done every 6 to 12 months, including a neurological workup. The procedure for evaluating tardive dyskinesia is discussed in Table 21-2.

An association appears to exist between drug potency and characteristics of undesirable effects, which provides a guide to understanding possible adverse effects. Table 21-3 summarizes this information.[17]

Other Side Effects

One example of andrenolytic side effects occurring frequently and therefore of particular concern to the daily evaluation of the patient by the nurse, the patient himself, and family is postural hypotension, which may be precipitated by any antipsychotic drug but in particular by thioridazine and chlorpromazine. This problem is evaluated by having the patient have his blood pressure taken in a sitting and lying position, both before and after the administration of the drug. It is important to instruct the patient to take his time in getting up and to be careful when stooping to avoid fainting. If the patient is working machinery, it is important that time be taken after drug ingestion so accidents can be avoided. Drowsiness is another feature that can inhibit daily activities. This side effect is usually controlled by taking the medication at night. Nasal stuffiness is another manifestation of andrenolytic side effects.

For men, impotence and inhibition of ejaculation or retrograde ejaculation occur especially with the use of thioridazine and mesoridazine. This can be useful for patients who are hypersexual but distressing for others. It is important to make sure that the sexual problems are not related to other factors than the drug.

Another important side effect is the reversal

TABLE 21-3. POTENCY OF ANTIPSYCHOTIC DRUGS AND RANGE OF ADVERSE EFFECTS

Low Potency	High Potency
Fewer extrapyramidal reactions.	More frequent extrapyramidal reactions.
More postural hypotension, more sedation.	Less postural hypotension, sedation.
Greater effect on the seizure threshold.	Less effect on the seizure threshold, cardiovascular toxicity.
Photosensitivity and skin pigmentation.	Fewer anticholinergic effects.
Rare cases of agranulocytosis.	Some cases of neuroleptic malignant syndrome.
Some cases of cholestatic jaundice.	

Adapted from Bassuk et al., 1983[7].

or blocking of administered epinephrine. This is most important for patients who for emergency reasons need epinephrine. Knowing that the patient is on antipsychotic drugs can alert the medical staff to use norepinephrine to counteract the blocking and potential paradoxical reactions.

Anticholinergic side effects include dry mouth, which can be helped with sugarless gum or gum drops or saliva substitutes.

Constipation is best dealt with by the use of stool softeners.

Cardiac changes, particularly rate problems such as tachycardia, are best attended to by periodically checking pulse and doing electrocardiograms (ECGs).

Vision can be blurred because of interference with the accommodation processes. If this symptom interferes with the patient's life, it is usually treated with physostigmine.

A potentially serious problem for men, and in particular men with benign prostatic hypertrophy, is urinary retention. Intake and output records are important in establishing urinary retention.

A most confusing state is the induction of atropine-like psychosis marked by confusion, incoherence, visual hallucinations, disorientation, and impaired concentration. This can be differentiated from the psychotic disorder under treatment if the nurse has become familiar with the most anxious state of the patient. This becomes a base-line measurement for the nurse by which to assess behavior change. The marked confusion and the acuteness of the symptoms plus the vivid visual hallucinations are different from the psychotic episode of schizophrenia, which usually does not manifest the same degree of confusion and disorientation. Symptoms are reduced by the use of physostigmine and withdrawal of the antipsychotic medication. Any onset of a psychotic episode needs to be fully evaluated by a physician with a review of drug therapy.

Hypothalamic side effects such as disturbances of menstruation, temperature deregulation, fever, and appetite change can all be addressed by having a daily program of evaluation and reporting.

Lowering of seizure threshold and production of seizures are usually associated with chlorpromazine and are dose-related. Being prepared is facilitated by screening for a history of seizure problems with the patient or family members.

Phototoxicity is another important potential side effect that is best avoided by protective clothing and staying out of the sun.

Nursing Management of Therapy with Anti-Parkinsonian Agents

Therapy with anti-Parkinsonian agents is directed at correcting a neurotransmitter imbalance within the CNS (a relative imbalance with dopamine deficiency and acetylcholine excess in the corpus striatum). The use of levodopa or amantadine enhances dopaminergic action. Centrally active anticholinergic agents are useful in inhibiting acetylcholine (Table 21-1).

Anti-Parkinsonian agents reduce the incidence and severity of akinesia, rigidity, and tremor. In addition to suppressing cholinergic activity, these agents may also inhibit the reuptake and storage of dopamine, thereby prolonging the action of dopamine.

Peripheral anticholinergic side effects, e.g., urinary retention, tachycardia, etc., frequently limit the dosages that can be instituted in therapy. Figure 21-2 shows the relative time range for onset of a variety of side effects.

In spite of somewhat limited efficacy, anticholinergic anti-Parkinsonian agents are widely used in the therapy of drug-induced extrapyramidal syndromes. There is, however, no evidence to support giving these drugs prior to the onset of symptoms. It is also important to eventually withdraw them from the medication regimen. This is possible since many of the symptoms they address subside within 3 to 6 months.

Most important is the recognition of the toxic effects or the anticholinergic effects of these drugs when used with antipsychotic drugs, as detailed in the next two sections.

Anticholinergic Syndrome as a Consequence of Anti-Parkinsonian Agents and Antipsychotic Drugs

Causes. Acute overdose or excessive prescription of medications with antimuscarinic properties, especially when anti-Parkinsonian agents are combined with tricyclic antidepressants, other anti-Parkinsonian agents, some antipsychotics (especially thioridazine), many proprietary sedative-hypnotic drugs, many antispasmodic preparations, several plants, Jimson weed, and some mushrooms.

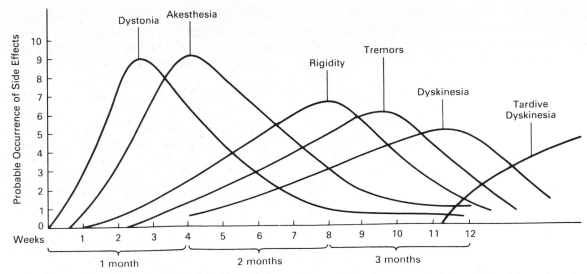

Figure 21-2. Probable time range in the occurrence of side effects that respond to anti-Parkinsonian drugs. (Adapted from DiMascio, A. (1978), with permission.[9])

Neuropsychiatric Signs. Anxiety; agitation; restless, purposeless overactivity; delirium; disorientation; impairment of immediate and recent memory; dysarthria; hallucinations; myoclonic seizures.

Systemic Signs. Tachycardia and arrhythmias; large, sluggish pupils; scleral injection; flushed, warm, dry skin; increased temperature; decreased mucosal secretions; urinary retention; reduced bowel motility.

Treatment. Adults and children: Physostigmine salicylate (neostigmine, pyridostigmine, etc.). The treatment may itself engender another imbalance; this time it would be a cholinergic excess. Familiarity with this syndrome is important.

Physostigmine-Induced Cholinergic Excess

Neuropsychiatric Signs. Confusion; seizures; nausea and vomiting; myoclonus; hallucinations, often after a period of initial CNS improvement when physostigmine is given to treat the anticholinergic syndrome.

Systemic Signs. Bradycardia; miosis; increased mucosal secretions; copious bronchial secretions; dyspnea; tears; sweating; diarrhea; abdominal colic; biliary colic; urinary frequency or urgency.

Treatment and Prevention. Atropine sulfate (CNS and systemic action) 0.5 mg per mg of physostigmine, intramuscularly or subcutaneously; methscopolamine bromide (Pamine); glycopyrrolate (Robinul).[18]

Effect of Anti-Parkinsonian Agents on Disease States

Although the anti-Parkinsonian agents are not contraindicated for patients with chronic liver or kidney disorders, these patients should be closely observed. Incipient glaucoma may be precipitated by these agents. When used to treat extrapyramidal symptoms caused by phenothiazine therapy, anti-Parkinsonian agents may exacerbate psychotic symptoms and precipitate a toxic psychosis. The possibility exists that the anti-Parkinsonian agents may mask the development of persistent extrapyramidal symptoms with prolonged phenothiazine therapy. These agents may impair mental or physical abilities required for the performance of potentially hazardous tasks.

Drug Interactions

Phenothiazines	Paralytic ileus (may be fatal), increased GI complaint
Barbiturates and alcohol	Enhanced CNS depression
Protriptyline	Increased mental confusion, anxiety, and tremor
Chlorpromazine	May reduce chlorpromazine levels 40 percent

Symptoms of Overdosage

Symptoms of overdose are similar in extent to those of antihistamine overdose, including dryness of mucous membrane; dilation of pupils; hot, dry skin; tachycardia; glaucoma; constipation; nausea and vomiting; mental confusion; convulsions; circulatory and respiratory collapse. Severe CNS depression is followed or preceded by stimulation. (See description of anticholinergic syndrome.)

Overdose Management

Overdose management consists of gastric lavage or emesis. Treatment should be symptomatic. Use of physostigmine salicylate will reverse the above-mentioned symptom of anticholinergic intoxication. Artificial respiration and oxygen therapy should be instituted if respiratory depression is present. Maintain normovolemic state with intravenous supplement and vasopressor agents.

Summary of Key Points Regarding Side Effects of Anti-Parkinsonian Drug Therapy

1. Anti-Parkinsonian drugs are better not started before the occurrence of side effects. Anti-Parkinsonian drugs have anticholinergic effects also and can compound the anticholinergic effects of the antipsychotic drugs.
2. Anti-Parkinsonian drugs usually do not need to be given more than 3 months beyond the starting of antipsychotic agents and the occurrence of extrapyramidal symptoms. By 3 months, most side effects abate.
3. Acute or increased agitation must be evaluated as a possible toxic effect of anti-Parkinsonian agents. In this case, the drugs must be stopped and the anticholinergic effects treated medically.
4. Tardive dyskinesia increases with anti-Parkinsonian drugs. When this side effect occurs, do not give anti-Parkinsonian drugs. Do not increase antipsychotic drugs. They mask the syndrome.

Nursing Management of Overdose with Antipsychotic Drugs

Although it is rare for a patient to overdose with antipsychotic drugs, this does occur. As indicated before, many times the problems of overdose have to do with drugs other than antipsychotics. Nevertheless, it is important to remember that antipsychotic drugs last in human tissue for a long period of time. Phenothiazines are detoxified in the liver, and where there is hepatic dysfunction, coma may be prolonged. In the case of hypotension, treatment is very difficult because of the beta-adrenergic blockade. *No epinephrine* or *isoproterenol* are to be given to raise blood pressure because these drugs have beta-adrenergic activity. Instead, ephedrine or norepinephrine (Levophed) should be used.[19] The medical management of overdose can be difficult. Other serious complications of overdosage are hypertension and hyperthermia, urinary tract infection with oliguria and renal failure, cardiac arrhythmias, skin lesions, and clinical relapse. Clinical relapse occurs mainly with the use of glutethimide, meprobamate, and tricyclic antidepressants.[20]

Treatment of overdose is best approached symptomatically. Gastric lavage is useful to decrease absorption of the ingested drug if initiated early post-ingestion. Maintenance of an adequate airway is also imperative.

Induction of emesis is not advised because a dystonic reaction could ensue, which would cause aspiration of vomitus.

The use of stimulants should be avoided as convulsions may be initiated as a result of a reduced convulsion threshold. Extrapyramidal symptoms may be treated with anti-Parkinsonian agents, barbiturates, or diphenhydramine.

If hypotension occurs, blood volume replacement measures to aid in the return to normovolemic state should be initiated. If a need for a vasoconstriction arises, because of dangerously low blood pressure, avoid epinephrine because anti-Parkinsonian agents tend to reverse the pressor action of epinephrine. The use of levarterenol or dopamine is indicated. These agents are not dialyzable.

Drug Interactions of Antipsychotic Drugs

Highlights of important drug interactions of antipsychotic drugs will be summarized in this section. (Table 21-4).

Antipsychotic drugs combined with other CNS agents have a cumulative depressant effect. For example, antidiarrheals and antacids reduce absorption of phenothiazines; antipsy-

TABLE 21-4. POTENTIAL ADVERSE INTERACTIONS AMONG PSYCHOTROPIC DRUGS

I. *ANTIANXIETY DRUGS*
 A. *Meprobamate*
  1. *With phenothiazines*
   Additive effects; and when given with piperazine, phenothiazines have been reported to cause grand mal seizures.
  2. *With antidepressants (both tricyclics and MAOIs)*
   Mutual potentiation—especially of sedation.
 B. *Benzodiazepines*
  1. *With phenothiazines*
   Mutual potentiation, especially of sedative effects; possible antagonism at limbic level (i.e., effects on aggressive behavior).
  2. *With antidepressants*
   a. *Of tricyclic class*—may potentiate anticholinergic effects; may potentiate sedative effects; simulation of organic damage—particularly with amitriptyline.
   b. *Of MAOI class*—may have potentiation of hypotensive actions (with feelings of light-headedness) and additive sedative-hypnotic actions.

II. *ANTIPSYCHOTICS* (phenothiazines)[a]
 A. *With antianxiety drugs* (see I, B, 1. above)
 B. *With antidepressants*
  1. *Of tricyclic class*—additive depressant effects; atropine-like side effects may enhance likelihood of toxic psychoses. Interfere with one another's metabolism and thus may elevate plasma level concentration of both drugs.
  2. *Of MAOI class*—inhibit phenothiazine metabolism. Increased likelihood of extrapyramidal side effects and of hypotension; reduces MAOI effects.

 C. *With antipsychotics* (other phenothiazines)
  Additive effects; long-term, high-dose; concomitant use may increase the possibility of tardive dyskinesia.

III. *ANTIDEPRESSANTS*
 A. *With antianxiety drugs* (see I, A and B above)
 B. *With antipsychotics* (phenothiazines) (see II, B above)
 C. *With antidepressants*
  1. *Of tricyclic class*—may have potentiation of sedative effects; may have antagonism of actions via enzyme induction causing increased metabolism.
  2. *Of MAOI class*—severe reactions may occur; symptoms noted include: excitation, hyperpyrexia, profuse sweating, severe headaches, convulsions, hypertensive crises, intercranial hemorrhage (leading to fatalities). Toxic psychoses have also been noted.

IV. *ANTI-PARKINSONIAN DRUGS*
 A. *With antidepressants*
  1. *Of tricyclic class*—potentiation of anticholinergic effects (dry mouth, constipation, paralytic ileus, damage to glaucomatous eyes). May produce, at toxic levels, agitation, confusion, psychoses, convulsion, and hyperpyrexia.
  2. *Of MAOI class*—potentiate anticholinergic effects such as tremors, profuse sweating, and neurological symptoms.
 B. *With antipsychotic drugs*
  Additive anticholinergic effects; serum levels of phenothiazines and haloperidol are lowered with concomitant reduction of clinical effectiveness of antipsychotics.

[a] Documentation that butyrophenones or thioxanthenes have interactive effects such as those listed has not been found.
MAOI = monoamine oxidase inhibitor.
Adapted from Dimascio, A. (1978)[9].

chotic agents may inhibit guanethidine; and chlorpromazine inhibits metabolism of propanolol. Another important consideration is that haloperidol (Haldol) and methyldopa may cause disorientation, aggressiveness, and assaultiveness.

Interactions of other drugs with antipsychotic agents are listed below.

Antacids
Studies indicate that the concurrent administration of chlorpromazine and alum or magnesium gel-type antacids results in significantly lower serum levels of chlorpromazine.

Haloperidol
When given in combination with anticoagulants haloperidol reduces the prothrombin time, causing an enhanced anticoagulant effect.

Phenothiazines and Thioxanthenes
These lower the seizure threshold in some patients, thereby necessitating an increase in seizure-controlling medications.

Anti-Parkinsonian Drugs

These usually decrease the extrapyramidal side effects of the antipsychotic agents. If the anti-Parkinsonian agent is prematurely withdrawn, a precipitation of extrapyramidal symptoms may occur.

Antipsychotic Agents and CNS Depressants

Together these cause additive CNS depression. Also, because barbiturates affect liver function, there may be a need for an increased level of antipsychotic agents.

Monoamine Oxidase Inhibitors

Used with antipsychotic agents, these may cause an additive hypotensive effect.

Tricyclic Antidepressants

Concurrent administration of tricyclic antidepressants and phenothiazines may increase the effects of either type of drug, necessitating lower doses of each agent.

Epinephrine

Epinephrine will have a paradoxical effect on blood pressure, i.e., lowering, in the presence of antipsychotic agents. Use ephedrine or norepinephrine.

Propranolol

Chlorpromazine inhibits metabolism of propranolol, resulting in increased hypotension.

Impact of Other Disease or Altered Physiological States

In view of the previously mentioned side effects of antipsychotic drugs, it is useful for the nurse to concentrate holistically on other ongoing disease processes unique to the patient.

Patients suffering from pulmonary insufficiency should be watched for signs of bronchopneumonia. It has been postulated that lethargy and a decreased sense of thirst resulting from central inhibition may lead to dehydration, reduced pulmonary ventilation, and hemoconcentration.

PSYCHIATRIC–MENTAL HEALTH NURSING PRACTICE REGARDING ANTIPSYCHOTIC DRUGS

Since antipsychotic drugs impact on practically every organ system in the body, it is important for the nurse to understand the major objective of drug intervention. Side effects must be distinguished from the targeted symptoms. An early nursing assessment combined with the basic medical assessment provides a base line of information for the nurse by which to monitor behavioral changes. This major principle is relevant to all drug therapy. In addition to the behavioral assessment of the nurse, there is that of the physician and, in the area of psychotropic drugs, the use of laboratory tests, such as blood levels, to monitor toxicity and to check on compliance, as well as a broad spectrum of laboratory tests to measure the impact of the drug on organ functions of the liver, kidney, heart, and the hemopoietic system.

Many severely and chronically disturbed patients are in service systems, both inpatient and community, that are medically underserved. That is, there are limited numbers of physicians and nurses. Therefore it is imperative that the nurse take the initiative, when necessary, to establish adequate protocols for the health surveillance of patients on drugs. In addition, the nurse may also be the one to activate various types of programs for drug education for the patient, family, and auxiliary mental health personnel.

General guidelines for the initiation of drug therapy with patients diagnosed as schizophrenic or acutely psychotic (no organicity) are based on ruling out major drug reactions. Dosage ranges are wide because of the high therapeutic index. Usually the patient is given a small test dose of the drug to rule out severe hypotension, oversedation, or severe allergic responses. These occur early in drug treatment. Chlorpromazine 50 mg, or its equivalent with other antipsychotic drugs, is used as a test dose. If the patient has no untoward reaction, he is usually started on a schedule of small, daily divided doses in the range of 60 to 1200 mg of chlorpromazine or its equivalent. Doses are gradually increased until a dose is reached at which the side effects are unacceptable. At this point, the dose is reduced carefully to the highest dose at which there are minimal side effects and continued symptom improvement.

Within 5 to 10 days, symptoms are usually in control, and the patient has developed a tolerance to the acute side effects. Dosage schedules can then be rearranged. Most patients like to take one dose at bedtime. This allows the patient to carry out his daily regime, and if there are mild side effects, these will occur during sleep.

Positive drug response should occur within 3 to 6 weeks. If there has been no improvement, and noncompliance is not the issue, the patient may require a drug from a different class or just a different drug. Variability of response is primarily a function of the individual. Usually there are approximately 10 to 12 percent of those diagnosed as schizophrenic who do not respond to drug treatment.

Rapid Neuroleptization

In the acute treatment phase of psychosis, some physicians use extremely large doses of antipsychotic drugs early in treatment. This approach is called *rapid neuroleptization* or *digitalizing* treatment. Although the purpose is to achieve rapid remission of psychotic states and early discharge from the hospital, studies do not support the efficacy of this approach over the standard regimen of gradually increasing drug dosage to effect. Furthermore, the rapid approach is associated with an increase in untoward reactions.

High-potency drugs are preferable if the rapid neuroleptization regimen is adopted. The usual reasons for using this approach are that a patient is highly excited or dangerous.[21] In this case, the nurse must be prepared to monitor the administration of drugs and the response of the patient. Emergency supplies and their use in case of drug reactions and side effects must be known. While the high-potency drugs are preferred, since they are less likely to produce hypotention and seizures, chances of extrapyramidal side effects are increased.

Usually the procedure followed is administering haloperidol, 2.5 to 10 mg, intramuscularly every 30 to 60 minutes until the patient's behavior is controlled. A maximum dose should be 30 mg/30 min and 100 to 120 mg/day. Once control is established, the dosage is reduced to the lowest effective oral dose.[22] This approach requires the close coordination of nursing and medical efforts.

After the cessation of the acute phase, usually 4 to 12 weeks, the dose of a drug can be slowly lowered to a maintenance dose that is often one half to one fifth of the highest dose needed to control symptoms. Patients often ask how long they have to be on drugs. Usually, with people who have had an acute psychotic episode, there is a strong possibility that once they have gotten over the acute phase and stabilized, they can be slowly removed from drug therapy. When people have had a recurrent psychotic episode, long-term intermittent maintenance may be required. People (and this includes children) who are maintained on long-term maintenance therapy run the risk of tardive dyskinesia.

Whenever a patient is taken off a drug, it is usually necessary to remove the drug gradually. In addition, time must be taken between the administration of a new drug or somatic therapeutic intervention. This is because these drugs tend to have a prolonged effect in the body because of the breakdown of the drugs or their mode of storage in the body. Only severe side effects warrant rapid removal of the drug, and this is best done under the direction of the physician. At these times, the management of the side effects as well as the impact of drug withdrawal requires medical management.

In many states, patients can refuse drug treatment even though they are hospitalized. Also, patients in the community, because of a variety of personal factors, may become annoyed or disenchanted with drug therapy and may attempt to remove themselves. It is imperative that the nurse make it clear to these patients that they have a right to refuse treatment; but if they once start a regimen, they must work closely with the nursing and medical staff if they wish to discontinue drug therapy. All patients must be adequately informed as to the risks and gains assumed by drug intervention, and they must give their permission for therapy.

In summary, maintaining people on a useful dose of medication while they remain in the community calls for special education. Educational programs for the patients, the family, and the community support providers can aid proper drug maintenance. Among this group may be the employers of patients who are on medication. Group methods are useful in monitoring dosage effectiveness and side effects. Some drugs, such as fluphenazine (Prolixin), are prepared in suspensions, which when injected, last over a two-week period.[23–24]

The relationship between the medical team and the patient must be positive in preparing the patient to reduce or withdraw from antipsychotic drugs. There may be an exacerbation of symptoms after removal of the drug, which would necessitate a return to the drug. This return can be very demoralizing, and a supportive relationship is necessary to mitigate the patient's emotional response to remaining on drugs.

The patient, nurse, and physician and the patient's family and, where appropriate, the work setting, must work together. Written information for patients, families, and employers; group presentations for family and patients; teaching what the objectives of drug intervention are and how to self-monitor; and group monitoring programs—all aid in effective and successful drug intervention.

From the basic review of nursing implications with regard to antipsychotic drugs and some of the most frequent side effects discussed above, the following general nursing practice principles can be stated:

- Nurses must continually study and discern how to distinguish side effects from the disordered state.
- Nurses are responsible for collaborating with the patient, physician, and family on various levels of education regarding drug intervention and the establishment of policies and procedures.
- Nurses are responsible for assessing the psychological and cultural meanings associated with drug therapy for the patient and the family. (For example, a large dose of drug does not necessarily indicate that a patient has a chronic problem or will need to be on drugs the rest of his life. This is the type of misconception that can interfere with the patient's recovery and his relationships with his family, and if the patient works—with his employer.)
- Nurses and physicians are responsible for making sure the patient and the family are sufficiently informed of the risks and benefits expected from drug therapy.

In concluding the section on antipsychotic drugs, we present in detail a study of management of patients with neuroleptic malignant syndrome.

THE NURSING MANAGEMENT OF NEUROLEPTIC MALIGNANT SYNDROME*

Neuroleptic malignant syndrome (NMS) is often an underdiagnosed, potentially lethal complication of treatment with major antipsychotic drugs.[25] This syndrome was first described in 1968 by Delay and Deniker.[26] More recent discussions of NMS in the literature may be related to the increasing use of neuroleptic agents in the past decade. Major tranquilizers are being used more extensively in a wider variety of settings including psychiatric facilities, general hospitals, and nursing homes. The serious nature of this illness cannot be understated. Evidence indicates that as high as 20 percent of patients identified as having NMS soon die from its effects.[27] Because of the greater use of neuroleptics, nurses must become more knowledgeable about NMS, its symptoms, and treatment.

NMS can occur at any time during treatment with a neuroleptic medication.[28,29] Certain predisposing factors have been found to increase the potential for NMS. These include: physical exhaustion; dehydration; and an infectious process in a compromised organic state.[30,31]

Signs and Symptoms

Nurses play a critical role in the important early assessments of patients who exhibit signs of NMS.[32] The four cardinal signs of NMS that nurses can observe are muscular "lead-pipe" rigidity, hyperthermia, disturbance of consciousness, and autonomic dysfunction.[33]

Muscular Rigidity
NMS is often first recognized as an acute dystonic reaction that involves the whole body. Concurrent symptoms may include postural instability, bizarre posturing, tremors, sialorrhea (excessive drooling), and masked facies.

Nursing Interventions. Promptly recognize and report symptoms, hold further doses of the neuroleptic agent, closely monitor the muscular

---

* This section from pp. 392 to 397 was written by Lois K. Novikoff, John L. Adam and Irene McGeady.

rigidity, help the patient to be comfortable and to maintain correct body alignment to prevent possible muscle contractures, offer support and reassurance to the patient and family.

Hyperthermia

Body temperatures range from 38.1°C to 42°C and are frequently accompanied by diaphoresis and decreased renal functioning, which can lead to rapid dehydration.

Nursing Interventions. Provide cooling blankets and alcohol baths to reduce fever; administer antipyretic medication; restore fluids through intravenous therapy as soon as possible; closely monitor urinary output.

Autonomic Instability

The patient may become tachycardic (120 to 180) and exhibit unpredictable blood pressures (70/ 50 to 180/130). In addition, respiratory status may be compromised with symptoms of dyspnea and tachypnea (18 to 40).

Nursing Interventions. Monitor vital signs frequently; be aware of and report signs of urinary incontinence.

Altered Consciousness

Level of consciousness in the patient may range from being alert to appearing dazed, lethargic, stuporous, or sometimes comatose.

Nursing Interventions. Monitor the patient's level of consciousness and report any changes as they occur; assess the patient's orientation and amount of confusion and provide for the patient's safety.

In addition to these interventions, the nurse may be required to administer certain medications. Some of these include anticholinergic agents, dantrolene sodium to reduce muscle stiffness, and dopamine agonists, e.g., amantadine, carbidopa-levodopa (Sinemet), or bromocriptine, which act to neutralize the effects of the neuroleptic by activating dopamine receptors. In addition to providing supportive nursing care for the patient's physical needs, it is essential that the nurse respond to the psychological needs of both the patient and family as a way of providing total care. The patient with NMS is often frightened, confused, and unable to verbalize his needs, fears, and concerns. The nurse must respond by establishing trust with the patient, providing emotional support and reassurance, as well as conveying a caring sensitivity to the patient and family. The nurse plays a critical role in helping both the patient and family to better understand and cope with this medical crisis.

Clinical Vignettes

─── CASE ONE ───────────────────────────────

Carol, a 17-year-old black female, was brought to the emergency room via ambulance, accompanied by her mother. Mother reported that the patient had not slept for 2 days and had refused to eat or drink for 24 hours. The patient's abrupt behavioral change also included suspiciousness, complete withdrawal, hallucinations, and persecutory delusions. Carol's behaviors indicated an acute psychotic episode. She was admitted that night to the adolescent psychiatric unit for a complete psychiatric evaluation. All presenting features continued and the patient remained awake the night of admission. On day one, she became physically combative during the routine medical workup and continued to refuse anything by mouth. The patient was begun on haloperidol (Haldol) 2.5 mg TID and received the first two doses intramuscularly that evening. The following morning the patient was observed lying across her bed with her legs rigidly extended to the floor and her neck and head pressing against the wall as a result of muscular rigidity. Her mouth was protruding with the tongue visibly fixed and the gag reflex was absent. She was incontinent of urine and was unresponsive to both verbal and painful stimuli. Respirations were shallow and tachypneic, temperature was 38.8°C, and the patient was tachycardic (140). Level of consciousness was strikingly altered with fluctuation of alertness. The AM dose of Haldol was held and a physician was immediately notified. Prompt institution of medical treatment and workup was begun. This included IV therapy, blood gases and cultures, lumbar puncture, CT scan, x-ray and consults from neurology and infectious disease. All test results were within normal limits with the exception of an elevated creatine phosphokinase (CPK) (consistent with NMS).

In the early stages of recovery, respiratory, renal, and cardiovascular functions were monitored constantly for signs of decompensation. Level of consciousness was continuously assessed for degrees of unresponsiveness and alertness. Autonomic instability caused frequent episodes of tachycardia, diaphoresis, hyperpyrexia, and labile hypertension. Vital signs were monitored every 4 hours. The patient received IV therapy for the first 72 hours for dehydration and absence of gag reflex. Hypertonic involvement of pharyngeal muscles resulted in intermittent dysphagia with inconsistent intake of fluids and food an ongoing problem. Alterations in urinary function fluctuated from frequent incontinence to prolonged retention, which required catheterization. This necessitated strict I & O for the next three weeks, with close monitoring of food and fluid intake, output of body waste, body temperature and electrolyte balance. Following the initial lead-pipe rigidity, the patient exhibited symptoms of catatonia accompanied by prolonged periods of posturing, which precipitated ankle edema and the development of a carpal flexion of the right hand. Frequent position changes, elevation of extremities, and ambulating the patient were effective interventions in reducing the edema. Range of motion exercises and use of a hand splint were initiated to prevent permanent contractures of the right hand. Carol remained mute for almost three weeks and required total care. This included feeding, offering frequent fluids to maintain hydration, toileting, bathing, oral hygiene, and skin care after incontinence.

To respond to the psychological needs of the patient, nursing staff communicated with Carol in a way that assumed comprehension despite her changeable level of alertness. All medical procedures were carefully explained to her before implementation and staff remained with her to provide support. A core group of staff was formed for consistency of care and to establish a safe and trusting environment for the patient. The use of touch became a therapeutic tool in diminishing feelings of isolation, fear, agitation, and helplessness. Family members were encouraged to become active participants in the patient's recovery and care.

By week four, mutism and posturing ceased, vital signs were stable, and the patient resumed independent ADL. Psychotic symptoms resolved, and the patient prepared for discharge with residual immobility of the right hand. Discharge teaching focused on early recognition of recurring psychotic symptoms and the risks and contraindication of future use of neuroleptic drugs. Outpatient physical therapy and use of the hand splint continued for 6 weeks. Carol is at present performing at her level of functioning prior to the psychotic episode and has regained full use of her right hand.

CASE TWO

Ms. Cass was a 17-year-old female brought to the emergency room. Her family was frightened by her running about the house, destroying property, and threatening violence to the family. To their knowledge, the patient had not eaten anything for 2 weeks because of her fears that the food was poisoned. The patient was 6 weeks postpartum at the time she came to the hospital. Upon arrival at the hospital, the patient was noted to have foul-smelling lochia and a temperature of 37.7°C. Shortly after her admission to the psychiatric unit, Ms. Cass became violent. Supportive nursing interventions were ineffective and the patient was placed in a quiet room for her own safety. A treatment regimen was quickly instituted that included the use of the neuroleptic haloperidol (Haldol). By the end of her third hospital day, the patient had received a total of 90 mg of Haldol. Some of the extreme violent behavior had dissipated by this time, and there was less talk of the food being poisoned. Nursing staff was able to stay with her and encourage intake. By the third day, however, nursing staff noted other marked changes in Ms. Cass's behavior. Her loud and fearful verbalizations were replaced by grunts. She became more regressed, to the point of crawling on the floor. When the patient was able to rest, the staff observed uncontrolled rhythmic flexion and extension contractures. These behaviors quickly changed to hyperreflexia with a lead-pipe rigidity in all extremities. Nursing staff remained with her during these developments, monitored vital signs frequently and offered comfort measures to the patient. The patient's vital signs were elevated, with pulses of 120 to 130, temperature of 38.3°C, and respirations of 20 to 30. An irregular pattern of blood pressures was noted, although the readings remained within the normal limits.

The patient was transferred to an intensive care unit to treat her deteriorating physical condition and to determine the diagnostic cause of these changes. All neuroleptic medication was discontinued. Intravenous therapy was instituted to increase hydration. Dantrolene and diazepam were used to treat the muscle stiffness. Nursing staff remained constantly with the patient to assess her physical condition, carry out the medical treatment, offer comfort measures, and monitor her emotional state. Primary nurses in psychiatry worked along with the intensive care nurses to keep in touch with the patient's family members. Nursing staff frequently provided the family with information about the patient's physical condition and responded to their concerns and anxieties by listening and offering support.

The patient remained in the intensive care unit for 1 week. Once medically stable, she returned to the psychiatric unit with the diagnosis of NMS. The patient continued to be fearful and exhibited disorganized thought processes. Eventually individual psychotherapy and milieu therapy were effective for the patient and she was discharged home in the following weeks.

NURSING DIAGNOSIS
Impaired Physical Mobility Related to Neuromuscular Impairment

ASSESSMENT

- Body rigid with extensive body dystonia
- Prolonged periods of posturing
- Carpal flexion of right hand

GOALS

- Patient will not experience complications of decreased mobility.
- Patient will return to optimal level of mobility.
- Patient will regain full range of motion in affected joints.

INTERVENTIONS

- Hold further doses of neuroleptic medications.
- Monitor muscular rigidity.
- Position patient in correct anatomic alignment to prevent complications.
- Provide ROM exercises to right hand and encourage active ROM when she is able.
- Assist patient with ambulation.

NURSING DIAGNOSIS
Hyperthermia Related to Neuroleptic Medications

ASSESSMENT

- Temperatures above 38°C
- Respirations shallow and rapid
- Exhibiting labile hypertension and diaphoresis
- Renal functioning ranging from periods of incontinence to urinary retention
- No p.o. intake for at least 24 hr. prior to admission

GOALS

Patient's temperature will remain within normal range (less than 37.3° C).

INTERVENTIONS

- Apply appropriate cooling measures such as cooling blankets, alcohol baths, or cool sponge baths.
- Monitor urinary output.
- Offer fluids frequently.
- Restore fluids via IV therapy.
- Monitor temperature and other vital signs very frequently.

NURSING DIAGNOSIS
Fear Related to Sensory Impairment

ASSESSMENT

- Exhibiting mutism for three weeks
- Appears very frightened and unable to respond verbally
- Exhibiting tachycardia, diaphoresis, and tachypnea
- Fluctuating levels of consciousness

GOAL

Patient will verbalize and identify her fears to the nurse.

INTERVENTIONS

- Help patient to identify what she perceives as the danger.
- Encourage her to express perceptions and feelings about what she is experiencing.
- Assess patient for physiological signs of fear and anxiety (e.g., increased heart rate, increased respiratory rate, dilated pupils, diaphoresis).
- Explain to patient what is happening to her in terms of the NMS.
- Tell patient what to expect when explaining all medical procedures and remain with her during these procedures.
- Use a consistent group of nursing staff as a means of establishing a trusting relationship with Carol.

NURSING DIAGNOSIS
Alterations in Family Processes Related to Illness of Family Member

ASSESSMENT

- Family has many questions about patient's state of health and her response to medications
- Family very concerned and supportive of patient

GOALS

- Family members will verbalize their concerns and questions to the nurse.
- Family members will participate in patient's care to help her regain wellness.
- Family members will offer support, encouragement, and reassurance to patient.

INTERVENTIONS

- Offer support and reassurance to the family.
- Listen to the family's concerns, answer their questions, and provide information about NMS.
- Involve family in patient's physical care.
- Encourage the family to provide verbal support and reassurance to patient.

ANTIDEPRESSANT DRUGS

Identifying Depression

It is important that the nurse be familiar with the symptoms of depression in order to evaluate the appropriate drug treatment.

Depressive states can be classified under three general headings: (1) schizophrenia-related affective disorders; (2) bipolar affective disorders; and (3) unipolar affective disorders.

Theoretical views of the etiology of depression include the following models:

1. Loss and lowered-self-esteem models.
2. Early-deprivation models.
3. Psychoanalytic-deficit models.
4. Cognitive set, disordered-thinking models.
5. Learned behaviors: (a) modeling; (b) gain-reinforcement.
6. Biochemical amine models (Fig. 21-3).

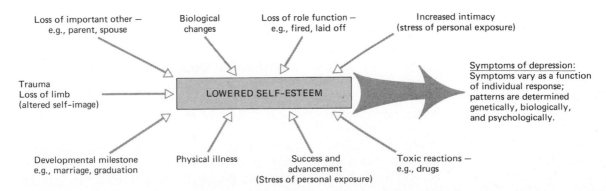

Figure 21-3. Etiologic possibilities of depressive states. (Adapted from Carlos Neu's lecture entitled, "Clinical Use of Antidepressant Drugs," In Hartman C. R. Di Mascio, A. (1978)[9])

Schizophrenia-Related Affective Disorders

The depressive symptoms associated with schizophrenia include the following clear symptoms of schizophrenia: delusions of being controlled or thought broadcasting; thought insertion or withdrawal; the presence of hallucinations that are not related to the depression; voices carrying on a conversation, commenting on the behavior of the individual; the presence of these hallucinations and delusions for more than one month without depressive symptoms; and marked thought disorder. There is no manic behavior, but there is a history of chronic asocial behavior. As a subclassification, depression with schizophrenic symptoms occurs in an under-30 population more frequently than in a population 40 years old or older.[34]

A second state classified under schizophrenia consists of depression in patients with histories of chronic asocial behavior but not overt psychosis. This state is referred to as a schizoid-affective disorder. It is not included in *DSM-III-R*. In general, schizophrenia is not a protection against depression, and at times antidepressants combined with antipsychotic drugs can be helpful. In the early stages of schizophrenia, depression may occur. In this case, treatment with antidepressants alone is usually not helpful and in some instances may precipitate or aggravate psychotic symptoms.

Bipolar Affective Depressive Disorders

Bipolar affective disorders are those depressive states that are associated with a prior history of mania or clear hypomania. Bipolar depression will be discussed in connection with the use of lithium later in this chapter. Here, the important distinction is that bipolar depression is responsive to lithium, whereas unipolar endogenous depressive states usually are not; rather they respond more specifically to tricyclics and monoamine oxidase (MAO) inhibitors.

Unipolar Affective Depressive Disorders

The unipolar depressive disorders are divided into endogenous depressive states (single-episode or chronic), situational depressive states, and demoralization. In the depressive states, tricyclics, tetracyclics, and MAO inhibitors have been most useful. In chronic depressive states, the use of drugs is more questionable. Research is at present being conducted on long-term use of antidepressants in the prevention of intermittent endogenous depressive states.[35]

Endogenous Depressive States. Single-episode endogenous depressive states are marked by a dysphoric mood or loss of interest or pleasure in all or almost all usual activities and pastimes. There is sleep- and appetite-pattern disruption including symptoms of loss of energy, fatigability, and tiredness. There can be psychomotor retardation or agitation, decrease in sexual drive, feelings of self-reproach, difficulty in concentrating, and suicidal ideation. The best drug response has been in depressive states that appear as a dramatic change for the individual or those that show ego-alien symptoms.[36]

In chronic depressive disorders, the individual has at least a 2-year history of a depressive syndrome, although the degree is not sufficient to call it severe.

During depressive periods there is the appearance of symptoms of a severe depression state. Some clinical research holds the possibility that treatment with antidepressants may be of some use. Some patients have a characterological manifestation of depression that is chronic and includes unhappiness, disatisfaction, weeping, preoccupation with losses or unpleasantness, and feeling short-changed. They may evidence dramatic attention-seeking behavior; avoid personal blame; act in a demanding, complaining, clinging, irritable, and anxious manner, and are full of self-pity. These behaviors are not restricted to a particular personality profile.[37]

The more the symptoms move from severe depressive episodes to the more chronic characterological symptoms, the less useful are the drugs. Most responsive are those depressive states that are endogenous as defined by the severe symptom complex outlined above, which is marked by vegetative reactions.[38]

Situational Depressive States. Situational depressive states are marked by a clear precipitant. The individual manifests signs of depression and sadness. These states are often grief reactions associated with the death of an important person. Symptoms include tearfulness, brooding, preoccupation with the loss, feelings of tension, inability to shift one's thoughts from the loss or situation, loss of appetite, and insomnia. However, the capacity for pleasure and interest in activities outside the person are maintained. The affective state is not fixed. Usually, depressions of this type are self-limiting, but on occasion they can become symptomatic of an endogenous depression.

Demoralization. Demoralization is an important depressive state to distinguish. It most often derives from an endogenous state. Symptoms of despair remain, yet many of the symptoms of an endogenous depressive state, such as sleep disturbance, weight loss, and diurnal variation (worse in the morning, better at night), have disappeared. Psychotherapy and guidance are needed here rather than medication.[39]

What may be happening is that an individual has developed a negative cognitive set toward himself because of the physiological symptoms of the depressive episode. Psychotherapeutic intervention is needed to reduce the possibility of chronicity.

Whatever the possible etiology of depression, the outstanding characteristic in depressive states is a lowering of self-esteem. This lowered self-esteem may be understood by a person as depression, or it may be experienced as simply not feeling oneself, being tired and irritable, or as not being functional in work or play with family or friends. A person may simply complain of feeling physically ill. Figure 21-3 depicts the possible sources of lowered self-esteem and its relationship to depressive symptomatology. The lowered self-esteem may be primary or secondary to a depressive experience.

Antidepressant Drug Action

Certain symptom patterns in depression are more responsive to certain drug interventions than others. This clinical observation has led to some major hypotheses about neuroreceptor site activity and depressive states. Tricyclics are thought to have their primary antidepressant activity associated with the inhibition of the re-uptake process of norepinephrine, resulting in increased norepinephrine at the receptor site. This inhibition of re-uptake activity may also extend to other biogenic amines. There are alterations in central catecholaminergic and serotonergic activity and in metabolism, which may be related to depression.

Tricyclics are potent anticholinergic agents, and some researchers think this activity may also play an important role in the antidepressant activity, though other anticholinergic drugs such as atropine or anti-Parkinsonian drugs have not been useful in the treatment of depression. One perplexing problem of tricyclics is that even though there is an immediate increase in norepinephrine, there is a time lag in clinical response.

The MAO inhibitors have both peripheral and central neuronal action. The inhibition of MAO within the cell reduces the metabolism of norepinephrine and other endogenous amines and exogenous monoamines, thus increasing their concentration. MAO inhibitors also potentiate the action of amphetamine-like compounds, sympathomimetic amines used in the treatment of allergies, and anticholinergic agents used in the treatment of Parkinson's disease. Some MAO inhibitors may cause hypotension as well as provide some relief from angina pectoris. They can also antagonize some of the pharmacological and biochemical effects of reserpine (used to treat hypertension). When used in conjunction with food containing tyramine, they can cause severe hypertension and stroke (food high in tyramine: cheddar cheese, wine [chianti], chicken liver, smoked salmon, raisins, figs).

A careful medical work-up is essential in the treatment of a depressed patient as in all psychiatric states. This health base line is necessary because of the increased danger in using psychotropic drugs arising from their anticholinergic properties. Once physical illness is ruled out, as are other possible toxic reactions, a decision can be made to use antidepressants. Special consideration must be given to the following: How severe is the depression and how serious is the suicidal threat? A base line of behavioral information is needed before a selection of a drug is made. If there are symptoms of psychosis, an antipsychotic drug may be given in combination with an antidepressant. If psychotic symptoms increase, the antidepressant must be stopped and only antipsychotic drugs given. Although antidepressants do not differ in clinical efficacy, they do differ in their ability to cause sedation. If there is a history of previous episodes of mania and depression, lithium or antipsychotic drugs may be needed to manage the acute mania. A history of previous positive or negative responses to a trial of psychiatric drugs in the patient or in the patient's immediate blood-related family is also useful in the selection process.[40]

In addition to treatment of depression, antidepressant drugs have provided an important model for understanding drug action in the brain in terms of neuroreceptor activity. These investigations have led to a clearer clinical classification of depressive states. This classification is important in that certain antidepressant drugs are more useful in certain clinical states than are other drugs.

Catecholamine Theory of Depression

The early catecholamine theory of depression proposed by J. Shildkraut hypothesized that certain depressive states are caused by a depletion of catecholamines at receptor sites and that elation or mania is caused by excesses of catecholamines at receptor sites.[41] This theory is quite complex with the inclusion not only of catecholamines but also indolamine (serotonin), other biogenic-amines, hormones, and ionic changes. The depletion (or excess) can be caused by insufficient release of neurotransmitters, alterations of chemical affinity at the receptor, excessive metabolic breakdown at the synaptic cleft, failure of re-uptake, or failures in the metabolic processes within the presynaptic neuron, such as an excess of MAO with the destruction within the presynaptic cell of norepinephrine, an important neurotransmitter whose depletion has been associated with certain depressive states.[42]

The receptor theory demonstrated by the catecholamine hypothesis depicts four different neuroregulators functioning in the brain. They are: the noradrenergic synapse, the dopaminergic synapse, the serotonergic synapse, and the least defined gabaminergic synapse. The latter has been linked to the hereditary disease Huntington's chorea. Although glutamic acid is found throughout the brain, its function is not clear. However, depressive states and schizophrenic states have been linked with receptor site excesses and depletions of norepinephrine (noradrenergic), dopamine (dopaminergic), and serotonin (serotonergic). Neurons emanating from the spinal cord and cranial nerves and nerves innervating peripheral organs transmit either by acetylcholine or by norepinephrine. It is not known how many different types of neuroregulators exist in the brain.

Current thinking underscores that a cogent theory of depression must integrate various levels of observations. Observations need to be made at the chemical, anatomic, and behavioral levels. Even with regard to chemical consider-ations, although changes in monoamines may be significant, a variety of relationships between the parts of the central nervous system and their unique physiology must be considered.

Clinical Treatment of Depression

Agents that are employed in the clinical treatment of depression are tricyclics, tetracyclics, trazodone, and the MAO inhibitors (Table 21-5). The term *heterocyclic* has been used as a major classification, and includes the tricyclics, tetracyclics, and trazodone. This categorization is based on the amine uptake-blocking properties of the drug rather than the chemical structure.

These agents are most effective in the treatment of endogenous depression. Although the exact mechanism of antidepressant effect has not been identified, effective activity has usually been associated with the "biogenic amine hypothesis." This theory states that depression is due to a reduced activity of one or more of the endogenous monamines (norepinephrine, serotonin) in the brain. It is felt that the antidepressant agents favorably affect the dysfunctional activities of the monamines, thereby normalizing their biogenic activity. This theory does not totally express the antidepressant activity of many other compounds, and other as yet unfound mechanisms may play a part in their activity.

The MAO inhibitors have a more nonspecific activity and enhance the action of epinephrine, norepinephrine, and serotonin by blocking out enzymatic activates in their neurotransmitters.

The tricyclic agents are generally preferred over the MAO-type agents because of the high risk of hypertensive crisis found with MAO-type agents when certain foods and drugs are combined with them.

Tricyclic antidepressants are structurally related to phenothiazines and have similar side effects. In contrast to the phenothiazines, which act in dopamine receptors, the tricyclic antidepressants block the re-uptake of norepinephrine and serotonin by the presynaptic neurons in the CNS (Table 21-6).

Since re-uptake terminates amine activity, inhibition of re-uptake enhances activity at the receptor site. These effects appear to play a role in the antidepressant activity of these agents.

These compounds can be characterized by specific amine re-uptake blocking activity. Ami-

TABLE 21-5. ANTIDEPRESSANT DRUGS

Antidepressant Agents	Generic Name	Daily Dosage Range (mg)
[a]A. *Tricyclics*		
1. Iminodibenzyl derivatives (dibenzazepines)		
a. Tofranil	Imipramine	75–300
b. Tofranil-PM	Imipramine pamoate	75–300
c. Pertofrane, Norpramin	Desipramine	50–300
d. Asendin	Amoxapine	75–100
e. Ludiomil	Maprotilene	75–225
2. Dibenzocyloheptine derivatives		
a. Elavil	Amitriptyline	75–300
b. Pamelor	Nortriptyline	50–200
c. Vivactil	Protriptyline	10–50
3. Dibenzodiazepine derivatives		
a. Sinequan, Adapin	Doxepin	50–300
[a]B. *Tetracyclics*		
a. Surmontil	Trimipramine maleate	75–150
C. Monamine oxidase inhibitors		
1. Hydrazine derivatives		
a. Marplan	Isocarboxazid	30–50
b. Nardil	Phenelzine	10–75
2. Nonhydrazine derivatives		
a. Parnate	Tranylcypromine	10–30
[a]D. *Miscellaneous*		
1. Etrafon, Triavil	Perphenazine-amitriptyline	
2. Desyrel	Trazodone	200–400
E. *Miscellaneous*		
1. Lithane, Eskalith	Lithium carbonate	750–2500

[a] Heterocyclics. Term is meant to incorporate emerging antidepresant drugs where the amine uptake-blocking properties are emphasized rather than chemical structure.

TABLE 21-6. AMINE UPTAKE-BLOCKING ABILITY OF HETEROCYCLICS

	Side Effects			
	Anticholinergic	Sedation	Norepinephrine	Serotonin
[a]A. *Secondary amines*				
Amoxapine (can cause common extrapyramidal reactions)	**	***	***	*
Nortriptyline	**	**	***	*
Desipramine	**	**	****	0
Protriptyline	***	May produce stimulation	***	0
[b]B. *Tertiary amines*				
Amitriptyline	****	****	*	**
Imipramine	***	***	**	**
Doxipin	***	****	**	**
Trimipramine	***	****	**	**
C. *Tetracyclic amines*				
Maprotilene	***	****	****	0
Trazondone	0	***	0	****

Source: Table compiled by A. G. Abrams, 6/19/83.
[a] Secondary amines block the re-uptake of norepinephrine more than serotonin.
[b] Tertiary amines block the re-uptake of serotonin more than norepinephrine.
**** = very high; *** = high; ** = moderate; * = low; 0 = very low.

triptyline is the most active inhibitor of serotonin uptake; desipramine is the most potent inhibitor of norepinephrine uptake. The tetracyclic maprotiline acts only on norepinephrine activity. These different activities may have a bearing on the different levels of response that patients exhibit to different agents.

It has been suggested that endogenous depression may be caused by deficiencies of either norepinephrine or serotonin activity or utilization. Patients with low norepinephrine activity [low urinary excretion of 3-Methoxy-4-hydroxyphenylglycol (MHPG)] will probably respond well to the secondary amines because of their enhanced blockage of norepinephrine uptake. Conversely, patients with low urinary levels of 5-hydroxyindolacetic acid (a serotonic metabolite) should respond well to amitriptyline.

Toxicity and Side Effects of Antidepressant Drugs[43]

Overdose is a real problem with heterocyclics and MAO inhibitors. Special precaution must be used with patients with urinary retention, narrow-angle glaucoma, or signs of increased ocular pressure. Cardiovascular disorders, diseases of the thyroid, and diseases of the prostate are other conditions in which special care must be taken. Patients with convulsive disorders and organic brain syndrome must be monitored carefully. To reiterate, quiescent schizophrenia may be exacerbated and patients may have difficulty with operating cars and dangerous machinery. The safe use of tricyclics with pregnancy has not yet been established. When a patient has been on the drug for two months or more, withdrawal should be made slowly.

More common side effects of antidepressant drugs will be discussed by systems as follows:

Psychiatric Symptoms. Increased psychosis can occur in undiagnosed cases of schizophrenia. The depression is secondary to schizophrenia. The antidepressant drugs increase the symptoms of schizophrenia. At other times the psychiatric signs appear to be the result of psychosis when in fact they are the result of anticholinergic excess toxicity. These signs are anxiety, agitation, restlessness, purposeless overactivity, delirium, disorientation, impairment of immediate and recent memory, dysarthria, hallucination, myoclonus, and seizures. Accompanying this behavior are systemic signs of tachycardia and arrhythmias, large slow-to-respond pupils, scleral injection, flushed dry skin, increased temperature, decreased mucosal secretions, urinary retention, and reduced bowel motility. The treatment of these side effects is aimed at increasing cholinergic activity, often by administering a drug such as physostigmine.

Autonomic Nervous System Symptoms. The most common toxic symptoms of the ANS are dry mouth, blurred vision, and constipation. Administering the drug at night and prescribing a stool softener and milk of magnesia for the constipation can help the patient cope with these symptoms. Less common symptoms are aggravation of glaucoma, urinary retention, flushing, and diaphoresis.

Central Nervous System Symptoms. Drowsiness is the most common side effect and bedtime doses handle this problem. If there is insomnia, administer the drug in a single dose in the morning. Jitteriness is also common. Decreasing the dosage or changing the drug may be necessary. Unlike the case of antipsychotic drugs, motor involvement is a less common side effect. Most common is muscle tremor, which can be reduced by a muscle relaxant. There can be seizures, twitching, dysarthria, paresthesia, palsies, ataxia, and sudden falls.

Cardiovascular System Symptoms. Postural hypotension, dizziness, tachycardia, and palpitations are not unusual in the beginning of the use of tricyclics. Teaching the patient to avoid sudden movements helps deal with these symptoms. Any cardiac symptom or ankle edema must be evaluated immediately. Hypertension may be another side effect deserving medical evaluation.

Dermatologic Symptoms. An uncommon side effect is a rash and itching. If this occurs, stop the medication. Photosensitivity requires the use of protective clothing and care in exposure to the sun.

Ophthalmologic Symptoms. Aggravation of glaucoma is a common side effect with known cases of glaucoma. Consultation with an ophthalmologist is the best way to proceed.

Gastrointestinal System Symptoms. Nausea and heartburn are not uncommon side effects. Symptomatic treatment and the taking of drugs after meals should reduce the symptoms. If not, stop the medication. Less common side effects are vomiting and anorexia. Medication is usually stopped, but small meals may be tried.

In addition to the above list, there are a number of disparate symptoms that must be evaluated in terms of their individual degree of severity. These include tinnitus (ringing in the ears), bad taste in mouth, weight gain or loss, impotence, peripheral neuropathy, galactorrhea, and endocrine changes, particularly estrogen effects.[44]

Use of MAO Inhibitors

As indicated earlier, MAO inhibitors are a second choice to heterocyclics in the treatment of depression because of their dangerous interaction with food substances. There are a number of toxic effects that must be noted with MAO inhibitors. The acute hypertensive reaction with tyramine is most serious and is to be prevented by restricting foods produced by fermentation, such as beer, wine, and cheeses. In addition, certain yeast products can cause hypertensive crises. This hypertensive danger is carried further in certain drug interactions. Certain proprietary drugs sold over the counter for colds and sinus trouble, such as phenylephrine (Neo-Synephrine) and decongestant inhalers, can have serious drug interaction effects. In addition, L-Dopa (a drug used in the treatment of Parkinson's disease) and other drugs that are converted into sympathomimetic amines can have interaction effects that lead to hypertensive crises (Table 21-7). Another rare but more serious problem is that of parenchymal hepatotoxic reactions. These reactions are more serious than the obstructive jaundice associated with antipsychotic drugs and heterocyclics.

Weekly laboratory tests and evaluation of serum bilirubin transaminase activities should be done, as well as restricting the use of these drugs with patients with chronic liver problems. Also, MAO inhibitors must not be given to patients with acute myocardial infarction because when used in combination with barbiturates, these drugs are most dangerous and can result in severe respiratory depression.

In summary, antidepressant drugs are most useful in the severely depressed patients when management of suicidal potential is essential. However, because of the low margin of safety of these drugs, outpatients need to be monitored carefully and frequently to decrease the chances of lethal overdosage. For those patients who are suicidal only *one week's* supply of antidepressants should be prescribed at a time. In milder forms of depression, there is some question as to the efficacy of these drugs in comparison with psychotherapy and supportive measures. Some comparative studies suggest that the immediate results of drugs and psychotherapy are the same, with the edge being given to drugs, but that in recurrent depression, drugs combined with psychotherapy are most efficacious.

Dosage and Monitoring of Antidepressants

When initiating the dosage of heterocyclic antidepressants, the object is to move slowly to a dose that can be tolerated by the patient. Usually doses are divided between the morning and afternoon for those drugs that tend to have sedative effects. It is useful to arrange an increase so that a single dose can be administered at bedtime. Thus, the side effects may occur during sleep, freeing the individual from such annoying side effects in the daytime. Most tricyclics can be administered in amounts up to 250 mg per day for effect and gradually reduced to 75 to 150 mg for maintenance. Protriptyline is an exception (10 to 50 mg). If one drug does not work, it is wise to withdraw the drug and try another.

Drug Interactions of Antidepressant Drugs

Heterocyclics and MAO Inhibitors. Together these can precipitate hypertensive cases. If an MAO inhibitor is replaced by a heterocyclic, allow 14 days minimum before initiating the heterocyclic.

Antihypertensives
Some heterocyclics inhibit action of antihypertensive guanethidine and clonidine hydrochloride.

Anticholinergics
Antidepressants and anticholinergic drugs such as anti-Parkinsonian types potentiate the atropine-like effect.

CNS Depressants
Heterocyclics potentiate CNS depressants.

Thyroid
Heterocyclics and thyroid together cause enhancement of antidepressant response. Tachycardia and arrhythmias may develop.

Beta-blockers
Beta-blockers are inhibited by heterocyclics.

Phenothiazines
Phenothiazines inhibit metabolism of heterocyclics and increase blood levels.

Overdose and Management

The main symptoms of overdose are CNS depression, respiratory depression, and cardiac arrhythmia. Physostigmine salicylate is used to remove CNS and cardiac symptoms.

Electroconvulsive Therapy

If drugs do not work or if there are severe cardiac problems or other endangering physical disorders, the safest and most effective intervention for depression is electroconvulsive therapy (ECT). This method is useful in the elderly and has become increasingly safe with the use of proper relaxant drugs and with adequate control over voltage and recovery. However, if ECT is used, the individual must be withdrawn from all antidepressant medication.[45]

Psychiatric Nursing Management of Patients on Antidepressant Drugs

Although newer antidepressants are coming on the market with the expectation that their side effects and toxicity will be less than that of the tricyclics and MAO inhibitors, nursing activities as well as medical practices are most important. The heterocyclics and the MAO inhibitors, compared to antipsychotic drugs, have a higher incidence of severe anticholinergic and adrenergic effects on the body systems. These reactions can be fatal; therefore, it is imperative that a physical examination be carried out before prescribing a drug. Of utmost importance is a careful cardiac history. A differential diagnosis is required regarding the type of depression, since underlying bipolar and schizophrenic states can be exacerbated.

The following assessments and tests are now being used to help monitor and decide on antidepressant intervention.

There must be a careful review of other medications being used by the patient. And to guard against suicide there must be a cooperative and safe interpersonal context in which to start drug intervention. Overdose can be fatal.

The physical examination should include: an ECG to check for both ventricular arrhythmias and evidence of cardiac abnormalities; tonometry to check for glaucoma; assessment for prostatic disease in men; ruling out thyroid disease; and comprehensive blood work.

Once medical clearance is given, a schedule of medication must be drawn up with gradually incremented doses. This is particularly true when starting patients on drugs that have moderate to very high anticholinergic effects.

If the patient is under 60 years of age, the following steps are reecommended: (1) Take a base-line blood pressure before medication and one hour later; (2) have the patient lie down and measure blood pressure; and (3) repeat with the patient standing up, waiting 2 minutes. If the systolic drops 30 mm or more or the diastolic drops 20 mm or more, postural hypotension is present, and the doctor is to be consulted as to whether to start the drug.

Usually the first daily dose is about 75 mg divided into three equal doses. The maximum dose is usually 150 mg arrived at by the end of 1 week (6 days). Usually the second dose consists of 50 mg in the morning, none at noon; rather, increases in dose of medication occur at time of sleep.

Another method has been to start out with 25 mg at bedtime and 25-mg increments every day until the maximum dose has been reached. It will take approximately 2 weeks once the maximum dose has been reached to achieve drug effect. It is this time lag that is dangerous with the depressed and suicidal patients.

With men it is particularly important to check for side effects and possible urinary obstructions. The nurse must ask questions or attend to the client's reports regarding problems in urination, such as dribbling, incontinence, or pain.

Constipation is a frequent side effect, and stool softener should be started if needed.

TABLE 21-8. INTERACTIONS BETWEEN PSYCHOTROPIC AND OTHER DRUGS

Drug	Interacting With	Clinically Significant Interaction	Clinical Effect of Interaction
Neuroleptics			
	Anticholinergics		1. Delayed onset of neuroleptic effect in acute oral dose
			2. May alter neuroleptic blood levels
		✔	3. Increased anticholinergic effect
			4. Possible increased risk of hyperthermia
	Antacids Cholestyramine Activated charcoal Kaolin Pectin		1. Oral absorption delayed
	Lithium		1. May reduce chlorpromazine plasma levels and clinical effect
		✔	2. May increase CNS toxicity
	Phenytoin		1. May increase phenytoin toxicity
			2. Decreased plasma levels and effect of neuroleptics
	Narcotics	✔	1. Increased sedation
		✔	2. Analgesia augmented
		✔	3. Hypotension augmented
		✔	4. Respiratory depression augmented
		✔	5. Anticholinergic effects augmented by meperidine
	Benzodiazepines		1. Increased CNS sedation
			2. Decreased akathisia
	Cyclic antidepressants	✔	1. Increased sedation
		✔	2. Increased hypotension
		✔	3. Increased anticholinergic effect
			4. May increase clinical effect of neuroleptic
			5. Possible increased risk of seizures
	L-dopa	✔	1. May exacerbate psychosis
		✔	2. Decreased anti-Parkinsonian effect of L-dopa
	Amphetamines	✔	1. May exacerbate psychosis by counteracting effects of neuroleptics
	Coffee Tea		1. Precipitates chlorpromazine in stomach; may delay clinical effect
			2. May counteract sedation
	Barbiturates	✔	1. Increased sedation
	Nonbarbiturate hypnotics	✔	2. Decreased clinical effect of neuroleptic
	Insulin Oral antidiabetic drugs		1. Neuroleptics increase blood glucose and may alter required dose of diabetic medication
	Iproniazid	✔	1. Hepatic toxicity and encephalopathy
		✔	2. Decreased neuroleptic effect
	Reserpine Clonidine Guanethidine Bethanidine Debrisoquine	✔	1. Decreased antihypertensive effect
	Ammonium chloride		1. Decreased clinical effect of neuroleptics

TABLE 21-8. (*continued*)

Drug	Interacting With	Clinically Significant Interaction	Clinical Effect of Interaction
	Phenylpropanolamine		1. Ventricular arrhythmias with thioridazine 2. May increase sedation
	Propranolol		1. Increased neurotoxicity 2. Increased neuroleptic effect 3. Seizure and cardiopulmonary arrest (case report)
	Dichloralphenazone Rifampin Dioxyline Griseofulvin Phenylbutazone Carbamazepine		1. May decrease effect of neuroleptic by increasing metabolism
	Chloramphenicol Disulfiram MAO inhibitors Oral contraceptives Acetaminophen		1. May increase effect of neuroleptic by increasing metabolism
	Epinephrine	✔	1. Hypotension augmented
	Coumarin Phenindione		1. Generally may increase bleeding 2. Haloperidol may decrease bleeding via enzyme induction
	Methyldopa		1. Reversible dementia with haloperidol 2. Increased sexual desire with chlorpromazine
	Hydralazine Minoxidil		1. Enhanced hypotensive effect
	Succinylcholine		1. May prolong apnea with ECT
	Enflurane Isoflurane Anesthetics	✔	1. Profound hypotension with phenothiazines
	Indomethacin		1. May cause severe drowsiness with haloperidol
	Bromocriptine		1. Effects of bromocriptine are antagonized
Cyclic antidepressant			
	Cimetidine Methylphenidate Acetaminophen Oral contraceptives Chloramphenicol Isoniazid MAO inhibitors	✔	1. Inhibits metabolism, increasing blood levels and toxicity of antidepressants
	Disulfiram		1. Inhibits metabolism, increasing blood levels of antidepressants 2. Possible induction of psychosis and confusional state
	Guanethidine Debrisoquine Bethanidine	✔	1. Decreased antihypertensive effect 2. Decreased antidepressant effect
	Clonidine		1. Decreased antihypertensive and antidepressant effect 2. Potential hypertensive crisis with imipramine (case report)

TABLE 21-8. (*continued*)

Drug	Interacting With	Clinically Significant Interaction	Clinical Effect of Interaction
	Thiazide diuretics Acetazolamide		1. Hypotension augmented
	Quinidine Procainamide	✓	1. Cardiac conduction prolonged
	Methyldopa		1. Increased agitation, tremor, tachycardia
	Propranolol		1. Decreased antidepressant effect
	Coumarin anticoagulants	✓	1. Increased bleeding
	Neuroleptics		1. Antidepressants may increase plasma level of neuroleptic
	Phenytoin Barbiturates Nonbarbiturate hypnotics Dichloralphenazone Rifampin Doxycycline Griseofulvin Carbamazepine Phenylbutazone	✓	1. Induces hepatic metabolism, decreasing clinical effect of antidepressants
	Anticholinergic drugs		1. Increased anticholinergic toxicity
	Triiodothyronine (T₃) Lithium		1. Possible potentiation of antidepressant effect
	Activated charcoal Kaolin		1. Helpful in overdose by decreasing absorption
	Estrogen		1. Decreased therapeutic effect of imipramine 2. Lethargy, headace, hypotension 3. Akathisia
	Testosterone		1. Paranoid psychosis with aggression
	Halothane Enflurane Anesthetics		1. Tachycardia with imipramine
	Phenytoin Phenylbutazone Aspirin Aminopyrine Scopolamine		1. Increased antidepressant effect by displacement from protein binding sites
	Epinephrine	✓	1. Hypotension augmented
	Local anesthetic dissolved in epinephrine	✓	2. Increased bleeding in nasal surgery
	Benzodiazepines	✓	1. Increased CNS sedation, increased confusion, decreased motor functions 2. Increased suicide risk
	Phenothiazines		1. Increased tricyclic levels 2. Possible ventricular arrhythmias with thioridazine with combination of drugs
	L-dopa		1. Increased agitation, tremor, rigidity are possible 2. Decreased plasma levels of antidepressants via impaired gastrointestinal absorption
	Alcohol		1. Increased sedation

TABLE 21-8. (*continued*)

Drug	Interacting With	Clinically Significant Interaction	Clinical Effect of Interaction
MAO inhibitors			
	Amphetamines Ephedrine Metaraminol Levarterenol Methylphenidate Phenylephrine Pseudoephedrine L-dopa Dopamine Mephentermine Chlorpheniramine Novacain (dissolved in epinephrine)	✔	1. Increased blood pressure
	Cyclic antidepressants	✔	1. May have enhanced clinical effect 2. Conflicting reports on toxicity—hyperpyrexia, excitability, muscle rigidity, convulsions, coma; use with caution 3. Weight gain
	Meperidine	✔	1. Excitation, sweating, hypotension. Use other narcotics; can be life threatening
	Succinylcholine		1. Phenelzine may prolong apnea with ECT
	General anesthetics Anticholinergics Sedative-hypnotics Antihistamines Benzodiazepines		1. May enhance CNS depression
	Insulin Sulfonylurea Phenformin		1. Increased hypotension
	Thiazide diuretics Hydralazine Phenothiazines Reserpine		1. Increased hypotension
	Guanethidine		1. Decreased antihypotensive effect
	Methyldopa		1. Excitation, visual hallucinations with pargyline
	Alcohol		1. Decreased MAO inhibition 2. CNS system depression
Lithium			
	Indomethacin Piroxicam Sulindac Ibuprofen	✔	1. Increased lithium effect and toxicity due to decreased renal lithium clearance
	Phenylbutazone Naproxen Zomepirac	✔	1. Increased lithium effect and toxicity due to decreased renal lithium clearance
	Thiazide diuretics Phenylbutazone Spironolactone Triamterene Amiloride		1. Increased lithium effect and toxicity due to decreased renal lithium clearance

TABLE 21-8. (*continued*)

Drug	Interacting With	Clinically Significant Interaction	Clinical Effect of Interaction
	Neuroleptics		1. Decreased neuroleptic blood levels 2. Decreased nausea and vomiting from lithium 3. Increased neurotoxicity (may be severe)
	Phenytoin		1. May increase neurotoxicity of both drugs
	Theophylline Acetazolamide Aminophylline	✔	1. Increased renal excretion of lithium, decreasing its effect
	Succinylcholine Pancuronium Decamethonium	✔	1. Prolonged apnea with ECT
	Amphetamines		1. May increase amphetamine "high"
	Benzodiazepines		1. Hypothermia associated with diazepam (case report)
	Potassium iodide		1. Increased likelihood of hypothyroidism
	Sodium bicarbonate Sodium chloride Urea Mannitol	✔	1. Increased renal excretion of lithium, decreasing its effect
	Tetracycline Spectinomycin	✔	1. Increased lithium effect and toxicity due to decreased renal lithium clearance
	Carbamazepine		1. Increased neurotoxicity of both drugs 2. Increased polyuria, ataxia, and dizziness due to antidiuretic property of carbamazepine
	Cyclic antidepressants		1. May increase lithium neurotoxicity 2. May increase lithium tremor
	Ketamine	✔	1. Increased lithium toxicity resulting from sodium depletion
	Digitalis		1. May cause cardiac arrhythmia by depleting intracellular potassium
	Furosemide	✔	1. Increased lithium toxicity resulting from sodium depletion
	Insulin		1. Insulin dosage may need adjustment early in lithium treatment due to altered glucose tolerance
	Mazindol		1. Increased lithium toxicity
	Norepinephrine		1. Decreased pressor response to norepinephrine
Benzodiazepine	Cimetidine Isoniazid Disulfiram Oral contraceptives		1. Increased toxicity of diazepam and chlordiazepoxide due to inhibition of metabolism
	Rifampin Phenytoin		1. Decreased clinical effect due to induced hepatic metabolism
	Antacids Anticholinergics		1. Delay in oral absorption

TABLE 21-8. (*continued*)

Drug	Interacting With	Clinically Significant Interaction	Clinical Effect of Interaction
Carbamazepine	Digoxin		1. Increased digoxin levels
	Alcohol Neuroleptics Narcotics Antihistamines Sedative-hypnotics	✔	1. Increased CNS sedation
	Cyclic antidepressants		1. Increased CNS sedation 2. Increased amitriptyline levels
	L-dopa		1. Possible decreased effect of L-dopa
	Lithium		1. Inhibits diuresis and polyuria associated with lithium
		✔	2. In combination, may increase ataxia, feelings of unreality, dizziness
		✔	3. Neurotoxicity with normal levels of both
	Haloperidol		1. May decrease carbamazepine levels and vice versa
	Cimetidine Erythromycin Isoniazid	✔	1. Increased carbamazepine levels 2. May produce somnolence, lethargy, nystagmus, dizziness, nausea, vomiting in combination
	Propoxyphene	✔	1. Increased carbamzepine levels 2. May produce headache, dizziness, nausea, ataxia
	Clonazepam		1. Clonazepam levels decreased by carbamazepine
	Charcoal		1. Binds carbamazepine; good for use in overdose
	Phenytoin		1. Decreased carbamazepine levels, but carbamazepine does not effect phenytoin levels
	Phenobarbital Primidone		1. Decreased carbamazepine levels
	Corticosteroids Coumarin anticoagulants Doxycycline Oral contraceptives		1. Decreased effect of carbamazepine
	Verapamil		1. Increased carbamazepine toxicity, especially neurotoxicity

(From Glassman, R., & Salzman, C. Interactions between psychotropic and other drugs: An update. *Hospital and Community Psychiatry*, 1987, *38*(3), 237–242, with permission.)
CNS = central nervous system; ECT = electroconvulsive therapy; MAO = monoamine oxidase.

Dry mouth, blurred vision, dizziness, and other mild symptoms are often offset by having the client take the medication before sleep.

Blood pressure and antidepressant drug levels must be checked weekly until stabilization.

Since treatment will usually extend over a period of years, the medical examination should be repeated every six months on people over 60 and at least once a year for those younger. A client should be asymptomatic for at least 6 months prior to discontinuation of medication.

Medication should be decreased very slowly and the client closely observed for increasing signs of depression.

MAO inhibitors have significant adrenergic effects. MAO is responsible for destroying many substances within the body. When MAO is blocked, there is a buildup of these properties. This is why food intake becomes most important with these drugs. Foods that encourage the release of epinephrine and norepinephrine and foods that contain tyramine and tryptamine are to be avoided, as well as sympathomimetic drugs. Fermented foods of all types, yeast products, chocolate, pickles, cheddar cheese, Camembert cheese, beer, wine, and coffee can all precipitate a hypertensive crisis. Examples of drugs to be avoided are cough and cold preparations, benzadrine, and amphetamines.

Symptoms of hypertensive crisis (which is rare with cooperative drug management) include occipital or temporal headaches of sudden onset accompanied by a stiff neck, sweating, chills, restlessness, nausea, vomiting, and blurred vision. Chest pain may accompany this syndrome. Blood pressure can go as high as 350/250 mmHg. There can be intracranial bleeding and death. Phentolamine 5 mg IV is definitive therapy. Nitroglycerin sublingual tablets are also often effective.

Starting slowly and giving MAO inhibitors in divided doses can be done—except that these drugs are not given in the evening because they tend to cause insomnia.

Since antidepressants are often used with the elderly, certain precautions need to be taken. The elderly are more responsive than younger patients to both therapeutic and adverse drug effects because of their slower metabolism and excretion rates. Thus they need smaller doses as increments, and there is an increased possibility of drug interaction issues. Also, older people are often on drugs for other reasons. Furthermore, anticholinergic drugs are to be avoided because confusion and arrhythmias are likely to occur in this population.

Particular attention needs to be paid to the psychiatric conditions that can be precipitated by both the tricyclics and the MAO inhibitors. When these drugs are given to someone with an underlying schizophrenic or bipolar disorder, symptoms of schizophrenia and mania can be exacerbated.

Young adults, such as Helen, age 27, present the type of situation in which severe depression can mask additional complex problems:

Helen had been seen at age 25 for short-term counseling because she had broken up with her boyfriend. Helen wanted short-term counseling rather than long-term. She did report that her father had been institutionalized years before for mental illness and that she had many issues regarding her family but did not want to deal with them. She did well in the counseling. She got a new job and started dating, at which point she terminated the counseling.

Six months later she contacted the nurse. She was profoundly depressed. The precipitants were a request to get married and the stress of a new job. She was evaluated in a mental health clinic for drug intervention and possible hospitalization. She refused to consider the latter. She had her boyfriend, mother, and brother as support, and everyone agreed they would help her at home.

She was started on a tricyclic antidepressant. She had changed jobs and was working as a service operator for an automobile towing service. Her depression lifted somewhat, but she began to complain that she could not remember the instructions and directions of people stranded on the highway. Laboratory tests were made, and it was found that she had a toxic level of the drug. It was slowly reduced; however, the problem of concentrating persisted. Helen took herself off the drug. By this time, her thinking process tended to be more concrete. She became suspicious and irritable, as well as frightened. With great difficulty arrangements were made to admit her to the day hospital. While in the hospital, and no longer on the drugs, although they were prescribed, she became much more aggressive, grandiose, and deluded. She left the hospital against medical advice but did agree to come to the clinic. One week later, she came in most excited, claiming that she was a borderline patient and hypomanic. She bolted from the room and went to the streets. For the next week the staff heard indirectly from her. Other clinics in the city heard from her as well. She was deluded, seeking help and treatment, and then rejecting the efforts. Eventually, she was placed on an antipsychotic drug and lithium.

In the initial drug evaluation, there was concern that Helen's personality was such that, although she did not have a prior history of psychosis or manic episodes, there was the possibility of an underlying schizophrenic disorder. This proved to be true after the initiation of antidepressant medication.

The complexity of Helen's situation underscores how a working relationship is essential, given the possibility that underlying disorders are initially not apparent because of profound states of depression. If such disorders are exacerbated, the relationship becomes the important link to management of a treatment change.

Current Chemistry, Laboratory Tests, and Psychiatric Nursing Practice

There is a newly evolving field of chemistry and laboratory tests being used in psychiatric practice. The nurse's role is to familiarize herself with the tests and with the necessary preparation of the patient so he will cooperate with the collection of samples. In addition, the educative aspects of nursing care continue with regard to the drugs and the symptoms of the patient. A brief description of the tests follows.*

List of Tests
- Antidepressant drug levels (tricyclic and tetracyclic).
- Platelet monoamine oxidase (MAO) activity.
- Urinary MHPG levels.
- Cortisol, base-line levels.
- Desamethasone suppression test (DST).
- Urinary-free cortisone (UFC) levels.

Description of Procedures for Testing[46,47] Plasma Levels of Antidepressant Drugs.

Serum lithium levels have been routinely monitored for years. More recently, plasma levels have made it possible to measure other antidepressant drugs. Because of mainly individual differences in metabolism, there are marked differences of plasma levels of these drugs. In addition, error in following the prescribed format for drug intake as well as possible noncompliance has been determined by an examination of plasma blood levels. Furthermore, in older people, there can be a higher drug plasma level on smaller doses. All of these factors are important in establishing the chemistry analysis of drug levels in the management of a patient on drugs. More information has been gathered on blood levels of imipramine and nortriptyline. The laboratory tests alone are insufficient in determin-

---

* Abstracted from J. J. Shildkraut's "Description of the Psychiatric Chemistry Laboratory," Massachusetts Mental Health Center, 74 Fenwood Rd., Boston, Mass., 1983.

ing drug effect. Close and careful clinical appraisal is necessary. Determining plasma levels of antidepressant drugs help with the following:

1. To identify those patients who develop very high plasma levels on low doses.
2. To document the therapeutic plasma level in an individual patient at the time of clinical response as a guide to treating future episodes.
3. To document compliance or possible short-term metabolic changes in patients who respond and then relapse on a given dose.
4. To explore causes for failure to respond to a standard dose of an antidepressant drug.
5. To investigate possible causes for the occurrence of pronounced side effects of small drug doses.

The following antidepressant drugs are being evaluated with regard to plasma levels: amitriptyline, nortriptyline, imipramine, desipramine, protriptyline, doxepin, amoxapine, and maprotiline.

Plasma levels are determined on a sample of blood drawn 10 to 14 hours after the last dose of antidepressant. It takes 24 to 48 hours for the results. These levels are not yet fixed to certain base line criteria. Rather the amount and the assessed clinical response of the patient are pooled for a conclusion regarding effectiveness of treatment.

Platelet MAO Activity. This investigation is primarily theoretical at this time. As yet, specific plasma levels of MAO inhibitor antidepressant drugs are not considered to be clinically useful. The test is being carried out because research studies have found differences in pretreatment base-line platelet MAO activity in various subgroups of depressed and schizophrenic patients as well as in patients with other psychiatric disorders. Since other drugs can affect MAO platelet activity, blood should be drawn under drug-free conditions. Special handling of the blood is necessary. Heparin must not be used in the collecting agent, and the whole blood must arrive in the laboratory no later than 4 hours after venipuncture. The specimen should be on ice but not frozen. It takes about a week for the results.

Urinary MHPG Levels. Urinary MHPG depressive disorders have a wide clinical and biologic order of signs and symptoms as well as etiologic considerations. Recent studies suggest that this heterogeneity may be associated with differences in catecholamine metabolism.[48,49]

Many longitudinal studies of individual patients with bipolar manic–depressive disorders have confirmed that urinary MHPG levels vary with alterations in affective states, and that MHPG excretion is lower during depressive episodes and higher during manic or hypomanic episodes than during periods of clinical remission. Some current studies suggest that there may be at least three subtypes of unipolar depressive disorders that can be discriminated on the basis of differences in MHPG levels and that in these patients, pretreatment urinary MHPG levels can aid in predicting differential clinical responses to certain antidepressant drugs.[50,51] Other studies have shown that patients with a low MHPG level respond more favorably to imipramine rather than amitriptyline. Again, the current use of this test must be placed in a complete clinical context.

MHPG is measured in the urine. The fraction of MHPG in the urine that comes from brain function is very small and must be differentiated from MHPG formed by other body organs. A 24-hour urine specimen is required, from which an aliquot of a 24-hour specimen is required. Sometimes three 24-hour specimens are required with three separate, sequential aliquot 24-hour specimens needed.*

The following dietary restrictions are necessary: Beginning the day before the urine is collected, not more than a total of three cups of coffee, tea, or cola beverage and no alcoholic beverages should be drunk. In addition, no psychoactive medications should be taken. It takes about one week for results.

Dexamethasone Suppression Test (DST). Based on a theory that some depressions are associated with the limbic system and the hypothalamus, many indirect tests have been derived to assess this relationship. At this point in time, the DST is a promising test, but the DST *is not a random screening test for depression.* Depression and increased cortisol have been linked. Dexamethasone, when ingested the day before, should normally produce a decrease in cortisol. Therefore, it is suspected that

in people who do not show this decrease, a depression or impending depression may be occurring. However, many drugs and conditions can give false readings. Phenytoin, barbiturates, tricyclic antidepressants, MAO inhibitors, lithium carbohydrate, and benzodiazepine have no effect on the DST.[52] Unfortunately, some patients are being placed on antidepressant drugs without a thorough consideration of their clinical picture. The test is not meant to be used in this manner.

The usual procedure for this test is to collect blood samples at 8 A.M., 4 P.M., and 11 P.M., on day one prior to the administration of dexamethasone. At 11 P.M., after the blood is drawn, a 1 mg dose of dexamethasone is administered and blood is drawn at 8 A.M., 4 P.M., and 11 P.M. of day two. Bloods are analyzed for cortisol levels. The test takes at least 48 hours for results.

Urinary-free Cortisol (UFC). This is a rather new and promising test that is used in the diagnoses of Cushing's disease. A 24-hour aliquot of urine is required. It is essential to list all of the medications a patient is on since many affect cortisol levels in a predictable fashion. In addition, urine samples containing radioactivity from any source are not acceptable. This is particularly important with patients undergoing treatment for other diseases that require radiation, isotopes, etc. There are no dietary restrictions for this test.

Separate aliquots of the same 24-hour urine can be submitted for both urinary MHPG and urinary-free cortisol. The total volume must be noted for each test. This test requires about 48 hours for results.

The nurse will note that all of these are new tests in psychiatric practice and therefore still quite experimental. Also they take time and money. Therefore some practical steps taken by the nurse can be most useful. First, enlist the cooperation of the patient and family. Take time to explain the specimen collection procedures, making sure the patient understands and will cooperate. Next, the laboratory will need the following information: the patient's full name, address, and date of birth; the physician's full name and address (this is important for outpatient studies); phone numbers; *clinical diagnosis:* current medications and any other drugs such as alcohol. Also give exact details of the date and time that the specimen is collected, type of specimen, and the test required.

---

* *Aliquot* is a mathematical term meaning an exact, proportional measurement of a whole.

MOOD STABILIZERS

Identifying Mood Disorders

Affective disorders are characterized by a disturbance in mood. Mood is a prolonged emotion that colors the individual's social, affective, and behavioral experiences.[53] Mood refers to the pattern presentation of depression or euphoria. These disorders of mood include mania and depression, as well as cyclothymic and dysthymic disorders. Often the terms *bipolar disorder* and *unipolar disorder* are used. A diagnosis of bipolar affective disorder is made when the individual has experienced at least one manic episode. This individual may also have suffered many major depressive episodes. A diagnosis of unipolar disorder describes that individual who has had depressive episodes but has never experienced a manic episode.

Manic episodes are marked by an elevated expansive mood. Symptoms of mania include highly increased physical, social, and sexual activity; marked irritability; felt pressure to talk; flight of ideas; grandiosity, which may be delusional; and a decreased need for sleep. In hypomanic episodes the mood disturbance is not sufficiently severe to cause marked impairment in social or occupational functioning or to require hospitalization.[54]

Symptoms of depression have been described previously.

Clyclothymic disorder is characterized by alternating affective states of euphoria and depression, but they are not of sufficient intensity, severity, and duration to meet the criteria for major depressive or manic episodes. In dysthymic disorder the symptoms are not of sufficient severity and duration for a major depressive episode, and there have been no hypomanic periods.

There are two types of medication currently being used in the treatment of mood disorders: lithium preparations and anticonvulsants.

Lithium as a Treatment for Mood Instability

Lithium is widely recognized and used as a major treatment for affective disorders. In the past, it was believed that lithium's action was specific to mania. However, more recently lithium has also been used for the treatment of depression, cyclothymic, and dysthymic disorders. When lithium is used for the treatment of mania, the person may be aware of a slowing down of his thought processes, but this is achieved without the sedating effect noted when antipsychotic drugs are used. Lithium takes 7 to 10 days at therapeutic blood levels to have any effect; therefore, antipsychotic agents are often used to bring about more immediate sedation and control of manic symptoms. Lithium is used for maintenance therapy to prevent the recurrence of the affective disorder.[55] When beginning treatment with lithium, the dosage must be adjusted carefully and slowly. Since lithium is excreted through the kidney, any impairment in renal function necessitates a withdrawal of the drug.

Lithium is usually administered in 300-mg tablets or capsules. It is readily absorbed into the system when taken orally and is eliminated almost entirely by renal excretion. However, sodium diuresis and deficiency of sodium tend to increase the retention of lithium and hence its toxicity. The mechanism of action is not yet clear. Some speculations deal with the electrolyte balance across membranes including neurons. Other hypotheses deal with antagonistic actions at synapses mediated by catecholamines in the brain. This includes inhibition of the release of norepinephrine and dopamine as well as alteration in intake and retention activities.

Unlike most drugs, the dosage range of lithium is not indicative of clinical effect (Table 21-9). Rather, daily blood levels must be taken when starting the drug, then taken weekly and monthly for maintenance. Generally speaking, 300 mg to 600 mg are given three times a day to reach lithium serum levels of between 0.5 to 1.5 mEq/L of serum. Lethal dosage is between 2 and 7 mEq/L. Toxic dosage can be at 1.5 mEq/L or less.[56]

Lithium Toxicity

Therapeutic levels of lithium closely approximate toxic levels. Manifestations of lithium toxicity are noted by body system below.

Psychiatric Symptoms. The psychiatric symptoms include mental retardation, somnolence, confusion, restlessness and disturbed behavior, stupor, and coma.

Central Nervous System. The central nervous system symptoms include anesthesia of

TABLE 21-9. LITHIUM DOSAGE

Brand Name	Dosage	Adult Lethal Dose
Eskalith	Initial: 600 mg (1200–1800 mg/day) until serum lithium level is reached—between 1.0–1.5 mEq/liter for therapeutic effect.	2–4 mEq/liter
Lithane Lithonate	Same. Maintenance: 300 mg t.i.d. (600–1200 mg/day)—maintain serum lithium level between 0.5–1.5 mEq/liter.	5–7 mEq/liter

the skin, incontinence of urine and feces, slurred speech, blurring of vision, dizziness, vertigo, epileptiform seizures.

Cardiovascular System. The cardiovascular symptoms include pulse irregularities, fall in blood pressure, electrocardiograph changes, peripheral circulatory failure, and circulatory collapse.

Gastrointestinal System. The symptoms of the gastrointestinal system include anorexia, nausea, diarrhea, thirst, dryness of mouth, and weight loss.

Other symptoms noted include polyuria, glycosuria, general fatigue, lethargy and tendency to sleep, and dehydration (Table 21-10).

The nursing management of toxic states is by the withdrawal of lithium. Lithium serum levels fall rapidly once the drug is discontinued. Treatment includes replacing water and restoring electrolyte balance by forcing fluids. Dialysis usually is not necessary.

Since diuresis decreases the tolerance to lithium, exercise on hot days with marked sweating may necessitate the reduction of the total daily dose of lithium. Chronic ingestion of lithium includes a diabetes-insipidus-like syndrome and thyroid disturbances sometimes causing goiter and necessitating thyroid therapy or removal of the drug. Both hypo- and hyper-

thyroid conditions have been reported. There may be elevated white blood cell counts. The effects on the kidney itself are the most serious consequences of long-term therapy. Renal function tests must be done. In patients with mild thyroid, or with kidney, heart, and seizure conditions, lithium must be used cautiously, and there must be constant monitoring of the physical status.

Uses of Lithium

Lithium is used to prevent the recurrence of depressions in bipolar illness. It is also used in prophylaxis of recurrent unipolar depressions and to control mood swings in emotionally unstable character disorders and explosive and aggressive outbursts in impulsive character disorders. The main use is in manic (bipolar disorders), where it is about 80 percent effective. Because it takes time between the administration of the drug and the control of manic symptoms, antipsychotic drugs are given with the drug.

TABLE 21-10. LITHIUM TOXICITY AND SIDE EFFECTS

Lithium Concentrate (mEq/L)	Signs of Lithium Toxicity at Different Serum Levels
<1.5	Nausea, vomiting, diarrhea, thirst, polyuria, lethargy, slurred speech, muscle weakness, fine hand tremor.
<2.0	Persistent GI upset, coarse hand tremor, mental confusion, hyperirritability of muscles, ECG changes (moderate), drowsiness, uncoordination.
>2	Ataxia, giddiness, large output of dilute urine, serious ECG changes, tinnitus, blurred vision, clonic movements, seizures, stupor, severe hypotension, coma. (At this concentration, fatalities are secondary to pulmonary complications.)
>3.0	Beginning of breakdown of many organ systems in the body.

Note: Treatment of toxicity: Gastric lavage, hemodialysis (rapidly effective). ECG = electrocardiograph; GI = gastrointestinal.

Drug Interactions with Lithium

Sodium Bicarbonate, Acetazolamide, Urea, Mannitol, Aminophylline

All these drugs *increase* renal clearance of lithium.

Thiazide Diuretics, Furosemide, Ethacrynic Acid

All these *decrease* renal clearance of lithium and may lead to lithium toxicity.

Indomethacin

Indomethacin and other nonsteroidal anti-inflammatory agents can increase plasma levels of lithium by 30 percent to 60 percent, which may lead to toxicity.

Mazindol, Phenytoin, Methyldopa, Thioridazine, Carbamaze

All these drugs increase CNS toxicity of lithium.

Haloperidol

An encephalopathic syndrome with irreversible brain damage has occurred in a *few* patients treated with lithium and haloperidol.

Chlorpromazine

Lithium may lower chlorpromazine levels in blood and brain.

Psychiatric–Mental Health Nursing Practice with Lithium

A major nursing responsibility is the monitoring of lithium blood levels. This is necessitated by its very narrow therapeutic index and the consequences of the drug's buildup as a result of its patterns of excretion and binding. The dosage level of lithium does not determine its clinical effect; rather it is the blood level. Frequent assessment of blood levels is required until stability is reached, and then monthly evaluation of blood levels are sufficient.

Many people will experience side effects, even after just several hours of the first administration of the drug. Nausea, resting tremor of the hands, and slight abdominal discomfort are early symptoms. When antipsychotic drugs are used in conjunction with lithium, they are apt to mask side effects and signs of lithium toxicity because of their antinausea properties. Even

with frequent blood level assessment, there is great personal variation as to when the side effect or signs of toxicity will occur. Any attempt to equate symptoms with blood levels must be understood as a general position; each client must be evaluated as an individual.

Mild side effects and signs of toxicity are usually registered with levels below 1.5 mEq/L. These are: muscular weakness or fatigue, polyuria, polydipsia, nausea, diarrhea or loose stools, fine hand tremor while resting, and a metallic taste in the mouth. These symptoms often occur with rising blood lithium levels approximately 1 hour after receiving the medication. This can often be prevented by taking lithium with food at mealtime. In this way, lithium absorbtion from the G.I. tract is slowed and blood lithium levels rise at a rate the individual can better tolerate.

Moderate symptoms are shown with levels between 1.5 to 2.5 mEq/L. These are: severe nausea, vomiting, diarrhea, mild to moderate ataxia, incoordination, dizziness, sluggishness, giddiness, vertigo, slurred speech, tinnitus, blurred vision, increasing tremor, muscle irritability or twitching, asymmetrical deep tendon reflexes, and increased muscle tone. Some people show even more toxic effects at these levels. The clinical picture is usually more important than the blood level.

Severe and toxic symptoms are shown with levels of 2.5 to 7.0 mEq/L. These are: coarse tremor, dysarthia, nystagmus, fasciculations, visual or tactile hallucinations, oliguria, anuria, confusion, impaired consciousness, dyskinesia, grand mal convulsions, coma, and death.

The best intervention is prevention. Lithium has an average serum half-life of 24 hours; the serum will gradually clear if no more lithium is given. Supportive measures need to be taken in severe and toxic states. Unfortunately, when serum levels are greater than 5.0 mEq/L and the individual survives the toxic reactions, there is apt to be a permanent aftereffect, such as dementia or cerebral ataxia.

Most side effects are reversible with a decreased dose and an increase in the time from onset of treatment. However, if the side effects do impede the patient, other measures may be necessary. For example, nausea can be offset by giving the drug with meals. Fine motor coordination may require the use of another drug such as propranolol (Inderal).

Toxicity can occur for many reasons. Aside from overdosing, either through error or intention, dehydration caused by excessive heat, fever, or exercise, can cause a buildup of lithium through the loss of sodium. The other extremely important cause of lithium buildup and toxicity is renal disease. The kidneys are a prime source of excretion of the drug. *The importance of these latter points cannot be sufficiently underscored.* The need for client and family cooperation and for thorough drug education is illustrated in the case of a young woman who was started on lithium without clear instructions. Her mother received no information regarding the drug. The girl developed the flu, and although she was vomiting and having diarrhea, she continued with the drug, only to develop a toxic condition and go into renal failure and tragically die.

Severe toxicity is a medical emergency. Some physicians believe that at 3.0 mEq/L or more, patients should be started on hemodialysis, or peritoneal dialysis when the other is not available. Some attempts have been made to induce osmotic diuresis with mannitol or urea or theophylline.

Gaining the cooperation of the patient for the blood-level assessment is challenging. Blood must be drawn between 10 and 14 hours after the last dose of lithium for a base-line measurement. This requires that the patient remember not to take the lithium and not to come in and have blood drawn before the 10-hour limit. This is the only way to avoid false readings. It also points out that it is difficult to get an immediate lithium level that reflects accurate buildup levels—thus the importance of clinical symptoms in making an initial decision.

When these nursing points are combined with the preceding information regarding drug interaction and the interplay of lithium with other disease states, such as thyroid problems, heart problems, and the drugs used to treat them, safe and very rewarding results can be derived for patients who have bipolar depressive disorder.

Anticonvulsants as a Treatment for Mood Instability

Since the early 1980s, anticonvulsants have been used in the treatment of affective disorders. Though not all of the anticonvulsants have been found to be efficacious, carbamazepine (Tegretol) and valproic acid (Depakene) have shown some promising results. These drugs have been used successfully in the treatment of neuro-psychiatric disorders, especially temporal lobe epilepsy (TLE), in which a large component of the illness manifests itself in behavior problems.[57]

More frequently, anticonvulsants are being used to treat affective disorders either as a single treatment or in conjunction with lithium. Studies have shown a 50 percent success rate in treating individuals whose illness appears to be refractory to lithium.[58]

The current literature that addresses the use of the anticonvulsants in the treatment of affective disorders does not indicate that these patients had electroencephalographic (EEG) abnormalities, although in some patients nonspecific wave abnormalities were noted. Both manic and depressive symptoms have improved with therapeutic levels of carbamazepine and valproic acid.

Action

The neurophysiologic action of carbamazepine or valproic acid is not known. However, as a result of their use in TLE and what seems to be behavioral improvement in all patients who have taken these medications, it is believed that the drugs induce alterations in the limbic system, which is responsible for thought and perception. Also, these anticonvulsants seem to suppress reaction at the synapse level.

Dosage

Like lithium, the dosage of medication is based on blood level. The therapeutic range for carbamazepine is 4 to 12 μg/ml and valproic acid 50 to 100 mg/ml. Of note is that when the medication is given in conjunction with antipsychotic drugs, the individual may experience resurgence of psychotic symptoms. This is due to the fact that anticonvulsants induce liver metabolism; hence, both drugs (neuroleptic and anticonvulsant) are metabolized and excreted more rapidly, leading to a decline in blood levels of the antipsychotic drug as well as the anticonvulsant drug.

Side Effects

Side effects include dizziness, ataxia, clumsiness, drowsiness, slurred speech, and diplopia. These are common and frequently occur early in treatment. Once the liver has begun metabolizing the drug, these symptoms disappear. If they continue, a blood level evaluation should be obtained and the dosage should be lowered. If heart block has been noted, base-line ECGs should be done. Routine white blood counts (WBC) should be drawn throughout treatment with anticonvulsants. Decreased WBC in all indices have been noted. Pruritus and exfoliative dermatitis have also been reported.

Drug Interactions

Nursing Management

Table 21-11 shows reactions of carbamazepine and valproic acid with other drugs. Base-line complete blood counts with differential, ECG, and a careful history regarding hepatic and renal function should be completed before beginning a trial of carbamazepine or valproic acid. Levels should be adjusted upward carefully to avoid initial side effects. Patients should be observed for colds, fevers, and flu-like symptoms. These drugs should not be administered to individuals within 2 weeks of receiving MAO inhibitors.

Summary

Though anticonvulsants are not a first-line choice for the treatment of affective disorders, they should be seriously considered for those patients whose illness is refractory to lithium treatment or those patients who have previously required long-term prophylaxis with neuroleptics. Current literature indicates treatment with carbamazepine and valproic acid can be extremely fruitful when patients are monitored carefully.

ANTIANXIETY AGENTS

Identifying Anxiety Disorders

The next group of disorders under discussion are the anxiety disorders. Like depression, anxiety is a human experience that touches everyone to a lesser or greater degree. It is part of the human condition and is associated with change and stress. It is part of learning, it is part of play, it is part of joy, and it is part of adversity. As a state, it has subjective characteristics (of the person) as well as bodily responses to the tension. Most often we experience anxiety as an unpleasant uneasiness, tension, or apprehension. Bodily signs are extensive and, as such, require scru-

TABLE 21-11. INTERACTION OF CARBAMAZEPINE AND VALPROIC ACID WITH OTHER AGENTS

Drug	Agent	Clinical Manifestations
Carba-mazepine (Tegretol)	Alcohol	Increased incidence of CNS depression
	Lithium	Increased CNS toxicity
	MAO inhibitors	Exaggerated side effects of carbamazepine
	Phenobarbital	Decreased effect of carbamazepine resulting from increased breakdown by liver
	Valproic acid	Decreased effect of valproic acid resulting from increased breakdown by liver
Valproic Acid (Depakene, Depakote)	Alcohol	Increased incidence of CNS depression
	Aspirin	Increased effect of valproic acid resulting from decreased plasma protein binding
	Benzodiazepines	Increased effect of benzodiazepine resulting from decreased breakdown by liver
	CNS depressants	Increased incidence of CNS depression

(Adapted from Loebl, S., & Spratto, G. R. *The Nurse's Drug Handbook.* New York: Wiley, 1986, pp. 462, 469.)
CNS = central nervous system.

tiny as to more definitive reasons for the tension. For example, thyrotoxicosis, clinically, has signs and symptoms that parallel an anxiety state (including feeling jittery, keyed up, muscle tightness, palpitations, tremulousness, dread, and emotional lability, to name a few).

As in psychosis and depression, a framework for assessment is essential for understanding drug interventions. In general, anxiety that is severe (panic) and that may be associated with certain physical problems needs to be reduced. Antipsychotic and antianxiety drugs are most important in the reduction of these states. It is essential to recognize the basis of the anxiety and to address the causal factors. Antianxiety drugs have time-limited benefits, and their essential usefulness is to reduce immediate aspects of anxiety, such as narrowed perception, disruption of thinking, and distracting muscular and autonomic symptoms of tension that interfere with the person's taking charge of his situation. In the case of anxiety associated with physical illness, reduction is essential so that more specific interventions can have a chance to work. For example, when an individual has a heart attack, fear associated with the attack and excitability over what is going on around the person do not permit the relaxation and rest necessary for the heart muscle to regain its equilibrium. Antianxiety drugs may prove most useful at these critical times.

Recognizing these general characteristics of anxiety states and intervention, the following principles must be observed in assessing anxiety:

1. Anxiety is an essential dimension of the human condition.

2. Symptoms associated with anxiety can be understood as emanating from social or psychological events, somatic events, or psychological reactions to somatic events.
3. Anxiety of an intense nature must be reduced by some effective means because it is disruptive to rational thinking and problem solving.
4. Interruption of intense anxiety is a temporary intervention. Drug intervention as well as other methods have a short-term effect. Understanding the sustaining factors of anxiety offers the only framework for more enduring intervention.
5. Continued use of drugs to manage anxiety has many ethical considerations because these drugs tend to be abused and in some cases can lead to addiction.

Psychophysiological and clinical evidence suggest that a continuum exists, with people emphasizing somatic symptoms at one end and psychological symptoms at the other end (see Table 21-12).

The list of signs and symptoms, as shown in Table 21-12, can be grouped as to their subjective level of awareness. Shader and Greenblatt offer the following framework for assessing anxiety[59]:

TABLE 21–12. EXAMPLES OF ANXIETY SYMPTOMS ON A CONTINUUM FROM SOMATIC TO PSYCHOLOGICAL COMPLAINTS (MOST PEOPLE REPORT A MIXTURE OF SYMPTOMS.)

Somatic States	States In Which Complaints Are Somatic But May Be Understood As Psychologically Induced Or Connected		States Most Usually Understood As Psychologically Distressing
Abdominal cramps	Diarrhea	Palpitations	Apprehensive
Anorexia	Dizziness	Sweating	Anxious
Breathlessness	Dry mouth	Syncope	Dread
Chest pains	Faintness	Tightness in chest	Fearful
Choking sensation	Flushing	Vertigo	Fright
Easily startled	Giddy	Butterflies in stomach	Impending doom
Tachycardia	Headache	Choked up	Overexcited
Pupils dilated	Muscle tension	Jittery	Restless
Hyperpnea	Nausea	Shaky	Scared for no reason
Urge to urinate	Pallor	Tense	Threatened
Vomiting			Troubled
Weariness			Worried
			Phobic
			Wound-up
			Terror
			Panic

Situational anxiety describes reactions to a variety of stressful events from test taking to major surgery. The anxiety is specific to the event. Basically this type of anxiety is handled by preparations for the event. However, if the fear is underscored by low self-esteem and marked irritability, other approaches need to be instituted such as desensitization, psychotherapy, and drugs, mainly to enlist the person in other interventions.

Phobic anxiety is a form of situational anxiety. It can be of a direct nature, i.e., fear of flying; or it can be less obvious, such as fear of open spaces (agoraphobia) or moths. In the latter types, the object and situation feared are more symbolic than real. Behavioral modification, drugs, and psychotherapeutic approaches have been useful. It is thought that the best way to avoid recurrence is to have the person gain an understanding of the evolution of his phobic anxiety.

Anticipatory anxiety or extreme fear or panic is associated often with phobic states. What is meant here is an individual's escalating response to his own sense of anxiety, whether it is emanating from an event, situation, or object. The range and characteristics of anticipatory anxiety vary from a mild sense of anticipation (of the anxiety state itself), to hypervigilance, to panic.

Free-floating anxiety is a state that cannot readily be connected to a precipitating event or a fear-inducing stimulus. This type of anxiety can last from minutes to hours to days. It may be linked to painful memories or conflictual feelings that are quickly suppressed. There may be general, unfounded fears of illness.

Traumatic anxiety is associated with unusual events, such as rape or national disasters (bombings, tornados). The events are not expected. Sometimes the stress is prolonged and life-threatening, and the person either cannot or does not wish to remove himself from the circumstances of stress. Symptoms associated with this type of anxiety are restlessness, irritability, headaches, sleep pattern disturbances, nightmares, and an overactive startle reflex. In prolonged cases, distrust, isolation, feelings of inferiority, and social withdrawal may also occur. If there is a possibility that a person has been injured, care must be taken to identify any type of head or body injury or internal bleeding before drugs of any kind are given. Removal from the stress, rest, opportunity to ventilate, and medication carefully considered are essential in the treatment of traumatic anxiety.

Psychotic terror is the extreme sense of anxiety associated with psychotic symptoms. If visual hallucinations are dominant, toxic psychosis may be present. Antipsychotic drugs are usually indicated as well as control over the environment to reduce stimuli. Anxious depression is often difficult to diagnose because the anxiety can be intermittent, and although antianxiety drugs can be useful, they tend to potentiate the anticholinergic properties of antidepressants. However, doxepin is an antidepressant that seems to have antianxiety properties. Since there is a long life to antianxiety drugs, care must be used when prescribing them for the elderly. Excessive tissue storage of drugs plus the potentiation of anticholinergic properties in other drugs can be most harmful to the older person.

Anxiety associated with medical conditions is another important category. With care, antianxiety drugs can be most useful once a clear diagnosis and understanding of the physical problems have been arrived at. Of prime importance is the need for a thorough health assessment and physical examination before any type of drug intervention is made.

Antianxiety Drugs

Sedatives and hypnotics constitute one of the largest and most popular categories of drugs. This class of drugs includes the benzodiazepines, barbiturates, chloral hydrate, meprobamate, and a few others (Table 21-13).

The purpose of sedative therapy is to reduce anxiety or tension *without* interfering with the normal day-to-day activities of the patient. A low degree of sedation can usually alleviate the anxiety associated with neuroses or the anxiety that often accompanies somatic disease. Sedatives are generally more appropriately used in emotionally disturbed or neurotic patients than in those instances where patients exhibit psychotic tendencies.

There are excellent derived benefits in the use of antianxiety drugs in acute or chronic distress. Even in a situation in which a patient presents symptoms of pain, the antianxiety agents can bring about a degree of relief, despite the fact that these agents have little analgesic activity.

The true usefulness of these agents depends to a large degree on the patients' general attitude toward the use of drugs. Some patients

TABLE 21–13. Antianxiety Drugs

Anti-anxiety Agent	Generic Name	Daily Dosage Range (mg)
Benzodiazepines:		
Librium	Chlordiazepoxide	10–100
Valium	Diazepam	6–40
Serax	Oxazepam	30–120
Halcion	Triazolam	0.225–0.5
Restoril	Temazepam	15–30
Altivan	Lorazepam	0.5–2
Substituted propanediols (glycol or glycerol derivatives):		
Equanil, Miltown	Meprobamate	600–1200
Miscellaneous:		
Atarax	Hydroxyzine	200–400

will even respond well to a placebo regimen, based on how much value they place on "the need to take a drug to get better."

In the choice of an antianxiety agent, the state of the patient is usually the deciding factor. There are numerous antianxiety agents with essentially equitherapeutic effect but with widely differing levels of side effect, of degree of dependence (psychological or physical), and of margin of safety, as well as variable interaction with other ongoing therapies. Newer compounds, such as the benzodiazepines, are far safer for the potentially suicidal patient than are the barbiturates because of their wider margin of safety, e.g., toxic versus therapeutic dose.

Antianxiety Drug Action

Although antianxiety drugs act at all levels of the central nervous system, it is the recticular activating system that is especially sensitive to the depressant effect of these agents. Therefore the drugs must be carefully evaluated for side effects. The sedative-hypnotic effect is typified by the barbiturates. Even normal therapeutic doses can impair motor performance, judgment, and the ability to perform intelligent tasks. It is unclear whether these agents act at cellular or synaptic levels, and many theories are expounded as to their mechanism of action.

Many antianxiety drugs stimulate the production of hepatic microsomal enzymes and have been referred to as "enzyme inducers."

Their inducing ability forms the basis of their interactions with this class of agents. A patient receiving a barbiturate who also has been stabilized on an anticoagulant will need a higher dose of anticoagulant (approximately 38 percent) because the barbiturate increases the amount of hepatic microsomal enzyme available to metabolize the anticoagulant.

Benzodiazepine has strong anticonvulsant, hypnotic, and muscle-relaxant qualities. Although there is some evidence indicating a decreased turnover of dopamine and 5-hydroxytryptamine, which blocks stress-induced acceleration of norepinephrine turnover in the brain, the exact drug action on pre- or postsynaptic sites is unknown. What is known about the antianxiety drugs clinically is summarized in a review of the literature by Greenblatt and Shader.[60] Benzodiazepine derivatives are consistently superior to placebos in the short-term treatment of neurotic anxiety, but there is no evidence supporting the superiority of one benzodiazepine to another. There is a suggestion of reduced incidence of sedation with certain drugs in the antianxiety group of drugs. In studies comparing the clinical effects of benzodiazepines and barbiturates, the benzodiazepines proved more effective with fewer side effects, lethality, or addiction. In comparing benzodiazepines with antipsychotic drugs, studies indicated that in anxious psychotic states, antipsychotic drugs are superior. In the treatment of elderly patients with symptoms of agitation and emotionality, antipsychotic drugs are superior, with evidence that benzodiazepines cause deterioration. In nonpsychotic or nonorganic anxious states, benzodiazepines are equal if not superior to antipsychotic drugs and are far more useful because there is no risk of tardive dyskinesia. Benzodiazepines have also been found to be superior to placebos in the management of anxiety associated with somatic diseases including gastrointestinal, cardiovascular, or rheumatic disorders.

Despite the proliferation of many benzodiazepine agents, there has not been a breakthrough in the treatment with drugs of the most troublesome if not most disabling peripheral symptoms of anxiety: tachycardia, palpitations, tremulousness, diaphoresis, hyperventilation, and many others. As indicated in the discussion of anticipatory anxiety, these symptoms can be self-perpetuating and sometimes lead to panic. This has led to experimentation with beta-adrenergic blocking agents. To date, studies do not confirm the superiority of drugs in this class to benzodiazepines or placebos in chronic states of anxiety manifested by somatic symptoms.

Propanediols have become less important in the treatment of anxiety because their effect is questionable; they are highly addicting and they are lethal in overdose.

Antihistamines are another group of drugs that need more investigation as to their use in treating anxiety. Studies that are available support benzodiazepines over antihistamines. Antihistamines have weak, nonspecific central nervous system effects. They do have anticholinergic effects that can lead to complications, but they have a useful place with anxiety-related pruritic dermatoses.

Toxicity and Side Effects of Antianxiety Drugs

Benzodiazepines are safe drugs if one is concerned with overdoses. Toxic effects are rare, but where there is some indication that an individual has paradoxical reactions to drugs, care must be taken. Increased irritability or excitement can be due to a paradoxical reaction. The potentiation of anticholinergic properties when other drugs are used with antianxiety drugs underscores one of the major problems. Since benzodiazepines are so widely used, drug interaction must be watched for. Their high usage may cause tolerance and subsequent addiction. The other groups of drugs—propanediols, antihistamines, and beta-adrenergic antagonists— have not been demonstrated to be as useful in the treatment of anxiety states.

In summary, antianxiety agents are most effective in acute to severe symptoms of neurotic anxiety and in anxiety associated with somatic diseases. Treatment should be carried out over a short period of time because of the risk of psychological dependence and addiction with withdrawal symptoms. Antianxiety drugs have questionable use in persons with chronic symptomatology and characterological problems, but research is being conducted in these areas.

Psychiatric–Mental Health Nursing Practice with Antianxiety Agents

Antianxiety drugs have been discussed as to their advantages over barbiturates in the reduc-

tion of anxiety. However, their low lethal potential from overdose, the lower risk of physical dependency, and their lower interference with the metabolism of other drugs have led to a rather widespread and careless use.

There are specific issues to be considered with the benzodiazepines. First, these drugs, in their breakdown in the liver, tend to have a long half-life. They are converted into metabolites, which are stored in the liver. This means that the long-acting effects of the benzodiazepines can be accumulated over time and will not be rapidly excreted from the body. This is most important with the elderly because the drugs can become toxic. Therefore it is preferable that older people be treated with lorazepam or oxazepam, which have no active metabolites and are quickly excreted.

The other aspect of this metabolite breakdown is that the people who develop not only a habit but a dependency on the antianxiety drugs suffer withdrawal symptoms up to two weeks after the last dose is taken.

Effect is not what distinguishes one antianxiety drug from another; rather it is the duration of action. Short-acting drugs are lorazepam and oxazepam. The others are relatively long-acting. Short-acting antianxiety drugs have to be given in divided doses for effect, whereas the others can be given once a day at bedtime.

Because antianxiety drugs have a strong addictive effect, they must not be used with other central nervous system depressants and alcohol. They also have a strong propensity for drug interaction, and clients on antianxiety drugs must be warned of the danger when they receive other medications.

Antianxiety drugs must not be prescribed for people who are addicted or alcoholic, except under supervision with regard to withdrawal from the primary addictive substance. Also, since these drugs are more often used by people in their homes, it is important to keep them away from children.

Antianxiety drugs do not cure anxiety. This is most important to make clear to people. The psychological and organic causes must be addressed. These medications are aimed at assisting a person in a short-term manner, helping him regain healthy sleep and activity patterns. Prolonged use has no therapeutic effect; rather an elaborate defense is established that diminishes the individual's own resources.

Summary

Various categories of psychotropic agents have been discussed. The numerous drug effects can be understood in terms of the specific drug classification. Principles of neuroregulation and the hypotheses of how alterations in neuroregulation influence motor, affective, and cognitive behavior become the foundation of clinical pharmacology. Although physicians are responsible for prescribing drugs, the nurse assumes a critical role in monitoring the effectiveness of drug intervention. Because all psychotropic agents have noxious to dangerous physiological effects, the nurse is in a critical position to educate patients and family to the expected effects of this intervention. In this way, cooperation can be enhanced for maintenance, and serious toxic reactions and side effects can be responded to readily.

Drugs are an important intervention, but they are limited in long-term problems. Other modalities must be used in conjunction with drug therapy. Behaviors affected by drugs are not always specific to the major disruptive symptomatology. The risk of adverse reactions to long-term drug intervention must be understood by the nurse, patient, and family. Informed consent is essential. Clearly understanding why a drug is being given is the only way these ethical considerations can be addressed. Drugs should never be used as a substitute for constructive human involvement.

Questions

1. Describe two important principles of drug action.
2. How is neurotransmission within the autonomic nervous system carried out?
3. Discuss tardive dyskinesia.
4. Identify common and severe side effects of overdose with antipsychotic drugs.
5. List the drugs and dosage commonly prescribed for:
   a. Depressive states including schizophrenia-related depressive disorders, bipolar disorders, and unipolar disorders.
   b. Psychotic states.
   c. Anxiety states.
6. Name the four cardinal symptoms of neuroleptic malignant syndrome.
7. Name three predisposing factors to neuroleptic malignant syndrome.

REFERENCES AND SUGGESTED READINGS

1. Schatzberg, A., & Cole, J. *Manual of Clinical Psychopharmacology*. Washington, D.C.: American Psychiatric Press, 1986, p. 12.
2. Task Force on Nomenclature and Statistics of the American Psychiatric Association. *DSM-III-R*. Washington, D.C.: American Psychiatric Association, 1987.
3. Shader, R. (Ed.). *Manual of Psychiatric Therapeutics*. Boston: Little, Brown, 1975.
4. Greenblatt, D., & Shader, R. Psychotropic drug overdose. In R. Shader (Ed.), *Manual of Psychiatric Therapeutics*. Boston: Little, Brown, 1975, pp. 237–268.
5. Ibid.
6. DiMascio, A., & Shader, R. I. *Clinical Handbook of Psychopharmacology*. New York: Science House, 1970.
7. Shildkraut, J. J. The biochemistry of affective disorders: A brief summary. In A. Nicholi, Jr., (Ed.), *The Harvard Guide to Modern Psychiatry*. Cambridge, Mass.: Harvard University Press, (The Belknap Press) 1978, pp. 81–92.
8. Shader, op. cit. (1975).
9. Hartman, C.R., & DiMascio A. *Drugs and Behavior: An Introduction to Psychopharmacology*. Chestnut Hill, Mass.: TV lecture series produced by Boston College, 1978.
10. Barchas, J. D. *Psychopharmacology: From Theory to Practice*. New York: Oxford, 1977.

11. Bassuk, E., Schoonover, S., & Gelenberg, A. *The Practitioners Guide to Psychoactive Drugs* (2nd ed.). New York: Plenum Medical Book Co., 1983.
12. Baldessarini, R. J. Chemotherapy. In A. Nicholi, Jr. (Ed.), *The Harvard Guide to Modern Psychiatry*. Cambridge, Mass.: Harvard University Press (The Belknap Press), 1978, pp. 387–432.
13. Kahn, A., Jeffe, J. H., & Nelson, W. Resolution of neuroleptic malignant syndrome with dantrolene sodium: Case report. *Journal of Clinical Psychiatry*, 1985, *46*, 244–246.
14. Zulbenko, G., & Pope, H. Management of a case of neuroleptic malignant syndrome with bromocriptine. *American Journal of Psychiatry*, 1983, *148*, 1619–1620.
15. Greenblatt & Shader, op. cit.
16. Bassuk, Schoonover, & Gelenberg, op. cit., p. 127.
17. Ibid. p. 125.
18. Baldessarini, op. cit., p. 417.
19. Ibid., pp. 387–432.
20. Greenblatt & Shader, op. cit., pp. 237–268.
21. Bassuk, Schoonover, & Gelenberg, op. cit., pp. 154–156.
22. Ibid., p. 156.
23. Stadnyk, A., & Glezoz, J. Drug-induced heat stroke. *Canadian Medical Association Journal*, 1983, *128*, 1619–1620.
24. Masters, C., & Spitler, R. Neuroleptic malignant syndrome. *Journal of Psychosocial Nursing*, 1986, 24; *9*, 12–15.
25. Henderson, V., & Wooten, G. Neuroleptic malignant syndrome: A pathogenetic role for dopamine receptor blockade? *Neurology*, 1981, *31*, 132–137.
26. Greenberg, L., & Gujavarty, K. The neuroleptic malignant syndrome: Review and report of three cases. *Comprehensive Psychiatry*, 1985, *26*, 63–70.
27. Birkhimer, L., & DeVane, C. The neuroleptic malignant syndrome: Presentation and treatment. *Drug Intelligence and Clinical Pharmacy*, 1984, *18*, 462–465.
28. Ibid.
29. Mueller, P. Neuroleptic malignant syndrome. *Psychosomatics*, 1985, *26*, 654–662.
30. Ibid.
31. Caroff, S. The neuroleptic malignant syndrome. *Journal of Clinical Psychiatry*, 1980, *41*, 79–83.
32. Ibid.
33. Smego, R., & Durack, D. The neuroleptic malignant syndrome. *Archives of Internal Medicine*, 1982, *142*, 1183–1185.
34. Shildkraut, J., & Klein, D. The classification of depressive disorder, a review of supporting evidence. In R. Schader (Ed.), *Manual of Psychiatric Therapeutics*. Boston: Little, Brown, 1975, pp. 39–62.
35. Shader, R. I., & DiMascio, A. (Eds.). *Psychotropic Drug Side Effects*. Baltimore: Williams & Wilkins, 1970.
36. Berger, P. Antidepressant medication and the treatment of depressions. In J. D. Banchas et al. (Eds.), *Psychopharmacology: From Theory to Practice*. New York: Oxford, 1977, pp. 174–207.
37. Ibid.
38. Ibid.
39. Shader, op. cit. (1975).
40. Ibid.
41. Shildkraut, J. J. The catecholamine hypothesis of affective disorders: A review of supporting evidence. In D. S. Segal, (Ed.), *Foundations of Biochemical Psychiatry*, Boston/London: Butterworth, 1976, pp. 167–180.
42. Ibid.
43. Berger, op. cit.
44. Greenblatt & Shader, op. cit.
45. Berger, op. cit.
46. Shildkraut, J. J., et al. Depressive disorders and emerging field of psychiatric chemistry. In L. Grinspoon (Ed.), *Psychiatric Update: The American Psychiatric Association Annual Review* (Vol. 11). Washington, D.C.: American Psychiatric Press, 1982.
47. Shildkraut J. J. Biochemical discrimination of subgroups of depressive disorders based on differences in catecholamine metabolism. In I. Hanin & E. Usdin (Eds.), *Biological Markers in Psychiatry and Neurology* (Vol. 1). New York: Pergamon Press, 1982, pp. 22–23.
48. Shildkraut, op. cit.
49. Ibid.
50. Ibid.
51. Shildkraut, Depressive Disorders, op. cit.
52. Schlesser, M. A. Hypothalamic-pituitary-adrenal axis activity in depressive illness: Its relationship to classification. *Archives of General Psychiatry*, 1980, *37*, 737.
53. American Psychiatric Association. *DSM-III-R*. Washington, D.C.: American Psychiatric Association, 1987, p. 213.
54. Ibid., p. 217.
55. Gerson, S. The treatment of manic-depressive states. In R. Shader (Ed.), *Manual of Psychiatric Therapeutics*. Boston: Little, Brown, 1975, pp. 101–104.
56. Ibid.
57. Ballenger, J. C., & Post, R. M. Carbamazepine in manic-depressive illness: A new treatment. *American Journal of Psychiatry*, 1980, *137*,
58. Dalby, M. A. Behavioral effects of carbamazepine. In *Advances in Neurology* (Vol. 11). New York: Raven Press, 1986, pp. 331–341.
59. Shader, R., & Greenblatt, D. The psychopharmacological treatment of anxiety states. In R. Shader (Ed.), *Manual of Psychiatric Therapeutics*. Boston: Little, Brown, 1975, pp. 27–38.
60. Greenblatt, D. & Shader, R. Drug interactions in psychopharmacology. In R. Shader (Ed.), *Manual of Psychiatric Therapeutics*. Boston: Little, Brown, 1975, pp. 269–280.

Chapter 22

Milieu Therapy

Ann Bertrand-Clark

Chapter Objectives

The students successfully attaining the goals of this chapter will be able to:

- Define the terms milieu, therapeutic milieu, and therapeutic community.
- Trace the development of the milieu concept and its implications for psychiatric mental health nursing practice.
- Describe the role of the psychiatric nurse as a manager of the milieu.

The terms *milieu, therapeutic milieu,* and *therapeutic community* are used often in the psychiatric–mental health literature. Sometimes, they are used interchangeably to describe the same concept. Redl, a leader in the psychiatric treatment of children and adolescents in residential settings, addressed the issue by challenging his colleagues to define the term.[1] Nearly 10 years later, the concept of milieu continued to pose problems of clarity. Treischman and his colleagues chose to sidestep the issue in their book on the use of milieu therapy with children in a residential treatment facility.[2] In 1981, Devine sought to clarify the terms, but ended by using the terms, milieu therapy and therapeutic community in an identical manner.[3] Before further discussion of milieu therapy is undertaken, an attempt will be made to bring clarity to the issue and the terms by looking at the history and origins of environmental strategies in the treatment of individuals with psychiatric disorders.

HISTORY

Devine cites Phillipe Pinel as an originator of the notion of the therapeutic community.[4] The French physician coined the expression *moral treatment* to describe his program of therapy for the mentally ill. In the early nineteenth century, William Tuke began a similar program of treatment in England. Dorothea Dix and the Quakers popularized moral treatment in the United States in response to inhumane treatment of the mentally ill in large state hospitals.[5] Artiss credits Harry Stack Sullivan as "experimenting with varying the milieu" as a method of treatment as early as 1929.[6] However, it is Maxwell Jones that most authors cite as a "founder" of the therapeutic community, and it was he who popularized the use of the term in reference to the treatment method at his British hospital.

Jones began using trained staff and volunteers in his setting in response to the dearth of psychiatrists in England following World War II. His population of patients consisted of individuals with character disorders, and the central focus of his program was to control acting-out behaviors and to emphasize the learning or rehabilitation of social skills.[7] Herz noted that Jones' program was geared toward patients who had a limited understanding of the effect of their behavior on others and questioned whether or not it was reasonable to assume that such a program is or should be effective with different groups of patients.[8] Another British psychiatrist, Zeitlyn, questioned whether the therapeutic community was effective at all.[9]

However, in spite of such questions, the popularity of therapeutic communities spread, and soon few, if any, hospitals treating psychiatric patients, regardless of the nature of their problems, failed to claim that their services used this approach to treatment. Spurring this phenomenon was the appearance of such books as Goffman's Asylums in 1961. Goffman showed that in a large state hospital the staff did not interact with the patient "society" or effectively address intrastaff conflicts.[10] He also demonstrated that the structure of the hospital milieu directly affected the symptoms, behavior, and course of improvement of the patients. Other concerns that fed the milieu movement included issues of abuse of authority, authoritarianism in general, the effects of institutional dependence on patient behaviors such as regression, failure to accept responsibility, and withdrawal, and custodial care rather than treatment, and staff boredom.[11-13]

NURSING ROLES

Devine notes that nurses have moved from a custodial role to a teaching role within the last thirty years.[14] However, nurses are also responsible for limit-setting activities and the execution and management of nursing care. Nurses in advanced practice roles may, in addition, supervise care given by professional and technical staff, use group and family therapy treatment

modalities, act as consultants or liaison team members and act as case managers. Carino has suggested that an additional role for clinical specialists in the milieu may be that of milieu manager.[15] Specifically, this means that the clinical specialist acts as a monitor for the milieu as a whole, plans and executes strategies affecting the setting in conjunction with the nurse–manager and staff members, and evaluates the efficacy of implemented interventions.

THERAPEUTIC COMMUNITY, THERAPEUTIC STRATEGY, OR NEITHER

The word milieu is taken from the French and means either a place or environment. It is from the latter term that the term milieu takes on meaning, for the environment here has the additional connotation of a social or cultural setting. Cumming defined therapeutic community as "all programs that use group techniques to help the patient to understand and control his own emotional impasses."[16] This definition of therapeutic community fits the prototype established by Maxwell Jones. Cumming distinguished the therapeutic community from milieu therapeutic strategies by referring to the latter term as "those that aim at developing in the patients both diffuse and specific skills . . . both social and instrumental competence." Examples of such "social and instrumental" strategies include teaching problem-solving skills, rehabilitation of social skills, and the use of occupational and recreational therapies. However, as Cumming indicates, such strategies can also be found in "therapeutic communities."[17]

Visher and O'Sullivan defined milieu therapy as "a careful structuring of the social and physical environment of a psychiatric treatment program so that every interaction and activity is therapeutic for the patient."[18] In nursing, Skinner differentiates between milieu therapy "as a treatment or as a philosophy." As a treatment, milieu therapy aims at "structuring" the environment with the goal of producing behavioral change; as a philosophy, it is "a belief in the value of free self-expression and group process as a therapeutic approach."[19] Devine wrote that therapeutic community "can be described as an attempt to utilize the environment itself as an instrument of treatment."[20]

Maxwell Jones never actually defined the

terms. Instead, Jones referred to the use of staff and group modalities as techniques to encourage socially acceptable behavior.[21] Indeed, in a 1973 article Jones and Bonn wrote, "It is our contention that the term 'therapeutic community' has been misunderstood, overused and misapplied."[22] He denies that the term "implies a specific treatment methodology that must exist in pure form." With such disclaimers coming from one of the founders of the milieu movement, it's not surprising that confusion over the terms and the nature of their meanings continue.

For the balance of this section the terms milieu therapy and therapeutic community will be used synononymously. Such a decision is not made lightly, for there are unexplained dimensions to both terms. For example, Redl questioned what "therapeutic" as an adjective meant.[23] He suggested several meanings ranging from "don't put poison in their soup" to "re-education for life." However, milieu therapy and therapeutic community are part of the common parlance in the psychiatric–mental health specialty. In general, both terms may be conceived of as environmental strategies, and they will be referred to as such in the interest of clarity and providing a base line for further study.

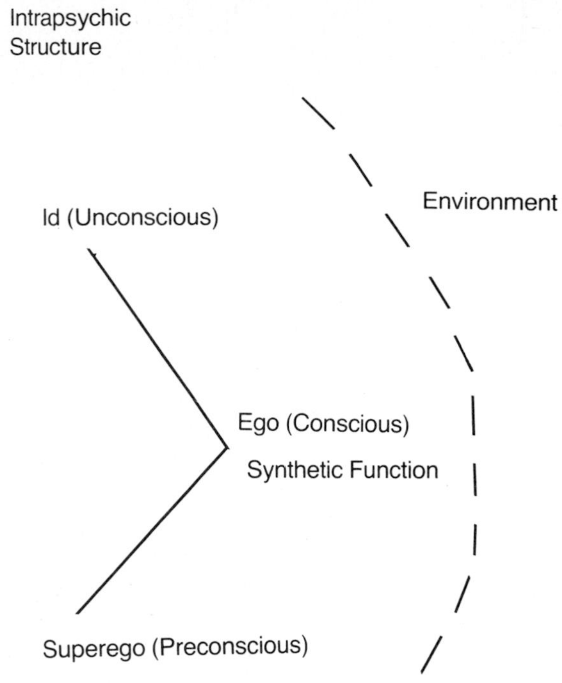

HOW IT WORKS (THEORETICALLY)

Essentially, milieu therapy is based on the various structures and functions of the ego, especially that of the synthetic function.[24,25] Before beginning to discuss how milieu therapy works, a brief review of psychoanalytic theory and ego structure and functions is in order.

The Synthetic Function

The synthetic function of the ego is a derivation of psychoanalytic theory and was first proposed by Nunberg.[26] Psychoanalytic theory is a developmental theory derived from the work of Sigmund Freud and is focused on personal–emotional development.[27] A central feature of this theory is that persons are motivated by irrational instincts and impulses. It is hypothesized that within the person intrapsychic structures—the id, the ego, and the superego—evolve (Fig. 22-1). The id, or unconscious, is the source of instinctual (libidinal) energy; the ego, or conscious, is the mediator between competing intrapsychic demands and between the psyche and the external world; and the superego, or preconscious, is the source of guilt or "conscience." In the late 1930s ego psychologists, whose primary interest is object relations, began to extend Freudian theory to include the area of interpersonal relationships.[28,29] Thus, Langer writes[30]:

Figure 22-1. Relationships among intrapsychic structures and the environments.

A core hypothesis is that intrapsychic conflict between id desires and ego and id desires and ego and superego restraints, and/or conflict between the individual and society leads to personal crises or intrapsychic disequilibrium.

The ego is hypothesized to have various functions in its role as mediator. Among them are the synthetic function. Nunberg defined the synthetic function as the ego's ability to "assimilate alien elements (from within and from without), and [to] mediate between opposing elements and even [to] reconcile opposites and set mental productivity in train."[31] Thus, according to Cumming and Cumming, "the ego grows through a series of successfully resolved crises, each of which disturbs a temporary equilibrium but leads to reorganization at a higher level."[32] Therefore, according to psychoanalytic theory, one hypothesis about the effect of environmental intervention might be the support and modification of the synthetic function.

Competing Views

Other theorists have considered the cultural and interpersonal influences on personal development.[33-35] These theories are derived from somewhat different views although Erikson's work clearly builds on Freudian (psychoanalytic) theory. Essentially, these theorists view environmental factors—either in combination with biologic endowments or alone—as affecting ego development. Therefore, environmental alteration will be expected to influence both the person's view of himself and his social milieu.*

Assumptions

Skinner lists seven assumptions on which every milieu program is based.[36] These are:

1. Health in each individual is to be realized and encouraged to grow.
2. Every interaction is an opportunity for therapeutic intervention.
3. The patient owns his own environment.
4. Each patient owns his own behavior.
5. Peer pressure is a useful tool.
6. Inappropriate behaviors are dealt with as they occur.
7. Restrictions and punishment are to be avoided.

In addition, Cumming states that another assumption is ". . . the *whole person* will benefit from treatment of *part* of his problem."[37] These assumptions clearly seek to establish ground rules for the community, and adaptations of these are to be found in the philosophies or community rules of most treatment programs. However, assumption 3, concerning "ownership" of the environment, requires a footnote. Although Skinner refers to ownership, it is worth noting that most programs exercise some discretion in the organization of program activities. At most,

this assumption addresses the right of patients to participate in the planning of activities and identified patient-governed activities.

Goals

Although goal setting in milieu therapy differs in various settings, four basic assumptions underlie the milieu design: (a) all patients have strengths, (b) patients can constructively influence their own treatment and the treatment of others, (c) successful treatment is dependent on pervasive therapeutic staff involvement, and (d) all levels of hospital personnel can offer therapeutic influence.[38] The milieu exists to facilitate social learning, interchange, and support as new behaviors are learned.[39] Theoretically, once behavior that has been targeted for change is identified, new behaviors must be learned so that alternative behavior is possible. Thus, the teaching of psychosocial skills such as problem solving, effective interpersonal relationship skills, and relaxation techniques, provides the person with substitute behaviors to replace less effective or dysfunctional choices.

A review of the literature in this area reveals eight possible goals:

1. To increase or decrease affect.
2. To increase awareness of the effect of behavior on others.
3. To arouse interest in the surroundings.
4. To provide opportunities for socialization.
5. To encourage a sense of responsibility.
6. To decrease regression.
7. To provide opportunities for participation in unit activities and management.
8. To increase interaction between staff and patients.

PROBLEMS IN THE USE OF ENVIRONMENTAL STRATEGIES

Numerous problems have been identified with the use of environmental strategies. What follows is an overview, not an exhaustive list. Rather, this discussion is aimed at spurring thought about and consideration of the general use of milieu-oriented interventions.

Administrative issues that have been identified are generally related to authority issues. The questions of who is "in charge" and who

---

* Readers are referred to Cumming and Cumming[25] for a more detailed analysis.

is responsible for what are at the heart of many issues that are associated with the use of environmental strategies. Among the most frequently encountered problems are those that relate to "power struggles" between both patients and staff and among the staff.[40-44] If responsibility is to be delegated, some amount of authority must also be delegated. If "every encounter" between patients and staff is potentially therapeutic, who is the "final authority" on therapeutic decisions?[45]

A second concern is related to the targeted population. Does every patient benefit from the milieu? Cumming writes: "A fault . . . is that identical treatment is used for all kinds of patients."[46] Is there a kind of "generic" milieu that will work for all groups of patients? Jones worked out his program for patients with character disorders who did not consider the effect of their behavior on others[47]; does it follow that all patients will benefit from "confrontation"? Johnson and Parker believe that "overuse of confrontation" is one of the "antitherapeutic effects" of milieu therapy.[48] The question is: are individual differences taken into consideration when "setting limits" on behavior and "confronting" patients? Finally, is it worth reflecting on whether or not environmental strategies work at all? Devine notes that there are problems with the process of studying the effects of environmentally based interventions; concepts are unclear and research reports indicate that it is not clear whether it is the strategy or the additional staff attention that is responsible for positive outcomes.[49]

IMPLICATIONS AND CONSIDERATIONS

What follows is a brief summary of the implications and considerations related to environmental strategies. Again, it is not a detailed discussion, but rather a summary of issues that have been raised about the use of environmental strategies. The concerns tend to cluster in five areas: administrative issues, economic issues, physical space and time considerations, staff supervision, and ethical questions. Although the categories are discussed individually, it is wise to keep in mind that these areas are interrelated.

Administrative Issues

Cumming wrote ". . . an administrative structure that permits, facilitates, or even demands,

the necessary structures" is a crucial element in the use of environmental strategies because of the implicit issue of authority.[50] Authority—who has it, how it is perceived and used, and how it is delegated—is at the heart of many of the issues related to the use of milieu therapies. The organizational structure at every level must lend support to the effort, for delegation of authority is the essence of an egalitarian therapeutic community. If the community is not to be egalitarian, the philosophy and decision-making structures must be adjusted, and the amount and kind of responsibility patients and staff will have must be clarified. Other considerations under this category include criteria for admissions, screening procedures for both the type and number of patients to be admitted, and program goals. In essence, it is the philosophy and practice of the administrative structure that must be considered so as to insure coherence in the design and execution of environmental strategies.

Economic Issues

In this era of cost containment and decreased length of stay, the number and kinds of patients admitted may not be determined as selectively as in the past. Hospitalization may be seen as a "stabilization" period or a brief period for adjustment of medications or other aspects of the treatment regimen. If the setting is an outpatient center, patients may have a limited number of visits or a specified period of time for which they are covered by insurance or other third-party payer. The number of clients may affect not only the kind of program offered but also the number and category of staff available to implement the strategies.

Physical Space and Time

It is almost impossible to coordinate multiple meetings and individual and group therapy time if there is a limited number of rooms available. Other considerations involve the population to be served, the number of patients to be served, staff:patient ratios, and the nature of the activities that are planned. An additional concern is whether or not there is enough time for patients and staff to process painful or other significant situations that have occurred. Individuals require time to reflect on their responses and reactions, and if this time is not available, the event may remain as a source of difficulty until resolution and closure take place. It seems redundant to add that environmental strategies require planning and "processing" time; however, this is a vital factor to include in planning and designing programs.

Staff Supervision

Countertransference reactions and staff values and skills often pose difficulties in the execution of environmental therapies.[51,52] Nowhere is this more evident than in settings with child–adolescent populations. Staff who work in this area may have values related to their own family experiences about how children or adolescents should be treated, or they may have unresolved issues related to authority figures.[53] Close involvement with parents may raise other issues for staff related to their own unresolved experiences; this is especially true if volatile issues such as sexual abuse or trauma are concerned.[54] It has been suggested that supervision of staff can be one avenue to decreasing such work-related issues since it acts as an approach to clarifying treatment problems and facilitating individual growth by reflecting on problematic reactions and responses.[55] However, this kind of supervision also requires time, and it must

occur on a regular basis, for if it occurs only when there are problems, an atmosphere of tension and hostility rather than growth and understanding may result.[56] Finally, although this issue has been discussed in relationship to the care and treatment of children and adolescents, it applies equally to those staff members who care for all age groups.

Ethical Questions

Ethical questions and considerations are ubiquitous in the use of environmental strategies. They begin with whether or not environmental strategies are effective. Issues related to "community rules" like body searches, right to refuse treatment, violence and abuse of patients and staff, and the ethics of behavior modification strategies form a very short list of concerns. There is much that is unknown about the long-term effects of behavioral interventions, and as previously stated, there are many obstacles to the conduct of research in this area. This is not to say that environmental strategies should not be used, only that it is rare to encounter any discussion of the ethical questions involved in their use. They are raised here to remind readers of their existence and to promote thought and discussion.

Summary

This section has reviewed the history of environmental strategies, lack of conceptual clarity in defining the various terms attached to environmental treatment modalities, and nursing roles in the "therapeutic community." A discussion of problems associated with the use of these strategies was presented, and associated implications and considerations were reviewed.

Questions

1. How did the concept of therapeutic milieu develop?
2. Describe the nursing student's role in the therapeutic milieu.
3. In your clinical setting, how do the psychiatric nurses manage the milieu?
4. How does the psychodynamic concept of ego interface with the milieu concept?

REFERENCES AND SUGGESTED READINGS

1. Redl, F. The concept of a "therapeutic milieu." *American Journal of Orthopsychiatry*, 1959, 29, 721–736.
2. Treischman, A. E., Whittaker, J. K., & Brendtro, L. K. *The Other 23 Hours*. Chicago: Aldine, 1969.
3. Devine, B. A. Therapeutic milieu/milieu therapy: An overview. *Journal of Psychosocial Nursing and Mental Health Services*, 1981, 19(3), 20–24.
4. Ibid.
5. Ibid.
6. Artiss, K. L. A narrow view of what is therapeutic. *International Journal of Psychiatry*, 1969, 7, 201–203.
7. Jones, M. *A Study of Therapeutic Communities*. London: Tavistock Publications, 1952.
8. Herz, M. I. The therapeutic milieu: A necessity. *International Journal of Psychiatry*, 1969, 7, 209–212.
9. Zeitlyn, B. B. The therapeutic community: Fact or fantasy? *British Journal of Psychiatry*, 1967, 113, 1083–1086.
10. Goffman, E. *Asylums*. Chicago: Aldine, 1961.
11. Zeitlyn, op. cit.
12. Herz, op. cit.
13. Islam, A., & Turner, D. L. The therapeutic community: A critical reappraisal. *Hospital and Community Psychiatry*, 1982, 33, 651–653.
14. Devine, op. cit.
15. Carino, C. Lecture given to graduate students at the University of Pennsylvania School of Nursing, Philadelphia, April, 1987.
16. Cumming, E. Therapeutic community and milieu therapy strategies can be distinguished. *International Journal of Psychiatry*, 1969, 7, 204–208.
17. Ibid.
18. Visher, J. S., & O'Sullivan, M. Nurse and patient responses to a study of milieu therapy. *American Journal of Psychiatry*, 1970, 127, 451–456.
19. Skinner, K. The therapeutic community: Making it work. *Journal of Psychiatric Nursing*, 1979, 17(8), 38–44.
20. Devine, op. cit., p. 20.
21. Jones, op. cit.
22. Jones, M., & Bonn, E. From therapeutic community to self-sufficient community. *Hospital and Community Psychiatry*, 1973, 24, 675–680.
23. Redl, op. cit., pp. 724–725.
24. Cumming, op. cit.
25. Cumming, J., & Cumming, E. *Ego and Milieu*. New York: Atherton Press, 1963.
26. Nunberg, H. *Practice and Theory of Psychoanalysis*. New York: International Universities Press, 1951, pp. 120–136. (Originally published in 1931.)
27. Langer, J. *Theories of Development*. New York: Holt, Rinehart & Winston, 1969.
28. Rappaport, D. An historical survey of psychoanalysis. *Psychological Issues*, 1959, 1, 5–17.
29. Blanck, R., & Blanck, G. *Beyond Ego Psychology: Developmental Object Relations*. New York: Columbia University Press, 1986.
30. Langer, op. cit., p. 24.
31. Nunberg, op. cit., p. 122.
32. Cumming & Cumming, op. cit., p. 13.
33. Sullivan, H. S. Socio-psychiatric research: Its implications for the schizophrenic problem and for mental hygiene. *American Journal of Psychiatry*, 1931, 10, 977–991.
34. Fromm, E. Individual and social origins of neurosis. *American Sociological Review*, 1944, 9, 380–391.
35. Erikson, E. *Childhood and Society*. New York: Norton, 1950.
36. Skinner, op. cit., p. 39.
37. Cumming, op. cit., p. 208.
38. Wolf, M. S. Review of literature on milieu treatment, *Journal of Psychiatric Nursing*, 1977, 15(5), 27.
39. Ibid.
40. Zeitlyn, op. cit.
41. Cumming, op. cit.
42. Herz, op. cit.
43. Johnson, J., & Parker, K. Some antitherapeutic effects of a therapeutic community. *Hospital and Community Psychiatry*, 1983, 34, 170–171.
44. Berlin, I. N., Critchley, D. L., & Rossman, P. G. Current concepts in milieu treatment of seriously disturbed children and adolescents. *Psychotherapy*, 1984, 21, 118–131.
45. Johnson & Parker, op. cit.
46. Cumming, op. cit., p. 207.
47. Jones, op. cit.
48. Johnson & Parker, op. cit.
49. Devine, op. cit.
50. Cumming, op. cit., p. 206.
51. Ibid.
52. Berlin, Critchley, & Rossman, op. cit.
53. Ibid.
54. Kohan, M. J., Pothier, P., & Norbeck, J. Hospitalized children with a history of sexual abuse: Incidence and care issues. *American Journal of Orthopsychiatry*, 1987, 57, 258–264.
55. Berlin, Critchley, & Rossman, op. cit.
56. Ibid.

Chapter 23

Individual Psychotherapies

Ann Wolbert Burgess

Chapter Objectives

The students successfully attaining the goals of this chapter will be able to:

- Describe the major individual psychotherapies.
- Compare brief individual psychotherapy models of care.
- Describe the role of the psychiatric nurse and psychotherapy.

One of the psychiatric nursing standards addresses the practice of conducting individual psychotherapy. To acquaint the beginning student with the variety of models of psychotherapy, this chapter will focus on short-term models. The practice of talking therapy began with psychoanalysis, and since Freud's time, numerous variations on the talking therapy model have been evolved. Social and economic factors have placed constraints on the time and number of sessions. Currently, short-term models of psychotherapy are a necessary part of the services available to patients.

Sullivan defined psychotherapy as primarily a verbal interchange between two individuals: one an expert, the other a help seeker. These two individuals work together on the patient's life problems in the hope of achieving behavioral change.[1]

It is very important to distinguish diagnostic interviews from ongoing therapy and to allow for the possibility, from a diagnostic interview, of "no therapy necessary."[2] Interventions and technical procedures performed during the evaluation process are quite different from the technical aspects of the psychotherapeutic process. During the evaluation, the nurse must consider the interaction of the patient's diagnosis, ego strength, physical health, and other selection criteria and the different treatment options.[3,4]

PRINCIPLES OF THERAPY

There are several psychotherapeutic principles that are critical in the process of psychotherapy. These are described below.

Transference

Every individual in an interpersonal transaction brings to that transaction certain ways of looking at life and perceiving other people that have been determined by his past experiences. These past experiences often distort the way in which the individual perceives his current reality. Thus, as a result of his past experience, an individual may feel that all authority figures are rejecting, punitive, or authoritarian, and thus, he may react to current authorities with distorted perceptions and expectations. These unconscious distortions constitute the phenomenon of transference.

Countertransference

Most often, a therapist tends to be idealized because she or he is identified with the patient's wishes and hopes that the therapist will be a perfect parent, who will help him most effectively. Therapists have their own backgrounds and experiences that may result in certain distortions. When these distortions are carried through into the therapeutic process and influence the ways in which therapists perceive their patients or behave toward them, these distortions constitute what are referred to as countertransference reactions.

Thus the therapist also brings conscious and unconscious attributes into the psychotherapeutic interaction. Real attributes—warmth, genuineness, empathy, knowledge, appearance, emotional maturity, personal style, etc.—play a significant role in the patient–therapist interaction. Add to these the therapist's own emotional needs, ambition, and value systems, as well as any countertransference distortions that may be present, and one can begin to appreciate the complex variables that enter into the patient–therapist relationship. The way in which this patient–therapist matrix evolves and is shaped in any individual therapeutic encounter is the basic foundation on which the therapeutic process rests and upon which a positive or negative therapeutic outcome depends.

Release of Emotional Tension

Given this basic matrix of the therapeutic relationship, a number of other important things also take place in the psychotherapeutic process.

To begin with, the ability of the patient to confide and express feelings to a person whom he trusts and counts on as being supportive, understanding, and ultimately helpful is an important factor in reducing emotional tension in the context of expectancy and hope. The greater the trust in the therapist and the greater the hope and expectancy of receiving help, the greater the sense of relief.

Acquisition of Insight

The therapist—by virtue of the questions asked, manner of confrontations and interpretations, or by what is focused on or ignored, and by verbal as well as nonverbal reactions—begins to convey to the patient a certain cognitive framework upon which the therapy is going to be based. Cognitive teaching, whether explicit or implicit, is an inevitable part of every psychotherapeutic process, because once a therapist tells a patient the rationale behind the process, she sets up a cognitive framework. In effect, the psychodynamic therapist imparts to patients that their problems have evolved over the course of personal development in relationship to significant people; this process creates certain distortions in the perception of life and of self. Therapy will try and uncover those causes, and in the process of uncovering those causes, the patient will begin to feel better.

Gestalt therapists tell their patients that their problems are due to a failure to be sufficiently aware of their feelings, and that in the course of their work they will learn to express their feelings better, and that this will make them feel better. This, too, is a cognitive framework. Behaviorists who tell their patients that they have acquired certain inappropriate habits as a result of faulty conditioning are also setting up a cognitive framework upon which their psychotherapeutic approach depends.[5]

In all therapies, there exists a certain amount of cognitive learning that gives the patient an intelligible, meaningful, and rational framework for understanding why and how this problem has developed. Also, in the course of confrontations and interpretations, all therapists also convey both their therapeutic objectives and their value systems to the patient.

As pointed out by Marmor, the therapeutic objectives of most psychotherapists in our culture are essentially similar and reflect our culture's normative ideals.[6] All basically aim at enabling their patients to have meaningful and satisfying social and sexual relationships, to work and love effectively, and to become productive and responsible human beings.

Operant Conditioning

In the course of pursuing these objectives, a certain amount of learning, or operant conditioning, takes place. This occurs through the kinds of responses that the therapist makes to the patient's verbal or behavioral expressions. Certain behaviors are approved, others are disapproved. This is not always explicit. The approval may be a shrug of a shoulder or an expression of the eyes. It may be in the interpretation of what is considered healthy or unhealthy behavior.

One type of therapy learning that takes place is what Franz Alexander called the corrective emotional experience. By virtue of the fact that the therapist responds differently, more objectively, more empathetically, or more realistically to the patient's emotional or behavioral expressions, the patient receives a different kind of emotional experience from what he may have received from the significant authorities in his past life. These corrective emotional experiences occuring within the matrix of the patient–therapist relationship are important elements in the therapeutic process.

Identification with the Therapist

Another factor observed in the therapeutic process is the degree to which patients, consciously or unconsciously, tend to model themselves after the therapist, gradually incorporating some of the explicit or implicit values that they are being exposed to. This kind of modeling is called identification by analytic psychotherapists, while learning therapists call it social learning. There is no doubt that it is one of the most important ways in which human beings learn from one other.

Suggestions and Persuasion

Another factor that occurs in all therapies is suggestion and persuasion. Whenever a therapist presents his rationale for his therapy and implies or explicitly states that the patient will feel better as a result of following that therapeutic model—whether it be psychodynamic, Gestalt, or behavioral—that therapist is using suggestion. The patient's expectation of being helped, the implicit assumption that this help will be forthcoming if he complies with the therapeutic program, and every indication received in therapy that certain patterns of behavior are more desirable or "healthy" than others involve implicit, if not explicit, elements of suggestion and persuasion. The greater the faith of the patient in the therapist, the greater the degree of idealization or positive transference, the greater is the impact of these suggestions on the patient.

Rehearsal and Adaptation

Finally, for therapeutic change to become really consolidated, for things to be learned, a certain amount of rehearsal and repetition has to take place. This rehearsal can be explicit, as in certain behavioral therapies; it can be implicit, as in the so-called working-through process of dynamic psychotherapy; or it can be deliberate, as in the giving of homework assignments. But regardless of how it is done, the things that are learned in the psychotherapeutic process have to be generalized, and the patient must be able to express these new adaptive techniques of behavior in other aspects of his life—to his family, his friends, his associates.

MODELS OF PSYCHOTHERAPY

Short-Term Therapies

Short-term therapy or brief models of psychotherapy have a time limit for treatment. One model, crisis intervention, is discussed in a separate chapter. Other models to be discussed here include brief dynamic psychotherapies: focal, short-term anxiety-provoking, time-limited, and brief adaptation-oriented therapy; and cognitive therapies. Feminist counseling, introduced in the 1970s as part of the Women's Liberation Movement is also discussed.

Focal Psychotherapy: Malan
The focal psychotherapy work of David Malan was influenced by Michael Balint from the Tavistock Clinic in London and is an example of applied psychoanalysis.[7] Malan emphasizes the

importance of choosing and maintaining a narrow focal area to be dealt with in a brief period of time. The time factor is given in terms of a date rather than in terms of the number of sessions. Practically speaking, this prevents the need for the patient and therapist to keep count of the number of sessions and rather, provides for a beginning, a middle, and an end to treatment.

In addition to the focal work, the patient must have a capacity to think in feeling terms, demonstrate high motivation, and exhibit a good response to trial interpretations made during the evaluation phase. Malan does not necessarily exclude patients with serious psychopathology; in fact, several of the patients he describes in his writings show significant degrees of pathology.

Patients may be excluded from treatment if, upon evaluation, problems are foreseen that can impair the ability to form an effective therapeutic alliance within a short time period or if motivation is not high. The ability to identify a focal area is very important. Identifying the precipitant factors, early traumatic experiences, or repetitive patterns can point to the area of internal conflict present since childhood and to the focus for treatment. According to Malan, the greater the probability that the conflict area will manifest itself in the transference, the more positive the outcome will be.[8]

Malan is less concerned with technique than with the importance of choosing the focus. He employs all the usual technical procedures of psychoanalytic psychotherapy and emphasizes the importance of making interpretations of the transference and connecting these to current and past relationships. This "triangle of insight" (the transference, the current relationship, and the past relationship) leads to the patient's cure. Overall, the goal is to clarify the nature of the defense, the anxiety, and the impulse that the patient is experiencing and to link these to the present, the past, and the transference. Once the defense and the anxiety are clarified, the link to the past can be made.[9,10]

Short-term Anxiety-Provoking Psychotherapy: Sifneos

At the same time that David Malan was undertaking his research in London, Peter Sifneos was studying brief psychotherapy at the Massachusetts General Hospital in Boston.[11] Many of Sifneos's conclusions are similar to those of Malan; however, there are some differences.

Patient selection is an important criterion for Sifneos because of the anxiety-provoking nature of his brief therapy techniques. He distinguishes anxiety-provoking therapy from anxiety-suppressing therapy, commonly referred to as supportive psychotherapy.

The criteria for patient selection include above-average intelligence and a history of at least one meaningful relationship with another person. The patient who has had such a relationship will be able to withstand the anxiety produced by the therapy and to develop a mature relationship with the therapist. This criterion tends to exclude patients with narcissistic disorders. In addition, the patient must be highly motivated for change, not just for symptom relief, and to identify a chief complaint. The patient's ability to identify one conflict area and to postpone work on others is an indication of his ability to tolerate anxiety. Sifneos is clear on his assessment of motivation. He defines motivation as including the patient's ability to recognize symptoms as psychological, a tendency to be introspective and honest about emotional difficulties, and a willingness to participate in the treatment situation. In addition, motivation includes curiosity, a willingness to change, a willingness to make reasonable sacrifices, and a realistic expectation of the results of psychotherapy. Sifneos focuses on the Oedipal conflict and does not expect a good outcome in dealing with other areas.[12]

After a good rapport and therapeutic alliance is established, Sifneos recommends using anxiety-provoking confrontations to clarify issues regarding the patient's early life situation and present-day conflict. The therapist is to avoid areas such as passivity, dependence, and acting out, which might lead to extensive regression. The sessions are 45 minutes in length and the usual course of treatment is 12 to 16 sessions. The aggressive confrontational style of this therapy underscores the importance of excluding preoedipal problems and the importance of the therapist's countertransference reactions related to being aggressive.[13]

Time-Limited Psychotherapy.

James Mann writes in the preface of his book, *Time-Limited Psychotherapy*, that in 1964 he met with the director of residential education at the Boston University School of Medicine Division of Psychiatry to find a solution to the problem of long waiting lists for treatment.[14] The model of the treatment at that time was to enter patients into long-term psychotherapy, which reduced the numbers of patients that could be seen at the clinic. A plan was devised to institute a program of 12 therapy sessions, or a time-limited psychotherapy model. Because of the resistance to this new treatment, a training program for psychiatric residents was instituted using a one-way mirror for easing the concept into reality.

Basic assumptions for Mann's model include the following:

Time Linkage. All significant human behavior is linked with time. A study looking at the concept of time in a normal group of children ranging from age 3 to 6 and found that when they learned to tell clock time, external factors became increasingly important.[15] Prior to that point, diurnal rhythm (the concept of the day as a unit of 24 hours) was described in terms of immediate personal experiences, that is, eating, sleeping, etc. The conclusions of the studies were that the concept of time is the result of the interaction between the child with his private experiences and rhythmic needs and an external world with external physical forces (light, dark, cold, etc.) and significant adults, all of whom have their own rhythmic patterns.[16]

Timelessness. The past continues its active existence in the unconscious at every point in the now of a person's life. The timeless quality of the unconscious was elaborated by Freud and analysts who followed him. Bonaparte observes that in adolescence, life seems to be spread out in a limitless expanse and death does not seem to exist. She wrote, "We destroy time from the moment we begin to use it . . . for in living our time we die of it."[17] She continued to identify five situations in which the pleasure principle prevails and time can cease to exist:

1. Dreams in which we guard the illusions of childhood and defeat time by immersing ourselves in the infinite time of childhood.
2. Daydreams in which fairy-tale fantasies of omnipotence dominate, and reality and time are conquered.
3. The intoxication of love, which, with its remarkable idealization of the loved object, allows the lover to transcend time, to vow eternal love, and to ignore reality.
4. Intoxication from drink or drugs, which is used to minimize or erase reality and allow full reign to the pleasure principle.
5. States of mystic ecstasy, which are not unlike the ecstatic states experienced by drug users and lovers. In all three, but particularly in the mystic states, subjective feelings of eternity are projected and given an objective existence, which effectively conquers time.

If one can eliminate time sense, one can also avoid the ultimate separation that time brings—death. As Mann points out, people are aware inwardly of growing older.[18] The pursuit of timelessness, of eternity, is dramatically accented by the usual portrayals of Time as an old man with a scythe and Death as a grinning skeleton with a scythe. We seek to avoid destruction by avoiding time. There is a tremendous investment in trying to avoid aging. There is the nostalgic reflection on the past. Fashion trends repeat. Or as Bonaparte observes, "In all human hearts there is a horror of time."[19]

Time-limited psychotherapy revives the anxieties of time. It brings fresh flame, to quote Mann, to the "conflict between timelessness, infinite time, immortality and the omnipotent fantasies of childhood on the one hand, and time, finite time, reality, and death on the other hand."[20]

Conceptual Framework. The conceptual framework for Mann's time-limited therapy is based on psychoanalytic concepts of unconscious determinants of thoughts, feelings, and actions and their relation to maturational phases of personality development as well as to the elaboration of structural elements (id, superego, and ego). Additionally, adaptation always implies defense.

Mann emphasizes the experience of loss and anxiety as related to the separation–individualization crisis. This phase includes the maturational and developmental processes occurring during the period from about age 3 months through the third year of life. It is during this phase that the child differentiates his internal representation of himself from that of his mother. The separation–individualization phase directly determines the course of ego development. In turn, this determines the adequacy of the adaptive modes that emerge as a means of managing relationships with others. The therapeutic task is mastery of separation anxiety which lies in the ambivalence experienced originally in the mother–child relationship.

Mann believes that the selection of the central issue is the critical event. It is the vehicle through which the patient is engaged for the work of therapy. Mann looks for a central issue that is developmentally and adaptively relevant and has been recurrent over time. The central issue formulated in terms of time, affect, and an image of the self is evoked in the transference. Time-limited psychotherapy is intended to resolve this present and chronically endured pain and the patient's negative self-image. Mann carefully words the central issue. In the case of a 41-year-old depressed woman who was preoccupied with any degree of lateness by her husband and children, Mann and Goldman suggested the following central issue: "You've encountered extreme life situations and have managed them remarkably well . . . yet you fear and have always feared that despite your best efforts you will lose everything."[21] In a 31-year-old married man attempting to get a college degree who was consumed with a fear of failing, they suggested the central issue: "Because there have been a number of sudden and very painful events in your life, things always seem uncertain, and you are excessively nervous because you do not expect anything to go along well. Things are always uncertain for you." The selection of a central issue include the following dynamic themes: (1) independence versus dependence; (2) activity versus passivity; (3) adequate self-esteem versus diminished self-esteem or loss of it; and (4) unresolved or delayed grief.

The treatment agreement and guidelines include an intake interview of two to three sessions and a formulation of the central conflict in terms of the current distress or problem. The patient's general psychological state is assessed and a tentative diagnosis made. A plan is made for best distribution of the 12 sessions. The amount of time in a session may vary, e.g., 24 20-minute sessions or 12 50-minute sessions. Certain patients are excluded: these include persons with acute psychotic reaction, acute decompensation, or profound depression. Identification of a termination date is used as a technique to increase anxiety in respect to loss as well as defenses against loss. The termination date is quickly repressed by the patient and the intensification of defenses against separation or loss serve to highlight much of the nature of the present central issue, its past history, and the means employed to master it.

Generally, the first three to four sessions see rapid symptomatic improvement. There is a rapid mobilization of a positive transference. Then, symptoms, character traits, and life-styles that have served to defend against awareness of the conflict contained in the central issue reappear or take on new strength. The remaining sessions focus on helping the patient develop a new coping style.

Brief Adaptation-Oriented Psychotherapy: Davanloo

Brief adaptation-oriented psychotherapy was developed out of the tradition of psychoanalysis, psychoanalytic psychotherapy, and ego psychology. There is a time limit in brief adaptation-oriented psychotherapy of a maximum of 40 sessions, once a week. The therapeutic goal is to change the major maladaptive pattern of the patient. The therapist cannot change a patient's environment or world but can work with the patient to help change the way in which the patient responds to the environment, that is, to alter the patient's defense organization and character.[22]

Pollack and Horner define adaptation as the integration of beliefs, wishes, needs, and impulses with the demands of the external world and the demands of the superego.[23] The core issue of adaptation is internal and external reality. A knowledge of reality and acting in accordance with it leads to the achievement of a maximum amount of gratification with a minimum amount of pain.[24] The failure of this integration by the ego may result in maladaptive patterns of behavior, which can lead to the formation of personality disorders.

Adaptation takes place under the guidance of the ego. It is an approach that explores ways in which the ego deals with wishes, beliefs, needs, and impulses. As such, brief adaptation-oriented psychotherapy focuses on rigid, enduring patterns of perceiving, relating to, and thinking about the environment that include the following[25]:

1. The wish to be "special," and the belief that one has to accommodate to the other in order to be special. This may lead to a loss of assertiveness and the undermining of the possibility for success.

2. The wish to succeed, which may generate the fear of competitiveness and fear of being envied by others. This can lead to the maladaptive behaviors of passivity, inaction, and dependency.

3. The wish to be taken care of, which leads to feelings of shame and loss of self-esteem. The maladaptive defense can be playing caretaker to everyone else, leading to resentment that one is not being taken care of in return.

4. The fear that one's aggression or self-assertion will lead to the loss of wished-for love. This may lead to withdrawal from conflict as soon as it appears and to overly compliant behavior.

To expose the specific major maladaptive pattern in order to understand ways in which it operates in the present, especially within the patient's important relationships, the questioning of the patient concerns the following: (1) the wish; (2) the beliefs associated with the wish; (3) the consequences of the wish; (4) conflicts between wishes; and (5) the defensive posture brought on by the conflicts.

The method of the therapist is to continually require the patient to look further into the various elements and not to be satisfied by general statements that blur the real nature of the wishes and beliefs. The working hypothesis is that examination of the patient's distortions will enable the patient to understand the maladaptive pattern and correct it.

The goal in this short-term dynamic psychotherapy is to promote the development of the unconscious therapeutic alliance, defined as the patient's spontaneous materials. This information can only be accessed when the characterological armor is punctured. Davanloo emphasizes the need to push at the patient's characterological defenses, including language, body posture and demeanor.[26] Statements are challenged and create the crisis for the patient in the "here and now" with the therapist. Also, there is active focusing of the treatment, rather than the strict use of the patient's free associations as they relate to the core problems. The techniques used to avoid regression and to focus the interaction promote intense patient–therapist interaction, which require constant exploration of the patient's ambivalent feelings toward the therapist.

The therapist's first goal is to quickly challenge the patient's characterological resistances through a systematic analysis of the defenses. The patient responds to this with anxiety and further defenses designed to prevent the therapist from entering his inner world. Concurrently, the patient responds with intense ambivalence: longing for closeness with a strong therapist to help fight the conflicts as well as experience of the therapist as an intruder into his inner world. This ambivalence resonates with the early ambivalence with care givers: the wish for the strong caring parent, versus the fear of an intrusive, controlling parent. By not allowing the patient to regress, unlike psychoanalysis, the responsibility for the therapeutic work is placed on the patient, and both conscious and unconscious therapeutic alliances are enhanced during this process.

Cognitive Therapy: Beck

Cognitive therapy's philosophical origins are rooted to the Greek Stoic philosophers, Zen of Citium (fourth century B.C.), Chrysippus, Cicero, Seneca, Epictetus, and Marcus Aurelius, who emphasized that one's emotions are based on ideas.[27] Cognitive theory derives from the conflict model around core dynamic issues, assuming internal conflict and that psychological disturbances frequently involve habitual errors in thinking or cognition.[28]

Cognitive therapy has been developed and researched by Beck and represents a short-term psychotherapy in which specific cognitions (thoughts or images) or schemata (silent assumptions) account for the onset and persistence of symptoms. The first part of treatment is directed toward reducing symptoms (often anxiety or depression) that are derived from these cognitions.

Cognitive therapy is an active, time-limited, structured approach to depression and other psychiatric disorders. Therapy, on an average, lasts 15 to 20 weeks with sessions scheduled weekly or biweekly depending on the severity of the depression. Follow-up visits are at times recommended during the year, after termination of the regular weekly sessions. Cognitive therapy focuses on "here-and-now" problems with minimal attention paid to childhood or family recollections. The major focus is on exploring the patient's thinking and feeling during therapy and between therapy sessions without interpreting the unconscious.[29]

The following case integrates the central position of Beck's cognitive therapy and nursing diagnoses and nursing interventions.

───── CASE EXAMPLE* OF BECK'S COGNITIVE THERAPY ─────

Mrs. Clara Potter is a 30-year-old white female who had a postpartum depression following the birth of her only son 1 year ago. She was hospitalized for 3 weeks in a psychiatric hospital because of severe depression, taking Sinequan, and was doing well up until 1 month ago. At this time the patient resumed her job as a cook at a church. She reduced her Sinequan to 50 mg from 125 mg at night time. Mrs. Potter at present is dysphoric, sleeps excessively, cannot sustain any enthusiasm, and feels guilty regarding her son. She berates herself as worthless. She admits to vague suicidal ideation but denies having a plan to hurt herself. Assessing Clara Potter from the family perspective, one would consider Mrs. Potter as a part of a greater organization, her family and family of origin. A genogram would be constructed to analyze family dynamics and family issues and themes (Figure 23-1).

Cognitive theory would view Clara Potter as an individual focusing on her alterations in cognitive processing or restructuring. Cognitive therapy is a collaborative process, and this collaboration begins at the first therapy session by sharing expectations and goals for treatment with the patient. The session can begin by eliciting Clara Potter's automatic thoughts about the cognitive therapy treatment ("Can you tell me what thoughts you had about coming here today?"). This introduces the patient to the use of automatic thoughts while eliciting pertinent information.

Cognitive therapy is quite structured as compared to other therapies, with goals for each session determined, a review time at the end of each session, homework assignments and review and particular agendas set. Beck proposed three concepts to explain the theory of depression.[30] These include (1) the cognitive triad; (2) schema; and (3) cognitive distortions. According to Beck depression disturbances are activated by three major patterns by which one views oneself, one's world and one's future in an idiosyncratic way.[31] The negative view of self was quite evident with Clara Potter when she stated "I don't feel good about myself. I'm a disappointment." The person's self-esteem is often poor and depressive patients are often self-critical, as was Mrs. Potter. Patients often regard themselves as undesirable and worthless and tend to reject themselves. Second is the negative view of the world or one's experiences. The patient often sees his life filled with burdens, obstacles, or traumatic situations. The last component is the negative view of the future as evidenced by Clara Potter when she said "I'm afraid I'll never get better." Hopelessness is common, and patients presume that things will never improve. Patients anticipate failure and doom, seeing ahead only hardship and frustration.[32]

Schema is another critical ingredient in the cognitive model, and this was strikingly evident with Clara Potter. The schema the patient holds or employs will determine how she will structure different experiences. One's schema constitutes the basis for differentiating and coding stimuli that one confronts, according to Beck, and these schemata are often recipes for depression.[33]

Schemata are active rules that govern our day-to-day behavior. They might be characterized as an awareness, our conscious. Some schemata are dormant and only govern our behavior under stress. Our goal is to understand the patient's schemata. It can be said that the first goal in cognitive therapy is to understand the patient's distortions. These will be Clara Potter's directional signals, which point to her schemata, and then we can understand

* This case was contributed by Susan M. Franklin.

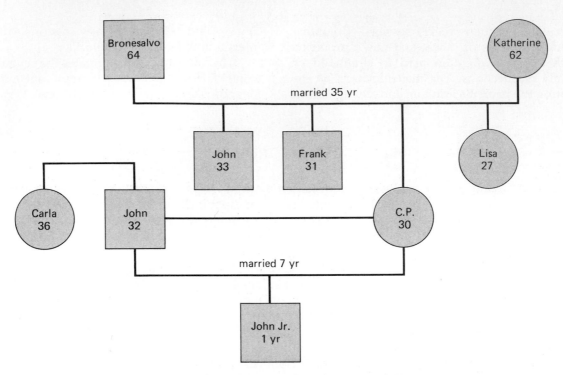

Figure 23-1. Family genogram for Clara Potter.

the rules she lives by. The focus in cognitive therapy is to determine what keeps the patient the way she is, not why she is, and by understanding and interpreting Mrs. Potter's schemata, one can work to help her to find more adaptive ways of dealing with them.

Early in the initial interview, Clara Potter stated that she felt like a failure. She said that she "felt guilty" that she was unable to keep her house clean and care for her son since going back to work last month. She said, "Other people can do it, why can't I?" The schemata Clara Potter lives by are "My worth is dependent on my role as a wife and mother," "You're no good unless you fulfill these roles," and "A woman's place is in the home," etc. These were kept in mind to be tested out throughout the interview and sessions of therapy.

The third concept of depression is idiosyncratic thinking patterns or "faulty information processing," ways in which people distort experiences, which contribute to the depression.[34] Examples of thinking errors evident with Mrs. Potter were personalizing, magnifying, self-blame, and overgeneralizing.

A beginning stage in cognitive therapy is the assessment of why the patient has the problem. The nurse-therapist attempts to train the patient in modifying his cognitions, an educational role, and help the patient restructure negative thoughts. One helps increase the patient's problem-solving repertoire and assists him to identify problems more clearly. There is an actual goal with each session.

Homework is an integral part of cognitive therapy. Homework enhances communication between patient and therapist, and continual homework completion by the patient promotes continued patient improvement after treatment termination.[35] Examples of homework are daily records of dysfunctional thoughts, activity schedules, and bibliotherapy.

Clara Potter will be seen weekly for approximately 15 to 20 sessions.

The goal of cognitive therapy is not just relieving stress but to focus on the cognitive content of the depression. The nurse determines where the distortions come from and what fuels the distortions, such as in the schemata. In cognitive and family therapy one can be said to play the role of investigator. In cognitive therapy one investigates the patient's distortions, schemata, and cognitive content.

NURSING CARE PLAN
Clara Potter

HUMAN RESPONSE

Diminished ability to think or concentrate.

NURSING DIAGNOSIS

Alteration in thought content related to depression as evidenced by suicidal ideation

SHORT-TERM GOALS

1. Patient will not harm self.
2. Patient will have increase in ability to concentrate.
3. Patient will have decrease in suicidal ideation.

LONG-TERM GOALS

1. Depression relieved.
2. Able to think and concentrate clearly.
3. Patient will have minimal suicidal ideations and be able to challenge these dysfunctional thoughts.

INTERVENTIONS

1. Elicit automatic thoughts about self and suicide.
2. Provide weekly review of depression symptoms.
3. Provide options and alternatives.
4. Have patient complete daily dysfunctional thought record.
5. Encourage ventilation of feelings.
6. Assist patient with problem-solving techniques.
7. Suggest healthy coping mechanisms.
8. Involve patient in treatment plan.

HUMAN RESPONSE

Feelings of worthlessness or excessive or inappropriate guilt.

NURSING DIAGNOSIS

Alteration in meaningfulness and self-concept as evidenced by statements of guilt, low self-worth and hopelessness.

SHORT-TERM GOALS

1. Increase patient's self-esteem.
2. Decrease feelings of guilt.

LONG-TERM GOALS

1. Patient develops feelings of self-worth.
2. Self-esteem has increased.

INTERVENTIONS

1. Encourage patient to verbalize positive feelings toward self.
2. Encourage patient to elicit positive automatic thoughts re: self-esteem.

3. Assist patient in learning association between thoughts and feelings.
4. Assist patient to have good personal hygiene.
5. Provide activities that patient can accomplish and succeed in.
6. Give positive feedback on patient's improvements and accomplishments.
7. Dispel feelings of catastrophe.
8. Teach re-attribution technique.
9. Involve patient in treatment plan.

HUMAN RESPONSE

Inability to perform self-care and care of others.

NURSING DIAGNOSIS

Alternation in role relationship: potential for disturbance in family functioning as evidenced by feeling overwhelmed in role of wife and mother.

SHORT-TERM GOALS

1. Patient will increase self-care abilities.

LONG-TERM GOALS

1. Patient will be able to care for self.
2. Patient will be able to fulfill adequately role as wife and mother.
3. Development of stable family relationship and level of previous functioning in family.

INTERVENTIONS

1. Elicit cognitive distortions and automatic thoughts about self-worth, role as wife and mother.
2. Challenge cognitive distortion.
3. Develop replacement imagery.
4. Cognitive rehearsal of coping.
5. Involve husband in treatment plan.
6. Provide patient education about cognitive therapy.

HUMAN RESPONSE

Poor appetite, decreased every day past 30 days.

NURSING DIAGNOSIS

Alteration in nutrition and body requirement related to decrease in seeking and securing food as evidenced by 10-pound weight loss over past 1 month.

SHORT-TERM GOALS

1. Patient will eat one half of each meal daily.

LONG-TERM GOALS

1. Patient will regain lost weight.
2. Patient will be maintained on balanced daily diet.

INTERVENTIONS

1. Obtain diet history to determine food preferences and eating habits.
2. Consult dietary department for additional assessment.
3. Make available favorite foods at meals and snacks.
4. Observe food and fluid intake. Offer fortified liquid nutrition. Have patient monitor intake and output.
5. Weigh patient on regular basis (self-weight).
6. Explore patient's automatic thoughts about eating and appetite.

HUMAN RESPONSE

Hypersomnia

NURSING DIAGNOSIS

Alteration in rest and sleep hygiene as evidenced by early morning awakening and sleeping long hours during day.

SHORT-TERM GOALS

Patient will sleep less during day.

LONG-TERM GOALS

Patient will resume prior sleep patterns.

INTERVENTIONS

1. Obtain previous and present sleep patterns.
2. Provide activity and stimulation during day.
3. Provide information and educate patient on relaxation techniques.
4. Discourage use of caffeine products.
5. Encorage warm milk or decaf before retiring.

EVALUATION

Evaluation of the nursing interventions is essential and occurs during the process of termination. Termination will expectedly be handled by some patients with doubt and some may question their ability to function well once therapy is terminated. Evaluation of treatment is made explicit. Termination begins upon meeting Clara Potter, and she is encouraged to discuss this during therapy. These doubts will be handled by having Mrs. Potter challenge her dysfunctional thoughts regarding termination. Because cognitive therapy has such a strong educational component, it is to be expected that Clara Potter will be better equipped to function because of the many cognitive and behavioral coping skills that have been added to her repertoire. She will be better able to care for herself because of her increased knowledge and understanding of self. If she were treated from the family perspective, her better sense of self would be in relation to her family of origin. Clara Potter will be evaluated on a continual basis in terms of decreases in subjective stress and symptoms and improved adaptations. After the short-term course of therapy, Mrs. Potter will be given cognitive and behavioral techniques to assist her to improved functioning and health.

Feminist Counseling*

Definition

Feminist counseling defies quick definition, for it may take a variety of forms and approaches to mental health problems. Whatever the form, however, it has a common philosophical base. Feminist counseling begins with the clear assumption that problems that are experienced as personal are also social and political. That is, social and political institutions, socialization processes, and cultural expectations are a primary source of psychological dysfunction in women, and active use of this awareness is essential to the counseling process. A primary goal of feminist counseling is the integration of the personal and the political, enabling the client to redefine reality and to expand available choices. This philosophical base is a radical departure from traditional approaches to therapy, which have reinforced the separation of personal problems and social and political issues and have advocated "adjustment" rather than change.

Critical Components

A number of critical components, which are now considered by many to be basic to the therapy process, have emerged from the experiences of feminist counselors. One of the most important is a *consumer orientation*. The mystique and magic long-attributed to therapy have been perpetuated by professionals who have been reluctant to share real information with clients. The consumer orientation, which is increasingly prevalent throughout the health care system, emphasizes the right of consumers to the knowledge necessary to make informed choices about their own health care.

A feminist counselor has a clear responsibility to educate and share information with her clients and with the public at large. A well-informed person is best able to seek the most appropriate source of help, formulate reasonable expectations, ask the right questions, and evaluate outcomes of therapy. Feminist counselors believe that questioning the goals, techniques, process, and outcomes of therapy should be valued and encouraged in clients. The use of written or verbal contracts is common to reduce vague, conflicting, or unrealistic expectations, and a feminist counselor relies heavily on her clients' critical evaluation of the therapy process.*

The emergence of self-help groups, the increased coverage of mental health issues in the public press, and the public validation of clients' rights to demand accountability in other parts of the health system have all contributed to an increasingly informed client group. Nevertheless, the percentage of therapists in the mental health field who possess a consumer orientation to their practice remains small indeed.

Feminist counseling is built upon *a strong belief in people's innate tendency toward growth and change*. There may be a wide variety of approaches that facilitate this growth process, but gimmick therapies and primary reliance on chemical intervention are discouraged. The counseling process itself, in fact, is seen as only one component in the growth process and is relatively ineffective without concomitant changes in other realms of the client's life and environment.

Self-definition is always a predominant issue in feminist counseling. A review of this culture's socialization process clearly demonstrates the fact that most women are trained to define themselves in terms of others—e.g., daughter, wife, lover, mother. Opportunities for women to clearly identify and develop their own individual strengths, talents, capabilities, and interests have been greatly limited. Sex-role stereotyping has, in fact, created formidable barriers to women seeking to move beyond prescribed roles. A major component in feminist approaches to therapy is that of consciousness-raising—enabling clients to view realistically the real and artificial barriers to their self-definition and to their full participation in life.

As a basis for effective and realistic self-definition, one needs first to have a clearly developed sense of trust in one's own feelings, ideas, and abilities, as well as in those of others. Many women, in accepting commonly held female stereotypes, have internalized these views of themselves as inferior and not to be trusted. The more we have complied with stereotypical expectations, the less we rely on ourselves and our perceptions of our needs and feelings. Thus, most women need planned opportunities and encouragement to get in touch with elements of

---

* This section through page 446 is written by Gretchen E. LaGodna.

* For examples of contract use, see S. Adams & M. Orgel, *Through the Mental Health Maze*, Washington, D.C.: Health Research Group, 1975; or *Women and Psychotherapy: A Consumer Handbook*, Federation of Organizations for Professional Women, 1981, Washington, D.C.

self-hatred, anger and rage, sexuality, and other misrepresented parts of themselves. In addition, self-definition almost invariably calls for a reappraisal of one's body image.

The focus on self-definition means that issues that have long been interpreted in traditional ways are deliberately viewed differently. For example, many individual differences and deviations from socially accepted norms are viewed as "maladjustments" by traditional therapists but may be encouraged and reinforced as strengths by feminist counselors. Such things as creativity or independent solitary life-styles might easily fall in this category. Likewise, the role of sexuality in one's life may take a wide variety of healthy forms. Right of choice has never been viewed as a possibility by a great majority of women.

The initial expectations and settings in which therapy takes place have long been recognized as influential in counseling processes and outcomes. This is no less true in feminist counseling. The counselor–client relationship is viewed as an exchange in which both parties have something valuable to offer the other. Since most traditional therapy involves the model of male therapist–female patient, the setting often recreates all the status and power issues present in the larger world. For this reason it is felt by feminist counselors that those working with women should also be female. There is *an effort to minimize status and power differences as much as possible.* Because any situation involving a helper and a person seeking help implies some power differential, this minimal differential should be openly acknowledged and should be used as a learning tool.

The *economics of therapy* has become a recognized social and political issue, and most feminist counselors have sought new ways to make therapy more widely available to all without sacrificing themselves in the process. Consonantly with the consumer orientation, many feminist therapists have established a policy of making the initial session one of evaluation for both counselor and client. Thus, this session is often provided free or at partial cost. The most widely accepted approach to the cost of therapy is the establishment of a sliding fee scale, with an individual determination for each potential client. Some feminist counselors have developed systems in which fees are tied to therapy outcomes. Others have developed alternatives to the traditional economic basis of money for service, such as the trading of skills, services, or time.

The economics of therapy has resulted in a dilemma for many counselors who believe that their skills should be highly valued as well as widely available.

Approaches to Feminist Counseling

Neither nurses nor clients can afford to continue supporting the caveat emptor philosophy of the psychiatric–mental health system. In addition to educating the public, we must do much to reeducate the present mental health professionals, to educate new ones differently, and to develop and support nontraditional alternatives to currently prevailing treatment modalities.

Prevention

A feminist orientation has a primary focus—the *prevention* of psychological dysfunction. Psychiatry, like other branches of medicine, has long been oriented to pathology and illness rather than to prevention and health. Nursing, on the other hand, has a historical tradition of focusing on health and wellness. People should be fully educated about normal growth and development, the handling of stress and life crises, the mental health threatening aspects of society and of the individual's environment, the skills of problem solving, the normalcy of grief, and a myriad of other influential life experiences. Nurses, with a basic holistic approach to clients, have unlimited potential to contribute to the prevention of crisis and mental illness. With a traditional focus on patient teaching, nurses can use these skills very specifically in the counseling process.

Group Approach

The gathering of people in small groups has been a critical factor in the origin and growth of the women's movement in this country. Consciousness-raising groups have been recognized as powerful change agents and necessary supportive networks for women questioning the impact of social expectations on their lives. What has been learned through the experience of consciousness-raising has provided important guidelines for the utilization of the small group as a feminist counseling approach. In fact, the *small group approach* is felt by many to be the most effective tool in feminist counseling. The small group is the only modality in which women have the opportunity to validate personal experiences, meet their needs of affiliation, and raise their social awareness. Most important, the group provides a supportive network in which to explore painful experiences and to change behavior.

As women share and compare their life experiences in a group context, it becomes impossible to continue to support notions of personal "problems" or inadequacies. Instead, as the social and external origins of such problems become apparent, women begin to trust their own perceptions, assert their own needs, and explore their own potential. A feminist counseling group can be therapeutic without the assumption that all the participants are "sick." The feminist counselor, then, works toward the obsolescence of her role of responsibility in the group.

Some small groups are structured around *skills training*, such as self-defense, assertiveness, meditation, training in creative arts (music, dance, art), and other kinds of specific developmental efforts. These efforts are particularly significant, for they often develop untapped potential or new behaviors that have previously been discouraged in women. As a woman's behavior repertoire and skills increase, her self-concept also changes in the direction of a more realistic self-appraisal.

Body Image

Traditional approaches to therapy have done little to bridge the mind/body gap or to enable women to develop a *more positive and realistic body image*. Nurses are perhaps the one professional group in the mental health field who are educated to be acutely aware of the intimate relationship between mind and body. The intricate balance between physiological and psychological processes has long been a critical basis of nursing practice, and nurses approach their clients fully expecting that an imbalance in one will have reverberations in the other. As Ruth Wu describes so clearly, the steady state of human adaptive systems requires both behavioral stability and physiologic homeostasis.[36]

Unfortunately, there has developed a wide gap in the mental health field between those within the medical model who focus almost exclusively on the physiological aspects of emotional problems and those who deal exclusively with the cognitive realm. A number of feminist counselors have taken the lead in insisting upon an *integration of the cognitive, behavioral, emotional, and physical aspects in therapy*. Anne Kent Rush, a pioneer in body therapy, points out that since a great deal of the oppression of women has been biologic, body therapy techniques are critical to feminism. She states:

As a result of centuries of negative programming, we have a great deal of healing to do on our bodies and our body images. . . . The term *body therapy** does not mean the exclusion of mental aspects of the personality but refers to the inclusion of physical aspects.[37]

Use of a combination of biofeedback, bioenergetics, body work, and other specific techniques is designed to help people reintegrate the psychological and physical. By clearly focusing on both the psychological and physical areas, the client gains an awareness of her internal bodily cues, begins to trust them more, and learns to use them in responding to external stress and problems.

Political and Social Change

An important principle espoused by most feminist therapists derives from the belief that the *personal is also political*, and that there are no solely personal solutions to the mental health problems of women. The principle that emerges is that a feminist counselor must actively work for political and social change in those institutions that have controlled and shaped women's lives in unhealthy ways. Just as feminism encourages diversity in the development of people's lives, feminist counselors have followed diverse paths in the pursuit of social and political change, from both within and outside the existing system. The nurse who is also a feminist counselor is in a unique position to identify discriminatory and growth-limiting practices in the health care system and to take steps leading to constructive change.

The approaches to counseling used by feminist counselors often vary widely in technique, emphasis, and setting, but the underlying assumptions and the outcomes sought remain constant. The primary goal of feminist counseling is always *change* rather than adjustment.

---

* Italics added.

Summary

The short-term individual psychotherapy models have to be understood within the context of the goal of the patient. Several types of brief psychodynamic therapy were discussed. The psychodynamic therapies organize around core dynamic issues derived from the psychoanalytic system. This system assumes a model of internal conflict and a resolution of these conflicts, especially the oedipal conflict. The therapy forces separation and individualization. The women's movement and the development of feminist counseling have gone hand in hand, and many nurses in independent practice are feminist counselors. Issues discussed as critical to feminist counseling include a consumer orientation, the integration of personal and political aspects, a reevaluation of the influence of social and cultural expectations, an emphasis on self-definition, and an integration of cognitive, behavioral, emotional, and physical aspects in therapy.

Questions

1. Briefly define several short-term psychotherapy models.
2. Compare and contrast these models.
3. Compare and contrast feminist counseling with traditional counseling.
4. Survey a group of individuals about their criteria for selecting a therapist and solicit their thoughts and reactions regarding a feminist nurse counselor versus a psychiatrist or psychologist.

REFERENCES AND SUGGESTED READINGS

1. Sullivan, H. S. *The Psychiatric Interview.* New York: Norton, 1954.
2. Frances, A., & Clarkin, J. F. No treatment as the prescription of choice. *Archives of General Psychiatry,* 1981, *38,* 542–545.
3. Ursano, R. J., & Dressler, D. M. Brief versus long-term psychotherapy: A treatment decision. *Journal of Nervous & Mental Disease,* 1974, *159,* 164–171.
4. Ursano, R. J., & Dressler, D. M. Brief psychotherapy: Clinician attitude and organizational design. *Comprehensive Psychiatry,* 1977, *18,* 55–60.
5. Marmor, J. The psychotherapeutic process: Common denominators in diverse approaches. In J. K. Zeig (Ed.), *The Evolution of Psychotherapy.* New York: Brunner/Mazel, 1987, p. 169.
6. Ibid.
7. Balint, M., Ornstein, P., & Balint, E. *Focal Psychotherapy.* Philadelphia: Lippincott, 1972.
8. Malan, D. H. *A Study of Brief Psychotherapy.* New York: Plenum, 1975.
9. Ibid.
10. Ursano, R. J., & Hales, R. E. Brief individual psychotherapies. *American Journal of Psychiatry,* 1986, *143,* 1507–1517.
11. Sifneos, P. *Short-Term Psychotherapy and Emotional Crisis.* Cambridge, Mass.: Harvard University Press, 1972.
12. Ursano & Hales, op. cit.
13. Ibid.
14. Mann, J. Time-Limited Psychotherapy. Cambridge, Mass.: Harvard University Press, 1973, ix.
15. Schecter, D. E., Symonds, M., & Bernstein, I. The development of the concept of time in children, *Journal of Nervous Mental Diseases,* 1955, *121,* 301–305.
16. Ibid.
17. Bonaparte, M. Time and the unconscious. *International Journal of Psychoanalysis,* 1940, *21,* 427.
18. Mann, J., op. cit., p. 7.
19. Bonaparte, op. cit.
20. Mann, op. cit., p. 10.
21. Mann, T., & Goldman, R. *A Casebook in Time-Limited Psychotherapy.* New York: McGraw Hill, 1982.
22. Pollack, J., & Horner, A. Brief adaptation-oriented psychotherapy. In A. Winston (Ed.), *Short-Term Dynamic Psychotherapy.* Washington, D.C.: American Psychiatric Press, 1985, pp. 42–60.
23. Ibid.
24. Hartmann, H. [Ego psychology and the problem

of adaptation] (D. Rapaport, trans). New York: International Universities Press, 1958.

25. Pollack and Horner, op. cit., pp. 47–48.

26. Davanloo, H. *Basic Principles and Techniques in Short-Term Dynamic Psychotherapy*. New York: Spectrum, 1978.

27. Beck, A. T. Cognitive therapy, In *Comprehensive Textbook of Psychiatry*, 4th ed. H. I. Kaplan & B. J. Sadock (Eds.), Baltimore, Md.: Williams & Wilkins, 1985, 1432–1438.

28. Beck, A. T. Cognitive therapy, In *The Evolution of Psychotherapy*, J. K. Zeig (Ed.), New York: Brunner/Mazel, 1987, pp. 149–163.

29. Ibid.

30. Freeman, A., & Greenwood, V. *Cognitive Therapy: Applications in Psychiatric and Medical Settings*. New York: Human Sciences Press, 1987.

31. Beck, A. T. *Depression*. Philadelphia: University of Pennsylvania Press, 1967.

32. Ibid, p. 255.

33. Beck, A. T. *Cognitive Therapy of Depression*. New York: Guilford Press, 1979, p. 13.

34. Ibid., pp. 14–16.

35. Ibid., p. 272.

36. Wu, R. *Behavior and Illness*. Englewood Cliffs, N.J.: Prentice-Hall, 1973, p. 90.

37. Mander, A. V., & Rush, A. K. *Feminism as Therapy*. New York: Random House, and Berkeley, Calif.: The Bookworks, 1974, pp. 55–56.

Chapter 24

Crisis Theory and Intervention

Ann Wolbert Burgess

Chapter Objectives

The students successfully attaining the goals of this chapter will be able to:

- Define an emotional crisis.
- Give examples of six classes of emotional crises.
- Outline the principles of crisis intervention.

Nurses are in daily contact with people who are in crisis. The patient who is hospitalized is in a dispositional crisis because his normal life-style is disrupted. A family member dealing with news of the death of a loved one is facing a traumatic crisis. The stress of hospitalization or the possible loss of job can predispose a person to a situational crisis. Crisis is a time when a person can either gain strength psychologically or regress to a mentally ill health level. Gerald Caplan, a crisis theorist, has defined an emotional crisis as follows[1]:

Crisis . . . [is] a psychological disequilibrium in a person who confronts a hazardous circumstance that for him constitutes an important problem which he can for the time being neither escape nor solve with his customary problem-solving resources.

Psychiatric nurses have the opportunity to practice primary prevention of mental illness specifically by intervening in patients' crisis situations. It thus becomes crucial that nurses be able to diagnose crisis situations and to plan appropriate interventions.

CRISIS THEORY

Over the past several years, social scientists and mental health clinicians have been studying the effects of crisis on individuals, families, and communities. Crisis theory traces its historical roots back to the work of Eric Lindemann, who designed a program to prevent unresolved grieving among survivors and relatives of those who had perished in the Coconut Grove fire of 1943.[2] Gerald Caplan and his colleagues continued the work and research of Lindemann

449

through the fifties and sixties.[3] The work of nursing leaders Aguilera and Messick in the field of crisis theory development has further advanced the state of knowledge into the eighties.[4]

The Coping Process

An understanding of crisis theory must begin with the concept of homeostatic balance and the relationship of coping processes to stable psychological functioning. The principle of homeostasis is borrowed from physiology and is defined as the need to preserve stable chemical or electrolyte balances within the body necessary to sustain life. When these balances are upset, self-regulatory mechanisms are triggered that help to return these balances to healthy levels for the individual. Crisis theory is based on this principle applied to psychological functioning.[5]

For each individual, there exists a reasonably consistent balance between affective and cognitive experience. However, this homeostatic balance may vary considerably from person to person. The primary characteristic of this balance is its stability for the individual, a stability that is "normal" for that person and that becomes a frame of reference against which to evaluate changes in the person's psychological functioning. A healthy homeostatic balance requires stable psychological functioning with a minimum of dysphoric affect, the maintenance of a reasonable cognitive perspective on experience, and the retention of problem-solving skills.

However, each and every day, experiences are encountered in which homeostatic equilibrium is disrupted, and negative and uncomfortable affect results. Often this increase in affective discomfort is accompanied by diminished cognitive capabilities. Caplan defines these experiences as "emotionally hazardous situations."[6] An emotionally hazardous situation occurs when a shift or change in the individual's psychosocial environment alters relationships with others or expectations of the self in ways perceived to be negative. The rise in stress that results from emotionally hazardous situations motivates the individual to bring into play coping mechanisms or problem-solving behaviors that help to reestablish the usual and stable homeostatic balance for the individual and the dysphoric affect is consequently diminished or eliminated.

Coping processes are those psychological self-regulatory mechanisms that, when used by the individual, facilitate a return to homeostatic balance after the impact of an emotionally hazardous situation. As such, they are crucial to the emotional well-being of the individual and are essential in maintaining stable functioning. Coping begins at the moment of birth and continues until the interruption of death. Most individuals through development and experience learn a repertoire of coping behaviors that are used as responses to various types of emotionally hazardous situations. Coping mechanisms, which encompass a wide range of behaviors, are defined as:

Those maneuvers used by individuals to reduce, to control, or to avoid unpleasant emotions in order to re-establish a state of homeostatic balance and facilitate return to normal functioning for the person.[7]

Coping behaviors occur at various levels of awareness of the individual using them, and these may be used simultaneously as responses to stressful situations. Perlman describes three basic levels at which coping behaviors are used: (1) the unconscious level of coping that includes mechanisms of ego defense; (2) the preconscious coping mechanisms, which are those almost automatic responses to stress that can be quickly brought to conscious awareness; and (3) the conscious coping behaviors that are in full awareness and that are used selectively as the result of an active decision process.[8] In crisis intervention, because of its focal and time-limited nature, interventions are planned primarily at the levels of conscious and preconscious coping.

By the time adulthood is reached, most individuals have developed a range of coping behaviors, some of which are adaptive and some that are less than adaptive. Maladaptive or immature coping responses are typically used in those situations in which the individual feels vulnerable. At best, coping is the process of mastery of a particular problematic situation. At worst, coping behaviors serve primarily to protect a vulnerable sense of self without mastery of the situation. Coping behaviors cannot be dichotomized into categories of adaptive or maladaptive; they should be viewed as a continuum with behaviors manifesting various levels of adaptiveness depending on the person and the situation. When the individual encounters a situation in which there is significant psychological threat and great personal vulnerability, coping behaviors are more likely to be self-protective than oriented toward mastery.

Responses to Stress

Stress, as defined by Caplan, is a condition in which there is a marked discrepancy between the demands made on an individual and the individual's capacity to respond, the consequences of which will be harmful to the individual's future.[9] The term *demands* refers to the loss or the threatened loss of appropriate levels and quality of essential information and energy.

Four interrelated phases are used by Caplan to describe an individual's response to a stressful event.[10] Phase 1 is behavior that changes the stressful environment or enables the individual to escape from it. Phase 2 is behavior to acquire new capabilities for it. Phase 3 is intrapsychic behavior to defend against dysphoric emotional arousal. Phase 4 is intrapsychic behavior to come to terms with the event and its sequelae by internal readjustment.

Phase 1

The task in Phase 1 is to act directly on the source of threat in order to reduce it and its consequences or to find ways of physically escaping. This behavior requires being goal-directed and problem-solving-oriented in the world of reality.

Combating this task may cause deterioration of the person's usual coping skills and cognitive problem-solving capacities. The magnitude of this change is related to the intensity of emotional arousal and dysphoria. What appear to occur are disorders in attention, scanning, information collecting, access to relevant memories that provide association for significant meaning to perceptions, judgment, planning, the capacity to implement plans, and the capacity to evaluate feedback. The result is that the individual's usual orderly process of externally oriented instrumental ego function is disrupted. This occurs at a time when it is important that he or she be able to operate at the maximum to solve the crisis. Although there is no clear understanding of this condition, Caplan believes that the cognitive deficit is linked with the neuroendocrine processes of emotional arousal, which initially stimulate improved cognitive functioning but, above a fairly low threshold, cause increasing disorganization.[11]

A second symptom of stress is a deterioration in clarity of the individual's self-concept. Not only does the person lose orderly access to memories that lend meaning to perceptions of the outer world but he also loses access to memories that help evaluate the self-representational system.

The capacity for effective problem solving is influenced by the person's expectation that he is likely to succeed in achieving at least part of the desired goals. This capacity depends on remembering previous successes in situations of similar stress. This memory provides the thrust to move ahead and by necessity requires positive feedback and support.

Inherent in problem solving is perseverance and an awareness that a certain level of pain and discomfort is likely to be involved in the task. Also, there must be the realization that others are capable of tolerating the discomfort.

Phase 2

A stressful situation overburdens a person's normal response capabilities. A great deal of work has been done in the area of anticipatory education and training in generic skills to assist people to operate effectively in situations of frustration and confusion where novel responses are necessary for unexpected problems. People also can be trained in the wide range of discomforts that may be experienced. Such training assists people to withstand the affective discomfort that stressful situations impose.

The use of social support is highly regarded by Caplan in crisis management situations. This support operates as a set of auxiliary ego functions for the stressed individual.[12]

Phase 3

Emotional arousal and associated dysphoria, such as conscious feelings of anxiety, anger, grief, and depression, are inevitable complications of psychological stress. They are likely to be reduced by externally directed action that the individual believes will result in reducing the threat or evading it or its consequences. However, the emotional discomfort will usually also require some form of direct relief. This is accomplished by the use of usual coping mechanisms, the most frequently used being denial, selective inattention, and isolation. When these ego defenses are working, they reduce not only the dysphoria but the associated neuroendocrine changes. Whether or not this process helps master the stress event will depend on the degree to which the situation of increased comfort, and probably also of increased cognitive effectiveness, is then used by the person to further efforts to change and improve the environmental situation.[13]

Phase 4

The nature of the intrapsychic work that needs to be accomplished by an individual in coming to terms with a threat or loss has been extensively discussed in the literature. This process may take considerable time, and it represents the end goal of emotional congruence experienced by the individual in terms of thinking of the stressful event and managing his feelings and behaviors.

Corollaries of Crisis Theory

Beyond this overview of crisis theory, there are a number of corollaries to crisis theory that are helpful in understanding emotional crises in more depth and that provide a foundation for crisis intervention. Ten basic corollaries identified by Baldwin are as follows[14]*:

1. Because each individual's tolerance for stress is idiosyncratic and finite, emotional crises have no relationship per se to psychopathology and occur even among the well-adjusted.

Emotional crises are more or less normative events that are experienced by almost everyone at some point during the life-span. Each individual has a specific tolerance for stress depending on general level of adjustment, the internal and external resources available to that person, the flexibility of learned coping mechanisms, and the degree and type of stress being experienced. Emotional crises may be experienced by the well-adjusted when stressful situations are encountered in particular areas of personal vulnerabilities (i.e., in those areas where coping behaviors are weak or absent) at critical points in time. It is true that the less well-adjusted individual is likely to experience more emotional crises than those with better levels of adjustment. However, an individual experiencing an emotional crisis cannot be assumed to

be significantly maladjusted or to manifest psychopathology based solely on the existence of an emotional crisis.

2. Emotional crises are self-limiting events in which crisis resolution, either adaptive or maladaptive, takes place within an average period of 4 to 6 weeks.

When an emotional crisis occurs, the individual becomes highly vulnerable as a result of the intense state of unpleasant affective arousal, and the question in responding to emotional crises is not whether the crisis will be resolved; it will. The only question is whether the crisis will be resolved in an adaptive manner that will contribute to greater emotional maturity and stability of functioning in the future, or whether it will be resolved in a maladaptive fashion that will render the individual more vulnerable and prone to more crises of a similar nature in the future. Caplan has stated that the vast majority of crises are resolved within a period of 4 to 6 weeks because in most instances the individual cannot tolerate a crisis state for longer than that period of time.[15] Even regressive, maladaptive, or neurotic coping behaviors share the quality of partially reducing stress (without resolving the situation) and therefore may be learned in lieu of more adaptive coping behaviors if the resources necessary for adaptive crisis-resolution are unavailable or unused.

3. During a crisis state, psychological defenses are weakened or absent, and the individual has cognitive and/or affective awareness of material previously well defended against and less accessible.

By definition, an individual experiencing an emotional crisis is not coping effectively with a present stressful situation. Coping occurs at several levels[16]; and during a crisis, failure to cope may be present at any or all levels. One result of coping failure is enhanced awareness of feelings and memories from the past that are helpful in understanding the crisis at a psychodynamic level. Often these data are not accessible to the individual, and by extension to the therapist, when that individual is not in a crisis state. The individual, because of this heightened affective and cognitive awareness, has an opportunity to deal with these past experiences as part of the crisis resolution process. However, in many instances, motivation during the crisis state is directed to return to a precrisis state in which this

---

* Reprinted with permission.

material is again suppressed or repressed rather than to using the accessibility of this material afforded by the crisis to work toward a deeper and lasting resolution.

4. During a crisis state, the individual has enhanced capacity for both cognitive and affective learning because of the vulnerability of this state and the motivation produced by emotional disequilibrium.

During a crisis state, the individual needs support and help, often manifested as increased dependency, and these needs must be understood and met as part of the crisis intervention and resolution process.[17,18] Because of the distress experienced by the individual in crisis, there is an enhanced capacity to learn new coping behaviors or problem-solving skills and to modify previously learned but maladaptive coping responses in the direction of increased adaptiveness. The net result of increased dependency and the motivation produced by painful emotional disequilibrium is an enhanced receptivity to help from others and the capacity to learn at both cognitive and affective levels more quickly than during noncrisis states.[19] Learning that occurs during a crisis state tends to last, and those coping behaviors adopted during the crisis tend to be repeated during stressful situations in the future. It is this enhanced capacity for learning that represents both the danger and the opportunity that are frequently associated with emotional crises.

5. Adaptive crisis resolution is frequently a vehicle for resolving underlying conflicts that have in part determined the emotional crisis and/or that interfere with the crisis resolution process.

Because of the affective and cognitive awareness that often accompanies crisis states, unresolved conflicts and traumas from the past that have been reactivated by a present experience can be identified and at least partially resolved as part of the crisis intervention process. Often these reactivated experiences create the disproportionately intense affective states that determine the failure to cope with a present situation. Hoffman and Remmel have defined these reactivated but unresolved experiences that are part of many emotional crises as the *precipitant* (in contrast to the precipitating event).[20] The precipitant surfaces when there is currently experienced a situation that is somehow analogous to a past trauma or conflict, or

when there is anticipation of such an experience. As part of helping the individual to respond more effectively to a present situation, the individual is helped to face and resolve the underlying conflicts or traumas that are present. Frequently, fear of facing a present stressful situation directly is determined by fear of facing past traumas or conflicts. It is this fear that is often found to motivate and support use of maladaptive coping responses. Without an understanding of and response to the precipitant of the crisis, adaptive resolution may be significantly impeded, and an opportunity for personal growth and maturation of the individual may be lost.

6. A small external influence during a crisis state can produce disproportionate change in a short period of time when compared to therapeutic change that occurs during noncrisis states.

Because of the vulnerability and receptivity to help produced by a crisis state, the individual in crisis has an opportunity to move therapeutically at a faster pace than would be possible when a crisis state is not present. The result is that gains made during crisis therapy may be disproportionately great when compared to therapeutic movement occurring during noncrisis states. Rapoport summarizes this aspect of crisis therapy succinctly when she states: "A little help, rationally directed and purposefully focused at a strategic time, is more effective than more extensive help given at a period of less emotional accessibility."[21] However, for such gains to be made, the individual in crisis must accept the opportunity for change that is brought by the crisis state. If this opportunity is not used effectively for growth, a disproportionate change in the direction of maladaptive learning may occur that will require great therapeutic effort to modify once the crisis state has passed. It is this capacity for rapid and disproportionate adaptive change (and the prevention of similar maladaptive change) that is part of the economy of crisis therapy from the perspective of both therapist and client.

7. Resolution of emotional crisis is not necessarily determined by previous experience or character structure but rather is shaped by current and perhaps unique sociopsychological influences operating in the present.

In crisis intervention, the resolution is not

necessarily determined by the past. When an individual is in crisis, previously used responses to stress are either inadequate or ineffective as coping behaviors. Often these responses are characterological in nature and part of the character armor of that individual. These may be long-standing and deeply ingrained patterns of behavior that may ordinarily be quite strong and very rigid. However, because these responses are not effective in the present crisis situation, preexisting characterological patterns do not determine the outcome of crisis resolution or the behaviors that bring such resolution. It is the individual's social and psychological resources and the adequacy of help received during this period of personal vulnerability and psychological defenselessness that are primary determinants of crisis resolution rather than past learning or character structure per se. Further, in those individuals with strong characterological defenses, it is during a crisis state that change must be facilitated quickly before that awareness is again sealed over and accessibility to psychodynamic material is lost and with it the stress that is a primary motivation for change. In such individuals, it is sometimes more therapeutically economical to attempt change only during crises when there is emotional openness and motivation for change.[22]

8. Inherent in every emotional crisis is an actual or anticipated loss to the individual that must be reconciled as part of the crisis resolution process.

In assessing emotional crises, it is assumed that there is an actual or potential loss to the individual that must be conceptualized and responded to as part of the therapeutic strategy for crisis intervention and resolution.[23] Strickler and LaSor are more specific in stating that in every crisis there is a loss involving: (1) self-esteem; (2) nurturance; or (3) sex-role mastery.[24] They believe that one of these losses is usually dominant in any given crisis, although elements of all three may be present to some extent. At another level, there is additional loss to the individual as part of adaptive crisis resolution. As part of the new learning that occurs during crisis intervention, there is loss of old and familiar, albeit maladaptive, responses to stress or to meeting personal needs that are given up as growth occurs. Identifying and reconciling these losses as part of the crisis resolution process reduces resistance to change. The process of adaptive change involves risk to the individual, and

to the extent that losses to the individual can be responded to as part of the process of change, the risks of growth can be more readily accepted.

9. Every emotional crisis is an interpersonal event involving at least one significant other person who is represented in the crisis situation directly, indirectly, or symbolically.

An emotional crisis is never a completely intrapsychic phenomenon even though the locus of stress that precipitated the crisis may be primarily internal. Emotional crises always have an interpersonal dimension that must be assessed and understood prior to the intervention and resolution process. The significant others involved in the crisis may be from the present or from the past or both. These individuals may be directly or indirectly involved in the present situation. Sometimes significant others are part of the precipitant of the crisis and help to understand the relationship of past traumas or unresolved conflicts to a present stressor.[25] At other times, significant others are represented psychodynamically as introjects, or in the form of values or behaviors that have been adopted by the individual in crisis from a significant other. In these instances, others exist primarily within the individual in crisis at a symbolic level but remain powerful determinants of the crisis that must be understood before an effective intervention can be made. Identification and clarification of the interpersonal dimension of an emotional crisis are essential to effective crisis assessment and necessary to the plan for adaptive crisis resolution.

10. Effective crisis resolution prevents future crises of a similar nature by removing vulnerabilities from the past and by increasing the individual's repertoire of available coping skills that can be used in such situations.

In many instances, crisis intervention and adaptive resolution have past, present, and future components. The primary emphasis in crisis intervention is resolving a present problematic situation that the individual is unable to cope with effectively. However, in order to resolve such a situation, the precipitant of the crisis must be identified when present and worked through as part of helping the individual in crisis to cope with the problem situation that has reactivated these past conflicts or traumas. There is selective attention to the past in crisis intervention in response to the precipitant. Yet, response to and work with the precipitant that links present to past also has future connotations. As the precipitant is resolved, the decreased vulnerability to that precipitant allows the individual to experience future similar situations more easily. Further, the new coping skills that are a key aspect of resolving the present situation also become a buffer against future crises of a similar nature. Optimally, the individual who has successfully and adaptively resolved a crisis will experience future similar situations only as emotionally hazardous situations for which there are available and effective coping behaviors that can be used to reestablish homeostatic balance quickly.

CRISIS MODEL FOR ASSESSMENT, DIAGNOSIS, AND INTERVENTION

Crisis work involves five major component parts that together create an in-depth understanding and intervention of the crisis. Each of these components in the crisis model is discussed below along with a rationale relating it to the tenets of crisis theory. See also Table 24-1 for a summary of this model.

The Therapeutic Alliance

People experiencing stress of crisis proportions often feel frightened and vulnerable. Part of establishing a therapeutic alliance is to help the individual feel safe, secure, and that he or she will be listened to with respect. The nurse directly provides or helps mobilize appropriate support for the client. In addition, the nurse helps the patient to restore a realistic perspective of the crisis situation and to define viable options or courses of action available. The personal resources of the patient are assessed and identified as essential to the development of adaptive response to the crisis.

Assessment of the Emotional Crisis

The Precipitating Event
Crisis theory is based on the interaction between an individual and a stressful situation. Understanding in detail the precipitating event that

TABLE 24-1. CRISIS MODEL FOR ASSESSMENT, DIAGNOSIS, AND INTERVENTION

I. The Therapeutic Alliance
  A. Anchor for safety
  B. Establish rapport
  C. Elicit personal resources
II. Assessment of the Emotional Crisis
  A. The precipitating event
  B. Psychodynamic issues in the crisis
  C. Present coping responses
  D. Precrisis functioning
  E. Related areas of patient assessment
III. Diagnosis and Intervention by Level of Crisis
  A. Class 1: Dispositional Crisis
  B. Class 2: Transitional Crisis
  C. Class 3: Traumatic Stress Crisis
  D. Class 4: Developmental Crisis
  E. Class 5: Crises Reflecting Psychopathology
  F. Class 6: Psychiatric Emergencies
IV. Therapeutic Crisis Work
  A. Explore the crisis event through thoughts, feelings, and actions
  B. Conceptualize dynamic meaning of the crisis
  C. Unlink the sensory and perceptual components of the crisis
  D. Process the cognitive component of the crisis
  E. Store the crisis event in past memory
V. Termination
  A. Review of coping and adaptive behaviors postcrisis
  B. Discussion of available resources
  C. Validation of the meaning of the crisis intervention

resulted in a failure to cope and an emotional crisis is a necessary part of crisis assessment. This information helps to structure and focus the intervention process. It cannot be assumed that the patient is aware of or understands the relationship of the precipitating event to the emotional crisis, and creating this understanding may be an important aspect of helping the patient organize the crisis experience. Several aspects of the precipitating event warrant closer scrutiny and exploration by the nurse.

Time and Place of the Precipitating Event. Sometimes patients easily define the time and place of the event that precipitated the crisis. However, this is not always the case, and in many instances the patient has not defined the event that evolved into the crisis or its emotional meaning. Defining the event and placing it in the framework of the patient's recent experience is important. Sometimes the event is quite subtle and is difficult to detect even by a skilled therapist. However, there is always a situational trigger for the crisis that, when conceptualized, is helpful to both patient and therapist in understanding the crisis.

For patients with little or no psychological-mindedness or capacity for insight, defining the time and place of the precipitating event may be difficult. However, with such patients, examining emotional cause-and-effect relationships can be very helpful and often is part of the psychological education that becomes part of the crisis assessment process. At other times, the precipitating event will not be evident even with close scrutiny of the patient's recent past. In such instances, the course of crisis intervention is initiated on the basis of available information, and it is not uncommon that the precipitating event becomes clearer during the course of crisis resolution.

Interpersonal Dimensions of the Problem Situation. It is extremely important for the nurse to assess not only the time and place of the precipitating event but also the interpersonal parameters of the situation. Sometimes significant others from the past are involved in the present crisis because conflicts or traumas associated with them are reactivated by a present situation. The interpersonal dimension of a crisis often represents an actual loss or potential loss to the patient. It is the defending against such losses, or attempting to replace them, that determines many maladaptive coping responses to problem situations and precipitates the crisis.

Affective Response to the Precipitating Event. Reacting to the precipitating event, the patient experiences disruption of homeostatic balance. This disruption is characterized by a rise of unpleasant or dysphoric affect that intensifies with time because there are no effective coping responses available to reduce it. The longer this situation (i.e., the crisis) continues, the more intense this disruptive affect becomes and the more incapable the patient becomes in retaining perspective of the situation, defining viable courses of action, and mobilizing problem-solving or coping skills. It is frequently very helpful early in the crisis assessment process to encourage the patient to express such affect and

thereby defuse (at least temporarily) some of the intensity of the crisis.

However, the nature of the dysphoria being experienced by the patient is also important in crisis assessment. It helps to determine whether any emergency measures must be taken to ensure patient welfare. The patient may be experiencing guilt, anger, anxiety, or depression, or may have already decompensated. The nature of patient stress is diagnostic and often reflects a particular type of vulnerability that has been instrumental in producing the crisis. The nurse needs to elicit a description of the affective experience of the crisis, in the patient's own words for future reflection during the crisis work.

Patient Request. In crisis intervention, the patient seeks the help of the nurse with often implicit expectations for the helping process. The nature of the help that the patient seeks (i.e., the psychological request) may be directly or indirectly communicated and may be healthy or quite regressive in nature. Assessing this request, always present in a patient contact, is of importance in understanding the crisis and the patient's response to a particular stressful situation and in planning an appropriate intervention process (see Chapter 12).

If the patient's request is not accurately understood and acknowledged early in the assessment process, there is a much higher dropout rate from therapy. The nurse, in acknowledging the patient's request, must make a decision about whether to grant it. If the therapeutic decision is not to grant this request, this becomes an area of negotiation and part of the assessment transaction between therapist and patient. Patient requests may be summarized as follows:

1. Request for support. Patients frequently request support from the nurse, but support may take a number of forms: control (please take over), reality contact (help me know I am real), succorance (take care of me), personal contact (always be there), confession (take away my guilt), and ventilation (let me get it off my chest).
2. Request for therapy. In those patients who are directly or indirectly requesting therapy, two different types of requests are encountered: clarification (help me put things in perspective), and intrapsychic (help me deal with my past).
3. Request for an authority figure. Several

types of requests are indicated when patients seek an authority figure: medical (I need a physician), administrative (I need your legal power), social (do it for me), advice (tell me what to do), and education (teach me what I need to know).

4. Other requests. Sometimes patients make requests outside of these major areas, two of which are not uncommon: community triage (tell me where I can get what I need) and nothing (I want nothing).

There may be a hierarchy noted to the requests. If the initial request of the patient is defined and responded to effectively, there is a shift that is progressive (i.e., from sicker to healthier for that patient). On the other hand, failure to respond to the patient's request may lead to subtle negotiations over regressive requests that move from healthier to sicker for that patient. How the initial request is handled, even when presented quite indirectly, is often influential in determining the outcome of crisis intervention.

The Psychodynamic Issues in the Crisis

Many emotional crises are determined, at least in part, by unresolved conflicts or traumas from the past that are reactivated or brought again to awareness by a particular event. The psychodynamic component of the crisis, the precipitant, is frequently instrumental in producing a failure to cope and will impede adaptive crisis resolution unless addressed as part of the crisis intervention process.

Although not all crises have psychodynamic determinants, most do involve antecedent factors reactivated by the precipitating event. When this is the case, the patient experiences an emotional overreaction that is often surprising in its intensity. The precipitating event has activated a dormant vulnerability of the patient, and the intensity of the affect produced is often overwhelming and confusing. When this occurs, usual coping behaviors become inoperable, and the patient may use coping responses that are orientated more toward ego-protection than toward mastery of the situation.[26]

It is the task of the nurse, when a precipitant is detected, to help the patient to respond adaptively to the present situation while using the situation simultaneously to address and work through the reactivated conflicts and traumas from the past.

Detecting and working through the precipitant is perhaps the most challenging aspect of crisis intervention. The precipitant may be activated in two basic ways: (1) by an experience that is somehow *directly analogous* to a past conflict or trauma; or (2) by an event that activates *anticipatory fear* of experiencing a past trauma again. When the latter is the case, coping responses are mobilized to avoid anticipated pain and to provide protection of the self.

There are a number of ways that the nurse can explore the crisis situation for clues to the precipitant. Some of the strategies are the following:

1. Defining similarities between current patient affect and affect recalled from past painful experiences (When have you felt this way before?).
2. Exploring situational similarities between the present experience and past experiences that remain painful and unresolved (When has this type of experience happened before?).
3. Detecting specific types of interactions that remind the patient of past pain (Who are you reminded of in this situation?).
4. Time of onset of the crisis as an anniversary reaction (Is this time of the year reminiscent of a past stressful experience?).
5. Determining the worst possible outcome of the present situation and relating it to past experiences (What would be the worst outcome now and has such an outcome happened before?).
6. Linking the patient's present coping behavior for possible secondary gain and comparing to past unresolved issues (How is your current response helping you and has that helped in the past?).
7. Reviewing past maladaptive coping behaviors (Have you had prior difficulty dealing with stress?).
8. Examining the present problem within the context of the patient's fear of being similar to a significant person with whom there is an ambivalent relationship (Who have you known that reacts like this to stress and are you like that person?).
9. Exploring dream and nightmare material that occurred in close proximity to the precipitating event for significant links of past to present (What have you been dreaming about at night?).
10. Inquiring whether there have been recent

memories, feelings, or thoughts that have emerged unexplained into consciousness (What types of thoughts have popped into your mind recently?).

Understanding the precipitant is important in crisis assessment and inquiry into this area is essential. When the precipitant cannot be defined in the crisis assessment process, using the basic strategy of crisis intervention by helping to modify responses to a present stressor often reveals the precipitant.

Present Coping Responses

When an emotionally hazardous situation has evolved into an emotional crisis, there has been a failure to cope. Assessing the coping behaviors the patient is using in response to a present stressor leads to more complete understanding of the crisis. It also helps to differentiate adaptive from maladaptive coping responses for the patient and to differentially reinforce them. Assessing the patient's present coping strategies also provides an opportunity to psychologically educate the patient about emotional maturity and the differences between adaptive and maladaptive coping responses.[27]

Coping mechanisms encompass an incredibly wide range of human behavior. They can be simple or complex, direct or indirect, cognitively based or affectively oriented, manipulative or nonmanipulative, active or passive, intrapsychic or interpersonal, verbal or nonverbal. Coping responses occur at the fully conscious, the preconscious, and the unconscious levels of awareness.[28] At the unconscious level, coping behaviors are synonymous with ego-defense mechanisms.

It is a basic task of the crisis therapist to assess the patient's coping responses at all levels. However, the thrust of crisis therapy centers on definition and modification of coping responses at the preconscious or fully conscious levels. In some respects, a major goal of effective crisis intervention is to bring coping behaviors operating at the preconscious level (i.e., just beyond awareness) to the conscious level and then to modify them. This involves defining and conceptualizing the implications of these responses in a collaborative process with the patient. Frequently, discussion of the differences between adaptive and maladaptive coping responses becomes part of this aspect of crisis assessment. The crisis therapist reinforces and encourages

adaptive patient coping responses but discourages use of those responses that are maladaptive or otherwise inappropriate.

Once the patient's present coping behaviors in response to the stressor have been conceptualized, a functional analysis of any maladaptive coping responses being used is initiated as part of crisis assessment. This process is very helpful in more fully understanding the crisis and the sources of patient resistance to modifying maladaptive coping responses, and ultimately in defining the precipitant of the crisis. This functional analysis is also an important aspect of patient education and is often part of crisis assessment. There are several steps in this analysis.

Examining Patient Gains Through Use of Maladaptive Coping Responses.
The functional analysis of coping responses begins with an examination of what the patient psychologically obtains and avoids through use of these responses. The patient, through use of maladaptive responses, usually avoids personal responsibility and gains a modicum of (at least temporary) security or safety. However, these gains are not directed toward healthy resolution of the problem situation. Typically, there are other payoffs from the use of maladaptive coping behaviors. For example, patients may obtain revenge, nurturance, attention, control, or temporary stress reduction through use of maladaptive coping. In addition, patients may avoid confrontation, anger, loss, or feelings of failure through use of these same behaviors. It is frequently helpful, once maladaptive coping responses have been defined, to specifically discuss with the patient the psychological gains that use of these mechanisms bring.

Defining Alternative, More Adaptive Coping Responses.
The second step in the functional analysis is defining with the patient more adaptive coping responses to the crisis situation. Patients often have at least some idea of "what needs to be done" to resolve the crisis situation, but they may need help from the therapist to conceptualize these responses clearly and to develop a sound rationale for their use (i.e., to define why more adaptive responses are more helpful than maladaptive ones). Sometimes, with patients who have little or no psychological-mindedness, the therapist must take the initiative to define more adaptive responses to a problem situation. Conceptualizing and devel-

oping a rationale for more adaptive coping behaviors is an important part of helping the patient learn more about emotional maturity in general and about more adaptive ways to respond in a given problem situation in particular.

Risk Analysis of Adaptive Coping Responses. Once adaptive responses have been defined, the central question becomes: "Why is this patient not using these responses?" For some the answer is simple: "They have not thought of them, or they had no rationale for such responses." For many others, however, the use of adaptive coping responses involves psychological risk. It is the inability to directly accept these risks that determines the maladaptive responses on one hand, and that produces resistance to their modification on the other. Examining the risks, and by implication the fears of the patient, frequently leads to definition of the precipitant of the crisis.

There are two types of risks that patients fear in "giving up" maladaptive responses: internal (or intrapsychic) risks and external (or interpersonal) risks. Either or both types of risks may be operational in any given crisis. The crisis situation, and the patient's responses to that situation, must be explored in terms of both types of risks. Often, these risks may be similar to what is being avoided through the use of maladaptive coping responses, but the risks may also involve differences. By defining the risks, the therapist and patient gain a deeper understanding of the subjective meaning of the crisis to the patient and the basis for patient resistance to change, when present. Understanding these aspects of the use of maladaptive responses is essential in planning effective interventions that encompass present problem solving blended with therapeutic response to patient resistance and to the dynamics of the precipitant of the crisis.

Precrisis Functioning

It is necessary in crisis assessment to understand the patient's psychological functioning in the period just before the crisis occurred. Such assessment provides a base line against which to evaluate the impact of the crisis on the client. In addition, this base line becomes the criterion against which successful crisis resolution (i.e., restoration of the patient's precrisis level of functioning) is determined.

The level of adjustment of the patient before the crisis is important in evaluating the crisis itself. By determining the normal or usual functioning of the patient, valuable clues about relevant issues and about the psychodynamic determinants of the crisis are often obtained. Although a complete or formal history is not part of crisis assessment, the patient's psychological functioning on a variety of interpersonal dimensions in the precisis period (i.e., in the 6 months prior to the crisis) is important. This 6-month period becomes the framework against which the crisis is evaluated.

In some ways, the particular dimensions on which the patient's precrisis functioning is assessed vary with the clinical population and the individual patient. However, several themes are important in this assessment, and each is related to understanding more completely the "why" of the crisis.

The Patient's Usual Repertoire of Coping Behaviors. The range and quality of the patient's usual coping responses are important parts of assessing the patient's precrisis functioning. Some patients have only a single coping behavior in response to stress (e.g., to attack or to withdraw). Others have developed a range of coping responses that are selectively used in different situations. In addition to the range of coping behaviors the patient typically has available, the therapist must also gain a sense of the maturity of these responses. In some patients, there are many coping behaviors available, but these may be neurotic, regressive, or otherwise maladaptive. It cannot be assumed that because the patient uses a variety of coping behaviors that these are healthy.

In this assessment, it is often productive to inquire of the patient how particular situations are dealt with. For example, the clinician may directly ask what the patient's responses are to anger, to disappointment, to loss, or to failure. The patient's responses help to elaborate the range and adaptiveness of coping behaviors usually used, but in addition they also provide insight into the patient's awareness of or conscious use of these coping mechanisms. Are these mechanisms primarily operating at the preconscious level of awareness, or is the patient selectively using them in response to the requirements of particular situations? This knowledge helps the therapist become more aware of the impact of the crisis on the patient's usual mode of functioning, and it also helps the therapist to begin formulating a tentative intervention strategy.

The Patient's Emotional Style and Communication Skills. The patient's general level of emotional awareness is important to understand when assessing an emotional crisis. Some patients are aware of and experience easily a full range of emotions and their emotional life is very rich. Yet, for others, there may be limited awareness of emotions in general, or selective blocking from awareness of specific emotions. For example, for some patients in crisis, it is not uncommon to find there is a lack of emotional awareness of anger, even when warranted. Instead there is only the experience of depression. Therefore, assessing the patient's general emotional awareness and specific emotional blocks is often of value in understanding an emotional crisis.

On the other hand, it is also important to assess how the patient deals with emotion interpersonally. This is the patient's emotional style, and it may vary considerably from patient to patient. For example, some patients may be extremely expressive emotionally, to the point of being volatile and losing emotional control under certain circumstances. At the other extreme are those who characteristically "bottle up" their emotions and do not express them except in very limited ways, if at all. Others may use a very intellectual style of response to emotions. Understanding this usual emotional style of the patient helps to put the crisis situation in perspective. This assessment also provides the crisis therapist with clues regarding the ability of the patient to relate emotional responses to particular events (i.e., the patient's psychological-mindedness).

The Patient's Existing Social Support System. The patient's "connections" to others and the nature of these relationships are important aspects of the patient's precrisis functioning. The most basic dimension of the patient's social support system is the number of relationships that the patient has formed. In addition, the depth of these relationships is also useful information to obtain. Some patients may have many acquaintances but no real friends to count on. Others may be very gregarious and have formed many and deep relationships. Assessing these relationships helps the therapist to determine on whom the patient can count for support during the crisis intervention and resolution process.

It is also helpful to explore the patient's social skills and level of social initiative. Can this patient form new relationships and take the first step in socially relating to others? Or is this a patient who is withdrawn and who relies on others for social involvement (i.e., to provide invitations, social activities, etc.)? Another related factor is the time the patient spends alone, and whether that time alone is by choice or by default. Some patients need alone time, and they create time for this each day. Others, particularly those with poor social skills, spend time alone because they have no one to relate to. As a result, they become quite lonely and depressed because of their social isolation. The patient's social support system is often directly or indirectly related to the crisis situation and can either help or hinder adaptive crisis resolution.

The Patient's Personal Vulnerabilities. Everyone has emotional vulnerabilities. In certain situations, a patient may exhibit emotional overreaction and the inability to respond maturely and appropriately. For most individuals, such situations occur infrequently or are of minor importance. However, for some individuals there are areas of vulnerability that have a significant influence on their adjustment and on their ability to cope with the vicissitudes of life effectively. To understand the nature of the patient's vulnerabilities is frequently of great help in understanding the issues involved in an emotional crisis.

Although it is "normal" to have some areas of vulnerability, it is usually in these same areas that effective coping behaviors have not been fully developed. As a result, individuals are prone to experience crises related to an area of weak or absent coping responses. Asking the patient to define those situations that cause difficulty coping or where emotional overreactions are likely to occur is helpful in assessing precrisis functioning. These situations often involve issues that are also inherent in the event that precipitated the emotional crisis and that may be related to the psychodynamic determinants of the crisis as well (i.e., the precipitant).

The Patient's Self-Report Personality Description. A last area of precrisis functioning to be assessed is the patient's self-image. This self-report may be defensive or disparaging, or it may reflect a balanced awareness of personal strengths and weaknesses. For a variety of reasons, individuals are more aware of their negative qualities and weaknesses than of their assets and strengths. The adjectives used in self-descriptions by patients are often quite helpful in gaining an understanding of the patients' ego-strengths, as well as a perception of their personal deficits that may be involved in the crisis.

There are several ways that a self-description can be obtained from the patient. For example, the patient may simply be asked to describe himself using a very open-ended question. Or the patient may be asked to provide a self-description through the eyes of significant others (e.g., a friend, spouse, parent, etc.). Sometimes it is appropriate to ask about very specific aspects that the therapist feels may be contributing to the crisis (e.g., body image, masculine or feminine identity, parental role, etc.). This description should be directed toward the patient's self-image before the crisis. This provides another dimension of contrast to the patient's self-concept during the crisis. Not infrequently, from such a description the therapist can help define personal strengths of the patient that can be mobilized to aid in crisis resolution.

Related Areas of Patient Assessment
To gain additional information about the etiology of an emotional crisis and to ensure adequate patient care, several areas of inquiry are part of *every* crisis assessment. Although not directly derived from crisis theory, these aspects of crisis assessment are part of the therapist's responsibility to understand and to use in making therapeutic decisions.

Among the most important of the related areas of patient assessment that must be addressed during the crisis assessment process are the following.

Suicide Assessment. Every patient in crisis is experiencing emotional turmoil and painful disequilibrium. The crisis therapist must inquire (of *every* crisis patient) about suicidal ideation, plans, and history of previous attempts or gestures. Patients usually do not volunteer this information, but they readily respond to questions when directly asked. When suicidal ideation or plans are detected, other factors related to increased suicidal risk must also be assessed. When significant risk is determined, appropriate action is taken as part of the crisis intervention process. The therapist assumes responsibility for decision making when the patient cannot. Interventions may include a no-suicide contract, admission to an inpatient unit, or mobilization of support from other persons or from appropriate community resources.

Drugs Currently Used. The patient's pattern of drug use and the nature of the drugs being used are important in crisis assessment. This information provides clues regarding the patient's coping responses to stress, life-style, and general level of functioning. Prescribed medications, street drugs, and over-the-counter medications must all be reviewed. It is not infrequent that symptoms experienced by patients in crisis are produced or aggravated by drugs the patient is currently using. When the drugs being used by the patient are unknown, particularly prescription drugs, it is often helpful to review information about possible side effects in the *Physician's Desk Reference*. Other references are available for street drugs and over-the-counter medications.

Recent Medical History. The patient's medical history for at least the 6 months preceding the emotional crisis should also be an area addressed during crisis assessment. Recent illnesses or traumas may have weakened the patient's ability to cope. In addition, it is not uncommon for illnesses or hospitalization to reactivate significant issues that produce or contribute to an emotional crisis. Sometimes, symptoms from a previous trauma resurface unexpectedly to produce a crisis. This is frequently seen in rape victims or in those involved in natural disasters where symptoms dissipate but reappear later.

Recent Psychiatric History. In crisis assessment, it is often productive to inquire about recent contacts with mental health facilities or professionals, as well as with alternate services. The nature of the problems that prompted contact with those services is important, and discussing these contacts also provides clues about the patient's past use of therapy, general attitudes toward mental health professionals, and issues that may be involved in the present crisis situation. At times, patients will contact crisis therapists because of a crisis in their on-going therapy, and these crises can be discussed within the context of the continuing therapeutic process.[29]

Mental Status. The mental status of any crisis patient should be assessed either informally or formally as needed. Often, patients presenting in crisis clinics or emergency services are in acute distress, and a mental status examination is necessary to access the level of functioning and to make appropriate decisions for treatment. Although not all patients require a formal mental status examination, the therapist must be skilled in its use and must be able to apply it more informally in less acute crises within the general context of crisis assessment.

Diagnosis and Intervention by Level of Crisis

The lack of a classification of emotional crises has been a significant gap in the development of crisis theory. If a present-oriented crisis resolution is needed, a classification system for different types of crises must be developed in order to understand crises in the present and to provide direction for planning effective intervention strategies. Such a classification is presented on the following pages.

Class 1: Dispositional Crises

The definition of a class 1 crisis is a problem in which the emotional distress results from a current explicit problem confronting the patient. The problem is well defined by the patient. The problem may be external (e.g., being assigned a roommate who has an entirely different lifestyle and philosophy of living), or the problem may be internally focused (e.g., a suspected pregnancy). The problems are well within the range of usual human experiences.

The nurse responds to the patient in ways peripheral to the therapeutic counseling role in that the intervention is not primarily directed at the emotional level. For example, the approach may be to provide educational information, make a referral to a specific agency, provide administrative leverage to the situation, or encourage the support of family and friends rather than professional intervention.

A dispositional problem confronts the patient with a sense of immediacy. For example, a family member reveals the stress caused to the family as the result of an alcoholic family member. Providing information to the client about local treatment options such as Al-Anon and other groups is a type of intervention in a dis-

positional problem. In another example, a college student learns that financial assistance has been eliminated from the school he is attending, causing disruption to his or her study concentration. The nurse may provide a referral to the financial aid office or other administrative avenues to assist the student. And in another example, a person is hospitalized for elective surgery. Often the intervention here is educational as well as supportive to attend to specific questions and concerns regarding the surgery.

CASE EXAMPLE*

Michael, a single, 27-year-old, black male, and semi-professional employee of the hospital, came to a mental health clinic to discuss concerns about "his sister." Michael was the oldest son of five children, all girls, ranging in age from 19 to 26. Four of the five children, including Michael, were successfully career-oriented and living independent of the parental system. Michael's concerns were regarding his youngest sister, who within the past 4 months resigned her position as a salesclerk and withdrew from her part-time studies at a local community college and moved back into the parental home to reside after living with a girl friend for approximately 1 year. Sister stated desire to "get her act together," however spent most of the day isolated in the house and evenings socializing with peers of an "inferior" nature, against parental wishes. Michael was concerned his sister was abusing substances. Family relationships became increasingly emotional and strained as parents and siblings responded to daughter's actions. Despite the increasingly tense living conditions at parents' home, the sister refused to leave and seemed to have become dependent upon parents to meet all financial, emotional needs. The client was concerned about his sister's numerous phone calls to him for help and parents' well-being. He was requesting information regarding family counseling as well as information about mental health facilities in the area offering treatment for substance abuse.

At the time of this clinic visit, Michael, although concerned and somewhat anguished about his family's well-being, was coping well within his limitations. After reiteration of the issues involved and clarifying the situation, specific information regarding his requests were provided. The interview was then terminated with no provisions for follow-up visits.

Class 2: Transitional Crises

The second class of crises involves the transitional crises. Transitional life problems occur

---

* The case examples for the six levels of crisis are contributed by Robin Perilstein.

over which the patient may or may not have substantial control. The defining features distinguishing these crises from dispositional crises relate to the psychological meaning of the life problem and its interaction with a change in role relationships or role status. One example of a transitional life problem affecting a change in role status involves becoming a parent, which adds a new role to existing role responsibilities and requires greater capacity for giving than being the recipient of care and comfort. Midlife career changes or returning to work also add a new role component or alter an existing role identity. The transitional phase of marital separation or divorce moves an individual from one role back to a former role or nonmarital status. Also the death of a spouse changes the role status to widow or widower. There are also transitional problems moving from one age level to another, i.e., moving from infancy to childhood, to adolescence, to adulthood, and finally to the role of elder. Another transition problem would be the development of a chronic illness or change in body image, which involves a possible role change concerning employment and the ability to work.

In many cases, there has been substantial forewarning and time for psychological acknowledgment that the transition is forthcoming and, optimally, time to prepare for the

changes that result. However, when coping and adaptation fail, therapeutic interventions are necessary to mobilize the patient, to provide support, and to repair or strengthen coping to the desired functional level.

The patient may seek psychological assistance at varying stages during a particular life transition. Help may be sought prior to, during, or after the life transition has taken place. The nurse responds to the patient, using specific interventions and skills, and the intervention is directed at the emotional level.

Intervention Strategy. The primary task of the nurse is to develop with the patient an in-depth understanding of the changes that have or will take place and to explore the psychological implications of these changes. Support is provided as needed, and anticipatory guidance is used to help the person plan adaptive coping responses to problems that have resulted from a life transition or anticipated problems that the patient will encounter as a result of the transition. Recently, there has been a trend toward the use of group approaches to help those experiencing various types of life transition (e.g., preretirement group, a Lamaze group for childbearing, and group approaches to college orientation).

──── CASE EXAMPLE ────

Robin, a woman in her late twenties, with three young children, had recently decided to divorce her husband after more than 12 years of marriage. She was referred to the counseling center by her private physician after complaining of constant fatigue, decreased appetite, and decreased sleep. Upon presentation, the patient discussed the need to evaluate her marriage, determine where things went wrong, and her role in the dysfunction. The patient realized and accepted eventual finalization of the termination of the marriage, but expressed tremendous feelings of guilt related to defeated expectations in the raising of her children within a "normal" family environment. The patient and her husband were the first marital couple within both extended families to undergo divorce proceedings. Although support was provided by patient's extended family and friends, the husband exacerbated Robin's feelings by initially pressuring for reconciliation and later manipulating the actual divorce by remaining in the marital home with the patient and children, as well as filing for full custody of the children. A fear of losing her children was expressed. Assessment indicated a cooperative, depressed, well-adjusted, well-educated individual reacting to a crisis situation. Intervention focused on evaluation and clarification of the relationship, responsibility for the evolved dysfunctions, alleviating fears of losing her children, in conjunction with feelings of guilt, and the development of alternative coping mechanisms to assist her through the ongoing process (especially in relation to the signs and symptoms of depression). Anticipatory guidance was eventually employed regarding issues of the marital loss, life as a single parent, and the development of other emotional support systems. After 3 months of continued therapy and positive results, patient verbalized desire to terminate;

however, she requested information regarding support groups for single parents. Such information was provided.

Class 3: Traumatic Stress Crises

Traumatic stress crises are emotional crises precipitated by externally imposed stressors or situations that are unexpected and uncontrolled. These experiences are outside the range of usual human situations (i.e., class 1). Such crises are emotionally overwhelming to the persons directly involved. The problem is clearly identified by the patient. Psychological assistance may be sought immediately following the impact of the stressful event, or there may be a time delay. The nurse responds to the patient by using acute crisis intervention techniques.

Examples of traumatic stress crises include situations that cause sudden and unexpected disruption. The sudden or untimely death of a family member or spouse triggers an immediate grief reaction. The sudden loss of job or status disrupts an individual's life plans and career. Another example is a person who learns of a diagnosis involving terminal illness. Natural disasters involving floods, earthquakes, blizzards, or drought can create severe stress. Acts of human aggression such as war produces war combat stress; and crimes of rape, assault, and murder set into motion a series of psychological responses for the victim and his family.

Usual coping behaviors are rendered ineffective due to the sudden, unanticipated nature of the stress. There may be a refractory period during which the patient experiences emotional paralysis and coping behaviors cannot be mobilized.

Intervention Strategy. In this type of crisis, the patient has usually functioned in a reasonably stable fashion prior to the sudden impact of the traumatic stress. The general intervention strategy is to provide or mobilize support for the patient during the refractory period (i.e., the time between the impact of the precipitating stress and the ability to mobilize coping behaviors), which may be more prolonged in this type of crisis than in any other. Following the refractory period, the patient is helped to emotionally acknowledge a situation that has usually not been encountered previously and for which no specific coping behaviors have been learned. Particular attention is given to helping the patient to acknowledge and express negative emotions that result from the stressful situation. Anticipatory guidance is used to aid the patient in planning for and coping with changes that result from the traumatic situation.

CASE EXAMPLE

Susan, a 26-year-old nurse and single parent of two elementary school children, came to a counseling center on her own cognition, after being physically assaulted in her home by two teen-agers in a robbery attempt three days before. Susan's children were home at the time of the assault and witnessed the attack of their mother. During the assault, Susan's initial screams alerted the neighbors, who in turn contacted the police. Upon their arrival, Susan was found sitting on the sofa, nurturing her two crying children, while her neighbor was placing ice packs on the numerous facial areas where she had been beaten. Susan refused police and medical assistance, insisting she would be fine and that her main concern was for the well-being of her children. She denied any sexual assault. In the days that followed, Susan's emotional condition worsened, even with the provided support of her mother and friend. She was experiencing decreased sleep, decreased appetite, intermittent crying spells, and a fear of being left alone. Mother was caring for the children in the patient's home. After assessment, it was determined that Susan's emotional reactiveness was being exacerbated by preexisting fears of being hurt and taken advantage of by men. Supportive therapy was provided within a safe and secure environment to initiate more adaptive methods by coping with the stressors and the ultimate depression. Susan was also encouraged to express feelings and concerns related to the critical event, as well as the alleviation of fears in being left alone. Later, the patient was able to begin the development of alternative coping mechanisms with regard to issues of trust with men. A referral for victim counseling was also helpful to Susan.

Class 4: Developmental Crises

Developmental crises result from attempts to deal with an interpersonal situation reflecting a struggle with a deeper (but usually circumscribed) issue. These developmental or maturational life issues have not been psychologically resolved adaptively in the past and thus represent unsuccessful attempts to attain emotional maturity. Several factors may account for a failure to resolve a life issue. One factor is that the individual may have had to deal with a stressful event to the detriment of achieving maturation of the normative life issues. Another factor involves the confrontation of the reality that a life goal cannot be realized, and this causes stress on the normal coping patterns. The nurse's task is to identify the key developmental issues involved as well as the impact of the current stressor.

There are a wide range of general examples of developmental problems with focal issues involving dependency, value conflicts, sexual identity, capacity for emotional intimacy, responses to authority, or the ability to attain reasonable self-discipline. Other examples include trauma situations that have created lags in the person's developmental progress such as deprived or abusive parenting experiences. Often there is a repeated pattern of specific relationship difficulties that occurs over time in those presenting with this type of problem.

It is important to note that every type of emotional crisis involves an interaction of an external stressor and a vulnerability of the individual. However, it is in class 4 problems that there is a shift from a primarily external locus of stress that produces the crisis to an internal locus determined by the unique psychodynamics of the individual and/or preexisting psychopathology that becomes manifest in particular problematic situations.

Intervention Strategy. Developmental problems may be encountered at any time during the life cycle and are not specific to any particular time of life. Basic intervention strategy is to help the patient to identify and conceptualize the underlying and unresolved developmental issue that has been instrumental in producing the crisis situation (i.e., the precipitant of the crisis). Emphasis is then placed on helping the patient to respond to the present problematic situation more adaptively while simultaneously aiding in the resolution of the determinant of the developmental conflict. It is in this type of crisis that the nurse has an excellent opportunity to blend present interpersonal difficulties with a focal psychodynamic issue (with its etiology in the past) into a productive growth experience for the patient during the intervention process. If the response in developmental problems is only to the manifest problem of the patient, while the developmental precipitant is ignored, the opportunity to prevent future similar crises may be lost. Rosenberg, writing on the treatment of developmental crises, has defined a very effective treatment model for this type of crisis that incorporates many of the concepts of crisis theory and practice.[30] Students will benefit from reading this text.

───── CASE EXAMPLE ─────

Marla, a 23-year-old graduate student, came to the counseling center with complaints of persistent nausea, intense feelings of sudden anxiety, and inability to concentrate on her studies for the past 3 weeks. After initial assessment, it was learned that Marla's fiancé of 1 year, whom she was living with, was going to break off the engagement if Marla had not made decisive plans for marriage. Marla was ambivalent in making this commitment. This was her first long-term relationship. It was also learned that Marla was having difficulty balancing the life-style she was leading with those moral, ethical, and religious values of her family. She verbalized feelings of guilt and disloyalty because of this predicament. Marla was raised in a devout Catholic environment. Her fiancé was Jewish. Underlying the presenting issues of conflict were Marla's difficulties in differentiating herself from her family.

With much support, Marla was assisted in realizing and conceptualizing the underlying issues that had motivated her discord. What resulted was an ability to emotionally differentiate self. Marla was then capable of making decisions for her life based on what she determined was appropriate. Therapy also dealt with aiding Marla in developing effective coping skills to deal with potential defeated expectations with regard to parents. Family meetings were also encouraged. Referrals to alternative therapists were provided in order to continue growth and development.

Class 5: Crises Reflecting Psychopathology

Crises reflecting psychopathology include emotional situations in which preexisting psychopathology has been instrumental in precipitating the crisis. Or the situation may involve a state in which the psychopathology significantly impairs or complicates adaptive resolution. The nurse needs to be able to diagnose the psychopathology and to adapt the intervention to include appreciation of the personality or characterological aspects of the patient.

Examples of crises reflecting psychopathology would include patients presenting with borderline adjustment, severe personality and characterological disorders, schizophrenia, and substance abuse behaviors. The traditional diagnostic categories of the *DSM-III-R* are essential to know in working with such a patient and family.

CASE EXAMPLE

Steven, a 23-year-old employed maintenance worker, came to the counseling center with complaints of increased alcohol intake during his lunch hour, causing him to "act strange" and feel highly embarrassed among his coworkers. The alcohol use was an ongoing problem for Steven, who could not understand reasons for his recent exacerbation over the past 2 weeks. His strange behavior was a great concern to him as he was fearful of losing his job and his friends. After initial assessment, it was learned that Steven had a long history of being generally passive, with poor social adjustment skills. Steven also could not cope effectively with virtually any form of confrontation. He described similar incidents in the past accompanied by bizarre delusional thinking, suggestive of a preexisting psychopathology.

After additional assessment to determine potentiality of other involved dynamics that might have triggered the crisis, intervention was provided. Negotiation of specific behavioral tasks revolving around substance abuse was developed and discussed so as to alleviate his fears and concerns. The patient was highly receptive to this modality. Following this crisis intervention, recommendation was given for continued long-term psychotherapy (patient was already in therapy and was unable to contact his therapist, who was out of state) to assist with more in-depth conflict.

Class 6: Psychiatric Emergencies

Psychiatric emergencies involve life-endangering situations in which the individual's general functioning has been severely impaired. The individual is rendered incompetent or unable to assume personal responsibility and is unable to exert control over feelings and actions that he experiences. Nurses need to be confident of their skills and abilities to manage the out-of-control behavior of the patient or to have adequate assistance available.

Examples of life-endangering crises include acutely suicidal persons, drug overdoses, reactions to hallucinogenic drugs, and alcohol intoxication. Individuals experiencing acute psychosis are also classified as psychiatric emergencies as well as people with uncontrollable anger and aggression. In general, these persons are dangerous to themselves as well as to others.

Intervention Strategy. The psychiatric life-endangering crises are difficult types of crises to handle as there may be less than complete in- formation about the situation available, the pa- tient may be minimally helpful or disruptive, and there is great urgency in understanding the situation in depth in order to begin effective treatment. One of the major settings for psy- chiatric emergencies is the emergency depart- ment of a general hospital.

—— CASE EXAMPLE ——

May, a 25-year-old single female with two children, was brought to the Emergency Room by ambulance with an overdose of tranquilizers and alcohol. She was admitted to the In- tensive Care Unit for 24 hours and then transferred to the mental health unit. She was placed on suicide precautions.

This young woman had recently been fired from her job. She had lost her home and had been living with various friends but had no place of her own. The father of her children, who had been helping her, had been sent to prison and was no longer going to be able to help her. May's family of origin lived out of state and was also unable to help her. This patient was extremely depressed and felt desperate. She felt there was no solution to her problems.

May received milieu therapy, individual psychotherapy, and group therapy. The social worker looked at the various social programs available to May and also looked into finding temporary housing for the family.

Therapeutic Crisis Work

Most crisis intervention takes place in 1 to 8 ther- apy hours, and the time required for therapist and patient to move through this sequence var- ies within these limits. Further, completion of each stage in movement toward crisis resolution may also vary from patient to patient. The stages with the therapeutic tasks are outlined below.

Explore the Crisis Event
The crisis event is explored both in detail and in terms of the patient's thoughts, feelings, and actions. The patient is encouraged to acknowl- edge and to express feelings generated by the crisis situation. The therapist helps the patient to restore a realistic perspective of the crisis sit- uation and to define viable options or courses of action available.

Conceptualize Dynamic Meaning of the Crisis
It is important to define the emotional meaning of the precipitating event that produced the cri- sis. The patient is helped to conceptualize the precipitant or psychodynamic meaning of the crisis situation that links present to past (when this component of a crisis is present). The ther- apist obtains from the patient agreement on a concise statement of the core conflict or problem that has produced the crisis.

Unlink the Sensory and Perceptual Crisis Components
Limited relevant background information is ob- tained from the patient to help in understanding more fully the crisis situation. The patient is helped to develop an awareness of those feel- ings that impair or prevent use of adaptive cop- ing behaviors in response to the crisis situation and to work through feelings that support mal- adaptive coping responses (i.e., resistance), which prevent adaptive crisis resolution.

Process the Cognitive Component of the Crisis
Therapist and patient agree on a tentative ther- apeutic strategy or plan to attain the goals nec- essary for crisis resolution. The therapist defines and directly supports patient strengths and adaptive responses to the crisis situation. The patient is supported in and helped to respond

directly and appropriately to the crisis situation in terms of both issues and feelings (e.g., direct communication with significant others involved is encouraged).

Store the Crisis Event in Past Memory

Part of the crisis resolution is "therapeutic forgetting." For this task, the therapist directly teaches or helps the patient to develop new or more adaptive coping responses or problem-solving skills that will assist in moving the thoughts of the crisis to past memory. The therapist prevents diffusion of the therapeutic process away from the focal problem and the goals defined for crisis resolution.

In addition to facilitating patient movement through these stages of crisis work, the therapist must also accept goals for crisis intervention that are different from those of longer-term psychotherapy. It is *not* the task of the nurse to effect major changes in the patient, to deal with *all* the patient's problems, to restructure personality, or to resolve deep-seated conflicts or chronic problems. There is a single general goal for crisis intervention that becomes the sole criterion for success in this form of therapy. This goal is to facilitate return of the patient in crisis to at least a precrisis level of functioning as quickly as possible, even though this level of functioning may not be optimal for that individual. Any gains made by the patient beyond restoration of precrisis levels of functioning is a therapeutic bonus that will be helpful in preventing future crises.

Termination

Termination is part of the therapeutic and evaluative process. The therapist elicits and responds to patient termination issues but does not prolong the therapeutic process because of them. Changes are reinforced in patient coping behaviors and affective functioning and these changes are related to adaptive resolution of the problematic situation.

As part of termination, the therapist evaluates with the patient goal attainment or nonattainment during the crisis intervention process. Anticipatory guidance is used to help integrate adaptive change and to help prepare the patient to meet future similar situations more adequately. The patient is provided with information about additional services or community resources needed, or a direct referral for continuing therapy is made as appropriate.

In addition to the general goal of crisis intervention, there are several subgoals that are part of successful crisis resolution:

1. The individual in crisis is prevented from using or learning maladaptive coping responses or regressing, thereby avoiding maladaptive crisis resolution.
2. The individual in crisis is aided in learning new and more adaptive coping responses that will result in reintegration at a more mature and stable level of functioning in the postcrisis period.
3. The individual in crisis is helped to use the crisis experience to become aware of and to resolve underlying conflicts or ambivalence that are manifest in and determine the crisis.
4. The individual in crisis is helped to integrate changes resulting from adaptive crisis resolution at both cognitive and affective levels to expand his repertoire of available coping skills.

In summary, every crisis involves an individual responding to a stressor within a particular psychosocial context. By structuring crisis assessment to emphasize the individual in a stressful situation, the interaction of that person's coping responses and the situation stressor become the focus that is established for the patient. The message to the patient must be clear: "There is a problem you are encountering that is solvable, and it is central in importance." This is in lieu of the message: "You have problems and you need psychotherapy."

Crisis assessment requires this shift in emphasis when interviewing the patient. Many patients become discouraged when their presenting problems are not addressed early. Particularly distressing to them is therapist concern about past problems rather than about current difficulties. The emphasis in crisis work is on the "here-and-now" problem, and this is attractive to many patients. However, although crisis assessment is very present-oriented and limited, it does not neglect or deny the psychodynamic implications of the crisis situation.

In crisis therapy, the question is not whether an emotional crisis will be resolved. The crisis *will* be resolved in a reasonably short period of time, usually in an average of 4 to 6 weeks. The real question is whether the crisis will be resolved in an adaptive fashion that results in enhanced maturity and stable functioning or in a maladaptive way that increases patient vulnerability and future crises. When using the crisis model, the nurse must proceed with the intervention on the basis of less than complete information about the patient.

Summary

This chapter traces the history of crisis theory and identifies the relationship between homeostasis and an emotional crisis that calls forth coping processes. Caplan's four interrelated phases are included to describe an individual's response to a stressful event. Baldwin's ten corollaries of crisis theory are discussed and the process of crisis intervention. A typology of emotional crises include: dispositional crises, transitional crises, traumatic stress crises, developmental crises, crises reflecting psychopathology, and psychiatric emergencies.

Questions

1. Describe a patient example involving an emotional crisis.
2. Identify the six types of emotional crisis and give a brief example.
3. Where do people with psychiatric emergencies receive care in your community?

REFERENCES AND SUGGESTED READINGS

1. Caplan, G. *Principles of Preventive Psychiatry*. New York: Basic Books, 1974, p. 53.
2. Lindemann, E. Symptomatology and management of acute grief. *American Journal of Psychiatry*, 1944, *101*, 141–148.
3. Caplan, op. cit.
4. Aguilera, D. C., & Messick, J. M. *Crisis Intervention: Theory and Methodology*, 4th ed. St. Louis: Mosby, 1984.
5. Engel, G. L. Homeostasis, behavioral adjustment and the concept of health and disease. In R. R. Grinker (Ed.), *Mid-Century Psychiatry*. Springfield, Ill.: Chas. C. Thomas, 1953, p. 51.
6. Caplan, op. cit.
7. Burgess, A. W., & Baldwin, B. A. *Crisis Intervention Theory and Practice*. Englewood Cliffs, N.J.: Prentice-Hall, 1981, p. 25.
8. Perlman, H. H. In quest of coping. *Social Casework*, 1975, *56*, 213–225.
9. Caplan, G. Mastery of stress: Psychosocial aspects. *American Journal of Psychiatry*, 1981, *138*, 414.
10. Ibid., pp. 414–415.
11. Ibid.
12. Ibid.
13. Ibid.
14. Baldwin, B. A. Crisis intervention: An overview. In A. W. Burgess & B. A. Baldwin (Eds.), *Crisis Intervention Theory and Practice*. Englewood Cliffs, N.J.: Prentice-Hall, 1981, p. 29.
15. Caplan, op. cit. (1974).
16. Perlman, op. cit.
17. Hirschowitz, R. G. Crisis theory: A formulation. *Psychiatric Annals*, 1973, *3*(12), 36–47.
18. Wolkon, G. H. Crisis theory, the application for treatment, and dependency. *Comprehensive Psychiatry*, 1972, *13*, 459–464.
19. Schwartz, S. L. A review of crisis intervention programs. *Psychiatric Quarterly*, 1971, *45*, 498–508.
20. Hoffman, D. L., & Remmel, M. L. Uncovering the precipitant in crisis intervention. *Social Casework*, 1975, *56*, 259–267.
21. Rapoport, L. The state of crisis: Some theoretical considerations. *The Social Service Review*, 1962, *36*, 211–217.
22. Paul, L. Crisis intervention. *Mental Hygiene*, 1966, *50*, 141–145.

23. Hitchcock, J. M. Crisis intervention: The pebble in the pool. *American Journal of Nursing*, 1973, *73*, 1388–1390.
24. Strickler, M., & La Sor, B. The concept of loss in crisis intervention. *Mental Hygiene*, 1970, *54*, 301–305.
25. Hoffman & Remmel, op. cit.
26. Silverman, W. H. Planning for crisis intervention with community mental health concepts. *Psychotherapy: Theory, Research and Practice*, 1977, *14*, 293–297.
27. Baldwin, B. A. Crisis intervention, Parkinson's Law and structure in psychotherapy. Unpublished paper.
28. Perlman, op. cit.
29. Skodol, A. E., Kass, F., & Charles, E. Crisis in psychotherapy: Principles of emergency consultation and intervention, *American Journal of Orthopsychiatry*, 1979, *49*, 585–597.
30. Rosenberg, B. N. Planned short-term treatment in developmental crisis. *Social Casework*, 1975, *56*, 195–204.

Chapter 25

Trauma Therapy

Carol R. Hartman and Ann Wolbert Burgess

Chapter Objectives

The student successfully attaining the goals of this chapter will be able to:

- Identify concepts important in trauma therapy.
- Describe the major intervention principles in trauma therapy.
- Describe defense mechanisms employed during traumatic events.

While the impact of experiencing childhood sexual abuse has been well documented by clinicians, social scientists, and feminists, less well advanced have been treatment models for child victims or adult survivors.[1-5] Although there is little dispute that conceptual frameworks are critical for intervention strategies, this area of model development is neglected in the clinical literature. The conceptual framework of traumatic-event processing was developed for a research project because of the lack of explicated or tested frameworks for understanding the linkage between child sexual victimization and level of adjustment.[6] During the research design phase, we were not aware of any related models, and our confidence in this model came from clinical and interview experiences with victims and victimizers.[7-9]

CONCEPTUAL FRAMEWORK

The past two decades have seen a phenomenal increase in research from brain science; the cognitive sciences of philosophy, psychology, artificial intelligence, linguistics, anthropology, and neuroscience; information theory; and stress response syndromes.[10-15] The contributions from the various disciplines provide the basic assumptions for the model for information processing of trauma.

The model assumes the basic constructs of information processing of a living system. These concepts and propositions state that experiences are processed on a sensory, perceptual, and cognitive level. The sensory level is the basic registrant of experience in the individual. The perceptual level is the beginning classification of sensory processing. The cognitive phase represents the larger organization of experience into meaning systems. The construct of memory is applicable to each level of information processing.

The psychosocial stressor of child sexual abuse is the unit of information under discussion. The DSM-III-R lists the severity for this type of stressor as "extreme," thus the designation of child sexual abuse as a trauma. Horowitz, researching the impact of trauma and response to stressful stimuli, identified a general stress response syndrome as (1) a clustering of disturbing psychological phenomena of intrusive and repetitive imagery associated with the memories of the traumatic event; and (2) avoidant strategies employed to keep associations to the trauma out of awareness.[16] The presumption was made that traumatic information is kept in active awareness until it can be placed in distant memory and that trauma resolution occurs when there is sufficient processing for the information to be stored, e.g., the event is remembered, the attendant feelings are neutralized, and the anxiety generated by the event is controlled. When a traumatic event is not resolved and either remains in active memory or becomes defended by a cognitive mechanism such as denial, dissociation, or splitting, the diagnosis is generally post-traumatic stress disorder (PTSD). The central feature of PTSD, which is the stress pattern resulting from traumatization, is that the individual reexperiences the original trauma both unconsciously and consciously.

The four major phases of the information processing of trauma (IPT) model (Fig. 25-1) outline factors associated with the impact of the trauma.[17,18] Intervention is an optional phase.

Pretrauma Phase

The pretrauma phase identifies parameters of the child's makeup and social context that can have a possible effect on the child's management and the resolution of sexual abuse (e.g., development in terms of age, personality, sociocultural factors, family structure and interaction with child, and history of prior trauma). Research on the influence of the parameters is not definitive in predicting outcome. Rather, these parameters serve to mediate that which is

particular to the general stress response syndrome.

Trauma Encapsulation Phase

The trauma encapsulation phase focuses on the mechanisms used by the child to regulate the ongoing sexual activities (abuse) and responses. Three components—input, thruput, and output—constitute the primary trauma experience.

Input

Input pays attention to the offender's behavior (e.g., victim's relationship to offender, entrapment and access to child, use of force, control used, occurrences and sexual activities, and method of ensuring secrecy). These offender behaviors are received, transmitted, and processed by the sensory, perceptual, and cognitive domains of the child.

Thruput

Thruput includes the coping and defensive mechanisms employed by the child to deal with the anxiety, fear, and other reactions invoked by the abuse. During the encapsulation phase, various defenses may be called upon. They are dissociation, denial, fragmentation of self, arousal disharmony, repression, and splitting. These defenses with their particular behavioral and experiential dimensions are noted by clinicians.

Dissociation is a general process in which the mind fragments psychic integrity in the service of survival by disengaging from an ongoing trauma. Sensory dissociation is marked by a total numbing of a body part; perceptual dissociation is noted in dimming of sensory cues such as a muffling of sound, a narrowing and distancing of the perceptual field; cognitive dissociation is noted in the experience of being somewhere else, floating above the trauma scene.

Denial is the total discounting that something has happened, that one has a negative emotional reaction to an event. In children, there can be denial of the abuse or denial that it was upsetting in any way.

Repression is the keeping from conscious awareness all aspects of a traumatic event. It is more comprehensive and basic than denial. A most dramatic observation of this defense is the

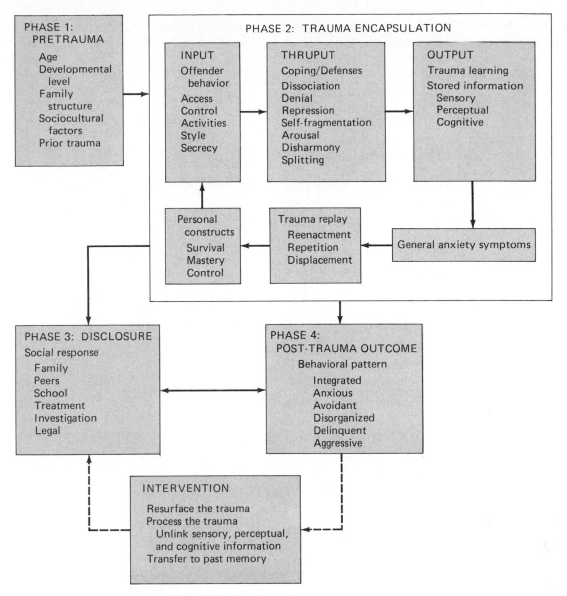

Figure 25-1. Information processing of trauma model.

lifting of repression with the child having a full-fledged recollection of the abuse.

Fragmentation of a sense of self implies disruption of integrative personality functions that result in knowledge of self. For example, an awareness of one's capacity to aggress is blocked; consequently, the child is unaware of assaulting another child. A sense of competency is compromised; the child identifies with his inability to master a particular situation but does not recognize the ability to handle other situations. Self-appraisal is distorted. The ability to move from experience in a flexible manner, using memory, making connections between different levels of experience, and evolving an integrated sense of self are compromised.

Arousal disharmony is the disruption of the capacity to regulate states of excitement and calmness. This phenomenon is noted in the numbness state that ensues to block sensory overload during the traumatic event. This leaves the individual blocking the anxiety generated by the trauma while at the same time cutting the person off from regulated ranges of arousal generated in nontraumatizing situations. In sexual abuse of children there is a premature excitation of sexual sensations compounded by fear and confusion. There are incongruent commands from the offender that disrupt the child's naturally unfolding, sensory-regulating capacities. One consequence of this is excessive masturbation without awareness.

Splitting is the polarization of a complex unit of behavior, perceptions and cognitions manifested in responses to self and other. In psychoanalytic terms, it is a conflict between the demand of the instinct and command of reality. The rift never heals, but instead increases with time.[19] In the sexually abused child, splits are noted in the good versus bad parent, the good versus bad child, the loved versus hated child, the trusted other versus the betraying other.

During thruput, these defensive operations shape the primary meaning of the abuse as well as shape the structure of how the abuse information is processed, stored, and represented through affect and nonverbal behavior.

Output

The third component of the trauma encapsulation phase, output, is the primary trauma learning, which is the charged sensory, perceptual, and cognitive memory base of the event. Trauma learning is an important anxiety-management mechanism. Of the three domains, the sensory and perceptual often override the cognitive in the registration of the abuse. All the information associated with the trauma learning results in an important feedback loop of intermediate outputs. These looping outputs have a reinforcing quality. Because of short-term anxiety reactions, they do not neutralize the anxiety; they are general anxiety symptoms. For example, the child develops new fears, onset of bed-wetting and soiling, irritability, regressive behavior, tics, startle response, and physical complaints. **Trauma replay** is the manifestation of specific actions, reactions, and activities that directly represent the trauma learning linked to the behaviors developed during the trauma itself. A series of fixed behaviors emerge, and the three manifestations of trauma replay presented in the model are descriptions to sensitize an observer to these phenomena.

Reenactment is reliving the event.

Repetition is noted in the victim's play with others. There is a repeating of acts toward another person, usually a child, that resemble the abusive event.

Displacement is the symbolic representa-

tion of the abusive act as in doll play, drawings, dreams, or fantasy construction.

The feedback loop also contains the dynamic individual meaning the trauma holds for the child. *Dynamic* is used to underscore the shifting meanings that arise from the victim's as well as the victimizer's behaviors. The interplay of cognitive efforts to mediate the trauma are grounded in personal constructs. First are constructs dealing with the recognition of danger and survival strategies associated with the reenactment of the trauma. The second level of construct and meaning formation deals with preliminary mastery over actions, reactions, and transactions that occur during the trauma and is represented in the various replay patterns. The third level of construct formation centers around control over anxiety induced by specific memories of the trauma and is more often manifested in displacement replay of the trauma. It is at the third level that attributions emerge. These attributions focus on cause, predictability, and significance of events to others as well as to self. These influence coping capabilities.

Nondisclosure presumes encapsulation of the primary trauma learning. Over time, the child, left to his own devices, reformulates the trauma through the defensive operations used to survive, the general anxiety symptoms, and the emerging meaning structures attached to the trauma. Behavior and learning problems are not associated by others with the sexual abuse and often compromise the child's development. The event is sealed from ongoing daily life. However, to the degree that the anxiety remains charged (non-neutralized), relationships, social and academic achievements, a sense of right and wrong and of self can be distorted. There is disturbance in the self-comforting, caring, and protective functions of the child's self-system. Attachment to others and social values are distorted or weakened. There is distortion in a personal sense of pleasure.

Phase two (trauma encapsulation) emphasizes the looping-back principle in an active system. Continued abuse is registered and modified in this process. We theorize that the powerful aspects of this primary trauma learning are linked to dominance of the sensory and perceptual domains over the cognitive domain.

Disclosure

Phase three of the model is disclosure and contains the social meaning or secondary trauma impact. This disclosure phase takes into consideration what happens if the child tells of the abuse. In this phase the child fields the reactions of his social network by revealing the sexual abuse. The social network includes family, peers, and associates as well as staff of the helping professions and justice system. This secondary learning can result in a reformulation of the trauma.

Outcomes

The fourth phase includes outcomes for the child in terms of behavioral response. Descriptively, in the *integrated* pattern, the child has no trauma-related symptoms, demonstrates the ability to recall the event in detail and with minimal distress, has an offender-oriented causal attribution to the sexual abuse, has an age-appropriate adjustment to social network, and is future-oriented in a positive manner. In the *anxious* pattern, acute physical symptoms have become chronic. Children are notably distressed when reminded of the event, feel guilty and blame themselves for the victimization, are unable to protect themselves, have unstable social relationships, become depressed, and are oriented to the past. In the *avoidant pattern*, the child is psychologically well defended against talking of the abuse and may deny that it happened or claim no memory of it. Children present a stoic demeanor, are afraid of the offender, and may develop avoidant behaviors such as running away and substance abuse. Peer and family relationships may be terminated and minor antisocial acts may surface. In the *disorganized* pattern, there are marked cognitive or psychotic symptoms accompanied by loss of personal maintenance. There is restricted personality development and the trauma is split off and buried in delusional and fixed sexualized thinking patterns. In the *aggressive* pattern, children assimilate and master the anxiety from the abuse by exploiting others and by adopting an antisocial position toward peers, school, and family. A delinquent pattern is first noted and can advance into criminal behaviors that include sexual and aggressive acts.

Intervention may be available at the time of disclosure or years later. The model of intervention depends on the theoretical orientation of the clinician and the timing of the disclosure.

PRINCIPLES OF EVALUATION AND INTERVENTION

This section describes evaluation and intervention principles used in play therapy to assist in eliciting the structure of the trauma learning.

Anchoring for Safety

The concept of safety has to be addressed and established when working with traumatized children. Part of the introduction of the child to the interview requires clinicians to use those skills necessary for the child to view the therapist as warm, safe, trusting, and sincere. This context of safety has to be reinforced by those caring for the child. Parents need to be advised on how to begin to establish safety with their child when this has been eroded by the abuse experience.

This principle has its roots in the IPT model. The encapsulation phase results in the loosening associations the child might have to a safe, caring, protective world. The energy that has been used in attachment to others and to the world of people and values is ruptured. The description in the model alerts the therapist to the difficult task of reestablishing a connection between caring adults and the child. The protest behaviors noted in the child give the therapist a reference point for recognizing the power of what has been learned during the trauma and its primacy over ongoing environmental efforts to reduce the anxiety and terror. Children often sense efforts on the parts of caring adults and will attempt to reduce tension by adopting a quasi-positive state. When this occurs, the dissociation of the trauma is noted in the child's almost automatic fear reactions to internal and external stimuli associated with the trauma event.

Establishing Stress-Reducing Resources

Personal inner resources of the child need to be established, recovered, and strengthened. These resources address the sensory, perceptual, and cognitive domains and include relaxation, humor, separating past from present, use of positive imagery, and developing mastery, control, and self-confidence.

This principle acknowledges the arousal disharmony noted in the encapsulation phase. It requires that the therapist attend to the pattern of disruptive behavior manifested by the child. For example, in dealing with hyperactive or acting-out behavior, the child is helped to learn that activity can be increased and then be relaxed. This skill will help the child manage the tension associated with more direct recall and recounting of the trauma itself. For the child who is avoidant and anxious, the use of quiet music and relaxation gives the child a means of dealing with anxiety-laden stimuli.

Surfacing the Trauma

This principle is applied within the ability of the child to control the degree of detail, using the safety parameters and the personal resources to comfort and reduce anxiety.

This principle is based upon the recognition that various defenses have been employed for the child to survive the abuse. Implicit is the assumption that the child made decisions to inhibit certain behaviors and to produce other behaviors. Surfacing the trauma is done to resurrect those behaviors inhibited by the child. The inability to neutralize the trauma rests in part on the child's lack of recognition that what he did do was important, rather than a reconstructed assumption that he did nothing or was responsible for what happened. The "fixed state" of the non-neutralized aspects of memory constructs occurs because the cognitive appraisal is limited by the age of the child or by the distortion perpetrated by the offender. Consequently, the sensory and perceptual domains dominate the learning, and the child experiences an inability to move from a highly noxious affective state. This state is induced by any cues associated with the event. Recognizing this, the child and the therapist need to institute any of the stress-reducing resources that have been developed.

Processing the Trauma

Closely associated with the resurfacing of the trauma is trauma processing, which has various levels of activity. What happened during the abuse is to be recalled as well as what did not

happen but did go on in the mind of the child: What the child did and what he did not do but wanted to do and why he was unable. This processing helps to integrate the fragmented experiences of the trauma and underscores the resourcefulness of the child to survive. Part of the processing is the unlinking or the conscious effort to assist the child in recognizing that the behaviors used to protect are no longer necessary because the child is now safe. The unlinking is done at the three levels of domain: sensory, perceptual, and cognitive. The trauma experience is neutralized in regard to its fear-induced symptoms and later in regard to the aggressive behaviors manifested in repetition and displacement.

Transfer of the Processed or Integrated Trauma to Past Memory

The child is introduced to strategies to reduce and categorize what is necessary to remember and to forget as well as how to remember and recall from memory with personal control over the associated anxiety.

Terminations

The last principle attends to reviewing the child's verbal reformulation of the trauma, includes termination of the therapeutic relationship and plans for telephone follow-up for additional monitoring of the child's progress.

CASE EXAMPLE

Tina [a pseudonym], a three-year-old girl, began nursery school the third day in September. She was an only child of middle-class parents. Initially she liked going to school; then suddenly she no longer wanted to attend school. Her parents thought this change in behavior was due to separation anxiety, as this was her first time away from her parents and home.

By the second week of September, Tina was not only reluctant but balked at going to school. Her parents noted a series of new behaviors over the next 4 weeks. She began bed-wetting, screaming "No, don't touch me!" in her sleep, and having nightmares. She ran through the house hitting at her parents; she threw food on the floor. While being dressed, Tina would cry, "Stop hurting me." Tina became unusually violent with her pet cat, hitting, kicking, or catching it in a neck hold. She began calling it "Pusswiggle." Her male dolls were rejected; she only played with female dolls. She frequently used the bathroom and complained of pain, especially during bathing. Her mother noted the child's red, irritated, and swollen genital area, which she treated with an ointment. Tina would rub her genitals while watching television or being read to and while sitting in her father's lap.

Five weeks later, Tina was taken on an emergency basis to her physician. As the regular physician was busy, a substitute doctor examined Tina. During the examination, Tina was extremely frightened of the male doctor and refused to part her legs. The doctor said Tina was "too raw to examine" and was unable to determine the cause of the genital injury, suggesting that perhaps Tina was not wiping herself adequately after urinating and advised that she stop wearing underpants while at home.

One morning 6 weeks after beginning nursery school, Tina asked her mother to rub between her legs "because it felt good." She was specific in taking her mother's finger to rub her, and she told her mother that Joey ("a big boy at school") played the "wiggle game" with her ("He puts his finger in and plays wiggle"). The mother learned Joey, a 5-year-old boy of recently separated parents, was not in his age-level class due to "hyperactivity and immaturity."

The Extended Evaluation: Four Play Sessions

The therapists introduced themselves to Tina and her parents as psychiatric nurses who work with children who have had various types of life experiences. Tina was asked how she understood the visit ("To talk about [school]"). A selection of play and art materials were available for Tina to inspect, and gradually the session began focusing on the use of animal stories for projective storytelling and an initial developmental assessment. Tina could provide her first name and address, color of her house, name of her school, the identification of animals, colors, animal facial features, and the distinction through visual constructs between a truth and a lie (e.g., how many eyes, what am I wearing, etc.).

Using animal pictures for projective thoughts, Tina was asked about the sex of the bear. Tina labeled the male bear as a female because "that what she wants." When asked what would make the animal a boy bear, the child looked alarmed and said, "I don't want it to be a boy bear." She manifested sadness in her tone and facial expressions. Her voice and lower lip dropped and she frowned as she said that the big bear helping the little bunny with its clothes was a "bad bear."

The use of play dolls and a schoolhouse provided the following dialogue regarding the school event and the boy's behavior toward Tina.

THERAPIST: What does the teacher say?

TINA: Sit down; stand up.
THERAPIST: We're at [school] and the teacher has left the room. The little boy comes to play. What is his name?
TINA: Joey
THERAPIST: Let's play.
TINA: I want to touch you down there. [Takes girl doll and uses boy doll's hand to touch the girl's genitals.]
THERAPIST: What does the little girl say?
TINA: She cried and told her teacher: "Joey touched my bottom."
THERAPIST: What did the teacher do?
TINA: She put him in another place to sit.
THERAPIST: What did Joey do with the other kids?
TINA: Hit them with a stick. He was a bad boy. He hit kids. They would play in the cubbyhole.

Joey, the boy in Tina's nursery school with whom she played, was discussed directly. Tina was upset that Joey had hurt her, and she showed the therapist (using the anatomically correct dolls) how Joey put his finger in her vagina. She also reported with her voice rising, eyes widening, and speech racing that Joey would go after little boys in the nursery school, pull down their pants, and run a comb or other object over the boys "bums and the front." When Tina saw the penis on the anatomically correct boy doll, she asked in a very natural way what it was and why was it there. When demonstrating with the boy doll what Joey did to her, she left his clothes on. As Tina related witnessing of Joey's aggression against the smaller children, she clenched her fists and pulled at the toys, throwing them to the floor.

When Tina was asked how the abuse could occur without anyone knowing, she replied that no grown-ups were present. On the other hand, she said that her teacher stopped Joey and made him sit still. Thus, it is unclear whether any adults witnessed the abuse. It was speculated that Tina was frightened and focused on Joey's behavior and was unaware of who else was present. The play with dolls revealed the amount of Tina's fear and aggression and the sexualization of peer relationships.

Tina was explicit in what had happened to her. She related that Joey was a bad boy for what he did to her, that she was in a new school, and that she had made a friend, Susan, at the school. Prior to starting school she asked her mother if there would be big boys at the new school. She continued to talk about Joey as a bad boy.

Tina mentioned her cat and said she wouldn't do anything to hurt the animal. Yet she continued to corner and torment the cat and her parents were active in rescuing the cat and separating the cat from Tina. During the first session, Tina was not confronted with her behavior toward the cat. Instead, storytelling was used to emphasize how upsetting it is to have something happen when parents cannot stop an event and protect their little girl. Through reciprocal storytelling and play, Tina was encouraged to tell her parents when something bothered her and was told that she needed to keep no secrets from her parents.

Tina was attracted to the anatomically developed Barbie dolls and ignored the nondeveloped baby dolls. She asked for help in dressing and undressing the dolls. She avoided the male Ken dols, and she dressed the male dolls in female clothing. Given her avoidance, her recent move to another nursery school, and her lack of new male friends, intervention was attempted to neutralize her belief that when one boy does something bad, all boys do the same thing.

During her second play session, Tina talked about Joey, confirming what she had revealed in the first session. She was more enthusiastic about her new school and new friend. She immediately played with the Barbie dolls, dismissing the Ken dolls by saying, "Ken has a bad, scary face, but the Barbie dolls have pretty faces." Toward the end of the session she was able to approach the male doll in play and cautiously hold it, but she did not bring it close to her body as she did the Barbie doll. She limited the male doll's power and influence by making Barbie, rather than Ken, drive the doll's car. Some resolution seemed to have occurred, as evidenced by her showing somewhat more trust in the male doll. In addition, Tina was excited about her father's coming to the session.

Tina was spontaneous in her stories about school. She did not like talking about what happened at her first school, although she said that "the [previous school] was a dumb school; the boys were rough; Joey used to be my friend; he was messing up people's hair; sometimes he made me angry." Tina did admit during both the first and second session how scared she was when Joey hurt her and the other children.

Another intervention was dealing with Tina's anger with her parents. Tina had been irritable and would not let her parents touch her or cried if they did. She was both angry and frightened that her parents had not known about the abuse and had not been able to protect her from it.

By the third session, Tina was easily engaged in conversation and was willing to play. There was warmth in her approach to the male doll. She put the mother and father dolls together with the baby dolls, and the doll family went off in their car with the Barbie driving. This was understood as some reestablishment of the protective bond, but the play activity demonstrated some continuing feelings of separation, anxiety, and lack of protection. No interpretation was made to the child.

During the third session, Tina pulled all the dolls out of the box. She again talked only about Susan in the context of her new school and did not mention the teachers. She continued to be divided over the nursery school experience, wanting to talk about it but still avoiding the subject. Not wanting to talk about Joey increased with each session. What was presented were incidences where the event was being acted upon in daily life, such as hitting the cat.

A continued symptomatic area was Tina's aggression toward her cat. Tina was repeating her own experience by cornering the cat and poking at it with a toy stick. In the session, using a toy cat, Tina was shown and told that hurting the cat was like what happened when she was trapped by the bigger boy and no one was there to protect her. She did not need to be mean to the cat anymore because she had told her parents that she was angry that they could not protect her.

Part of the intervention was to link Tina's anger toward others in relationship to the trauma. During these interpretations, Tina would nod her head "yes" while pushing the therapist's hand away with her hands—a mixed message. This was Tina's ambivalent reaction to, on the one hand, the relief provoked by the interpretation but the countering issue of anxiety being invoked by uncovering the trauma. In this third play session, it was emphasized that it was important to tell her parents when bad things were happening so that she could be safe and protected. Also, intervention was aimed at separating the past event (danger) from the present (safety) by emphasizing that Joey was no longer present and hurting her.

In the fourth and final evaluation play session, Tina arrived happy with a new doll family and anxious to play. When asked if she had any memories of Joey, she stated she did not want to talk about it anymore and suggested playing the piano (e.g., taking conscious control of the trauma memory).

The themes that emerged in Tina's play were gender anxiety, abandonment, and protection. She asked for the Ken doll but did not use it in the doll play. Tina conversed with a toy Santa Claus about wanting a Ken doll but also had Mrs. Claus in the scene. In other play, Tina gathered all the women dolls in a tight cluster so that no one could be alone; she was startled to find one doll sitting by herself and quickly drew her into the group.

Her first story drawing included a cat, angry that someone had stolen her orange. The mother cat got mad at whoever stole the orange and the father cat broke the thief's leg. This spontaneous reference to the cat, to something happening to the cat, and to the cat's parents punishing the offender parallels Tina's reenactment to her own cat. In this last session, Tina's mother was encouraged to join actively in the session. It was interpreted to Tina that she must have been very scared and angry that mother and father could not protect her from Joey.

Later in the session, Tina played with a puppy. There appeared to be both affectionate and aggressive elements in this play. The puppy took Tina's playfulness as a cue for more exuberant play. This was monitored so that Tina and the puppy could be safely aggressive with each other and to show how protection can accompany aggression. During this time Tina had to use the bathroom and needed assistance (she allowed one therapist to accompany her). In her excitement, she jumped off the toilet and wanted to go outside without her tights and pants. There was nothing compelling outside the bathroom to attract her interest. This behavior suggested an impulse toward exhibitionism, which raised a question as to whether there was more sexualized behavior on the part of Joey that she had witnessed than had been revealed up to that time.

Between sessions, Tina's mother reported the following incidents. At church, several boys were running around and this scared Tina. She asked her mother to take her to the bathroom even though she did not need to use it, telling her mother, "The boys are too rough." She also expressed fear of playgrounds because of boys playing rough. In reading a story with her mother about parents bringing home a new baby and a little sister coming down the stairs to see the baby, Tina asked, "Who was taking care of the little girl while the parents were out of the house?" And in playing with the new friend, the girl told Tina's mother that Tina threw things at her, stuck out her tongue, took her pants off to "show her bum," and kept her pants off. A few days later, Tina cut her finger. She hid her hand and asked her father for some food; when she opened her hand her father saw the bloody finger. To bring this theme of protection into the session, one of the therapists drew a little dog in the woods with a cut paw. When Tina was asked what the little dog did, she said the dog went home and told its mother. It appeared that Tina understood that parents want to be told if anything hurts. Whether Tina fully trusted that she could tell her parents about bad things was a question still unanswered.

APPLICATION OF MODEL TO CASE

The application of the model to this case unfolds during the assessment and intervention as follows.

Pretrauma Phase

Tina was a bright, attractive, 3-year-old child who demonstrated age-appropriate language and play activities. She was in good physical health and from an intact family who communicated their positive feelings for their child. There were no prior traumas to Tina. The implications of this information is that Tina does not have pretrauma life events that in any way would predict more vulnerability to trauma. In

fact, one would expect that the trauma would be managed or not have as negative an impact.

Trauma Encapsulation Phase

The fact that Tina did have a distinct trauma response (e.g., information from the parents and the play sessions) supports the propositions of the encapsulation phase. In particular there was a dominant sensory and perceptual learning that occurred during the trauma that became determinant of symptomatic behavior, e.g., her strong avoidant behavior of male dolls, her fear and anger toward them and separating them out from her play, as well as her negative reaction to father were in juxtaposition to her ability to explain the classmate's sexual aggression. The point is that the fear and avoidance of the male in play and in her daily life were not associated to the assault; rather, the learnings from the trauma were carried into nontrauma situations while at the same time she held a recollection of the details of what had been done to her by the little boy, e.g., the symptomatic behavior derived from the trauma learning. This suggests that the concept of trauma replay has to be understood as types of psychological states that can occur independent of one another or simultaneously.

There was no information available on the schoolmate Joey; thus, the input of his behavior was reconstructed from the trauma replay and direct details as follows. The classmate, 2 years older, enticed her through play and she could not escape. He had access through the school. The entrapment was her lack of protection by adults at the school. He poked at Tina's genitals with toy sticks while hiding under a table; secrecy was used by seeking concealed areas in the school to "play house."

The general anxiety symptoms include: onset of bed-wetting, irritability, startling easily, genital soreness, and temper tantrums. The protest behavior of not wanting to go to school and avoiding playing with males at school and in play were direct expressions of a generalized fear of males.

The three types of trauma replay were noted through the following: Father's attempts to remove her coat or help her dress triggering screaming, crying, and resisting were reenactment, i.e., what happened in the past was going on now. Aggression toward the cat and toward her female playmate were repetition, i.e., she was physically involved in acting out both the role of aggressor and victim with other animate objects. The content of frightening dreams and nightmares and her avoidance and disdain for male dolls during spontaneous play were displacement. In this model, we are using this construct of displacement to refer to inanimate, symbolic representations of the trauma and ideational representations, such as dreams.

During the encapsulation phase, Tina acted out her dilemma at school by being angry with her parents and in particular her father. This anger at her father, particularly when he attempted to remove clothing, alerted the clinician to the trauma replay. The anxiety and displacement of resistant and angry behavior toward the male figure underscores that the abuse was carried out by a male.

This angry behavior at her father was becoming more or less routine when she expressed the sexualization to her mother. The most obvious expression of the encapsulation of the trauma was the drive disharmony, marked by her aggressive behavior and open sexualized interest. Splitting was noted in Tina's denial of her aggressive acts and presentation as "I'm a good girl" ("I'm not mean or hurt people—only bad boys do this") versus her aggression toward her cat and the female playmate.

The drive disharmony shaped the splitting of Tina's sense of herself as a good girl who does not hurt others. There was a lack of acceptance and integration of her aggressive acts as well as an impulsiveness to these acts. She was not testing to find the limits of her behavior but rather exploded into aggressive acts toward the cat or picking on a smaller child.

Disclosure

The disclosure of the abuse was met with positive, prompt, sensible action by the parents.

The mother quickly recognized that her anxiety and upset response to the disclosure was responded to by Tina's becoming silent. As she relaxed, Tina spontaneously revealed details. Tina's mother learned, by watching the therapists, how to manage new details of the abuse, in her terms, modeling "benign curiosity."

Outcome

While the four sessions had the major objective of an evaluation, there was a therapeutic thrust to the process. First, the establishment of safety and trust was essential, not only with the therapist but with Tina's parents. The initial play of Tina around the abuse and being forced to go to nursery school despite her protests had to be addressed, not only for the fundamental welfare of the child but to enable the evaluative process to proceed. The avoidance, fear, and anger that were manifested both in spontaneous play with dolls and in response to specific requests for demonstration of what happened became the focus of interpretive efforts on the part of the evaluators. In particular, the theme of helplessness, anger, and perplexity in not knowing that the parents could not observe what was going on in the nursery school were addressed. This was done through play and dialogue and used at various points in the evaluation when Tina would resurrect behavior either at home or in the session that indicated she was anxious, upset, and fearful of not being protected.

The conclusion of the extended evaluation was that Tina demonstrated an avoidant behavior pattern with traits of aggressive and sexualized play. Her removal from the nursery school and the evaluation interrupted the primary trauma learning. Efforts to neutralize the drive disharmony were instituted in the evaluation sessions and continued at home by the parents.

Summary

This case illustrates the organization of a 3-year-old girl's defensive style derived from a 6-week period of unwanted sexual aggression by a 5-year-old male schoolmate. Case analysis recommends that clinicians both inquire and evaluate children's sexual activities commonly labeled "normal sex play and curiosity" to rule out exploitation by one child of another. Rather than play, one of the children may be coping with ongoing sexual trauma. Failure to suspect, identify, and interrupt abuse between children places a child at risk for developing defensive personality structures, unregulated arousal patterns, delayed social and academic learning, and an impaired sense of self. The psychiatric diagnosis of post-traumatic stress disorder and the nursing diagnosis of rape trauma syndrome apply.[20]

In summary, we have presented an assessment and intervention model for understanding the process by which young children cope with intrapsychic sexual trauma. Two additional steps in model development would be to develop measurements for the key processes that block, link, or solidify symptomatic behaviors and to test outcome response to different interventions.

Questions

1. Autognose your feelings regarding a child victim of sexual abuse and a child perpetrator.
2. What legal action would you suggest for this case example?
3. Apply the principles of intervention to a clinical case you have worked on or heard about.
4. How do the phases of information processing of trauma relate to other life crises?

REFERENCES AND SUGGESTED READINGS

1. Herman, J. L. *Father-Daughter Incest.* Cambridge, Mass.: Harvard University Press, 1981.
2. Conte, J. R., & Shore, D. A. *Social Work and Child Sexual Abuse.* New York: Haworth Press, 1982.
3. Finkelhor, D. *Child Sexual Abuse.* New York: Free Press, 1979.
4. Finkelhor, D. *Sexually Victimized Children.* New York: Free Press, 1984.
5. Rush, F. *The Best Kept Secret: Sexual Abuse of Children.* Englewood Cliffs, N.J.: Prentice-Hall, 1980.
6. Burgess, A. W., Hartman, C. R., & McCormack, A. Abused to abuser: Antecedents to socially deviant behaviors. *American Journal of Psychiatry,* 1987, *144,* 1431–1436.
7. Burgess, A. W., Hartman, C. R., McCausland, M. P., & Powers, P. Response patterns in children and adolescents exploited through sex rings and pornography. *American Journal of Psychiatry,* 1984, *141,* 656–662.
8. Burgess, A. W., Hartman, C. R,., Ressler, R. K., McCormack, A., & Douglas, J. E. Sexual homicide: A motivational model. *Journal of Interpersonal Violence,* 1986, *1,* 251–272.
9. Burgess, A. W., Hartman, C. R., Wolbert, W. A., & Grant, C. A. Child molestation: Assessing impact in multiple victims. *Archives of Psychiatric Nursing,* 1987, *1,* 33–39.
10. MacLean, P. A. *Triune Concept of Brain and Behavior.* Toronto: Toronto Press, 1975.
11. Gardner, H. *The Mind's New Science.* New York: Basic Books, 1985.
12. Shannon, C. E. A symbolic analysis of relay and switching circuits (Master's thesis, Massachusetts Institute of Technology, 1937). *Transactions of the American Institute of Electrical Engineers,* 1938, *57,* 1–11.
13. Figley, C. R. (ed.). *Trauma and Its Wake.* New York: Brunner/Mazel, 1984.
14. Horowitz, M. J. *Stress Response Syndromes.* New York: Jason Aronson, 1976.
15. Van Der Kolk, B. A. *Post-Traumatic Stress Disorder: Psychological and Biological Sequelae.* Washington, D.C.: American Psychiatric Press, 1984.
16. Horowitz, op. cit.
17. Burgess, Hartman, McCausland, & Powers, op cit.
18. Hartman, C. R., & Burgess, A. W. Child sexual abuse: Generic roots of the victim experience. *Journal of Psychotherapy and Family,* 1986, *2,* 83–92.
19. Freud, S. [Splitting of the ego in the defensive process]. In J. Strachey (Ed. and trans.), *Collected Papers* (Vol. 5). New York: Basic Books, 1959. (Originally published, 1938).
20. American Psychiatric Association. *Diagnostic and Statistical Manual* (3rd ed., Rev.). Washington, D.C.: American Psychiatric Association, 1987.

Chapter 26

Family Work in Nursing Practice

Gloria Edelhauser Shapiro

Chapter Objectives

The students successfully attaining the goals of this chapter will be able to:

- Demonstrate the ability to identify the structure and functions of a family.
- Demonstrate the ability to describe basic components of family assessment.
- Demonstrate an understanding of basic concepts that elucidate family functioning.
- Demonstrate the ability to identify and describe an example of the following basic family interventions: prevention of future dysfunction, intervention in life-cycle crises, and identification and referral of problem families.

INTRODUCTION

All individuals are members of a family and bring some aspects of their family context to other relationships. Nurses encounter families and family influences in every area of clinical practice. Acquiring knowledge of basic family principles enhances the effectiveness of all nursing practice.

Nurses are in a key position to work toward preventing dysfunction, to intervene in normal life-cycle crises, and to identify and refer troubled families to a family therapist. A working knowledge of family concepts will guide the nurse in assessing how well a family is functioning and what level of intervention is appropriate. It is useful for the generalist to understand the premises and language of the specialist so that care can be coordinated. This chapter will: (1) review the historical development of the field of family therapy; (2) describe assessment concepts for the nurse generalist and for the specialist; (3) present an overview of intervention models; and (4) discuss the role of nurses in family work and research about family phenomena.

HISTORICAL DEVELOPMENT

Traditional practice of mental health professionals has focused on understanding the intrapsychic life of an individual and on fostering insight and emotional growth in a dyadic relationship between therapist and client. However, as twentieth-century thought has evolved to a more systemic view of the natural world, the attention of behavioral scientists and many clinicians has turned to the study of the individual in his network and to the complex and subtle ways in which families and other social networks function as interconnected systems. Many therapists have begun to broaden their perspective and look at *patterns of interaction* between people. The notion that people are not isolated and are constantly reacting to and interacting with others in the family has become a new basis for fostering growth and change.

The best-known pioneer in the family movement in mental health is Nathan Ackerman, originally a psychoanalyst and child psychiatrist, who published a paper in 1937 that underscored the importance of the family.[1]

In the early 1950s, many clinicians were meeting with frustration and poor results in the individual treatment of schizophrenia and delinquency in children. The research of the period primarily focused on families who had a schizophrenic member. Clinicians working with patients who exhibited schizophrenic symptoms began to notice that often when the identified patient improved, another family member would become symptomatic. A new perspective evolved that viewed the symptomatic member as bearing a problem for the entire family. Hoffman observes that "Bateson's 1952–1962 research project on communication [indicated] that a change in a family depended very much on the interplay between deviation and the way deviation was kept within bounds 'in a specific family'."[2] While more recent research has clarified the biologic etiology of schizophrenia, Bateson's work with schizophrenics built a framework for examining the influence of social context in understanding individual behavior.

In 1957, the family movement gained recognition at the annual American Orthopsychiatric Association meeting at which a Family Research Panel presented their work for the first time at a national professional conference. Momentum began to pick up. In 1960, Jackson published *The Etiology of Schizophrenia*, and Murray Bowen published *A Family Concept of Schizophrenia*.[3,4] Around 1960, another family movement pioneer, Salvadore Minuchin, began work in Pennsylvania at the Wiltwyck School for Delinquent Boys. Later, Minuchin moved on to Philadelphia, where he developed a therapeutic model (structural family therapy) for treating poor urban families.

Around the same time, Nathan Ackerman founded the Family Institute in New York. Two years later, Ackerman and Don Jackson collaborated to produce the field's first journal, *Family Process*.[5] Other notable early family researchers and clinicians included Gregory Bateson, Richard Fisch, Jay Haley, Paul Watzlawick, John Weakland, Don Jackson, and Virginia Satir in California; Murray Bowen in Washington, D.C.; Theodore Lidz in New Haven; Carl Whitaker in Atlanta; and Ivan Boszormenyi-Nagy and James Framo in Philadelphia.

As clinical research advanced, it became clearer that the behavior of the symptomatic person was only part of larger repeating patterns in which the symptom was noted to be a response to family behaviors, and those behaviors were observed to occur in reaction to the symptom. Circularity displaced "linear thinking" as an explanatory model. Linear thinking assumes that one behavior *causes* another; circularity assumes that behaviors are part of a repeating pattern, without assigning cause or effect. Therefore, interventions were devised to alter or disrupt the patterns rather than cure an isolated symptom.[6] With change from focusing on the individual to working with families, there has been movement away from only identifying mental "illness" to also assessing functioning within a family.

In the late 1960s and early 1970s, the family movement came into its own as a major treatment modality in mental health. As the field grew, a number of different schools of thought and clinical application developed. Among them are systems therapy, structural therapy, and strategic therapy. At present, the family movement is still growing, and an increasing number of mental health professionals are integrating family therapy into their work.

ASSESSMENT

Assessment Concepts for the Generalist

Functions of the Family

The family is the basic unit in the structure of human social organization. A family may be defined as a group of people united by blood, marriage, or other bonding.[7] It provides an environment for contact, interaction, and intimacy. It is a system of interconnected and interrelated parts that is greater than the sum of its parts. Like other natural systems, the structure and process of a family can be identified and understood.

A family functions as a subsystem within the larger community and is organized around the regulation, support, nurturance, and socialization of its members.[8] The family "serves as a mediator between the needs of [its members] and the forces, demands, and obligations of society."[9] The family must accommodate to the culture and also must transmit that culture to its members.[10] The emphasis placed on different functions can vary in different cultures, and the manner in which functions are carried out may be culturally determined. Families teach people the basic skills of how to care for themselves, how to communicate thoughts and feelings, how to be responsive to others and share resources, how to follow rules and set limits, and how to make decisions and solve problems. A family must also teach its members how to be close to others without losing individual identity, how to be different and separate without being isolated, and how to balance belonging with independence. Of all the influences on an individual, the family has been described as the greatest potential resource as well as the greatest potential source of stress.[11]

Adaptation to change is a basic requirement of human survival. All families must deal with constant change from within and from without. Within the family are life-cycle changes of births, deaths, illnesses, marriages, puberty, and separation. Each person is constantly evolving in his own developmental cycle and sense of identity. From without, the family is faced with numerous societal forces: Political crises, changing neighborhoods, wars, racial discrimination, and economic depressions only begin the list of stressors. The family must provide continuity in the midst of change and maintain a connectedness over generations while solving the problems and needs of today. The task for a family is to achieve a state of balance that can adapt to and even encourage change.[12]

In assessing family functioning, the nurse may use the following questions as a guideline:

1. Is the living environment safe?
2. Is the family maintaining adequate nutrition, health, and shelter?
3. Is the family able to generate adequate economic resources to meet its material needs?
4. Are all family members at appropriate stages of growth and development for their phase in the life cycle?
5. Are there appropriate rules for guiding behavior both within the family and outside?
6. Does the family have a viable method of resolving conflicts? Does it allow for interaction of differences?
7. Can family members work together to meet their goals?
8. Are members able to look to one another for support and for love?
9. Are the children learning skills of daily living?
10. Do family members have workable decision-making methods and problem-solving skills?
11. Do family members have a peer group outside of the family?
12. Do family members have a healthy balance of time with the family and time with others?

It is especially important to look at the relationship of the parents. They set the tone and furnish the foundation of stability for a family system. Are they caring with each other, or do they fight to make contact? Can they resolve conflict? Can they function as a team to exert appropriate authority in their family?

Each family will have different areas of strengths and weaknesses in its overall ability to function. Some families will have overt symptoms of dysfunction. Functioning will vary, depending on the amount of stress the system is subjected to at any given time, so one must look at the number and intensity of stressors. A family's ability to respond to a crisis will depend on the balance of resources and degree of stress at a particular time.

Skills by Which a Family Achieves Its Goals

In each family there are basic skills that members must have to move toward goal attainment. These skills include communication, cooperation, decision making, and problem solving.

The most basic interpersonal skill in a family is communication. Without an exchange of information, ideas, and feelings, a family cannot function well. Communication is the basic mechanism for human contact; it is a link between family members and between the family and others. The basic aim of any communication is for the receiver to get the same meaning from a message that the sender had in mind. Both verbal and nonverbal communication are important and powerful.

In the assessment of communication patterns in a family, the nurse must keep in mind that each family has its own unique patterns that have evolved in the context of cultural influences over time. Above all, as each pattern is identified, one should remember the following key questions: How well does it work? What is gained and what is lost?

The following questions are offered as guidelines for looking at family communication:

1. Who talks to whom? Are communications person-to-person, or do they involve a third person?
2. Do people give clear messages of their thoughts, wishes, needs, and feelings, or do they expect others to magically "know"?
3. Can people speak freely and candidly? Are some or all family members interrupted? Who interrupts whom?
4. Do people listen to one another? Can they repeat what they have heard?
5. Is there congruence between verbal and nonverbal messages? (Does a mother say, "I love you" to a child but recoil from a hug?)
6. Do people use dysfunctional forms of communication, such as "blaming, placating, distracting, or intellectualizing"?[13]

Effective communication makes it possible for a family to make decisions and solve problems. Like any other living system, the family and its members need feedback about their performance in order to modify their responses for successful adaptation to the changing environment.

Decision making and power in a family are closely related. The way decisions are made in a family will be one indication of how power is distributed among its members. Power is also expressed in families by those who have the ability to seek or block intimacy.[14] Dysfunctional family patterns often include confused communication and avoidance of power issues.[15] Minuchin believes that in a healthy family, there must be a power hierarchy in which parents and children function within different levels of authority.[16] T. E. Horton points out that the decision-making process is affected by coalitions in the family and that such coalitions are dysfunctional when they involve people from different generations.[17]

In assessing the distribution of power in a family, one can keep in mind the following questions:

1. Do family members share in some way in decisions, appropriate for their age and stage, or do one or more members make all decisions?
2. How do family members find out about key decisions?
3. Do family members have a chance to say how they feel about decisions that directly affect them?
4. Do family members feel that they can make a difference in the life of the family?

Concepts for the Specialist

People who specialize in working with families have begun to identify a number of dynamic concepts that elucidate the lives of all families. These concepts are the tools that guide a family therapist's observations in assessing families. They help a therapist determine what is going on in a distressed family so that a plan for intervention can be developed.

Circularity

The concept of circularity is a new way of thinking about human behavior. When applied to family assessment, it transcends the traditional understanding of cause and effect. This idea arose from the practice of viewing families through a one-way screen through which clinicians observed family communications and behaviors. Over time many "circular" patterns were observed with the behavior of the symptomatic person emerging as only part of a larger repetitive pattern.[18] In such a cycle, the symptom is maintained by the very behaviors that seek to solve the problem.[19]

An example of circularity is a wife whose continued suspicious questioning of her husband only reinforces his silence, which only serves to reinforce her jealousy; it becomes a vicious circle.[20] Such a relentless pattern traps all the participants. To look for causality presents the same dilemma as the classic "chicken and egg" question. Interactional events can be seen as simply "moments" in circular patterns.

Several terms may be used to describe family interaction. For example, a single action is a *move,* and a string of two or more such moves may be called a *sequence.* Sequences may be *cyclic* and the most important sequences are those that are *recurrent.*[21]

All families experience a variety of stresses that trigger vicious circles in interpersonal relationships. What is different in families with members in the deepest trouble is the way these vicious circles continually repeat, without ever allowing the family to change.[22]

Psychopolitics

Kantor and Lehr employ a conceptual model that identifies the specific types of moves that can be made in patterns of family interaction. They call their model psychopolitics, and it uses a four-player "part" system as a means for describing and analyzing interpersonal family processes. Observing numerous natural family interactions, they noted that there were only four types of roles that any individual could assume in interacting with others. A person could play the part of *mover* by initiating an idea or action; he could respond as a *follower* by supporting another or going along; he could act as an *opposer* by disagreeing with the idea of a mover or refusing to go along in some way; or a person could function as a *bystander* by watching the others or giving them nonjudgmental feedback about their actions or about the situation.[23]

People meeting for the first time have the same basic options at their disposal; that is, the potential for parts remains the same no matter how many persons are present in the social field. In families, patterns and sequences of moves tend to develop, and some members tend to play one part or a certain combination of parts more frequently than others.[24] The important factor is flexibility. Ideally each family member should be able to play any of the four parts with ease, depending on what is most appropriate and useful in a particular situation. Problems occur when people can only play some of the parts or when certain people or certain situations evoke a stereotyped response, for example, the daughter who always opposes her father regardless of what he says or does. The most serious problems arise when one or more family members can only play one part, like the anorectic adolescent who can be seen as a "stuck opposer."

Boundaries

The concept of boundaries is a metaphor used by family therapists and other systems thinkers to talk about the ways in which people regulate contact and interchange in a social system. A boundary can be thought of as a physical, emotional, or interpersonal space that separates parts. Every living system has boundaries. An example in the physical world is the cell membrane. The membrane is the barrier that sur-

rounds and contains the material that makes a cell. This barrier separates the cell from the outside world and regulates the inflow and outflow of products necessary for the cell's survival. Boundaries also occur between people. There is a boundary between the family and the outside world, and within the family between groupings of family members (subsystems) and between individuals (Fig. 26-1).

Within the family, boundaries function to maintain individual identity, to regulate emotional intimacy, to define rules of relating, and to manage the flow of resources and information. To work well, these boundaries must be clear and at the same time flexible. Each family member must be able to function without undue interference, and each one must have healthy contact with others in the family. For example, the boundary around the parents allows children to have access to the parents but excludes them from spouse intimacy and parental functions.[25] Parents, in their own relationship, share emotions, conversations, and activities with each other that would be inappropriate to share with children. For example, a family has a "boundary dysfunction" if a mother is telling her 9-year-old son about her marital problems and is using his advice to try to correct them.

Successful negotiation of self-boundaries in relation to the family has been called differentiation by Murray Bowen.[26] He has emphasized that in the healthy development of self, it is important that each individual learn to weigh family expectations and patterns and to cull out what works for himself, rather than unthinkingly accepting or uniformly rebelling against family ways. A person who has achieved mature self-identity in relation to the family will be able to let family members know what he believes, wants and needs, and what he can offer others. Bowen believes that a differentiated person will be goal-directed and will use reason instead of making choices determined by the flow of emotion in the family.

When boundaries surround groups of individuals in a family, *subsystems* are formed. Subsystems are defined by commonalities of generation, function, gender, or interests. Each family member simultaneously belongs to a number of different subsystems. In each subsystem a person learns different skills and learns about the experience and use of different levels of power. For example, the sibling subsystem can be thought of as a "social laboratory" where children can experiment with peer relationships without undue interference from their parents.[27]

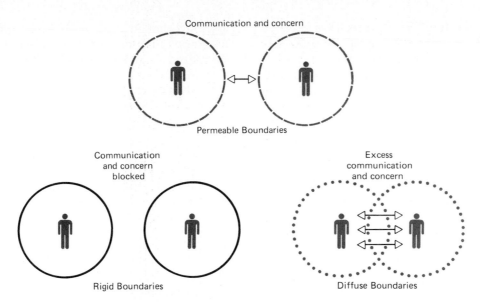

Figure 26-1. Concept of boundaries.

Boundary Dysfunctions

Boundary regulation can go awry in families and other human relationships in a variety of ways. A blurring of boundaries between the self and others is called fusion.[28] In all relationships there is a pull for togetherness. If the pull is too strong and the togetherness becomes extreme, each individual loses the clarity of his unique identity. One should not confuse fusion with closeness. Closeness permits sharing but without the loss of self-boundaries. People who become "fused" function as a single emotional system; neither individual feels "whole" without the other and different feelings and responses to the outside world are not tolerated. In a fused relationship there is often an imbalance of functioning. In a fused dyad, one person may overfunction and the other may underfunction; one person may assume too much responsibility and the other too little for managing his life. An example would be a passive spouse whose assertive partner makes all the decisions regarding family life and household management. The death of the overresponsible member of this dyad could be crippling for the spouse.

In all relationships there is constant negotiation of closeness and distance. During times of stress, people tend to respond by moving toward fusion, which functions to manage anxiety. Fusion is an expected phenomenon in a family's life; the crucial factor is whether a person can restore healthy boundaries when the stress subsides.

When fusion threatens to engulf individuality, it is a natural response for a person to react

by "distancing." However, when a true separateness has not developed, emotional fusion can continue to exist even when there is considerable geographical distance.

Fusion can characterize relationships between any number of people in a family system. When it becomes a widespread pattern throughout a family, it has been called enmeshment. Minuchin describes a family as enmeshed when it is not clear who belongs in what subsystem.[29] In an enmeshed family there is an excess of communication and concern between people, which usually results in an overload of emotions for the family members. For example, in such a system, the whole family might be in an emotional upheaval if a child brings home one poor paper from school.

Another effect of enmeshment, which Minuchin emphasizes . . . is to weaken the boundaries that allow subsystems to work. In brief, the boundary between the nuclear family and families of origin is not well-maintained; the boundary separating parents from their children is frequently invaded in improper ways; and the roles of spouse and parent are never clearly differentiated. . . . Finally the children are not differentiated on the basis of age or maturation level, so that the sibling subsystem cannot contribute properly to the socialization process.[30]

At the other end of the continuum of boundary regulation is dysfunction resulting from excessively rigid boundaries. It is the opposite of fusion and enmeshment. Minuchin uses the term disengaged when a family's boundaries are so rigid that the communication of information, thoughts, and feelings between people is seriously limited, and the protective functions of the family are handicapped.[31] Members of such a family are so separate that they are isolated from one another; mutual support is unavailable; and responsiveness to the other is lacking.

Although an entire family may have a disengaged pattern of interaction, the more usual pattern is to have different subsystems with varying degrees of disengagement. It is normal for families to have some degree of enmeshment and some disengaged subsystems at various points in the family life cycle. The important consideration is the degree of enmeshment or disengagement. When children are very young, the parent-child relationship is naturally enmeshed; and as children grow up, parents and children need to become more disengaged.

Concept of Triangles

Another concept that describes a normal phenomenon in family life is that of triangles. It is a common organizing principle among family therapists that is used to assess patterns of family closeness and distance. A triangle, or three-person group, has been described as the basic stable unit of an emotional system.[32] A two-person system is thought to be stable as long as there is no experience of anxiety. However, few people can relate personally with one another for very long without some anxiety. When anxiety is felt, a dyad becomes stressed, and then a third focus of attention is brought in to divert or to decrease the tension.

Triangles can occur even when a third person is not present. Distance between two people can be created by talking about a third person rather than about themselves. Some couples have trouble talking if the discussion is not about their children, in-laws, or friends.

The phenomenon of triangulation offers emotional stabilization through diversion rather than through direct resolution of issues within a dyad. For example, in a family where the parents are emotionally estranged from one another, in their aloneness they may overinvolve a child in their emotional distress.[33] Usually triangles are made up of a comfortably close twosome and a less comfortable outsider.[34] The contact between members of any dyad can appear either harmonious or conflictual in nature because some people maintain close contact through fighting.

People in families are members of many triangles. Some triangles will cross generational lines and will involve the extended family. Family triangles are functional when the positions regularly change; that is, who is close or who is the outsider does not remain fixed. For example, in a functional triangle that includes a father, mother, and daughter, the mother and daughter may spend time together and share ideas and feelings, while the father assumes a distant position. At another time the father and daughter share a special time together, and the mother is involved elsewhere. At another time, the husband and wife are close as a couple and the daughter is the outsider. There is a constant flow in this three-person system (Fig. 26-2).

In families with a symptomatic member therapists have observed that the triangle that appears most frequently is a coalition between two people of different generations at the expense of the third person.[35] A dysfunctional triangle can be exemplified by a triangle that again includes a father, mother, and daughter. But this time the mother and daughter are always close, and the father remains in a distant position. Any effort made by the father to make contact with his daughter or move closer to his wife is either overtly or covertly blocked by his wife or daughter, and any attempt by the wife to move closer to her husband is blocked by him or their daughter, and so on. Each person in a dysfunctional triangle plays a part in keeping the positions fixed.

According to Hoffman, Bowen associates pathology with rigidity and suggests that although all families create triadic patterns, these patterns will become more rigid when the family is facing a change or undergoing stress, and will be more flexible in periods of calm.[36]

Closeness and apartness are both important aspects of family relationships, but it seems that these processes in a distressed family are always triadic, because no closeness, or any apartness either, is ever comfortable between two people.[37]

Hoffman further notes that Bowen believes that there can be positive repercussions on others in a family if someone can achieve a more flexible position in a family triangle, even if it is a distant one. Bowen sees networks of triangles as deeply linked and reactive to one another. As in a spider's web, a touch at any spot will vibrate across the web. Thus, in a family, change in one corner may activate unpredictable responses in another corner, and this may help to free persons long caught in inhibiting positions, including the person initiating the change.[38]

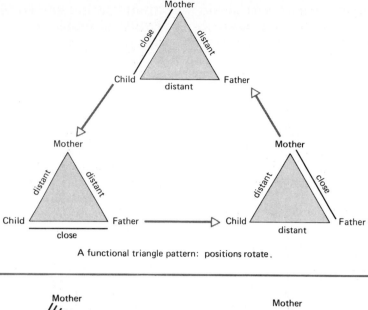

A functional triangle pattern: positions rotate.

A dysfunctional triangle: positions remain fixed.

Figure 26-2. Triangles.

INTERVENTION: THE GENERALIST AS HELPER

Nursing practice takes place in a variety of settings and reaches across the life-span of families. A nurse has the opportunity to have contact with members of families during some of the most stressful times of their lives—at births, illnesses, and deaths. At such times, families are more open; they may be more willing to ask for or accept help, and they may be more able to make changes in their usual manner of functioning.

Prevention of Dysfunction

For the nurse to implement preventive interventions, she must be knowledgeable about the nature and impact of life-cycle events and be able to identify dysfunctional responses. Preventive interventions include teaching families about: normal life-cycle changes, normal growth and development of individuals, normal ex-pected responses to change, and the value of mutual support and open communication. Family members need to know that anxiety increases at times of transition and trauma and that anxiety often decreases when feelings are appropriately acknowledged and shared.

Intervention in Life-Cycle Crises

There are a variety of interventions that nurses can implement in families with a prior history of healthy functioning who are experiencing a developmental or situational crisis. The nurse can help families identify the nature of the particular crisis they are experiencing, can open communication about stressful issues among appropriate family members, and can support family members in problem solving. In some families the nurse may need to help the members to strengthen diffuse boundaries by fostering the cessation of inappropriate sharing or inappropriate actions between generations. In other families the nurse may support the relaxation of overly rigid boundaries by fostering communication between members who are isolated. In all families the nurse can facilitate relationships by helping members to talk directly with each other.

The following interventions illustrate the type of therapeutic work that may be done. In a family with a new baby, the nurse may help the parents solve how to arrange needed time alone. In a recently divorced family, the nurse may help a mother who has become overinvolved in the life of her child to establish more appropriate distance and to generate some adult activities and relationships. In a family having difficulty with adolescent children, the nurse may help the family to negotiate fair and appropriate rules and expectations. The nurse can help the couple with a newly retired member to renegotiate their roles and grieve over the losses involved in changing.

In settings oriented toward physical care, nurses can foster mutual support and sharing of feelings and information in families. Nurses should include patients in all planning and can help patients to appropriately involve their families. Nurses can also help other professionals become more aware of family members and to include them in the overall plan of care.

Identification and Referral of Troubled Families

The identification and referral of seriously troubled families is an important part of nursing practice.

In all settings of practice, nurses should be able to assess family functioning so that families with dysfunctions can be identified and referred to a family therapist. Supporting a troubled family until the referral is completed is essential. Families needing services are those who are not able to cope with everyday stresses, those who are having difficulty adjusting to major illnesses or disabilities, or those who exhibit serious symptoms of distress. These symptoms include:

1. Psychosis in any member.
2. Alcoholism in any member.
3. Physical abuse.
4. Sexual abuse.
5. Psychosomatic disorders.
6. Anorexia or bulimia.
7. Suicide gestures or attempts.
8. "Acting out" behavior in any member.
9. Depression in any member.

Clinical Illustration of a Family Intervention

—— CASE EXAMPLE OF MR. ROBERTS: DEPRESSION ————————————

I. Medical Diagnosis (upon admission to a medical–psychiatric inpatient unit): Depression, status post right posterior parietal CVA, rule out metastasis from colon cancer.
II. Patient Summary
   A. Personal and Family History: Mr. Roberts is a 78-year-old married man of Eastern European descent. As a young man he entered the family business as a textile merchant and enjoyed extreme success throughout his career. He retired at the age of 77. He is the youngest in a family of five sons and two daughters; only one sister is currently living. Throughout most of his adult life he was romantically involved with two women, dividing his time between them for about 20 years. He married one of the women when it was discovered that she had cancer; she died shortly thereafter. He then married the other, his wife for the past 18 years. He did not have any children in either marriage.
   B. History of the Problem: Mr. Roberts had a colostomy for colon cancer about 6 months prior to admission and suffered a stroke while recovering from his surgery. The stroke left him with some perceptual and cognitive deficits, some reversible muscle weakness, and possibly caused increased depressed mood. He reports feeling depressed since his retirement and the death of a valued business associate. Since his surgery he has lost nearly 50 pounds, has had appetite and sleep disturbance and extreme irritability. He has been home for about 2 months and has refused to care for himself. He will not touch his colostomy. Though able to walk, he either stays in bed or sits in a wheelchair. His wife has hired a home nurse's aid to help with Mr. Roberts' care. The two of them have done everything for him including holding his penis while he urinates. Mrs. Roberts has been so overwhelmed by his demands and frightened by his irritability that she and the nurse's aide have sedated him at the time that the aide departs so he will sleep until her return in the morning. His wife reports that since the stroke, her husband has begun to use profane language and has become ag-

gressive, assaulting her at times. He has not been able to tolerate being alone for any length of time. His wife currently is exhausted and clearly overwhelmed.

C. Nursing Diagnosis.
1. Ineffective Family Coping, Disabling
2. Depression, Reactive (situational)
3. Body Image Disturbance

NURSING CARE PLAN
Depression

ASSESSMENT

A   Problem # 1
S   "I can't do anything myself. I'm used to having someone do everything for me."
O   Patient wishes to stay in bed wearing nightclothes. He calls for staff when he needs to urinate to ask them to hold the urinal and his penis. Though physically capable of self-care, he wants to be bathed and dressed by staff. When the nurse's aide employed by the family visits, she holds his water glass and accedes to his demands surrounding elimination. She approaches the staff frequently to ask for personal care items so she can tend to him. She visits every day, coming in arm-in-arm with Mrs. Roberts, who literally leans on her for support. The nurse's aide interacts with the family and others as if she, too, were a family member. Mrs. Roberts accedes to all of her husband's demands (which increase when she is present); she seems afraid to say no or suggest any alternative.

NURSING DIAGNOSIS

Ineffective Family Coping, disabling for the patient and spouse.

GOALS

Long-Term
1. The family will alter their pattern of reinforcing Mr. Robert's helplessness so he will cease to underfunction.
2. Patient's wife will resolve her guilt and anger toward her husband and only assist him in activities that he is incapable of doing alone. She will cease to overfunction in the dyad.
3. The nurse's aide who has "joined" the family will assume an appropriate role. She will support the family members emotionally and will assist with Mr. Robert's rehabilitation in a manner that builds autonomy and function.

Short-Term
1. Patient will become aware of rehabilitation rationale and will tolerate others saying no to requests for help in areas that are within his capabilities.
2. Wife and nurse's aide will become knowledgeable about rehabilitation philosophy and approach.
3. Wife and nurse's aide will be able to differentiate activities patient can do independently, activities patient needs some assistance with, and activities that patient cannot do for himself.
4. Wife and nurse's aide will be able to say no to the patient when appropriate.
5. The couple will meet with the family worker and primary nurse to discuss changes in their life and relationship.
6. Patient will carry out tasks surrounding urine elimination: he'll hold his penis, use the bathroom, pull his pants up and down.
7. Patient will dress and undress himself and care for his clothing, including doing laundry with minimal assistance.
8. Patient will wean from wheelchair and begin to use walker for ambulation.
9. Patient will eat meals in dining room with other patients.
10. Patient will bathe himself with minimal assistance.

INTERVENTIONS

1. Teach patient about rehabilitation philosophy, and rationale for doing things himself.
2. Help patient to assume self-care activities of which he is capable, starting with most basic (i.e., urine elimination). Add one activity every day or every other day depending on patient's tolerance. Stay with patient during care activities at first to offer emotional support.
3. Build alliance with wife and nurse's aide and then begin to teach them that "doing for" the patient may not be the best way to help, even when he asks.
4. Offer nurse's aide and wife clear guidelines for when to help, how much to help, and when and how to say no to Mr. Roberts without withdrawing support.
5. Support Mr. and Mrs. Roberts' attendance at family meetings. Collaborate with family worker to facilitate couple's adaptation to life changes.

NURSING CARE PLAN
Depression

ASSESSMENT

A   Problem #2
S   "What's the use of doing anything. I can't do anything anyway."
O   Patient has been an active, competent person throughout his life. He now presents himself as helpless to carry out even the most basic tasks of daily living. He is reluctant to leave his wheelchair to ambulate with a walker even though the physical therapist has assessed that he has adequate strength. He asks others to put on his clothes and fasten his pants. He is resistant to leaving his room; he avoids interaction with other patients. He has always been an avid sports fan and now shows no interest in sports events on TV or the sports page in the newspaper. His appetite is poor and he has trouble getting to sleep without medication. He demonstrates generalized irritability and exhibits rage toward his wife.

NURSING DIAGNOSIS

Reactive Depression (situational).

GOALS

Long-Term
1. Patient will be free of vegetative signs of depression, i.e., appetite disturbance, sleep disturbance, compromised energy.
2. Patient will accept and adapt to his limitations and function fully to his potential. He will become reinvolved in relationships and previous areas of interest in a positive fashion.

Short-Term
1. Patient will increase his autonomy and esteem by assuming responsibility for basic activities of daily living within his capabilities.
2. Patient will attend therapeutic groups and milieu activities to decrease withdrawal and isolation.
3. Patient will eat part or all of three meals a day.
4. Patient will begin to develop a healthy sleep pattern.
5. Patient will begin to participate in TV sports viewing.
6. Patient will grieve over his loss of work-related roles and loss of physical function.
7. Patient will become knowledgeable about his specific deficits and realistic capabilities.
8. Patient will cease directing excessive anger toward his wife.

INTERVENTIONS

1. Offer patient firm direction and emotional support to begin doing his own ADL, one activity at a time. Allow patient opportunity to talk about what it's like to carry out the activities.
2. Negotiate schedule of groups and activities with patient and assist him in getting to the groups at the outset.
3. Assist patient with menu selection and getting to dining room for meals.
4. Discourage naps and staying in bed during daytime hours; discourage extremely early bedtimes.
5. Invite patient to view sports on TV and initiate discussions of sports events.
6. Facilitate patient reminiscing about work life and physical capabilities before his surgery and stroke.
7. Teach patient about the specifics of his limitations and capabilities. Encourage expression of feelings about losses.

NURSING CARE PLAN
Depression

ASSESSMENT

A   Problem #3
S   "I never do anything with my colostomy."
O   Mr. Roberts has never applied the ostomy appliance or emptied the bag in the 6 months since his colostomy procedure. He has "state-of-the-art" equipment that is easy to apply and to manage; the care is within his ability. He appears to have an aversion to viewing the ostomy area of his body.

NURSING DIAGNOSIS

Body Image Disturbance: Specifically nonintegration of change in bowel function and appearance of abdominal area.

GOALS

Long-Term
1. Patient will accept colostomy as a "normal" part of his body.
2. Patient will assume complete care of his colostomy.

Short-Term
1. Patient will become familiar with the ostomy equipment.
2. Patient will discuss the components of ostomy care with the staff.
3. Patient will routinely observe ostomy care by the staff.
4. Patient will touch ostomy area and equipment.
5. Patient will assist staff with emptying the ostomy bag.

INTERVENTIONS

1. Encourage patient to express thoughts and feelings about the change in his body.
2. Discuss ostomy care in a matter-of-fact, normalizing manner.
3. Offer patient the opportunity to handle the ostomy equipment but do not pressure if he seems reluctant.
4. Increase invitations for patient's involvement in ostomy care as his tolerance increases.

PROCESS RECORDING OF A SESSION WITH MR. ROBERTS*

Mr. Roberts	Nurse's Thoughts Feelings	Nurse's Actions	Nurse's Interpretatons
1. "I need you to give me a shower today. My wife or Diane always does it at home."	2. I have to find a way to avoid taking on the role of his wife or Diane.	3. "I understand you are used to your wife and Diane giving you a shower, but we need to try something a little different. I can assist you with this but I'd like you to try to do as much as you can yourself."	4. Mr. Roberts wants to re-create his family dynamics in the hospital.
5. "I can do it. It's just easier if you do it for me."		6. "Helping people be independent is one way we help people feel better about themselves."	
7. "I already feel okay about myself. I don't need that kind of help."	8. I feel frustrated with his opposition, and I realize this is one of the ways he manipulates his family. I want to avoid getting into a struggle with him. I know he's angry with me.		9. He is overtly denying his dependency needs and displaying his opposition; this is a rudimentary step toward autonomy.
11. "Never mind. I'll wait for Diane. She'll do it for me."		10. "Can you tell me what kind of help you do need?"	12. He is falling back on his old strategy of triangling in another woman to get his needs met.
		13. "I understand that Diane is helpful to you at home, but here in the hospital it is important to work with us."	

494

14. "All right, but it's going to take me a long time."

15. He can respond to a firm approach, but he isn't going to make it easy.

16. I want to reinforce his doing things for himself.

17. "I have plenty of time set aside to work with you on this right now."

18. I am feeling relieved that he is less oppositional.

19. "OK, we can go step by step. What is your usual routine at home?"

20. "First I need to take off my shirt." [minimal effort to undo the buttons] "I can't seem to do it. Will you do it for me?"

21. I know he can do this himself; I've seen him. I have to resist giving in to his helplessness.

22. Mr. Roberts is attempting to get me to nurture him.

23. "I know I've worked with you other times when you've been able to do this on your own. Why don't you give it another try?"

24. "I am trying."

25. I wonder if it's a mistake to confront his lack of effort. I think we're starting to struggle: better to try another approach.

26. "We can work on this together. If you show me which button is hardest, I can help you start."

27. "This top one is the hardest; see, I just can't get it."

28. Relieved that this worked.

29. "That's great. I realize that was hard, but it's good you can keep trying even if it doesn't work the first time."

30. Mr. Roberts needs some show of nurturance before he can engage in any independent behavior. He's afraid of being abandoned if he acts too independently.

* Appreciation is expressed to Mr. Roberts' primary nurse, Karen Duvall, and to his associate primary nurse, Greg Graham, for contributing the process recordings. The history and care plans were based on their nursing documentation in the patient's chart.

PROCESS RECORDING OF A SESSION WITH THE NURSES'S AIDE

Diane	Nurse's Thoughts Feelings	Nurse's Actions	Nurse's Interpretations
1. "I'm so glad he is finally here. He has been such a problem at home. He is so demanding and won't do anything for himself."			
	2. Impressed by the intensity of her feelings. I now realize how much she was involved.	3. "I can appreciate how difficult that must of been."	
4. "Is he ever going to get better? Because I've had it, and it's making his wife really ill too."	5. I think she's going to need a lot of support.	6. "Maybe it would be helpful for me to go over some of the things we feel will be helpful to Mr. Roberts right now."	7. She has adopted the perspective of a family member
8. "Does he do anything for himself here?"		9. "We encourage him to do as much as possible for himself."	
10. "You mean he doesn't get angry and make you do it?"	11. No wonder it's been so hard at home.	12. "I'm not sure what you mean 'make me do it'."	
13. "Well, it's like he can do stuff for himself, but he's so stubborn. He'll say he can't, and when I won't do it he gets real angry."	14. I feel wary of her. She seems really angry.	15. "It must be hard to have him get so angry."	16. She knows she's being manipulated but probably doesn't know how to change things.
17. "What do you do when he does that?"	18. I hope that Diane is engaging with us and is willing to adapt to our treatment plan. I realize she needs a lot of education and support in dealing with a person who is so depressed and dependent.		19. She seems open to new alternatives because of her extreme frustration.
	20. I hope she will be able to understand what we're trying to do.	21. "When people have had a lot of losses, they can feel hopeless and less able to help themselves in ways they	

could before. He may feel very badly about his stroke and ostomy. One way to help people have a better image of themselves is to help them be as independent as possible. We are working on a gradual step-by-step process to help Mr. Roberts practice all the skills he has. This will create more of a balance between what's still there and what has been lost. What's most useful when he says he can't is to acknowledge how hard it is but to encourage him to go on trying. It won't change overnight but will be a gradual process. It's important to be consistent and we would appreciate your hlep with this plan when you visit."

22. "I'm willing to try anything to make things better at home. I just know it can't go on as bad as it was. He is driving us both crazy; I worry about his wife the most."

23. She seems very involved with both Mr. Roberts and his wife. She really seems to have taken on caretaking for them both and is probably feeling overwhelmed. I feel very concerned. We need to have an alliance with Diane or she'll sabotage the treatment.

24. "We would appreciate your support. We'll post a current care plan in his room so we'll all be aware of how to be helpful. Sounds like it would be helpful for you to gain some distance from his demands and anger. I'm sure that it was an awful burden at home. You can always let the staff take the blame for the plan if he's angry because you won't do everything he wants."

25. At least on the surface she appears to be responding to "joining" the treatment team. She has a strong need to be a caretaker.

PROCESS RECORDING OF A SESSION WITH MRS. ROBERTS

Mrs. Roberts	Nurse's Thoughts Feelings	Nurse's Actions	Nurse's Interpretations
1. "I just can't go on like this. I'm not well myself and his demands are impossible."		2. "I can hear that it must of been awful. What has been the hardest for you?"	3. She is in clear need of some support.
4. "He can't stand to be alone anymore. He wants me to be with him every minute. If I go to the kitchen or even to the bathroom, he'll be calling me every 2 minutes to come back. I care about him, but I just can't tolerate this."	5. I feel sorry for her because of the overwhelming nature of his demands.	6. "Having worked with Mr. Roberts here and having experienced some of his demands, I can see how frustrating it must have been 24 hours a day. Was there anything at all that was working for you in dealing with him?"	
7. "The only relief I got was when he was asleep."		8. "One thing that we've found helpful is to establish firm limits on what Mr. Roberts can expect from us."	9. She can't say no to her husband.
10. "He's like a baby. He wants everything done for him. This has all happened since the stroke."	11. I am impressed by how desperate she has been feeling. Maybe a possible explanation for his behavior will offer her some hope.	12. "It has been our experience that when people experience losses that they haven't been able to grieve for, it can often cause them to be very depressed and regressed."	

498

13. "What is the treatment for that? How can it ever get better?"

16. "He won't. We've tried. He's never taken care of his ostomy. Sometimes he pretends it's not there and wants to use the toilet like he used to, but of course it's impossible."

20. "If he could be less depressed, that would be wonderful and it would help me feel better too."

14. I need to engage his wife or it will be hard to treat Mr. Roberts.

17. I don't know if I can get her to change her behavior with her husband. She seems pretty stuck, but its worth a try.

15. "One thing we can do is encourage him to talk about how he feels about the stroke and ostomy."

18. "I've talked with Diane and we are working on a step-by-step way to help Mr. Roberts do more for himself. This gradually will include helping him to get used to caring for the ostomy. We hope that we can help Mr. Roberts accept the changes in his body. We know that when people are depressed they feel better if they can care for themselves and if they can express their feelings."

21. "If we all work on this plan together it will be much more effective."

19. She has fused with her husband in his hopelessness.

22. She wants to have hope.

Owing to excellent nursing work with the family, Mr. Roberts left the hospital using only a walker for assistance in ambulation and assuming nearly full responsibility for nearly all of his activities of daily living. His depression was markedly improved and he had begun to socialize.

Clinical Illustration of a Group Intervention with a Family Focus

The Family Study Group as outlined below is an example of an application of some family concepts to clinical work.* It was designed for use in an acute inpatient or day-treatment milieu where group work is a major treatment modality.

This group consists of seven sessions, six of which are organized around structured exercises to facilitate the exploration of different aspects of family experience. The primary purpose of the group is that of data collection and assessment for the clinicians and to serve as a catalyst for work on family issues for the clients. The group may meet two or three times a week.

Family Study Group

Session I   Goals are discussed and a contract is formulated. The leaders teach patients about genograms and how to construct one. Specific symbols and their meanings are reviewed, and a genogram is illustrated on an easel pad or blackboard. (A "famous" example or historical family can be used.)

Session II   Previous group session is reviewed. Patients construct a genogram of their family and "introduce" one family member to the rest of the group. Leaders encourage clients to tell a story about the family member. Often a relative from a past generation is chosen, and humorous anecdotes can set a comfortable tone for the group. More anxious or reticent members can simply choose three to five adjectives to describe their family member. This session is an icebreaker for sharing about families.

Session III   Previous group session is reviewed. Patients enrich their genograms by adding more information (nicknames, occupations, geographical location, dates of important events, health problems, etc.). The patients then work on a group task: constructing a list of "characteristics" that can be found in family members, e.g., the most fun, the biggest gossip, the neatest, the smartest, the stingiest, the best listener, etc. The group then discusses what attributes fit their own family members. A strong sense of commonality among families is often generated in this session.

Session IV   Previous group session is reviewed. Patients use colored pencils to construct a communication "traffic pattern" on their genogram by drawing lines to indicate who talks to whom. Thick lines or multiple lines indicate a lot of communication; a dotted line (or different color) can indicate minimal contact. Patients then share the results of their work with one another. This exercise makes the genogram come alive; patients may begin to notice patterns they may never have been aware of before. Clinicians can begin to

* The Family Study Group was designed by Gloria E. Shapiro. Group leaders who contributed to the evolution of the group are Carolyn Alper, Maureen Riley, Terry Newman, Margaret Gasnick, and Paula Chasan. Appreciation is expressed to Peggy Nast Hayes, cosupervisor of the group for its first 2 years.

see the "real" family structure.

For one patient on an inpatient unit, this session proved to be a turning point in her therapy. She had been hospitalized for depression, apparently precipitated by the death of a great aunt with whom she had only occasional contact. She was not making progress and her therapy was somewhat unfocused; it was a confusing clinical picture. When she drew her "traffic pattern," it became startlingly clear that all the family members with whom she had communicated were now deceased, the last to die being her great aunt. When specific grief work became the focus of her treatment, she began to improve.

Session V Previous group session is reviewed. Patients construct a "time line" by drawing a long line; and starting with their birth, they mark all important events in their own life and in their family that have occurred during their life-span. Changes in the life cycle of the individual and the family are highlighted by this exercise. Patients are encouraged to discuss their perceptions of how changes have affected them and other family members. Ideas about change and stress are explored.

Session VI Previous group session is reviewed. Patients participate in the task of developing a group definition of "what is a family" based on their learning from each of the previous sessions. This is the least structured exercise and serves to integrate the group experience as a whole. This session facilitates a great deal of sharing among group members as each exercise has brought them closer together

in their exploration of an intimate area of their lives. Patients have often commented at this point that "this group feels like a family."

Session VII Previous group session is reviewed. This is an evaluation session where patients give feedback to the group leaders about the group as a whole and any parts they wish to cite as particularly useful, difficult, etc. Group members terminate with the other members and with the leaders. Many members have requested to keep their materials, so leaders should prepare duplicates.

Post-group follow up If there is an individual and/or family therapist involved with the patient, a post-group meeting is arranged by one of the Family Study Group leaders with the patient and other therapist(s). The patient uses this meeting to present "what they learned in the group" to bridge the therapeutic work.

Although the study group is primarily intended for the assessment phase of treatment, therapeutic work around family issues may begin in the group. The sense of universality that patients experience when they see that others have pain and stress in their families, as well as resources, has decreased patients' anxiety and sense of shame about their own "crazy" families. A number of patients have reported that the group has been a turning point in their treatment as crucial issues came into focus.

INTERVENTION: THE SPECIALIST AS HELPER

Nurses who have advanced training in family therapy may intervene in families in a more complex manner. Therapeutic intervention in family therapy has four phases: (1) contracting; (2) assessment; (3) working on problems; and (4) evaluation. In applying the nursing process to families, one needs to remember that each family coming for help brings its own structure, emotional tone, expectations, and rules. Some of these elements may not be working for the family, but they are familiar and comfortable patterns. Participation in a process of change is frightening, uncertain, and may be painful. Throughout such an experience a family needs strong external support. The therapeutic process should maximize a family's strengths while working on problems.

Contracting

Contract negotiation is important in beginning the therapeutic process. It defines the boundaries of the therapeutic situation, sets up a framework of guidelines and expectations, and creates an environment that is safe. The contract will make it possible for the family members to engage in the risk taking involved in family problem solving and change. Contracting needs to be a process of negotiation between the family and the helper, and the elements agreed upon in the contract should reflect the parameters needed by both parties in order to work together.

The first task in contracting involves negotiating the general boundaries of the therapeutic relationship, and the second involves negotiating specific outcome goals and a specific number of sessions. A typical family therapy contract may include the following general guidelines:

1. The frequency, length, and number of sessions for the assessment, and agreement on a proposed number of total sessions.
2. The persons who will attend the sessions and any expectations regarding absences.
3. Expectations for participation (for example, no violence, no one speaks for another, etc.).
4. Expectations for behavior outside sessions during the course of therapy (for example, no retaliation for feelings or ideas shared in the sessions, no violence, no illegal activities, family members will do "homework" agreed upon in sessions, etc.).
5. Mutually negotiated goals.

Assessment

The following considerations are important in assessing the length of treatment. Short-term work (under 20 sessions) is most appropriate for families who (1) have a history of functioning well before the current difficulty; (2) are experiencing difficulty in dealing with a transition in the life cycle; (3) are reacting to a painful trauma; (4) are action-oriented rather than thinking-oriented in problem-solving style; or (5) are oriented toward basic needs and short-term goals in their life-style.

Long-term work is called for when a family has functioned at an extremely chaotic level. This type of family usually benefits from intensive work for a period of time and then less frequent contact for long-term support and crisis intervention.

Specific foci for intervention in a family are identified in the assessment process. During this phase the nurse generates data by constructing a genogram, observing the family's interactions, and discussing with each member how he sees the problem.

Working on Problems

The goal of working with troubled families is to effect change. Chasin and Grunebaum identify three modes through which people can change: understanding, transformation (altering behavior patterns), and identification (imitation). They believe that the therapy of any family involves all three of these approaches and that a therapist cannot avoid providing some understanding, some direction, and some model for identification in working with families.[39]

In using the understanding-oriented approach, the therapist interprets past influences and illuminates current patterns to enrich the family's knowledge about the origin and nature of its present predicament. The work could focus on assisting family members to see the historical forces that shape their behavior; it might be to assist them in learning the interactive sequences that work to frustrate one another's needs; or to help them become aware of their own internal experience and that of other family members.

If transformation is the primary mode of change employed, the therapist strategically directs the family to modify and correct its dysfunctional moves, sequences, and structure. The therapist might intervene by creating specific tasks to alter family interaction; or present instructions aimed at changing style and language of communication, changing sequences, or altering family structure.[40]

A strategic therapist may try to push the family system away from equilibrium, forcing it to search for a different solution.[41] Many families improve because the therapist has blocked their usual pathways and necessitated their finding new ones.[42]

In using identification and reinforcement to facilitate change, the therapist acts as a model with the active involvement of older family members to promote new identifications and relax the grip of troublesome identifications and destructive loyalties among family members.[43]

Hoffman suggests that therapists interacting with families need to attend to the important matters of: To whom does he speak? Who is allowed to speak? Whom does he elevate? Whom does he challenge? Which persons does he bring together? Which does he push apart? With whom does he make a coalition? With whom does he not? It is by such moves that the therapist begins to restructure the relationship system in the family and to alter the context that supports the symptom.[44]

Evaluation

The final phase of the therapeutic process is evaluation and termination. The nurse and family need to look back upon the work that has been done. Were the goals accomplished? What did each family member learn in the process? What has changed? What was helpful? What did not help? New issues or problems should not be explored at this time, but a mechanism for additional work in the future may be set up for families who need further intervention.

NURSING RESEARCH

Nursing research regarding family phenomena is beginning to emerge as an important area of study. To date, most of the nursing studies have focused on issues surrounding perinatal experiences in family life.

Romona T. Mercer and three other nurse researchers have developed three theoretical models for studying the effect of antepartum stress on families, which should prove invaluable to nurses doing perinatal research.[45]

Linda R. Cronenwett has examined network structure and social support in couples having their first baby. In one of her studies she looked at the differences between men and women regarding "changes in network structure, need for support, satisfaction with available support, access to support from network members and conflict in [relationships]."[46]

Other notable areas of study in nursing research are: the health of bereaved parents, adjustment in parents of children with epilepsy, spouse support of patients with myocardial infarction, and health promotion for families of hospitalized patients.[47–50] All these studies have significant implications for nursing practice for they enable nurses to broaden their view to include the needs of the entire family.

THE NURSE'S ROLE

The generalist nurse's role in working with families can be organized into three basic areas: (1) prevention of dysfunction; (2) intervention in life-cycle crises; and (3) identification and referral of troubled families. For psychiatric specialists in nursing who wish to practice family therapy, there are graduate programs and special training institutes for the development of advanced skills.

Integrating family oriented nursing practice into every nursing speciality is a challenge for all clinical nurses.

Summary

Nurses should understand the basic concepts of family dynamics, develop basic skills in family assessment, be able to intervene in life crises, and be knowledgeable about resources for family treatment. In all settings, the nurses can support patients while fostering healthy family functioning. Nurses can facilitate the inclusion of families in planning and can help other professionals become more aware of family members and their needs.

Questions

1. Define boundaries in a family system and give an example of enmeshment and disengagement in a family system.
2. Define the process of triangulation in families. Give an example of a dysfunctional triangle.
3. What are three patterns of behavior that would alert the nurse to impaired family functioning?
4. Name three types of interventions that nurses may make with families in a variety of practice settings.

REFERENCES AND SUGGESTED READINGS

1. Ackerman, N. W. The family as a social and emotional unit. *Bulletin of Kansas Mental Hygiene Society*, 1937, 12, 1–3, 7–8.
2. Hoffman, L. *Foundations of Family Therapy: A Conceptual Framework for Systems Change.* New York: Basic Books, 1981, p. 11.
3. Jackson, D. (Ed.). *The Etiology of Schizophrenia.* New York: Basic Books, 1960.
4. Bowen, M. *A Family Concept of Schizophrenia.* New York: Basic Books, 1960.
5. Guerin, P. Family therapy: The first twenty-five years. In P. Guerin, Jr. (Ed.), *Family Therapy.* New York: Gardner Press, 1976.
6. Hoffman, op. cit., p. 7.
7. Horton, T. E. Conceptual basis for nursing intervention with human systems: Families. In J. E. Hall & B. R. Weaver (Eds.), *Distributive Nursing Practice: A Systems Approach to Community Health,* Philadelphia: Lippincott, 1977, p. 102.
8. Ibid.
9. Ibid.
10. Minuchin, S. *Families and Family Therapy.* Cambridge, Mass.: Harvard University Press, 1974, p. 46.
11. Carter, E., & Orfandis, M. G. Family therapy with one person and the therapist's own family. In P. Guerin, Jr. (Ed.), *Family Therapy,* New York: Gardner Press, 1976, p. 196.
12. Fogarty, T. Systems concepts and the dimensions of self. In P. Guerin, Jr. (Ed.), *Family Therapy.* New York: Gardner Press, 1976, p. 149.
13. Satir, V. *Conjoint Family Therapy.* Palo Alto, Calif.: Science and Behavior Books, 1967.
14. Hoffman, op. cit., p. 195.
15. Ibid., p. 97.
16. Minuchin, op. cit., p. 52.
17. Horton, op. cit., pp. 112–113.
18. Hoffman, op. cit., p. 6.
19. Ibid., p. 271.
20. Ibid., p. 272.
21. Chasin, R., & Grunebaum, H. A brief synopsis of current concepts and practices in family therapy. In J. Pearce & J. Friedman (Eds.), *Family Therapy: Combining Psychodynamic and Family Systems Approaches.* New York: Grune & Stratton, 1980, p. 4.
22. Hoffman, op. cit., p. 64.
23. Kantor, D., & Lehr, W. *Inside the Family.* San Francisco, Calif.: Jossey-Bass, 1975, p. 177.
24. Ibid., pp. 181–182.
25. Minuchin, op. cit., p. 54.
26. Bowen, M. Therapy in the practice of psychotherapy. In P. Guerin, Jr. (Ed.), *Family Therapy.* New York: Gardner Press, 1976, pp. 69–75.
27. Ibid., p. 57.
28. Guerin, P., Jr., & Guerin, K. B. Theoretical aspects and clinical relevance of the multigenerational model of family therapy. In P. Guerin, Jr. (Ed.), *Family Therapy,* New York: Gardner Press, 1976, p. 94.
29. Minuchin, op. cit., p. 55.
30. Hoffman, op. cit., p. 72.
31. Minuchin, op. cit., p. 34.
32. Carter and Orfandis, op. cit., p. 197.
33. Napier, A. Y., & Whitaker, C. A. *Family Crucible.* New York: Harper & Row, 1978, p. 84.
34. Bowen, M. Theory and practice of psychotherapy. In P. Guerin, Jr. (Ed.), *Family Therapy,* New York: Gardner Press, 1976, p. 75.
35. Hoffman, op. cit., p. 106.
36. Ibid., p. 30.
37. Ibid., p. 135.
38. Ibid., p. 31.
39. Chasin & Grunebaum, op. cit.
40. Ibid., pp. 11–13.
41. Hoffman, op. cit., p. 341.
42. Ibid., p. 78.
43. Ibid., p. 10.
44. Ibid., p. 264.
45. Mercer, R. T., May, R. A., Ferketich, S., & DeJoseph, J. Theoretical models for studying the effect of antepartum stress on the family. *Nursing Research,* 1986, 35, 339–345.
46. Cronenwett, L. R. Parental network structure and

perceived support after birth of first child. *Nursing Research*, 1985, 34, 347–352.

47. Miles, M. S. Emotional symptoms and physical health in bereaved parents. *Nursing Research*, 1985, 34, 76–81.

48. Austin, J. K., McBride, A. B., & Davis, H. W. Parental attitude and adjustment to childhood epilepsy. *Nursing Research*, 1984, 33, 92–96.

49. Hilbert, G. A. Spouse support and myocardial infarction: patient compliance. *Nursing Research*, 1985, 34, 217–220.

50. Hathaway, D., Boswell, B., Stanford, D., Sneider, S., & Moncrief, A. Health promotion and disease prevention for the hospitalized patient's family. *Nursing Administration Quarterly*, 1987, 11(3), 1–7.

Chapter 27

Working with Groups

Ann Wolbert Burgess

Chapter Objectives

The students successfully attaining the goals of this chapter will be able to:

- Define the role of the psychiatric nurse in conducting group therapy.
- Explain the concept of hypothesis building and the group process.
- Describe the benefits of time and silence in group process and the early behaviors of group members.
- Explain the importance of think analogies and group process.
- Explain the value of summarizing statements to conclude the group meeting.

Groups assume a key role in the organization structure of a society. The importance of the group process for coping and adapting in our society has heightened the need for nurses to develop skills in group approaches to patient care. There are several reasons for the increased group method of intervention. First, group intervention is effective and appeals to both patients and practitioners; it can be combined with individual therapy; and the same number of therapists can treat more people.

Second, group intervention has come to be regarded as a replacement for individual therapy for selected patients and may be equally or more effective than individual therapy in many instances. It also may be the preferred intervention. And third, with the waning of natural social groups such as the extended family and the increase of single-parent homes, the need for small group network has emerged to counter social isolation.

Both group therapy as a traditional psychiatric treatment intervention and new contemporary methods of group work are being credited as being therapeutic and responsive to the sociocultural needs of people.

Material in this chapter is intended to (1) inform nurses of the scope of group therapy as defined by the Division of Psychiatric and Mental Health Nursing Practice; and (2) increase the nurse's skill and understanding of traditional and contemporary group methods and the role of the group leader.

HISTORY

The concept of group therapy has been greatly expanded in the past decade. Carl Rogers has called the intensive group experience movement "one of the most rapidly growing social phenomena in the U.S. . . . perhaps the most significant social invention in this century."[1] Group work has been influenced by many persons and some of the early pioneers are described as follows.

Pratt

Joseph Pratt, a Boston internist, first introduced therapy with a group in a medical setting in 1905. Pratt would meet once or twice a week with 20 to 30 patients, all of whom had tuberculosis. He would lecture about the disease and the method of cure, and he was generally supportive and encouraging about the prognosis. Patients who had responded successfully would tell the group how they had been helped. The positive therapeutic results were transferred to other groups of patients.

Marsh

In 1919, L. Cody Marsh, a minister and psychiatrist and familiar with Pratt's work, began to use the group method of treatment with a group of institutionalized mental patients. Weekly meetings were held at which Marsh lectured on a variety of topics pertaining to mental illness. Marsh also arranged discussion groups with all hospital personnel who came into contact with patients, e.g., nurses, doctors, social workers, and attendants. He was one of the first psychiatrists to recognize that every encounter a patient had within the hospital setting had therapeutic potential. In this sense he was a pioneer in the concept of the hospital as a therapeutic community.

Lazell

Concurrent with Marsh's work, another psychiatrist, E. W. Lazell, was gathering schizo-phrenic patients in groups and lecturing to them about schizophrenia. He concluded that patients improved because, in part, their fears were reduced as a result of education. He also believed that the socialization process, defined most simply as patients getting to know one another, accounted for the positive changes he observed.

Moreno

In 1925, Jacob L. Moreno, a psychiatrist, introduced the technique of psychodrama. He encouraged the acting out of problem situations in a group setting to achieve a heightened awareness of the patient's actual conflict and its possible resolution.

Freud

In 1921, Sigmund Freud published *Group Psychology and Analysis of the Ego*. He differentiated the leaderless group (a mob capable of great excesses) from the leader-centered group (a potential vehicle capable of diminishing anxiety). In the psychotherapy group, which has a leader, members identify with one another and have a common bond to the central figure, who is seen as a parental surrogate. Members react to each other as siblings within the family; as a result they have mutualities of both love and hate.

Lewin

Kurt Lewin focused on "group dynamics," a term coined by him in 1939, in the same way that Freud focused on individual dynamics. To Lewin, acts of the individual cannot be explained on the basis of an individual's psychodynamics but must be explained on the basis of the nature of the social forces, the field to which the person is exposed. Lewin defined the concept of *group pressure*, whereby influence is brought to bear on a particular member of the group to the extent that the member's behavior can be altered. In turn, the individual member influences the group, and together they form a gestalt or whole. While the group includes individual members, it functions as a unit.

GROUP THERAPY IN PSYCHIATRIC NURSING PRACTICE

The statement on Psychiatric and Mental Health Nursing Practice defines the scope of practice in group therapies as follows:

In group therapy, the dynamics of collective interaction are purposefully utilized to foster exploration of adjustive patterns and to discover more effective and realistic behavioral alternatives. When the group is used as a primary treatment modality, the nurse-therapist selects the participants on the basis of each individual's needs and potential for constructive participation in the experience. Decisions about overall composition of the group take into account individual client assessments, specific goals and structure of the group, and known principles of group composition.[2]

In convening the therapy group, the nurse leader establishes the formal elements of the sessions: time, place, frequency, duration, and the norms by which the group will function. The therapist influences and uses the group process to develop a working, cohesive unit that is capable of attending to the progress and goals of both the individual members and the group as a whole.

In the role of group therapist, the nurse uses knowledge of behavior at the intrapersonal, interpersonal, and small group levels. Development of group therapist skills requires specific and extensive preparation in this modality, including both graduate level of study of relevant theory and supervised clinical experience. The specialist in psychiatric and mental health nursing with the appropriate qualifications may also function in other capacities related to group therapy, such as group therapy supervisor for professional nurses and others who conduct groups, consultant in group therapy, teacher of group therapy in formal classes, and coordinator of workshops or seminars on the group process and the leadership role.

Types of Group Therapies

In a small survey reported by Irvin Yalom, a bewildering array of group approaches was disclosed: psychoanalytic groups; crisis groups; psychodrama groups; Synanon; Recovery, Inc.; Alcoholics Anonymous; marathon encounter groups; marital couples groups; family therapy groups; traditional T-groups; multimedia groups; and Gestalt therapy groups. Yalom emphasized that many of the groups are designated as therapy groups; others straddle the blurred boundary between personal growth and therapy.[3]

If we review the groups according to their curative factors instead of on the basis of what the titles of the groups imply, we see that the array of group therapies seems a bit more organized. Yalom categorizes groups with similar goals as: (1) groups that aim for providing support, suppression, and inspiration (Recovery, Inc., and Alcoholics Anonymous); (2) groups that aim for the restoration of functioning and the reinstitution of old defenses (groups on acute, rapid-turnover psychiatric wards); (3) groups that aim for the maintenance of reality testing and prevention of ward friction (groups on long-term psychiatric wards); and (4) groups that aim for the building of new defenses and changes in coping style and characterological structure (groups of patients with neurotic and characterological problems).[4]

Therapists, depending on their professional training and personality style, will master a particular system of therapy that fosters the growth of the curative process in clients. Of extreme importance is that, in addition to the presenting method of operation and appeal, there is a basic framework to the therapy and an organized method for promoting growth in clients. Yalom identifies the curative factors of group therapy, that is, how group therapy helps clients, in the following categories. These categories, in rank order of preference of group therapy patients, resulted from a study conducted by Yalom.[5]

1. *Interpersonal learning (input)*. The group's teaching me about the type of impression I make on others; learning how I come across to others; other members honestly telling me what they think of me; group members pointing out some of my habits or mannerisms that annoy other people; learning that I sometimes confuse people by not saying what I really think.
2. *Catharsis*. Getting things off my chest; expressing positive and negative feelings toward another person or toward the leader; being able to say what was bothering me instead of holding it in.
3. *Group cohesiveness*. Belonging to and being accepted by a group; continued close contact with other people; revealing embarrassing things about myself and still being

accepted by the group; feeling along no longer; belonging to a group of people who understand and accept me.

4. *Insight*. Learning that I have likes or dislikes for a person and reasons which may have little to do with the person and more to do with my hang-ups or past experiences with people; learning why I think and feel the way I do; discovering and accepting previously unknown or unacceptable parts of myself; learning that I react to some people or situations unrealistically; learning there are reasons I am the way I am, which has to do with my early life.

5. *Interpersonal learning (output)*. Improving my skills in getting along with people; feeling more trustful of groups and other people; learning about the way I related to the other group members; the group's giving me an opportunity to learn to approach others; working out my difficulties with one particular member in the group.

6. *Existential factors*. Recognizing that life is at times unfair and unjust; recognizing that ultimately there is no escape from some of life's pain and from death; realizing I still face life alone; facing the basic issues of my life and death and thus living my life more honestly and being less caught up in trivialities; learning I must take ultimate responsibility for the way I live my life.

7. *Universality*. Learning I'm not the only one with the same problem; seeing that I was just as well off as others; learning that some others have some of the same bad thoughts and feelings I do; learning that others had parents and backgrounds as unhappy or mixed up as mine; learning that I'm not very different from other people gave me a "welcome to the human race" feeling.

8. *Instillation of hope*. Seeing others getting better was inspiring to me; knowing others had solved problems similar to mine.

9. *Altruism*. Helping others gives me more self-respect; putting others' needs ahead of my own; forgetting myself and thinking of helping others, giving part of myself to others; helping others and being important in their lives.

10. *Family reenactment*. Being in the group was like reliving and understanding the family in which I grew up; helped me to understand family hang-ups; [the] group was like my family and helped me understand past relationships.

11. *Guidance*. The leader suggesting or advising me to do something; group members suggesting or advising me to do something; someone in the group giving me a definite suggestion about a life problem; group members advising me to behave differently with an important person in my life.

12. *Identification*. Trying to be like someone in the group: seeing that others could take risks; adopting mannerisms or the style of another group member or the group leader.

TRADITIONAL GROUP THERAPY

Group therapy is defined as a form of intervention in which carefully selected persons are placed in a group, guided by a trained therapist, for the purpose of changing the maladaptive behavior of the individual member.

Traditional group therapy is predicated on the assumption that people are consistent in their stylistic manner of behavior whether they are in a formal setting such as a group or in an everyday informal setting such as a family scene. Because people behave in characteristic styles, a formal gathering is one mechanism whereby people can be helped to become more aware of their interaction and coping patterns, including their strengths and their weaknesses. One of the roles of the nurse-therapist in group therapy is to help patients understand their characteristic manner of relating by examining their interactions with the leader and other group members.

Patient Preparation

In group therapy, the patient is prepared for the group experience. The preparatory session consists of explaining the processes to which the patient will be exposed, emphasizing the need to be open and honest with fellow patients, and alerting the patient to the possibility that he may not like all of the other members, nor they the patient; but that by examining the interaction that evolves, self-knowledge will increase, and in the process more adaptive ways of thinking, feeling, and behaving will develop.

Patients who receive a preparatory session are more likely to develop positive feelings about being in a group, have a lower dropout rate, more communication, and a greater sense of cohesiveness than those who are not so prepared.

Patient Selection

Careful selection of patients and careful group organization are essential clinical responsibilities. Group psychotherapy cannot be applied as a blanket form of psychiatric treatment for all types of emotional disorders, although a great variety of patient populations have been exposed to the method. To determine a patient's suitability for group psychotherapy, the therapist needs a great deal of information gathered in an individual session.

There are key dynamic factors to consider in selecting patients for traditional group therapy. The dynamics of the patient, including commonly used defense mechanisms, current and past relationships to peers and to authority figures need to be assessed and are discussed as follows.

Authority Anxiety
Patients whose primary difficulties center on their relationship to authority and who are very anxious in the presence of authority figures often do better in the group setting than in the dyadic or one-to-one setting. They gain support from the peer group and are thus aided in dealing with the therapist more realistically.

Adolescents often manifest authority anxiety, and for that reason, are often viewed as good candidates for group therapy. For the adolescent who has not had a peer group experience, a normal stage of adolescent development, such a choice is especially apt; therefore, the screening interview should include a careful history of attitudes toward parents, teachers, and other adults, but equally important, of the adolescent's participation in clubs and gangs. A clear indication for group therapy is the adolescent who gives a history of isolation, withdrawal, and no exposure to peers.

Patients with authority anxiety may be blocked, anxious, resistant, and unwilling to verbalize thoughts and feelings in the individual setting, generally for fear of censure or disapproval from the therapist. They often welcome the suggestion of group psychotherapy to avoid the scrutiny of the dyadic situation.

Peer Anxiety
The patients who have destructive relationships with their peer group or who have been extremely isolated from peer group contact generally react negatively or with increased anxiety when placed in a group setting. For example, some patients whose early development was characterized by sibling rivalry and whose hostilities toward or from their siblings were overwhelmingly intense may be unable to tolerate a group and may leave it. For those patients whose nuclear problem is rooted in the sibling relationship, the group can provide the corrective emotional experience necessary for relationship improvement. However, the group leader needs to evaluate the patient's ability to tolerate the degree of anxiety and discomfort that will be produced. The reality of having other patients with whom they can interact often leads to greater insight than does a verbal reconstruction in individual psychotherapy.

For the child who was raised without siblings, the group may provide anxiety because the patient's central position is jeopardized—perhaps for the first time if the adult life-style is organized so that the patient remains the center of attention. Within the group, those patients demand to have their narcissistic needs gratified by the therapist; but the group setting demands that sharing occur, and such a setting may represent the first time the only child has been in such a position, one that may be very stressful. On the other hand, the only child may see the group as providing the sibling experience that was always denied. In either case, that of the only child who is unwilling to share or the only child who longs to share, the group setting rather quickly causes those dynamics to unfold and be subject to examinations and ultimate resolution.

Defense Mechanisms
Defense mechanisms are mental processes that a person uses for protection from consciously experiencing anxiety; they enable that person to cope with a variety of internal and external stresses. The following defense mechanisms lend themselves particularly well to the group method of intervention.

Projection. Patients who use the defense mechanism of projection (the attribution to others of impulses that they find unacceptable in themselves) are good candidates for group therapy. These patients persistently blame others for their own inadequacies and failures and distort the realities of the outside world. They are reluctant to talk about their own motives and avoid introspection that may lead to the uncovering of their own thoughts. In a one-to-one setting these people may be unable to establish a working relationship because of their tendency to project onto the therapist thoughts and feelings, generally negatives ones, that interfere with and are not available for reality testing.

Projection can be dealt with in the group setting by the other group members, who constantly confront such patients with their distortions as they are directed toward them or the therapist. Such group processes force introspective analysis to occur, and the projective mechanism is thereby eroded. One of the problems to be faced by the therapist is that often patients using that defense mechanism make accurate observations about others, because they may be especially sensitive to finding in others the same faults as they themselves possess. Thus, their observations about others may be accurate. Accordingly, the therapist cannot assume that the patients' observations are incorrect but must make sure that the project members take responsibility for the same character traits in themselves that they note in others.

Repression, Denial, and Suppression. The defenses of repression, denial, and suppression are especially well suited for examination in group therapy. When these defenses are delineated in the screening interview, the therapist should consider the advantage of group treatment. When one member recalls an event, other group members may recall repressed material; this process is inherent in every group that has as one of its goals a revealing or disclosure of historical events.

Suppression, the conscious witholding of information about oneself because of fear, anxiety, guilt, shame, or embarrassment is one of the mechanisms attended to by the group. One issue common to all groups involves self-disclosure. The effectiveness of group therapy is often contingent upon the ability and willingness of the group members to be open and disclose information about themselves. The issue involves trust, and questions group members ask themselves include: Can I trust the group, the leader, myself? Can I dare to let others know what I am thinking, feeling, and doing?

The issue of self-disclosure—that information about oneself that a person is willing to reveal to others—is an important area of research. Some studies have looked at disclosure in terms of the child-rearing process, personality types, the interviewing process, intimacy and family communication, adolescent patterns of communication, marriage relationships, and stigma.[6–12]

Part of the decision that must be made by individual group members is what experiences or issues are appropriate to bring to the group. Goffman's classic analysis of stigma and of the management of spoiled identity is particularly useful for group leaders in analyzing disclosure of certain types of events that groups members have experienced. Goffman uses the term *stigma* to indicate "an attribute that is deeply discrediting" in a certain social context.[13] Goffman distinguishes between cases where the stigma is known to others already or evident immediately (the individual is discredited), and cases where the stigma is not known by others and not immediately perceivable (the individual is discreditable). As Goffman states,

When an individual's differentness is not immediately apparent, and is not known beforehand . . . then . . . the issue is . . . that of managing information about his failing. To display or not to display; to tell or not to tell; to let on or not to let on; to lie or not to lie; and in each case, to whom, how, when, and where.[14]

The issue becomes "the management of undisclosed discrediting information about self."[15] Thus, a specific skill of group leaders is helping group members to deal with the information revealed in a manner that is therapeutic to the person disclosing.

Traditional group therapy designates at least one person as leader, that is, the group therapist. Various styles of leadership exist as well as principles of group operation. In general, the leader assumes responsibility for the following tasks:

1. Organization of the group. The rules for organizing the membership of the group and the conduct of the meetings are identified in the *Statement on Psychiatric and Mental Health Nursing Practice* guidelines on group therapy.[16]

2. Themes of the meetings. A considerable amount of data can be generated in group therapy meetings if members feel that they can trust the group and that there is respect for human dignity and confidentiality of issues. The task of the nurse is to make sense out of the data through the process of conceptualization and to reflect the themes in a meaningful way back to the group. Notes kept of the meeting, whether by group members or the leader, are one source of data that can be reviewed weekly. Recurrent themes and their dynamic or symbolic meaning are noted for current or future reference.

   Themes can be anticipated or predicted on the basis of a general knowledge of human behavior. For example, it might be speculated that members' behavior around holidays or vacation time would vary. Group members might feel happy or sad, in anticipation of the group meeting. The thoughts, feelings, and behavior of group members would have added meaning relevant to the individual's past experiences with special events. The nurse–leader usually confirms or refutes the accuracy of the predicted behavior with the group.

3. Facilitating group interaction. Characteristic behavior patterns become most apparent when people engage in meaningful conversation and dialogue. Affect or emotional response heightens the opportunity to respond to other group members as one did to important people in the past. The task of encouraging group members to increase their interactions with each other may necessitate the leader's assuming a less verbal rule. The timing of remarks and the responses made to the group are important leadership skills. Becoming comfortable with silences is helpful to allow the natural evolution of group content. Stalls can occur if the nurse reponds too quickly or offers premature interpretations to the group. The stall warning for the leader is immediately answering a client's question without allowing the affect in the group to develop.

4. Linkages between themes. Important group content may be disguised or referred to in a symbolic manner. Group therapists are advised to pay special attention to early remarks made in a group meeting in hopes of forecasting significant issues for the group. Because the content may be disguised, the linking of themes and the decoding of content are the work of the leader.

5. Autognosis. Being attentive to one's own thoughts, feelings, and actions during a group meeting is an essential skill for the group leader. Autognosis, as discussed in Chapter 1, is the process whereby one reads one's own feelings and reactions in order to better understand the current situation.

   Group therapists disagree on the issue of sharing their feelings with the group. Those favoring disclosing one's feelings openly believe this sharing communicates the universality of affective states and serves as a model for the group. Those therapists not in favor, such as Rutan and Alonso, believe patients gain more if affective input by therapists is kept to a minimum.[17]

6. Psychodynamic component. Psychodynamic theory believes that the client's reason for entering group therapy (e.g., his "problem") is part of his characterological structure and will be repeated in the group in an overt or covert manner. The task of the nurse is to assess the problem initially, keep these "presenting problems" uppermost in mind throughout the group process, formulate the group dynamics, observe the reemergence in the group, and time the reformulation of the problem in the group setting for understanding by the group.

7. Concluding a group session. Various methods of concluding a group session may be used. A summary statement by the nurse that pulls together the thoughts and feelings of the group is one technique. This type of conclusion terminates group discussion but provides the group members some affective and cognitive structure. Initially, this technique may be initiated by the leader, but as the group develops, individual members may share in this task. A second type of leader response is to announce the fact that the session is terminated at the end of the meeting time. This statement provides closure to the time structure but not to any cognitive or affective resolution. Group members are simply told the time is up and that the group will meet at the same time the following week.

The leader may use this type of response as a matter of personal style or when there is insufficient content to summarize. The burden is placed on group members to summarize the meeting to themselves or to bring their thoughts and feelings to the next session.

THE THERAPEUTIC PROCESS IN GROUP WORK

A discussion of the factors that assist in the therapeutic process of group work may be separated into the following three categories: (1) actional factors consisting of reality testing, ventilation, catharsis, abreaction, and group pressure; (2) emotional factors consisting of cohesion and transference; and (3) cognitive factors consisting of universalization, intellectualization, and spectator therapy (imitation and identification). The group processes that are believed to account for therapeutic change are listed and discussed by Sadock as follows.[18]

Actional Factors

Reality Testing
The group setting provides a reality-testing forum for the objective evaluation of the individual's self and the world. Any transaction between two people contains six potential interactions: (1) what each person wants the other to think the person is; (2) what each thinks himself to be; and (3) what each is in actuality. In a group of eight people, these complexities may seem difficult to resolve, but through the process of consensual validation, the group defines the beliefs and actualities for each of its participants. When one member's perception of another is distorted, others in the group are able to bring their own observations to bear on the misperception. As a result, a constant assessment of reality takes place.

Within the group, honest and open communication, which is encouraged by the therapist, helps the group maintain that assessment. Some theoretical frameworks suggest therapists be open about themselves, thus acting as models for that standard. Those who hold a more traditional view of leadership suggest that therapists remain sufficiently apart from the group to maintain objectivity. That does not mean that they may not use examples from their own lives to illustrate certain points, but they must be constantly aware of the impact of such revelations on particular group members.

The group recreates the family setting for many patients and may produce a revival of previous familial tensions and conflicts. Accordingly, it is common for patients to see other members as surrogate fathers, mothers, and siblings. Those reactions may be elicited because the surrogate figure actually may resemble the original family member, either physically or behaviorally. In successful reality testing the patient is able to separate reactions that are appropriate to current stimuli from those that are carry-overs from past conflicts. The therapist may attempt to elicit the association from the individual or make the interpretation directly in an effort to bring such associations to consciousness, e.g., patient A is relating to patient B as the competitive sister.

Ventilation and Catharsis
Ventilation is the open expression of one's innermost thoughts and secrets. Catharsis is the evocation of feeling tones and affects that may be attached to the ventilated thought or secret. Ventilation allows for the amelioration of guilt feelings and anxiety through confession and provides the group with important information about the person's thoughts, feelings, and problems. It also stimulates in other members associations that may bring repressed material to awareness.

Each group develops its own mix of ventilatory and cathartic process, the mix depending on the composition of the group, the leadership style, and the theoretical framework.

Abreaction
Similar to catharsis, abreaction is the reliving of past events and the emotions associated with them; it is a more heightened process than catharsis in that the discharge of affect is greater. Moreover, it is associated with increased insight, because the patient is able to recognize the link between current irrational attitudes and previous emotional states. Abreaction also brings about an awareness, often for the first time, of degrees of emotion previously blocked from consciousness. While it is often a highly therapeutic experience, it may produce an unavoidable sense of distress in all concerned as the process unfolds.

Motor abreaction is the experiencing of an unconscious impulse through physical activity. It is known that emotional states may manifest themselves in physical ways. Hysterical paralysis, psychosomatic illness, and anxiety states are some examples.

Emotional Factors

Cohesion

Working groups are marked by some sense of cohesion. Members feel a "wellness," a sense of belonging. They value the group, which engenders loyalty and friendliness. They are willing to work together and to take responsibility for one another in achieving their common goals. They are also willing to experience a certain degree of frustration to maintain the group's integrity. A cohesive group is one in which members are accepting and supportive and have meaningful relationships with one another.

Individual group members are often evaluated using the measure of cohesion. The cohesive member is willing to take on responsibility for effective group functioning by participating actively in the meetings, by working hard to achieve difficult goals, by attending meetings regularly, and by remaining within the group for a long period of time. The cohesive member is willing to attempt to influence others and to listen to differences of opinion. Also, that member is willing to adhere to the standards of the group and to encourage others to do the same. It stands to reason that the more effectively the therapist can increase a member's cohesion in the group, the more probable is a successful outcome for the patient.

Transference

An unconscious process, transference refers to feelings, attitudes, and wishes originally linked with significant figures in an individual's early life that are projected onto new persons in the individual's life. In group therapy, when this happens between an individual member and the leader, other group members will often help the individual member recall earlier treatment by a parent or significant other that was similar to the experience in the group. Through this process, the client is assisted in seeing the distortion and in experiencing reality.

Cognitive Factors

Universalization

In the group, members recognize that they are not alone in having emotional problems and that others may be struggling with the same or similar problems. This process of universalization is a major therapeutic aspect of group work. The simple sharing of experiences fills an important human need.

As group members sense that they are important in the lives of one another, they seek to be of help to each other. This process, called altruism by some and support by others, is characterized by the sacrificing of personal interests to the group. In so doing, the sacrificing member receives help in return, for heightened self-esteem is gained by offering advice, attempting to guide, or otherwise influencing a fellow member to a greater awareness of psychological functioning. Supportive members also strengthen their own identities as they separate their problems from those of others and learn to share themselves realistically.

The mechanism of universality and its derivatives—altruism or support, advice giving, and reassurance—are processes that continue throughout the life of the group.

Intellectualization

This process implies a cognitive awareness of self, others, and the various life experience, both good and bad, that account for current functioning. Not only does it connote more than a knowledge of personal history, it also implies that patients understand how they relate in the here-and-now. Feedback, in which each member confronts the others with immediate responses to events as they occur, is a learning experience. Confrontation groups, as used in drug rehabilitation groups, rely on the feedback mechanism extensively.

Interpretation

A derivative of intellectualization, interpretation also provides group members with a cognitive framework within which they can understand themselves better, whether that interpretation comes from the therapist or other group members.

Intellectualization does not necessarily lead to change; experiential factors must be added if effective learning is to take place. The concept of the corrective emotional experience, first formulated by Franz Alexander in 1946, combines both the intellectual and the experiential factors into a functional theoretical framework. The corrective process unfolds as the patient experiences the therapist or a fellow group member in a distorted manner, with the painful or pleasurable affects associated with that experience, and as the patient later recognizes through the transference phenomenon that the person acts in a manner different from what was expected (i.e., reality testing).

Identification

For the personality to develop into a healthy, functioning pattern, a person must be able to model himself on a person with sound psychological makeup. Many psychiatric patients have identified with faulty models. In individual therapy many patients attempt to learn new modes of adaptation by taking on qualities of the therapist. In the group setting a variety of other models are available and patients identify with certain qualities of these other members. That process of identification may occur either consciously by simple imitation or unconsciously and outside of awareness.

Other group mechanisms can be understood within the framework of identifications that take place between members. The sense of alienation is lost as patients develop feelings toward one another and toward the group as a whole. The group provides a sense of security, and a feeling of belonging develops. The mechanism of acceptance is therapeutic in that members realize that there is an appropriate place for differences of opinion. Arguments, the expression of hostility, and negativity do not disrupt the positive forces that link members of the group. For example, the group member exposed to parental arguments that led to dissolution of the family can find this mechanism of acceptance most beneficial.

GROUP INTAKE PROCEDURE AS AN ALTERNATIVE IN URBAN COMMUNITY SETTINGS

All clients entering an agency to request some type of mental health assistance talk with a staff member and present their reason for seeking services. This process is called the intake interview. Sometimes brief information is taken over the telephone from the patient, and the patient is then given an appointment with a staff member for the full interview. The traditional intake interview may require several meetings in order for the staff member to obtain the information needed to make an assessment, diagnosis, and intervention plan. This type of intake procedure usually occurs on an individual basis.

In contrast, a group intake procedure provides an alternative to the traditional individual intake interview. In this method, one or several staff members meet with a group of patients who are requesting services. In addition to discussing patient requests for services, treatment issues, clinical negotiations, orientation to clinic services, and policies and other community agencies are discussed.

Needs of the Low-Income Urban Populations

The search for tools and procedures to combat barriers to comprehensive mental health services in low-income urban populations began as the role of sociocultural factors in the prevalence of mental illness and the unequal distribution of mental health services became glaringly apparent. The use of intake groups as an orientation procedure to mental health services in community mental health center settings was studied by nurse-clinician Patricia L. Kelley, who attempted to broaden the use of mental health services by redefining the concept of mental illness and the goals of treatment in terms less culturally biased than those of the traditional psychiatric model.*

Class Factors

Three early epidemiologic studies established the significance of social class factors in mental illness and health. First, Hollingshead and Redlich demonstrated a distinct inverse relationship between social class and the prevalence of mental illness, with lower classes contributing a much greater percentage of patients, proportionately, than did the upper classes.[19] The evidence of Hollingshead and Redlich showed that a similar class relationship existed in terms of diagnosis and treatment of mental illness; that is, most lower-class patients were labeled

* This section on intake groups was written by Patricia L. Kelley.

severely disturbed or psychotic and were treated by institutionalization or medication. Conversely, most middle- and upper-class patients were seen as less severely disturbed, or neurotic, and were treated by psychotherapy on an outpatient basis. It is important to note that Hollingshead and Redlich defined lower class and low-income groups in terms of educational level, housing conditions, adequacy of income and employment, and stability of the family unit[20]; this system of economic classification has been widely accepted and used in mental health research.

In a 1962 study of a midtown Manhattan population, similar findings were made.[21] That is, "poor" groups showed proportionately more mental impairment and were less likely to receive satisfactory psychiatric attention. Finally, Ryan's extensive and careful survey of mental health needs and services in Boston between 1960 and 1962 added confirmation to the Hollingshead and Redlich study.[22] Ryan found clear evidence of two distinct systems of mental health services existing in Boston: one of good quality, well-staffed by highly trained professionals, serving people of high education, income, and resource levels, and a second of poor quality, inadequately staffed by less skilled personnel, serving people not so endowed socially and financially. The significance of these findings was heightened by the fact that Boston, at the time of the study, enjoyed a more than adequate level of mental health resources and had already exceeded the "ideal" goal of one psychiatric clinic for every 50,000 people.[23] "Two-class care" was not eliminated by additional manpower.[24]

Other less extensive but no less conclusive studies contributed further to the growing recognition of sociocultural barriers in the delivery of mental health services. Rosenthal and Frank and Hunt—all social scientists—pointed out the inappropriateness of the traditional intrapsychic treatment model for clients who were not "insight-oriented."[25,26] They found, as had Hollingshead and Redlich, that professionals selected for treatment only those patients who shared their middle- and upper-class values, thus "tailoring" the patient population to suit the treatment model. Clearly, the professional preference for verbal, educated patients who can profit from traditional techniques of intervention has contributed to the skewed distribution of mental health services.[27]

It is evident, however, that the problem is not that simple. Low-income patients themselves contribute to the imbalance through failure to seek available health services and through rejection or premature termination of treatment.[28,29] As Ryan and others have noted, people who live in poverty tend to define health in terms of the ability to function and work; thus, they are unlikely to seek aid until the problem has reached disabling proportions.[30,31] These observations indicated that the prevalence of severe disturbance found among low-income groups was not wholly attributable to professional bias in labeling; it arose, at least in part, from prolonged tolerance of less severe symptoms. This same group of authors concluded that an additional contribution was made to the prevalence of severe disturbance by the very conditions of poverty, which are themselves stressful and disorganizing. The contribution made by these factors to the unequal distribution of health services may be ameliorated by increased community education regarding early recognition of problems, as well as by increased professional education regarding the realistic stresses inherent in the condition of poverty.[32]

Among those low-income patients who do attempt to use clinic services, further self-selection has occurred through treatment refusal.[33] Some of this patient loss is attributable to the dominance of the psychiatric model and the focus on intrapsychic sources of disorder; patients familiar with the stress of limited resources and restricted opportunities seldom accept intrapsychic problem definition and treatment goals.[34] However, further investigation has shown that incongruent expectations concerning the method and process of treatment also play a significant role in the relationship between social class and accessibility to treatment.[35] Thus, researchers have extended their focus beyond the need for more flexible and socially oriented theoretical models to include the study of these additional barriers to equitable service delivery.

The medically oriented intrapsychic model of traditional psychiatric treatment has been labeled severely limited and largely unsuitable for community mental health practice.[36,37] Not only does this model constrain the therapist to a culturally biased definition of acceptable patients but it also fails to provide her with any meaningful way of relating to those patients who do not value "self-actualization" goals. Patients from lower classes, Reiff observed, are oriented toward the present, not the future; they are limited in opportunities and role flexibility and are struggling to achieve self-determination. The concept of realizing one's "full potential" through internal change is wholly irrelevant and unrealistic for them.[38] Many author-clinicians have validated this position.[39–41]

Responding to the Needs of Low-Income Populations

The importance of sociocultural factors in general and of economic stress in particular has generated a new perspective on the delivery of mental health services to low-income populations. Much attention has been devoted to the search for a more comprehensive and widely applicable model, capable of including social and environmental factors in the understanding and treatment of human problems. Four contemporary views have been described in the clinical literature in terms of (1) eclectic prescriptivism; (2) crisis intervention; (3) consumer approach; and (4) patient expectations.

Eclectic Prescriptivism

One group of authors focused on the importance of offering a broad range of intervention techniques aimed at helping patients gain control over their "problems of living."[42,43] Dimond and Havens formulated this approach as "eclectic prescriptivism."[44] In this system, the patient, as he presents himself, becomes the primary focus of treatment. The therapist must develop skillfulness in fully understanding the patient's point of view within the framework of the patient's sociocultural and environmental context. This done, the therapist can draw on his knowledge of a variety of treatment techniques for those measures likely to prove most suitable and beneficial for this particular individual's style and situation. Ideally, this model calls for a broader background in theories of therapy than many practicing professionals may have; however, Dimond and Havens pointed out that this is not essential. They observed that the significant innovation lies in placing the focus on the patient and modifying techniques to suit him rather than the traditional reversal of this focus.

Crisis Intervention

Another group demonstrated the successful use of a crisis intervention model in community

mental health programs. Meeting several of the desirable model criteria, that is, being individually focused, task- and present-oriented, cognizant of external variables and of brief duration, crisis theory is thought by many to offer the most effective approach for community work.[45] It may be argued that the majority of problems brought to a mental health clinic are long-standing, often chronic, in nature. However, as Caplan defined it, the essence of the state of crisis lies in the current failure of coping mechanisms and the resultant energy-mobilizing disequilibrium.[46] The chronicity of the problem and the history of successful or partial coping in no way diminish the distress experienced when the individual realizes that familiar resources are no longer adequate for the restoration of equilibrium. Thus, at the time of seeking professional aid, this individual is as accurately described by the state of crisis as is someone who has suffered an external crisis event, such as desertion or death.[47]

Consumer Approach

A third approach, currently gaining support, suggested a consumer orientation in mental health service delivery. In 1967, Levinson, Merrifield, and Berg studied the process of becoming a patient in a psychiatric clinic as affected by three existing models. The "diagnostic" or medical model focused on symptoms of psychiatric illness in selecting patients for treatment; the "suitability" model focused on patient attributes characteristic of "good" candidates for treatment; and the "applicacy" model focused on those patients most active and skillful in obtaining treatment. On the basis of their results, the authors concluded that all three could be incorporated and improved upon in a model they called "negotiated consensus." This model focused on the transaction between applicant and agent (patient and counselor) and defined as their joint responsibility a negotiated agreement concerning the nature and sources of the problem and the help to be received. Implementation of the model at their clinic resulted in dwindling waiting lists and the use of a much wider range of treatment modalities.[48]

Expectations

In addition to the differences in patient–counselor definitions of needs and goals as a result of professional adherence to the traditional conceptual model, incongruent expectations concerning the method and process of treatment have also played a part in the unequal distribution of mental health services.

The relationship between favorable expectations and successful treatment is evident throughout the recorded history of witch doctors, healing rituals, and miraculous shrines. Frank noted that even Freud acknowledged the significance of gaining the patient's "confidence" in any therapeutic relationship, but Freud went on to claim that psychoanalysis was not so dependent.[49] Through careful study, Frank and his colleagues have produced convincing evidence of the powerful role played by expectations in all forms of treatment, including psychoanalysis.[50]

Preparation of Treatment Through Intake Group Method

The enhancement of compatible treatment expectations through preparation of the patients has proven successful in several studies.[51,52] In general, such preparation serves to educate the patients in regard to the goals and process of treatment, so that they may anticipate and make use of the kind of help offered.

A number of studies demonstrated that group intake procedures offer an efficient way of avoiding waiting lists and facilitating prompt intervention in crisis.[53,54] Moreover, group methods have been found superior to individual intake models in several ways. McGee and Larsen found that group intakes were more economical of staff time, facilitated prompt identification of priority cases, and served as a screening situation for patient ability to use group therapy.[55] Allgeyer observed that the presence of a supportive, understanding peer group facilitated communication for disadvantaged, less verbal patients, and provided therapists with a rapid education in "accurate empathy."[56] The group intake experience also serves to reduce anxiety and encourage self-awareness.

Operational Rules for Intake Orientation Group

An intake orientation group generally includes a single meeting of 1 or 2 hours' duration attended by those patients who requested clinical services during the 2 weeks preceding the meeting. The average size of the group is five to seven people. The group may be led by more than one intake worker. Group discussion focuses on available clinic services, other community services (when appropriate), patient expectations and requests, preliminary contract negotiations, and the specific issues leading to the treatment request at that time. The meeting is designed to clarify clinic policies and procedures, provide a direct experience with treatment, establish the importance of patient–therapist involvement in treatment, and demonstrate professional respect of the problem and treatment.

SELF-HELP GROUPS AS A SUPPORT-INTERVENTION MODEL*

Intervention groups using the self-help or support model as a modality for response to various kinds of living situations have met with success and are increasing. Such groups have been helpful to those who are single parents, victims of child or adolescent sexual abuse, battered wives, homosexuals, runaway youths, or alcoholics, and those with many other types of problems as well. The self-help group model provides the patient with acceptance and understanding when other social support systems or facilities to help with people are inaccessible or (in some instances) nonexistent. In a self-help setting, it is easier to neutralize the stigma associated with some problems and to have the opportunity to discuss openly experiences with others who have similar problems. Discussing problems in a controlled and nonjudgmental atmosphere is the foundation for personal growth.

A self-help group consists of three to twelve (ideally five to seven) patients who share a problem and who meet regularly for the purpose of aiding one another to resolve that problem (or problems) and to learn to cope more adaptively. Most often, groups using this model meet for a set number of times so that the point of closure is known in advance. To maximize effectiveness, these groups may be organized by a nurse familiar with the type of shared problem identified by the group.

One type of peer support-intervention group now emerging involves adults (usually young adults) who were sexually abused as chil-

---
* This section, through page 523, was written by Hollis Wheeler.

dren. This type of group is helpful to such patients because they have experienced traumas that carry a social stigma, and few services have been designed to respond specifically to this type of problem. It is a problem that may affect self-esteem, general adjustment, and relationships for many years.

Organizational Considerations

The organizational mechanics for a self-help group are not difficult. The following guidelines were found helpful in organizing and implementing a group for patients who share in common previous sexual abuse in the form of incestuous relationships.

Publicity

A minimum of 2 weeks before the group is to begin, and preferably 3 to 4 weeks beforehand, publicity (e.g., newspaper ads or radio spots) can be arranged. Two weeks are usually needed for potential patients to weigh carefully the decision to join and to muster courage to make contact. Publicity should stress confidentiality and inform the potential group members that they can call in anonymously for more information if they desire. In addition, posters can be placed in such public locations around the community as grocery stores, laundromats, schools, and colleges. Area mental health facilities and professionals, another source of referrals, can also be informed of the group and its emphasis.

Location

Optimally, meetings should be arranged in a warm, comfortable, and private setting. It may be a house, a school, church, YWCA, or a woman's center that is in a central location. The location for meetings is determined before the first meeting in order for group time and energy not to be dissipated on this issue. Arrangements for refreshments are also helpful.

Screening

A screening contact before the start of the group is helpful in several ways. It provides a context to create expectations for the group, a chance to become acquainted with potential group members, and an opportunity to screen out those who are not ready for such an experience or who are otherwise inappropriate. Screening can be done over the telephone, but it is more effective in person. For those who are not ready for this type of helping experience, a referral is often necessary and appropriate. At times, a recommendation to obtain brief individual counseling as preparation for such a group is helpful and frequently welcomed.

Referrals

Before beginning the group, the nurse should identify and make contact with all available referral resources in the area. These may include specific professionals as well as facilities or programs that are sensitive to the particular type of problem and issues involved. Contact with referral resources is helpful not only for members who need additional work but also as a source of referrals to the group. The family physician can be extremely helpful here.[57]

Developing Guidelines

For effective functioning, a self-help group requires guidelines to structure and provide boundaries for the helping process. Necessary guidelines are discussed below.

Closing Membership

At the first meeting, a cutoff date for accepting new members is decided. Members are encouraged to arrive on time and to minimize interruptions during the group time (e.g., telephone or messages). It is also helpful to obtain members' home telephone numbers (if they are agreeable) to relate changes in schedules, problems, and so forth. First names may be used in the group if more informality (or anonymity!) is desired by the participants.

Outside Contacts

Another helpful guideline for the group to consider is that there be no discussion of other group members outside the group. This guideline depends on self-monitoring for enforcement but makes participants more comfortable. Group members who meet outside the group may be particularly cautioned against discussing the group or its members. This is helpful to avoid cliques or alliances and helps ensure that if an issue needs to be raised, it is done in the group.

Confidentiality

The group may decide on specific confidentiality guidelines, because these are extremely important to this type of group. Participants should be permitted to retain as much anonymity about their identities within the group as is comfortable. A decision about any record keeping, observers, or supervisors for training purposes must also be made.

Time Limits for Meetings

It is easy to run over the time limit for meetings when issues, feelings, and experiences suppressed for years begin to emerge. However, it is helpful to close the meeting on time whenever possible. This prevents participants from becoming physically and emotionally exhausted from the interaction. Members find it more helpful if left with the desire to meet again and continue the following week. Issues being discussed must be brought to a reasonable point of closure before the meeting is adjourned to prevent members from feeling they have been left hanging.

Possible Crises

It is not uncommon for one or more group members to experience an emotional crisis during the course of a self-help group of this type. The nurse may elect to give her phone number to group members with instructions to call if they become extremely distressed during the week. The release of long-suppressed memories and feelings often overwhelms a person's capacity to cope and produces an emotional overload and consequent crisis. The nurse must be sensitive to this and take preventive measures by giving the group members specific instructions on what to do if and when this occurs.

Termination

A termination date for the group is always established at the onset. As the termination date approaches, the nurse reminds the group of this fact so that members are able to prepare themselves for separation. Termination issues are anticipated and dealt with, with the guidance of the nurse. It is possible, but not always advisable, to extend the group meetings if there is strong sentiment to do so within the group membership.

Group Structure

Group members must decide on the basic dimension of structure; that is, the group must decide on a structured or unstructured format. As a general rule, as the size of the group increases, the need for structure also increases. Structure can be imposed in many ways and can be negotiated by the nurse with the group. One example of a structured format is allotting each member a specific length of time to talk, with members more or less taking turns during the course of the meeting. Conversely, an unstructured alternative is to ask all members to make sure they do not use excessive time for discussion and to encourage all members to participate and become involved. It is axiomatic that in an unstructured format, the nurse and the group must monitor the process closely.

The nurse may seek to establish an unobtrusive group leadership role so that after the first two or three meetings the group is able to guide itself. In the self-help group, beneficial effects accrue from interactions among members, and the nurse may function only as a low-key facilitator who steps in when the group "gets stuck" or "off the track" or when a problem becomes manifest. Sometimes the role of "facilitator," with the nurse present, can be rotated from one group member to another week by week, if participants decide on that format.

Disclosure of personal experience has not been made a prerequisite for group membership. However, individual members are gently and supportively encouraged to disclose as early in the group as they are willing, but without pressure to disclose prematurely. After initial apprehension, one group member breaks the ice, and once trusting relationships develop among group members, initial apprehension may evolve into a desire to share with the group. Generally, details of incestuous acts are the most difficult to discuss, and many women do not provide much specificity here. It is more important to share and discuss the feelings generated by these experiences than the acts themselves.

One interesting variation in the self-help group is to develop a group action project when the group meetings are about half over. Such a project serves two primary purposes: (1) It helps bring closure to the group by producing some product at its ending that all have been part of; and (2) it helps group members begin turning outward and to their futures after focusing inward during the group. One group decided to be interviewed by a journalist who submitted the resulting article about the group to a magazine for publication. Another group met periodically following the regular group meetings to discuss and write about their relationships with their mothers. Yet another possibility is for group members, with the help of the nurse, to initiate another group for others with similar problems.

Small Group Dynamics and Interventions

As the group begins, group members can be asked to define their hopes or expectations for the group. Questions not previously covered by the nurse in the introductory remarks can be answered. It is explicitly stated that each member's role includes supporting others in the group as well as to work on personal concerns for personal growth.

Although self-help groups usually select a common theme that involves personal experiences, some members may be apprehensive about discussing their experiences. It is often helpful to have one group member take the initiative to disclose her experience so that it can be supported by the group. Another option is to show a film specific to the theme as a means to begin group interaction and disclosure.

In creating expectations for the group members, some apprehension can be allayed by assuring members that (1) the group will take seriously and accept all they have to say; (2) the group wants to help and to hear what members have to say; and (3) the experience of sharing is therapeutic, particularly when that sharing is with others who have had similar experiences.

Another way to build confidence and rapport among group members is to spend some time focusing on the strength and courage all have demonstrated simply by deciding to join the group and attend the first meeting. It is also helpful to comment on the strength it takes to cope with a problem alone for a long period of time, and to congratulate them on taking a constructive new step to work out this problem in conjunction with others who share it.

It is often useful to close each meeting with a few minutes devoted to "debriefing." This helps patients to make an emotional transition back to their private lives and the real world outside. Someone may be asked to summarize what has been discussed in the meeting. In one group, one member asked everyone present to join hands and she reinforced everyone for something that had been accomplished as she went around the circle. These closure techniques may be substituted for "debriefing" in many instances, and members also find they build greater group cohesion as an added benefit.

Related Considerations

Several other points are salient for group members, and the nurse must be aware of and responsive to them. Because of the difficulty in breaking the silence about past experiences, group members may experience an increase in anxiety as the group meeting time draws closer each week. This is a normal response and to be expected, but it may create concern (and avoidance) in group members if they are not sensitized to this possibility in advance.

Further, members have typically been coping for years with their feelings and memories, and the group interaction may upset a stable, but perhaps not entirely adaptive, pattern of coping. Dealing with these issues in the group may cause some of their relationships to change. Often relationships become more tenuous as deep feelings are dealt with, and then change for the better. Members again can be sensitized to this possibility and can be advised to talk about such an eventuality with those they are close to.

The nurse must also anticipate that with the strong feelings involved in reviewing past experiences, emotional outbursts may occur in the group. Often strong anger, crying, or even self-destructive behaviors are seen. The nurse can handle these situations directly within the group, but must be aware that they may also occur outside the group after these feelings have been "opened up" following perhaps years of suppression or denial. A plan for handling such emergencies must be discussed with the group members so they will know who to call and how to obtain help.

As the group draws to a close, at least some members may desire (or need) to continue in some form of helping relationship. It is at this point that referral resources are very helpful. A knowledge of local facilities, programs, or helping resources can help to facilitate referrals. The nurse can provide names or instruct the group in making contacts with other resources, or she may become more actively involved in facilitating a referral quickly. Handling referrals is an important but easily neglected aspect of the nurse's functioning in a self-help intervention group, but it is an area of responsibility that is critical to the group.

COMPARISON OF GROUP MODALITIES

Nurses, in their work in psychiatric–mental health settings, may be called upon to provide a wide variety of group treatment modalities such as have been discussed. In order to determine the most effective model for the particular patient group, the three models will be compared.

The goals of traditional group therapy include changing individual attitudes, beliefs, emotional states, and behaviors that are assumed to be maladaptive or deviating from the norm. Whether treatment is focused on recovery from illness, modifying difficult behavior and emotional states, or discovering the underlying causes of symptoms, traditional group therapy centers on the individual and is adjustment-oriented. Therapy assumes that the individual is the object of change, that the person is responsible for the solutions, and that individual solutions are indeed possible. Diagnosis and intervention in therapy are based on clinical theories and research as well as on the clinical experience of the therapist.

The goals of group intake procedure are derived from principles of group treatment and the innovative concepts of the customer approach. This approach addresses the conceptual model barrier to comprehensive service through respect for the patient's definition of the problem and desired treatment goals. It allows consideration of social and environmental variables in understanding the problem, and requires the use of "eclectic prescriptivism" by opening the treatment contract itself to patient–counselor negotiation. Adherence to this model focuses on adjusting clinical services to patient needs, rather than the traditional reversal, and the model has proven effective in serving resistant urban populations.

In self-help groups, institutional structures, social norms, and individual attitudes and behaviors provide the framework for analysis. Through sharing, self-help groups assist people to understand and deal with personal problems as they are related to various social role factors.

Through this process, personal attitudes and behaviors, roles and relationships, as well as social policies and practices, become targets for change. The personal experiences of group members are considered the central ingredients for understanding problems and for devising solutions, both private and public.

In traditional group therapy, the structure of the therapist–patient relationship is hierarchical and relies on the expertise of a trained mental health professional. It is assumed that the therapist does not share the problems of the patient and will not reveal personal material. The therapist professes to be morally neutral and nonjudgmental. Authority and control are maintained by the therapist, who establishes therapy goals and interventions. Conversely, intake groups and self-help groups are based on equal sharing of resources, power, and responsibility. Intake groups maximize efficient use of staff time by eliminating nonattenders and through prompt identification of priority cases and facilitation of immediate intervention. Additional time is saved for both staff and patients through appropriate referrals to other agencies directly from the intake group.

The structure of self-help groups usually includes a nonauthoritative leader (or even no leader) and stresses principles of personhood and the authority of personal experience. The structure of the group inherently assumes and promotes people's abilities to be autonomous, self-directing, and competent. There is an assumption of shared experience and shared difficulties. Self-help groups emphasize being supportive and nonjudgmental toward group members' behaviors and attitudes but critically examine values and beliefs from a sociopolitical framework.

There are certain processes common to the three types of groups, including provision of a role model, sharing of personal experience, imparting of information, peer support, identifying commonalities, instillation of hope, and cohesiveness. However, traditional group therapy is designed to be a corrective experience based on exploration of individual factors and emphasizing interpersonal relationships within the group as a major factor in the change process. Intake groups encourage the patient's definition of the problem and opens to negotiation the nature and goals of treatment. Although the group leader does not negotiate the final treatment contract, the concept of negotiation is introduced, and the expression of expectations is urged and supported. Self-help groups are not viewed as a corrective experience or as a step in negotiating treatment but rather as a process of personal growth. Self-help groups also minimize the importance of interpersonal learning in the group; change occurs through people's increasing understanding of themselves as part of a larger social group and through viewing personal problems within the context of common social roles and social conditions.

Traditional group therapy and intake groups are conducted within conventional mental health institutions and social service agencies and professional offices. In contrast, self-help groups are organized through a wide range of formal and informal networks and organizations, many of which are identified with various social movements. Many of the small, multiservice alternative agencies through which self-help groups are formed share the characteristics of the self-help groups themselves: (1) their authority structure is collective or collegial; (2) emphasis is placed on personal growth and includes advocacy and social change as a focus for

activity and analysis; (3) a humanistic approach is used; (4) they are located in a range of settings, including private homes, churches, libraries, schools, and community centers; and (5) they are grass roots and work outside established institutions.[58]

In conclusion, it is important that nursing research be conducted toward clarification of these three types of group modalities. The results of such study would provide a basis for linkages and referrals between professional and nonprofessional services for people under stress. Once the relative utility of the various group method approaches is established, people will be able to choose among the modalities, using them separately or in conjunction with another, depending on the particular problem, goal, or personal preference. Ideally, the ultimate goal of all group approaches is to enable the individual to have the power to control his own life. It is hoped that the skills and resources of nurse-researchers will contribute and support this goal to enhance an individual's personal growth and promote meaningful social change.

Summary

This chapter describes and compares three models of group treatment: traditional group therapy, intake group procedure, and self-help groups. *Traditional group therapy*, identified as a major technique within the scope of psychiatric and mental health nursing practice, has specific organizational and operational rules for conduct. *Intake groups*, as a technique to use with low-income urban populations, is described as a way to overcome existing barriers to comprehensive service delivery in community mental health centers. *Self-help groups* are an alternative to traditional mental health services and serve many purposes. The groups often are designed to deal with individual as well as group issues involving psychological, social, legal, economic, political, and cultural components. Nurses can take a leadership role in all three of these modalities in their work with groups.

Questions

1. What are the differences among traditional group therapy, intake group orientation, and self-help groups?
2. What benefits of group therapy, intake groups, or self-help groups have patients described?
3. Talk with someone who has been involved with a group treatment method and present his or her view of the process.

4. Identify the socially stigmatizing experiences that are most responsive to the self-help group method.

5. Describe how the group process is or may be a useful concept in other nursing situations.

REFERENCES AND SUGGESTED READINGS

1. Rogers, C. Interpersonal relationships: Year 2000. *Journal of Applied Behavioral Science*, 1968, *4*, 265–280.
2. American Nurses' Association, Division on Psychiatric and Mental Health Nursing Practice. *Statement on Psychiatric and Mental Health Nursing Practice*. Kansas City, Mo.: American Nurses' Association, 1976, pp. 16–17.
3. Yalom, I. D. *The Theory and Practice of Group Psychotherapy*. New York: Basic Books, 3rd ed. 1985.
4. Ibid.
5. Ibid.
6. Doster, J. A., & Strickland, B. R. Perceived child-rearing practices and self-disclosure patterns. *Journal of Counseling and Clinical Psychology*, 1969, *33*, 382.
7. Jourad, S. M. Healthy personality and self-disclosure. *Mental Hygiene*. 1959, *43*, 499–507.
8. Jourad, S. M., & Jaffee, P. E. Influence of an interviewer's disclosure on the self-disclosing behavior of interviewees. *Journal of Counseling Psychology*, 1970, *17*, 252–257.
9. Gilbert, S. J. Self-disclosure, intimacy, and communication in families. *The Family Coordinator*, 1976, *25*, 221–231.
10. Rivenbark, W. H., III. Self-disclosure patterns among adolescents. *Psychological Reports*, 1971, *28*, 35–42.
11. Levinger, G., & Senn, D. J. Disclosure of feelings in marriage. *Merrill-Palmer Quarterly*, 1967, *13*, 237–249.
12. Goffman, E. *Stigma*. Englewood Cliffs, N.J.: Prentice-Hall, 1963.
13. Ibid., p. 3.
14. Ibid., p. 42.
15. Ibid.
16. American Nurses' Association, pp. 16–17.
17. Rutan, J. S., & Alonso, A. Some guidelines for group therapists. *Group*, 1978, 2(Spring), 11.
18. Sadock, B. J. Group psychotherapy, combined individual and group psychotherapy, and psychodrama. In H. I. Kaplan & B. J. Sadock (Eds.), *Comprehensive Textbook of Psychiatry*, 4th ed. Baltimore: Williams & Wilkins, 1985, p. 1409.
19. Hollingshead, A., & Redlich, F. *Social Class and Mental Illness*. New York: Wiley, 1958.
20. Ibid.
21. Srole, L., et al. *Mental Health in the Metropolis*. New York: McGraw-Hill, 1962.
22. Ryan, W. (Ed.) *Distress in the City*. Cleveland: Press of Case Western Reserve, 1969.
23. Joint Commission on Mental Illness and Health. *Action for Mental Health*. New York: Science Editions, 1961.
24. Ryan, op. cit.
25. Rosenthal, D., & Frank, J. The fate of psychiatric clinic outpatients assigned to therapy. *Journal of Nervous and Mental Disease*, 1958, *127*, 330–343.
26. Hunt, R. Social class in mental illness: Some implications for clinical theory and practice. *American Journal of Psychiatry*, 1960, *116*, 1065–1069.
27. Garfield, S. Research on client variables in psychotherapy. In A. Bergin & S. Garfield (Eds.), *Psychotherapy and Behavior Change*. New York: Wiley, 1971.
28. Miller, S., & Roby, P. *The Future of Inequality*. New York: Basic Books, 1970.
29. Braceland, F., & Lundwall, L. Dropping out of treatment: A critical review. *Psychological Bulletin*, 1975, *82*, 738–783.
30. Ryan, op. cit.
31. Valentine, C. *Culture and Poverty*. Chicago: University of Chicago Press, 1968.
32. Dunham, H. Community psychiatry. *Archives of General Psychiatry*, 1965, *12*, 303–313.
33. Miller & Roby, op. cit.
34. Lazare, A. Hidden conceptual models of clinical psychiatry. *New England Journal of Medicine*, 1973, *288*, 345–351.
35. Overall, A., & Aronson, H. Expectations of psychotherapy in patients of lower socioeconomic class. *American Journal of Orthopsychiatry*, 1963, *33*, 421–430.
36. Albee, G. Models, myths, and manpower. *Mental Hygiene*, 1968, *52*, 168–180.
37. Reiff, R. Social interventions and problems of psychological analysis. *American Psychologist*, 1968, *23*, 524–531.
38. Ibid.
39. Garfield, op. cit.
40. Hornstra, R., et al. Worlds apart: Patients and professionals. *Archives of General Psychiatry*, 1972, *27*, 553–557.
41. Levinson, D., Merrifield, J., & Berg, K. Becoming a patient. *Archives of General Psychiatry*, 1967, *17*, 385–406.
42. Ford, D., & Urban, H. *Systems Psychotherapy*. New York: Wiley, 1963.

43. Nader, R. Community mental health centers. *Behavior Today*, 1972, *3*, 3–6.
44. Dimond, R., & Haven, R. Restructuring psychotherapy toward a prescriptive eclecticism. *Professional Psychology*, 1975, (May), 193–200.
45. Aguilera, D., & Messick, J. *Crisis Intervention*, 4th ed. St. Louis: Mosby, 1984.
46. Caplan, G., & Grunebaum, H. Perspectives on primary prevention. *Archives of General Psychiatry*, 1967, *17*, 331–346.
47. Aguilera & Messick, op. cit.
48. Levinson, Merrifield, & Berg, op. cit.
49. Frank, J. The role of hope in psychotherapy. *International Journal of Psychiatry*, 1968, *5*, 383–395.
50. Frank, J., et al. Patients' expectancies and relearning as a factor in determining improvement in psychotherapy. *American Journal of Psychiatry*, 1959, *115*, 961–968.
51. Heitlen, J. Precounseling preparation increases the effectiveness of counseling. *Manpower Science Services Newsletter*, February 12, 1973, pp. 1–6.
52. Hoehn-Savic, R., et al. Systematic preparation of patients for psychotherapy. *Journal of Psychiatric Research*, 1964, *2*, 267–281.
53. Hare-Mustin, R. Extending clinical service through group intake procedure. *Journal of Community Psychology*, 1967, *4*, 362–368.
54. McGee, T., & Larsen, V. An approach to waiting list therapy groups. *American Journal of Orthopsychiatry*, 1967, *37*, 594–597.
55. Ibid.
56. Allgeyer, J. The crisis group—its unique usefulness to the disadvantaged. *International Journal of Group Psychotherapy*, 1970, *20*, 235–240.
57. Boekelheide, P. D. Incest and the family physician. *Journal of Family Practice*, 1978, *6*, 87–90.
58. McShane, C., & Oliver, J. Women's groups as alternative human service agencies. *Journal of Sociology and Social Welfare*, 1978, *5*, 615–626.

Chapter 28

Liaison and Consultative Issues in Psychiatric Mental Health Nursing

Ann Wolbert Burgess

Chapter Objectives

The students successfully attaining the goals of this chapter will be able to:

- Identify mental health concepts that are useful in general nursing settings.
- Identify the systems approach to liaison psychiatric nursing.
- Describe liaison psychiatric nursing as an expanded role in nursing.
- Contrast emotional crisis and psychiatric emergency.
- Describe the role of the psychiatric nurse in dealing with psychiatric emergencies.

The following example illustrates a patient reaction that is of great concern to practitioners of liaison psychiatric nursing, that is, the psychological reaction of the medically ill patient.

The intern and nurse stared wide-eyed as Mr. R., who had just been hospitalized for a massive coronary occlusion, ran down the corridor. Mr. R's aberrant behavior did not cease after he was chastised for his defiance of his doctor's orders to stay in bed. When the staff explained that bed rest was essential for recovery, Mr. R. proceeded to demonstrate his strength by lifting his bed. He did push-ups in front of the nurse's station. Angry warnings that he might kill himself were to no avail.[1]

INTEGRATING MENTAL HEALTH CONCEPTS

The field of liaison psychiatry emerged with the development of psychosomatic medicine as its theoretical base in the 1920s. Consultation liaison psychiatry is concerned with the study, diagnosis, treatment, and prevention of psychiatric morbidity in the physically ill; of psychological factors affecting physical conditions; and of somatopsychic and psychosomatic interactions. The field includes two major areas: (1) psychiatric consultation with patients; and (2) collaboration with nonpsychiatric health professionals in all types of medical settings.[2]

It has been emphasized that one half of ambulatory and at least one third of hospitalized patients have significant psychological reactions that accompany their medical illness or physical condition.[3] Liaison psychiatric services have emerged in medical centers to improve the hospital environment of the patient, to develop the team approach to psychological care, to impart psychological dynamics to nonpsychiatric caretakers, and to participate in studies to expand the understanding of the psychology of the medically and surgically ill.[4]

Liaison nursing is a subspecialty of psychiatric nursing. Nurses prepared to do liaison nursing have advance training at the Master's level. The focus is on persons with psychological problems associated with physiological illnesses and treatments.[5] It is important for the basic nursing student to know about the role of the liaison nurse in order to know under what circumstances and in what patient situations it is appropriate to ask for assistance.

The liaison model in the hospital and community is intended to (1) practice the three levels of prevention (primary, secondary, and tertiary); (2) focus on the consultant and milieu in addition to the patient; (3) participate in case detection instead of awaiting referral; (4) clarify the caretaker's status as well as the patient's (using the chart, the doctor, nurse, family, and patient as data sources); and (5) provide an ongoing educational program that promotes more autonomous functioning by medical, surgical, and nursing personnel with regard to handling their patients' psychological needs.[6]

CONCEPTUAL FRAMEWORK OF GENERAL SYSTEMS THEORY

A conceptual framework is needed to guide the nurse in assisting patients to obtain optimal health. The conceptual framework used in liaison nursing is largely based on general systems theory. This framework was chosen because it enables the nurse to deal with the complexities of the ill person within his social system, because it is general enough for wide use by nurses, and because it can be easily integrated into other frameworks.

The origin of systems theory is multidisciplinary. Health professions can make efficient use of systems for team planning and problem solving. A system is defined as a set of units with relationships among them. All living systems have boundaries. Boundaries determine the outer parameter of the system and constitute the interface between systems.[7]

Systems are hierarchically arranged. The organization unit that a liaison nurse primarily works with is defined as the *target system*. Everything that is larger or outside the target system is called the *suprasystem*, and any smaller units within the target system are called *subsystems*. The liaison nurse looks outward toward the suprasystem and inward toward the subsystem, while being primarily concerned with what is happening in the target system.

A simple diagram and example may clarify the ideas presented thus far. In Figure 28-1, the target system may be a specialized unit within a hospital that requires the consultation services of the liaison nurse. The suprasystem is the health care system such as a hospital, and the subsystems are specific patient groups such as preoperative patients on a surgical nursing unit. The figure is useful for taking a simplified look at the different levels of a system. A hierarchy of influencing forces that are relevant to the target system can be analyzed.[8] Similarly, when man is the target system, physiologically he is viewed as a complex adaptive system comprising biological subsystems. In liaison nursing, the primary target system is usually a specific patient (group) in relation to his (their) social system and environment.

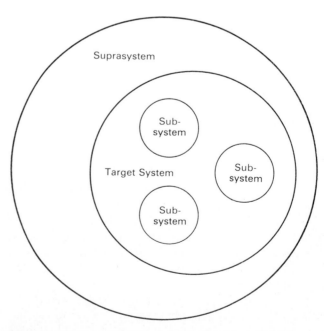

Figure 28-1. Schematic representation of three system levels. (From Stevenson, J. S., 1977, with permission.[7])

There are a number of key properties of an open system that nurses need to be aware of. Systems are characterized by some degree of *wholeness*. Every part of a system is so related to its fellow parts that a change in one part will cause a change in all parts and in the total system.

And yet, a system cannot be taken for the sum of its parts; indeed, formal analysis of isolated segments distorts the very object of interest. The liaison nurse assesses the patient, his illness, and the environment and its interrelatedness as a whole; whereas the patient's primary nurse may focus only on limited aspects of the disease or treatment affects.[9]

Negentropy is a process in open systems that leads to increasing order and complexity in the system. Negentropy is achieved by a systems process known as *feedback*. In feedback, information about systems output is monitored back into the system as information input. Feedback is the manner in which systems are related. Decisions in systems, then, are based on information input to the system as feedback. As information in the form of feedback adjustment increases, the probability of efficient decision making and steady state increases. It is the purpose and the goal of the open system to determine the state desired. All open systems seek some desired relatively steady state determined by a set of values, goals, ends, and purposes. Each system decides what adjustments it can make vis-à-vis the desired state, for there is always a cost-efficiency factor attached to such decisions in terms of materials, energy, and information.

Vickers has proposed four ways in which a system adjusts through feedback when usual responses fail. The system can: (1) alter itself; (2) alter the environment; (3) withdraw from the environment; or (4) alter its desired state.[10] These options can serve as a guide for the nurse liaison in assessing a system in distress. When the flexibility of a system is exercised beyond its limits, a stress is produced that constitutes a threat to the system. The system must then use its capacities for adaptation, integration, and decision making to reduce the stress and stabilize the system.

Fragmented knowledge characterized by a collection of isolated facts is not easily recalled and does not furnish a systematic way of viewing a situation. A general systems perspective permits the organization of a vast number of theories and concepts into a meaningful framework as a basis for making clinical judgments.

Concept of Adaptation

The concept of adaptation identifies humans as an integral part of a dynamic system that is constantly acting and reacting to incoming stimuli. Coping skills and adaptation strategies are key factors to be assessed. Illness, disability, hospitalization, and medical treatment are all stimuli that generally create discomfort. Patient status may threaten the individual's identity and self-concept. The person, in turn, must use coping mechanisms to deal with the discomfort. If these efforts fail, maladaptive behaviors frequently result, and in hospitals that have liaison services, a liaison nurse may be called to help with maladaptive behavior of the patient.

In the case cited earlier, Mr. R. had experienced a severe myocardial infarction. His subsequent behavior of running down the corridor, doing push-ups, and lifting the bed disturbed and annoyed the staff. Their attempts to set limits by reprimanding the patient made him more volatile. By working with the staff, the patient, and his wife, the liaison nurse was able to demonstrate that the hyperactivity was a defensive reaction to worries about being passive and feeling less masculine. The patient was told that the most difficult and manly job he would ever have was to stay in bed. He was asked to chart his vital signs and progress and to offer suggestions to the staff on his care. This plan helped the patient to put his thoughts into words instead of into actions.[11]

Concept of Anxiety

Anxiety—a feeling state of discomfort—is internally experienced as a threat to one's self or to one's sense of integrity. This feeling is a result of perceiving incoming stimuli in terms of previously experienced threatening events. For example, if a nurse prefaces her comments to a patient with the words, "I'm afraid I have bad news for you," the person will probably be flooded with anxiety because the message relates to a previous experience in which there was distressing news. The person will simultaneously react physically and mentally to the words. In addition, the person will attempt to maintain a steady balance in the face of the stressful stimuli.

A primary goal in liaison nursing is to support the person so that disequilibrium does not occur and so that a steady state is maintained. Support means helping the person identify and better cope with his feelings of anxiety. As long as the person can cope with the incoming stimuli, the anxiety level is manageable. If the coping mechanisms fail, the ego functions are affected, anxiety increases, and the person is in crisis. Uncontrolled anxiety precipitates an extremely vulnerable state. Liaison nurses must be especially knowledgeable in assessing anxiety and in determining what type of nursing intervention is needed.

PSYCHOSOCIAL REACTIONS TO ILLNESS

The liaison nurse is concerned with people who are experiencing an illness. "Illness" used here refers to an event experienced by people that manifests itself through observable or felt changes in the body, causing an impairment of capacity to meet minimum requirements for appropriate functioning.[12] The illness may be acute or chronic, and may require varying types of health care services, such as hospitalization, continuing care, or intermediate care in the community.

A person hospitalized for a physical condition has to deal with many feelings and reactions. Some reactions are the result of his feelings of helplessness at being confined in the hospital, his feelings of dependency at having to rely on other people for care, his feelings of inadequacy at not being able to do what he normally could and would do for himself, his feelings of anger at what has caused his present predicament, his feelings of anxiety over the uncertainty of the situation, or his feelings of sadness over the loss of his previous state of well-being and independence. Some factors contributing to his illness may be based on situations relevant to his family or community, his economic status, his ethnic background, his religious needs, or his employment situation.

When patients are overwhelmed by these reactions, they respond in a variety of ways: some may deny the seriousness of the illness; some may be excessively demanding; others may simply be outwardly depressed.

How a person copes with the reactions his illness provokes usually is dependent on his personality or character style, the nature of the illness, and how he perceives the illness. The impact of hearing about his illness and the environment in which he finds himself may compound the problem.

Everyone brings his own unique way of coping into a situation. In other words, the patient who has an ulcer does not react in a "typical ulcer personality way." If the person has previously used rationalization when he was under stress, he will bring rationalization into this situation. To a large extent his previous coping mechanisms and the impact of the illness will determine his method of coping.

When a patient perceives his illness as being a "life or death" situation, he is then more likely to use denial. A person with a broken finger may find the inconvenience of a cast annoying, but a broken finger to a baseball pitcher may be catastrophic. When any illness achieves major psychological significance, an adequate coping defense is needed.

The environment in which the patient finds himself will also affect his coping abilities. If he finds himself in an intensive care unit with many electrical devices attached to him, his defensive reaction will be much stronger than if he finds himself in a six-bed ward for convalescents. Coping mechanisms are used as protective devices by individuals who are overwhelmed by anxiety. The defenses may become pathological and may ultimately interfere with the patient's treatment.

Behavioral Patterns in Adjusting to the Illness

We find it useful to view the patient's reactions to his illness within four patterns of behavior: (1) shock and disbelief; (2) awareness; (3) reorganization; and (4) readjustment or change.

Shock and Disbelief

When first confronted with the news of serious illness, the person generally reacts with shock and disbelief. This behavioral response brings defense mechanisms into play. The nurse's ability to assess the defenses will help to identify the therapeutic route to take with the patient in formulating a patient care plan.

The patient needs to use his defense in this

phase because he is overwhelmed. The nurse must recognize this as an appropriate reaction. For example, the patient may say, "I don't believe I have a serious illness," or "I could not have diabetes. The tests must be wrong."

The nurse should not encourage denial or any defense—any more than a patient is encouraged to talk about his delusion in the psychiatric setting. It is more therapeutic not to focus on the defense but rather spend time with the patient and encourage him to talk and express his feelings about his illness.

A therapeutic response to someone who says that he cannot believe that he has a certain illness should be supportive: "It is hard to believe," or "What makes it so hard to believe?" The nurse supports and stands by the patient in the hope that he eventually can come to terms with the illness and can give up the defense by himself.

Some of the verbal responses and behaviors that demonstrate the common defense of denial are listed below.

"I don't have it."
"I had it, but not now."
"It's not serious."
"It isn't what they think it is. My heart isn't the problem; it 's my stomach."
Patient verbally agrees but acts in a way that the nurse knows is denial; e.g., he keeps smoking or overeating or drinking, which are contraindications for the illness.
Patient changes the subject.
Patient is evasive and does not talk about the issue.
Patient tries to get the nurse to talk about herself.
Patient is excessively cheerful and jokes about what is going on.
Patient goes from a specific topic to a general topic.

Denial may interfere with the prescribed treatment. For example, the patient may refuse to take radiation therapy for a tumor because he insists that it really is not there. Or the patient who has an enlarged liver may continue to drink alcoholic beverages even though he has been warned of the possible consequences. The patient's denial may be so great that he wishes to sign himself out against medical advice. The therapeutic task is either to try to reduce the patient's anxiety and defense mechanism of denial so that they do not interfere with the treatment or to encourage him to express his feelings in order to gain some awareness of his illness.

The nurse should autognose her own reactions in helping the patient during this behavioral phase because these may stall the therapeutic process in several ways. First, the nurse may become anxious while she is listening to the patient talk and therefore change the subject or deny that the patient should feel as he does. For example, the patient says, "I am afraid of the radiation treatments. I won't take them." The nurse who says, "Don't be afraid of them," or "You should do what the doctor says because he knows best," or "You should be thinking of going home," or "I am here to record the amount of fluids you have had today," is stalling the process of encouraging the expression of feelings.

Another stall may occur when the nurse, upon entering the room and finding the patient perspiring freely, asks, "Are you too warm?" If he asks, "Doesn't everyone perspire after taking the tests that I have just taken?" his response may be interpreted as going from the specific to the general. The nurse may unintentionally support this by continuing to talk in generalities. This keeps the subject of the patient's distress from being discussed. The difficulty the nurse is having is her inability to relate to and to help the patient bear the painful feelings that he has. A more helpful statement to the patient would be, "How did you feel about the tests you took this morning?"

Awareness

The second behavioral area in dealing with the news of a serious illness is when the patient develops awareness of the illness. Included in developing awareness are the feelings of anger, sadness, anxiety, or dependence. The patient still is not dealing directly with the reality issue of his illness.

The sign that a patient is moving into an awareness of his illness is seen when he makes such statements as, "If I have had this," or "If this has really happened, then what about . . . ?" There is neither complete acceptance nor acknowledgment yet, but there is a conscious attempt to deal with the reality that others see. This kind of verbal statement by the patient indicates that he is beginning to incorporate the news. This behavior is to be encouraged by the nurse.

It is in this phase that the patient often shows the feeling of anger. This may be because of the patient's feelings of helplessness, of having to depend on others, of not being independent and strong as he once was. The patient may be angry at having to give up his self-image as an independent person, or he may be wishing to be cared for but feels uncomfortable about directly expressing this wish.

The anger is often displaced onto anything that is available; for example, the water in the pitcher is not the right temperature, the wastebasket is not emptied, the food is cold, someone isn't coming to visit, or the nurse walks into the room.

Take another example. A surgical patient who appeared very angry and displeased at just about everything was a puzzle to the staff who tried in many ways to cheer her up. All efforts ended in failure until the day she had the gastric tube going to her stomach removed from her nose. After this the patient changed to a delightful person. When the staff asked her what had made the big change in her mood, she said that she was not aware of how dreadful she felt until the tube was removed and she realized how well she then felt.

It is important not to overlook the fact that people become quite angry and irritable when they are in pain or are hurt. And unquestionably, many physical nursing procedures can and do hurt. Some people get angry with the person who hurts them. They will react unfavorably to nurses because they hurt them by making them get out of bed when it is painful to them, by making them walk when they feel very dizzy, or by removing adhesive tape from a dressing that covers a sensitive area.

The stall in this situation occurs when the nurse takes the anger personally and withdraws from the patient. In order to prevent the stall, the nurse needs to identify the issue about which the patient is really upset. The therapeutic task is to help bear the feeling the patient is experiencing. Even if the nurse cannot identify what the patient is angry about, she should not take the anger personally unless she knows that she has specifically provoked the patient. She has to realize that the anger is not because of her and that she has to bear the feeling.

When the nurse can openly bear the content of the patient's complaint and not become angry, this acceptance will be therapeutic. For example, if the patient is complaining that the food is cold or that the nurses seem busy and do not answer his bell when he rings, the nurse may be helpful by listening and thereby acknowledge and accept the feelings of the patient.

There may be a clue in the patient's behavior that can help the nurse understand the patient. If the nurse does find a clue, she should not feel annoyed because the patient is so demanding or complaining; instead she can begin to try to find a solution to the problem. Dealing with the needs of the patient rather than with her own judgmental reactions is the goal for the nurse.

Reorganization

The phase of developing an awareness of illness blends progressively into the third phase, reorganization. It is at this time that the patient begins to ask questions. These questions may be masked or direct.

A question may be compared to an iceberg in that the manifest question may have little to do with what is really there and submerged beneath the surface. The manifest question usually does not tell the nurse precisely what is on the patient's mind. As a rule, the nurse is unaware of exactly what precipitated the question because she does not have access to all the thoughts that have prompted the patient to ask the question.

Sometimes the nurse deals directly and openly with the question because she thinks that a yes or no answer is indicated. Generally, it is more useful to reply to the patient, "You seem quite concerned about what is happening to you. I wonder what you have been thinking about or what your doctor has talked about." Or, "You are asking if you have emphysema. What makes you think that?"

To respond to the patient's question with statements such as, "Don't worry about that," or "You should ask your doctor about that," or by changing the subject are all potential stall situations to the therapeutic process. In order to correct the stall, the technique of asking and answering questions might be reviewed (see Chapter 17).

Readjustment or Change

The fourth behavior phase, the readjustment or change phase, follows the reorganization of the patient's thinking that allows him to ask questions about his illness. This phase is necessary for him because it helps him to continue with his personal life goals. The acceptance of the changes that must be made implies that the person has dealt with the pain of the news of his illness and that he has come to terms within himself by accepting the demands or modifications that will be involved in his life.

Coming to grips with the loss that is inherent in the illness situation may mean indulging in some fantasy or substitution, but ultimately the patient must give up what has to be given up. For example, if the patient's leg must be amputated and the patient lies in bed fantasizing that he still can be a great runner, he is going to trip and fall when he gets up because he hasn't come to terms with the reality of the lost leg.

Or if the patient is facing the possibility of the removal of an organ, contingent upon unfavorable biopsy reports, and persists in fantasizing that surgery will not be necessary, he is not facing reality. The patient needs to face what it would be like if surgery is required. If he doesn't, the reactions, for example, depression, will probably occur during the recovery period. In this phase the patient has to be prepared to integrate a new self-image to fit into and to feel comfortable with.

The problem for the patient in this phase is learning how to heal the pain received when he heard the news of the illness and how then to move on into the world of everyday living.

Mastery is a critical part of this behavior phase. As the patient becomes skillful in his situation and realizes his control, he regains a feeling of adequacy and security. It is at this point that nurses need to evaluate the amount and degree of nursing care needed in helping the patient to master his situation.

Stalls in the therapeutic process may occur in several ways. A stall may occur when routine, impersonal care is given to the patient. This problem may be seen in overcrowded institutional settings in which staff members are overworked and patients are neither motivated nor encouraged to change their situation.

A stall will also occur when nursing care is excessive and infantilizes the patient. Dependence is encouraged and the patient's efforts at mastery are inhibited.

Another stall situation may occur when the patient maintains the fantasy that prevents him from dealing with reality. For example, a 35-year-old man develops arthritis, takes to a wheelchair, and stays there because he cannot meet the demands of physical therapy or his reactions to his illness.

Patient Status

In assessing the patient's response patterns in adjusting to illness, it is important that the nurse have a good grasp of the reality of the patient's medical situation and the conditions under which the patient was admitted to the hospital. The liaison nurse, the nursing staff on the unit, and the patient's physician need to identify mechanisms for sharing communication among their various systems so that consistent, accurate, and up-to-date information is available. The liaison nurse may play a key role in assisting staff with the development of communication mechanisms for input and feedback.

Patients are temporary occupants in a hospital. They are at a distinct disadvantage in an established, highly organized, bureaucratic institution. Patients are anxious in their new setting, and they are separated from people who normally support their identity. Their being ill and hospitalized compounds the anxiety. It is to be expected that they will use defense mechanisms to suppress anxiety. The pressures of running an institution often encourage staff members to let a patient regress to a dependent position, which then allows the professional to make the decisions for the patient as to needs and nursing care. Social isolation may then develop quickly. Staff relationships are usually superficial, and patients are attended to on a priority of care basis. In order to avoid this potential stall situation, routinely scheduled nursing conferences designed to carefully review and evaluate patient progress can facilitate ensuring individualized patient care.

THE PROCESS OF LIAISON NURSING

There are two models that describe the liaison nurse's role. In the first model, the liaison nurse works directly on a specialty unit or clinic setting and is a part of the team that gives direct care to patients. In this role, the nurse is responsible for identifying patients who are in need of psychological support as an ongoing process. The liaison nurse is involved early in the course of the patient's treatment, and the patient is followed during the entire hospital course and after discharge if indicated.[13] This model will be discussed in terms of various clinical situations.

In the second model, the liaison nurse acts as a consultant to the specialty unit to help the staff clarify the problem. A referral is made to the liaison nurse by the staff. Generally, if a patient problem exists, the nurse will assist the staff in assessing the situation and support the staff as needed. The problems can be short- or long-term. Using this approach, the liaison nurse primarily assesses the key elements of the subsystems, the target systems, and the suprasystem. Generally, the target system is the nursing unit in which a specific patient and the staff are having difficulty relating to each other. The purpose of the consultation is ultimately to raise the standards of psychosocial care of patients. A liaison nurse can help staff nurses heighten their sensitivity to the patient's psychological needs and increase their tolerance for the patient's deviant or disturbing behavior.[14]

Referral

Once the referral is made, the nurse must identify *who* needs help, *who* is seeking it, *what* is the real problem, and *how* the intervention must be structured.[15]

When the nurse is employed by an institution, she must be aware that her actions have an impact on all levels of the system, including the institution, the specialty unit of care, the staff, the attending physician, and the patient. All levels of the system must agree on the purpose of the liaison service in order for it to be successful.

Assessment

The nurse has a variety of data available, for example, the patient's record, which includes age, sex, occupation, diagnosis, and orders. The order sheet may be analyzed in order to evaluate medications and to see if behavior reactions may be the result of drugs. Temperature rise may indicate delirium. Also the ways in which orders are written may alert the nurse to the fact that the patient's behavior is not matching the frequent changes in orders.

The manner in which physicians write orders may also indicate poor communication between the physician and nurse. Progress notes may show that nursing and medical observations are either similar or different, and they should be followed up by an observation of subsequent patient behavior.

Talking with staff provides useful background data. Asking strategic questions about subtle or obvious changes in the patient's behavior under varying circumstances may also provide helpful clues to understanding the patient.

Interviewing the Patient

The liaison nurse may or may not interview the patient directly. She may rely on the primary nurse's assessment of the patient. No matter who does the assessment, the following areas need to be included: the patient and the family's perception of the illness; the patient and the family's goals in the treatment process; the psychological, social, behavioral, and medical aspects of the illness; and the patient's strengths. In addition, the liaison nurse should assess the environmental context in which the problem is occurring and review the policies and procedures that keep the system functioning.

The entry to the patient is a very important step. Liaison staff make it a special point to be direct and open as to who they are and why they are called to see the patient. For example, the liaison nurse may say, "I was asked to see you because the nurses knew you must have been upset last night when you slapped Mr. Jones." Or, "The nurses are concerned about you. They saw you were worried about your surgery."

The remaining part of the interview, following the introduction, then deals with the concerns of the patient.

Patient's Perception of His Illness

The question, "What do you think is wrong with you?" will evoke a variety of responses from the patient. How the patient describes his illness in his own words is a significant point to record. As with the psychiatric patient, these words may tell you more than the several paragraphs that follow.

For example, if the patient says that he is in the hospital because of an ulcer, in what terms does he describe this? Does he use medical terminology, for example, "I have a duodenal ulcer." Or does he say that his stomach burns after he eats? Or does he say that the doctor told him he had an ulcer?

The patient might say he is in the hospital because of high blood pressure or that his wife thought he should come to have some tests in order to find out why he was tired all the time. These words help determine the patient's perception of his illness.

The Family's Perception of the Illness

During the assessment process the nurse can ask the patient how he thinks his family perceives his illness. If the patient's family does visit, it will be useful to ask each member directly what his or her own interpretation of the illness is, what impact this news has on each of their lives, and whether the family will be able to continue to function as a family unit.

Does the family want the patient in the hospital? Does the family feel that he should be in the hospital? Would the family rather have him home? Does the illness frighten and keep the family from visiting the patient?

The Patient's Goals for Treatment

How does the patient see the hospital helping with the illness? What does he expect from the hospital? What previous experiences has he had with hospitals, medical treatment, and nursing care? It is important to clarify the patient's misconceptions about his illness and the effects of treatment.

If the patient is having diagnostic tests, what does he plan to do when the results of the tests are known? Will he continue to do what medical judgment advises, and does he feel the need to be a part of the treatment process?

From a comprehensive health care standpoint, does the patient indicate any need for follow-up visits by a community health nurse to assess his readjustment back into the home and community setting? Does he see his hospitalization as an isolated experience? The inpatient nursing staff should include posthospitalization health care plans in every nursing assessment.

The Family's Goals in the Treatment Process

How does the family see its role in the treatment process? Do the members feel involved with the treatment the patient is receiving, and how may they be of support to the patient both in the hospital and at home? Do they see any need for comprehensive health care follow-up?

For example, if the patient has had a myocardial infarction, does the family see this as a frightening experience that may happen again? Are the family's feelings and reactions considered? Is the community health nurse or the home care coordinating service of the hospital of help to meet the family's needs?

Psychological Assessment

What is the dynamic issue for the patient in relation to his illness? Are his needs to be cared for uppermost in the patient's mind, or is his need to be in control of the situation more the issue? Does the patient feel he has "lost" because of the forced dependence, and does he become defensive because of this lowered self-concept?

What coping mechanisms is the patient using to deal with the stress of the news of the illness? What defenses should be strengthened and supported?

What is the meaning of the illness to the patient? What does this illness do or not do for the patient? Does he respond positively to family and visitors and enjoy cards he receives, or does he leave his mail unopened? Does he get secondary gain from the illness?

Are there any unrealistic fears in connection with the illness? For example, does the patient's anxiety about having an intravenous pyelogram seem out of proportion to the procedure? Or does the patient who is facing cardiac catheterization seem cheerful and totally unconcerned?

Social Assessment of the Patient

What has the patient heard about the illness from friends or relatives? Does he know anyone who has had this illness? What experiences has he heard about? For example, if he is having a surgical procedure, what other men does he know who have had a similar operation and how does he relate this to himself?

Does the illness help the patient identify with an important person who has had the illness? For example, does the patient who has had a heart attack say, "Look at all the presidents who have had what I had."

When the family visits, what visiting style does it have? Do the members talk with the patient about the illness or do they avoid it?

Is the patient worried about finances?

What are his religious needs?

Behavioral Assessment

What behavior does the patient present? Is the patient aware that his behavior is different or changed because of the stress of hospitalization? How does the staff react to the patient's behavior?

Medical Assessment

What symptoms has the patient been having? How clearly can the patient describe his symptoms? Does he say he has pain in his stomach, or does he point to the area and describe it as either sharp or dull pain? Does he gloss over the symptoms or go into great detail during the interview?

Strengths of the Patient

What was the patient doing before he became a patient? Does he talk of his work, his family, his community involvement? Does he seem anxious to be back in that role again, or is he concerned only with the illness?

What questions is the patient able to ask the nurse? This can be an area of strength. It means that the patient wants to be involved in his illness and the treatment, and it is essential that the nurse support this strength.

Does the patient want to know what will be happening during the hospital course? What has been his reaction to the hospitalization so far?

How does the patient feel he will be able to deal with the illness? Does he say, "I know I can get through this; I have made it through other surgical experiences. This illness isn't going to get me down."

Assessment of the Environment

Components of the environment that are important to assess include: physical setting, organizational factors, human aggregate, and social climate. What is the physical setting of the unit like? Are multiple health services involved? How are the services organized to facilitate communication among the various staff? Are there adequate numbers of staff to deliver care? Do staff members have adequate education and preparation for their responsibilities?

Have specific policies been developed to enhance psychosocial care, such as preoperative teaching programs for surgical patients? What is the social climate of the unit? Are staff nurses encouraged to ask for assistance and to make suggestions, or are they expected to follow the rules and not question specific policies?

CLINICAL SITUATIONS

There are various clinical situations in which a liaison nurse may be called. They will be described briefly in the following pages.

The Newly Admitted Patient

The crisis of hospitalization begins the moment the person learns that he must be hospitalized, and it becomes most apparent as he sits before the admissions clerk. Being subjected to the impersonality of admission forms, questions, and the ritual of receiving the wrist band (the badge of patienthood), and observing an array of uniformed people with their professional aloofness are only the beginning. Vital signs, urine sample, weight, and history may be taken immediately and then followed by the order to remove one's clothing and put on the uniform of patienthood, the gown. The medical examination, serology, and chemistry testing follow.

The basis of the patient's anxieties is the threat of loss of identity. All procedures are done routinely by the staff, but the patient is alone and is often ignorant of the procedure. A primary nursing intervention to be provided by nurses is patient teaching. Presenting the facts prepares the patient to better handle his anxiety. Uncertainty surrounding the situation and what to expect can be reduced by sharing information.

The Patient with Undiagnosed Illness

The person who enters the hospital to find out the etiology of symptoms will undoubtedly experience many unsettling feelings and thoughts. Uppermost in the patient's mind is that something very serious might be found. The symptoms are a nagging reminder and may be overwhelming if the person thinks about them constantly. The stress of uncertainty weighs heavily on the mind of any patient.

The Preoperative Patient

The person facing surgery is usually preoccupied with the immediate aspects of surgery, the reason for the surgery, and the unknown element or the loss of consciousness during the surgical procedure.

The seriousness of the surgery or the potential for seriousness is important. For example, a person scheduled for a hemorrhoidectomy may be less preoccupied with the surgery itself than with what he has heard about the pain he will experience after the operation. Or a woman scheduled for a breast nodule biopsy will undoubtedly be under great anxiety regarding the outcome of surgery.

The preoperative patient is generally preoccupied with safety and survival issues; thus he has minimal energy to respond to external pressures. Learning is difficult because it requires cognitive input and the person is only thinking of the surgery. If the patient is in conflict about the surgery, emotional energy is doubly invested in worry.

The element of the unknown in terms of what might be discovered, or if one will recover from the surgery, registers with the patient. When people are faced with possible danger, an alternative to the surgery might be selected. It is not surprising that people do not always accept the physician's advice for surgery.

Preoperative tests may be viewed as legitimate assaults on the body. Gynecological exams, proctoscopy, cystoscopy, and cardiac catheterizations are all done while the patient is awake. These procedures are painful and the patient has to cope with his feelings and anxieties.

Methods to decrease anxiety regarding the unknown have been studied by Johnson and her colleagues. They found that when a person is about to encounter a new experience such as a diagnostic procedure, forewarning the person of the sensations to be experienced allows him to form an image of the impending event as it is experienced and thereby the person achieves cognitive control over the event. This type of information, with descriptions of typical sensations, significantly increased the rate of recovery from surgery.[16]

In cases of extreme stress, the liaison nurse may go to surgery with the patient. The goal is to condense the anxiety-producing experience and focus the patient's attention on one area so that he is not overwhelmed by many stressors at once.[17]

The Patient in Pain

Pain is a defensive reaction to alert the body that there has been injury or damage to the body. Pain may register psychologically, physiologically, or both ways. The sensory experience of pain is complex, and varying theories have been proposed regarding the etiology of pain.

The assessment of people experiencing pain may be made through the following areas: motor responses (movement of body, clenching of teeth, writhing, twisting); vocal responses (crying, screaming, groaning); verbal responses (asking for relief, complaining, cursing); social responses (withdrawal, changes in social manners or communication style); or the absence of overt behavior (hiding pain).[18]

Factors that influence a person's response to pain are personality style, race, culture, intellect, family, environment, occupation, and life-style.

Patients in pain are usually referred to the liaison nurse for three reasons[19]:

1. The patient's pain may be causing him to feel intense anxiety, which heightens the actual pain and hinders the action of routine analgesia.
2. The patient may feel very anxious and simultaneously experience uncontrollable pain. The staff can neither control the patient's pain nor identify its unremitting intensity and thus they feel helpless and frustrated. The liaison nurse then deals with the staff's reaction to the patient as well as with the patient's reaction to the staff and to his pain.
3. Another situation occurs when the patient has experienced chronic, persistent pain over a long period of time. The patient appears withdrawn, apathetic, depressed, and unable to sleep at night. The patient has had pain for so long that he is unaware that living can be different. The nurse needs to legitimize the patient's pain and contract with the patient to take regular doses of analgesics at specified times.

The secret to successful pain management lies in the nurse's ability to establish a trusting relationship with the patient to achieve common objectives.

The Pediatric Patient

The liaison nurse is called to work with children who are presenting serious problems to the pediatric staff. For example, infants who have a diagnosis of failure to thrive and shriek at human contact, children who have been rejected by parents, or children who experience stress severe enough to threaten personality structure are candidates for the liaison nurse.

The developing psyche in the child does not have the repertoire of defenses that the adult has to protect against overwhelming stress, such as stress caused by long periods of hospitalization, painful treatments, or isolation from family.

Childhood is a period of life characterized by helplessness, powerlessness, and authority figures. This situation may be intensified in the pediatric setting if the staff is rewarded in terms of getting the job done (a procedural orientation) rather than in terms of having a positive relationship with a patient (humanistic orientation).

The Seriously Ill Patient

In helping the patient to deal with his feelings and reaction to the news of serious illness, the nurse's therapeutic task is to provide those human elements essential in interaction with patients—being supportive and helping to bear painful feelings.

The emergence of depression is always a consideration to be observed. For example, in the first phase (shock and disbelief), upon hearing the news, the patient says, "I don't have a lump in my breast. That is just a gland swelling." In the second phase (awareness), the patient says, "It really provokes me to have to go without breakfast for these tests. Are you sure you know what you are doing? Nurse, could you please comb my hair? Nobody cares if I get breakfast or not [crying]." In this phase, the feelings of anxiety, anger, dependence, and sadness are all expressed.

In the third phase (reorganization), the patient says, "What does it mean to have a lump in my breast? Do I have cancer? What will happen to my breast?" The patient is asking questions and expressing anxiety, fear, and concern.

In the fourth phase (readjustment), the patients says, "I hear I have to have surgery on my breast. The doctor may have to remove it." The patient may be crying during this conversation.

It might be helpful to know that some patients pass very quickly through these stages, but others take a long time, even months. Some never go through the entire cycle. Although patients cannot be pushed into expressing their feelings, the nurse should be aware of the ways in which she can facilitate or stall these processes.

Adaptation to illness generally includes hope as well as a variety of defense mechanisms. Although the patient relinquishes control of his body, he still clings to hope, which generally means returning to his former life-style.

In summary, the nurse can be very effective in helping the patient to deal with the news and implications of a serious illness. Aiding in the healing process means helping the patient to become involved in mastering his illness and accepting his feelings. As he is able to make peace with that which must be, he then finds the strength to move on, which may include the process of dying.

If the situation is deteriorating from seriously ill to chronically ill, the alternative must be addressed. To many, chronicity is a hopeless state. Robinson describes this state:

> Patients crossing the boundary from acute illness to chronicity must realign their body image with the limitations of a chronic condition . . . they must redefine their social roles and functions. . . .[20]

During this period of redefinition, the person must define a new concept of self and a new concept of the environment as he will experience it. Personality integrity is a main goal in working with the chronically ill.

The Patient in an Intensive Care Unit

With the increase in medical specialization, many patients admitted to a hospital are treated in special care units. An intensive care unit is very different from other areas of the general hospital. It is usually a small area set aside to care for acutely ill people. Units may be called ICU, coronary care, special nursing care, critical care, or trauma units. The pace of the unit is tense and fast. Economy of movement is practiced by staff.

Life-supporting equipment is readily available. Many units are completely open so that all may be seen and heard. Artificial light is used so that patients are prevented from perceiving time changes.

Time loses all meaning. There is no way to orient a person to time. The unit is isolated from the rest of the hospital. Very often the staff is involved with nursing, monitoring, and hospital equipment instead of with the patient. The liaison nurse has to be able to provide direct care if she works in these units.

THE CLINICAL SPECIALIST IN THE EMERGENCY ROOM

The preceding discussion has focused on the role of the psychiatric nurse as liaison to patients within the general hospital setting. The clinical specialist in psychiatric nursing also practices in the role of liaison and consultant to specialty units. Two such settings—the emergency room and rural community mental health centers—are presented in this section to illustrate the role of the psychiatric nurse.

Emergency psychiatric situations are most often defined by someone other than the professional mental health worker, such as the family, patient, or agents of society.* Studies have shown that patients identified as "psychiatric emergency" have presented with various symptoms in the following order of frequency: depression and suicidal attempts, anxiety, intoxication, aggressive behavior, psychosis, confusion, excitement, bizarre behavior, and hysteria.[21] The following characteristics are common among this group of patients:

1. They manifest chronic multiple problems; that is, there is often a somatic–social problem as well as a psychological component to their presenting problem.
2. They are young adults.
3. They are of a lower socioeconomic level and tend to use the emergency room of a hospital as their primary care facility.
4. They are homeless, with meager personal and material resources and are crisis-oriented in their health care.

Where Is Care Delivered?

Psychiatric emergency care can be delivered in a variety of settings and contexts, including ambulances, police rescue squads, community mental health centers, walk-in psychiatric clinics, hot lines, mobile psychiatric units, neighborhood health centers, crisis centers, churches, homes, and streets. However, in many communities, the emergency room of the general hospital is the primary site for the delivery of psychiatric emergency services. This is due to the fact that the emergency room: (1) is open and available 24 hours a day and is accessible

when private practitioners and other community agencies are not; (2) has high visibility in the community and is well known to consumers; (3) is perceived as less expensive by the consumer; and (4) is needed because many patients have accompanying physical problems.[22]

The dramatic increase in the use of psychiatric emergency services in general has been another important factor in the increasing use of the emergency room. The increase in need and demand for crisis intervention and psychiatric emergency services over the past 20 years reflects a significant increase in the population of consumers of these services. In a historical context, the increase in need has been an outgrowth of changes in the organization and delivery of mental health services. There has been a shift in focus from state-hospital-based care to community-based care and a subsequent shift from custodial to therapeutic orientation in delivery of services. This shift has occurred primarily as a result of two events: (1) the increased capability of treating and maintaining patients in the community because of the advent and widespread use of major tranquilizers and antidepressants in the mid-1950s; and (2) passage of the Community Mental Health Care Act of 1963. This act acknowledged the importance of and defined the need for crisis emergency services and mandated that this component be included as one of the essential services provided by any newly created mental health center.

Who Are the Providers?

The psychiatric emergency service in a general hospital is usually located in or near the medical emergency service. Services are provided by an interdisciplinary team of professional mental health specialists and sometimes will include paraprofessionals under the supervision of the professional. The team may include all or some of the following members: psychiatrists, psychiatric nurses, psychiatric social workers, and clinical psychologists. Paraprofessional members may include mental health workers, technicians, and assistants. Team members will usually have a wide range of personal and professional qualifications and characteristics, which include:

1. A high degree of clinical expertise.
2. A broad range of clinical experience.
3. Advanced degrees in the mental health

fields of psychiatric nursing, psychiatry, social work, and psychology.

4. An ability to tolerate a great deal of stress and frustration, to function effectively, and to act decisively in a high-pressure, unpredictable, high-intensity situation.

For the purposes of this discussion, we will focus on the emergency room of the general hospital as the primary site of delivery of psychiatric emergency services and on the clinical specialist or psychiatric nurse as the primary provider of psychiatric emergency care in that setting.

Role of the Psychiatric Nurse

The psychiatric nurse in the emergency department has a variety of responsibilities. These include the functions of a consultant, educator, and facilitator, as well as providing direct services.

Consultant Role

Where psychiatric emergency services and medical emergency services operate out of the same space and closely interface with each other, the psychiatric nurse functions as a consultant to the medical staff. As the "mental health expert," she may be sought out to consult about any of the following: a difficult medical patient who is refusing treatment; a person who has overdosed on drugs and who is unmanageable and combative; an acutely intoxicated patient who is paranoid, hallucinating, and threatening to hurt himself; or a woman who is frightened about receiving an internal examination and the possibility of being pregnant. The psychiatric nurse may be asked to talk with the family and friends of a patient who has just had a severe heart attack, or with the mother of a patient who has died from an accidental drowning, or with a frightened, angry boy who has just witnessed his mother being stabbed.

For the purposes of this discussion we will refer to behaviors and behavioral changes that are a result of some type of biologic dysfunction. These behavior changes may be due to: (1) organic brain or cerebral dysfunction that is a result of some type of damage resulting from traumatic, vascular, infectious, metabolic, or neoplastic disease of the central nervous system (e.g., pneumonia, hematuria, cerebral laceration, meningitis, diabetes, CVA, etc.); (2) too

much of a drug (toxicity caused by alcohol or drug overdose); (3) too little of a drug (withdrawal); and (4) ingestion of drugs that have behavior-altering properties (hallucinogenic drugs such as LSD, mescaline, and THC).

Target indicators as to the possible presence of an organic problem are disturbances in memory and orientation, fluctuating and diminishing levels of consciousness, confusion, and disturbances in psychomotor functioning and intellectual functioning.

The most common behaviors in this category that are identified as "psychiatric emergencies" (and where there is a request for consultation) are those associated with alcohol intoxication and withdrawal, drug overdose and ingestion, and elderly patients with dementias and chronic brain syndrome who have become "unmanageable" at home or in a nursing home.

Often the behaviors can be—and are easily—mistaken for an indication of the presence of a "psychiatric problem." This is due to the fact that in some instances the presenting behaviors and symptoms closely mimic those found in various types of psychiatric disorders such as schizophrenia and mania. In these situations a thorough and complete work-up and evaluation (medical-neuropsychiatric) are essential so that the etiology of the problem can be accurately identified and the patient can receive the treatment necessary to alleviate the symptoms.

A patient who is withdrawing from alcohol may exhibit extreme paranoia and frightening hallucinations of a threatening, accusatory nature. These symptoms are very similar to the ones found in an acute episode of paranoid schizophrenia. The patient who is acutely intoxicated may become threatening, combative, assaultive, and exhibit suicidal ideas and behavior, all of which subside as he becomes sober and the toxins leave the body. The patient who has ingested hallucinogenic drugs will show signs of extreme excitement, restlessness, agitation, anxiety, fearfulness, confusion, and hallucinations. These behaviors and symptoms are similar to the hypomanic behavior present in manic-depressive illness.

Patients with temporal lobe epilepsy may have signs and symptoms similar to those found in schizophrenia (psychosis and affective disorders), including paranoia, delusions, episodic mood changes, irritability, depression, and mania. In addition, they often exhibit impulsive aggressive behavior with sudden outbursts of anger and excessive violence toward others.

Psychological intervention can increase the effectiveness of medical intervention during the medical emergency and can help prevent the development of more serious psychosocial problems after the medical emergency is under control. The psychiatric nursing staff should be seen as a source of emotional support for other staff in the emergency department. The emergency department is a stressful, anxiety-provoking work setting where staff is constantly surrounded with life-and-death situations and dealing with life-and-death issues. Therefore the medical nursing staff members need time to share and process their feelings and experiences, and an opportunity to get psychologically replenished and nourished as well. This ventilation and sharing of feelings usually occurs after the medical emergency has resolved because it is difficult to deal with feelings while one is in the heat of providing emergency treatment. The psychiatric nurse should assume a leadership role in helping the staff to recognize, legitimize, and meet this need.

Educator and Facilitator Role

During the medical emergency, psychiatric patients can arouse a great deal of discomfort in the medical staff. Patient behaviors often evoke feelings of anger, fear, anxiety, frustration, and resentment in the medical staff and can lead to rejection by them of both the psychiatric patients and the various psychiatric staff members. This stance interferes with the effective delivery of services. It may be partially caused by ignorance and a lack of information, understanding, and familiarity with the psychiatric patient on the part of the medical staff members. These patients sometimes exhibit loud, threatening, dangerous, abusive, disruptive, and frightening behaviors, including an assaultive manner, screaming, undressing, and sexual "acting out." Such patients often create a disturbance that can interfere with the delivery of medical services and can prove quite upsetting to other patients and staff. Medical staff statements and comments such as the following are quite common:

Mr. Jones is clearly crazy. Look at him and listen to his talking. He doesn't make any sense. How come he's not going to the psychiatric hospital?

Mr. Smith is screaming. He's going to get violent and hurt someone. Why don't you tie him up?

Mr. Brown is acting like an animal. When are you going to get him out of here?

In these instances, it is the responsibility of the psychiatric nurse to function as an educator and a facilitator in an effort to deescalate and neutralize the situation. This can be accomplished by the following:

1. Providing reassurance that you are in charge and assuming responsibility for controlling the situation.
2. Providing on-the-spot information regarding the status of the situation, an explanation of the patient's behavior, and the plans and rationale for intervention.
3. Offering recognition and validation of staff feelings and allowing for ventilation.
4. Being involved in the triage of all psychiatric patients at the point of arrival in the emergency department so that decisions and understandings can be reached jointly and collaboratively between the medical staff and psychiatric staff.
5. Organizing weekly joint staff meetings. This is a time for the staff to get to know one another, to ventilate, share information, register complaints, discuss mutual issues of concern, and engage in problem solving.

These measures will contribute greatly to developing a sense of mutual support, trust, and respect and thus make it possible for *all* staff to perform more productively and effectively in a very difficult work situation. Otherwise, antagonism and resentment will mount, and this can lead to the psychiatric patients and staff becoming isolated and ignored.

Direct Service Role

As a member of the psychiatric emergency service team in the general hospital, the psychiatric nurse also provides direct service. The psychiatric nurse, in this role, functions as a first contact and front-line mental health expert in the emergency department. She can provide immediate services to identified patients and families of patients. The psychiatric nurse also can act as a consultant and liaison with other hospital units regarding psychiatric emergency situations.

In conjunction with her role in an emergency department, the psychiatric nurse provides the following services: (1) evaluation, assessment, and management of psychiatric emergency patients; (2) consultation and liaison with other front-line mental health workers and community providers—e.g., initiating and receiving referral, transfer of information, requests for assistance and information; and (3) advocacy in securing needed follow-up services and facilitating transfers of patients (and information) from the general hospital emergency room to another agency or facility—e.g., setting up appointments, identifying contact persons, and introducing patients on the phone. Patients often present with the complaint of a sudden occurrence of a physical problem that needs immediate attention, e.g., partial paralysis, blindness, nausea and vomiting, amnesia, chest pain, or hyperventilation and shortness of breath. This type of conversion–reaction symptom is commonly seen in psychosomatic disorders. These symptoms function as a defense against painful feelings and are usually associated with acute anxiety states. Although these are not classically considered psychiatric emergencies, they often require psychiatric consultation.

CASE EXAMPLE

A patient came to the emergency room with the complaint of awakening with pain and stiffness in his neck, which became increasingly worse over the course of the day to the point of being unable to turn his head. The results of the medical examination and x rays were negative, and a psychiatric consultation was requested by the physician. In exploring the events surrounding the sudden onset of pain and stiffness, the patient stated he had had an argument with his mother the night before in which he had threatened her and come close to hitting her. He said he felt enraged and angry initially prior to and during the confrontation, and subsequently felt guilty and upset with himself over the way he had behaved. He had also been concerned and worried about an examination he was going to take that day for which he felt unprepared. The interview was useful in (1) helping the patient gain insight into his own feelings; (2) developing an understanding of his own process; and (3) establishing a connection between his feeling angry at his mother and afraid of his feelings and being unable to express these feelings, and the onset of his physical problems.

Grief Reactions. Behaviors exhibited in immediate and acute grief reactions are similar in many regards to those shown in depression states, e.g., expressions of guilt, anger, confu-

sion, disbelief, hostility, and sadness. Symptoms include crying spells, insomnia, withdrawal, screaming and banging, fainting, pacing, and praying. The psychiatric nurse will come into contact with these persons either at the time of the sudden death of a loved one or days or weeks later when they seek help because they are experiencing emotional difficulties.

CASE EXAMPLE ONE

A 32-year-old niece of a fire victim who had been treated in the emergency room and subsequently died comes to the emergency room one week after the death of her aunt requesting "to talk to someone because I'm not myself, I'm afraid of what I'm feeling, and it won't get better or go away. I don't understand what's happening to me." She stated she was preoccupied with seeing visions of her aunt and thinking about her constantly, had difficulty falling asleep and getting out of bed, was irritable and impatient with her three children, was crying and sad all the time, was withdrawn and wanted to be left alone, was unable to think about going back to work, felt that there was nothing worth living for except her kids, and was frightened that she might hurt herself.

CASE EXAMPLE TWO

Two female members (ages 17 and 20) of a large Portuguese family (12 siblings, 8 to 24 years old, and the mother and father) from the Cape Verdian Islands are brought to the emergency room by members of the extended family after news of the death of their 22-year-old brother by strangulation. The mother and father were away on vacation to the islands and were unreachable. Upon arrival in the emergency room, the 17-year-old was uncommunicative, unresponsive, totally mute and withdrawn, staring into space, not eating or drinking, and required being carried into the emergency room. The 20-year-old sister was also unable to verbalize her feelings, sobbing and screaming uncontrollably, throwing herself on the floor, thrashing about, and attempting to bang her head against the wall.

Physical and Sexual Trauma Reactions. Behaviors that are a result of acts of violence such as battering, rape, and sexual molesting result from the life-threatening aspect of the assault. The development of fears and phobias are major reactions. Symptoms include musculoskeletal tension, gastrointestinal upset such as lack of appetite or nausea, genitourinary disturbance such as vaginal or rectal discharge, headaches, nightmares, and mood swings. Victims of physical and sexual abuse are a target population for psychiatric emergency care (see Chapters 50 and 51).

In conjunction with her role as a nursing consultant to other hospital units, the psychiatric nurse will receive requests for (1) immediate evaluation of a patient's behavior when the individual has become a "behavior problem"—e.g., uncooperative, refusing medications or treatment, belligerent, argumentative, uncommunicative, threatening, and assaultive; (2) assistance with nursing management of "problem patients"; and (3) information and referral sources.

In summary, the goals of nursing intervention in providing a wide range of functions are as follows:

1. To evaluate and assess patient status and initiate appropriate interventions.
2. To support the staff, allowing for ventilation and processing of feelings.
3. To initiate and facilitate the process of problem identification and problem solving.

Nursing Process

The goal of *all* nursing interventions in the delivery of psychiatric emergency care is to initiate and institute measures that provide *immediate* relief and alleviate the emotional discomfort of the identified patient and that person's significant others. The nurse in this setting is often referred to as the "front-line" person and the "first contact." This means that she is accessible and available at the time the patient and family and other referring persons arrive at the hospital. As such, nurses will find it necessary to manage many aspects of the situation at once and to perform a number of tasks within a very brief time span. They must deal with the patient's feelings and behavior, the response and reactions of family members, and the concerns of the police, and so forth. Nursing tasks may include triage of patient and family, information gathering from referral sources, decision making regarding need for restraints or need for consultation with a psychiatrist, and liaison with the medical staff. Although the nurse works in consultation and collaboration with other team members and the psychiatrist, she may be the *only* mental health provider that the patient and family will have contact with during their emergency room visit. In these situations, the psychiatric nurse assumes responsibility for all aspects of psychiatric emergency care.

The Psychiatric Evaluation

The evaluation is an essential component of psychiatric emergency care. It provides a basis from which decisions about "what to do" and "how to effectively intervene" can be made. The nurse may conduct the evaluation alone or jointly or collaboratively with another team member. The evaluation process is an active clarification and decision-making process that contains the following steps: (1) collecting, sorting, and organizing data from a variety of sources; (2) assessing immediate needs and identifying immediate problems; categorizing and prioritizing those needs and problems that are acute or immediate and those that are chronic or long-term; and (3) formulating the "anatomy of the crisis" by answering the following questions:

1. What is the emergency nature of the crisis (i.e., what are the immediate concerns of patient, family, and others?)?
2. What are the stressors (i.e., what recent events occurred in the person's life to precipitate the present emotional response?)?
3. What is the person's "usual" behavior and mode of response and interaction?
4. Why now?

The evaluation should include the following aspects of the "total person" in interacting with his "total environment," thus using a holistic framework.

Psychological and Behavioral Status (also known as mental status exam). This refers to observations about the patient's present thoughts, feelings, and actions, as well as his past psychiatric history. It includes assessment of the patient's mood, judgment, insight, thought processes and content, orientation, memory, nature and extent of body movement, and thoughts about suicide or homicide. This information is sometimes obtained from those requesting the exam because the patient may be unwilling or unable to share feelings or reveal information about himself.

Social Relationships (Family, Peer) and Work Status. Patterns, recent changes, losses in significant relationships and work or career situation are all evaluated.

Biological Status. This is perhaps one of the most crucial parts of the evaluation. It includes a complete physical examination and medical or neurological work-up if indicated by the emergency room physicians so as to "rule out" any organic causes of the presenting behavioral and personality changes. The psychiatric nurse, because of her medical expertise and knowledge, is in a key position to obtain an accurate and complete history and make clinical observations that would assist the medical staff in accurately identifying the source of the presenting emotional problem. Some indicators as to the possibility of an organic-based problem are: (1) history of abrupt personality change without an identifiable precipitant; (2) history of high level of functioning and achievement; (3) rapid and periodic fluctuations in behavior during the exam; (4) history of central nervous system trauma or disease; and (5) history of drug or alcohol abuse.

The Nature or Origin of the Crisis Request. Often the request comes from someone other than the patient. The clinician should determine (1) what the nature of the request is; (2) who is making it; (3) why now; and (4) what the expectations of patient and family are, that is, what kind of help they want and what they want you to do. Clarification of the crisis request may reveal that the behavior observed was either misunderstood or inappropriate to a specific situation; it may be a request to remove an unwanted, difficult-to-care-for family member; it may be a request for support and collaboration by another agency or provider who has been involved in treating the patient; or it may be a request on the part of another person to provide protection for the patient because he can no longer care for himself.

The evaluation can take place in the waiting room, corridor, medical or surgical treatment room, or interview room—just so long as it is away from the main emergency room activity. The patient may be lying on a stretcher, sitting in a chair, or pacing the floor. The interview can last anywhere from a few minutes to several hours and can involve a lot of interaction or very little verbal communication. This will depend on the patient's and family's ability and willingness to verbalize their feelings and concerns, to respond to questions, and to tolerate contact and stimulation. For example, an extremely agitated, excited, threatening, paranoid patient or an intoxicated patient who is thrashing about and ex-

pressing suicidal feelings would be a poor candidate for a lengthy evaluation. Such a patient would need to be medicated to relieve the acute symptoms and then observed for several hours before an evaluation could take place.

Types of Therapeutic Nursing Interventions

Psychotherapeutic Interventions. Psychotherapeutic interventions include a variety of activities involving verbal communication techniques.

First, the psychiatric nurse should offer validation and recognition of the patient's positive qualities as well as acknowledging the feelings and behaviors he is exhibiting at present, thereby assisting him to make use of his residual emotional strengths and internal resources. The nurse should be aware that the patient may be unable to do this for himself, and by doing it for him, she is helping the patient to feel less overwhelmed, hopeless, and despairing. For example, she can say, "I can see that you are feeling scared and feeling as if you are unable to do anything to help yourself feel better; but you were able to see that you needed help right now with your problems and you came here to get it."

Second, the nurse should encourage ventilation and exploration of feelings and thoughts so as to assist the patient and his family in developing an understanding of what the problem is. This will help alleviate some of the emotional discomfort for both the patient and his family.

CASE EXAMPLE

A 32-year-old man was brought to the emergency room by ambulance. He had been present at the scene of a robbery and shoot-out and had barely missed being hit by a bullet as he was in the process of towing a car from the street. On arrival at the emergency room, he was extremely anxious and frightened, tearful, felt weak and faint, exhibited shortness of breath, was experiencing heart palpitations, was unable to talk, and afterwards expressed confusion as to why he had gotten so upset. His request was to rest in a safe place. He said he would be fine and for someone to call his girl friend and tell her to come and get him. After the nurse sat with him for a while, giving him coffee and cigarettes, he began to talk about his near-death experiences in battle in Viet Nam, his guilt and fears about killing and being killed, how he hadn't thought about it for a long time and just wanted to forget it and put it out of his mind; but hearing those gunshots and being that close to the robbery had brought back unusual flashbacks for him. He talked for a long time and cried; his somatic symptoms disappeared; and he left the emergency room with his girl friend several hours later.

The following techniques are helpful in encouraging ventilation and exploration:

1. Listen attentively so that the patient knows he is being heard.
2. Reflect back feelings; restate the affective quality and emotional meaning rather than asking questions related to content. For example, the nurse can say, "It sounds as if you are feeling pretty angry right now. Can you tell me what that means for you or what that feels like?" rather than saying, "Why do you think you are feeling angry?" "When did you start feeling angry?" or "How angry do you feel?"
3. State and restate the patient's feelings when he is unable to express them. This will provide ego strength to the patient. This is a particularly effective technique with patients who are having difficulty verbalizing their feelings, e.g., severely withdrawn patients. The nurse putting into words what the normal feelings would be in a given situation can provide a tremendous sense of relief and release and thus help the patient begin ventilating.

Third, the psychiatric nurse should offer reassurance by providing brief and clear information and by answering questions honestly and directly. For example, she should introduce herself, stating who she is, what her role is, what her intentions are, and her interest in helping. She should explain emergency room procedures and protocol, what is going to happen, and the sequence of events.

Fourth, the psychiatric nurse should indicate and facilitate a problem-solving process in which she can assist the patient and family toward mobilizing and employing their internal and external resources. Whenever and wherever possible the problem-solving process should be a negotiation between patient or family and nurse or clinician, and decisions regarding treatment and care should be arrived at through mutual exploration. Thus, by exercising power and control over his own destination, the patient is able to maintain some sense of self-esteem and effectiveness.

Pharmacological Interventions. The nurse is responsible for developing a familiarity and understanding of the therapeutic use of medications in the management and treatment of psychiatric emergencies. This means dispensing medications, observing and monitoring patients' emotional and physical responses to medications (including any side effects), and recording the use and effects of the medications. The major and minor tranquilizers (haloperidol [Haldol], chlorpromazine [Thorazine], thioridazine [Mellaril], chlordiazepoxide [Librium], diazepam [Valium]) are a form of chemical restraint and as such are frequently used in emergency situations to control severe agitation, excitement, anxiety, hypomania, and assaultive and suicidal behavior. In general, the primary initial intervention for behaviors related to forms of psychosis and manic-depressive illness is pharmacological followed by psychotherapeutic; whereas the primary intervention for less severe forms of anxiety (emotional problems with somatic symptoms, situational depression, and interpersonal crisis) is psychotherapeutic with medications used as an adjunct.

Physical Interventions. Touching can be an effective nonverbal means of communicating caring and concern, reaching out and establishing a connection and providing a reality contact. This may be useful for a patient who is unable to communicate verbally and who is frightened, scared, unsure of his immediate reality, or extremely withdrawn. This intervention should be used discriminatingly and done in a nonthreatening manner. It will not be helpful for patients who are paranoid, in panic, or assaultive because it may be felt as a threat, intrusion, or violation. Assessment for restraint use is necessary for the combative patient.

Providing for Basic Needs. Providing for basic needs means giving concrete material help in the form of food, clothing, shelter, and cigarettes, as well as human contact and caring through the act of giving something and "breaking bread." This is also a nonthreatening way of establishing initial rapport and decreasing a patient's fears and resistance. It is a means of providing immediate relief for the primary concerns of that segment of the patient population who have chronic psychiatric problems and are homeless, resourceless, and lonely and who have fallen "between the cracks" in the mental health system.

Initiating Referral and Facilitating Referral Process. The nurse plays an important role in establishing contact with the referral agency, in the transfer of information, and in getting feedback as to the outcome of the referral, e.g., did the patient follow through and was the intervention helpful? Referrals generally fall into the following categories: (1) psychiatric (inpatient and outpatient); (2) residential; and (3) nonpsychiatric (medical, legal, social service, and home care).

Manner of Intervention

It should be noted that nursing interventions occur with families, friends, and couples as well as with individual patients. The manner of intervention will depend on the nature and extent of the crisis; who is involved; the patient and family's request and desire to be involved; and cultural, racial, and ethnic factors. The "identified patient's" significant others may be included in the planning of the nursing process and the follow-up care plan. A family's availability and willingness to be involved in the care and support of the patient will have a great deal of influence on the treatment plan for that patient (for example, home care for outpatient treatment versus hospital care for inpatient treatment).

In order to enhance the therapeutic value of all nursing interventions, the psychiatric nurse should take the following steps: (1) communicate a message of caring, concern, and genuine interest so the patient feels seen and responded to as a total person in emotional pain, not simply a set of symptoms and behaviors to be dealt with and changed; (2) support and respect the patient's positive use of defense mechanisms, recognizing that he might need to use these mechanisms as a form of protection and a means of coping with his state of increased vulnerability and pain; and (3) be aware of her own expectations, assumptions, biases, limitations, and feelings in a given situation and with a given patient (anger, fear, rejection, disgust) and how these personal factors might be interfering with her ability to be "therapeutic." In some instances, the nurse may want to ask for help, remove herself from the situation, and review the case with a supervisor.

Legal Aspects of Mental Health Emergencies

There are legal aspects of psychiatric–mental health nursing that pertain to "psychiatric emer-gency" situations. The psychiatric nurse as the front-line, first-contact provider is often involved in (1) providing care and treatment to a patient against his will and without compliance (i.e., using medications after restraints); or (2) making a decision to hold someone in the emergency room for evaluation who wants to leave. The following situation is typical and will illustrate this point:

CASE EXAMPLE

A family called the police because the father suddenly went crazy, screaming and threatening to kill anyone if they came near him; he put his fist through the mirror and threw kitchen chairs against the wall. The patient arrived in the emergency room handcuffed and escorted by the police and his family. He was calm, cooperative, responding appropriately to questions, knew what had happened and what he had done, and stated he had gotten upset and lost his temper, that he was sorry, he was fine now, and sure it wouldn't happen again. His request was to have the handcuffs removed and to leave. This patient got increasingly agitated when told he had to remain in the hospital for an evaluation, and it was necessary to restrain him and hold him against his will until the evaluation could be completed.

As in this case, if the nurse establishes there is sufficient reason to be concerned about the patient being dangerous to himself or others based on historical information and prior behavior, she has the legal authority to temporarily hold the patient for evaluation. However, the nurse should obtain the psychiatrist's consultation and authorization as soon as possible. The nurse in this situation has the dual responsibility of maintaining the physical safety and protection of the patient and members of society, as well as respecting and protecting the patient's civil liberties.

In order for a nurse to preserve high standards of professional quality care and at the same time protect herself by operating within legal boundaries, she should:

1. Be familiar with what her liabilities and responsibilities are (e.g., use of restraints or medications; evaluating suicidal or homicidal behavior; initiating and providing treatments).
2. Understand the mental health laws in her state and their implications for nursing in this setting, i.e., standards for care; criteria

for commitment; confidentiality and when it can be waived. (Confidentiality can usually be waived when a crime has been committed or the intent to commit a crime has been established, or in cases of child abuse, etc.)

3. Be aware of and follow hospital policies and protocols.

4. Distinguish between legal matters and mental health matters. The nurse in this setting is often called upon by the police and medical personnel to make a legal determination. The clinician must always bear in mind that as a psychiatric nurse in the emergency room, she is a representative of the mental health care system and therefore assumes the responsibility for treating and caring for "patients." The nurse has authority in clinical matters only, which includes assessing the patient's emotional state and making recommendations for treatment. The clinician is not there to decide whether or not someone is a criminal and should be arrested. Likewise, mental competency is a legal issue and must be dealt with through the legal system.

5. Enlist immediate consultation and support from physicians and psychiatrists in cases where care is given without the consent of the patient.

6. Keep accurate and complete records documenting physicians' orders—what was done, what time, and why (restraints). Records should include direct quotes and statements from the patient as well as a description of the patient's behavior (rather than interpretation and labeling).

THE RURAL COMMUNITY MENTAL HEALTH NURSE

In the last three decades, the role dimensions of the psychiatric nurse have greatly expanded.* As a result of the mental health legislation of the early 1960s, the scope of psychiatric nursing has changed considerably. The psychiatric nurse has been challenged to create and implement new patterns of care for persons with psychological and emotional problems, as well as to

---

* This section through page 550 is written by Melva Jo Hendrix.

become actively involved in the prevention of mental illness. The work environment has expanded from the confines of institutions to the often diffuse boundaries of the community. As the role and the environment of the psychiatric nurse have changed, so has the title of the nursing care giver. Over the decades, the titles referring to nurses working in the psychiatric-mental health settings have ranged from *psychiatric nurse* to *community psychiatric nurse*, to *psychiatric–mental health nurse*, and finally to *community mental health nurse*.[23] The responsibilities have changed and broadened from a role of patient supervision on hospital wards to a multifaceted role in the community, with a major emphasis on populations at risk.

The community mental health ideology is based on the premise that locating mental health centers within the community will make services more accessible, thus enhancing the quality of care provided and promoting use of services. In addition, it was believed that community facilities would mitigate the stigma attached to mental illness, and clients would be able to maintain contact with their families. Finally, a portion of the responsibility for treatment and prevention of emotional problems would be given to the community.

Certain demographic, geographic, and cultural characteristics of rural areas make implementation of this model more difficult than in their nonrural counterparts. Rural populations differ from urban populations in many ways. Average income, employment rate, and health status are all lower for rural populations. Despite the high level of need, the ability to ameliorate mental health problems in rural areas has been limited. In rural areas there exists a greater likelihood of inadequate services, housing, and transportation, *and* an inadequate tax base. The geographic and topographic character of rural areas creates additional barriers. Inadequate roads, long and often tortuous distances that must be traveled by both those seeking help and those who provide it, and the psychological barriers of people living in relative isolation make the delivery of mental health care difficult if not impossible at times.

Added to these difficulties is the fact that certain cultural values generally more prevalent in rural areas further influence acceptance of mental health services. In a study reported by the National Institute of Mental Health, rural residents, when compared to the population as a whole, were found to be more conservative, religious, puritanical, work-oriented, asthetic, ethnocentric, isolationist, authoritarian, and family-centered.[24] Given these characteristics, it is apparent that the role of the community mental health nurse in rural areas is one of significant challenge and diversity.

Rural Community Mental Health Nursing Defined

The rural community mental health nurse must necessarily be a generalist. She must possess a variety of skills and be willing to practice in diverse settings. Flexibility, imagination, and innovation are needed in order to make optimal use of existing resources. Above all, the rural community mental health nurse must be willing and able to assume several areas of responsibility, each of which is equally demanding. The role of the community mental health nurse can be delineated in the following ways: clinician, consultant and liaison, educator, and change agent. Although functions within these roles are similar, and in fact often overlap, each role is significant in its own right and worthy of further exploration.

The Nurse as Clinician

The primary role of the community mental health nurse, as with most nurses, is that of clinician. Clinical expertise is necessary not only for effective performance of all other roles but also for establishing credibility as a knowledgeable professional in the community as well as within the health care team. As a clinician, the rural community mental health nurse must be knowledgeable in a number of areas such as human ecology, the developmental life cycle, social systems change theories, and crisis intervention.

Within the rural community mental health setting, the nurse is often involved in a variety of clinical activities. Most frequently the nurse acts as the team's dispenser and monitor of medication, which is central to the management of many chronic psychiatric patients. Other activities might include: making home visits, conducting medication groups, or supervising day-care programs. In recent years, an increasing number of mental health nurses have assumed the role of primary therapist with a regular caseload of clients. In rural community mental health centers, involvement in counseling and therapy currently constitutes a major portion of the nurse's total responsibility. The nurse is likely to be involved in the screening and evaluation of clients, as well as in providing counseling services to individuals, groups, and families.

In many rural communities, some forms of counseling may be difficult or impossible to conduct because of the familiarity people have with each other's lives and families. For example, it would be unlikely that group therapy could be used effectively since many people fear that personal disclosures would not be kept confidential. The speed and relative ease with which information travels in rural areas creates further difficulties when the problem of confidentiality is compounded by that of community and family disapproval. Family therapy and often individual therapy with a woman or a child are difficult in rural areas where husbands and fathers, who are the major decision-makers, may disapprove of their families' participation in therapy. Disapproval is not necessarily directed at the mode of therapy or the therapist, but there is a stigma attached to the very act of seeking help. Perhaps nowhere else is the belief that one should deal with one's own problems as prevalent as in small rural communities. Consequently, the individual who does seek professional help for emotional problems risks being viewed as "weak," or worse, being labeled as "crazy."

Although it may be very frustrating and often difficult to contend with rural values, prevailing practices and beliefs must be respected if the community mental health nurse is to develop and maintain the trust of the community. Generally accepted goals of therapy must often be modified when working within the rural setting; for example, the goal of therapy for an abused wife might simply be to help her understand that being beaten by her husband is not a normal part of married life and that it is appropriate to be angry. Furthermore, since many rural women are totally dependent on their husband for financial security, it might be difficult to encourage them to be autonomous because they have few acceptable financial alternatives available to them.[25]

Rural values also influence the efficacy of long-term reconstructive therapy. A basic orientation to the here-and-now makes the rural resident less interested in realizing his potential than in gaining relief from specific problems. Recognizing these factors, the community mental health nurse must make use of innovative and creative approaches to assist the client in realizing specific therapeutic goals.

The Nurse as Consultant and Liaison

The nurse's role in community mental health is not restricted to clinical therapeutic activities. The shortage of mental health professionals in rural areas has added impetus to the movement of community mental health nurses toward more diversified roles. One important role that mental health nurses in rural areas have begun to assume is that of consultant. Mental health consultation can be defined as a communication process between a mental health professional and an independent person, group, or institution (consultee), designed ultimately to benefit clients of the consultee.[26]

Nurses are the members of the mental health team most suited to serve as consultants in rural areas. Nurses are associated with physical health and illness, and they tend to be viewed by the public as "helping professionals." In general, they are more readily accepted in rural communities than are social workers, psychologists, and psychiatrists. This acceptance, plus a broad physiological and pharmacological knowledge base, affords the community mental health nurse a unique opportunity to collaborate with a variety of individuals and agencies. Through consultation with the health and human service agencies, the schools, and the courts, much indirect service can be provided to the community. Examples of mental health consultation common in rural areas include working with local teachers who wish to develop drug-prevention programs in the schools, or collaborating with community hospitals and nursing homes to assist personnel in recognizing and dealing more effectively with patients who have emotional problems. Perhaps the most direct form of consultation provided by the community mental health nurse consists of answering questions and educating team members about medications and other aspects of the client's health care.

Closely related to but different from the role of consultant are the functions of the nurse as liaison. For reasons discussed earlier, the rural resident is unlikely initially to seek help from the identified mental health agency in the community. Studies have shown that 50 percent of rural residents with emotional problems never seek treatment. Those who do most often turn to the community primary care physician, fam-

ily members, or minister for assistance.[27] Understanding this practice, the community mental health nurse can play an important part in establishing linkages between key agencies or individuals and the community mental health center.

Developing a system of coordination within the rural community requires significant skill and political strategy. The first step necessary in establishing these links is gaining the trust of the people. In rural communities, personal trust supersedes issues of competence. A person is seen as a useful professional only if she is seen as a trustworthy individual.[28] To facilitate the development of trust, it is beneficial to begin contact with local professionals on a specific and problem-solving basis; help must be offered to the courts, schools, and other agencies on their long-standing and recognized problems. When convinced of the concrete service potential of mental health professionals, rural leaders will usually respond with cooperation.[29]

As liaison, the mental health nurse must also endeavor to establish working relationships with the native healers in the community. "Native healers" include informal counselors such as folk doctors and lay midwives. These individuals know the community and often have valuable insights and influence. Rather than attempting to supplant these natural healers, the community mental health nurse must work cooperatively with them through consultation, education, and planning.[30]

The community mental health nurse who serves in the capacity of the consultant or liaison must necessarily be patient, reliable, and nonjudgmental in order to inspire trust and confidence. Nevertheless, once a communication network has been established, the nurse can begin to educate individuals and the community to accept as well as make use of the available mental health services.

The Nurse as Educator

The American Nurses' Association *Standards of Psychiatric–Mental Health Nursing Practice* states that psychiatric–mental health nursing is directed toward "both preventive and corrective impacts upon mental illness and is concerned with the promotion of optimal mental health for society, the community, and those individuals and families who live within it."[31]

In keeping with this definition, the community mental health nurse must necessarily focus on prevention within the community, which begins by identifying high-risk populations and then providing educative or therapeutic services *before* psychological function is seriously impaired. Focusing on the community as client does not imply neglecting particular needs of individual members. Rather, a community focus demands a broader approach that acknowledges both those individuals currently seeking mental health intervention and those who may eventually need intervention if certain deleterious circumstances continue.

As educator, the rural community mental health nurse faces significant challenges. First, she must be prepared to "sell" the concept of mental health to the community because of the fear and stigma attached to mental illness. Second, the educational process itself is directed toward a change in behavior, and generally speaking, it is change of any kind that rural individuals find difficult to accept or believe possible. Acknowledging and accepting these challenges, the rural community mental health nurse can look forward to a role that encompasses a broad array of educational endeavors. Opportunities range from teaching individuals or families in the clinic or home, to the organization of a health fair within the local school or community.

At the individual level, the community mental health nurse might teach patients to recognize the signs and symptoms of their particular problem and the side effects of the medication prescribed to treat that problem. Teaching in the area of physical health is also important in rural areas since many of the individuals who visit mental health centers have had little or no prior health instruction. Nurses are educated to assess the health and nutritional status of individuals, to detect abnormalities, and to provide health teaching to all their patients. In fact patient teaching is mandated by many state nurse practice acts.

In addition to teaching individual patients, the rural community mental health nurse must often provide instruction to the other members of the mental health team. In casual collaboration, as well as during formal work, the nurse acts as a valuable source of general health information. Nurses are more likely to view patients holistically; therefore, it is often she who identifies or further explores areas of somatic complaint not previously noted by the other team members.

At the community level, the mental health nurse might plan and implement programs for high-risk groups such as teen-age mothers or victims of rape. She also provides programs aimed at educating other non-mental-health professionals in the community, such as police officers, who are in daily contact with groups considered to be at risk. For example, scarcity of resources in rural areas often results in less than desirable placement for many persons, particularly the chronically mentally ill. These individuals are frequently arrested and jailed because of the shortage of facilities and a lack of understanding on the part of the police. The rural nurse can plan programs to instruct local law enforcement officials in the early recognition and appropriate referral of persons with emotional problems.

The Nurse as a Change Agent

Effecting behavioral change is the underlying goal of all psychiatric–mental health nursing practice. Thus, acting as a change agent is one of the most important and all-encompassing roles of the nurse in rural communities. Activity within this role runs the gamut from assisting individual patients to change through the provision of supportive therapies, to the formation of coalitions to affect health care legislation. In addition to skills necessary to function in the roles of clinician, consultant and liaison, and educator, the rural community mental health nurse must have a capacity for understanding human behavior and possess keen problem-solving abilities in order to accurately assess specific problem areas and then effect changes in these areas.

The target for change in rural areas may be an individual, a couple, a family, or other groups with potential or identified problems. Any subsystem of the community that impinges on the mental health of an individual, couple, family, or group might also be a target for change. For example, when working with an adolescent demonstrating self-destructive "acting out" behaviors, the target for change might be the client's school, peer group, or the family system within which he lives. Also targeted for change might be the mental health agency or other service agency, the political hierarchy of the community, or state and national legislative bodies that plan health policy.

Although the rural community mental health nurse does not always possess a great deal of formal power within the organizational structure, as one of a few health professionals in the area where she works, the nurse has a unique opportunity to influence the system favorably in regard to the promotion of health and mental health services. Participating in community organizations such as school boards, ad hoc task forces, and planning committees provides a direct means of input at the community level. Perhaps nowhere as much as in rural areas can the nurse participate in and influence community decision making.

In addition to participating in change at the community level, it is important that the nurse become involved in the larger political arena. Most state agencies have task forces composed of a variety of care givers and community leaders that address particular needs. These task forces can be influential in the development and passage or defeat of legislation affecting specific populations. Nurses who participate in groups such as these can serve as strong advocates for community services as well as gaining experience in the political process.

Summary

This chapter discussed liaison psychiatric nursing services within the hospital setting to help nurses integrate psychiatric–mental health concepts into nursing care. The theoretical framework for liaison nursing is based on general systems theory. The clinical situation often determines which patients are to be referred to the liaison nurse; they are identified as the newly admitted patient, the patient with undiagnosed illness, the preoperative patient, the patient in pain, the pediatric patient, the seriously ill patient, and the patient in intensive care. Some management aspects of patient care are included, although not all hospitals have liaison services.

The second part of the chapter describes the outpatient setting of the emergency department of a general hospital where many patients are taken for emergency crisis care. The issues of the consumers of psychiatric emergency care, the providers of care, the role of the psychiatric nurse in an emergency setting, a typology of behaviors, the nursing interventions, and the legal aspects of mental health emergencies are described.

The problems faced by the rural community mental health nurse who seeks to help, to educate, and to change are frequently compounded by geographic, economic, and cultural factors over which she has little or no control. Facilities are often inadequate, and community members may initially be skeptical, fearful, and resistant to the services offered by the nurse. Yet, nowhere is the knowledge of skill or the community mental health nurse so needed as in the rural areas.

Although there are numerous limitations and frustrations inherent in rural community mental health practice, there are also important rewards. Autonomy and independence as well as increased responsibility and latitude are advantages of rural community practice commonly acknowledged by nurses. Furthermore, being one of a few professionals in the rural community offers the possibility of gaining substantial influence. Opportunities for creative planning and implementation of programs are also significant. Because of the small number of health and human service agencies, a holistic approach and continuity of care are often facilitated. Also, the size and stability of the rural community allow clients to be followed long after they leave treatment. In short, the nurse who chooses rural community mental health nursing can largely define her role to suit the needs of the particular community as well as her own professional interests.

Questions

1. Why has liaison nursing become an important component of nursing care in general hospital settings?

2. How does the process of liaison nursing differ from the process of general nursing?
3. Talk with a seriously ill patient and report on his feelings about the illness.
4. Identify one additional mental health concept that can be part of liaison nursing but is not so identified in the text.
5. Identify several situations in which you would ask for the assistance of a liaison nurse.
6. What differences are there in the types of care given in a community mental health clinic?
7. How would you deal with an assaultive and combative patient?
8. What are three key skills in working with psychiatric emergencies?
9. What are the legal aspects of psychiatric emergency care?
10. How are the mental health needs of people living in rural areas in your state being met?
11. What clinical and educational background do you believe essential for practicing rural mental health nursing?
12. Talk with a patient who lives in a rural area and inquire about the type and nature of the health services provided.

REFERENCES AND SUGGESTED READINGS

1. Strain, J. J. Liaison psychiatry: Treating psychological reactions of the mentally ill. *Medical World News Review*, 1974, 1(2), 42.
2. Pasnau, R. O. Consultation-liaison psychiatry at the crossroads: In search of a definition for the 1980s. *Hospital and Community Psychiatry*, 1982, 33, 989.
3. Strain, op. cit.
4. Ibid.
5. Robinson, L. *Psychiatric Nursing as a Human Experience*, 3rd ed. Philadelphia: Saunders, 1983.
6. Strain, op. cit., pp. 42–43.
7. Stevenson, J. L. *Issues and Crisis During Middlescence*. New York: Appleton-Century-Crofts, 1977.
8. Ibid.
9. Samter, J., Scherer, M. F., & Shulman, D. Interface of psychiatric clinical specialists in a community hospital setting. *Journal of Psychiatric Nursing*, 1981, 19, 28.
10. Vickers, G. Is adaptability enough? *Behavioral Science* 1959, 4, 219.
11. Strain, op. cit., p. 43.
12. Wu, R. *Behavioral Illness*. Englewood Cliffs, N.J.: Prentice-Hall, 1973.
13. Jones, P. Psychiatric liaison nurse for neurosurgery: An innovative approach to management of chronic pain. *Journal of Neurosurgical Nursing*, 1978, 10(4), 164.
14. Lipowski, Z. J. Liaison psychiatry, liaison nursing, and behavioral medicine. *Comprehensive Psychiatry*, 1981, 22, 556.
15. Robinson, L. *Liaison Nursing: Psychological Approach to Patient Care*. Philadelphia: Davis, 1974.
16. Johnson, J. E., et al. Sensory information, instruction in a coping strategy, and recovery from surgery. *Research in Nursing and Health*, 1978, 1(1), 4–17.
17. Robinson, op. cit. (1974), p. 117.
18. Copp, L. A. The spectrum of suffering. *American Journal of Nursing*, 1974, 74, 492–493.
19. Robinson, op. cit. (1974), p. 117.
20. Ibid., p. 178.
21. Talbott, J., & Monroe, R. The organization of psychiatric services. In R. A. Glick (Ed.), *Psychiatric Emergencies*. New York: Grune & Stratton, 1976, pp. 261–262.
22. Ibid., pp. 265–266.
23. Lancaster, J. *Community Mental Health Nursing: An Ecological Perspective*. St. Louis: Mosby, 1980, p. 7.
24. Flax, J. W., et al. *Mental Health and Rural America: An Overview and Annotated Bibliography* (National Institute of Mental Health, DHEW Publication No. ADM 78-753). Washington, D.C.: U.S. Government Printing Office, 1979, p. 10.
25. LaGodna, G. E. The single rural woman: Invisible struggles. *Advances in Nursing Service*, 1981, 3(2), 17–23.
26. McClung, F. B., & Strunden, A. A. *Mental Health Consultation to Programs for Children: A Review of Data Collected from Selected U.S. Sites* (National Institute of Mental Health, DHEW Publication No. HSM 72-9088). Washington, D.C.: U.S. Government Printing Office, 1972.
27. Berry, B., & Davis, A. E. Community mental health ideology: A problematic model for rural areas. *American Journal of Orthopsychiatry*, 1978, 48, 673–674.

28. Jeffrey, M. J., & Reeve, R. E. Community mental health service in rural areas: Some practical issues. *Community Mental Health Journal*, 1978, *14*, 59–62.
29. Berry & Davis, op. cit., p. 678.
30. Leininger, M. Some anthropological issues related to community mental health problems in the U.S. *Community Mental Health Journal*, 1971, *7*, 234–241.
31. American Nurses' Association. *Standards of Psychiatric-Mental Health Nursing Practice*. Kansas City, Mo.: American Nurses' Association, 1973.

Chapter 29

Psychological Testing and Psychological Assessment

Selina Kassels

Chapter Objectives

The student successfully attaining the goals of this chapter will be able to:

- Define the psychometric tradition of measuring behaviors that are standardized and objective.
- Define quantitative and qualitative types of analysis.
- Identify the diagnostic role of the clinical psychologist on the mental health team.
- Understand and use psychological test reports included in the record of the patient.

The psychological testing process includes assessment and measurement. This chapter is designed to help students better understand the process so they can become discriminating in the use of such services and comfortable in collaborating with the psychologist for referral and treatment planning.

Communication is the heart of any effective consultation. Thus an important goal of this chapter is to facilitate the healthy interchange and communication between psychiatric nurses when they are referring patients for testing or when they are reviewing the results of testing. The presentation here is designed so that nurses can learn what kinds of questions psychological testing can address and how to use the reports.

THE SCIENTIFIC AND CLINICAL RATIONALE OF PSYCHOLOGICAL TESTING

Psychological testing is frequently imbued with a mystique. Such mystique leads to an initial overvaluing and subsequent devaluing of psychological tests.[1] Realistically, a skilled psychologist often elicits additional information beyond that obtained from clinical interviewing. Psychologists qualified to administer tests are those who have had specialized training in the administration and interpretation of psychological tests. Typically, they hold a Ph.D. in clinical or counseling psychology or a Psy.D. degree and are licensed as psychologists in the state where they practice.

When psychological tests were first widely introduced in psychiatric clinics and hospitals after World War II, the role of the psychologist was largely that of a diagnostician. Today psychologists serve multiple roles on both the mental and medical health care teams. They fill roles of psychotherapists, administrators, consultants, and researchers. But the use of psychological tests and assessment tools remains a distinctive domain of psychologists and differentiates the role they play of making specialized contributions in diagnosis.

Specialized contributions of psychologists result from scientific and clinical rationale, underlying test construction and from the knowledge base that the psychologist applies in interpreting the test results. The rationale for psychological testing rests upon: (1) the psychometric tradition that enables psychologists to devise standardized approaches to measuring human behavior; (2) the projective hypothesis that provides a rationale for understanding and interpreting individual differences on *unstructured* tasks; and (3) the hypothesis-testing model that guides the psychologist in collecting and interpreting test data on a given patient.

Cronbach has described the two traditions (psychometric testing and projective techniques) that have influenced the development and use of psychological tests. A psychological test is defined by Cronbach as a systematic procedure for comparing the behavior of two or more persons. Tests may measure by assigning scores to aspects of an individual's functioning or yield verbal descriptions of behavior. The term "assessment" is frequently used to describe the process of using a whole battery or assortment of techniques to understand the personality of a given individual and to distinguish such a comprehensive evaluation from the process of psychometric measurement.[2]

The Psychometric Tradition

The psychometric approach to testing is based on the ideal of science that strives to measure physical reality and to describe objects by numbers. This tradition assumes that all people possess the same traits, but in different amounts, and it strives for accurate comparison of different individuals on a dimension of personality or intellectual functioning. The psychometric tradition encouraged the development of procedures for measuring behavior that are standardized and objective. According to Cronbach, a standardized test is one in which procedure, apparatus, and scoring have been fixed so that precisely the same test can be given at different times and places.[3] A test is objective when every observer assigns the same score to an individual's performance. In order to develop measuring tools, it is necessary to create the standard units of measurement against which all individuals are compared. Standards are created by collecting norms, that is, large samples of behavior that can become the standard against which the future assessment of individuals is compared.

Self-report personality questionnaires are a commonly used example of standardized, objective psychometric instruments. They may take the form of questionnaires, inventories, or adjective checklists presented either in paper-and-pencil format or in a computerized format. Questionnaires and inventories can be used to assess one or more related personality traits, such as anxiety or depression, or to assess an aspect of psychological functioning, such as attitudes toward authority, assertiveness, sexual activity, marital problems, etc. A questionnaire cannot become an instrument that is used in comparing individuals until it has been demonstrated to be both reliable and valid. Reliability and validity are the two concepts that describe how accurate tests are as measuring instruments. A test is reliable to the extent that it always measures the same thing; it is valid to the extent that it measures what it purports to measure. Establishing the reliability and validity of psychometric instruments is a complex, technical issue—one that is critical to developing a sophisticated technology for measuring individual differences and to interpreting test scores.[4]

The Projective Hypothesis

The approach to personality assessment that Cronbach calls "impressionistic interpretation" relies more on projective techniques than objective tests.[5] In contrast to objective tests, "projective" procedures are those that present the subject with relatively unstructured stimuli or undefined tasks. Projective instruments are usually called techniques, rather than tests, because they are not designed as precise measuring tools but as procedures that permit the examiner to make observations and inferences about the subject. When a psychologist uses projective techniques in personality assessment, he is attempting to gather comprehensive impressions and to sample a wide range of personality processes that can yield a verbal description of personality functioning. The projective techniques are used to address the question of what personality structure or organizational principles can explain or predict the subject's behavior.

An underlying assumption called the "projective hypothesis" provides the rationale for the use of projective procedures and for their unique contribution to personality assessment.[6] It is assumed that the relative lack of structure and ambiguity of projective procedures allows the individual room to "project" aspects of his underlying personality structure (needs, wishes, feelings, and motivations) in the way in which he organizes, responds to, and deals with the test materials. It is also assumed that ambiguous and unstructured situations are those most likely to arouse emotion in individuals, so that projective techniques are the methods most useful for eliciting samples of individual's functioning when emotionally aroused. Thus the projective procedures afford data on the unique aspects of an individual's personality and contribute to an understanding of how he might function when he is emotionally involved.

Originally, projective techniques were thought to tap primarily the unconscious motivational structure of the individual and that the unconscious motivations were the major determinants of how an individual perceives his world and reacts to situations. Bellak clarified the concept of "projection" as it is used in personality assessment and distinguished this concept from the concept of projection as a defense mechanism.[7,8] The phenomena tapped in a projective procedure are the subjective distortions in perceptions of the external world that are introduced by a person's needs, wishes, and feelings, be they conscious or unconscious, acceptable or unacceptable to the ego. Only hypothetically can there be purely objective perception of the world, especially of interpersonal relationships. Almost everything individuals experience or perceive is thus a reflection of their personality and is organized by their subjective wishes.

The two separate traditions of psychological testing result in many internal controversies regarding the establishment of reliability and validity of projective and psychometric techniques, and they raise the question whether concepts of validity and reliability apply to the procedures or to the interpretations of test findings. It is generally concluded that projective techniques are evaluated in terms of their utility and that their usefulness is highly related to the skill of the examiner using them.[9]

Hypothesis-Testing Model of Test Interpretation

The two traditions of psychological testing are synthesized by clinical psychologists trained as both scientists and practitioners. Science and intuition are blended as the psychologist gathers data during administration of tests and as the test findings are interpreted. The test battery is often viewed as an opportunity to sample psychological functioning under different stimulus conditions, ranging from structured intelligence tests to unstructured projective tasks.[10] The assessment situation is conceived of as an experiment in which data are collected and hypotheses are tested to determine which best explains the data and answers the referral questions.[11] The processes of test interpretation are described as combining logical analysis and intuition to form inferences about the data. All information is tested and checked against all available data. This view of interpretation is further elaborated in the section on analysis and interpretation of test data later in this chapter.

PSYCHOLOGICAL ASSESSMENT: THE PROCESS FROM BEGINNING TO END

Part of the mystique of testing stems from the lack of opportunities for nursing staff, or other mental health professionals, to actually observe a patient being tested. In order to preserve conditions that standardize test administration and maintain validity, the tests are individually administered and rarely can be observed, even through a one-way mirror. There are also strict ethical limitations officially adopted by the American Psychological Association restricting the sale and distribution of test materials since the validity of testing would be compromised by any extensive dissemination of the materials.

Much of the sense of mystery in test administration vanishes when it is recognized that testing is very similar to an interview situation, except that the situation is more structured. During a clinical interview, the clinician frequently uses open-ended questioning and varies the questions or stimuli to develop whatever emerges as important content in the patient's associations. The essential contribution of testing is that it presents each patient with the same tasks and stimuli so that responses given by all the patients can be systematically compared. The examiner is also expected to be warm but relatively neutral and nonresponsive so as to have relatively minor effects on actual test conditions. Since examiners do vary in their personalities and professional images, such neutrality is difficult to achieve in practice, and examiners are at least expected to recognize the degree to which their functioning influences the results they obtain from patients.

Clarifying the Referral

In describing the process of testing, it should be noted that the assessment process begins before the psychologist initially meets with the patient. Communication with referring clinicians is essential. Besides talking with clinicians, the psychologist may review the patient's chart. Psychologists rarely test "blind" without any prior information about the patient, although such procedures were common when psychodiagnostic testing was first establishing its reputation as an independent profession. However, such procedures are no longer necessary to establish the worth of testing; also such procedures do not enable the psychologist to develop a comprehensive assessment using all the available data that can enhance treatment planning and increase the understanding of the patient.

Preparing the Patient for Testing

Before meeting the psychologist, the patient is likely to request an explanation for the referral and the purpose of testing. Communication is essential so that the referring clinician sufficiently prepares the patient for testing and facilitates cooperation but does not inadvertently arouse the patient's anxiety about the procedure. Simple explanations are likely to be most effective. It may be explained to patients that the purpose of testing is to assist the clinician in understanding their mental health problems. During the testing they can expect that the psychologist will talk with them about their problems and their past history and will administer different kinds of tests. Some of the tests may include simple arithmetic problems, defining

words, etc., but many will be tasks that are probably unfamiliar. The psychologist will be able to explain the tests further and can answer specific questions. Most patients are relatively familiar with psychological testing because of media presentations; few are surprised to learn that their test battery includes some projective tests. If patients do press for information about the "unfamiliar tasks," they could be told the testing might include tasks in which they will be asked to use their imaginations. Providing more specific information may only generate increased anxiety.

In requesting information from the nurse about testing, patients are implicitly asking for help in managing the anxiety surrounding being evaluated. If encouraged to verbalize anxiety, a common concern is, "What if I don't know any of the answers? It will show I'm a dummy." Such a patient may need reassurance. The patient may be told that no one is expected to know all the answers, and it is important just to share his thinking with the psychologist. Worrying about being perfect, or knowing all the answers, may be a concern that the patient sustains in everyday life, and if anxiety persists after this brief reassurance about the tests, he should be encouraged to talk only about the issues of perfectionism, not about the testing.

Another common concern expressed by patients is the fear that the testing will show "I'm nuts." To explore such anxiety supportively with the patient, the nurse might ask the patient to explain further what "being nuts" means. It is helpful to restate such concerns in terms of possible feelings of being confused, of having difficulty in distinguishing between what is real versus unreal, or other issues that are reflected in the patient's explanation of his anxiety. Depending on the specific functioning of the patient, nurses can then manage such situations as they would if these feelings emerged in a clinical interview. For example, it would be helpful for many disturbed patients to accept that their thoughts are confused, that confused thinking could be part of the problems that brought them to the hospital, and that the tests would be another way in which the staff is trying to understand their problems. Patients should be encouraged to feel comfortable in expressing all their thoughts and concerns to the psychologist, emphasizing that the psychologist is best able to answer their questions about the tests and that sharing what is on their minds is the way in which they can best cooperate with their treatment, even if their thoughts seem unusual.

Administering the Test Battery

Establishing good rapport with a patient is essential to the process of psychological testing, as it is to any clinical interviewing. Therefore, upon first meeting the patient, the psychologist will essentially proceed as any clinician would to ensure that the patient feels comfortable in the test room and views the psychologist as a member of the team who is contributing to the overall treatment plan. Typically, the psychologist will briefly orient the patient to the purpose of the tests, estimate how long the process will take, establish any special needs the patient has for hearing or vision, or medical limitations.

As mentioned, administering a full test battery is a lengthy procedure (3 to 5 hours), so that more than one session may be scheduled. For example, testing may be scheduled for morning and afternoon, with a break for lunch. The goal of the psychologist will be to establish rapport that is supportive and respectful to the patient but reasonably neutral. The psychologist does not want to encourage the patient to develop any transference (either positive or negative) that could bias responses to the test.

The administration of tests has been standardized to increase the reliability and validity of the tests. The psychologist is responsible for adhering to any standardized instructions, yet he may modify administration when it is necessary to preserve rapport or to prevent the patient from becoming so stressed by the testing that it precipitates a crisis that is countertherapeutic for the patient. Thus, much clinical judgment is employed during testing, especially with severely disturbed patients.

Sometimes patients will become very upset during their testing, but such reactions should not be misconstrued as an indication that the testing was too stressful for the patient. Especially on an inpatient service, testing can often be the stimulus that evokes a catharsis that is quite beneficial in overcoming a stall in the psychotherapy. With some borderline patients, testing can precipitate a brief regression, but such a reaction essentially becomes part of the data that are needed in order to clarify a differential diagnosis and to understand the severity of the patient's psychopathology.

In summary, the nurse needs to recognize that the psychologist is making many decisions during the test administration. Any concerns the nurse may have about the patient's ability to tolerate testing, or concerns about the patient's reactions to the testing, should be communicated to the psychologist so that there can be dialogue about the patient's needs and any reaction to the testing.

Communicating Testing Results

Patients often ask if they will or can learn the "results" of their psychological tests. Even if the patient has not initiated this question, it is the role of the psychologist to inform the patient of procedures for discussing the findings either directly with the psychologist or with the referring clinician after the psychologist has communicated with the clinician. Several issues will be involved in deciding on the procedures for informing the patient of the results, including the patient's relationship to the referring clinician and the nature of recommendations that result from the psychological testing. It is the responsibility of the psychologist as a consultant to respect the patient's legal and ethical right to feedback about testing and to respect the right and responsibility of the primary therapists to communicate with the patient in a manner that enhances and preserves their relationship to the patient. Any potential conflicts in these issues can usually best be addressed when the psychologist communicates his results to the referring clinician. The nurse's role is to communicate the types of concerns and questions the patient asks about the testing and not to reveal any privileged information.

REFERRAL QUESTIONS

Psychodiagnostic assessments can be used to answer almost any question about diagnosis, treatment, or prognosis. They can be used to give an overall assessment of the patient's functioning and are occasionally used for this purpose, especially on first psychiatric admissions to teaching hospitals that have large psychological testing services augmented by psychological interns. Since psychological testing is an expensive service (consuming approximately 10 hours of a psychologist's time), the current climate of cost-effectiveness combined with increasing specialization of mental health services emphasizes the importance of using psychological assessments when they can contribute to answering questions that are not conclusively answered otherwise, even after interview information and case history data have been collected. Generally, psychological testing is most useful in answering a specific referral question, and communication between referring clinician and psychologist can often clarify the specific issues that the psychologist is being asked to address. Some of the most commonly posed referral issues are discussed below.

Assisting in Differential Diagnosis

Data from psychological testing often can be used to assist in determining a differential diagnosis and to explicate the relationship between presenting symptoms, diagnosis, and prognosis. A referral question about differential diagnosis may implicitly or explicitly ask for assistance in understanding the level and severity of a presenting symptom or complaint and in understanding the role that the complaint plays in the overall context of the patient's functioning. For example, is acute anxiety part of an anxiety syndrome or a sign of incipient psychosis?

Test data can also reveal latent psychoses that are difficult to detect clinically, for example, the emergence of an incipient psychosis in an individual with decompensating premorbid obsessive-compulsive personality disorder. Test data can be used to differentiate the level of pathology (neurotic, psychotic, etc.) and the typical personality style that is part of the more enduring personality structure. Thus test data supply information that frequently affords a diagnostic impression of the clinical syndrome recorded on Axis I of the *DSM-III-R* and of the underlying personality disorder that is recorded on Axis II (see Appendix).

Differential diagnoses are derived by noting both presence and absence of test data that are consistent with alternative diagnoses. For example, in making the differential diagnosis between schizophrenia and major affective disorder, the examiner examines test data for the degree and kind of disruption in thought processes; for the presence or absence of psychomotor retardation on performance tasks; for the presence or absence of Rorschach imagery connoting wintry, desolate, isolate, barren scenes;

for the presence or absence of several constellations of test scores; and for responses that are consistent or inconsistent with schizophrenia or mood disorders.

Assessing Suicidality or Homicidality

During clinical interviews, patients will frequently acknowledge that they are suicidal or afraid of losing control of their aggressive impulses. In requesting psychological testing, the clinician is seeking further information that the patient may not be able to reveal about the degree of risk to harming self or others. Testing seeks to clarify the intensity of suicidal thoughts and the degree to which the patient may be likely to act on such impulses. Data that can bear on such questions may include establishing whether suicidal thoughts are occurring in an acutely psychotic individual who is receiving command hallucinations. Testing can also clarify whether the suicidality is acute or chronic, and whether such thinking is exacerbated by projective test stimuli that elicit associations of loss or rejection.

Recent research has documented that psychological tests have limited validity in predicting violent behavior and that a past history of violence is the best criterion for predicting future violent behavior.[12] Thus, clinical psychologists are justifiably cautious about accepting referrals that ask for an assessment of homicidality. Although testing is not the best tool for predicting future behavior, it can contribute valuable information about understanding the intensity of aggressive impulses, the dynamic conflicts that fuel rage reactions, and the deficits in reality testing that lower judgment under stress and increase the likelihood of impulsive behavior. Testing may also be useful in uncovering the constellation of seething rage, paranoid ideation, and potential explosiveness that can be masked clinically in a very guarded, paranoid patient. Recent developments in neuropsychological testing have also expanded the potential for detecting subtle patterns of cortical dysfunction that are associated with some aggressive outbursts. Thus, neuropsychological workups, along with a developing specialty in forensic psychology, promise to expand the contribution that psychologists can make to assessing violent or criminal behavior.[13]

CASE EXAMPLE

Sally Norman was a 20-year-old college senior majoring in philosophy and literature. She was hospitalized because of increasing depression and suicidal ideation. She denied precipitants associated with recent losses and had consistently functioned well academically and socially during college. She realized that her thinking was deviant, and she stated that she was very despondent about her future, that she saw nothing to live for, and therefore believed that it was "logical" to choose to die. The psychological testing was requested to explore the intensity of her depression and suicidality, as well as to contribute to assessment of dynamics and diagnosis.

Psychological test results were useful in contraindicating any presence of major depressive episode. Sally denied many of the features associated with severe depression. For example, she denied loss of interest in people and denied feeling sad. Her performance on visual-motor tasks was accurate and efficient; her speech was fluent and spontaneous; associations and responses flowed smoothly—all indicators that ruled out either psychomotor retardation or agitation. The content of projective test responses revealed much human movement. Her verbalizations were animated, reflecting a high level of energy and vitality.

The test results clarified that Sally's depression was associated with marked feelings of hopelessness and with a punitive superego. This combination of personality variables warranted viewing the patient's suicidality with serious concern, even though she was not impulsive, psychotic, or visibly impaired in her social and academic functioning. The test results helped to focus on the issues of self-esteem and impairment in interpersonal relationships that could illuminate the patient's despair, sense of hopelessness, and despondency about her future. Sally could be understood as a young woman who had developed a "false self" designed to comply with the expectations for her to function as a model student and successful daughter and had split off genuine negative feelings associated with having dependency needs gratified or frustrated. She had reached a potential identity crisis since the demands of transition from college student to young adult were stirring up unresolved issues of separation and were confronting her with her lack of self-definition. Because of her rigid superego, Sally was prone to flagellate herself for a sense of "failing" when she compared her own pessimism about the future to the optimism of her classmates. The test results pointed to the importance of helping her to define her current life crisis and to recognize that long-term outpatient psychotherapy was indicated to help her resolve separation issues and free her from bonds of functioning out of a "false self."

It was not likely that there would be any major change in either the patient's expression of feelings of hopelessness or her tendency to blame herself for her problems during short-term hospitalization, since both stemmed from deeper characterological problems. However, intervening to help the patient develop a firm initial alliance with an outpatient psychotherapist could significantly reduce the risk of her acting on suicidal thoughts and feelings. Sally Norman needed to recognize that her alienation was taken seriously and that she was encouraged to share and express her genuine needs and feelings in a therapeutic relationship.

Assessing Ego Strengths and Weaknesses

Frequently clinicians request psychological testing in order to assess one or several aspects of a patient's ego functioning. Such requests are again implicitly or explicitly requesting information that can help the clinician determine the patient's capacity to benefit from psychotherapy. Frequently, psychologists are asked to assess the level of reality testing and the degree of impulse control. Such specific requests are very useful in focusing the referral. However, in order to answer such a specific question, the psychologist must derive an overall assessment of ego functioning from the test data by formulating a picture of the defense structure and character traits used in control of impulses and a general picture of the interplay between impulses, controls, actions, and thoughts. Psychological test data, by providing a comparison of a subject's psychological functioning on both structured and unstructured tasks and under emotionally arousing as well as neutral conditions, can yield a comprehensive picture of such aspects of ego functions as reality testing, judgment, sense of reality, autonomous and synthetic ego functioning, thought processes (memory, attention, concentration), and regulation of primary and secondary processes.

CASE EXAMPLE

Bob Evans was a 17-year-old referred for psychological evaluation two weeks after his graduation from high school. A female classmate had accused him of harrassing her, making threatening phone calls to her, and stalking her at her home because she refused to date him. Psychological testing was requested by his parents to assist in evaluating his emotional stability and judgment.

The psychological test results indicated that Bob

was not imminently psychotic but that he could distort reality temporarily when he was under stress and that he had inappropriately feared ridicule from all his classmates when he was unable to secure a date from a female classmate. Bob did show significant patterns of emotional immaturity and instability. He felt vulnerable, insecure, confused about his identity as a young man and inclined to deny and project his feelings of inadequacy. Much of his energy was directed into defending against his anxieties. In order to compensate for feelings of inadequacy, he compulsively jogged, lifted weights, bragged about episodic heavy drinking, and related in a cocky manner to young women. Despite his cocky veneer, he was excessively timid in relating to women, inhibited about expressing sexual feelings, and rigidly eschewed any violent behavior. He was not likely to present as a danger for "acting-out" violent behavior toward women.

With the test results, Bob's parents were reassured that their son was not likely to act to harm others and they would dissuade neighbors from seeking any legal action. The evaluation itself had impressed upon Bob the seriousness and inappropriateness of his recent behavior and response to rejection. However, he was unable to acknowledge that such behavior indicated a need for counseling and maintained that the female classmate was exaggerating his threats. On the basis of test results, he was encouraged to enter psychotherapy to deal with concerns about starting college and developing intimate dating relationships. However, Bob denied he needed help at that time and maintained that he could cope with his problems by avoiding hassles with girls and devoting more of his time to time-consuming athletic activities and jobs.

This case illustrates how psychological testing can highlight the defense patterns and coping mechanisms that a patient uses. Increasing compulsive defenses would possibly temporarily lower Bob Evans' anxieties—primarily by rationalizing his avoidance of heterosexual encounters—but would not address the underlying conflicts that could be predicted to resurface at a future time.

Evaluating Depression or Other Affects (Such as Anger, Anxiety)

Requests for such evaluations occur either when the clinician suspects the patient is masking such a problem or when the patient does present with manifest depression or anxiety and more information is needed about the role of these affects in the overall personality functioning. Underlying depression can often be detected in

projective test responses when patients may be consciously denying they are depressed and presenting with somatic complaints or other masked depression. When patients are presenting with anxiety disorders, testing can help clarify the intensity of the symptoms, the degree to which task functioning and cognitive functioning are affected, and the type and effectiveness of defenses and coping mechanisms used to manage the anxiety. Testing can also be useful in ferreting out evidence of a post-traumatic stress disorder. Projective test stimuli may elicit recollections of traumatic events that the patient is avoiding in daily life and may reveal a constellation of signs of the post-traumatic stress disorder (such as complaints in concentrating, diminished responsiveness, estrangement in interpersonal relationships) that otherwise present as a vague depression, which could elude treatment.

Evaluating the Effectiveness of Treatment

This problem is frequently an implicit basis for initiating a test referral. However, it is more frequently communicated explicitly when there is sufficient trust between clinician and psychologist. The purpose of this chapter is to help psychiatric nurses view such a request as a legitimate basis for a professional consultation with a psychologist and to view psychological testing as a resource that potentially can contribute additional data that may or may not lead to a revision in treatment planning. Essentially, a psychologist who receives a direct request framed around assessing the effectiveness of the patient's current treatment begins by discussing the case with the clinician. The consultation includes reviewing all existing data, administering a complete psychological test battery, and extensively discussing all results and recommendations with the referring clinician and team. In practice, this author approaches such consultations by developing a comprehensive picture of the patient's personality structure and dynamics. Then clinical experience as a psychotherapist can be applied to formulate hypotheses about transference and countertransference issues. When reviewing existing data of clinicians and discussing the case with the team, the consultation becomes focused around possible impasses that have resulted from discrepant formulations of the patient's psychological functioning.

Such a consultation process becomes possible in an inpatient milieu when the psychologist is familiar with the milieu and with the staff–patient interactions and can hypothesize about how patients may be eliciting countertransference from the unit as a whole. The referral for psychological testing can be an implicit or explicit request from the unit staff for the psychologist to serve in a consulting function and to help them see the patient more objectively. An example of a case illustrating the use of such psychological test consultation to an inpatient staff follows.

CASE EXAMPLE

Jim, a 15-year-old, exceptionally bright adolescent, was admitted following a suicide attempt and after running away from home because of quarrels with his parents. He presented continual management problems on the ward because he demanded explanations for every rule, found loopholes in ward policies, defied staff, and was rallying other patients to engage in rebellious behavior. The staff increasingly viewed him as a manipulative adolescent and became split about how many privileges to give him, whether he needed tighter or looser controls, and whether he was sincerely motivated for treatment.

Psychological testing was requested and confirmed evidence of a very superior IQ score. Although Jim could use his superb reasoning abilities on structured, neutral tasks, he became disorganized and close to psychotic in functioning on unstructured, projective tasks, which aroused more affect than he could handle. His anxiety escalated rapidly, and reality testing disintegrated very significantly under conflicts, especially with authority figures.

Such results of psychological testing were used in helping staff understand and manage the patient's "provocative" behavior on the unit. By understanding the patient's potential for regression and his level of pathology, the staff could recognize the need for firm limits in managing his attempts to provoke power struggles with authority figures. They could also view such conflicts as a manifestation of the patient's profound fear of losing control rather than merely manipulative expression of adolescent behavior.

Evaluating Intellectual Functioning

In educational settings, parents and teachers frequently request psychological testing to determine intelligence, abilities, and aptitudes in order to provide guidance for children who are having difficulty in their academic functioning. In most mental health settings, referral questions are rarely limited to intellectual evaluation alone; usually intellectual evaluation is incorporated with broader psychodiagnostic questions of how cognitive functioning interacts with emotional components of personality. An evaluation of intellectual functioning without a complete psychodiagnostic testing battery is likely to be requested when mental health clinicians have some indication that a patient sustains intellectual limitations and they are seeking further information about how such limitations may afffect treatment planning. For example, an individual who has a history of placement in special classes is reported to be a "borderline intelligence" and presents with complaints of loneliness. Dispositional planning involves considering whether such a patient can benefit from referral to a supportive psychotherapy group held in a clinic or whether the patient requires referral to programs in a sheltered workshop setting. Such questions may be partially addressed by intelligence tests that can reveal the pattern of specific intellectual strengths and weaknesses of the patient, his level of concrete thinking, expressive versus receptive language difficulties, social judgment, etc.

DESCRIPTION OF TESTS USED IN A PSYCHODIAGNOSTIC BATTERY

Hundreds of instruments and procedures for measuring psychological functions have been devised and can be employed in assessing various aspects of abilities, cognitive functioning, or personality functioning.[14] Most of these instruments are used in behavioral research rather than clinical practice. The traditional psychodiagnostic battery is likely to consist of the various instruments described below, which are traditionally administered individually to test cognitive and personality functioning in structured and unstructured situations. The clinical and research literature has provided a rich body of interpretation around responses from these tests, which also perpetuates their use in traditional clinical practice. The following descriptions are not meant as an exhaustive list of tests but rather as an attempt to acquaint psychiatric nurses with some of the psychological tests that will be most widely used in psychodiagnostic assessments of their patients.

Wechsler Adult Intelligence Scale (WAIS or WAIS-R)

The WAIS is the most widely used instrument for assessing intelligence. (The 1982 revision and restandardization is referred to as the WAIS-R.) It consists of 11 subtests (6 verbal and 5 performance or nonverbal tests) and takes about 1 hour to 1½ hours to administer. The subtests will be described, since they are frequently referred to in descriptions of intellectual functioning contained in psychological test reports.[15]

The six verbal subtests of the WAIS include:

Information
This subtest consists of a list of questions of increasing difficulty that tap the fund of general information, scientific information, and contemporary affairs information (location of countries, capitals, etc.).

Comprehension
Items are presented that measure ability to make practical judgments in everyday life, deal with facets of the environment, and interpret proverbs.

Arithmetic
Arithmetic problems are read to the patient by the examiner and require solution without paper or pencil.

Similarities
This test consists of pairs of concepts expressed in single words in which the examiner asks in what way they are alike.

Digit Span
The examiner reads a series of numbers, and the subject is asked to repeat digits forward and backward.

Vocabulary
This test consists of a list of words, which are presented to the subject visually and auditorily, and the subject is asked to "tell the meaning of some words."

The WAIS performance subtests include:

Digit Symbol
This test consists of a set of nine symbols that are paired with the numbers one through nine, in a visible key. The subject is required to fill in the appropriate mark for rows of numbers and told not to skip any.

Picture Completion
This test consists of pictures of familiar objects or scenes that are incomplete. The subject has to identify the essential missing element within a 20-second time limit.

Block Design
The subject is required to reproduce geometric designs using colored cubes. This is a complex task that requires the subject to accurately perceive, analyze, and synthesize the design and then reproduce it.

Picture Arrangement
This test consists of a series of pictures presented in scrambled order that tell a story. The subject is asked to put the pictures in the correct order so that they tell a logical story.

Object Assembly
This test consists of puzzles containing six or seven pieces, which are cut-up figures. The subject has to arrange the pieces together without prior knowledge of what they make.

The Rorschach (Rorschach Inkblot) Test

The Rorschach test is the most widely used projective assessment technique. It consists of ten inkblot plates with such unstructured form that they permit innumerable interpretations. The subject is asked to tell the examiner what they might be, look like, or remind him of. There is no time limit, although the examiner records initial reaction time of response to each plate and total time of responding. The administration is designed to elicit observations on how the subject approaches the task, for example, whether subject turns cards, etc. Typically, the administration is divided into phases of response followed by inquiry. The inquiry can be administered after each card, but generally it is delayed until free responses have been given to all cards. The examiner's inquiry is moderately structured to elicit information necessary for scoring, for example, information about the location of the responses.

Proper use of this instrument requires extensive training, supervised experience in interpretation, and familiarity with an extensive body of clinical and research literature. Some approaches to complex interpretation will be discussed in the next section of this chapter. Administering the Rorschach can arouse intense anxiety in some psychiatric patients since this ambiguous unstructured task is analogous to the conditions most likely to elicit emotional arousal and to stress coping mechanisms. The trained examiner can provide the patient with support and make clinical judgments about managing any "acting out" that is evoked in the test situation.[16]

Thematic Apperception Test (TAT)

The TAT is another widely used projective task that requires a subject to make up a story about a picture visually presented to him. The standardized set of 20 pictures mainly consists of persons involved in doing things. The administration is not completely standardized, so different examiners may use different cards. Rarely is the complete set administered in a full test battery. The aim is to confront a subject with a great variety of pictured situations about interpersonal relationships so that data can reveal which situations and relationships are fraught with anxiety, personal implications, or conflict. The instructions ask the subject to develop a plot for the story, tell what the situation is, what events led up to it, what the outcome will be, and to describe thoughts and feelings of characters. Thus the task taps more directly than the Rorschach test into imaginative content of subject, eliciting conscious and unconscious expression of motivations and attitudes. It is difficult to determine the extent to which stories are true fantasy and to what extent they represent clichés. The rationale for interpretation is based on viewing the clichés as an expression of defenses, and interpreting stories with real involvement as expressing dynamics. Principles for interpretation will also be elaborated in a further section of this chapter. Subjects frequently enjoy this task since it can be approached with a playful, imaginative attitude. However, the task can prove frustrating for subjects who are constricted in fantasy life and thus find it difficult to comply with the instructions.[17]

Additional Projective Tasks Used in Test Batteries

Human Figure Drawings, or House–Tree–Person Drawings

The subject is given brief, unstructured instructions to draw a person and then a person of the opposite sex. Or as a variant of this technique, the subject is asked to draw a house, a tree, and a person. The subject is usually asked to describe the drawings and to make up stories for them. Validity and reliability of scoring and interpreting drawings are even more difficult to document than other projective techniques, so this technique is less widely used, except by practitioners who are comfortable with nonverbal expressive techniques. The drawings are interpreted as reflecting aspects of body image, self-image, and psychosexual development, and as indicating aspects of conflict and psychopathology. For example, the omission of limbs on a human drawing can indicate trauma or conflict.[18]

Sentence Completion Test

The Sentence Completion Test is slightly more structured than other projective tasks. It consists of phrases that the subject is asked to complete into sentences. It taps into more conscious attitudes about self and the world than other techniques. It is especially useful to administer to constricted, self-conscious subjects since it is one of the few projective tasks that can be administered without constant observation by an examiner. The style of verbalization and content of responses constitute data for interpretation.[19]

Objective Personality Tests

Minnesota Multiphasic Personality Inventory (MMPI)

The MMPI is one of the most widely used self-report personality inventories. Subjects are asked to indicate true or false for over 500 items. The items range from those tapping social and political attitudes to issues of health, psychosomatic symptoms, and manifestations of psychopathology such as delusions, hallucinations, and phobias. The MMPI provides scores on ten clinical scales, several additional new scales, and four validity scales that provide checks on carelessness, malingering, and special test-taking attitudes. It is easy to administer and has been so widely used in clinical and research settings that considerable data exist on norms and interpretations that can be correlated with individuals who show certain patterns of scores or profiles. The MMPI is likely to be included in screening batteries that seek to assess personality. It is also likely to be included in an individually administered test battery, especially when an examiner wishes to supplement projective personality test data or to gather data for determining a differential diagnosis.[20]

ANALYSIS AND INTERPRETATION OF TEST DATA

The amount of data obtained in administering a full battery of psychological tests is considerable. Although modes of analyzing and interpreting vary among psychologists, the process is not magical. It involves steps of categorizing the data, comparing the individual's performance to normative data for comparable populations, and formulating clinical interpretations that are consistent with dominant trends and patterns in the test data. A basic rule of interpretation is that isolated aspects of data are never interpreted apart from the context of all data obtained from that given battery. The psychologist is simultaneously analyzing and synthesizing the formal test data. Such data include test scores and content of test responses and the data derived from the subject's style of verbalizing and responding, including affective reactions that accompany responses. Also included are data from the interpersonal relationship that develops between examiner and subject, both the subject's observed behavior and the subjective responses that this elicits within the examiner. Any given interpretation must be integrated with all available data from other levels before being presented as a final hypothesis or conclusion.

Since interpretation and analysis are such a skilled and complex process, the following section contains many examples that suggest and illustrate how the process can be used by psychologists. Such examples should not be regarded as providing definitive interpretations for given tests.

Interpreting Tests of Intellectual Functioning

Scoring

Analysis and interpretation of results on the WAIS begin with scoring responses using the standardized manual. Responses receive full, partial, or no credit, according to whether the response is accurate and meets qualitative criteria. For example, answers on vocabulary that give only minor uses of the word are scored partial credit. Each subtest of the WAIS yields a raw score, which can be converted into a scaled score from 0 to 10. The scaled scores of the six verbal tests and of the five performance tests are then summed separately to yield a verbal IQ and a performance of IQ, respectively. All 11 tests summed together constitute the Full Scale IQ. The WAIS and the WAIS-R currently yield what is termed a "deviation IQ," which allows any individual's score to be compared to his age peers.

Such objective scores provide a starting point for comparing individuals against group norms and for analyzing the pattern of variability of abilities for that individual. For example, since in the standardized norms, roughly two thirds of the population have verbal and performance IQs within 10 points of each other, a difference between the separate verbal and performance IQs is determined as significant in a clinical sense if it exceeds 15 points or more. Further interpretation of differences requires an analysis of the pattern of variability versus consistency of the subtest's scores, hypothesizing factors contributing to the intellectual deficits versus assets. At this point, the analysis proceeds by applying to the subtest score profile a possible range of interpretative hypotheses drawn from both research and clinical literature.

Qualitative Analysis

Although the WAIS is highly regarded for its psychometric properties that permit standardized scoring, it simultaneously yields a wealth of information that can be interpreted clinically and qualitatively.[21] The qualitative analysis of response content is an essential aspect of a sophisticated psychodiagnostic evaluation, indicating that individuals with comparable IQ scores can show widely varying patterns of cognitive functioning and varying degrees of psychopathology. In the qualitative analysis, the responses to comprehension items are scrutinized for indications of idiosyncratic thinking, disturbed perceptions, poor judgment, and various character traits. For example, the question, "What should you do if, while sitting in the movies, you were the first person to discover a fire?" could yield a range of responses from "Yell fire!" to "I don't know what I would do. I know I shouldn't yell fire." Such answers reflect differing degrees of impulsivity. Similarly, the patterns of success or failure on the Block Design items can be diagnostic both in terms of possible impairment of visual–constructive abilities and also in indicating character trends. Approaches to solving the problems can be chaotic or methodical. There can be bizarre arrangements of the blocks or careless errors in small details.

Interpreting Tests of Personality Functioning

The process of interpretation differs significantly between objective and projective tests. Objective tests are frequently so highly standardized that scoring is essentially a clerical task of tallying responses on different scales. The scoring and interpretation of the MMPI are so well standardized that the entire process has been computerized, using a program that tallies scores for different scales, analyzes the profile of patterns and totals of the scale scores, and prints out the interpretive hypotheses, which are systematically correlated with the individual's scores. Such analysis and interpretation are based on extensive research data that have collected norms for clinical populations.

Interpretation of objective tests is efficient as well as frequently impressive in reliability and validity; however, such tests alone can rarely provide the rich array of data that is required to answer referral questions. Projective test analysis and interpretation are generally more complex and vary depending on the level of experience and skill of the clinician. Like analysis of other psychological tests, analysis of projective data begins with the scoring of the data, although scoring systems for projective tests frequently require clinical judgment.

Interpreting Rorschach Responses

Several elaborate scoring systems have been devised for categorizing Rorschach responses.[22] All Rorschach scoring systems provide some summary codes for classifying how a subject responds to different aspects of the inkblot. The characteristics that are usually scored include:

Location. This score indicates where on the card the response was seen; that is, whether the subject uses the whole blot or focuses on large or small details, etc.

Determinants. These scores reflect what qualities of the blot were used in the response, and indicate what attributes of the stimuli the subject is responding to. For example, the subject can be using only the form per se, that is, the shape or contour of the inkblot, in their responses, or their response may be determined by only the color, or by a combination of form and color. Additional major determinants can include the shading, in which dark and lighter gradients in the blot suggest texture or dimensional depth. The subject can also project movement into the static blot, seeing animals or people dancing, or inanimate motion such as gusting winds. Movement, hence, becomes a determinant.

Content. Responses are also scored on the basis of the category of content (such as animals, humans, etc.).

Popular Original. This dimension scores whether the response is one frequently given (frequency being defined by norms collected for Rorschach responses) or is unique.

Form Level. One of the most important scoring characteristics reflects how accurately the response is seen, whether it fits the blot area.

Each of the scores and the combinations of, or ratios of, the scores within a Rorschach scoring system are tied to several interpretive hypotheses. The psychologist is required to simultaneously consider all possibilities and select those that are clinically useful because they fit with data from the total protocol. Rorschach interpretive hypotheses constitute a vast specialized body of psychological literature.[23–25] The interpretive hypotheses pertain to scoring categories, content, and sequence of responses.

An example of the interpretation of the scoring category of color determinants begins with the hypothesis that color scores are assumed to relate to an individual's responsiveness to environmental stimuli and to show how a person reacts to the emotional aspect of relationships to other people, which is a significant aspect of responsiveness to the environment. Thus an individual who combines color with good form is hypothesized to have the ability for controlled responsiveness to emotional demands in interpersonal relationships and can react appropriately to others and get along smoothly with others. Such a score becomes a sign of good emotional adjustment.

In contrast, if color completely determines several inkblot responses without any inclusion of form as a determinant, the psychologist may hypothesize that the patient has some impulsivity and difficulty in handling emotional impact of situations. This interpretation can be qualified depending on the frequency of color responses and the total context of additional scores.

Other scoring categories that can be considered simultaneously can yield hypotheses regarding the interpretation of additional personality variables such as the individual's way of managing needs for affection, his level of maturity, and the degree of tension and conflict.

Analysis of the content of the Rorschach responses and the sequence of responses yield hypotheses about the unique aspects of a person's functioning. The content of responses is examined for the convergence of themes within varying manifest responses. Interpretation of the sequence of Rorschach responses, combined with interpretation of the patient's attitudes to these responses, frequently yields hypotheses regarding the interplay of impulses, defenses, and adaptive strivings within the personality of the individual. During the sequence analysis, the examiner attempts to experience the subject's world and view it as the subject views it. Such interpretation cannot be standardized but requires the flexible use of all interpretive hypotheses. While doing this interpretation, the psychologist notes the patient's successive use of locations, the determinants, the test behavior, what is expressed versus what is omitted, and the interplay between themes in the content.

Interpreting TAT Responses

The interpretation of the Thematic Apperception Test is even less standardized than that of the Rorschach. It also focuses on integrating an analysis of themes expressed in the story content, with the analysis of sequence of responses, test attitudes, styles of verbalization, etc. Generally it is assumed that the subject is identifying with the figures in the picture. The heroes in the story can often express how the subject feels or perceives under a variety of interpersonal situations. Common themes and patterns are noted in responses to a wide variety of interpersonal situations. For example, when presented with a card that depicts a human figure slouched over a couch, the young adult male subject tells a story of a dejected man who is considering suicide because of loss of a job. The same subject responds to a card depicting a younger male and older male with a story depicting a critical boss chastising a sulky younger man for poor performance. The theme of threat surrounding a work situation suggests that the patient is fantasizing about a job loss or has experienced some actual loss related to work, which has been a vital blow to his self-esteem and has led to anger that is turned against himself. Such hypotheses, of course, would be confirmed only if they were consistent with other data in the test protocol.

Interpretations cannot be based upon a single response to a given test item or even upon the responses to two TAT cards. Any interpretative hypothesis must be integrated with all available data from other tests before being presented as a final interpretation or conclusion.

In summary, analyses and interpretations of psychological test data are based on the scientific research that establishes the reliability and validity of the testing instrument. Interpretation is a process of applying clinical experience and knowledge of test norms to an understanding of individual responses and articulating the specific pattern of personality traits and dynamics that are manifested by the test responses.

UNDERSTANDING TEST REPORTS AND INTEGRATING RESULTS INTO TREATMENT PLANNING

A psychological test report is frequently the major tool of communication between the psychologist and referring clinician. As a written document, especially when it is used in a hospital or institutional setting, it can attain significant legal and medical–legal status. However, all written communication is limited in serving as a communication tool to explore all the many subtleties and complexities of psychological functioning. Therefore, the report should, whenever possible, serve as a catalyst for further verbal communication between referring clinician and psychologist. The following section will describe the potential range of information that can be included in a report and, it is hoped, will encourage psychiatric nurses to initiate discussion when they have questions or would like to discuss further the implications of testing. Nurses should not be deterred by specialized test jargon in a report; it is the responsibility of the psychologist to discuss test findings in language that is comprehensible to all members of the mental health team.

The psychological report is written to address the referral question, to present data on which the psychologist is basing his conclusions, and to provide a sufficiently comprehensive description of the patient's psychological functioning that questions regarding treatment or dispositional planning can be generated and discussed.[26] The potential benefit of the report becomes limited if it is focused primarily on the test data or even solely on the referral problem. A test-oriented report that presents findings from each test sequentially may confuse the reader. The psychological report that limits data and conclusions only to the referral question may neglect data that are not known to, or understood by, the referring clinician, yet this data could lead to an expanded view of the patient's problems. Therefore, psychological reports are optimally organized in a format that presents major findings from tests, the conclusions that address the referral questions, and also a range of information that reflects the professional expertise of the psychologist. Briefer reports, of course, suffice on a busy clinical service. However, the best report would include most of the following sections and would highlight information relevant for treatment planning.

The initial section of the report includes identifying data, a list of the evaluation procedures and the tests used, and a description of the referral question.

The next section reviews background information. The extent of the information will vary depending on whether the psychologist is the only clinician doing an evaluation or is part of a team. Most of the background, which may include interview data elicited by the psychologist or case history data, will be focused on the referral question. For example, if the referral question requested an evaluation of the degree of depression, the psychologist may document recent behavioral changes noted by the patient and family such as weight loss, trouble concentrating, sleep difficulties, etc.

Similarly, this section is focused on observations that pertain either to the referral question, to interpreting the formal test results, or to explicating the relationship between patient and examiner. Conditions that could affect test results are described in this section, and factors such as the patient's cooperation and apparent motivation are reported. The observations are not merely descriptive but begin the integration of behavioral observations with other data. For example, noting that behavioral manifestations of anxiety fluctuated under different types of tasks or that the patient exhibited some bizarre behavior bears on additional data that address the issue of assessing ego strength.

The section on formal test results usually begins with a section on intellectual and cognitive functioning. This section contains a report of the obtained IQ scores, what they represent in functional levels, estimates of the differences between present functioning and potential abilities, and a discussion of a pattern of assets and deficits in intellectual functioning. The interplay between intellectual functioning and emotional or affective functioning is also discussed. Aspects of cognitive functioning that can be highlighted include how the patient perceives reality, examples of bizarre thoughts, fluctuations in concrete and abstract thinking, etc.

A major section of the report addresses personality functioning. A wide range of potential functions are assessed in a complete battery. The most useful reports are organized to address issues that relate to the referral questions and highlight aspects of personality functioning that capture the uniqueness of the subject. For example, this section frequently describes: (1) the nature of the patient's anxiety, whether he consciously experiences anxiety, "acts out," or somatizes the interplay between impulses and controls in the personality, or whether the patient is overcontrolled, etc.; (2) particular conflicts and tensions and how the patient deals with anger, guilt, dependency, sexuality; (3) self-image and self-esteem; (4) potential for self-destructive "acting out"; (5) the nature of the defensive structure and types of defenses used to manage respective affects; (6) how needs are met in interpersonal relationships; and (7) patterns of relating to significant others: parents, peers, authority figures, etc. In this section of the report, the formal test results should be integrated with life history so that conclusions begin to emerge about areas in which the patient is experiencing stress and about the relative strengths of the patient's coping mechanisms.

The summary restates findings in a few sentences and may include statements of diagnosis and prognosis. The recommendations highlight specific suggestions that will assist referral in treatment planning. For example, in assessing ego strength, findings that the patient sustains fragile defenses, variable reality testing, and has difficulty tolerating intense emotional stimulation all point to a recommendation that the patient would benefit from supportive psychotherapy rather than uncovering or depth therapy. Or recommendations for group or family therapy follow from findings that major areas of conflict are found in interpersonal relationships rather than in management of intrapsychic conflict. The possible recommendations are myriad.

On an inpatient service, the report ideally serves as a catalyst for a treatment planning conference or a treatment review in which the referring source, treatment team, and psychologist integrate the psychological test reports with additional clinical data and case history. On such a service, the psychologist who serves as a regular member of the team can become involved in continually interpreting the implications that the test results have for daily aspects of case management. For example, the patient who complains bitterly and refuses to attend therapy sessions is beginning to exasperate the nursing staff. Constant reminders of the patient's severe level of depression and illustrations of test responses can help nursing staff retain their empathetic and therapeutic stance to the patient and can prevent a countertransference response of rejecting patients who are manifesting resistance to treatment.

A case example of a psychological report can be found at the end of the chapter.

NEW DIRECTIONS IN PSYCHOLOGICAL ASSESSMENT

The field of psychological assessment has been expanding rapidly during the last decade, paralleling the increased scientific understanding of interrelationships between biologic and emotional factors in physical and mental health and paralleling the increased clinical collaboration between medicine and psychology in such fields as behavioral medicine. In their role as diag-

nosticians, psychologists are being asked to assist in differential diagnosis and assessment on a variety of medical services. For example, they may be asked to evaluate geriatric and neurological patients to determine decline in memory function, or they may be asked to assess stress-related life-style factors that influence prognosis of cardiac rehabilitation.

Medical settings pose a fertile field for the development and use of objective psychological assessment procedures. Medicine has a traditional belief in the necessity of clinical diagnosis and in the importance of systematic patient assessment. Psychometric instruments seek to standardize clinical evaluations and to ensure that a comprehensive data base is obtained. Many of the traditional psychometric tests that were useful in mental health or psychiatric settings do not necessarily answer the questions posed in assessing general medical patients. Moreover, psychometric tests that originally were devised to detect the presence or absence of organic brain damage do not address our current understanding of brain–behavior relationships. Both theoretical advances and the challenge of new referral questions are prompting the development of new techniques in neuropsychological and medical assessment.

Neuropsychological Assessment

Many psychiatric symptoms can be attributed either to organic or functional causes, or both. For example, disturbances in memory can be a symptom of either depression or dementia, or both. Until 15 years ago, traditional psychological assessment was used as a method for detecting the presence or absence of organic brain damage. However, a new field of clinical neuropsychology, a subspecialty of clinical psychology, has developed neuropsychological test batteries that are significantly more valid than the traditional assessment techniques for identifying patients who are organically impaired.[27]

Traditional psychological assessment batteries still remain useful as screening devices. However, a complete neuropsychological assessment is indicated whenever there is a request for differential diagnosis of higher nervous system dysfunction or whenever organic factors are thought to contribute to cognitive dysfunction or behavioral disturbance.

Referral Questions

By applying knowledge of brain–behavior relationships to assessment, neuropsychologists can assist in differential diagnosis, in evaluating the contribution of organic and functional factors, and at times in detecting the localization of lesions. When a person has documented evidence of brain lesions, testing is useful in determining the specific effects of brain lesions on behavior, cognitive functioning, emotional functioning, and social adjustment—information that is useful in planning rehabilitation programs.

Referrals for differential diagnosis may be initiated by neurologists who note symptom constellations such as headaches, numbness of limbs, nausea, and vomiting and who request testing as part of the work-up to assess whether there has been any change in the person's cognitive functioning that would specify localization of lesions or if there is any functional component to the patient's complaints. Conversely, mental health specialists refer when they suspect likelihood that the psychiatric disturbance has some organic basis. For example, complaints of word-finding difficulties, memory difficulties, concentration problems, and depression are noted by clinicians. The neuropsychologist may then be asked to discriminate the degree to which such complaints are attributable to clinical depression or dementia. Frequently patients with seizure conditions or alcoholism are tested with a neuropsychological battery to detect the degree to which such conditions affect their intellectual functioning.

Tests Used in Neuropsychological Assessment

Brain–behavior relationships can be assessed by noting deficits or disorders in a variety of intellectual, cognitive, and behavioral functions.

Neuropsychologists either use a uniform battery for all patients or conduct assessment through an individualized approach by administering a small core group of tests to all patients and then selecting further tests to elucidate the referral questions. Both these batteries and the individualized approach to assessment have advantages and disadvantages in providing sufficient or insufficient information and in their cost-effectiveness.

Two common neuropsychological batteries are the Halstead-Reitan neuropsychological test battery and the Luria-Nebraska neuropsychological battery. Both batteries comprehensively sample a range of behaviors and exemplify the psychometric tradition of using procedures that are standardized and objective. A number of neuropsychologists prefer the individualized approach to ensure that assessment can be tailored to provide an in-depth evaluation of specific impairments. Some prominent neuropsychologists are associated with individualized approaches and qualitative analysis. At this time in the development of neuropsychology, no single approach is dominant.

Both the batteries and the individualized approaches are designed to tap into a range of functions. Some examples of the range of functions and the tests that evaluate these areas include:

Intellectual Ability. WAIS-R, subtests from WAIS-R, or additions to the WAIS-R are typically administered in the battery.

Verbal Functions. Items assess receptive and expressive language. For example, understanding simple words and phrases, object naming.

Memory. Some areas assessed include verbal and nonverbal short-term memory; delayed memory, recall for complex geometric figures; recognition versus recall.

Sensory and Perceptual Functions. These include tactile discrimination, stereognosis, pitch and rhythm discrimination.

Abstract Reasoning and Concept Formation. Some widely used tests include Wisconsin Card Sorting, Raven Progressive Matrices, and the Halstead Category Test.

Psychomotor Performance. Unilateral and bilateral motor speed and coordination are assessed, as is verbal control of motor movements.

Attention and Concentration.

Ability to Shift Mental Set. Train-making test requires subject to connect an alternating sequence of numbered and lettered circles scattered on a page.

Writing Skills. Tests include writing to dictation, spontaneous writing.

CASE EXAMPLE

Ann Dobbin was a 57-year-old married mother who remained a diagnostic puzzle after 1 month of hospitalization. She was insecure, frightened, agitated, depressed, and responding poorly to antidepressant medication. Dementia was suspected. Her CT scan was negative, but the neurological exam was inconclusive, and neuropsychological testing was recommended for a more comprehensive evaluation.

Initial findings on the traditional psychological test battery documented patterns of intellectual dysfunction that could be attributable to either a major affective disturbance or dementia. For example, Mrs. Dobbin scored only in the low average range on her intelligence test. Since she had earned a college degree 20 years earlier, such functioning can be viewed as representing a significant decline in performance. She was also slow on motor tasks, had difficulty constructing puzzles, and showed variable attention, concentration, and memory on several tasks. More refined neuropsychological testing showed that the patient's difficulties were attributable to functional depression and were not associated with organic impairment. For example, when compared to other individuals her age, Ann Dobbin scored within normal limits on tasks of new learning, motor speed, abstract thinking, and visual memory. When asked to write a paragraph about anything that came to mind, she accomplished the task efficiently and without any errors in sentence construction. Her writing was creative and fluent.

After the neuropsychological evaluation had ruled out dementia, the patient's behavioral slowness and variable attention and memory could be entirely attributable to her psychogenic depression. The projective test data also indicated a constellation of dynamics and psychopathology consistent with clinical depression and passive–aggressive behavior. Ann Dobbin felt deprived, fearful of sustaining future losses, and unable to express the anger and sadness associated with past losses. She tended to wait for someone to discover her needs and provide for her. She also was denying conflicts about caring for her aging mother, who had Alzheimer's disease.

The results of psychological testing, combined with clinical data, yielded recommendations for review of medication and supportive counseling directed to helping the patient acknowledge and verbalize issues of loss, especially difficulties in caring for her aging mother. With the reassurance that all of the patient's difficulties could be attributed to her depression, the staff was more consistent in confronting the patient about passive–aggressive behavior and the underlying anger that contributed to the patient's helplessness and passivity. Ann Dobbin's depression gradually lifted so that within 3 weeks she had improved sufficiently to be discharged to her home.

Psychological Assessment in Medical Settings

The movement toward more psychologically oriented medical care reflects an increase of focus on interrelationship of mind and body, a concept that has growing acceptance in modern medicine. Physicians frequently turn to psychology out of frustration, seeking help in managing "difficult" patients. A biosocial model of medical care also requires that psychosocial events and the personality of the patient be appraised to provide a comprehensive data base for prevention and healing of medical symptoms.

Assessment in medical settings is an important new area for employing psychometric tools. Psychologists are currently in the process of developing tools that will be reliable, valid, and tailored to address questions posed in assessing general medical patients and specific target populations. The challenge continues to be one of developing self-report objective instruments that are brief, easy to administer, minimize fatigue, and maximize patient compliance in completing the questionnaire. Psychologists are being challenged to develop procedures that can be used for cost-effective screening of target populations and tools that can be used to supplement clinical interviews and individual consultations on medical services.

Referral Questions and Examples of Tests Used in Medical Settings

Screening for Mental Health Issues. Psychometric instruments can be used as an adjunct to a medical examination to gather data on medical history, to provide checklists for medical problems, and to screen for mental health problems.

The Cornell Medical Index is a 195-item true-false inventory that provides a comprehensive screening tool. The SCL-90 is a 90-item self-report symptom inventory of both medical and psychological symptoms. It was originally designed to reflect symptom patterns of psychiatric patients but has recently been used to assess distress levels in medical patients.[28]

Assessing Depression in Medical Patients. Mild depression and anxiety are associated with many medical conditions and surgical interventions. Such symptoms often spontaneously remit over the course of medical treatment or during recuperation from surgery, when individuals have sufficient social support and personality strengths to cope with their medical crisis. However, even mild depression may be a symptom of more serious emotional disturbance. So referral for mental health consultation needs to be considered whenever depression persists or is accompanied by marked changes in appetite, sleep disturbance, concentration difficulties, or marked changes in activity level. The Beck Depression Inventory is an instrument originally designed for research purposes to discriminate among levels of depression in psychiatric patients. It serves a similar function with medical patients. It is easy to administer, relatively short, and serves as a psychometric barometer of the severity and extent of depression, thus providing a useful assessment tool to determine clinical levels of depression in medical patients.

Assessing Relationships Between Life-Style Factors and Stress-Related Illness.

Life-styles, coping styles, and recent life events have been demonstrated to have significant impact on physical health. Current research studies are demonstrating complex relationships between stress and illness, ranging from the risk of developing cardiovascular health disease to the aggravation of chronic conditions such as asthma and arthritis. All these relationships are mediated by the effects of stress on the sympathetic nervous system and the endocrine and immune systems.[29]

Several personality questionnaires have been developed in conjunction with the research studies that established the correlations between extent of stress, life-style adaptations, and frequency of physical illness. Tools developed for research on group differences cannot predict individual risk of illness until validity is established, but the questionnaires still do contribute information that is useful in highlighting an individual's susceptibility to physical illness. Examples of these tools include the Jenkins Activity Survey and the Holmes–Rahe Schedule of Recent Experience.

The Jenkins Activity Survey is a 52-item self-report questionnaire developed to measure Type A behaviors by assessing the predisposition to react to challenging activities with speed and impatience, hard-driving competition, and job involvement. This questionnaire has been used for assigning individuals to cardiovascular health prevention intervention programs.[30]

More recent research is demonstrating that refinements in assessment of Type A behaviors, focusing on the patterns of hostility in Type A profiles, are necessary to increase the validity of predictions based on the relationship between cardiovascular risk factors and Type A behaviors.

Holmes and Rahe developed an objective self-report questionnaire to use in research that demonstrated the links between degree of stressors and frequency of subsequent illness. The Holmes–Rahe questionnaire has been widely publicized as a popular tool for assessing the significant events and stressors that occur in an individual's life during the previous 12 months. Despite its widespread use, the questionnaire can only demonstrate modest capacity to predict the connection between stress and illness for any given individual, since the amounts of adaptation and social adjustment required by significant life changes vary with the individual's perception of the meaning of the life changes. Despite the methodological issues surrounding this questionnaire, it remains a useful research tool and an example of a self-report instrument that pioneered in gathering psychosocial data on medical patients.

Recent studies have been made to devise psychometric instruments to gather comprehensive data on behavioral issues that affect health care. The Millon Behavioral Health Inventory (1982) includes scales to assess chronic tension, recent stress, attitudes of helplessness, hopelessness, willingness to plan for the future, level of social support, level of anxiety, and other scales to assess attitudes that increase the psychosomatic susceptibility of an individual or aggravate the current course of a disease. Several research studies have been instituted to establish the validity of the Millon Behavioral Health Inventory, and it has been shown to predict outcome in response to pain management interventions and response to presurgical counseling for coronary bypass surgery.[31,32] If the validity continues to be established, this questionnaire may become a widely used tool in psychological assessment of medical patients.

PSYCHODIAGNOSTIC EVALUATION

Patient   Tom Davis, an inpatient

Date of Birth   May 4, 1950

Dates of Testing	February 15 and 16, 1987
Tests Administered	WAIS-R, Rorschach, TAT, Sentence Completion Test, Human Figure Drawings, Bender-Gestalt, and MMPI.
Referred by	M. Jones, M.D.

BEHAVIORAL OBSERVATIONS AND CLINICAL IMPRESSIONS

Mr. Davis is a 30-year-old male, recently separated from his Vietnamese wife. He has a three-year history of weekend alcoholism and has been sober for several months. He was referred by Dr. Jones to rule out psychosis and rule out any early organic brain dysfunction from alcoholism. He initially presented as soft-spoken, cooperative but somewhat self-reproaching. He manifested some mild slowing of speech, indecisiveness, dysphoric mood, and marked constriction of affect that initially contributed to the impression he might be masking a deeper underlying disturbance. A significant change in his behavior occurred during the administration of the TAT. The patient indicated by subtle nonverbal behavior that he was deeply identifying with the story he had told to Card 8BM of a boy "thinking of going off to war and . . . a little afraid to face it but he knows he has to." When Mr. Davis was encouraged to share more of his personal associations to this projective response, he initially stifled his tears, then eventually began crying freely as he gradually revealed vivid memories of his Vietnam experience. The significance of his associations and issues are reflected in his feeling that he was "born and raised in Vietnam." He has guilt feelings about surviving. He strongly identifies with the civilian casualties of the war. He recalls traumatic memories when they are elicited by stimulus events that resemble events in Vietnam. For example, the sound of helicopters evokes vivid memories of flying over battlefields and witnessing brutal maiming and killing of civilians and seeing corpses of enemy forces. He experienced culture shock upon return to this country and has periodically had nightmares of battle scenes. He states that he has been able to open up somewhat to his wife about these issues but has felt ambivalent and conflicted about seeking other support. His primary fear is that once he begins to talk about the memories, he becomes obsessed with his thoughts and fears losing control in the sense of dwelling in the past. He denies that his memories of Vietnam stir up violent or aggressive impulses. But he does express strong concern about encountering potential social rejection and ostracization because of his participation in an unpopular war.

COGNITIVE FUNCTIONING

On the WAIS-R, Mr. Davis attained a Full Scale IQ of 118, pro-rated Verbal IQ of 112 (based on 5 subtests) and pro-rated Performance IQ of 119 (based on 4 subtests). His functioning falls within the High Average range and he is consistently functioning up to his potential with the exception of a decline in psychomotor speed on rote tasks.

There is no evidence of minimal organic dysfunctioning. Graphomotor functioning is well coordinated; visual organization skills are intact and above average; abstracting abilities are above average on both verbal and nonverbal tasks. Bender–Gestalt designs were reproduced accurately and neatly without any distortions. Immediate memory was accurate for retaining six digits forward and repeating five digits backward. Seven of the nine Bender designs were correctly recalled in a test for incidental visual memory.

Patient's level of cultural knowledge is excellent considering that his formal education was limited to high school. Social intelligence is also above average. Mr. Davis can quickly, intuitively grasp the essential cues that help him appraise social situations accurately. While his overall judgment is good, there is some evidence that he might act panicky in situations that evoke a sense of physical danger or harm to self.

In summary, the patient's cognitive functioning is intact in spite of a current overall high stress level. His combination of above average verbal and visual motor skills, along with good social intelligence, are assets that would generally lead to a higher level of educational or vocational achievement than he has currently attained. Thus, it can be speculated that some long-term characterological issues or situational-variables have led to a pattern of underachieving, which may be both reflective of and contributing to the patient's low self-esteem.

EMOTIONAL FUNCTIONING

The results of psychological evaluation are consistent with the diagnostic impression (Axis 1:309.81) Posttraumatic Stress Disorder, Delayed. Criteria include: (1) existence of stressor (war); (2) reexperiencing of trauma when there is association with environmental stimulus; (3) overall reduced involvement with external world shown by estrangement from others, a feeling of detachment, constriction of affect consistent with the quality of "psychic numbing"; (4) symptoms not present before trauma include exaggerated startle response, guilt about surviving when others have not, possible avoidance of activities that arouse recollection of the traumatic events.

The test results also suggest the presence of features consistent with a mixed personality disorder, although this diagnostic impression is provisional, given limited data about the extent of impairment in social and occupational functioning. Current and long-term functioning is characterized by extensive feelings of inadequacy and low self-confidence. His character structure appears to be derived from compromises in gratifying versus defending against dependent wishes. Thus, his depression is deeply integrated into his character structure and is revealed more through the lack of self-confidence than through depressive affect. The patient appears to use a variety of mechanisms to cope with his dependency conflicts, with a primary emphasis on establishing counterdependent relationships with his wife and children. He also exhibits some features of avoidant behavior and a pattern of subordinating his own needs to people he depends on.

There is no indication of psychotic thought disorder. The patient does maintain good contact with reality. He also has some significant ego strengths but has significant difficulty in integrating intense affect into his functioning. He is frightened that his feelings will overwhelm him, resulting in loss of control. Thus, he has stripped himself of strong affect by a combination of defenses, including distancing from others, intellectualizing, compulsive functioning, and some reaction formation, especially against aggressive impulses.

He has entertained suicidal ideation as a response to his recent loss and perceived suicide as primarily a mechanism for alleviating his emotional pain. Currently, he no longer is seriously considering suicide as an option for solving his problems. He wants to resume living, recognizes that it will take him a long time to grieve. In the past, he also was inclined to entertain an intensive passive wish to withdraw by merging into nature—a wish that may be expressed through his interest in fishing. When drawing a man, the patient drew himself going fishing. He discussed his enjoyment of this solitary pastime partly as a challenge to defy nature and also described an event where he nearly drowned by sinking into marshlands.

One of the main features of Mr. Davis' functioning is that he has experienced a long-term pattern of loneliness and a distance in interpersonal relationships that borders on detachment. Consciously, he dwells on feeling "used and rejected" by his wife. But the projective themes indicate loneliness was a chronic problem. The loneliness points to significant unresolved difficulties in relating to and separating from parents. Although many dynamics are unclear, there is indication that the patient attempted to adapt to needs and wishes of his parents, wanting their approval yet subconsciously feeling deprivation and lack of attention to his own wishes and need for individuation. As a young adult, it appears that his identity was largely a negative identity of wishes to be free from parental pressures and this wish may have unconsciously motivated his desire to go to Vietnam. He describes himself consciously as wanting to go far away and "somehow prove myself."

Doubts about masculinity are also an important dynamic in his functioning, pointing to the possibility of latent homosexual urges that are defended against by his marriage and possible reaction formation defenses. His Rorschach contains a productive record, rich in several well-organized responses that follow a repeated sequence. First, he sees affectionate, close interactions between males, but then subsequently perceives such images as "masks" or "cloaks" and other responses suggesting a fear of disclosing his impulses. On a conscious level, he depicts male authority figures as supportive. However, unconsciously, he perceives them as dangerous, intimidating objects that have to be appeased. Consciously, he sustains intense wishes to receive nurturance from female objects and he rationalizes his dependency wishes through taking the counterdependent role of provider. On a more unconscious level, he sustains some anger toward women, perceiving them as greedy—which may in part reflect a projection of his own oral dependent cravings.

SUMMARY AND RECOMMENDATIONS

Mr. Davis is a 30-year-old male recently separated from his Vietnamese wife. He has a history of weekend alcoholism and was referred for testing to rule out early signs of organicity and to rule out psychosis. His intellectual functioning is intact, falls into the High Average range, and does not show any signs of organic dysfunctioning. Given his intellectual assets, which are well maintained even under current stress, it can be speculated that he has a long-term pattern of underachieving, which both reflects and contributes to his low self-esteem. Therefore, some possible long-term interventions in facilitating his review of vocational goals are suggested as a mode of increasing his self-esteem.

The evaluation yields a diagnostic impression of (Axis 1:309.81) Post-Traumatic Stress Disorder, Delayed. There is also evidence of long-term issues with dependency, loneliness, unresolved separation from parents, and doubts about masculinity, which contribute to low self-confidence and long-term inadequacy feelings. He is not an imminent suicidal risk, is not psychotic, and does possess significant ego strength. Therefore, on the basis of test results, it is recommended that the patient's current marital crisis be viewed both in the context of his long-term issues and as a probable triggering of his delayed stress reaction. He needs to be referred for treatment that can address all of these issues, preferably a combination of couples therapy and individual psychotherapy. Vietnam veterans support groups would also be an important resource to provide the patient with peer group support and to address post-traumatic stress-related symptoms.

Summary

This chapter is designed to help students and practitioners of psychiatric nursing gain a deeper understanding of the process and techniques of psychological testing so that they can more effectively use the skills and contributions of psychologists in coordinating quality patient care. In their various and expanding roles in the mental health field, psychiatric nurses have a key function in initiating referrals for psychological testing, in preparing patients to cooperate with testing, and in using the test results in appropriate treatment planning. This chapter describes the role of the psychologist in administering psychological tests and the scientific method of interpretation of test results and report formulation.

Questions

1. Define the concepts of reliability and validity in tests and measurements.
2. Define the role of a psychologist on the mental health team and give an example of nursing collaborating with psychology.
3. Identify six different referral questions that may be addressed through psychological testing.
4. Identify three types each of objective and projective psychological tests.

REFERENCES AND SUGGESTED READINGS

1. Schafer, R. *Psychoanalytic Interpretation of Rorschach Testing.* New York: Grune & Stratton, 1954, pp. 6–73.
2. Cronbach, L. J. *Essentials of Psychological Testing.* New York: Harper & Bros., 1970, p. 21.
3. Ibid., pp. 24–29.
4. Anastasi, A. *Psychological Testing,* 3rd ed. New York: Macmillan, 1968, pp. 71–153.
5. Cronbach, op. cit., pp. 578–582.
6. Maloney, M., & Ward, M. *Psychological Assessment: A Conceptual Approach.* New York: Oxford, 1976, pp. 345–351.
7. Bellak, L. On the problems of the concept of rejection. In L. E. Abt & L. Bellak (Eds.), *Projective Psychology.* New York: Knopf, 1950, pp. 7–32.
8. Freud, A. *The Ego and the Mechanisms of Defense* (Rev. ed.). New York: International Universities Press, 1967.
9. Anastasi, op. cit., pp. 516–519.
10. Holt, R. R. Editor's foreword. In D. Rapaport, M. M. Gill, & R. Schafer, *Diagnostic Psychological Testing* (Rev. ed.). New York: International Universities Press, 1968, pp. 10–23, 32–37.
11. Renken, M. K. Psychological assessment and report writing. In C. E. Walker (Ed.), *Clinical Practice of Psychology.* New York: Pergamon Press, 1981, pp. 134–138.
12. Rubin, B. Prediction of dangerousness in mentally ill criminals. *Archives of General Psychiatry,* 1972, 27, 397–407.
13. Schoenfeld, L. S., & Lehman, L. S. Management of the aggressive patient. In C. E. Walker (Ed.), *Clinical Practice of Psychology.* New York: Pergamon Press, 1981, pp. 216–255.
14. Buros, O. K. (Ed.). *The 8th Mental Measurements Yearbook* (Vols. 1, 2). Newark, N. J.: Gryphon Press, 1978.
15. Matarazzo, J. D. *Wechsler's Measurement and Appraisal of Adult Intelligence,* 5th ed. Baltimore: Williams & Wilkins, 1972.
16. Rorschach, H. [*Psychodiagnostics*] (P. Lenkau & B. Kronenberg, trans.). Berne: Hans-Huber, 1942. (U.S. distributor, Grune & Stratton.)
17. Murray, H. A. *Manual for the Thematic Apperception Test.* Cambridge, Mass.: Harvard University Press, 1943.
18. Machover, K. *Personality Projection in the Drawing of a Human Figure.* Springfield, Ill.: Charles C Thomas, 1949.
19. Rotter, J. B., & Rafferty, J. E. Rotter incomplete sentence blank. In A. Weider (Ed.), *Contributions Toward Medical Psychology* (Vol. 2). New York: Ronald Press, 1953, pp. 590–598.
20. Welsh, G. S., & Dahlstrom, W. G. (Eds.). *Basic Readings on the MMPI in Psychology and Medicine.*

Minneapolis: University of Minnesota Press, 1956.

21. Zimmerman, I. L., & Woo-Sam, J. M. *Clinical Interpretation of the Wechsler Adult Intelligence Scale.* New York: Grune & Stratton, 1973.

22. Exner, J. E. *The Rorschach: A Comprehensive System* (Vol. 1). New York: Wiley, 1974.

23. Klopfer, B., Ainsworth, M., Klopfer, W. G., & Holt, R. R. *Developments in Rorschach Technique* (Vol. 1). New York: World Book Co., 1954.

24. Schafer, R. *Clinical Application of Psychological Tests.* New York: International Universities Press, 1948.

PART V

Clinical Syndromes and Human Responses

The use of the psychiatric diagnostic classification system continues to be debated in terms of usefulness to patient care. Some mental health professionals take the position that diagnostic classification leads to the labeling and stereotyping of patients. They feel that the patient's unique problems should be the primary and only concern of the helping staff. Therapeutic efforts are viewed as being geared toward patients and their problems in coping with other people and in society. They do not see any relevance in trying to classify patient symptoms or behaviors into diagnostic categories. When this concept is followed, intervention and treatment plans tend to be carried out on an intuitive basis, with justification in the art of mental healing.

Some psychiatric nurses feel that the psychiatric diagnostic categories, because they are medically oriented, are not relevant to the practice of psychiatric mental health nursing, and they advocate teaching by concepts of behavior patterns and adapting nursing care to these patterns.

An opposing position is taken by clinicians who feel there is a need for some logical ordering of patient difficulties, and through this process, clinical judgment regarding treatment plans and goals can be developed.

We prefer a convergence of approaches and agree that there need not be a conflict in using both psychiatric diagnoses and nursing diagnoses. In fact, the human responses listed in the *DSM-III-R* in the Appendix can assist in the development of additional diagnoses, and vice versa.

Paying attention to the immediate concerns of individuals as well as to their particular behavioral style is essential in psychiatric mental health nursing practice. The diagnostic categories are important because nurses continually deal with mental health professionals who do use the psychiatric terminology. Also, third-party reimbursement for services requires that a diagnostic label be provided before payment for care can be made.

Every clinical symptom and category can be regarded as an expression of psychic distress. The products of emotional distress are expressed through thoughts, feelings, and behaviors, and biochemistry in the form of dysfunctional patterns.

CHAPTER 30: INTEGRATING PSYCHIATRIC AND NURSING DIAGNOSES IN PLANNING CARE

This chapter discusses the mental health disorders from two perspectives, psychiatric diagnoses and nursing diagnoses, in terms of planning nursing care for psychiatric patients.

CHAPTER 31: CHILDHOOD DISORDERS

The various disturbances and dysfunctions that become evident in childhood are discussed, with nursing care plans outlined and illustrated by student process recordings.

CHAPTER 32: ADOLESCENT DISORDERS

The increase in adolescent disturbances in our society dictates the necessity for a separate chapter describing teen-age conflicts and disorders.

CHAPTER 33: EATING DISORDERS OF ADOLESCENCE: ANOREXIA NERVOSA AND BULIMIA

While there are sufficient differences in the clinical manifestations of anorexia nervosa and bulimia, this chapter focuses on the more generic problem of the eating disorder in adolescence characterized by a voluntary refusal to eat. The nursing interventions will be discussed from a behavioral model approach.

CHAPTER 34: TREATING THE DRUG ABUSER

The assessment and identification of the problems of the drug abuser are discussed in the context of current treatment models.

CHAPTER 35: ALCOHOLISM: A TREATABLE DISEASE

Alcoholism is an increasing concern in providing patient care. This chapter discusses the nursing management as well as community problems of dealing with the social problem of alcoholism.

CHAPTER 36: ORGANIC DYSFUNCTIONAL PATTERNS

Organic mental disorders constitute a heterogeneous group of abnormal mental states resulting from definable conditions of the brain. By evaluating the patient in terms of specific neuropsychological functioning, the nurse can plan and implement care.

CHAPTER 37: SCHIZOPHRENIC DISORDERS

Schizophrenic disorders produce marked disruptions of thinking, mood, sensorimotor functioning, and of behavior, and they lie at the most severe end of the spectrum of psychopathology.

CHAPTER 38: DELUSIONAL (PARANOID) DISORDERS

Delusional or paranoid disorders need to be understood as a separate clinical condition requiring careful assessment and intervention for protection of patient, staff, and community.

CHAPTER 39: MOOD DISORDERS

Mood disorders involve behaviors characterized by marked disturbances of emotional lability or affect. The range of affect is from pathological grief or melancholia to elated or manic states. Loss is an underlying issue with many patients suffering from mood disorders.

CHAPTER 40: ANXIETY DISORDERS

Anxiety, either confronted, avoided, or resisted, is the major affect addressed in this disorder. In addition, post-traumatic stress disorder is described with reference to the chapters on victims in the next section.

CHAPTER 41:
SOMATOFORM DISORDER

In somatoform disorders, physical symptoms are due to psychological rather than biologic factors.

CHAPTER 42:
DISSOCIATIVE DISORDERS

Alteration in the normally integrative functions of consciousness is the cardinal feature of dissociative disorders.

CHAPTER 43: SEXUAL DISORDERS

Sexual dysfunctional patterns include the paraphilias and psychosexual disorders with inhibited desire and other conditions.

CHAPTER 44: STRESS RESPONSE AND PHYSICAL ILLNESS

The relationship between emotions and biophysiological symptoms is explored. Psychosomatic nursing concentrates on the role of the psychosocial variables, not in causing dysfunctional patterns but in altering, through stress, individual susceptibility to illness.

CHAPTER 45:
DEVELOPMENTAL DISABILITIES

Our understanding of the complex phenomenon of mental retardation will increase to the extent that the many relevant etiologic factors are researched multilaterally. Nurses could significantly expand the knowledge base for the client management of the mentally handicapped by careful observation and documentation of biopsychosocial factors.

CHAPTER 46:
PERSONALITY DISORDERS

The character or personality of an individual is a consistent and stable pattern of behavior. The management of dysfunctions becomes a challenge for nurses in psychiatric mental health nursing.

Chapter 30

Integrating Psychiatric and Nursing Diagnoses in Planning Care

Ann Wolbert Burgess

Chapter Objectives

The students successfully attaining the goals of this chapter will be able to:

- Discuss development of psychiatric nursing diagnosis.
- Integrate psychiatric and nursing diagnosis in planning care.

The field of mental health recognizes four major classes of health workers: psychiatric nurses, psychiatrists, psychologists, and psychiatric social workers. These clinicians contribute to the care of the psychiatric client. Because the various clinicians work in the same agencies and institutions, it is important to have frameworks to facilitate clear communication for planning care.

Three major concepts guide this part of Clinical Syndromes: (1) a systems view of the psychiatric mental health field; (2) the integration of diagnostic labels in the planning of patient care; and (3) the nursing diagnosis and care plan. This chapter focuses on a suggested schemata for the integration of nursing diagnoses with psychiatric diagnoses (*DSM-III-R*).* See

---

* *DSM-III-R* stands for *The Diagnostic and Statistical Manual of Mental Disorders (Revised)* published by the American Psychiatric Association.

Appendix for *DSM-III-R* classification of Axis I and Axis II categories and codes.

Psychiatric nursing is concerned with human responses to both actual and potential mental health problems. This human response can be named the *coping process* and is based, in part, on theories relevant to stress and human growth and development. In addition, psychiatric nursing assumes a holistic approach by dealing with the entire person rather than with an isolated system or subsystem. This holistic approach calls for an integrated use of data, concepts, and techniques derived from the biologic, cognitive and behavioral, psychological, and social models to explain human behavior and to study and treat deviations from health. Psychiatric nursing brings knowledge of the human mind, as an area of science, to bear on human behavior and its vicissitudes.

This approach is a systems view and is based on the assumption that an appreciation of the pluralistic, multifactoral origin of psychological distress broadens the nurse's understanding and increases her therapeutic potential. The psychiatric nurse who thinks in systems terms is a true generalist in nursing, practicing in a specialty area with a view that is a highly effective way of treating psychiatric clients.

Illness, whether physical or psychological, should no longer be thought of as the fault of certain parts of the body, but rather as a reaction or mode of behavior of a living human organism in response to forces it encounters as it moves in space and time. To paraphrase a question written over 40 years ago by British psychiatrist James Halliday: If a pebble hits a pane of glass that breaks, was the pebble the cause of the pane of glass breaking, or was the brittleness of the glass responsible, or the nature and temperature of the surrounding medium, or the velocity with which the pebble was moving? The answer is clearly that it was the interaction of all of these factors and probably of others also.[1]

STRESS THEORY AND HUMAN BEHAVIOR

The following major principles of systems theory apply in part, at least, to human personality and behavior:

1. Humans are an active organismic system.[2] Such a system is capable of self-regulation, goal seeking, and growth and learning and is internally active as well as externally responsive.
2. Like all living systems, the human system is an open one, with permeable boundaries, permitting physical energy and information to pass from inside out and from outside in. It is this capacity to incorporate energy and information that enables humans, like other living organisms, to grow, learn, and reproduce over the course of time. The human brain is now considered to be analogous in many ways to an extraordinarily complex computer and information-processing apparatus.
3. Personality develops out of the interactions of the human biologic substrate with matter, energy, and information coming from outside the biologic system, that is, from

the physical environment, the nuclear family, the school system, peer groups, the community, the nation, and the culture at large. By the same token, the origins of psychopathology are now sought not from within the individual alone but rather from within his total system of relationships, including his physiology, nuclear family, and even patterns of culture.
4. Tensions, conflicts, or difficulties within any of these interacting systems can induce ripple effects in any or all of the other systems. For example, changing cultural values, which are themselves the result of numerous complex forces within other systems, may produce changes in government reactions, family attitudes, and individual psychodynamics. The current revolution in sexual mores is an example of the production of such reverberating effects within a number of systems on different levels.

Implications for Clinical Nursing

The importance of systems thinking for clinical nursing is that relieving stress in parts of the outer system can sometimes benefit the mental health of an individual more effectively than trying to modify his intrapsychic processes directly. For example, modification of dysfunctional family patterns and relationships can often help a troubled adolescent more expeditiously than attempting to treat the adolescent individually. By the same token, poverty, malnutrition, inadequate schooling, and various forms of prejudice and discrimination can leave scars on personality fully as deep as those left by absent parenting or a broken home. The recent research on the relevance of stressful life events not only to mental and emotional disorders but also to somatic pathology exemplifies this point.

An additional step in systems thinking states that the impact of all such stresses also depends on the specific context in which they are experienced. The context itself is a relative matter, changing at different times and in different settings. What is considered psychologically healthy in one era may not be considered so in another. Within a lifetime we have seen enormous changes in our sexual mores and patterns of sexual behavior, so that language and behavior once considered totally socially unacceptable in polite society are no longer regarded as exceptional by large segments of the population. Even in such a condition as process schizophrenia, in which the biologic factor is clearly of major importance, one must still raise the question of whether, in a particularly undemanding environment, such individuals would necessarily be regarded as ill. A child with a reading disability in our culture would not be regarded as having a problem in a society in which the written or printed word did not exist, just as color blindness would not be a defect in a society in which the ability to distinguish red from green had no functional importance.

Another implication of systems thinking is that the growing tendency to think in terms of distinct and sharply demarcated categories, as evidenced in the *DSM-III-R*, deserves some skeptical evaluation despite its pragmatic usefulness. In the field of mental disorders it is difficult to decide whether an individual is relatively normal or neurotic, or neurotic or psychotic, or schizophrenic or affective. This is not to say that there are no qualitative differences between various psychopathological states, but rather that there are no rigid lines of demarcation between them. Normalcy, neurosis, and psychosis should not be regarded as static and fixed entities but rather as dynamic and changeable states of behavior that are potentially reversible and the borders of which are often indistinct.

PSYCHIATRIC DIAGNOSIS: THE *DSM-III-R*

A diagnosis is a labeling method of communication. Diagnoses enable clinicians to communicate effectively with each other about their patients and to compare and contrast cases, one with another.

A psychiatric diagnosis is a medical way of labeling a patient's mental distress. The diagnostic process involves stressing relevant data, eliminating irrelevant information, and arriving at a conclusion that is pertinent to the case at hand.

The publication of the American Psychiatric Association called *The Diagnostic and Statistical Manual of Mental Disorders* (first edition published in 1952) serves as the accepted manual for mental health.[3] In the service of gaining more precision and therapeutic consequences, a revision of the 1980 third edition is now being field-tested and reviewed. This revised manual was developed over a period of seven years with the aid of over 100 specialists from various mental health disciplines.

DSM-III-R

The revision of the *DSM-III* began in May 1983 with the Board of Trustees of the American Psychiatric Association's approval of the appointment of a Work Group to Revise *DSM-III*. The members of the Work Group were selected to ensure a broad representation of clinical and research perspectives and included members from psychiatric nursing, psychiatry, psychology, and social work. During the process of developing *DSM-III-R*, two successive drafts (10/5/85 and 8/1/86) of the proposed revised diagnostic criteria were made available to interested professionals and were widely distributed for critical review. Final approval was given to the *DSM-III-R* for professional distribution in November 1986.

The basic features of the *DSM-III-R* include the following:

- Each of the mental disorders is conceptualized as a clinically significant behavioral or psychological syndrome or pattern that occurs in a person and that is associated with present distress (a painful symptom) or disability (impairment in one or more important areas of functioning) or with a significantly increased risk of suffering death, pain, disability, or an important loss of freedom. In addition, this syndrome or pattern must not be merely an expectable response to a particular event, e.g., the death of a loved one. Whatever its original cause, it must currently be considered a manifestation of a behavioral, psychological, or biologic dysfunction in the person. Neither deviant behavior, e.g., sexual, religious, or political, nor conflicts that are primarily between the individual and society are mental disorders unless the deviance or conflict is a symptom of a dysfunction in the person, as described above.
- There is no assumption that each mental disorder is a discrete entity with sharp boundaries between it and other mental dis-

orders, or between it and no mental disorder.

- The classifications are for mental disorders, not for people, e.g., a person with schizophrenia, not "a schizophrenic."
- While all the people described as having the same mental disorder are alike in that they have at least the defining features of the disorder, they may well differ in other important respects that may affect clinical management and outcome.
- A multiaxial system provides a biopsychosocial approach to assessment.
- The *DSM-III-R* is descriptive in approach in that the definitions of the disorders are limited to descriptions of the clinical features of the disorders. For the most part, etiology is unknown.

This revised edition of the *DSM-III* provides a common language with which all mental health disciplines may communicate about disorders for which they have professional responsibility. Psychiatric nurses care for patients who have a *DSM-III-R* diagnosis and thus need information about the diagnostic categories in order to plan nursing interventions.

Multiaxial Evaluation

A multiaxial system for evaluation is recommended to ensure that certain information is elicited for the planning of treatment and evaluation of outcome.

Mental Disorders. Axes I and II include all of the mental disorders. Axis II includes personality disorders and specific developmental disorders. All other mental disorders are assigned to Axis I. Part V of this text contains the disorders listed in Axes I and II.

Physical Disorders. Axis III is for physical disorders and conditions. The rationale for this axis is based on the tradition of separating those disorders whose manifestations are primarily psychological or behavioral from those whose manifestations are not. The manual uses the term *physical disorder* as a means to recognize the boundaries between the two classes of disorders—*mental* and *physical* disorders.

Psychosocial Stressors. Axis IV classifies the severity of psychosocial stressors. The addition of this axis represents an important evaluation criterion for assessing human response to stress. This axis provides a coding for the overall severity of a stressor judged to have been a significant contributor to the development, recurrence, or exacerbator of a *DSM-III-R* disorder. The rating is based on the nurse's assessment of the stress that an "average" person would experience from such a situation. This judgment considers the following: (1) the amount of change caused in a person's life by the stressor; (2) the degree to which the event is under the person's control and is or is not desired; and (3) the number of stressors, i.e., the intensity. The stressors need to have occurred within a one-year period to be so classified. The types of psychosocial stressors identified include the following broad categories: conjugal or family-related events; parenting; other interpersonal events; occupational events; living circumstances; financial, legal, and developmental phases; physical illness or injury; victimizations including natural disasters and human-induced violations, and other family factors and school events.

Global Assessment of Functioning (GAF).
Axis V provides for evaluation of the individual's highest level of adaptive functioning over the preceding year. This criterion is especially helpful for planning and evaluating treatment and predicting outcome. The level of adaptation must have been evidenced for at least several months and speaks to the strengths of an individual. Role functioning is very important to assess. In major psychiatric disorders this dimension often shows marked impairment. Usually measured in occupational terms, the cost to society of this impairment can be enormous. Also, the personal hardships endured by the family and patient make this an area of grave concern. Data on adaptive functioning are used prognostically and serve as a marker to which the individual usually hopes to return following an episode of mental disturbance or dysfunction.

Axis V provides for the nurse's overall judgment of a person's psychological, social, and occupational functioning on a scale, the global assessment of functioning scale (GAF scale), that assesses mental health–illness. The GAF scale is a revision of the global assessment scale (GAS) and the childrens' global assessment of functioning scale (CGAS), which are revisions of the health-sickness rating scale.[4–6]

Usefulness of the *DSM-III-R*. The *DSM-III-R* is intended as a teaching and learning resource. It is a methodological attempt to define, in terms of descriptive psychopathology, the vast range of mental disorders that are seen and encountered in clinical practice. Each diagnostic category is described systematically and comprehensively.

Skodal, Spitzer, and Williams clearly state that the *DSM-III-R* is not to be considered a textbook of psychiatry nor as the final word in the classification of mental disorders.[7] For example, the *DSM-III-R* does not discuss theories about etiology; rather it makes explicit that the etiology of the disorders is generally not known. It also states that much more is needed than a *DSM-III-R* diagnosis before an adequate treatment plan is designed. It is the hope of the Task Force that the *DSM-III-R* will pave the way for future studies to increase the knowledge base about mental disorders.

NURSING DIAGNOSES: RESPONSE TO HEALTH PROBLEMS

A nursing diagnosis is the conceptualization of the patient's health problems identified from the assessment process. Concepts are abstractions from observed events, as textbooks on research methods repeatedly remind us. As such, concepts are human creations. They do not simply exist "out there" in the world, waiting to be discovered. Rather, they are abstractions made by clinicians in their attempts to "make sense" out of what has been observed and recorded.

Traditionally, it has been felt that the term *diagnosis* has been dominated by the medical profession. However, the term *nursing diagnosis* has been in the nursing literature since 1963.[8,9] It is recorded that the idea of classifying clinical problems was introduced into nursing by Abdellah and others.[10,11] The original classification included 21 problems stated as therapeutic goals.

It was in October 1973 that the First National Conference on the Classification of Nursing Diagnoses was held. At this conference the first tentative list of nursing diagnoses was developed, and the pledge was made for nurses to continue to participate in its refinement and expansion.[12]

Nursing diagnoses are essential to the profession. Diagnosis allows nurses to communicate with each other and with other health professionals regarding similar clinical issues. It provides a frame of reference for discussion, specifically to focus on the care or intervention plan (see Chapter 13).

Nursing Diagnosis of Mental Health Problems

The definition of nursing, as stated in the 1980 ANA Social Policy Statement, is the "diagnosis and treatment of human responses to actual or potential health problems."[12] The ANA publication *Standards of Psychiatric–Mental Health Nursing Practice* outlines actual or potential health problems, and each specialty area defines its own list of health problems. The terminology used is *phenomena of concern*.[13]

Maxine Loomis, in defining the phenomena of concern to psychiatric mental health nurses as the physical, emotional, cognitive, family, social, and cultural human responses to actual or potential health problems, suggests using the diagnostic structure of the *DSM-III* to diagnose, treat, and cure clients with emotional disorders. She observes that the diagnosis and labeling of health problems in the *DSM-III* are based on a set of verbal, nonverbal, or affective behavioral manifestations.[14] This section will derive the nursing diagnoses from the behavioral criteria (e.g., symptoms or human responses) of the psychiatric disorders and will present the nursing care plan within this framework.

Nursing Diagnosis Debate

Nursing diagnosis is in an evolutionary state of development and, as such, the issue is exciting and open to healthy debate. It will be useful for students to read critical discussions that argue both for a taxonomy in nursing and in psychiatric nursing and against a premature effort.[15]

Several perspectives on nursing diagnosis have been offered in the past decade. The three major ones are:

North American Nursing Diagnosis Association (NANDA)
This group was the first to organize; it is an independent group and deals with the diagnosis itself and not with the overall classification system.

American Nurses' Association's Council on Psychiatric Mental Health Nursing

This is a group of clinical specialists in psychiatric mental health nursing who have been instrumental in generating standards of practice, supporting certification at two levels, and are now making contributions to efforts to develop a taxonomy of nursing diagnosis salient to psychiatric mental health nursing. The latter effort has, in part, been prompted by the implementations of DRGs within the psychiatric service setting and the increasing efforts to carry out research by psychiatric nurses. This group is at a preliminary stage of organizing phenomena of concern under the major categorical headings of biopsychosocial phenomena of concern.

Independent Nurse Clinicians and Researchers

Kim, McFarland, and McLane have described their pocket guide of nursing diagnoses as a clinical tool and a ready reference designed to affect the quality of patient care, diagnoses, and care plans.[16] They suggest that the nursing taxonomy system falls under general broad human response patterns.

Controversial Points

Although nursing diagnosis has been part of the nursing structure for almost 30 years, controversy continues. This controversy focuses on several major issues.

How to Categorize the Classifications.

NANDA has organized its diagnoses under functional health patterns; the Psychiatric Mental Health Nursing diagnoses are organized around biopsychosocial patterns, and Kim, McFarland, and McLane list their diagnoses alphabetically. There is diversity of opinion between those who feel the process of diagnosis is so new that the phenomena themselves need to be the focus of attention and others who believe that nursing diagnoses will be best derived from the conceptual basis of the categories of classification.

What Constitutes a Domain of Phenomena that is a Diagnosis.

The issues here emanate from the definition of nursing practice as the treatment and diagnosis of human responses to health and illness. This comprehensive statement of practice domain leads to generation of diagnoses in terms of the potential for illness and dysfunction and to diagnoses that focus primarily on dysfunctional patterns. There are no clear rules or conceptualizations of how the potential for dysfunction and dysfunctional patterns relate, and there is a gap when it comes to diagnoses relevant to human responses to health. Efforts to fill this gap have seldom been on a diagnostic level but rather on a conceptual level, where constructs such as hardiness and humor and health beliefs are emerging.

Methods and Identified Defining Characteristics of Diagnoses.

The validity of the defining characteristics and the reliability of the diagnostic phenomenon are continually under challenge and reevaluation.

Emphasis on Etiology in Relationship to Nursing Diagnoses with Regard to a Taxonomy.

Since there are usually divergent opinions as to the etiology of dysfunctional patterns, we find that nursing diagnoses are determined more by the theoretical considerations of cause than by empirical verification that certain behaviors cluster in a manner consistent enough to define a syndrome suitable for diagnostic consideration. This issue is fundamental to the arguments that nursing needs to focus on the phenomena and accurately describe similarities and differences between phenomena and response of phenomena to various interventions before we consider systems of classification. This position contends that classification constructs are derived from a thorough understanding of the structure, form, and processes of the phenomena under investigation.

Diagnosis Specific to Nursing or Applicable to Other Disciplines.

The singularness of a diagnosis to those phenomena that are the concern only of nursing as opposed to phenomena that overlap with areas of concern of medicine or disciplines other than nursing is another issue about which many disagree.

Duality of Diagnosis Subject.

A final area of debate is that some of the diagnoses fit an individual and other diagnoses assume a social structure, such as parent–child–family. This duality is confusing in terms of type of criteria used for diagnosing.

Psychiatric and Nursing Diagnoses

There needs to be a word of caution said about classification. Any classification of complex clinical phenomena is inherently arbitrary and reflects the universal urge to classify. Classification imposes on the data of observation a particular, human cognitive organization, which allows the observer to cope with the phenomena more comfortably. That imposed organization is neither unique nor necessarily correct. The same data can be viewed and organized in a logical fashion in many other ways. Classification is an effort to create formal structure according to the application of human logic, on the dual assumptions that there are an inherent and a similar order in the data. The activity of nosology is a mental process and cannot escape the conscious and unconscious biases of the classifier. Ultimately, nosology reflects a personal preference as to how data are to be interpreted. Classifications need not be true in the platonic sense and probably cannot be; however, they must be useful. This usefulness may be scientific, in the sense of generating testable hypotheses, or clinical, in the sense of influencing the management of the patient.[17]

In conclusion, for this psychiatric nursing textbook we use descriptive titles suggesting a problem list of the patient. For the beginning psychiatric nursing student, we use the diagnosis as a domain of problems and issues that are addressed through nursing intervention. Case examples will be included in the discussion of the clinical syndromes of the *DSM-III-R* with both psychiatric and nursing diagnoses used for deriving the nursing care plan.

Summary

Integrating psychiatric and nursing diagnoses for planning care is in the best interests of the psychiatric patient. This chapter outlines the issues inherent in the developing knowledge base called psychiatric nursing diagnoses. The following chapters in this section utilize both the *DSM-III-R* psychiatric diagnoses of behavioral defining characteristics and the nursing diagnoses for assisting the patient to regain adaptive functioning.

Questions

1. A physician says that nurses should not make diagnoses. How would you respond?
2. How are nursing diagnoses integrated with psychiatric diagnoses in your agency?

REFERENCES AND SUGGESTED READINGS

1. Halliday, J. Principles of aetiology. *British Journal of Medical Psychology*, 1943, *19*, 367–380.
2. von Bertalanffy, L. *General Systems Theory*. New York: Braziller, 1968.
3. American Psychiatric Association. *The Diagnostic and Statistical Manual of Mental Disorders*. Washington, D.C.: American Psychiatric Association, 1952.
4. Endicott, J., Spitzer, R. L., Fleiss, J., et al., The global assessment scale: A procedure for measuring overall severity of psychiatric disturbance. *Archives of General Psychiatry*, 1976, *33*, 766–771.
5. Shaffer, D., Gould, M. S., Brasic, J., et al., Children's global assessment scale (CGAS). *Archives of General Psychiatry*, 1983, *40*, 1228–1231.
6. Luborsky, L. Clinicians' judgments of mental health. *Archives of General Psychiatry*, 1962, *7*, 407–417.
7. Skodol, A. E., Spitzer, R. L., & Williams, J. B. W. Teaching and learning the *DSM-III. American Journal of Psychiatry*, 1981, *138*, 1581–1586.
8. Bonney, V., & Rothberg, J. *Nursing Diagnosis and*

Therapy. New York: National League for Nursing, 1963.

9. Komorita, N. Nursing diagnoses. *American Journal of Nursing*, 1963, *63*, 83–86.

10. Abdellah, F. G. Improving the teaching of nursing through research in patient care. In L. E. Heidgerkin (Ed.), *Improvement of Nursing Research*. Washington, D.C.: Catholic University of America Press, 1963, pp. 74–91.

11. Gordon, M., Sweeney, M. A., & McKeehan, K. Development of nursing diagnoses. *American Journal of Nursing*, 1980, *80*, 669.

12. American Nurses' Association Congress on Nursing Practice. *A Social Policy Statement*. Kansas City, Mo.: American Nurses' Association, 1980, p. 1.

13. American Nurses' Association. *Standards of Psychiatric Mental Health Nursing Practice*. Kansas City, Mo.: American Nurses' Association, 1982, p. 1.

14. Loomis, M. E., O'Toole, A. W., Brown, M. S., Pothier, P., West. P., & Wilson, H. S. Development of a classification system for psychiatric/mental health nursing: Individual response class. *Archives of Psychiatric Nursing*, 1987, *1*(1), 16–24.

15. Proter, E. J. Critical analysis of NANDA nursing diagnosis taxonomy 1. *Image*, 1986, *18*(4), 136–139.

16. Kim, M. J., McFarland, G. K., & McLane, A. M. *Pocket Guide to Nursing Diagnosis*. St. Louis: Mosby, 1987.

17. Cancro, R. History and overview of schizophrenia. In H. I. Kaplan & B. J. Sadock, Eds., *Comprehensive Textbook of Psychiatry*, 4th ed. Baltimore: Williams & Wilkins, 1985, pp. 634–635.

Chapter 31

Childhood Disorders

Maureen P. McCausland

Chapter Objectives

The students successfully attaining the goals of this chapter will be able to:

- Describe child psychiatric services from a historical perspective.
- Describe normal growth and development of children.
- Identify the range of emotional and behavioral disorders that may be present in children.
- Identify selected situational stressors that impact on children.
- Identify the scope of practice and settings of child psychiatric nursing.
- Apply the nursing process in the delivery of nursing care to children treated in a community mental health or inpatient psychiatric setting.
- Describe areas of future research in child psychiatric nursing.

HISTORICAL BACKGROUND

Juvenile delinquents were the first children in America to receive psychiatric attention. In the 1890s the courts became concerned about troubled youths, and Illinois established the first juvenile court. A study by Healy in 1909 of delinquency in Chicago concluded that pathological behavior was the product of multidimensional factors, including the family.[1] Later that year Healy founded the Chicago Juvenile Psychopathic Clinic. Neurological deficit, heredity, and organ impairment were deemphasized as causes of juvenile delinquency.

The field of child psychiatry was greatly influenced by the psychoanalytic school of thought. Freud emphasized the crucial nature of childhood experience in adult mental health.[2] Two European psychoanalysts, Anna Freud and Melanie Klein, influenced the development of child psychiatry in the 1920s. Anna Freud used play to communicate with children and to foster their understanding.[3] She rejected the concept of a transference neurosis in children because the original love objects, the parents, are still actively in the situation. The parents are not fantasy objects that can be transferred to the analyst. Klein pioneered the use of play therapy with children in a way that was similar to the use of free association with adults. She regarded the child's play as symbolic representation of unconscious content and interpreted it as such directly to the child.[4]

Psychology has also contributed to the development of child psychiatry. Jean Piaget, a Swiss psychologist, studied the development of the child's perceptual and sensorimotor systems.[5] The behaviorists, Pavlov, Watson, and Skinner, contributed the ideas of stimulus–response which have been used to modify troubled behavior in children.[6]

Historically educators have presented the idea that children require learning as well as caring if they are to fully develop their potential. Binet and Catell were pioneers in the field of measuring intelligence in children.[7,8]

Child guidance clinics were established in the 1920s and 1930s and extended services to children other than delinquents. The use of a multidisciplinary treatment team was introduced. Classically, child psychiatrists, social workers, psychologists, educators, and criminal justice professionals worked together to diagnose and treat the child, the family, and their environment.

Contemporary childrens' services are delivered by multidisciplinary teams in a variety of hospital and community settings. Consumers of services range from infants and mothers to older children and their parents or surrogate parents. The theoretical frameworks for interventions continue to reflect a variety of schools of thought and the various disciplines.

NORMAL GROWTH AND DEVELOPMENT

An understanding of the parameters of normal growth and development discussed in previous chapters provides an initial framework for assessing the child psychiatric patient. Concepts of health and disease in children are different from those applicable to adults, depending upon the child's capacities at a particular stage of development, the current nature of family transactional operations, and other factors.[9]

The developmental stages of the child exist on a continuum. Each stage is characterized by certain tasks or goals that must be mastered if the child is to successfully progress to the next stage. Psychoanalytic theory describes oral, anal, phallic, oedipal, latency, and preadolescent stages of psychosexual development, each period having erotic and aggressive characteristics.[10] Erik Erikson's theory of development includes eight stages of psychosocial development, which span the entire life cycle of the individual. His epigenetic stages of childhood include basic trust versus mistrust, autonomy versus shame, initiative versus guilt, industry versus inferiority, and identity versus role confusion.[11] Jean Piaget developed a framework of cognitive growth and development based upon the child's perceptual and sensorimotor systems. Four stages of cognitive growth and development are the sensorimotor period, the preoperational period, the period of concrete operations, and the stage of formal operations.[12] The three major schools of thought discussed above are presented in summary form in Table 31-1.

When using a developmental framework for assessing a child or adolescent, the nurse must remember that there is a wide range of variations within the "normal" developmental pattern. The rate of growth and developmental change varies with the highest rate of growth taking place between infancy and 3 years. Changes during latency are less dramatic. In puberty and adolescence, the rate increases sharply and behavior becomes labile again.

DISORDERS ASSOCIATED WITH CHILDHOOD

Nurses must be aware of the complex, multidimensional etiology of mental illness in children. The fact that emotional disorders of children usually have more than one etiologic factor cannot be stressed enough. In 1970 the Joint Commission on Mental Health of Children described an approach identifying the following five areas as at least some of the possible origins for such disorders.

(1) Faulty training and faulty life experiences; (2) surface conflicts between children and parents which arise from such adjustment tasks as relations among siblings, school, social, and sexual development; (3) deeper conflicts within the child (these are the so-called neuroses); (4) a difficulty associated with physical handicaps and disorders; (5) difficulties associated with severe mental disorders, such as psychoses. It is estimated that 80% of emotional problems are

related to the first two categories; 10% to the third category; and 10% to the fourth and fifth.[13]

The role of hereditary factors in the etiology of some of the above categories is a major research area. Any combination of the above factors may contribute to a psychiatric disturbance that may arise in a child in any phase of his development.

In this section the disorders of childhood will be presented in six major categories on the basis of the predominant area of disturbance. Implications for nursing care will be stressed.

Intellectual Disorders

Significantly subaverage general intellectual functioning resulting in or associated with deficits or impairments in adaptive behavior, with onset prior to age 18, is referred to as mental retardation.[14] The mentally retarded individual is likely to have substantial functional limitations in three or more of the following areas: self-care, learning, mobility, self-direction, capacity for independent living or economic self-sufficiency.[15]

The care of the mentally retarded child and family is discussed at length in Chapter 45.

Disruptive Behavioral Disorders

Behavioral disturbances of childhood are primarily of three types: attention-deficit hyperactivity disorders, conduct disorders, and oppositional defiant disorders.

Attention-Deficit Disorders

Attention-deficit hyperactivity disorders are characterized by signs of developmentally inappropriate inattention, hyperactivity, and impulsivity.[16]

The child suffering from an attention-deficit disorder does not complete tasks and has difficulty organizing and completing work. The child often gives the impression of not listening or that he has not heard what he has been told. Work is often messy and performed carelessly and impulsively.[17]

Performance at school is usually impaired. The group learning situation of the classroom tends to exaggerate attentional difficulties.

The child with hyperactivity often appears to be "bouncing off the walls." Gross motor activity, such as running, is usually present for extended periods of time in young children. The older child appears restless and fidgety. It is the quality of the motor activity that distinguishes this disorder from ordinary overactivity. Hyperactivity tends to be haphazard, poorly organized, and not goal directed.[18] A case example is given below:

Billy, a 7-year-old black male of African heritage, was admitted to an inpatient child psychiatric unit with a diagnosis of attention deficit with hyperactivity disorder. The student nurse caring for him described him as "almost out of control, just about bouncing off the walls. It's hard to have our special meeting. He runs around touching things, doesn't establish eye contact, and can't even remember my name."

Nursing interventions with Billy included establishing a therapeutic one-to-one relationship, limit setting on disruptive or dangerous behavior, and structuring play activities to include an opportunity for discharge of energy through the use of the large muscle groups. Two initial meetings between the child and his student nurse proved unsuccessful when conducted in a very small room filled with temptations. A fish tank, typewriter, and many types of toys were too distracting to permit sustained, meaningful interaction between patient and nurse. Feelings of frustration were evoked in the nurse and firm limit setting proved to have mild, punitive overtones. Future sessions that included trips to the local playground and the surrounding neighborhood facilitated communication and the discharge of energy after school.

Conduct Disorders

The essential features of a conduct disorder are a persistent, repetitive pattern of conduct in which either the basic rights of others or major age-appropriate societal norms or rules are violated. The conduct is more serious than the ordinary mischief and pranks of children and adolescents.[19]

The *DSM-III-R* delineates three specific subtypes of conduct disorders. These three subtypes and the distinguishing characteristics of each type are presented in Table 31-2. The presence or absence of aggressive conduct or social attachment to others are the key diagnostic features of each subtype.

TABLE 31-1. MAJOR STAGES OF GROWTH AND DEVELOPMENT: A COMPARISON OF FREUD, ERIKSON, AND PIAGET

Age	Psychoanalytic Freud	Ego Psychology Erikson	Failure of Stage Results in[a]	Age	Cognitive Piaget
	Oral	*Trust Versus Mistrust*			*Sensorimotor*
Birth to 1 year	Focuses on mouth as primary organ of gratification Trust and dependency issues are mastered	Trusts maternal figure and becomes able to allow her out of his sight without rage or fear	Chronic mistrust, dependency, depressive trends, withdrawal, shallow interpersonal relationships	Birth to 2	Practices primary reflexes (grasping, sucking) and coordinates them into new actions Gradually coordinates information from various sensory inputs
	Anal	*Autonomy Versus Shame and Doubt*			*Preoperational*
1–3 years	Anal sphincter control learned; Separation–individualization Autonomy begins	Develops self-esteem through limited self-control Establishes cooperation–willfulness, love–hate, self-expression–suppression ratios	Feelings of shame and doubt, fear of exposure, ritualized activity Later in life may be compulsive character type	2–7	Egocentric stage initially, replaced by social interaction at the end First symbolic substitutions Recognizes the difference between "I" and "me" and "you" and "yours" Perceptions dominate judgments and he operates on what can be seen directly
	Phallic	*Initiative Versus Guilt*			
3–5	Sexual organs take on new interest Oedipal wishes develop and lead to inevitable disappointment and conflicts Critical phase for early formations of gender identity	Prerequisites for masculine and feminine identity established Guilt and conscience develop Anxiety controlled by play, fantasy, and pride in new skills	Confusion of psychosexual roles, rigidity in interpersonal relationships Loss of initiative in exploration of new skills		
	Latency	*Industry Versus Inferiority*			*Concrete Operations*
5–12					

Focuses on learning Formation of same-sex peer groups	Wins recognition by doing Wants to learn by demonstration from others as well as learn by self Beginning of friendship and love outside the family, "best friends" begin Fight in games to work off hostilities	Feelings of inadequacy and inferiority: "I will never be good at anything"	7–11 Acquires basic, concrete understanding about groupings of objects Concepts of time, space, and number system still rudimentary Unable to relate logical groupings to one another
13–Adult *Adolescence/Puberty* Resurgence of sexual development accompanied by family triangle issues Sexual feelings towards parent of opposite sex are now unconscious Masturbation resumed with conscious sexual–romantic fantasies toward members of opposite sex Guilt feelings about such behavior often present "Love life" is characterized by restricted infatuations	*Identity Versus Role Confusion* Preoccupied with difference between what he appears to be in the eyes of others and own self-image Body image changes and secondary sex characteristics accompany physiological revolution Unpredictable wishes and mood swings from independence to dependence Heterosexual involvement Goal is independence and self responsibility *Intimacy Versus Isolation* Differentiates from family without complete withdrawal Clarification of self-identity and social role	Sense of inadequacy in controlling and competing Inability to establish a true and mutual psychological intimacy with another person Tendency toward self-isolation characterized by lack of warmth, spontaneity and honest exchange of emotional involvement	11–Adult *Formal Operations* Begins to understand causal thinking and scientific experimentation Inductive and deductive logic Expansion and exploration of cognitive capacities Beginnings of creativity

a Entries in this column are based on D. Aguilera and J. Messick, *Crisis Intervention: Theory and Methodology*, 5th ed., St. Louis: Mosby, 1986, pp. 191–211.

593

TABLE 31-2. THE DISTINGUISHING CHARACTERISTICS OF CONDUCT DISORDERS

Diagnostic Criteria for Conduct Disorder
   A. A disturbance of conduct lasting at least 6 months, during which at least three of the following have been present[a]:
      (1) has stolen without confrontation of a victim on more than one occasion (including forgery)
      (2) has run away from home overnight at least twice while living in parental or parental surrogate home (or once without returning)
      (3) often lies (other than to avoid physical or sexual abuse)
      (4) has deliberately engaged in fire setting
      (5) is often truant from school (for older person, absent from work)
      (6) has broken into someone else's house, building, or car
      (7) has deliberately destroyed others' property (other than by fire setting)
      (8) has been physically cruel to animals
      (9) has forced someone into sexual activity with him or her
      (10) has used a weapon in more than one fight
      (11) often initiates physical fights
      (12) has stolen with confrontation of a victim (e.g., mugging, purse-snatching, extortion, armed robbery)
      (13) has been physically cruel to people
   B. If 18 or older, does not meet criteria for Antisocial Personality Disorder.
Criteria for Severity of Conduct Disorder
   Mild: Few if any conduct problems in excess of those required to make the diagnosis, and conduct problems cause only minor harm to others.
   Moderate: Number of conduct problems and effect on others intermediate between "mild" and "severe."
   Severe: Many conduct problems in excess of those required to make the diagnosis, or conduct problems cause considerable harm to others, e.g., serious physical injury to victims, extensive vandalism or theft, prolonged absence from home.

Subtypes

Group Type	Solitary Aggressive	Undifferential
Predominance of conduct problems occur mainly as group activity with peers	Children make little attempt to conceal their antisocial behavior	May be more common than other two types
Aggressive physical may or may not be present	They are often socially isolated	Evidence of a mixture of clinical features that cannot be classified as either solitary aggressive type or group type
Usually these children claim loyalty to the members of their group.	Predominance of aggressive physical behavior, usually toward both adults and peers, initiated by the child (not as a group activity)	

[a] Items are listed in descending order of discriminating power based on data from a national field trial of the *DSM-III-R* criteria for Disruptive Behavior Disorders.
(From *DSM-III-R*, 1987, pp 53–56, with permission.[14])

The nursing interventions with two patients diagnosed as having conduct disorders from different subtypes are compared and contrasted in the next two nursing care plans.

It must be emphasized that the case of the child with a conduct disorder requires consistency in both primary providers on the milieu and limit setting on impulsive, egocentric, or aggressive behavior. Feelings evoked in the staff by such patients often include anger, fear, and frustration. Staff must have an opportunity to identify and express such reactions in supervi-

sion to prevent acting them out with the patient. Therapeutically, it is essential that patients feel and believe that staff can limit their inappropriate behavior.

Oppositional Defiant Disorder

This disorder consists of disobedient, negativistic and provocative opposition to authority figures. A striking characteristic is the persistence of such behavior even when it is destructive to the interests and well-being of the individual.[24]

The child projects the cause of the problem

onto others. His behavior rarely causes him to experience personal distress and is ego syntonic.

Treatment of the oppositional child requires a great deal of patience. The nurse continually accepts the child despite his negativistic and provocative behavior. The nurse attempts to structure a corrective life experience for the child. Gently pointing out the defense mechanisms used by the child gradually reduces the resistance to treatment.

CASE EXAMPLE

Arnold is an 8-year-old black male with a conduct disorder, group type, nonaggressive, and an attention deficit hyperactivity disorder. Arnold is courteous at times with elders but can be impulsive and disruptive in the milieu. He appears to be a very insecure child who has trouble expressing his thoughts and feelings verbally. Arnold is able to interact with peers on the unit and form relationships with members of the milieu. He often participates in lying and initiates physical fights with other peers.

NURSING CARE PLAN
Conduct Disorder, Group Type

NURSING DIAGNOSES

- Social interaction, impaired, related to inability to consistently form interpersonal relationships that respect the rights of others and behavior manifested by disobeying rules of unit, lying and stealing at school.
- Impulsivity related to hyperactivity and unpredictable behavior.

GOALS

Long-Term
1. Will avoid blaming or informing on peers by end of 9 months.
2. Will demonstrate age-appropriate behaviors that conform with guidelines at school and on unit by end of school year.

Short-Term
1. Will show concern for the welfare of companions by asking how someone is at the community meeting by end of 3 months.
2. Will gradually be able to show evidence of impulse control through:
   (a) Asking staff for objects he wants within 2 months.
   (b) Deferring immediate gratification of oral needs within 6 months.

INTERVENTIONS

1. Establish therapeutic nurse–patient relationship to model behavior that demonstrates concern for others.
2. Reinforce appropriate peer-group activities and do not reinforce blaming behaviors.
3. Reinforce appropriate behaviors. Set strict, consistent limits on inappropriate behaviors, e.g., taking toys from other children.
4. Set strict, consistent limits on disruptive behaviors including chair time or a quiet time as necessary. Collaborate with school to set consistent limits at school. Discuss plan to decrease special privileges when lying or stealing occurs.

─── CASE EXAMPLE ──

Kevin is a 7-year-old black male with a diagnosis of conduct disorder, solitary undersocialized, aggressive, attention deficit hyperactivity disorder, and gender identity disorder of childhood. He has difficulty forming relationships with others, is impulsive, and threatens violence toward both children and adults on the unit. Kevin has a gender identity problem and has reportedly enjoyed dressing in women's clothes since a very young age.

NURSING CARE PLAN
Conduct Disorder, Solitary Aggressive

NURSING DIAGNOSES

- Social isolation related to discomfort in interaction with peers.
- Potential for violence related to threatening both peers and adults.
- Role performance, altered, related to conflict in gender identity.

GOALS

Long-Term
1. Will form a minimum of one peer relationship by end of 6 months.
2. Formation of strong sense of masculine identity without evidence of aggression by end of 2 years.

Short-Term
1. Will participate in 1:1 relationship with primary nurse by end of 2 months.
2. Episodes of violent behavior will decrease to less than two times a week by end of 1 month. Patient will verbalize feelings associated with violent behavior by end of 3 months.

INTERVENTIONS

1. Encourage formation of age-appropriate "best friend" relationship with another patient.
2. Meet with patient for ½ hour two times a week for 30 weeks. Model caring and concern for patient. Set strict limits on any behavior that violates rights of the nurse or others.
3. Monitor behavior: at first sign of escalating verbal abuse or threats, assign chair time. If physical violence occurs, assign quiet-room time. Reinforce positive nonaggressive behavior through increased human contact with staff. Model appropriate verbalization of feelings and reward such behavior in Kevin.
4. Provide opportunity for symbolic representation of conflicts about gender identity. Limit inappropriate behaviors on unit, e.g., trying on girls' clothes. Provide appropriate male role models. Clarify appropriate distinctions between maleness and femaleness.

Emotional Disorders

The emotional disorders of childhood or adolescence are characterized by anxiety, ego deficits, or identity problems.

Anxiety Disorders
The *DSM-III-R* categorizes three types of anxiety disorders: separation anxiety disorders, avoidant disorder of childhood, and overanxious disorder.[20]

Separation Anxiety. Separation anxiety is a clinical picture in which the predominant disturbance is excessive anxiety on separation from major attachment figures or from home or other familiar surroundings. When separation occurs, the child may experience anxiety to the point of panic. The reaction is beyond that expected at the child's developmental level.[21]

Intervention with children suffering from separation anxiety is geared toward lowering the level of anxiety. Progress toward the treatment of the psychodynamic process of anxiety cannot be made when the patient is at the severe or panic level of anxiety. Traumatic early separations from the primary attachment object are often a part of the patient's clinical picture. Mastering the first developmental stage of basic trust is a beginning step in the treatment process. Nursing care should be provided by a minimum number of care givers. Gradual reassurance that those who leave often return is a major breakthrough for these children. Other interventions include attempting to reduce fears at night by having a staff member stay with the child until he falls asleep and removing other sources of fears such as animals. Such children often experience morbid fears of becoming lost or separated from loved ones. Play therapy and stories such as Hansel and Gretel provide an opportunity for symbolic expression of fears and mastery over the situation.

Avoidant Disorder of Childhood or Adolescence. This is evidenced by a persistent and excessive shrinking from contact with strangers of sufficient severity so as to interfere with social functioning in peer relationships, coupled with a clear desire for affection and acceptance, and relationships with family members and other familiar figures that are warm and satisfying.[22]

Nursing care of the child or adolescent with an avoidant disorder attempts to decrease the patient's anxiety and capitalize on the patient's ability to emotionally care for others. The patient should be protected from being thrust unassisted into new groups of people. Increasing the assertiveness and self-confidence of the patient is also a goal. Teaching age-appropriate socialization skills is necessary.

Overanxious Disorder. This disorder has excessive worrying and fearful behavior that is not focused on a specific object or recent stressor as determining characteristics.[23] Anxiety may be related to competence in areas such as school, sports, or peer relationships. The child may appear older than his chronological age because of "precocious" concerns. Treatment is concerned with the reduction of anxiety and strengthening of a sense of identity and self-esteem. Teaching the child age-appropriate play activities is necessary. Fostering peer-age friendships is appropriate.

Other Emotional Disorders of Infancy, Childhood, or Adolescence

Other emotional disorders often seen in child psychiatric settings are discussed below. See also Chapter 49 for a description of Infants and Mental Health.

Identity Disorder. This usually has an onset at late adolescence with severe subjective distress regarding inability to reconcile aspects of the self into a relatively coherent and acceptable sense of self. Long-term goals, sexual orientation, and group loyalties provoke uncertainty.[25]

Nursing care of the mild anxiety and depression that accompany the diagnosis is necessary. The nurse establishes a one-to-one relationship with the patient to promote a sense of worth and explore insecurities. The focus of the relationship is on increased independence in making decisions. Ambivalence about choices is worked through during treatment. Group support and treatment is also beneficial.

Physical Disorders

Eating disorders such as anorexia nervosa and bulimia are becoming increasingly common. Chapter 33 covers the diagnosis and treatment of these disorders in detail.

Enuresis

Enuresis is one of two physical problems encountered in child psychiatric settings. Enuresis is the repeated involuntary voiding of urine during the day or at night after an age at which continence is expected.[26] Studies indicate that etiologically this problem may have physiological, psychological, and hereditary roots. Because the etiology is unclear, staff must try to counteract the feelings of shame and guilt instilled by angry parents. Encouraging the child to take responsibility for his actions is often suggested. Fluids are restricted from after dinner until bedtime. The child is also encouraged to discuss his feelings of inadequacy. The child requires considerable support and firm expectations to achieve mastery of this problem.

Encopresis

Encopresis is the repeated voluntary or involuntary passage of feces of normal or near-normal consistency into places not appropriate for that purpose. The behavior is not due to any physical disorder.[27]

The nurse must begin to help the child explore the complex range of feelings he experiences along with soiling behavior. A goal is to help the child assume responsibility for cleaning up after an episode. The nurse must be aware of her own feelings and attitudes toward fecal soiling before she can be invested in a therapeutic intervention.

Developmental Disorders

Pervasive Developmental Disorders

Pervasive developmental disorders are characterized by distortions in the development of multiple basic psychological functions that are involved in the development of social skills and language, such as attention, perception, reality testing, and motor movement.[28] Pervasive developmental disorders may begin in infancy (autism) or later in childhood.

Nursing problems of such children are complex and require many levels of intervention. Emphasis on supporting ego development is central to care. The nurse attempts to promote appropriate behavior, decrease clinging, and reduce anxiety. Sensory stimuli may need to be reduced. The child must be protected from self-mutilating behavior. A change in the ward routine should be introduced gradually and carefully because this type of child is dependent upon a rigid routine.

Specific Developmental Disorders

This category includes disorders of specific areas not caused by another disorder. Each aspect of development in this category is related to biologic maturation. The etiology of such disorders is complex and may be biologic or nonbiologic.[29] Disorders may be centered around reading, arithmetic, language, or articulation.

The care of these disorders is often delivered by a specialized, multidisciplinary team. A complete neurological examination is especially important in these cases. Nurses provide the support necessary for patients to cope with their disability. Emphasis is on exploration of feelings, structuring situations in which the patient can gain mastery, and promoting peer relationships.

Situational Stressors

Children are not strangers to stress. Over a significant span of human history they have been more often the victims of stings and arrows of an uncaring society than the recipients of its beneficent protection.[30]

Currently children and adolescents are experiencing a variety of stressors that include child abuse and neglect, divorce and separation, chronic or acute illness, relocation, actual war, and threat of nuclear war.

The situational stressors of child abuse and neglect, sexual victimization, and chemical abuses are dealt with in other chapters of this text. The student is encouraged to review them.

Divorce and separation are experienced by many children in the United States each year. It has been estimated that in 1979 there was one divorce for every two marriages.[31] Over the years, the number and proportion of children involved in divorce has increased while the number of children per decree has decreased. Divorces now involve more than 1 million children under 18 annually.[32]

Wallerstein and Kelly studied the effects of divorce and separation on children longitudinally.[33] Their preliminary findings demonstrate that children have a variety of emotional responses, which include anger toward the parents, feelings of guilt, fantasies about reconciliation, and disruptions at school and with peers.

Nurses are in a key position to diagnose and treat the child's response to stressors such as divorce. It should be remembered that the child's developmental stage will interact with the situational stressor. Therefore, responses to similar stressors differ, in part as a result of variations in age. Wallerstein and Kelly, for instance, were able to determine age-specific responses to the divorce stressor. Preschoolers tended to regress behaviorally and worry about being abandoned by both parents. The early-school-age group, on the other hand, demonstrated moderate depression and was preoccupied with father's departure from the home.[34]

Crisis intervention services designed for children must incorporate the developmental perspective in order to deliver effective services.

SCOPE OF PRACTICE AND SETTING OF CHILD AND ADOLESCENT PSYCHIATRIC NURSING

Nurse generalists and nurse specialists may practice child psychiatric nursing. The registered nurse is a generalist who delivers nursing care to psychiatric patients.

The American Nurses' Association *Standards of Psychiatric and Mental Health Nursing Practice* delineates the following activities of the nurse generalist[35]:

1. Uses the nursing process as a framework to plan, implement and evaluate care.
2. Structures a therapeutic milieu.
3. Works collaboratively with patients to foster activities of daily living.
4. Provides health teaching.
5. Uses psychotherapeutic interventions to assist clients in regaining or improving their previous coping abilities.
6. Collaborates with other health care providers in the delivery of care.

Nurse specialists are nurses prepared at the Master's level or above in Psychiatric–Mental Health Nursing who are certified by the American Nurses' Association. The specialist may engage in the private practice of psychiatric and mental health nursing and provide individual, family, or group psychotherapy to adults, children, or adolescents. The specialist also participates with other members of the community in assessing, planning, implementing and evaluating mental health services and community systems that promote primary, secondary, and tertiary prevention of mental illness.[36]

Nurses in child psychiatric nursing practice in a variety of community and institutional settings. Inpatient, outpatient, and community-based programs are settings for the child psychiatric nurse. Nurses also function in a consultative role in the school, criminal justice, and social service systems.

THE NURSING PROCESS

The ANA Standards of Care and Standards of Psychiatric and Mental Health Nursing are based upon the nursing process.[37,38] Nurses use the process to collect data, formulate nursing diagnoses, develop interventions based on scientific rationale, and evaluate care.

A care plan developed by a senior nursing student during a psychiatric nursing rotation is presented below, directly following the case history. This nursing care plan was based on the nursing process. An example of a process recording of a student's session with Joy is also included.*

---

* The case history, nursing care plan, and process recording were prepared by Maureen Burke, a Simmons College nursing student, during her community mental health nursing course.

——— CASE EXAMPLE ———————————————————

I. Medical diagnosis (upon release from pediatric hospital): Conduct disorder, rule out psychotic disorder
II. Patient Summary
  A. Personal and Family History
    Patient is a 6-year-old interracial (black and white) female born 1-21-77. She lives with her mother, a 31-year-old black woman at present employed by the telephone company. Patient's mother and father severed contact before her birth. She knows nothing about him. Patient's relationship with mother is described in the charts as intense, intrusive, and physical. They would brush each other's hair, stroke each other's genital area, dress, bathe, and sleep together. At other times, however, they would have disagreements or struggles that would result in mother's screaming, swearing, and threatening physical violence. Maternal grandmother lives upstairs from patient and mother in a two-family house. Mother describes relationship with Grandmother as

close. Mother is the youngest of seven children and has never lived away from grandmother. At present there is a report of suspected child abuse filed on mother by a guidance clinic for sexual abuse. Mother admits to "inappropriate parenting" but denies abuse. She has relinquished temporary custody of patient to Department of Social Services, who is having a difficult time locating a weekend foster home.

B. History re Present Hospitalization:

The information available regarding patient's medical history is scant. At $3\frac{1}{2}$ years old patient was admitted to the hospital for vaginitis. A report of suspected child abuse secondary to sexual abuse was filed.

NURSING CARE PLAN
Conduct Disorder, Sexual Abuse

ASSESSMENT

A. Problem #1

S* "Here, this doll is the mother." [The doll with long blond hair and tan.] "My mother is sexy. She has short black hair, red lipstick, nail polish, black high heels, and very fancy clothes." "When my mother was young she had long blond hair. She tried very hard to be good."

O* In play, patient always used the tanned blond doll (the one most resembling her) to portray the mother. She always plays the mother, and whoever she is playing with portrays the 6-year-old daughter Joy. She is unable to describe her mother physically except for the cosmetic accessories she wears. She draws her mother with long blond hair, light skin, and accessories (make-up and jewelry) but no distinct physical features. She often dresses in provocative, seductive clothing. When she becomes angry, she swears, threatens physical abuse, and speaks in a voice imitating an adult black woman's. She often uses this "adult" voice when dealing with other children. She constantly asks others questions about herself and her feelings in an attempt to gain information. In addition, she frequently projects her feelings onto others. She sometimes refers to herself as "we" or "us" and other people as "girl," "boy," "him," "her," without associating a name.

Information in patient's chart as well as notes in the Nursing Communication Book supports these observations.

NURSING DIAGNOSES

- Self-concept, disturbance in personal identity related to impairment of self–mother differentiation.
- Self-concept, disturbance in self-esteem related to lack of eye contact, self-destructive behavior.

GOALS

Long-Term
1. Patient will be able to differentiate self as separate person from mother by end of May.
2. Patient will have concept of self as a person.

Short-Term
1. By Christmas, patient will use terms such as I, me, mine, when referring to self.
2. By Christmas, patient will be able to express or discuss anger and other emotions in her own voice rather than that of her mother.
3. With the assistance of staff, patient will now begin to refer to people (especially mother) by their proper names, thereby connecting a name with a face.

4. With the assistance of the staff, patient will begin describing people in terms of their physical and personal characteristics and not their accessories or material items.
5. By January, patient will be able to describe mother in terms of physical characteristics instead of material possessions.

INTERVENTIONS

1. Refer to patient and other people by name so that patient may begin to connect faces with names, the first step in identifying self and others as separate entities.
2. Discuss the different people on the unit in terms of personality traits and physical characteristics.
3. Encourge patient to do the same by asking direct questions that focus patient's attention on personal characteristics of others.
4. When patient refers to others in terms of material possessions or uses terms such as boy, girl, him, supply their name for her.

_____

* S = subjective; O = objective.

NURSING CARE PLAN
Conduct Disorder, Sexual Abuse

ASSESSMENT

B. Problem #2

S

O   Patient becomes so involved in play with dolls that she becomes oblivious to surroundings. She does not respond to questions unrelated to play unless they are repeated several times. Her voice mannerisms and expressions take on those of the doll (using the "mother" doll). She often asks if the dolls can speak or feel and sometimes insists they can. During the monopoly game, she became inappropriately concerned with the money, constantly asking what it can buy. She is very anxious about the cat. She fears that he will grow larger and attack her at night. She frequently asks questions about the differences between adults and children and demonstrates a very distorted image of what it means to be an adult. She often attempts to assign roles to people and to determine the corresponding expectations. Very often, however, these expectations have no basis in reality. According to her therapist, she is obsessed with the puppets he has and demonstrates great confusion in determining whether or not they are real. Themes of devil and monster possession frequently are brought out in therapy sessions.

When shopping with a counselor, patient was fascinated and frightened by costumes, gave them human characteristics and expressed the fear that they would "come after her."

The Communication Book and patient's chart support above data.

NURSING DIAGNOSIS

Thought processes, altered related to impaired reality-testing.

GOALS

Long-Term
1. By May, patient will be able to define general societal roles and corresponding expectations.
2. By May, patient will be able to distinguish between real and unreal by using proper reality-testing as evidenced by decreased confusion with dolls, puppets, etc.
3. By Christmas, patient will be able to distinguish between real and unreal in her play.

INTERVENTIONS

1. Constantly emphasize the difference between real and unreal, providing concrete demonstrations of how the conclusions were reached.
2. When in play with patient, emphasize that dolls, money, stuffed animals, etc., are not real.
3. Question patient as to what is real and what is not real in her environment. Ask her to substantiate.
4. Constantly assess patient's orientation (person, place, and time).
5. Discuss various roles of people in patient's environment—nurse, counselor, mother, therapist, child, and adult—and the expectations or significance of roles.
6. Set and enforce concise, realistic, consistent limitations with patient, providing explanations so patient can understand reasons for limitations.
7. Maintain frequent communication with other team members to ensure consistent implementation of interventions and to evaluate.

NURSING CARE PLAN
Conduct Disorder, Sexual Abuse

ASSESSMENT

C. Problem #3

S

O   Patient has questioned me regarding my sexual behavior. Patient has masturbated through clothing in my presence. In play with dolls, patient often dresses dolls in low-cut, tight-fitting, revealing clothing and has them speak and act in provocative, seductive manner. She is very interested in the "sexiness" of her wardrobe and expresses the desire to dress "sexy." She often asks questions concerning what is "sexy" and what is not. Also in play, the threats she voices as mother are often sadistic and sexual in nature. According to her chart and the Communication Book, she has engaged in inappropriate sexual behavior (masturbation, provocative advances, graphic verbalization) with other children. She has asked her male therapist to "take off his pants" and has voiced concern over being touched "down there" by male doctor.

NURSING DIAGNOSES

- Accessory to sex related to sexual abuse.
- Growth and development, altered, related to deviation in behavior, sexualization of interactions.

GOALS

Long-Term
1. Patient will establish healthy sexual identity appropriate for developmental stage.
2. Patient will be able to recognize and discuss feelings without first acting on those feelings inappropriately.

Short-Term
1. By end of November, patient will be aware of appropriate people to whom to direct questions regarding sexuality.
2. By semester break, patient will be able to bring up feelings and questions regarding sexuality without first acting on them.
3. By semester break, patient will be aware of inappropriate and appropriate sexual behavior.

INTERVENTIONS

1. Indicate to patient the appropriate people (counselors, nursing interns, therapist) to ask questions regarding sexuality. Be explicit as to what is meant by "questions regarding sexuality."
2. Answer all appropriate questions concisely, honestly, and in manner appropriate to patient's level of understanding. If question is not appropriate, inform the patient and give reason(s) why question is not appropriate.
3. Encourage patient through warm, receptive, sensitive approach to bring up sexual concerns.
4. Set and consistently enforce clear, concise limitations regarding sexual behavior.
5. Communicate verbally and nonverbally with other team members to ensure consistent implementation and evaluation.
6. Offer opportunities through symbolic play to work through feelings about her own sexual abuse.

NURSING CARE PLAN
Conduct Disorder, Sexual Abuse

ASSESSMENT

D. Problem #4

S

O   Patient's affect is not always consistent with the emotions she claims to be feeling, nor is it always appropriate to the situation patient is involved in.

Patient often laughs uncontrollably and in inappropriate situations.

Patient demonstrates mood swings without appropriate provocation. For example, she will become extremely angry and belligerent without external stimulus. In play, patient demonstrates extreme anger but often denies feelings of anger.

Patient expresses concern over her emotions. She has difficulty connecting the name of an emotion with the appropriate feeling. She constantly questions others about their feelings and often projects her own feelings to them.

Patient has great difficulty with and often refuses to discuss topics that generate any emotion. If pressed, she will retreat into fantasy or simply ignore question or statement or laugh inappropriately.

Notes from Communication Book and patient's chart support these observations.

NURSING DIAGNOSIS

Coping, ineffective individual, related to impaired ability to express emotions and inappropriate use of defense mechanisms.

GOALS

Long-Term
This problem is very much related to identity.
1. Patient will recognize feelings and, when appropriate, communicate these feelings to other people.
2. With assistance of staff, patient will employ appropriate methods of expressing and coping with feelings.

Short-Term

1. By Christmas, patient will express (not necessarily in an appropriate manner) feelings that are appropriate to situation.
2. Patient will be able to connect a behavior in others (e.g., a child on the unit screaming and "acting out") with a feeling (anger) regarding a certain situation (parents cancelling their visit) by Christmas.

INTERVENTIONS

1. Establish trusting relationship with patient so that she will feel comfortable expressing feelings.
2. Connect the label or description term for a feeling or emotion with situations that might arouse that feeling and with behaviors that might accompany it so that patient may begin to distinguish between different emotions and relate them to present experiences in her life.
3. Encourage patient by example and through warm, receptive approach and calm, controlled environment to discuss feelings.
4. Assure patient that feelings are valid and normal; they are neither good nor bad.
5. Relate various behaviors of patient to feelings she may be experiencing. Validate and encourage patient to expound upon or comment on observations.
6. Emphasize that patient must take responsibility for behavior.
7. Set and enforce reasonable limits for the expression of feelings.
8. Identify acceptable means of expressing and coping with feelings; provide rationale. Provide positive reinforcement when patient uses coping mechanism.
9. Communicate with staff to ensure consistent implementation and evaluation of the nursing care plan.

RESEARCH

The potential for nursing research in the area of child and adolescent psychiatry is practically limitless. Investigators who study the effectiveness of psychiatric nursing intervention are essential in a changing health-care delivery system environment that emphasizes cost containment.

Descriptions of several recent studies will indicate the range of possible area's for investigation. One study was designed to assess the inter-relationships between parents' and siblings' grief reactions following the death of a child or sibling.[39] A self-report questionnaire was used. This study is an excellent example of a study that investigates a situational stressor that child psychiatric nurses may encounter in their practice.

Findings demonstrated that parents' emotional distress was correlated with siblings' emotional distress and parented role dysfunction was correlated with siblings' behavior problems. The findings support grief theorists' assertions that children's unexpressed grief may be manifest as behavioral problems.

An early intervention program was designed by a child psychiatric nurse with a goal of reducing and preventing impairment to a child's social, emotional, and cognitive development.[40] The child psychiatric nurse who is knowledgeable about normal growth and development psychological assessment, counseling, and consultation is one mental health professional who is specifically prepared for this type of intervention.

A comparison of maternal lifetime psychiatric illness in cases of children with anxiety disorders and of children with other psychiatric disorders was made by Last and colleagues.[41] The study reports that 83 percent of the mothers of the clinic sample of children with separation anxiety disorder or overanxious disorder had a lifetime history of an anxiety disorder. However, approximately one half of the mothers presented with an anxiety disorder at the same time at which their children were seen for similar problems.

The need for seclusion rooms on a child psychiatric unit occupied another researcher, who reported on the experience of managing children in an eight-bed, acute short-term child

TABLE 31-3. PROCESS RECORDING

Perceptions and Patient Actions	Thoughts and Feelings	Nurse's Actions	Interpretations
1. I was sitting on the couch talking with Elaine, a 13-year-old patient who was home from school with a stomachache. Joy got out of class and came running down the hall toward me. She stopped directly in front of me, looked at Elaine and me with slightly angry expression, grabbed my hand and said, "Maureen, I'd like you to play a game with me."	2. Slightly uncomfortable because I knew that J. felt threatened because I was sitting next to E. and speaking with her.	3. Just a minute, Joy. I'm talking to Elaine right now.	4. J. has begun to regard me as *her* special person and feels threatened by my talking with Elaine. By grabbing me and demanding that I leave E. and play with her she is attempting to show E. that I'm "hers."
5. Joy sighs and stands there looking at me with no expression on face.		6. All right, Joy, what game shall we play?	
7. "Monopoly, Monopoly! Can we play Monopoly?"	8. Surprised at how quickly J.'s attitude changed.	9. "Sure. Elaine, would you like to join us?"	10. J. is relieved that I am directing my attention toward her—she has not "lost" me to E.
11. Joy: "Oh, no. She can't play. She has a stomachache. Just us will play."	12. I felt determined not to be manipulated by J. and not to contribute to E.'s loss of self-esteem by ignoring her presence or desire to play.	13. "Just because E. has a stomachache doesn't mean she can't play a quiet game of Monopoly. Even if she doesn't want to play, I'd like her to know that she's more than welcome to join us or to sit close and watch. Elaine, would you play?"	14. J. using E.'s stomachache as an excuse to exclude her. Attempting to manipulate me.
15. "Yes, Elaine, you can play if your stomach doesn't hurt too much."	16. Amused by J.'s turnaround.		17. Joy is attempting to ensure that she hasn't lost my affection by agreeing with me and inviting E. to play. She knows this will please me.
18. Elaine refused at first but then changed her mind and asked to join us.			
19. "Yes, Elaine. Sit here next to me." [Watching my face for signs of approval]	20. Very pleased that J. was behaving appropriately. Amused that she wanted E. to sit next to her, instead of next to me.	21. Smiled at both girls.	22. J. invites E. to play not because she wants her to but because she knows I want her to. She attempts to convey to E. that I am her special person by commanding E. to sit next to her, rather than next to me.

TABLE 31-3. (continued)

Perceptions and Patient Actions	Thoughts and Feelings	Nurse's Actions	Interpretations
23. After a few moments of the game, lunch was being served. Joy became very angry with Joan because she allowed Elaine to serve herself lunch but would not permit J. the same privilege.			
24. When Joan attempted to explain that E. is 13 and she has privilege of serving herself, J. began cursing and stuck up her middle finger at Joan. She was sent out and then returned to table.	25. Taken back by harshness of J.'s response.	26. Observed interaction between Joy and Joan.	27. J. expressing her anger the way she has learned to.
28. During lunch, J. was very restless at the table. She began stuffing large quantities of food into mouth, chewing it with mouth open, and spitting contents out.	29. Slightly nervous because this is the first time J. has ever deliberately provoked me.	30. "Joy, that is not appropriate behavior for the dinner table, and if you don't stop it right now you'll sit out."	31. J. angry at both Joan and me—demonstrating this by deliberately acting inappropriately.
32. J. laughed and continued behavior, watching me for my reaction.	33. My anxiety heightened but I was determined to enforce the strict limits that had been set.	34. "J., sit out."	
35. "F--k you." Jumped up from the table and stuck up her middle finger.		36. "I'll give you to the count of 3 to get into that chair or then you'll go to the Quiet Room." (QR)	
37. "F--k you! F--k you!" Dancing around chair with both middle fingers in air, laughing uncontrollably.	38. Anxious because I knew I was losing control and the staff, students, and other children were watching me to see how I'd handle the situation.	39. "All right, J., I can see you need to go to the QR."	
40. Laughing uncontrollably, bouncing off walls in block area.		41. "I can see you need me to escort you to the QR." Took patient by hand and walked (practically dragged) to QR.	
42. In QR Joy began slapping herself hard on the face and bending her fingers backwards: "I'll break my f--king fingers! I'll crack my f--king bones! I'll break my f--king skull!" [Still laughing]	43. Horrified at how out of control and angry she was. I knew (much to my dismay) that she would need to be restrained.	44. "Joy, I won't allow you to hurt yourself. I'm going to restrain your hands until you gain control and can be safe." Proceeded to firmly restrain hands behind her back.	

TABLE 31-3. (continued)

Perceptions and Patient Actions	Thoughts and Feelings	Nurse's Actions	Interpretations
45. "F--k you! Let go of my f--ing hands!" Started to whip head around, attempting to bang it on wall. "F--k you! I'll kill you, you f--king a--hole!"	46. Shocked at the anger in her threats but attempting not to convey this to J. Aware that I was sweating and that my heart was pounding at about 5 times its normal rate.	47. Keeping her arms behind her back with one of my hands I placed my other arm around her upper chest and pulled her close to me in order to contain her further. Said calmly in her ear: "Joy, you can swear at me, threaten me, even hit me, but I'm not going to let you go until I'm sure you'll be safe. I'm going to hold you until I can be certain you won't hurt yourself."	48. J. is testing me. She is out of control and determining whether or not I can contain her and keep her safe. The extreme anger she feels has been triggered by the events of the morning. Her anxiety is at the panic level and despite her protesting versus my intervening she is really desperately asking for my help.
49. Relaxed in my grip. Said in softer but very angry tone "I hate this f--king place. Let my f--king hands go. I won't hurt myself."	50. Relieved that at least physically she's regained control of herself.	51. "All right, you've calmed down. If you can promise me that you won't hurt yourself, I'll let you go and we can sit on the mat and talk. Can you promise me that?"	
52. I said I won't hurt myself, f--king goddammit."			53. J. is able to relax a little because she feels that I can at least keep her physically safe now. I am slowly allowing her to regain some control by making contact with her, i.e., asking her to promise not to hurt herself if I let her go.
		54. I release her and sat down next to her, very close to her but not touching her. "Joy, you are obviously very angry. Can you tell me why you're so angry?"	
55. She moved her body closer to mine but turned her face away from me. "I'm pissed at Elaine's stomachache. I'm f--king pissed off!" Patient speaking with "black" intonation.	56. At this point I felt so sorry for her I just wanted to hold her and tell her everything would be all right but I knew it wouldn't be appropriate. She's so used to relating only in a physical-sexual manner that I wanted to communicate with her without touching her (i.e., allowing her to press her body against mine).		57. J. displacing her anger—directing it toward a stomachache, something a lot less threatening than the actual source of her anger. Also, as J. feels more relaxed with me she attempts to press her body to mine. Sexual-physical contact is probably the only demonstration of any type of affection she's used to. She cannot, however, sustain eye contact—too invasive, unsafe.

TABLE 31-3. (*continued*)

Perceptions and Patient Actions	Thoughts and Feelings	Nurse's Actions	Interpretations
		58. "Well, a stomachache is not someone you can direct anger against. Are you angry with E. because she has a stomachache?"	
59. "She stayed home from school like a f--king baby and cried to everyone!. Everybody feels sorry for poor f--king E. She thinks she can take over meals and steal other people's special times. You let her, too! She needs to get her f--king self together."	60. My anxiety level was lower because J. was beginning to ventilate anger more appropriately.	61. "It sounds as if you're angry that E. received attention because she has a stomachache and that she has the privilege of serving herself because she's older. It seems as if you're also angry with J. and with me for spending time with E."	
62. "Yes . . . no, I'm not mad at you. Just get your f--king self together to be safe."	63. Feeling that she is projecting her feelings toward me and that more than E.'s stomachache has precipitated this display of anger.	64. "Joy, I am safe and I am together. I'm here now to help you to get together and be safe. Now what else is bothering you besides E.'s stomachache?"	65. J. projecting her feelings of being out of control, anxious and unsafe toward me in order to lower her own anxiety.
66. "Oh, sure, so you can beat the shit out of me! Talk to that Donna's f--king asshole! I'd like to f--king spit right in her face!" She begins to laugh and proceeds to spit on the mat.	67. Disappointed/ disgusted/sad that she would actually think I'd beat her for expressing her feelings. Also curious that she's bringing Donna's name up.	68. "Joy, I'll never beat you no matter what you do or no matter how much you swear, threaten, or try to hurt me. I'll keep coming back. I'll keep caring about you. I'll continue keeping you safe. Now, tell me about Donna. It sounds as though you are very angry with her."	69. Joy is asking for reassurance that I won't beat or punish her. Also she is revealing indirectly the real source of her anger—Donna who has become the symbol of *her* own *mother* on the ward. She has displaced rage and hatred for mother with Donna, which is much less threatening.
70. Joy's posture erect, body rigid, teeth clenched. She proceeded to recite a graphic litany of obscene sadistic and sexual things she intends to do to Donna.	71. I was horrified and shocked by what J. was saying but I was trying very hard to fight the revulsion and not convey this to J.	72. "You obviously have a lot of angry and hostile feelings re: Donna. What happened with her that makes you feel this way?"	
73. "She says them to me. She is a f--king mess! Don't you believe that bitch for a minute. She can't get herself together! She can't keep kids safe. She doesn't know what the f--k she's talking about! She f--king hates me, boy! I'm not safe! Nobody can keep me safe!"	74. Feelings of disgust and anxiety heightening as I realized that she was talking about her mother and not about Donna. The intensity of her fear and rage was frightening. I wasn't sure how I should respond. I didn't want to strip her defenses by disagreeing with her about Donna.	75. "I realize you're very angry, but Donna is very together. She would never hurt the children here. I really think you need to work out your anger with her. You have many concerns about being safe. It's good you're on full report. I'm going to recommend you stay on full report."	76. Again, J. is using Donna as target for anger. She feels that her mother will do those things to her, that her mother hates her, and that she is not safe with mother. She is indirectly asking (begging) me (and the staff) to keep her safe from her mother.

TABLE 31-3. *(continued)*

Perceptions and Patient Actions	Thoughts and Feelings	Nurse's Actions	Interpretations
77. Joy sighs and leans on me. "Can I eat now? I'm hungry and I want to get out of here."	78. Relieved that she's ventilated some anger and gotten herself under control. Aware that she's revealed a lot and has had enough time with me for one day.	79. "All right, if you do good chair time you may go back to the table."	80. By informing J. that she will stay on full report I am guaranteeing that we'll keep her safe. This relieves (or at least decreases) her anxiety for the time being. She is emotionally exhausted and wishes to end our discussion. Lunch provides the excuse she needs.
81. Did good chair time and went back to table.		82. Reported incident to staff nurses verbally and rest of staff via Commun. Book.	

psychiatric unit.[42] The techniques used to manage the children's behavior included the standard interventions of milieu therapy, such as processing, negotiating, avoidance of power struggles, and stress-reducing strategies. The author concluded that a coherent, safe and therapeutic milieu can be organized without a seclusion room.

A fifth study examined the effects of the presence of a severely disabled child in the family on psychopathology in nondisabled (normal) siblings.[43] The 5-year follow-up of 192 siblings and 284 controls aged 11 to 23 years showed a decline in mothers' perception of the siblings' functioning. Excess aggression, depressive affect, and social isolation were noted in the siblings. Depressive symptoms were also noted in the mothers of disabled children. It should be noted, however, that the rate of *DSM-III-R* major depression was not significantly different for either siblings or mothers of the disabled as compared with the controls.

Summary

This chapter examines child psychiatric nursing interventions from a developmental framework which is integrated with the *DSM-III-R*. The settings and roles of the psychiatric nurse are discussed. The nursing process and process recordings provide a conceptual schema for organizing patient data and the nurse's reactions to patients.

Questions

1. What is the advantage of using a developmental framework to assess a child or adolescent psychiatric patient?
2. What nursing interventions are appropriate to use with a 9-year-old male with a conduct disorder, socialized nonaggressive?
3. Identify two situational stressors impacting on children in the United States in increasing numbers.
4. A mother tells you that her 6-year-old son has begun soiling himself while at school. She asks your advice. What would you recommend?
5. Why is the technique of limit setting especially important in child psychiatric nursing?

REFERENCES AND SUGGESTED READINGS

1. Healy, W. *Twenty-Five Years of Child Guidance.* Chicago: Institute for Juvenile Research, 1934.
2. Freud, A. *Sexual Enlightenment of Children.* New York: Macmillan, 1963.
3. Freud, A. *The Psychoanalytic Treatment of Children.* New York: International Universities Press, 1965.
4. Klein, M. *The Psychoanalysis of Children.* London: Hogarth Press, 1932.
5. Ginsburg, H., & Opper, S. *Piaget's Theory of Intellectual Development,* 2nd ed. Englewood Cliffs, N.J.: Prentice-Hall, 1979.
6. Hall, C., & Lindzey, G. *Theories of Personalities,* 3rd ed. New York: Wiley, 1978.
7. Binet, A., & Binet, S. *The Development of Intelligence in Children.* Baltimore: Williams & Wilkins, 1916.
8. Catell, J. Mental tests and measurements. *Mind, 15,* 1890, 373.
9. Committee on Child Psychiatry. *Psychopathological Disorders in Childhood: Theoretical Considerations and a Proposed Classification* (Vol. 6, Report 62). New York: Group for Advancement of Psychiatry, 1966, p. 183.
10. Weeks, E., & Mack, J. The child. In A. Nicholi (Ed.), *Harvard Guide to Modern Psychiatry.* Cambridge, Mass.: Belknap Press of Harvard University, 1978, p. 497.
11. Erikson, E. Growth and crises of the healthy personality. In *Identity and the Life Cycle: Psychological Issues* (Monograph No. 1). New York: International Universities Press, 1959.
12. Ginsburg, H., & Opper, S. *Piaget's Theory of Intellectual Development,* 2nd ed. Englewood Cliffs, N.J.: Prentice-Hall, 1979.
13. Joint Commission on Mental Health of Children. *Crisis in Child Mental Health: Challenge for the 1970's.* New York: Harper & Row, 1970, p. 251.
14. American Psychiatric Association. *Diagnostic and Statistical Manual of Mental Disorders,* 3rd ed. (Rev.). Washington, D.C.: American Psychiatric Association, 1987, p. 36.
15. Rehabilitation Comprehensive Service and Developmental Disabilities Amendments of 1978 (PL 95-602). Washington, D.C.: U.S. Government Printing Office, 1978.
16. *DSM-III-R,* p. 50.
17. Ibid.
18. Ibid., p. 52.
19. Ibid., p. 53.
20. Ibid., p. 58.
21. Ibid., p. 59.
22. Ibid., p. 61.
23. Ibid., p. 63.
24. Ibid., p. 56.
25. Ibid., p. 71.
26. Ibid., p. 84.
27. Ibid., pp. 82–83.
28. Ibid., p. 33.
29. Ibid., p. 86.
30. Garmezy, N. Stressors of childhood. In N. Garmezy & M. Rutter (Eds.), *Stress, Coping and Development in Children.* New York: McGraw-Hill, 1983, p. 49.
31. Levitan, S., & Belous, R. *What's Happening to the American Family?* Baltimore: Johns Hopkins University Press, 1981, p. 29.
32. *Ibid.,* p. 60.
33. Wallerstein, J., & Kelly, J. The effects of parental divorce: Experiences of the child in later latency. *American Journal of Orthopsychiatry,* 1976, 46, 256–259.
34. Wallerstein, J. Children of divorce: stress and developmental tasks. In N. Garmezy, & M. Rutter (Eds.), *Stress, Coping and Development in Children.* New York: McGraw-Hill, 1983, pp. 279–280.
35. American Nurses' Association. *Standards of Psychiatric and Mental Health Nursing Practice.* Kansas City, Mo.: American Nurses' Association, 1982.
36. *Ibid.*
37. American Nurses' Association. *Standards of Nursing Practice.* Kansas City, Mo.: American Nurses' Association, 1973.
38. American Nurses' Association, op. cit. (1982).
39. Demi, A., & Gilbert C. Relationships of parental grief to sibling grief. *Archives of Psychiatric Nursing,* 1987, 1, 385–391.
40. Helmer, L., & Laliberté, M. Assessment groups for preschool children: A preventive program. *Archives of Psychiatric Nursing,* 1987, 1, 334–340.
41. Last, C., Hersen, M., Kazdin, A., Francis, G. and Grubb A. Psychiatric illness in the mothers of anxious children. *American Journal of Psychiatry,* 1987, 144, 1580–1583.
42. Irwin, M. Are seclusion rooms needed on child psychiatric units? *American Journal of Orthopsychiatry,* 1987, 57, 125–126.
43. Breslau, N., & Prabucki, K. Siblings of disabled children. *Archives of General Psychiatry,* 1987, 44, 1040–1046.

Chapter 32

Adolescent Disorders

Maureen P. McCausland

Chapter Objectives

The students successfully attaining the goals of this chapter will be able to:

- Describe the societal issues facing adolescents that may impact on their mental health.
- Describe normal growth and development of adolescents.
- Identify the range of emotional and behavioral disorders that may be present in adolescents.
- Identify selected situational stressors that impact on adolescents.
- Apply the nursing process and nursing diagnosis in the delivery of care to adolescents treated in community mental health or inpatient psychiatric settings.
- Describe areas of future research in adolescent psychiatric nursing.
- Identify the scope of practice and settings of adolescent psychiatric nursing.

Adolescence is a time of growth, challenge, transition, and stress both for individuals and their families. The adolescent is neither adult nor child. The successful completion of the developmental tasks of this stage are critical for the transformation from a child into a fully able adult.

Adolescence plays a profoundly significant role in the life of the individual and in society as a whole.[1] The adolescent is faced with physical and emotional changes. Multifaceted environmental and societal issues influence the adolescent. Adolescents in turn exert a strong influence in establishing the tone of our particular culture.[2]

This chapter will (1) provide a definition of adolescence; (2) discuss societal pressures affecting adolescents; (3) relate *DSM-III-R* diagnoses with nursing diagnoses and care plans; and (4) explore the role of the adolescent psychiatric nurses.

DEFINITION

A wide variety of definitions of adolescence exist and are related to the theoretical perspective that developed them. Biologists, psychologists, cognitive experts, and sociologists all address the issue of adolescence.

The American Psychiatric Association defines adolescence "as a chronological period beginning with the physical and emotional processes leading to sexual and psychosocial maturity and ending at an ill-defined time when the individual achieves independence and social productivity. The period is associated with rapid physical, psychological, and social changes."[3]

SOCIETAL ISSUES

Muuss reports on the secular trend, reflecting the idea that the children of today grow faster, experience the adolescent growth spurt earlier, reach puberty earlier, and attain their adult height earlier than before.[4] This secular trend is also evidenced by a decline in the age of dating and an increase in the number of adolescents engaging in physical intimacies and intercourse at an earlier age. The resulting sociomedical problems of increased incidences of venereal disease and illegitimate births in young persons are familiar to most providers of adolescent health care.

Adolescents and their families are at risk for a wide variety of social problems that have the potential to impact on mental health. Divorce and separation now affects one out of every two families.[5] Blended families with children from earlier marriages of both spouses are becoming more prevalent.

Drug and alcohol abuse by adolescents are receiving renewed media and professional attention. The psychiatric nursing implications of alcohol and drug abuse are discussed in Chapter 35.

NORMAL GROWTH AND DEVELOPMENT

Only recently has adolescence been recognized as a distinct period in the human life cycle. The term adolescence first appeared in the literature during the first half of the fifteenth century, but it was rarely used until the latter part of the eighteenth century. As a result of societal changes linked with the Industrial Revolution, passage of laws against child labor, and increased demands for prolonged education, adolescence emerged as a transitional period in the human life cycle.[6]

The developmental tasks and stresses of adolescence have been demonstrated to be monumental for many.[7] Adolescence represents a transition for the school-age child from a comfortable position as a dependent family member to a social position separate from the family. Adolescents must begin to take responsibility for their well-being and social behavior. Concurrently, marked anatomic and physiological changes as a result of physical and sexual development, coupled with the changing values in society and peer group pressures result in a unique and often stormy developmental period for the adolescent and his family.[8]

The criterion for attaining a comfortable and productive adult stage is the integration of a new body, new sexuality, new individuality, and new responsibility and control. This integration is, in turn, dependent upon the developmental aspects of separation from the family and behavioral control.[9]

The theoretical works of Erikson, Freud, and Piaget provide information that is very useful in adolescent psychiatric nursing.[10–12] Table 31-1 outlines the developmental tasks of adolescence as conceptualized by Erikson, Freud, and Piaget.

Both parents and children play a role in the developmental tasks of this stage. It is not surprising that changes in adolescent behavior may disrupt family systems, causing stress for many or all of the family members. It is not unusual for adolescents and their families to turn to the health care system for assistance at this time.

DEVELOPMENTAL DISORDERS

Mental Retardation

The mentally retarded adolescent demonstrates significantly subaverage general intellectual functioning, accompanied by significant deficits or impairments in adaptive functioning.[13]

The psychiatric nursing care of the mentally retarded is discussed in Chapter 45.

DISRUPTIVE BEHAVIOR DISORDERS

This subclass of disorders is characterized by behavior that is socially disruptive and is often more distressing to others than to the people with the disorders.[14] The subclass includes attention-deficit hyperactivity disorder, oppositional defiant disorder, and conduct disorder.

Conduct disorder and oppositional defiant disorder are discussed here in relationship to adolescents. Please refer to Chapter 31 for a discussion of attention-deficit hyperactivity disorder.

Conduct Disorder

The essential feature of this disorder is a persistent pattern of conduct in which the basic rights of others and major age-appropriate societal norms or rules are violated. The behavior pattern typically is present in the home, at school, with peers, and in the community.[15]

Three types of conduct disorders are differentiated: group, solitary aggressive, and undifferentiated. Table 31-2 shows the defining characteristics of each type of conduct disorder. The age of onset of these disorders is usually prepubertal, particularly of the solitary aggressive type. Postpubertal onset is more common among females than males.

Adolescents may have already experienced the juvenile criminal justice system before an inpatient psychiatric hospitalization is ordered. The psychiatric nurse must keep in mind that low self-esteem covered by a protective toughness usually accompanies a conduct disorder. Consistent limit setting, accompanied by a genuine caring, is essential for treating these patients.

Oppositional Defiant Disorder

A pattern of negativistic, hostile, and defiant behavior without the more serious violations of the basic rights of others that are seen in conduct disorders constitute the essential features of oppositional defiant disorder.[16]

The features of oppositional defiant disorder may be seen during the course of the psychotic disorders, especially schizophrenia or during manic, hypomanic, or major depressive episodes.[17]

EATING DISORDERS

Eating disorders including anorexia nervosa and bulimia nervosa typically begin during adolescence. Chapter 33 discusses the disorders and the nursing care.

GENDER IDENTITY DISORDER OF ADOLESCENCE, NONTRANSSEXUAL TYPE

The essential features of this disorder are persistent or recurrent discomfort and sense of inappropriateness about one's assigned sex, and persistent or recurrent cross-dressing in the role of the other sex either in fantasy or in actuality.[18]

IDENTITY DISORDER

According to Erikson, identity versus role confusion is a major developmental task of adolescence. Identity disorder is characterized by severe subjective distress regarding inability to integrate aspects of the self into a relatively coherent and acceptable sense of self.[19]

Self-doubt and doubt about the future are usually present, and take the form of either difficulty in making choices or impulsive experimentation. Negative or oppositional patterns are often chosen in an attempt to establish an independent identity distinct from family or other close people.[20]

SCHIZOPHRENIA

The onset of schizophrenia is typically during adolescence or early adulthood. The individual with this disease fails to achieve the expected level of social development. Characteristic symptoms involve multiple psychological processes.[21] Chapter 37 addresses multiple theories of the cause of schizophrenia and the nursing process in caring for the schizophrenic patient.

The first psychotic episode and the diagnosis of schizophrenia are usually very frightening for the patient and his family. Adolescent psychiatric nurses are in a key position to work with both individuals and families. The patient is typically dependent on nurses for physical as well as psychosocial care. Teaching about the disease, medications, and behavioral management is extremely important.

The local chapter of the Alliance for the Mentally Ill may provide excellent peer support for the patients' family.

─── CASE EXAMPLE ───────────────────────────────

Mark is a 16-year-old white male with a psychiatric diagnosis of schizophrenia. This is his first psychiatric hospitalization. The patient reports hearing voices "that tell me to jump from the roof." He is suspicious of nursing staff and lashes out violently without warning.

NURSING CARE PLAN

NURSING DIAGNOSES

- Altered thought processes related to command hallucinations and suspiciousness.
- Potential for violence related to suspicion of others and hallucinations.

LONG-TERM GOALS

1. By discharge the patient will function at highest level possible with or without assistance despite presence of disturbed thinking.
2. By discharge patient will identify warning signs that indicate loss of control and will use a constructive outlet to manage behavior.

SHORT-TERM GOALS

1. Patient will not harm self by end of 1 week.
2. Patient will report hallucinations to nurse by end of 2 weeks.

INTERVENTIONS

- Institute suicide precautions because command hallucinations are destructive.
- Instruct patient to report hallucinations to nurse.
- Assist patient with activities of daily living as necessary.
- Establish trusting relationship with patient.
- Assist patient to identify antecedents to behavior change related to agitation or anger.

SUICIDAL BEHAVIOR

National attention has been focused on the increasing rate of adolescent suicide. A rate of 5 per 100,000 in 1960 has grown to 12.1 per 100,000 in 1982 for people aged 15 to 24 years.[22]

Suicide is the leading cause for 25 percent of teen-agers' deaths. Boys have a higher rate (up to four times more) than girls, and it is estimated that the actual suicide rate is probably three times the reported rate.[23]

Suicide risk occurs among young people who are dealing with the crisis of adolescence, who are experiencing added social stressors, who lack strong external supports and are alienated from family and friends, and who feel hopeless and helpless about resolving their problems.[24]

Psychiatric nurses in inpatient, ambulatory, and community settings are in key positions to care for the suicidal adolescent, case find, and educate adolescents and their parents and teachers about the risk factors and warning signs of suicide.

SCOPE OF NURSING PRACTICE

Adolescent psychiatric nurses practice in a variety of traditional and nontraditional settings. Inpatient adolescent units, community-based programs, and ambulatory settings are just a few of the potential practice sites for professional nurses.

Using the *American Nurses' Association Standards of Child and Adolescent Psychiatric and Mental Health Nursing Practice* as a framework, nurses are involved in providing numerous interventions to and for their adolescent patients.[25]

Therapeutic Environment

The role of the milieu is extremely important when caring for adolescents. The nurse designs and participates in developing a therapeutic milieu through consideration of physical, social, psychological, and cultural variables.[26] The adolescent and his family are oriented to the milieu and the rationale for limit setting, restraint, or seclusion. Both patient and family are assisted to interpret the effect of interactions with staff and the other members of the milieu. The milieu should be goal-directed, therapeutic, and safe.[27]

Activities of Daily Living

Nurses are the major health care providers who interact with patients on a day-to-day basis around the tasks of daily living. Adolescents should be encouraged to collaborate in self-care as appropriate for their development. Daily situations should be used as a basis for therapeutic interactions.[28]

Psychotherapeutic Interventions

Nurses diagnose actual or potential health problems that impede the patient's normal, healthy development. Knowledge of phenomena such as anxiety, loss, guilt, conflict, grief, and anger is used to assist the adolescent and family in coping, adapting, and dealing constructively with feelings.[29] The psychiatric nurse uses herself in the therapeutic relationship to accomplish these goals.

Health Teaching and Anticipatory Guidance

Adolescents are a target population in need of education regarding normal development, developmental needs, mental health principles, and stress and coping. Societal issues mentioned earlier such as divorce, alcohol and drug abuse, and sexual development should be covered by providing anticipatory guidance.

Multifamily Group Therapy

Psychiatric nurses are potential group leaders for multifamily group therapy. The purpose of a multifamily group is to provide an opportunity for family members to talk about their situation, discuss their views and concerns, and to support and learn from others. Families may feel both relieved and guilty about their adolescents' hospitalization. The group experience provides a forum for working through those feelings.

NURSING RESEARCH

Research into the issues facing contemporary adolescents and their families offers an opportunity for nurses and other researchers to shed light on a major developmental and societal issue. Social support is a concept of particular relevance to adolescent psychiatric nurses. Kane[30] proposed a preliminary conceptual model of social support as a *process* of interaction through which the family develops versatility and resourcefulness rather than an outcome or a resource.

Suicide is addressed by researchers from both an epidemiological[31] and clinical[32] perspective in two recent studies. Nurses can use the findings from these studies to design suicide prevention programs specifically for at-risk adolescents.

Adolescence is often referred to as a time of crisis. Gutstein[33] reported on the Systematic Crisis Intervention Program which uses the opportunity of the crisis precipitated by the adolescent's life-threatening behavior to alter family myths that have led to network fragmentation. The observations and theoretical perspective of the author are valuable for adolescent psychiatric nurses.

Adolescents and their families often seek help in emergency rooms. Hillard, Slomowitz, and Levi[34] compared characteristics of 100 visits by adolescents to a psychiatric emergency service with those of 100 visits by adults. Adolescents were more likely to receive diagnoses of adjustment and conduct disorders, were equally likely to be in current treatment and required more time to evaluate than adults. Self-destructive ideation or behavior was present in 40% of the adolescents. Nearly all visits were judged to have represented genuine emergencies.

Recent attention has focused on the children of alcoholics. Bogdamiak and Piercy[35] reported the synthesis of years of clinical experience counseling adolescent children of alcoholics. A program that uses a combination of educational and therapeutic principles is recommended. Nurses should be familiar with the concerns of this target population because of the widespread prevalence of alcohol abuse in the contemporary family.

Summary

This chapter examines adolescent psychiatric nursing interventions from a developmental framework which is integrated with *DSM-III-R*. Nursing care is conceptualized using the nursing process and nursing diagnosis. The scope of nursing practice is also discussed.

Questions

1. Discuss various health promotion activities that can impact on adolescent suicide.
2. Explore the role of the nurse in the milieu of an adolescent inpatient unit.
3. Discuss strategies for limit setting with an adolescent with a conduct disorder, group type, and potential for violence.

REFERENCES AND SUGGESTED READINGS

1. Nicholi, A. The adolescent. In A. Nicholi (Ed.), *The Harvard Guide to Modern Psychiatry.* Cambridge, Mass.: Belknap Press of Harvard University Press, 1978, p. 519.
2. Ibid.
3. American Psychiatric Association. *A Psychiatric Glossary.* Washington, D.C.: American Psychiatric Association, 1975, p. 48.
4. Muuss, R. (Ed.). *Adolescent Behavior and Society: A Book of Readings,* 2nd ed. New York: Random House, 1975, pp. 1, 56.
5. Levitan, S., & Belous, R. *What's Happening to the American Family?* Baltimore: John Hopkins University Press, 1981, p. 29.
6. Muuss, op. cit., p. 56.
7. Lourie, I. The phenomenon of the abused adolescent: A clinical study. *Victimology: An International Journal,* 1977, 2, 271–272.
8. Bandura, A. The stormy decade: Fact or fiction? In R. Muuss (Ed.), *Adolescent Behavior and Society, A Book of Readings,* 2nd ed. New York: Random House, 1975, p. 25.
9. Lourie, op. cit., pp. 271–272.
10. Erikson, E. Growth and crises of the healthy personality. In *Identity and the Life Cycle: Psychological Issues* (Monograph No. 1). New York: International Universities Press, 1959.
11. Freud, S.
12. Ginsburg, H., & Opper, S. *Piaget's Theory of Intellectual Development,* 2nd ed. Englewood Cliffs, N.J.: Prentice–Hall, 1979.
13. American Psychiatric Association. Diagnostic and Statistical Manual of Mental Disorders, 3rd ed. (Rev.). Washington, D.C.: American Psychiatric Association, 1987, p. 28.
14. Ibid., p. 49.
15. Ibid., p. 53.
16. Ibid., p. 56.
17. Ibid., p. 57.
18. Ibid., p. 76.

19. Ibid., p. 89.
20. Ibid., p. 89.
21. Ibid., pp. 187–188.
22. Hollinger, P., Offer, D., & Ostrov, E. Suicide and homicide in the U.S.: A epidemiologic study of violent death, population changes, and the potential for prediction. *American Journal of Psychiatry*, 1987, *144*, 217.
23. Department of Health, Education and Welfare. *Healthy People* (Public Health Service Publication No. 79-5571). Washington, D.C.: U.S. Government Printing Office, 1979.
24. Gilead, M., & Mulaik, J. Adolescent suicide: A response to developmental crisis. *Perspectives in Psychiatric Care*, 1987, *21*(3), 97.
25. American Nurses' Association. *Standards of Child andAdolescent Psychiatric–Mental Health Nursing Practice*. Kansas City, Mo.: American Nurses' Association, 1985.
26. Ibid., p. 12.
27. Ibid.
28. Ibid., p. 13.
29. Ibid., p. 14.
30. Kane, C. Family social support: Toward a conceptual model. *Advances in Nursing Science*, 1988, *10*(2), 18–25.
31. Hollinger, P., Offer, D., & Ostrov, E. Suicide and homicide in the U.S.: A epidemiologic study of violent death, population changes, and the potential for predictors. *American Journal of Psychiatry*, 1987, *144*, 215–218.
32. Friedman, J., Asnis, G., Boeck, M., & DiFiore, J. Prevalence of specific suicidal behaviors in a high school sample. *American Journal of Psychiatry*, 1987, *144*, 1203–1206.
33. Gutstein, S. Family reconciliation as a response to adolescent crises. *Family Process*, 1987, *26*, 475–491.
34. Hillard, J., Slomowitz, M., & Levi, L. A retrospective study of adolescents' visits to a general hospital psychiatric emergency service. *American Journal of Psychiatry*, 1987, *144*, 432–436.
35. Bogdamiak, R., & Piercy, F. Therapeutic issues of adolescent children of alcoholic groups. *International Journal of Group Psychotherapy*, 1987, *37*, 569–588.

Chapter 33

Eating Disorders of Adolescence: Anorexia Nervosa and Bulimia

Constance M. Carino
Patricia Chmelko

Chapter Objectives

The students successfully attaining the goals of this chapter will be able to:

- Describe the clinical syndromes of anorexia nervosa and bulimia.
- Describe the nursing diagnosis of alterations in nutrition.
- Integrate psychiatric and nursing diagnoses in planning patient care in eating disorders of adolescence.

Disorders of eating and body weight, especially notable in adolescence, encompass a broad range of medical, nursing, psychological, and social problems. Patients do not usually come for psychiatric help with a chief complaint of weight or appetite disturbance. More commonly, they are referred to mental health clinicians by family physicians or internists who have seen the adolescent at the request of a parent.

The goal of this chapter is to discuss approaches to the clinical syndromes of anorexia nervosa and bulimia in terms of psychiatric and nursing diagnoses and nursing care plans.

THE CLINICAL SYNDROME OF ANOREXIA

Anorexia nervosa is a clinical syndrome characterized by a voluntary refusal to eat, usually explained by the patient saying that he or she is not hungry.[1] Females constitute 95 percent of those in whom the diagnosis is made. The age of onset can range from prepuberty to the thirties but generally occurs between the ages of 12 and 18. *The Diagnostic and Statistical Manual of Mental Disorders* (*DSM-III-R*) of the American Psychiatric Association lists the following criteria for confirming the diagnosis of anorexia nervosa[2]:

Diagnostic Criterias for Anorexia Nervosa

A. Refusal to maintain body weight over a minimal normal weight for age and height.
B. Intense fear of gaining weight or becoming fat, even though underweight.
C. Disturbance in the way in which one's body weight, size, or shape is experienced.
D. In females, absence of at least three consecutive menstrual cycles when otherwise expected to occur (primary or secondary amenorrhea).

Hilde Bruch, in her book *Eating Disorders: Obesity, Anorexia, and the Person Within*, states that impairment of psychological functioning can be recognized uniformly in almost all anorectic patients. Symptoms are[3]:

1. A disturbance in body image and body concept of delusional proportions.
2. Inaccurate and confused perception and cognitive interpretation of stimuli arising in the body, with failure of recognition of signs of nutritional needs as the most profound deficiency.
3. A paralyzing sense of ineffectiveness that pervades all thinking and activities.

Defining Characteristics of Anorexia

Body Image Disturbances
Body image disturbances are evidenced by the stubbornness and steadfast manner in which the anorectic patient defends her skeleton-like appearance as being normal, right, and not too thin. It is her only security against the dreaded fear of becoming fat. Development of a realistic body image is essential for the patient's recovery from anorexia nervosa.

Misperception of Bodily Function
Misperception of bodily function arouses the most concern as well as the most frustration. The term *anorexia* is really a misnomer. It refers to the patient's refusal to eat or abstinence from food, not to a true loss of appetite. The problem lies in the patient's inability to recognize hunger and nutritional needs. The problem is much more complex than just the refusal to eat. Eating behavior becomes disorganized, and unhealthy practices emerge. The patient becomes frantically preoccupied with food and eating, often restricting food intake to protein only. Many patients are gourmet cooks and will prepare lavish meals for family members while eating only a few morsels themselves. They will often take hours to finish the smallest meal, cutting everything into minuscule size. This dawdling and preoccupation with food are consistent with what is observed during the process of starvation.

In an experimental study in semistarvation carried out during World War II with a group of healthy young men, a characteristic pattern was observed. The men would toy with their food and dawdle for almost 2 hours over the meal. As the starvation progressed, there was no diminution in the desire for food, and food became the dominant topic of all conversation and thinking.[4] Victims of starvation will eat whatever they can find, in contrast to the starving anorectic who lives in a food-rich culture but, because of fear of losing control, rejects food. Anorectics will complain of feeling full after only a few mouthfuls of food. Others complain of feeling full just watching another person eat. This is explained in part by a poor sense of identity and the inability to differentiate themselves from others. It is important to clarify that in the very late stages of emaciation and starvation, a true loss of appetite can occur, resulting in severe nutritional deficiencies and a lack of interest in food. In an effort to keep weight low, anorectics often resort to self-induced vomiting, laxative, and diuretic abuse. Serious electrolyte disturbances, cardiac arrest, and arrhythmias may occur.

Hyperactivity
Hyperactivity is another manifestation of misperceived bodily function. The drive for excessive activity can persist until the patient becomes severely emaciated. Patients give subjective accounts of feeling alert and energized. Families often report that the patient will study for hours, late into the night. It is uncertain whether this is a result of hyperactivity or whether it is due to poor concentration and decreased energy. What used to be accomplished in a short time now takes hours to accomplish.

A Paralyzing Sense of Ineffectiveness
A paralyzing sense of ineffectiveness is experienced by these patients as a form of helpless-

ness. They perceive themselves as responding only to the demands imposed on them by others and not doing anything because they themselves want to. This helplessness is incongruent with reports of the patients' early growth and development. Typically, parents will describe their children as outstandingly good, obedient, eager to please, helpful at home, dependable, and excelling in school. A childhood of robot-like obedience has left these children ill-prepared for the tasks of adolescence since they are deficient in initiative and autonomy.

The onset of this illness is often precipitated by a new experience such as going to camp or college. Many patients can recall a remark made to them concerning their weight in the new environment. Weight loss becomes a symptom, an expression of an underlying fear of incompetence. The person gains a sense of competency and accomplishment by controlling her eating and weight.

THE CLINICAL SYNDROME OF BULIMIA

Bulimia nervosa, referred to as *bulimia* in the literature, is a clinical syndrome characterized by voluntary restriction of food intake followed by extreme overeating and then attempts to rid the body of food by self-induced vomiting and laxative abuse. In contrast to patients with anorexia nervosa, bulimic patients are somewhat older, more socially inclined, have fewer obsessive characteristics, and actually lose control of eating. Andersen defines the essential criteria for the diagnosis of bulimia as listed below.[5]

1. An irresistible urge to eat, leading to the ingestion of large quantities of food.
2. The use of self-induced vomiting or laxative or diuretic abuse to counteract the effects of binge eating.
3. The presence of a preoccupying morbid fear of becoming overweight.

The *DSM-III-R* lists the following criteria in order to confirm the diagnosis of bulimia[6]:

Diagnostic Criteria for Bulimia Nervosa

A. Recurrent episodes of binge eating.
B. A feeling of lack of control over eating behavior during the eating binges.
C. The person regularly engages in either self-induced vomiting, use of laxatives or diuretics, strict dieting or fasting, or vigorous exercise in order to prevent weight gain.
D. A minimum average of two binge eating episodes a week for at least 3 months.
E. Persistent overconcern with body shape and weight.

Defining Characteristics of Bulimia

Binging, a major characteristic of bulimia, suggests problems with impulse control. Concentration is impaired as a result of rumination, thoughts of food, or increased guilt feelings over a previous binge. Enormous quantities of high-caloric foods requiring little chewing are ingested. Binging occurs not because of a sensation of true hunger but often as a result of a lack of perceived satiety.

Bulimic patients often will exhibit many of the symptoms of anorexia nervosa. Generally, however, they do not appear emaciated, and weight loss is not as severe. The bulimic individual will strive to maintain an ideal weight for herself, which is often below what is considered to be a healthy weight. Maintenance of weight is achieved by avoidance of food in between bouts of binging, vomiting, laxative and diuretic abuse, and exercise.

The frequency and severity of binging vary greatly within the bulimic population. Some patients will have an episode of binge eating every 1 to 2 weeks, whereas others will succumb daily. Binge episodes may last from 15 minutes to 2 hours. There have been reports of binges lasting 24 hours followed by exhaustion. Laxative abuse varies from occasional use to 50 to 70 tablets daily. Vomiting may occur infrequently or after anything ingested.

Precipitants to binge eating are emotional stress, loneliness, and depression. The binge behavior only serves to intensify these feelings, further lowering self-esteem and impairing interpersonal relationships.

Vomiting

Bulimic patients rely on various methods to induce vomiting. The most common method is by insertion of the fingers into the mouth and throat to stimulate the gag reflex. This method sometimes results in ulcerations of the throat and scarring of the hands due to repeated forceful rubbing. Other patients will insert objects into their throats, such as a handle of a tooth brush.

Secretiveness

Bulimia is a secretive syndrome. Patients will conceal their symptoms from family and friends for prolonged periods of time. The ability to hide symptoms leads to the chronicity of the disorder. Behaviors frequently associated with bulimia are stealing and substance abuse. Some patients will steal food or money to support their binge habit. In these patients, stealing seems to be more of a problem with impulse control. Patients report substance abuse such as amphetamine use, as a means to control weight.

Depressive Symptoms

Depressive symptoms are generally present. Frequently the patients' outward appearance fails to reflect the severity of their feelings. Patients will subjectively report feelings of gloom, recurrent suicidal ideation, irritability, and impaired concentration.

THEORETICAL PREMISES

Although the diagnostic criteria have been refined in recent years, the causes of anorexia nervosa and bulimia, to a large extent, remain a mystery. The more accepted propositions for diagnosis are:

1. *Psychoanalytic Theory.* The development of anorexia nervosa implies a regression in psychosexual development to the oral or anal stage. It is an attempt to avoid adolescent sexuality by a return to these stages. "Typically, the anorectic shows such characteristics of these stages as stubbornness, obsessiveness, obstinancy, marked oral-anal fixation regarding eating, bowel and even bladder control. This regression is maladaptive and eventually leads in advanced cases to the adolescent or adult appearing childlike, losing secondary sex characteristics, finally being cared for and even fed by others."[7]

2. *Psychodynamic Theory.* Anorexia nervosa results from various ego deficits, and the pursuit of thinness is the struggle for control and sense of identity and personal effectiveness.

3. *Family Interactional Model.* The family interactional model developed by Minuchin proposes that the family "organizes" around the symptom (anorexia) and focuses so much on the disorder that it avoids other interpersonal conflicts. The child's symptoms thus serve to stabilize a dysfunctional family through the development of a psychosomatic illness. This type of family is described as having four transactional characteristics: enmeshment, overprotectiveness, rigidity, and lack of conflict resolution. The child plays a significant role in the family's pattern of conflict avoidance.[8]

4. *Behavioral Theory.* Behavioral theory is the most accepted theory of causation. Briefly stated, anorexia nervosa is viewed as a rejecting behavior and is reinforced by the attention it receives. The patient becomes the center of attention and learns to manipulate the environment for need gratification. Lack of success in meeting needs results in maladaptive behavior.

5. *Medical Theory.* Although the medical theory is a less accepted one, a possible cause may be in the hypothalamus (not a tumor but some type of "override") with subsequent weight loss, anorexia, and various chemical imbalances. Some proponents of this theory defend it by citing that amenorrhea develops before extreme weight loss in some instances. It is important to note that amenorrhea often develops as an emotional response to stress.

6. *Cultural Theory.* We live in a food-rich culture. Self-inflicted starvation would be an ineffectual tool in a setting of poverty and scarcity. Therefore self-starvation is usually found only under conditions of adequate food supply. It is not found in underdeveloped countries where threat of food shortage and famine exist. Our culture has been inundated with diet books, exercise programs, and self-improvement guides. Overweight, aging, and illness are considered moral weaknesses. This overconcern with bodily appearances may lead to various attempts at controlling the body by skipping meals, laxative or diuretic abuse, self-induced vomiting, and use of over-the-counter diet pills.

INDICATIONS FOR INPATIENT HOSPITALIZATION

Anorexia

The goals of treatment for the anorectic patient are weight gain, changing the patient's attitudes toward food, and the development of more effective coping skills to overcome the underlying conflicts. Hospitalization is definitely recommended when it becomes evident that these goals cannot be met in outpatient psychotherapy.

Specific criteria for admission are as follows:

1. Loss of 25 percent of body weight or more. Such weight loss leaves the patient physically and emotionally compromised. The patient is usually not responsive to psychotherapy and is in a life-threatening situation. Hospitalization is necessary for nutritional support and intensive psychotherapy.
2. Inability to cope with daily living. When patients cannot cope with daily living without resorting to the use of laxatives, diuretics, diet pills, or self-induced vomiting, even if weight is within the normal range, hospitalization is necessary to prevent serious electrolyte imbalances that could lead to medical complications and even death.
3. Family conflict. Often, there is a great amount of tension between the patient and the parents. Both sides are engaged in a power struggle surrounding the patient's eating behavior. Hospitalization can be effective in diffusing this power struggle by separating the patient from her parents. Also, individual family members can often gain a clearer perspective on the problem when the tension is reduced.
4. Severe depression with suicidal ideation. If the patient is experiencing suicidal ideation, hospitalization should be viewed as a necessary emergency measure. If the patient refuses to accept psychiatric treatment, the parents should be encouraged to take the necessary steps to commit the patient to the hospital for treatment as a lifesaving measure.
5. Obsessive–compulsive behavior. This is a behavior disorder marked by rumination, self-doubt, and repetitive acts, which impede effective functioning. It is very difficult to break this cycle. The patient will be more amenable to psychotherapy after receiving help in dealing with the obsessional thoughts and compulsive behavior. Hospitalization can offer an intensive approach to managing these symptoms.
6. Lack of motivation or cooperation. Anorexia nervosa should be viewed as a slow suicidal process. If the patient is unwilling to cooperate in outpatient therapy, a more active, intensive program is indicated.

Bulimia

Bulimia is a more recently recognized form of an eating disorder than anorexia. Prognosis is difficult to make since there is an absence of long-term follow-up studies. Treatment approaches should be aimed at normalization of eating behaviors by:

1. Eliminating or decreasing bouts of overeating.
2. Helping the patient accept a healthy weight.
3. Alleviation of depression.
4. Impulse control.

Hospitalization in a psychiatric facility is usually necessary to facilitate successful treatment. Hospitalization is essential if the risk of suicide is present or if medical complications develop due to diuretic and laxative abuse or purging.

PSYCHOTHERAPEUTIC INTERVENTIONS

Behavior Therapy

Behavior therapy attempts to alleviate specific behavioral problems as quickly as possible by controlling the learning behavior of the patient. Emphasis is placed on the overt observable symptoms of the patient. The theoretical model used is based on one of the many psychological learning theories developed in experimental laboratories. The three primary ways of altering behavior are:

1. Altering the antecedent situational events that precipitate a particular behavior (e.g., modifying the thoughts and feelings about food).
2. Altering the type of behavior that occurs in a particular situation (e.g., using a newly learned behavior to deal with the frustra-

tion of eating, talking to the nurse, or using relaxation exercises).

3. Altering the situational consequences to which the behavior leads. The idea is that certain behaviors are exhibited because they lead to satisfying results or because they enable the person to avoid painful consequences, e.g., the patient must learn to think and feel differently about her body and weight. Eating can become less anxiety-provoking when a patient can view it as a healthy behavior allowing more energy, promoting well-being, and functioning more effectively as an autonomous adult.

Behavioral Contract

This is an agreement that the patient makes with the therapeutic community (patients and staff) to change a maladaptive behavior. It is based on the principles of operant conditioning with positive reinforcement. The contract should be written by the treatment team with the patient's approval and written consent. If the patient does not agree to the use of the contract, it will be ineffective and the contract itself can become a source of power struggle. However, it can be a very effective tool in placing the responsibility on the patient for weight gain or changing other maladaptive behavior. The patient can gain a clear understanding of how she can effect weight changes. The patient can also begin to examine some of the false ideas held about food and gain a better understanding of the real relationships between food and weight.

Psychoanalysis

Psychoanalysis is a slow, tedious process. It emphasizes undoing repression and recovering lost memories, as well as the gradual integration of the previously repressed material into the total structure of the personality. Generally, this is not effective in treating anorexia nervosa. Effective treatment requires immediate emphasis on problems dealing with the outside world and not a narcissistic concentration on the body.

Insight-Oriented Therapy

An insight-oriented approach views anorexia nervosa as a symptom and would assume deeper conflicts. Emphasis is placed on dealing with the underlying issues or conflicts. Weight gain is only a part of the goal for therapy. Anorectic symptoms are an expression of ineffective coping skills. The goal of therapy is the development of healthier coping skills for dealing with stress. The type of insight gained should enable the patient to see herself objectively, thereby recognizing the perceptual distortions she has concerning her body. The role of the therapist is to assist the patient in looking at the difficulties she is dealing with. The therapist may make suggestions as to how the patient might approach a particular problem, but the patient must make the final decision in how to deal with the problem. Through this process the patient can achieve self-awareness.

Supportive Therapy

Supportive therapy is a more direct, confrontive, reality-oriented therapy. The goal of therapy is to assist the patient in becoming more self-reliant, independent, and mature. Direct suggestion is used by the therapist. The patient is given much positive reinforcement for using healthy defense mechanisms. The focus of therapy should not be weight and food issues but the development of interpersonal relationships and interaction with others.

Group Therapy

Group therapy can provide a very rewarding and growthful experience for the anorectic patient. It provides a safe forum for the patient to test out newly learned behaviors, to alleviate some of her fears by sharing her thoughts and feelings, and to reexamine her negative perceptions of self. The patient can develop a healthier self-concept by others sharing their perceptions of her. She can increase her self-esteem by having the opportunity to offer support and encouragement to others. The patient accomplishes this only by making the commitment with fellow group members not to discuss food and weight issues.

Family Therapy

Friedman and Kaplan outline the goals of family therapy as follows:

Family therapy derives from two fundamental propositions: First, the family is conceptualized as a behavior system with unique properties, rather than the sum of the characteristics of its individual members. Second, it is postulated that a close interrelationship exists between the psychosocial functioning of the family as a group and the emotional adaptation of its separate members.[9]

Families of anorectic patients are generally of small size and are female-dominated. Socio-economic status is middle to upper class, with a high proportion of patients coming from prosperous and professional homes. Age of parents at the birth of the anorectic child is generally higher than the norm, around 30 years of age. Marriages appear stable. Parents will emphasize the stability and happiness of their homes. On close observation, it can be recognized that parental encouragement for self-expression by the child is lacking. The child usually does not have the opportunity to make autonomous decisions or rely on her own inner resources.

The fathers, even though socially and financially successful, perceive themselves as second best and place a great emphasis on outer appearances. They expect good behavior and achievement from their children. The mothers are also success-oriented, many having had successful careers before having their children. Generally, they are conscientious in their role of mother. But they may feel thwarted in their aspirations, often living their lives through their children. Feeding histories for the anorectic child are negative for problems.

As mentioned earlier, this family is described as having four transactional characteristics: enmeshment, overprotectiveness, rigidity, and lack of conflict resolution.[10] **Enmeshment** refers to role confusion within the family. The tasks and roles of each family member are not clearly defined. Family members may expect others to know what they are thinking, or they may act on assumptions without clarifying what the other members are thinking. **Overprotectiveness** refers to an overconcern and overreaction to another family member's distress. Family members will quickly try to reduce the tension in order to protect the stressed individual.

In general, the goals to be achieved in family therapy include: resolving or reducing pathogenic conflict and anxiety within the matrix of interpersonal relationships; enhancing the perception and fulfillment by family members of one another's emotional needs; promoting more appropriate role relations between the sexes and the generations; and strengthening the capacity

of the individual and family as a whole to cope with destructive forces from within and from the surrounding environment.

INPATIENT NURSING CARE

The nursing approach to those patients with severe eating disorders is a holistic one in which the patient is conceptualized as a unified bio-psychosocial being who is in a continuous interaction with her environment.* This approach encompasses meeting the identified, individualized needs of the patient through an understanding and assessment of the interrelationship of psychological, physiological, social, and cultural processes. It also involves active participation in an interdisciplinary process, which facilitates the coordination of medical, nursing, social service, and occupational therapy goals and interventions.

Nursing Diagnoses

The nursing diagnosis most useful in planning care for the anorectic and bulimic patients seems to be the one titled Alterations in Nutrition: Less than Body Requirements, as determined by The National Conference Group for Classification of Nursing Diagnoses.[11] Interventions that are intended to aid in weight gain include the following:

1. Calorie counts as prescribed by physicians. These will be calculated by the patient and nurse at the meal.
2. Observation at mealtimes for structured support.
3. Initially, 90 minutes postprandial observations.
4. Monitor daily weight in hospital gown with arms at sides after emptying bladder to ensure accurate weight. It is important that this intervention be consistent.
5. Evening snack to be provided that is 10 percent of the patient's caloric requirement; 90-minute postprandial observation.
6. Structured support at mealtimes.
   a. Assist patient to avoid focusing on food.

* Acknowledgment is made to the Inpatient Psychiatric Nursing Staff at the Hospital of the University of Pennsylvania for their work in the development of a Standard of Care for the anorectic patient.

b. Avoid power struggles with patient.

c. Assess level of control and independence, e.g., ability to consume meal within a prescribed period of time.

d. Coaching techniques for helping the patient to eat:

1. Implementation of relaxation techniques.
2. Encourage patient to imagine or think more pleasant thoughts rather than somatic thoughts.
3. Provide pleasant environment for meals.
4. Reality testing regarding calorie intake.

7. Act as a role model to assist the patient to improve judgment about normal and abnormal eating behaviors.

8. Provide support and positive feedback for accomplishments made in normalizing eating habits and behaviors.

9. Provide supplemental feedings during mealtime when caloric intake is inadequate.

10. The daily required caloric intake is determined on an individual basis.

a. The total caloric intake for breakfast and lunch should be approximately two thirds of the total daily required calorie intake.

b. The evening snack should be approximately 10 percent of the total daily required calorie intake.

Additional nursing diagnoses related to anorexia and bulimia include:

1. Alterations in bowel elimination: constipation.
2. Ineffective family coping: disabling.
3. Alterations in nutrition: potential for more than body requirements.
4. Self-care deficit: feeding.
5. Disturbance in self-concept.
6. Sensory perceptual alterations.
7. Sexual dysfunction.
8. Sleep pattern disturbance.
9. Alterations in thought processes.
10. Spiritual distress.
11. Role disturbance.

Nursing Intervention

The goals of nursing interventions are directed toward assisting the patients to: (1) normalize their eating behavior; (2) develop realistic perceptions (attitudes) of their body and food; (3) develop adaptive coping mechanisms to deal with their perceptual distortions; (4) obtain a beginning identification and understanding of

---

TABLE 33-1. NURSING INTERVENTION CHECKLIST FOR ANOREXIA AND BULIMIA

Protocol for _____
                    (Name of Patient)

INSTRUCTIONS: Check as applicable—include date begun and date discontinued

___ 1. Menu will be selected by dietitian.
___ 2. Menu will be selected by patient.
___ 3. Meals will be eaten on hospital unit under observation.
___ 4. Meals will be eaten on hospital unit.
___ 5. Patient will be observed for 90 minutes after meals.
___ 6. Patient will be observed for 60 minutes after meals.
___ 7. Patient will not be observed after meals.
___ 8. Patient will use bathroom under observation during 90-minute observation.
___ 9. Patient will use bathroom only under observation.
___ 10. Patient will remain in lounge during waking hours, under observation.
___ 11. Patient will consume designated number of calories.

Date	Calories
___	800
___	1000
___	1200
___	1400
___	1680
___	1800
___	2000
___	2200
___	2400
___	2600
___	2800
___	3000
___	3200

___ 12. Passes and privileges are contingent on compliance with this protocol.
___ 13. Patient may use pass but will eat all meals in the hospital.
___ 14. Patient may eat meals outside the hospital.
___ 15. Patient will begin to eat meals outside the hospital with a staff member.
___ 16. Patient will be fed through a Dobbhoff tube the designated number of calories. The tube feedings will be given during the evening and night (8 P.M. to 8 A.M.) under observation.

their underlying issues and conflicts; (5) develop adaptive interactions and relationships with family and other support systems; (6) identify strengths in order to enhance self-worth and self-esteem; and (7) use a comfortable, non-threatening environment (milieu) in which to practice new behaviors and explore sensitive or painful issues.

Case histories and nursing care plans of an anorectic patient and a bulimic patient are given next. Table 33-1 provides a checklist of nursing interventions.

CASE HISTORY OF ANOREXIA NERVOSA

This was the first psychiatric hospitalization for this 22-year-old white, single female with anorexia nervosa. Her chief complaint: "I want to gain weight but I'm afraid I'll look gross."

The patient gives a history of a 40- to 50-pound weight loss gradually over the past 4 years secondary to "dieting." The patient denies purging, laxative, or diuretic abuse. She admits to occasional binging followed by increased guilt and rigid dieting. The patient dates the onset of dieting to a period of time just prior to moving out of her parent's home 4 years ago to attend school to become a courtroom reporter. She relates that she had been dating a group of friends at that time who teased her about being fat. She feared she would lose control and would continue to gain weight after she gained 5 pounds, going from 110 to 115 pounds 4 years ago. She subsequently began dieting, losing roughly 10 to 15 pounds a year over the past 4 years, resulting in the current weight on admission of 69 pounds (59 percent IBW).

There is no history of psychiatric hospitalization or medical hospitalization for malnutrition. The patient was in outpatient psychotherapy for 3 months in high school, focusing on problems with older sisters. The patient has been in irregular outpatient psychotherapy since the onset of anorexia nervosa, which began 4 years ago. The patient has had no therapeutic trials of antidepressants or major or minor tranquilizers. She denied drug abuse and denies any history of suicide attempts or self-mutilating behavior. Past medical history is unremarkable. The patient's mother has a history of high blood pressure, and the patient's maternal uncle has a history of alcoholism and depression.

The patient has had amenorrhea for the past 4 years. She exhibits bilateral pitting edema of the shins and feet.

The patient has lived with her parents and 26-year-old sister for the past year. The patient has another sister, aged 29. The patient lived independently 3 years prior to returning home, while she was in school to become a court reporter. The patient has had 2 years of community college. The patient reports considerable conflict with her family since early childhood. She describes herself as always being concerned with living up to her own perfectionist standards and feeling guilty about not pleasing her parents. She describes herself as being unable to take initiative at home and letting her parents do many day-to-day tasks for her, such as making her bed. She feels fearful that she will not make the "right decisions" on her own and may also hurt her parents by becoming more independent.

Mental status examination shows the patient to be a cachectic white woman with a weak voice and considerable lethargy. Thinking is goal-oriented; mood is depressed; affect restricted. She denies delusions, hallucinations, ideas of reference, suicidal or homicidal ideation. She has some peculiar magical thinking regarding her relationship with her sisters being "unlucky." Sensorium—she is oriented $\times 3$; memory is intact; insight and judgment are fair.

The important findings upon physical examination were marked cachexia. Patient has +2 pretibial edema bilaterally. Weight is 69 pounds.

The patient was treated with individual, group, and adjunctive therapies; she was placed on behavioral protocol for weight gain. Weight loss during the first 3 weeks of hospitalization (hiding food, noncompliance with protocol) necessitated the placement of Dobbhoff feeding tube. Focus of psychotherapy included distortion of body image and conflicts with family over autonomy.

NURSING CARE PLAN
Anorexia

NURSING DIAGNOSIS

Alternation in nutrition.

GOALS

1. Weight gain.
2. Normalization of eating behavior.
3. Adequate hydration.
4. Maintenance of ideal body weight.

INTERVENTIONS

1. Behavioral protocol for weight gain.
2. Record intake and output.
3. Daily weights.
4. 90-minute observation after meals.
5. Supervise meals to ensure adequate caloric intake.
6. Provide emotional support and understanding to help patient overcome fear of gaining weight.

NURSING DIAGNOSIS

Thought processes impaired.

GOALS

1. Behavior will reflect reality-based thinking.
2. Improvement in judgment and decision making.
3. Improved concentration.

INTERVENTIONS

1. Patient teaching regarding importance of nutrition to adequate mental functioning.
2. Encourage patient to reality test her distorted body image by comparing self to an average female counterpart.
3. Encourage patient to check out her perceptions of self with others and look at the areas of discrepancy.
4. Impress upon patient the seriousness of restricting food.

NURSING DIAGNOSIS

Moderate anxiety.

GOALS

1. Will verbalize feelings of anxiety rather than somaticizing.
2. Will not feel shame or guilt after eating.

INTERVENTIONS

1. Encourage verbalization of feelings.
2. Provide outlets for increased energy via normal amounts of exercise and relaxation techniques.
3. Reinforce realistic notions regarding food and its relationship to weight gain.

NURSING DIAGNOSIS

Self-esteem disturbance.

GOALS

1. Strengthen autonomy.
2. Acceptance of self and limitations.
3. Begin to establish independence.
4. Will refrain from self-negating verbalization.

INTERVENTIONS

1. Assist patient in reexamining negative cognitions of self.
2. Help patient identify her strengths and limitations.
3. Encourage patient to begin making decisions for self.
4. Help patient explore her need to be perfect.
5. Family meetings to improve communication style and to determine what does happen when the patient begins to act autonomously.

CASE HISTORY OF BULIMIA

The patient is a 19-year-old single, white female with no prior psychiatric admissions but has had an eating disorder for 4 years, diagnosed as bulimia. Her chief complaint: "I want to stop binging and using laxatives. I'm so ashamed."

The patient is the youngest of three children with two siblings who are both males and older. One brother, age 22, was diagnosed as being hyperactive as a child but is now enrolled in college. Both parents are alive and well. The patient's mother is extremely thin and very concerned with physical appearances.

The patient is a sophomore in college, at present on academic probation. She lives in an apartment near campus with four roommates. Patient consumes 3 to 5 mixed drinks or glasses of wine 3 to 4 nights a week. She reports occasional marijuana use and uses cocaine via the nasal route once or twice a month.

The patient states that her problems began about 4 years ago, in the summer between the 11th and 12th grade, when her mother began to criticize her for her weight, which was approximately 135 pounds. Patient is 5' 5" tall. The patient states that she felt angry that her mother wanted to control her weight, but she complied in trying to lose weight. The patient did this by binge eating, followed by self-induced vomiting. At this point the patient began seeing a therapist. Within 6 months the problem appeared to be resolved. Then, after several months, the problem began again in an identical fashion with no clear stressor. The patient was able to keep the eating habits a secret, at least from her parents. During her first year of college she missed many classes because she was involved in binging and purging or was too depressed over her eating behavior. The patient ended up on academic probation. With the start of the new school year, her symptoms worsened. She began using laxatives 3 to 4 times a week (as many as 75 at one time) along with diuretics and over-the-counter diet pills. Her vomiting increased to 5 to 10 times per week. The patient's weight fluctuated between 105 and 116 pounds. The patient felt guilty and ashamed. She also felt angry toward her mother, blaming her for the start of her problems with eating. Prior to seeking inpatient psychiatric treatment, the patient began stealing articles (books, jewelry, money) from her roommates to support her eating habits. Her father is involved in legal proceedings to make restitution to the injured parties.

NURSING CARE PLAN
Bulimia

NURSING DIAGNOSIS

Potential for fluid volume deficit.

GOALS

1. Adequate hydration.
2. Moist mucous membranes.
3. Normal vital signs.
4. Good skin turgor.
5. Maintenance of ideal body weight.

INTERVENTIONS

1. Record intake and output.
2. Record daily weights.
3. Observe and record skin integrity.
4. Monitor vital signs.
5. Monitor weekly electrolyte levels.

NURSING DIAGNOSIS

Alteration in nutrition.

GOALS

1. Normalization of eating behavior.
2. Patient will consume appropriate number of calories daily.
3. Patient will refrain from vomiting and laxative and diuretic use.

INTERVENTIONS

1. Provide emotional support during meals.
2. Encourage patient to use staff support and talk about the feelings, especially when she has the urge to binge.
3. Observe patient during meals and for 90 minutes after to prevent vomiting or binge eating.

NURSING DIAGNOSIS

Moderate anxiety.

GOALS

1. Improvement in sleep pattern.
2. Normal activity level.
3. Improved attention span.
4. Absence of somatic complaints after eating.

INTERVENTIONS

1. Promote relaxation through deep-breathing exercise and visual imagery.
2. Encourage patient to focus on one activity or one thought at a time.
3. Encourage patient to develop hobbies and leisure activities.
4. Assist patient in expressing feelings verbally rather than use of somatization.

NURSING DIAGNOSIS

Ineffective individual coping.

GOALS

1. Will demonstrate effective individual coping.
2. Will demonstrate appropriate participation in society.
3. Appropriate use of defense mechanisms.
4. Will refrain from self-destructive behavior.

INTERVENTIONS

1. Assist patient in identification of strengths.
2. Help patient identify problem areas and begin problem-solving techniques.
3. Develop therapeutic relationship to facilitate patient's expression of anger, fear, and anxiety.
4. Assist patient in role definition and setting appropriate expectations of self.

NURSING DIAGNOSIS

Self-esteem disturbance.

GOALS

1. Patient will develop a more positive self-concept.
2. Will refrain from self-negating verbalizations.

INTERVENTIONS

1. Nurse use of self as significant role model for patient.
2. Help patient reexamine negative cognitions of self.
3. Encourage eye contact during conversations.
4. Refer to OT groups that provide opportunity for patient to work on social skills.
5. Provide safe and nonthreatening arena for patient to practice risk taking.

─── CASE EXAMPLE* ───────────────────────────

Jennifer Downs, a 15-year-old high school sophomore, was referred to the crisis center with her parents by the police. During the past 3 months Jennifer had become withdrawn, isolative, and secretive from family and friends. One day, after school, Jennifer was caught shoplifting laxatives and ipecac syrup from a local drugstore. On arrival at the police station, Jennifer's parents found her crying uncontrollably and they agreed to seek counseling for her.

Jennifer arrived at the crisis center with her parents, both of whom were supportive of her seeking help and concerned over her recent behavior. Jennifer's general appearance was of a neatly groomed, attractive adolescent who appeared her stated age. Her affect and mood were dysphoric and slightly anxious.

During the initial interview Jennifer explained why she was seeking help. She was tearful at times and avoided eye contact. Jennifer stated her life has been a mess since the breakup with her boyfriend 4 months ago. She explained that this was her first serious boyfriend and that they had gone out for 6 months prior to the breakup.

* This case and nursing care plan are contributed by Eileen D. Taggart.

Jennifer stated she felt let down and rejected. She began to feel lonely, depressed, fat, and ugly. She lost interest in her friends and family and spent much of her time alone crying. Shortly thereafter, Jennifer had her first binge episode.

Jennifer stated she would binge at home late at night when her family was asleep. She began to notice that she was putting on weight but was unable to stop the binging, which was now taking place almost on a daily basis. Jennifer tried unsuccessfully to induce vomiting. She then turned to laxatives and ipecac to purge after her binges.

After her mother began questioning the family about the rate at which food was being consumed in the home, Jennifer began to binge in the grocery store on the way home from school. She stated it was fairly easy to binge in the store because it was so busy no one seemed to notice her. Jennifer admitted to stealing laxatives and ipecac on other occasions before being caught.

Jennifer throughout the interview expressed feelings of guilt and remorse not only for the binging and stealing but for lying and hiding her problems from her family.

NURSING CARE PLAN

ASSESSMENT

The hazardous event was the breakup with the boyfriend. The precipitating factor was her arrest for shoplifting. Jennifer perceived the breakup as her fault. She then began to act out in ways that reinforced her feelings and perceptions of self, which were inconsistent with her usual patterns of behavior. She also did not use her available support systems.

Diagnosis, according to the *DSM-III-R*: Axis I is 307.51 Bulimia Nervosa.

NURSING DIAGNOSES

- Impaired self-esteem.
- Impairment in solitude and social interaction.
- Alterations in conduct/impulse control.

GOALS

Through joint collaboration, Jennifer and her therapist formulated goals of treatment which would ultimately return her to the precrisis state or better.

Long-Term Goals
1. Jennifer will eliminate binge–purge eating patterns.
2. Will verbalize self-confidence and self-acceptance.
3. Will utilize familial and social supports.
4. Will eliminate impulsive and potentially self-destructive behaviors.
5. Will develop increased ability to cope with future life changes and stress.

This will be reviewed at the time of the follow-up session.

Short-Term Goals
1. Jennifer will decrease binge-eating patterns, establish regular nutritional eating patterns, maintain normal bowel elimination without laxatives by the fifth session.
2. Will verbalize feelings of guilt, anger, and rejection; express acceptance of present body weight and physical appearance; and identify personal strengths by the sixth session.

   3. Will reestablish social relationships with friends and improve communication with her family by the fourth session.
   4. Will control impulsive behavior such as binging in the supermarket and stealing by her second session.

INTERVENTION

   1. Jennifer will meet weekly with the therapist for 1 hour, for a total number of six sessions.
   2. A follow-up will be scheduled to further assess and evaluate Jennifer's status in regard to her current problem-solving abilities.
   3. Jennifer's family will be included in at least two sessions, once at the start of treatment, the other at the close of the initial treatment. The family will also be invited to participate in the follow-up session.

EVALUATION

Jennifer acknowledged that the plan could be renegotiated at any time. The effectiveness of treatment would be determined by Jennifer meeting the above stated goals.

Summary

Although the clinical syndromes of anorexia nervosa and bulimia are currently receiving a great deal of scientific and clinical interest, there are only minimal research findings that predict successful outcomes. The most effective approach to date gleans intervention strategies from the behavioral model. This approach does not negate individual, family, and group approaches, but it gives direction for the maintenance of the individual in a therapeutic milieu. The work of the Task Force of the National Group for Classification of Nursing Diagnoses gives guidance for the development of adequate assessment tools and standardized care plans. Ultimately, outcome criteria should be available for prediction and testing.

Questions

   1. What are some similarities and some differences between the psychiatric disorders of anorexia nervosa and bulimia?
   2. Talk with some adolescent patients about their belief patterns on eating and dieting. List the beliefs and compare them with your colleagues.
   3. How would you explain either anorexia nervosa or bulimia to a parent of an adolescent hospitalized with the disorder?

REFERENCES AND SUGGESTED READINGS

   1. American Psychiatric Association. *Diagnostic and Statistical Manual of Mental Disorders*, 3rd ed. (Rev.). Washington, D.C.: American Psychiatric Association, 1987, p. 67.
   2. Ibid.
   3. Bruch, H. *Eating Disorders: Obesity, Anorexia and the Person Within*. New York: Basic Books, 1978.
   4. Ibid.
   5. Andersen, A. Psychiatric aspects of bulimia. In A. Andersen (Ed.), *Directions in Psychiatry*. New York: Haterleigh, 1981.
   6. *DSM-III-R*, p. 67.

7. Richardson, T. Anorexia nervosa: An overview. *American Journal of Nursing*, 1980, *80*, 1470.

8. Liebman, R., Minuchin, S., & Baker, L. An integrated treatment program for anorexia nervosa. *American Journal of Psychiatry*, 1974, *131*, 432–436.

9. Kaplan, H., & Sadock, B. *Comprehensive Textbook of Psychiatry*. 4 ed. Baltimore: Williams & Wilkins, 1985.

10. Liebman, Minuchin, & Baker, op. cit.

11. National Conference Group for Classification of Nursing Diagnosis. St. Louis: Washington University, 1983.

Chapter 34

Treating the Drug Abuser

Christine Vourakis
Gerald Bennett

Chapter Objectives

The students successfully attaining the goals of this chapter will be able to:

- Describe social and political perspectives on drug abuse and the factors creating changes in patterns of drug abuse.
- Identify the major issues involved in drug-abuse prevention.
- Examine the legal and professional issues of the chemically impaired nurse.
- State the major theories of drug abuse.
- Define the terms psychological dependence, tolerance, and physical dependence.
- Describe the drugs that are commonly abused.
- Explore the special challenges of working with the dual diagnosis patient.
- Discuss the use of nursing diagnosis in assessment of the patient diagnosed with a psychoactive substance abuse disorder.
- Evaluate the total rehabilitative needs of the patient diagnosed with a psychoactive substance abuse disorder.
- Describe nursing management factors in working with drug abusers, including hallucinogenic crises and drug-induced delirium and delusional disorders.
- Define types of treatment models.

INTRODUCTION

The misuse or abuse of psychoactive drugs continues to be a major health problem in the United States and throughout the world. Although in recent years we have seen a slight downward trend in the growth of drug abuse, there is indication that this downward trend is leveling off. Cocaine has been especially problematic with a resurgence of its popularity in the early 1980s. This popularity has escalated of late, with the routine processing of cocaine into purer and more convenient forms of the drug. For example, free-based cocaine is an inexpensive, readily accessible, and more purified form of cocaine. It has the opportunity to create dependency problems in a much wider segment of the population, especially those who are younger and less affluent, and is showing signs of doing just that.

The governments of countries world wide have joined the war on drugs. The United States has been instrumental in organizing the international community to participate in curtailing the production, processing and transportation of illicit drugs, particularly cocaine, heroin, and marijuana. Efforts to eliminate illicit drug supplies have shown us that the war on drugs will not be won in a single battle but will require constant and vigilant attention. The problem is not one of illicit drugs alone. Many people suffer from the consequences of using prescription drugs (legally obtained), alcohol, nicotine, and caffeine. It reminds us that although we must continue directing resources toward decreasing the drug supply, at some point the bulk of our attention will most appropriately be directed toward issues surrounding demand for drugs in our society.

The health professions have simultaneously expanded and heightened their participation in addressing substance abuse in our society. The nursing profession, in particular, has moved to recognize addictions nursing as a specialty area of practice. The American Nurses' Association Division on Psychiatric and Mental Health Nursing Practice, in recognition of the unique needs of the substance abuser, recommended that the practice area of addictions nursing be considered a specialty area in nursing. As a result, a scope-of-practice statement delineating guidelines for practice and specialty development was published in 1987.[1]

The nurse may encounter clients with psychoactive substance use disorders (PSUDs) in one or a combination of several clinical roles and a variety of clinical settings. For example, a staff nurse on an acute psychiatric unit may find that the patient admitted with an acute psychosis has no history of mental illness but has been taking high doses of amphetamines. Or the nurse working with a residual schizophrenic in the community may find that cannabis abuse is a serious threat to an already marginal adjustment to life outside the hospital. Some psychiatric nurses specialize in working with drug abusers during early assessment, detoxification, initial treatment, or long-term rehabilitation. Drug abuse is so pervasive in our society that nurses in general practice and in nonpsychiatric specialities also encounter patients with health disruptions that may be traced to or are associated with psychoactive substance consumption.

Problems of drug abuse should not be considered in isolation from alcohol abuse. Drug abusers have a wide choice of drugs available to them, and many adopt a pattern of multidrug use. Alcohol, readily available and legal, may be used when illicit drug supplies are diminished or in combination with other drugs to soften or enhance a current drug experience. It may also be used to ease the withdrawal or "come down" syndrome at the cessation of a drug-taking "marathon." For example, it is common for opiate and stimulant abusers to report regular alcohol abuse. It is obvious, therefore, that alcohol plays an important role in patterns of multidrug use, albeit often a secondary one. Thus the topics covered in the next chapter on alcohol abuse are essential to understanding the complex clinical picture that polydrug abusers present.

The self-help model has gained increasing popularity as a method of drug-abuse treatment incorporated into both inpatient and outpatient programs. Peer counseling is a self-help approach that attempts to minimize or eliminate the hierarchical relationship between patient and counselor. This approach is now making its way most noticeably in nontraditional programs. The current trend in drug treatment is increasingly toward expecting the patient to assume an active role in problem identification and solution. The counselor's role, ideally, is one of offering support and facilitating the patient in achieving his goals. However, in reality, many patients require a great deal of professional or paraprofessional involvement and guidance before they are able to pursue self-help in a serious fashion. Nevertheless, collaboration and encouragement of client decision making at some level should begin early, increasing in complexity and scope over time.

CONCEPTUAL MODEL

Orem's self-care nursing model provides a framework of care for clients with PSUDs.[2] It is particularly suited to this population because assessment is oriented around the patients' ability to meet their own self-care needs. The overall aim of care for clients with PSUDs is for them to ultimately assume responsibility for maintaining a life-style without abusing drugs. This goal is achieved by encouraging patient participation in treatment planning early on, with gradual assumption of leadership over their own care. Use of this model is demonstrated in the nursing intervention section.

SOCIAL AND POLITICAL ISSUES

The Domestic Scene

A recent estimate of the cost of drug abuse (excluding alcohol) in the United States each year was placed at $46.9 billion based on data available from 1980.[3] This figure took into account treatment costs, reduced productivity, lost employment, and the involvement of drug abuse in crime. Since the cocaine epidemic did not hit with full force until several years after 1980, it is likely that the costs have moved dramatically upward in this decade.[4] In fact, it was the cocaine epidemic, and Nancy Reagan's long-standing commitment to stopping drug abuse among youth, that led to drug abuse becoming a top public policy issue in 1986. The political momentum culminated when President Reagan signed into law the Drug Enforcement, Education and Control Act, providing $1.7 billion for drug law enforcement, treatment, and prevention. Like the previous wars on illicit drugs in the United States, the new law included measures to limit the availability of illicit drugs and decrease the demand for these substances.[5]

The objectives of the dual approach designed to cut supply and demand are to discourage casual experimentation with controlled substances, to bring the addict to treatment through arrest or hardship, and finally to help the addict learn to live without unprescribed drug use. It was the federal government's commitment to these objectives that fostered the tremendous growth in the drug abuse field during the 1970s, a time that has been described as the "drug abuse decade."[6] The breakdown in federal funds for treatment and law enforcement has tended to be roughly equal over time.[7]

The Drug Enforcement Administration (DEA) of the Department of Justice is responsible for enforcing the laws regulating controlled substances. Essentially DEA is in the business of limiting the supply of illicit drugs and illegally obtained prescription drugs. Nurses are in compliance with the Controlled Substances Act when they take special precautions to account for each dose of drugs such as meperidine and diazepam. The National Institute on Drug Abuse (NIDA) of the Department of Human Services leads the federal effort to decrease the demand for illicit drugs through research, prevention, and treatment.

Some significant changes in federal drug-abuse policy accompanied the Reagan Administration's "new federalism." In the prevention and treatment areas, NIDA lost a great deal of influence when drug-abuse funds were lumped into the Alcohol, Drug Abuse and Mental Health (ADAMH) Block Grant. The intent of the block grant funding strategy was to transfer from the federal to the state level the power to make allocations for specific programs.

The Reagan Administration has placed emphasis on the creation and operation of regional antidrug forces. These task forces have operated in Boston, New York, Baltimore, Atlanta, Miami, Chicago, St. Louis, Houston, Denver, San Francisco, Los Angeles, and San Diego. The South Florida Task Force, based in Miami, was the first of these collaborative efforts by local prosecutors and agents from the DEA, Internal Revenue Service, Customs, and the Federal Bureau of Investigation. DEA and related law enforcement agencies do not prevent the eventual distribution of large quantities of illicit drugs, but they do succeed in making these drugs high-priced and risky to traffic, possess, and use.

When physical, financial, legal, personal, or social pressures come to bear on the addict, or when the addict wishes to "kick" for any of a variety of reasons, a system of treatment services is in place in the United States that was largely developed through the leadership of NIDA during the 1970s. The 1980s have seen a substantial increase in the development of private treatment programs to provide services to adolescents and adults. The cocaine epidemic had the effect of bringing large numbers of middle-to-upper-class clients to treatment who could afford private inpatient and outpatient programs.[8] The public perception of drug addiction as a problem associated with lower socioeconomic status was challenged by the increasing numbers of professionals, athletes, entertainers, and others with cocaine problems.

One of the most controversial approaches to decreasing drug abuse in the work place and schools is urine drug screening. In 1986, President Reagan made drug screening the center-piece of an initiative to stop drug abuse among federal employees and called for similar screening programs in the private sector. This set off a wave of newspaper and magazine articles about the pros and cons of drug testing, including technical, legal, and ethical issues. Proponents claim that current testing procedures are reliable, that employers are within their rights to demand a drug-free work-place, and drug testing is the best way to achieve this end. Opponents argue that usual testing procedures are unreliable, urine drug screening violates the right to individual privacy, and it is a waste of money that could be spent on law enforcement to limit the supply or on education to decrease demand.[9] It is expected that court cases related to drug testing will eventually lead to a ruling from the Supreme Court on the legality of the practice.

George Lundberg, editor of the *Journal of the American Medical Association* (*JAMA*), called mass routine or random drug screening in the work-place "chemical McCarthyism."[10] Students are invited to debate this issue for and among themselves. In particular, students may wish to consider whether they would support or oppose the use of urine drug testing among nurses as an approach to discouraging drug use in the profession.

The International Scene

The use of psychoactive drugs for spiritual and medicinal purposes has been practiced in many areas of the world for centuries. A recreational style of drug use was evident in China during the eighteenth century in the form of opium smoking. Approximately a century later, the Chinese identified a problem of drug abuse among the population. It is unclear what factors created the transition from drug use to drug abuse. What we do know is that an opium drug-abuse problem in China was noted in concert with the organization of the production and transportation of opium for economic and political gain.[11]

The British, early in the nineteenth century, using their political and military power, organized a market for the Asian opium drug trade. Through the British East India Company, the opium trade enabled them to raise 15 percent of the revenue needed to maintain their Indian Colony. Since that time a global economy has been established through the production and distribution of illicit drugs.[12,13]

The first major international effort to reduce global drug abuse occurred in 1909 at the Shanghai Conference. The widespread phenomenon of opium smoking, especially its spread to Americans in California from Chinese immigrants, prompted the State Department to take action. The convening nations agreed on the need to control opium and its derivatives, especially morphine. Agreements in principle were duplicated at a larger conference at the Hague in 1911. Actual steps to control drug production, distribution, and consumption were not clearly delineated, although producing countries, e.g., India and China, agreed to reduce and regulate poppy growth.[14]

Later investigations revealed that the market for opium remained buoyant. The British were involved in processing morphine from opium and distributing the derivative to the Eastern countries. Their exports increased from five and one-half tons in 1911 to fourteen tons in 1914. India, China, and Persia were growing poppies at a high rate but were reporting a reduction in growth. The revenue produced from the drug trade inhibited development of any real change in the patterns. Countries in Latin America, Southeast Asia, and Southwest Asia, major providers of opium, cocaine, and marijuana, have for over a century based their economies on the production of these drugs. Other countries have joined in and have profited from the processing and distribution of illicit drug substances.[15,16]

A powerful network of production and distribution of illicit drugs among the countries of the world continues into the present. This is evidenced by the current level of illicit drug consumption in the United States. Over 90 percent of the illicit drugs consumed in the United States are produced in other countries.[17] The cost of controlling the importation of these substances is prohibitive. In addition, our law enforcement efforts have had relatively little impact on the flow of drugs across our borders. Unfortunately, in many cases the production and distribution are not significantly discouraged by the governments of the countries involved. As a result, the international treaties and conferences over the years have not had real long-term impact on controlling drug abuse world wide.

It is obvious that a system of cooperation and support among all the countries of the world is necessary for long-term control of drug abuse. Two respected international organizations in a position to assist in the struggle, the United Nations (UN) and the World Health Organization (WHO), have been active in illicit drug control since the 1940s. The UN directs its efforts at reducing the supply and demand for drugs, coordinating crop substitution projects in producing countries, enforcing crop control agreements, and supporting research. WHO primarily focuses on issues related to health. In the area of drug abuse, its activities are aimed at preventing and reducing the health consequences of drug abuse. The activities of the organization therefore include the assessment and classification of potentially harmful drug substances. WHO also functions in a more specific manner by convening scientific and study groups of experts throughout the world to generate and disseminate knowledge on drug abuse. In addition, WHO coordinates drug-related projects among a group of cooperating countries.[18,19]

A growing concern, enhancing worldwide participation in combating drug abuse, is the escalating drug-abuse problem in producing countries. "For example, while Pakistan reported a negligible heroin addict population in 1980, a recent Pakistani study estimated the addict population to be as high as 300,000 persons in 1985."[20] World concern is further exemplified by the first worldwide "International Conference on Drug Abuse and Illicit Trafficking (IC-DAIT)" called by the Secretary-General of the UN. The eight-day conference in Vienna drew hundreds of people from 138 countries around the globe. The conference emphasis was on reducing drug supply, with a display of the latest equipment and technology for drug detection and seizure. By the last day of the conference the participants made an agreement to continue to work together and further agreed on a variety of options for reducing supply and demand.[21]

The Reagan Administration's emphasis on the prevention and inhibition of the spread of drug abuse includes efforts in the international arena. The United States has operated on the belief that international drug supplies must be curtailed in order to expect success from efforts to control drug abuse in the United States.[22] To this end President Reagan put forth his plan for international narcotics control in the *1984 National Strategy for Prevention of Drug Abuse and Drug Trafficking*. A summary of this plan, including appropriate department or agency re-

sponsibilities, as noted in the Government Accounting Office (GAO) report is presented here:

1. The Department of State is responsible for coordinating all U.S. drug control efforts, diplomatic initiatives, and bilateral and multilateral assistance for crop control and interdiction overseas.
2. The Drug Enforcement Administration is the lead agency for drug law enforcement. It provides technical assistance and training (funded by the Department of State) to foreign drug law enforcement officials and promotes the collection and sharing of international narcotics data.
3. The Agency for International Development (AID) provides development assistance to source countries to generate alternative sources of income and employment and improve living standards in narcotics-producing areas. AID also attempts to inform opinion leaders and the general public of source countries about the adverse effects of drug production and abuse.
4. The U.S. Information Agency provides public affairs supports through its posts in U.S. embassies in countries where illicit drug production or trafficking has been identified as a priority issue.
5. The Department of Agriculture, through the Agriculture Research Service, assists in crop substitution programs and research in agricultural alternatives to narcotics crops and offers advice on herbicidal eradication programs.
6. The Central Intelligence Agency provides strategic narcotics intelligence and is responsible for coordinating foreign intelligence on narcotics matters.
7. The National Institute for Drug Abuse provides technical information to international health service officials on treatment and prevention practices and epidemiologic methods and findings.
8. Units within the Departments of Justice, State, and Treasury are concerned with offshore banking practices and extradition treaties.[23]

The Reagan Administration's 1984 plan for international drug control has met with little success in limiting the available supply of illicit drugs in the United States. More recent efforts have been directed toward controlling demand, including the encouragement of massive drug testing.[24] Although issues related to demand need greater emphasis in the United States, the international community must continue to put greater emphasis on supply and demand through a cooperative effort on an ongoing basis.

DRUG-ABUSE PREVENTION

There appeared to be more support for drug-abuse prevention programs during the latter 1980s than at any other point in American history. There was concern that the transfer of funding authority from the National Institute on Drug Abuse (NIDA) to the states in 1981 might leave the prevention field without adequate support. However, those who have studied the status of drug-abuse prevention programming following the inception of block grant funding to the states have concluded that the combination of local, state, and federal support is impressive and will probably grow in the future.[25,26]

Standard V-B of the American Nurses' Association *Standards Psychiatric-Mental Health Nursing Practice* states that health teaching is an essential nursing function.[27] Nurses, with their background in both the biologic and behavioral sciences, are uniquely prepared to provide drug teaching and counseling in formal prevention programs and informally in the routine practice of other clinical roles when the issue of drug use is relevant.

Nurses in schools, camps, private clinics, and community agencies involving young people are in an excellent position to develop formal drug-abuse prevention programs. However, before launching such a program, the nurse should be knowledgeable about the approaches and techniques that have been shown to be more effective in changing attitudes toward drug use. It is known that "drug horror stories" and other scare tactics only serve to damage the professional's credibility with the young population. It is also known that programs designed for children and adolescents should not focus on providing drug information as such.[28] In fact, sharing information about the potential "highs" available through drug use may stimulate an interest in or a desire for drug use that was not present before the teaching took place. Rather than information, either in the form of "horror stories" or as an objective presentation of the actions and side effects of psychoactive drugs, children and adolescents need teaching and guidance related to coping with drug use choices.[29]

A general "life skills" program is often the best approach, with an emphasis on developing personal values and decision-making skills. The expected outcome of this approach is an in-creased ability on the part of young people to say no when faced with the issue of drug use. The "Just Say No" campaign is the most popular drug education strategy. It places emphasis on dealing with the peer pressure often involved in drug-use initiation. A recent study indicated that a limitation of this approach is that it may detract from parents' recognizing the strong influence they have on their children's behavior.[30] When a drug-using peer group has gained sufficient influence with a child or adolescent to initiate drug use, more involvement by parents is likely to be more effective as a first step in stopping drug use than learning refusal skills. Those who do not want to say no have little motivation to learn the skills for saying no. Increased involvement by parents is the most potent approach to limiting the influence of peer groups.

Although values-clarification and refusal-skills approaches to drug-related health teaching can be recommended over informational approaches, the evidence from studies of all types of drug education thus far shows no consistent relationship between education and actual drug use. Hanson agrees with the National Commission on Marijuana and Drug Abuse that there should be a moratorium on drug education programs until studies identify an approach that clearly is associated with decreased drug use following participation.[31,32] We suggest that the nurse involved in drug education and counseling should be discriminating in the strategies selected for a given target group, should always include a means for evaluation of a program's effectiveness, and should be able to defend a given program based on the most recent research findings or the potential value of an innovative idea.[33]

Two examples of drug education are briefly described here. The first example, the Ombudsman program in Charlotte, North Carolina, sought to target children for values clarification who were experimenting with drugs rather than those who had never tried them.[34] In the second example, Blizard and Teague reported on a program that was planned for adolescents who had been found intoxicated or in possession of drugs at school.[3,5] This program focused on exploring alternatives to drug abuse for achieving "highs." Both programs demonstrated limited success. Participation in the Ombudsman project was related to a decrease in "hard" drug use, and the program focusing on alternatives to drug use led to an increase in awareness of such alternatives. The target groups for these programs, children or adolescents who had already tried drugs or had gotten into trouble with them, may offer a better "payoff" for drug education than young people who are abstainers or have had no problems with drugs. This possibility is related to a larger debate between a "health promotion" policy or a "problem prevention" approach to drug education. The "health promotion" perspective emphasizes programs for normal populations, particularly children, and the "problem prevention" perspective highlights the need to target efforts toward people with problems of various kinds throughout the life-span. Room makes the case for the "problem prevention" approach as the most effective means of discouraging drug abuse in people who are at risk for abuse.[36]

Drug education in the course of routine nursing practice in various roles and specialities is an area in which investigation is needed. For example, the growing body of knowledge that points to the harmful effects of drugs on fetal development places special responsibilities on maternal–child nurses to engage their clients in drug-abuse teaching and counseling. A question for research is: What techniques are effective in decreasing drug use during the childbearing year? Another question is: To what extent do decreases in drug use during the childbearing year carry over into the parenting years? McKay gives a comprehensive treatment of substance abuse during the childbearing year for the interested reader.[37]

Another example is the psychiatric–mental health nurse working with chronic schizophrenic clients in an attempt to promote their community adjustment. It is unfortunate that many of these clients are at risk for alcohol and other drug abuse as a means of recreation, anxiety reduction, or escaping negative feelings related to loneliness. Bakdash has proposed an approach for working with the "dual problem" (substance abuse and chronic psychiatric illness) that includes helping clients learn to manage negative feelings without resorting to street drugs or alcohol abuse.[38]

One final example of the psychiatric–mental health nurse's potential role in drug education is related to the recent emphasis on "stress management" in our society for working people. Whether in the mental health center, community college, church, or occupational setting, stress management classes are being planned in increasing numbers, and the community mental health nurse is likely to be involved as a teacher or consultant for such classes. Since alcohol and other drugs are major stress-reduction resources for many adults, teaching skills such as relaxation or meditation may in part contribute to drug-abuse prevention since they may be viewed as substitutes for the "happy hour," tranquilizer use, or marijuana smoking. Again, these speculations and suggestions related to drug education in the context of nursing practice have not as yet received the attention by researchers that is clearly needed.

THE CHEMICALLY IMPAIRED NURSE

No discussion of drug abuse in a nursing textbook would be complete without addressing what has come to be called the problem of the impaired nurse. When one considers the long history of concern about drinking and drug use among nurses, it is remarkable that it was only in 1982 that the American Nurses' Association House of Delegates adopted a resolution calling for programs to identify, confront, and offer treatment to chemically dependent nurses.[39] Most nursing licensure suspensions and revocations are directly related to substance abuse. Meperidine, diverted from clinical use in the hospital, is the most common drug of abuse among chemically dependent nurses. Before this decade most nurses caught diverting controlled substances for their own use were arrested. It was not unusual for an arrested nurse to be taken from the hospital in handcuffs and to serve a prison term following conviction. Despite the severity of these consequences, there was a "conspiracy of silence" surrounding the problem of drug and alcohol dependence among nurses. It was something that was not talked about or accepted as a possibility except in the individual cases where there was overwhelming evidence showing repeated theft of drugs on a unit.

Since the 1982 American Nurses' Association resolution on impaired practice many of the state nurses' associations have implemented peer-assistance programs that are called into action when a nurse is suspected of drug abuse. While the practices differ from state to state, there is often close cooperation between the peer-assistance program, the hospital reporting the problem, the state board of nursing, and drug law enforcement authorities in presenting the impaired nurse with an option of treatment and recovery. Naegle listed several behavioral patterns suggestive of chemically impaired practice:

- Frequent absenteeism and tardiness after days off
- Frequent absences from work for illness or personal "emergencies"
- Aberrant behavior in the work setting such as irritability, mood swings, frequent absences from the unit
- Decreased productivity or job shrinkage
- Sloppy charting, errors and irregularities in relation to medication dispensing
- Frequent job changes or requests to work in areas with little supervision
- Inability to perform psychomotor skills because of intoxication or tremors[40]

Peer-assistance programs usually have a hotline available for nursing peers and managers to call if they observe these patterns in a colleague. Assistance is provided by confronting the impaired nurse using procedures designed to assess the problem further to determine if a drug problem exists, protect the rights of the public, recognize the addiction as an illness, and provide for the nurse's needs for treatment and recovery.

The following is a case history of a drug-addicted nurse reported by Jefferson and Ensor[41]:

Betty was an orthopedic nurse who sustained a back injury while lifting a heavy patient. She began taking diazepam (Valium) for the pain. In the course of taking the drug, she found that she felt more relaxed and better able to cope with the daily frustrations of her job. She obtained several prescriptions for Valium on the pretense of her back problem until one physician questioned her need for it and wouldn't write the prescription for her. She had increased her daily intake substantially by this time, so she found it necessary to feign other illnesses to receive some kind of central-nervous-system-depressant medication. During one visit to the emergency room, she was given meperidine (Demerol) for the migraine headaches she described. After that she feigned other illnesses and took whatever she could get her hands on. Only when the prescription source became inadequate did she begin to forge prescriptions and steal from the unit where she worked. Even when she went as far as taking patients' medications, she didn't see herself as addicted. She didn't even believe that what she did was really wrong; she rationalized that she needed the mediation more than the patients did anyway.

Peer-assistance programs provide a structured confrontation for the impaired nurse, usually referred to as an intervention. The intervention generally involves an administrative supervisor, members of the peer-assistance team, family members, and colleagues. The impaired nurse is brought by the supervisor or family member to a group meeting at which the pattern of impaired practice is presented with a mandate that it not be allowed to continue. Drug addiction is discussed as a disease, and the need for treatment is emphasized. The existing consequences of the drug problem are presented, including position and license being in jeopardy, laws being broken, and family problems. This is all presented in a caring yet firm manner, with the expressed expectation that the impaired nurse will enter drug treatment immediately. Such an approach is usually very effective in getting the impaired nurse into treatment because at this point her license is on the line. It is only later that most nurses in treatment begin to recognize that the license was a relatively minor issue when weighed against the emotional, physical, and spiritual deterioration suffered.

As impaired practice interventions increase throughout the country, there is a growing interest in nurses with substance abuse disorders as a special treatment population. Most major cities have inpatient and outpatient programs designed specifically for impaired health professionals, and programs that focus on assisting nurses in recovery are not uncommon. Estes describes a comprehensive approach to group treatment of nurses recovering from substance dependence. It appears to be particularly useful to have nurse therapists lead these groups. "The sharing of a common professional background with those under treatment provides an immediate and ongoing avenue for conveyance of understanding and reality testing."[42] Groups led by nurse therapists, whether providing peer support in a self-help format or psychotherapy, are an essential component of peer-assistance programs.

THEORIES OF DRUG ABUSE

Experimentation and occasional use of illicit drugs are common phenomena among a significant portion of the population and, in most cases, do not lead to a pattern of chronic abuse and dependence. Drug abusers, however, in relation to their style and frequency of drug taking, eventually exhibit disruptions in some part of their personal environment (e.g., interpersonal relationships, work patterns, or physical health). There is no actual prototype for the drug-dependent person. These individuals are a diverse group emerging from all socioeconomic levels and cultural groups. A next-door neighbor may have a drug problem.

The numerous theories explaining the causes of drug abuse reflect the diversity among people with drug problems. No single theory is suitably flexible to explain the varied and complicated phenomena of drug abuse and dependence. Generally, the theories fall within three categories: psychological, sociological, and biologic. The categories tend to capture the main themes within each theory. However, some of the theories are linked to more than one category; for example, a biologic theory of drug dependence cannot ignore the voluntary initiation of drug use and its psychological components. Theories from within each of the three categories were selected to illustrate the varying conceptualizations of drug abuse etiology. A brief description of the selected theories follows.

Psychological

The psychological theories of drug abuse identify the individual as the primary source of the problem and consider the environment as a secondary factor. The person is perceived as disturbed in some fashion and therefore unable to cope with a variety of environmental influences. These theories attempt to offer a reasonable explanation for the occurrence of drug abuse among various members of a given community. People who grow up in the same environment, or even within the same family, as a drug abuser may not necessarily develop drug-abuse problems.

Interactional Theory

An interactional theory developed by Ausubel identifies the chronic narcotic addict as an individual with an inadequate personality who finds the effects of narcotics adjustive for personality deficiencies. The euphoria felt provides an immediate sense of gratification and boost to the ego. The theorist recognizes the role of accessibility to drugs and a permissive social network as secondary predisposing environmental factors in the development of drug abuse.[43]

Existential Theory

A psychological theory with an existential perspective designates the individual's life experiences and emotional state as precursors to drug abuse. The person's personality structure in interaction with drug-taking behavior therefore leads to addiction. A psychopathological state may be exhibited, e.g., chronic anxiety, whereby the person is lacking in pleasurable sensory experience. It is frequently the case that the individual lacks the motivation or skills to actually seek a variety of pleasure-producing life experiences.[44] The continuation of drug abuse seems plausible in a situation where other alternatives for pleasure are not perceived as available.

Psychoanalytic Theory

The psychoanalytic perspective includes theoretical formulations of drug-abuse origins. A popular psychoanalytic theory views the ego of the addict as severely impaired. A significant amount of psychopathology is present, and ego functions such as rational decision making, establishment of a sense of self, and drive mediation are limited. Heroin addicts frequently present with lifelong histories of difficulty in handling impulses and feelings associated with aggression. It is hypothesized that heroin is used to subdue their aggressive impulses. Another notion is that heroin assists addicts to cope with the emptiness felt as a result of repression of dependency and nurturance needs.[45]

Learning Theory

Although physiological factors are recognized as important in maintaining addiction patterns, psychological factors are given prominent importance when viewed from a learning theory perspective. In general, learning theory follows a particular order. Initially there is an intense stimulus situation, which is followed by tension or anxiety. The drug abuser diminishes this anxiety by taking drugs and may in addition experience pleasure from drug effects. The anxiety is viewed as a secondary reenforcer in this model, since the drug-taking behavior has its own inherent reenforcements. The cycle is repeated when a stimulus situation reemerges.[46]

A ratio of destructive:constructive factors determines the likelihood of drug-abuse behavior. The greater the destructive part of the ratio, the greater the risk of drug abuse. The factors primarily consist of personality components and habits. The degree of reinforcements relative to these factors alters the ratio toward either the destructive or constructive direction.[47] Drug abuse and its continuation are therefore perceived as learned behavior. Psychological factors reinforced through interaction with the environment are central to the theory.

Sociological

The sociological theories generally place great emphasis on environmental factors contributing to drug abuse. The origins of drug abuse may be traced to families, underprivileged slum areas, drug-abuse subculture, roles, and social settings. A few of these will be discussed. Most of the theories specify the drug abuser as either an equal contributor to the development of a drug-abuse life-style or secondary to the prevailing social and environmental influences.

Family Theory

Stanton, well known for his work with drug-abusing families, offers a family theory of drug abuse. He identifies several features of drug-abusing families leading to a homeostatic model of addiction. Traumatic loss is one feature and is characterized by the premature death of a family member or the loss of kinship ties experienced by American immigrants. In families experiencing traumatic loss, there is a tendency for parents to turn to their children to fill emotional gaps and thus impede the individuation process that occurs as the children progress through adolescence.[48]

Fear of separation is a feature of both the addict and the family. There is a tendency for the drug abuser to grow away from the family as successful treatment ensues. The family panics at this point and a crisis occurs. The addict is drawn into the situation and reverts back to drug-abusing behavior. The family crisis seems to disappear as the drug-abusing behavior is reestablished.[49]

The next two features are the addict–family context and the family structure. The addict–family feature refers to the rather close ties between addicts and their families. Compared to non-drug-abusers, these addicts tend to maintain excessively close ties to their families of origin. The family structure feature of drug-abusing families typically reveals an overinvolved relationship between the parent of the opposite sex and the drug abuser. This pattern of family relationships interferes with the addict's emotional development and eventual separation.[50]

In sum, the foregoing discussion of drug-abusing families reveals excessive involvement among members and consequent difficulty in allowing children to grow up and individuate.

Subculture Theory

The theory of a drug subculture attempts to offer an explanation for youthful involvement in a pattern of drug abuse. The concept of culture refers to the grouping of people, primarily according to their social values and norms. A dominant culture in the United States is middle-class culture. The emergence of subcultures, e.g., peer culture and drug subculture, involves groups with social values and norms that may depart significantly from the traditional middle-class culture.[51]

Generally, the peer culture carries the values and norms of the middle-class culture. However, peer subgroups within the peer culture may alter norms and values depending on the composition and tolerance of a particular group. Participation in the peer culture precedes the young person's entry into the drug subculture. Movement into the drug subculture and adoption of the conduct norms and values depend on the person's predisposition to unorthodox behavior.[52] Adolescents and young adults, therefore, prone to unconventionality, may be attracted to peer groups with more deviant norms and values. These groups are more likely to be involved with and tolerant of drug-abusing behavior.

Role Theory

A role theory of drug dependence identifies three factors that when present promote a high incidence of drug abuse[53]:

1. Access to dependence-producing substances.
2. Disengagement from prescriptions against their use.
3. Role strain or role deprivation.

Role is defined as a group of behaviors that are associated with a certain status or position in society. Role strain occurs when the person recognizes an inability to fulfill the expectations of a role. Role deprivation refers to the effect of the loss of an important role relationship.[54]

It is hypothesized that individuals who are taking on new roles in society, e.g., an adolescent, parent, employee, or spouse, will experience role strain. In addition, conflicting expectations within a given role set contribute to role strain. Groups who experience role strain are vulnerable to an increased incidence of drug abuse, especially if the other two prongs of the theory are present. On the other hand, if role strain is decreased, drug access declines, and the social milieu opposes drug abuse, then the subgroup is likely to discontinue the behavior.[55]

Relapse is a common phenomenon among many recovering drug abusers, and the role theory perspective provides a rationale for its occurrence. The development of roles in society is viewed as a dynamic process. As the ex-addict takes on the nonuser's role, the likelihood of role strain is high. Several attempts to incorporate the nonuser's role may be necessary until the drug abuser feels comfortable.

Physiological

The physiological theories of drug abuse are concerned with the chemical interaction of drug substances with the human body. These theories generally recognize the environmental influences in drug abuse. However, the primary source of the problem is identified as within the biologic system of the individual or as a result of the interaction between the individual's biologic system and drug substances. Two of the physiological theories of drug abuse will be discussed in this section.

Genetic Theory

Although most of the evidence indicating genetic factors in the development of substance abuse comes from alcoholism research, it is hypothesized that genetic factors underlie drug abuse as well. The genetic theory postulates that individuals are born biologically predisposed to drug abuse. A number of genes as opposed to a single gene may be inherited to predispose the individual.[56] The strength of these inherited genes in combination with an environment ori-

ented toward drug abuse is believed to influence the degree of dependency.

Opiate Receptor Theory

The opiate receptor theory is based on the belief that there are specific areas or receptors in the central nervous system that opioids tend to gravitate toward and bind with to create their effects. The discovery of these opiate receptors led scientists to explore the possibility of naturally occurring endogenous opioids. Opiate-like substances were eventually discovered and named endorphins.[57]

Endorphins behave similarly to exogenous opioids, binding to the same receptor sites. Recent evidence links endorphins to the development of tolerance to or dependence on opiates in humans. The data are inconclusive at this time, but a rapid improvement in the abstinence syndrome in narcotic withdrawal has been demonstrated in addicts treated with one subgroup of endorphins. Although this theory has only evolved in the past 10 years, it holds exciting prospects for understanding the phenomena of dependence and tolerance and abstinence in opioid addiction.[58]

PSYCHIATRIC DIAGNOSIS OF DRUG DISORDERS

The psychiatric diagnosis of drug disorders is in a state of transition and refinement. The *DSM-III-R* introduced some important changes in taxonomy from that used in the *DSM-III*.[59] Given the ongoing debate regarding the most appropriate terminology and classification system for drug disorders, it is likely that more change is in store before a lasting consensus is achieved. Despite the changes in the taxonomy, research has shown a high level of agreement between the previous and current systems in identifying individuals with drug disorders.[60]

In the *DSM-III-R* classification, there are two types of disorders directly related to drug use: the psychoactive-substance-induced organic mental disorders and the psychoactive substance use disorders. The former type refers to the direct pharmacological effects of drugs on the central nervous system (CNS) such as intoxication, withdrawal, and delirium. The latter type refers to maladaptive behavior patterns that are associated with compulsive psychoactive drug use. Whereas alcohol is included as a psychoactive substance of abuse in the *DSM-III-R* classification, it will not be covered here. The next chapter focuses on alcohol abuse and alcoholism.

Psychoactive-Substance-Induced Organic Mental Disorders

The *DSM-III-R* recognizes ten classes of substances other than alcohol as commonly associated with substance-induced mental disorders: (1) amphetamines and related stimulants; (2) caffeine; (3) cannabis; (4) cocaine; (5) hallucinogens; (6) inhalants; (7) nicotine; (8) opioids; (9) phencyclidine (PCP) and related substances; and (10) sedatives, hypnotics, and anxiolytics. Examples of psychoactive-substance-induced organic mental disorders involving these drugs are withdrawal syndromes after ceasing repeated use of sedatives, opioids, nicotine, amphetamines, or cocaine. Other examples are cocaine, amphetamine, PCP, hallucinogen, or cannabis intoxication.

Depending on the circumstances and the particular drug used, the consequences of the substance-induced organic disorders may be minor or quite severe. For instance, consider the constrast in potential consequences between cannabis intoxication in an individual's home and cannabis intoxication while driving a car or operating heavy machinery. The delirium that may follow ingestion or withdrawal from some drugs can also pose serious problems for the user. Hallucinogenic crises and drug-induced delusional disorders are discussed later in the chapter. Although psychoactive drug intoxication is common in our society, cases of intoxication that are diagnosed as an organic mental disorder are not. In fact, the diagnosis of substance-induced organic mental disorder is typically made in persons who exhibit a use pattern indicating a psychoactive substance use disorder (PSUD) as well.

Psychoactive Substance Use Disorders

Nine classes of substances other than alcohol are commonly associated with PSUDs: (1) amphetamines and related stimulants; (2) cannabis; (3) cocaine; (4) hallucinogens; (5) inhalants; (6) nicotine; (7) opioids; (8) phencyclidine (PCP) and related substances; and (9) sedatives, hypnotics, and anxiolytics.

There are two types of PSUDs: substance

dependence and substance abuse. Substance dependence is characterized by "a cluster of cognitive, behavioral, and physiologic symptoms that indicate that the person has impaired control of psychoactive substance use and continues use of the substance despite adverse consequences."[61] The diagnostic criteria for psychoactive substance dependence are listed below.

Diagnostic Criteria for Psychoactive Substance Dependence*

A. At least three of the following:
1. Substance often taken in larger amounts or over a longer period than the person intended.
2. Persistent desire or one or more unsuccessful efforts to cut down or control substance use.
3. A great deal of time spent in activities necessary to get the substance (e.g., theft), taking the substance (e.g., chain smoking), or recovering from its effect.
4. Frequent intoxication or withdrawal symptoms when expected to fulfill major role obligations at work, school, or home (e.g., does not go to work because hung over, goes to school or work "high," intoxicated while taking care of his or her children), or when substance use is physically hazardous (e.g., drives when intoxicated).
5. Important social, occupational, or recreational activities given up or reduced because of substance use.
6. Continued substance use despite knowledge of having a persistent or recurrent social, psychological, or physical problem that is caused or exacerbated by the use of the substance (e.g., keeps using heroin despite family arguments about it, cocaine-induced depression, or having an ulcer made worse by drinking).
7. Marked tolerance: need for markedly increased amounts of the substance (i.e., at least a 50 percent increase) in order to achieve intoxication or desired effect, or markedly diminished effect with continued use of the same amount.
   Note: The following items may not apply to cannabis, hallucinogens, or phencyclidine (PCP):

---

* From *DSM-III-R*, pp. 167–168.

8. Characteristic withdrawal symptoms (see specific withdrawal syndromes under Psychoactive Substance-induced Organic Mental Disorders).
9. Substance often taken to relieve or avoid withdrawal symptoms.

B. Some symptoms of the disturbance have persisted for at least 1 month, or have occurred repeatedly over a longer period of time.

Criteria for Severity of Psychoactive Substance Dependence

- **Mild:** Few, if any, symptoms in excess of those required to make the diagnosis, and the symptoms result in no more than mild impairment in occupational functioning or in usual social activities or relationships with others.
- **Moderate:** Symptoms or functional impairment between "mild" and "severe."
- **Severe:** Many symptoms in excess of those required to make the diagnosis, and the symptoms markedly interfere with occupational functioning or with usual social activities or relationships with others.*
- **In partial remission:** During the past 6 months, some use of the substance and some symptoms of dependence.
- **In full remission:** During the past 6 months, either no use of the substance, or use of the substance and no symptoms of dependence.

Most patients with problems serious enough to be seen in a drug treatment setting will meet the criteria for severe substance dependence. It is important to note that patients are not given a general substance dependence diagnosis but are determined to meet the criteria for dependence on one or more of the drugs listed earlier. In addition, there is a category for polysubstance dependence and a category for dependence on a drug not specified in the diagnostic manual. The following case example illustrates the psychoactive substance dependence syndrome in a patient dependent on cocaine.

A 32-year-old stockbroker calls a crisis hotline after losing his job and being confronted with his wife's

plans for divorce. He wants to know where the next Cocaine Anonymous (CA) meeting will be held and says it's a matter of life and death. After moving to the city only 2 weeks ago, he began a cocaine "run," never reporting to work for his new job. At this time he is "crashing," out of cocaine, out of money, and frantic to find a CA meeting. He describes himself as a cocaine addict who found recovery through CA 4 months ago in another city. Before going to CA he had been using cocaine for 2 years, reaching the point of spending most of his time getting and using the drug. The "crash" is described as "hell," "unbearably painful," and "the worst bottom ever." "I thought I could get by here for a while on my own, without the CA group, I guess I was setting myself up for a slip. I thought one line of coke wouldn't amount to anything. Besides no one here knew I was an addict. Can you believe that? I set myself up! After the first line, I brought a big bag of crack home and smoked it for a week. I hardly stopped to eat. I'm a real case."

Although not commonly encountered in a treatment setting, a substance abuse diagnosis is included in the *DSM-III-R* for individuals showing a maladaptive pattern of drug use without meeting the criteria for dependence.

Diagnostic Criteria for Abuse

A. A maladaptive pattern of psychoactive substance use indicated by at least one of the following:
1. Continued use despite a persistent social, occupational, psychological, or physical problem that is caused or exacerbated by use of the psychoactive substance.
2. Recurrent use in situations which are physically hazardous (e.g., driving while intoxicated).
B. Some symptoms of the disturbance have persisted for at least 1 month, or have occurred repeatedly over a longer period of time.
C. Never met the criteria for Psychoactive Substance Dependence for this substance.[62]

The following case example describes a person who shows a pattern of abuse with cannabis.

John Danforth, a 26-year-old truck driver, tried some marijuana offered by a fellow driver who said it would take the "drag" out of the long day on the road. John had used marijuana several times during high school with friends when it was offered, but he had never had his own supply and did not think of himself as a pot user. To his delight, John found that the marijuana did take much of the boredom out of the long

---

* Because of the availability of cigarettes and other nicotine-containing substances and the absence of a clinically significant nicotine intoxication syndrome, impairment in occupational or social functioning is not necessary for a rating of severe Nicotine Dependence.

drive and bought a bag for his own use. He began to smoke one "joint" each day to "break up the trip." This continued for 5 weeks until a manager found a small bag of marijuana under the driver's seat of the truck during a routine safety check. John was confronted with this, suspended from duty for a week, and told he would be fired if it happened again. John was so upset by the incident that he followed the manager's advice to see a counselor in the company's employee assistance program.

Physiological Tolerance and Withdrawal

While there is less emphasis on physiological tolerance and withdrawal as primary symptoms of dependence in *DSM-III-R* than in *DSM-III*, most clients in treatment will experience a withdrawal syndrome of some type. Tolerance occurs when, after a drug has been repeatedly used, the dose of the substance must be increased in order to achieve the desired effect. Tolerance appears to be mediated through the adaptation of CNS cells to the presence of the increasing dose. Once this adaptation has taken place, abrupt cessation of drug use may begin a withdrawal syndrome. The drugs that *DSM-III-R* identifies as being capable of causing a withdrawal syndrome are: alcohol, amphetamines, cocaine, nicotine, opioids, and sedatives, hypnotics, or anxiolytics. Withdrawal syndromes differ in their character and seriousness depending on the particular drug or, commonly, the several types of drugs the client has been using.

It is important to recognize that the problems of substance dependence may not come up in a psychiatric context but rather in the management of other conditions such as accidents, hepatitis, HIV infection, malnutrition, venereal disease, pneumonia, tuberculosis, skin infections, and pregnancy. Thus, the student should keep in mind the *DSM-III-R* classification in the evaluation of drug use patterns of patients in all clinical settings. If a patient's problem is suggestive of substance dependence, a psychiatric–chemical dependence consultation is indicated. The *DSM-III-R* system is purely descriptive; it does not have a particular theoretical bias, and it does not provide prescriptions for intervention.

Since the student rarely has the opportunity to work with a range of patients having a variety of drug-specific disorders as outlined in the *DSM-III-R*, it will be helpful to briefly discuss the major categories of drugs (excluding alcohol, caffeine, and nicotine) with a case example for each type. The source for most general information on the pharmacology of the drugs is "The Substances of Abuse," in *Substance Abuse: Pharmacologic, Developmental and Clinical Perspectives*.[63] An in-depth discussion of most drugs of abuse may be found in this text.

DUAL DIAGNOSIS

The Dual-Diagnosis Patient

Dual-diagnosis patients meet the criteria for at least one drug disorder and a major mental illness, such as one of the psychotic, mood, or anxiety disorders. These patients are an enormous challenge to diagnose and treat successfully. Few treatment facilities are prepared to respond to the special treatment needs of this population. The following case example illustrates a dual-diagnosis patient.

Tim was a 26-year-old father of two at the time of his admission. He had lost both his marriage and his job as a salesman as a result of heavy alcohol and marijuana use that had increased over a period of years. After 2 weeks in an inpatient alcohol treatment program, he attempted to hang himself. He was quickly transferred to a psychiatric unit and diagnosed as having a major affective illness, bipolar type. The severity of his depression eventually led to his involuntary commitment to the state hospital.[64]

Dual-diagnosis cases are not unusual. In one state hospital where McKelvy, Kane, and Kellison developed a special program to identify and treat dual-diagnosis patients, it was found that 60 percent of patients entering the hospital had significant substance abuse problems and major mental disorders. The guiding rule with these patients is to provide a program of recovery that addresses both their drug disorder and mental illness.[65]

DRUGS OF ABUSE

Amphetamines

Amphetamine drugs are synthetic compounds derived from ephedrine. These drugs are racemic amphetamines ("uppers," "bennies," "peaches"), and dextroamphetamine ("speed," "meth," "crystal," "whites"). There are also a number of amphetamine-like drugs (anorectics) and over-the-counter appetite suppressants (Dexatrim, etc.) that may be abused in a fashion similar to the amphetamine drugs.

Amphetamines are potent CNS stimulants. Feelings during amphetamine intoxication range from alertness, euphoria, and optimism to being on edge, "wired," and "strung out." Amphetamine psychosis, often indistinguishable from paranoid schizophrenia in clinical presentation, occurs in some abusers. Repetitive behavior is commonly seen in amphetamine addicts. This behavior may be purposeful in terms of school or occupation, or it may seem nonpurposeful, such as taking a radio apart and putting it back together again for no apparent reason.

Medical complications of amphetamine abuse include cardiac arrhythmias, hyperthermia, hypertension, bruxism, and malnutrition. Amphetamine abuse in the extreme is seen in the "speed freak" who injects dextroamphetamine over a period of several days, sleeping little or none at all during the "run." A deep but often disturbing sleep or "crash" follows the run, along with several days of depressed activity until another run begins.

Tolerance develops rapidly in compulsive amphetamine users, particularly if the intravenous route of administration is used. A predictable withdrawal syndrome begins after cessation of chronic amphetamine use. Depressed mood, fatigue, and disturbed sleep are the main features of the syndrome. Suicide is a real danger during the withdrawal period.

CASE EXAMPLE

Sam Selden is a 32-year-old suspended police officer who lives with his wife and one child in an upper-middle class suburb of the city. Sam's wife, whom he met in college, comes from a wealthy midwestern family and has been used to having many of the finer things in life. Sam, who barely makes enough to get by as a police officer, was convinced by his in-laws that he should provide "decent" housing for his family and a comfortable environment. Sam has been doing this for the past few years by working full time as a police officer and moonlighting in odd jobs, mostly special security positions. In order to keep up this pace, Sam was taking amphetamines in large quantities. At first he received his supply from a local physician, but after about 6 months, the physician refused to renew Sam's prescription. After going through several doctors with the same results, Sam

went to the street for his supply. Sam had been in on several drug busts, so the street contacts were easily made. Eventually Same became obligated both in a professional and personal way: The street dealer required Sam to alert him to any planned bust that would affect him. The police department became suspicious of Sam's actions and instituted an internal investigation. Through this investigation, set up by an internal affairs board, Sam was arrested by an undercover state police investigator. He has yet to appear before the police trial board.[66]

Cannabis

The cannabis class of substances includes marijuana, hashish, and hash oil. Tetrahydrocannabinol (THC), the most potent active ingredient in cannabis, is very difficult to synthesize in clandestine laboratories and is rarely available on the street. If a person claims to have used THC, he probably has been using PCP, lysergic acid (LSD), or anticholinergics such as atropine or scopolamine. However, the THC content of marijuana smoked in the United States has increased considerably over the last 10 to 15 years as a result of the increasing sophistication of marijuana farming as an industry. The relaxing of inhibitions seen in cannabis intoxication can lead to bizarre behavior or aggressive expression of anger. Marijuana is the name given to a collection of dried leaves, flowers, and stems of the plant *Cannabis sativa*. Hashish, generally referred to simply as *hash*, is a concentrated block of resin from the plant. If hashish is boiled in a solvent and the solid matter is filtered out, a potent "hash oil" results.[67] Cannabis intoxication may be mild or trully hallucinogenic, depending on the THC content of the substance consumed. Mild intoxication is often described as a pleasant, dreamy state. The enjoyment of food, music, conversation, or sex may be perceived as enhanced. As the THC content is increased, as it is in hashish and hash oil, the potential for a negative experience increases.

It was estimated that in 1979 alone, 50 million pounds of marijuana were smuggled into the United States. Deducting 10 percent for government seizures, these shipments and street sales generated about $22.5 billion in the underground economy. When one compares this figure to the $16 billion earned annually by the cigarette industry, the enormous demand for marijuana is placed in dramatic perspective.[68]

The scientific community is generally split over the potential hazards to health that cannabis use entails. One interpretation of the controversy is that it is related to the mind–body dichotomy in Western scientific disciplines. Psychosocial research has consistently shown that cannabis use cannot be directly related in a causal manner to crime, use of "hard" drugs, or a general "amotivational syndrome." On the other hand, biologic researchers, using animal models of high-dose cannabis consumption, have concluded that the drug leads to direct and harmful alterations in the respiratory, reproductive, and nervous systems.[69]

In the late 1970s, the movement to decriminalize cannabis led by the National Organization for the Reform of Marijuana Laws (NORML) seemed to be gaining political credibility. At one point, Robert Dupont, former director of the National Institute on Drug Abuse, and former President Carter supported marijuana decriminalization. In fact, as late as 1980, Johnson and Uppal wrote that there was "no antimarijuana equivalent to NORML; thus, no continuing or contending forces are in dispute, as on the abortion issue (National Organization for Women versus Right to Life)."[70] As it turned out, the potential for a serious antimarijuana movement was underestimated.

In the late 1970s and early 1980s, attention began to focus on the consequences of widespread "pot" use by preteens and teen-agers. This issue led to one point of consensus in the marijuana controversy: Regular use of this potent psychoactive substance is hazardous to normal development in children and adolescents.[71] Parents' action groups organized at the national level as the National Federation of Parents for Drug-Free Youth (NFP) became formidable political opponents of NORML and the cannabis paraphernalia industry.[72,73] These groups resisted decriminalization efforts in the state legislatures and also supported a model law written by the DEA that had the effect of outlawing the sale of drug paraphernalia. The Reagan Administration, and particularly Nancy Reagan, have given their support to a hard line against marijuana decriminalization.

CASE EXAMPLE

Dave Moore was only 17, but for the past 2 years much or most of his life had revolved around buying, selling, growing, and smoking marijuana. A tall, handsome young man with a pallid complexion and unruly and uncombed, shoulder-length hair, he was invariably dressed in torn, dirty jeans and T-shirt. Dave's appearance was almost as irritating to his parents as was his constant use of marijuana. They also quarrelled with him over his not going to school, his use and abuse of the family car, and his demands for money. He would say he needed money for the car for one purpose (for example, looking for a job or going to a school function) but would use the money to buy "pot" and to drive around with his friends while high. Dave had violent fights with his family, particularly with his mother. In addition to destroying things in the house, he was verbally abusive to his mother and had hit her on occasion.[74]

Whether as a result of the impact of the concerned parents movement, drug abuse education, changing values of youth, or a combination of these and other factors, marijuana use is showing a significant decline in the high school population. A national study of substance use among high school seniors found the number of students admitting to daily marijuana use climbed from 6 percent to 11 percent between 1975 and 1978. After 1978 daily marijuana use among high school seniors began steadily decreasing, reaching a low of 5 percent of all seniors in 1984.[75]

Cocaine

Cocaine is the principal psychoactive ingredient of the South American coca plant, *Erythroxylon coca*. Chewing the leaves of this plant has been a custom of the natives of Peru and Bolivia for centuries. The leaves may be easily converted to coca paste, which is used for the production of cocaine hydrochloride, the white crystalline powder available on the illicit market in North America and Europe. In the late 1970s, "free-basing" became popular in the United States. This process has been described as "freeing" cocaine from its hydrochloride salt "base." Cocaine hydrochloride is dissolved, a product such as baking soda is added, and a resulting precipitate is filtered off and dried. These granules are then smoked in a free-basing pipe. Larger chunks of free-base available on the street are called "crack." Smoking cocaine free-base leads to rapid addiction not substantively different from injecting the drug.

Cocaine is a stimulant with a short half-life. For instance, the euphoric rush that the free-base smoker gets will only last about 1 minute, with the feeling of being "high" lasting about

10 minutes. Whether the drug is being snorted, smoked, or injected, the abuser must readminister frequently to achieve the desired effect. This feature of cocaine abuse is prized by recreational or social users. They are able to have their drug experience within a clearly defined period of time. For the cocaine abuser, the constant need to procure and administer expensive cocaine results in an almost total preoccupation with the drug. Cocaine dependence has become pandemic in the 1980s, spreading from South America to North America, Western Europe and Asia.[76]

CASE EXAMPLE

Susan Stein is a 35-year-old secretary and mother of 2 young children. After a divorce several years ago, she began dating a manager in her company who introduced her to cocaine. At first she would use cocaine only occasionally at a party. She found the drug gave her the best feeling she had ever experienced. Over time she began to look forward to the cocaine parties as an escape from the pressures of her work and family life. She relied more and more on her mother to care for her children on weekends while she went on cocaine binges. Soon she found it difficult to make it to work on Mondays, and finally she was fired for poor attendance. It was only after Susan had not worked for several months and used cocaine daily that her mother convinced her to see a therapist about her problems.

Hallucinogens

Hallucinogens include natural and synthetic drugs that produce sensory illusions, and more rarely, hallucinations or delusions. Peyote, containing natural mescaline, is used by the Indians of northern Mexico and members of the Native American Church for long-established religious ceremonies. Such use is not considered "abuse" by *DSM-III-R* criteria, and the Native American Church has been exempted from the Controlled Substances Act in regard to ceremonial use of peyote. Psilocybin and psilocin are natural hallucinogens derived from mushrooms.

Lysergic acid diethylamide (LSD), a semi-synthetic substance produced from lysergic acid found in a fungus of rye, and synthetic mescaline are the most used and abused hallucinogens. A fascinating account of the synthesis of LSD may be found by the interested reader in Albert Hofmann's book *LSD: My Problem Child*.[77] This book, by the researcher who not only first produced the substance but also was the first to experience its psychic effects, explores the basic question concerning psychoactive substances in our age: How can psychoactive drugs be used in modern society so that the quality of life is enhanced rather than diminished? As for LSD, Hofmann concludes that despite its potential for psychological harm, it also offers a unique experience to spiritual seekers, artists, and some persons engaged in psychotherapy. He believes his "problem child" still has the potential to become a "wonder child" in certain contexts. The potential for useful applications of LSD and other hallucinogens continues to be noted by neuroscientists.[78] Senay, a drug-abuse specialist who has also considered the question of possible therapeutic effects of hallucinogens, concludes that these drugs may be too powerful and unpredictable to have accepted psychiatric uses.[79]

CASE EXAMPLE

A 21-year-old woman was admitted to the hospital along with her boyfriend. He had had a number of LSD experiences and had convinced her to take it to make her less constrained sexually. About half an hour after ingestion of approximately 200 mg, she noticed that the bricks in the wall began to go in and out and that light affected her strangely. She became frightened when she realized that she was unable to distinguish her body from the chair she was sitting on or from her boyfriend's body. Her fear became more marked after she thought that she would not get back into herself. At the time of admission she was hyperactive and laughed inappropriately. Her stream of talk was illogical and her affect labile. Two days later, this reaction had ceased. However, she was still afraid of the drug and convinced that she would not take it again because of her frightening experience.[80]

Inhalants

The vapors of gasoline, glue, paint, paint thinners, spray paint, typewriter correction fluid, or spray-can propellants may be inhaled to produce intoxication. Users are called "sniffers." Although there are adult cases, most sniffers are adolescents with multiple problems living in poverty. A recent study suggests users are just as likely to be girls as boys, and use is more common among junior high students than in the high school population.[81]

The psychoactive effects of inhalants are traced to the hydrocarbons contained in these substances. Heavy use is associated with renal and hepatic complications.

CASE EXAMPLE

John is 11 years old and a gasoline sniffer. His mother found him passed out in the alley near their apartment with a gasoline-soaked rag covering his face. She took him to the emergency room, where he recovered. He told the nurse he and his friends liked the smell of gas and sniffed it sometimes. The nurse encouraged him to talk more about the gas sniffing and learned it had been going on every few days for several months. An appointment was made for John the next day at the local community mental health center.

Opioids

The opioid drugs may be subdivided into the opioids of natural origin, the semisynthetic opioids, and the synthetic opioids. The principal natural opioids are opium, morphine, and codeine. Opium is the dried juice scraped from the oriental poppy pod, *Papaver somniferum*. Morphine and codeine are the active ingredients in opium, morphine being the most potent. Semisynthetic opioids include heroin, hydromorphine (Dilaudid), and oxycodone (contained in Percodan). These drugs are derived by chemical modification of the natural opioids.

Heroin is the most notorious of the opioids in the United States. Heroin addicts are generally considered to be the "hardest core" of the drug culture. It is often incorrectly stated in textbooks that heroin was first discovered and marketed as a cure for morphine addiction. In actual fact, heroin was first produced by the English chemist C. R. Ala Wright in 1874 when he was exploring the effect of combining a number of acids with morphine. In 1898, a German pharmacologist, Heinrich Dresser, named the drug diacetylmorphine "heroin," meaning heroic or powerful, and promoted it as a treatment for coughs, pneumonia, and tuberculosis. Trebach points out that a drug with such claims was bound to demand the attention of American physicians at the turn of the century when tuberculosis and pneumonia were the two leading causes of death in the United States.[82] Since 1900, heroin has passed through stages of being an over-the-counter drug for coughs, a controlled substance only to be prescribed by physicians, and an illicit substance with no legal medical use. There has been some discussion in recent years about legalizing the use of heroin for administration to terminal cancer patients.

The synthetic opioids are produced in the laboratory without opium products but are pharmacologically similar in action to the natural and semisynthetic drugs such as heroin. Meperidine and methadone are examples of completely synthetic opioids.

The opioids are the most potent and effective pain relievers known and have relatively few destructive effects on normal physiological processes in comparison to alcohol. However, their high potential for abuse and dependence have made them problem drugs among some groups in our society. These groups are diverse, including health professionals, entertainers, and the alienated poor in urban areas. Of all people in "straight" society, health professionals have the greatest risk of becoming addicted to opioids, particularly meperidine.

Intravenous users of heroin or other opioids experience a "rush" of euphoria, which usually lasts less than 1 minute. Heroin is the preferred opioid of abuse by addicts because it provides the ultimate rush experience. Heroin crosses the lipid blood–brain barrier more easily than morphine. Snorting, injecting under the skin ("skin popping"), and simply swallowing are other routes of administration that produce a less intense "euphoric drowsiness," a feeling that most addicts would describe as being "high." Repeated use of opioids leads to tolerance and physical dependency.

Opioid addicts using the intravenous route of administration (most do) are engaged in a very risky practice. Risks include overdose, hepatitis, and other infections from impure drug products and contaminated equipment. Intravenous drug abusers are also at risk for the much-feared Acquired Immune Deficiency Syndrome (AIDS).[83]

Opioid overdose is a medical emergency and requires prompt hospitalization. Support of vital functions and administration of an opioid antagonist are indicated.[84]

CASE EXAMPLE

Pam was "busted" for possession of heroin. She claims the police stopped her for a traffic violation and found her in possession of the drug. She is only seeking treatment because of the "bust"—she has no history of previous arrests. Now she wants "to get off drugs" and get off probation. She doesn't see methadone treatment as being on drugs. She has tried to quit heroin twice before, the first time when she was pregnant—"Tried to get off for the kid." And then there was a second attempt that failed after 1 month, 1½ years ago. She has been told about methadone programs by friends who talked about the "convenience" of having reliable methadone. Her daughter is now 3 years old and is "real neat."

Phencyclidine

Phencyclidine hydrochloride (PCP), a synthetic white crystalline powder, poses a classification dilemma. It has hallucinogenic effects in some users and additional CNS depressant effects in others. The drug's erratic course and unpredictable effects have led R. S. Burns and S. E. Lerner to suggest that PCP may represent a new class of psychoactive drugs.[85] It was introduced in 1967 as an experimental anesthetic agent; however, bizarre behavior in postoperative patients precluded its continued use with humans. Later in the same year it appeared illegally in the drug community in San Francisco. Initially, its frequent negative effects delayed its acceptance with drug users in major cities. However, in recent years it appears the drug has attained widespread use among youthful drug abusers throughout the United States.[86]

Effects of PCP vary with dosage, previous experience with the drug, and route of administration. It may be injected, insufflated, ingested, or—most commonly—smoked after sprinkling it on marijuana, parsley, or a similar substance. The general characteristics of low-to-moderate dose intoxication (approximately 1 to 10 mg) are subjective responses ranging from euphoria to panic. Typical physiological manifestations of low-to-moderate dose are nystagmus, ataxia, increased blood pressure, and decreased peripheral sensations. At higher doses (10 mg or more) the most characteristic psychological effect is amnesia. The most serious physical effect of high-dose intoxication is CNS depression, which may lead to coma and death. Chronic abusers appear to develop tolerance and psychological dependence. Major problems resulting from PCP abuse are violent outbursts, medical emergencies associated with acute phencyclidine overdose, and phencyclidine psychosis.

A 16-year-old male, acting belligerent and combative, was brought to the hospital from a party where he was drowsy but responsive to verbal stimuli. There were abrasions on his right arm and face. Over the next 3 hours he became verbally abusive, belligerent, and uncooperative and was transferred to the county hospital. Initially violent, he alternated between periods of sleep and moaning. Toxicology screen obtained at this time revealed a phencyclidine urine value of 1.1 mg/ml. Over the next 15½ hours the patient became alert and oriented and was subsequently discharged.[87]

Sedatives, Hypnotics, and Anxiolytics

The category of sedatives, hypnotics, and anxiolytics includes drugs frequently prescribed in clinical practice. These drugs, including barbiturates, chloral hydrate, meprobamate, methaqualone, and the benzodiazepines, share with alcohol the psychoactive property of being central nervous system depressants. Nurses frequently administer low-to-moderate doses of these drugs to relieve anxiety or to induce sleep. Opioid and stimulant users often medicate themselves with depressants to ease withdrawal or to calm their thoughts or feelings. A danger in using barbiturate or barbiturate-like drugs for these purposes is the high potential for a progressive tolerance that requires more and more of a drug to achieve the desired effect.

The National Commission of Marijuana and Drug Abuse suggested in 1973 that "barbiturate dependence may be the modern equivalent of the hidden opiate dependence of the late 19th century."[88] The Commission reported that of the 214 million psychoactive drug prescriptions in 1970, 28.6 percent were for barbiturate and barbiturate-like drugs. Prescriptions filled for minor tranquilizers accounted for 38.8 percent, which brings the total percentage for this drug category to 67.4 percent, or more than half of all psychoactive drug prescriptions in 1970. These trends in drug prescription and drug use appear to continue in the 1980s. Probably a million or more Americans abuse sedative–hypnotics, and it has been estimated that 30,000 are dependent on them. Sedative–hypnotic overdoses, both accidental and intended, account for the largest number of overdose deaths in the United States.[89]

Sedative–hypnotic withdrawal and sedative–hypnotic overdose are serious medical emergencies that require prompt professional management. As tolerance develops, a sedative–hypnotic user may increase the daily dose up to 20 times the level considered therapeutic. It has been established for some time that physical dependence on secobarbital or pentobarbital develops in doses of 900 mg to 2.2 g per day for longer than 30 days. However, predicting the dosage level and required length of use to establish physical dependency to the nonbarbiturate sedative–hypnotics is not well supported by research at the present time. The best practice for the clinician is to suspect the possibility of physical dependency in any person who has been taking sedative–hypnotics on a regular basis. There is no harm in finding that physical dependency does not exist when it is suspected as a possibility; however, there can be serious consequences, including death, for an addicted person who abruptly stops intake of depressants without detoxification.

The withdrawal symptoms induced by abrupt cessation of sedative–hypnotic drug intake have been collectively termed the *general depressant withdrawal syndrome*. Depending on the extent and length of addiction, this syndrome may be limited to anxiety or may progress to seizures or delirium. The onset of the syndrome varies among the short-acting and long-acting CNS depressants.

The short-acting drugs, such as chloral hydrate, have a timing of withdrawal onset similar to alcohol, usually within 6 to 12 hours after the last dose, peaking within the first or second day of abstinence. Examples of short-to-intermediate-acting drugs are secobarbital, pentobarbital, and amobarbital. Since these drugs and their active metabolites take longer to leave the body, the withdrawal symptoms during the first day of abstinence may be mild, but a severe withdrawal reaction can be expected on day 2 or 3 if an addict goes without appropriate detoxification. The benzodiazepines are long-acting drugs and produce withdrawal symptoms that do not peak until approximately 1 week after the last dose.

CASE EXAMPLE

Mary Lang, an attractive woman of about 40, is married and the mother of two beautiful children, an adolescent girl and a 12-year-old boy. Mary has a problem—she is dependent on drugs. It started slowly, when the children were younger and the days were terribly long. Wanting to appear relaxed and loving to her husband, she would take a tranquilizer before he came home from work. It helped; the minor irritations of the day didn't seem quite so important, and she was ready to listen eagerly to her husband's tale of his day. Soon though, one tranquilizer wasn't enough; the children became difficult earlier in the day, so she would take a pill to deal with them more calmly. As time went on, she became dependent on drugs. Her children stopped bringing friends home from school even though Mary promised them that she'd "behave." Her husband became increasingly angry at her and threatened to leave if she didn't improve. As a result, she spent less time at home, and she needed tranquilizers to deal with her loneliness.[90]

Designer Drugs

Designer drugs are synthetic analogues of popular controlled or illicit substances such as phencyclidine, meperidine, fentanyl, and methamphetamine. Although the designer drugs are not included in the *DSM-III-R* classification system, the student should be aware of the increasing hazards to health posed by these substances. Fentanyl analogues, called "China white" or "synthetic heroin," are many times more potent than heroin and have been associated with over 100 overdose deaths.[91]

The designer drugs were originally developed as a way for clandestine drug producers to circumvent the laws governing controlled and illicit substances. Technology has advanced to such a degree that new variations of established drugs can be readily synthesized in illegal laboratories. Not only is the development of synthetic analogues cost-effective but producers have in many cases been able to avoid confrontation with law enforcement agencies, primarily because these drugs were too new to be declared illegal. The Anti-Drug Abuse Act of 1986 banned analogues similar to any controlled substance; however, designer drugs continue to be distributed on the street and pose a great risk to users.

ASSESSMENT AND PSYCHOACTIVE SUBSTANCE USE DISORDERS

In 1980 the American Nurses' Association published *Nursing: A Social Policy Statement*, in which nursing is defined as the diagnosis and treatment of human responses to actual or potential health problems.[92] Since psychoactive substance use disorders are a major health problem in our society, and the nurse's charge is to promote health as well as to intervene when health problems are present, a drug history should be an integral component of the assessment of individuals, families, and communities in all health care settings. Although the purpose of this section is to present the assessment of the patient with a PSUD admitted to a drug-abuse or psychiatric treatment setting, a brief discussion on assessing patients in other health care settings will be offered first.

Nonpsychiatric and Drug-Abuse Health Care Settings

Nursing school graduates who choose to work in nonpsychiatric health care settings need guidelines for assessing patients with PSUDs. Effective case finding and appropriate follow-up depend on the nurse's understanding of PSUDs, an awareness of community resources (described later in the chapter), and the ability to establish a trusting relationship with the patient. In addition, the nurse must be able to gather and evaluate relevant data. Is it not surprising, then, that the assessment of patients with potential or actual PSUDs is a challenging task for the nurse?

The psychiatric diagnosis of PSUDs may be rather straightforward in the patient admitted to a drug-abuse treatment program, especially when the drug problem is known to the patient and staff. However, the difficulty in assessing PSUDs increases with patients admitted to other health care settings. Chychula presents a detailed drug assessment tool for the nurse to use as part of the health history data gathering in a variety of primary care settings. In addition, she offers tips on how to approach patients to enhance establishing a rapport during the interview. This is followed by ideas for beginning intervention when a drug problem is confirmed.[93]

PSUDs, in some cases, are more apparent but not necessarily easier to address when patients are admitted with secondary consequences such as overdose, withdrawal, and drug-induced psychosis; hepatitis or abscesses are also common from injecting drugs with contaminated needles. Familiarity with the physical consequences of PSUDs as identified by Ciske

provides the nurse with valuable clues for continuing with an in-depth drug-abuse or -dependence assessment.[94] Williams discusses the primary and psychological aspects of care and health maintenance needs of parenteral drug users.[95] Nurses working in primary care settings may find her guidelines useful.

An important related issue to bring up here is the problem of AIDS in intravenous (IV) drug users. Approximately 17% of people diagnosed with AIDS are IV drug users.[96] The route of drug administration is important information to obtain during the assessment of patients with PSUDs, particularly in light of the AIDS epidemic. Nurses working in areas serving this population will be involved in health teaching (e.g., the safety hazards of improperly cleaning and sharing needles and syringes) and assessing patients with PSUDs for AIDS-related problems. An accepting attitude and genuine concern over their presenting problems may assist the establishment of rapport with patients. One study indicated a positive rapport was established with drug-using women presenting in an emergency room when nurses employing a "personalized nursing" approach respected the autonomy of the patient. This is particularly noteworthy, since over half the women diagnosed with AIDS are IV drug users.[97]

Psychiatric and Drug-Abuse Health Care Settings

The immediate tasks of the nurse when admitting the patient with a PSUD to the inpatient or outpatient facility is to begin to establish a bond between the client and the treatment community. The patient may be ambivalent about treatment and is at risk for leaving before completing the program. Staff are challenged to create an environment supportive to the patient, who is often frightened and uncertain during the early stages of recovery. The assessment of the patient is therefore conducted in concert with establishing a trusting relationship. It does not matter what type of program the patient is admitted to or the length of stay, a commitment to changing a drug-using life-style may be enhanced by staff attitudes and skills.

A nonjudgmental attitude in the nurse may encourage the suspicious and fearful client to give an honest account of drug use. Two major concerns of drug users are trouble with the police and suffering withdrawal in jail. If the patient is unable to be interviewed for drug use, available family or friends should be contacted. Keep in mind that family and friends may want to protect the patient and therefore require a trusting relationship with the nurse, as well. The following drug history information would be helpful for further assessment:

1. Identify drug(s) used (including alcohol).
2. Pattern of use for each drug:
    a. First use
    b. Length of time used
    c. Variation of use
    d. Variation of amount used
    e. Route of administration
    f. Last dose and amount consumed.
3. History of withdrawal symptoms.
4. History of complications from drug use.

If the patient happens to be an experimenter (one time or infrequent use) an appropriate referral is to a drug education program (drug education programs should be screened to determine if they offer assistance in assertiveness training, building self-esteem, and developing recreational alternatives. Each patient, particularly youthful drug experimenters, should receive an individual assessment to determine the need for drug information).

One difficult problem is psychotic behavior precipitated by drug use. In some cases hallucinations or other psychotic behaviors are a result of an untoward reaction to the drug itself. In other cases an exacerbation of psychotic behaviors in a person with a history of mental illness may be precipitated by drug use. The dual-diagnosis person is one who has both a diagnosis of a mental disorder and a drug-abuse or -dependency disorder. Unfortunately, even occasional use of illegal drugs by psychiatric patients may alter the course of their illness or adversely effect their treatment regimen; therefore (according to the *DSM-III-R* criteria, discussed earlier) a diagnosis of substance abuse is applied. As noted earlier, dual diagnosis is fairly common, with M. J. McKelvy, J. S. Kane, and K. Kellison estimating that over half of psychiatric admissions have a concomitant problem of substance abuse or dependence.[98]

Whenever possible it is helpful to determine whether the patient is having an untoward reaction to a drug, is a dual-diagnosis patient, or is displaying the symptoms of a psychiatric disorder and has not abused drugs. If the psychosis is prolonged and differentiation is not possible,

efforts should be directed toward ameliorating presenting symptoms. At times, even if a dual-diagnosis problem is obvious, exploration of which disorder is primary may be fruitless. Efforts would be better spent addressing both disorders concurrently.[99] The usual approach with these patients is initially to stabilize the psychiatric condition. Once the patient is alert and oriented, the drug problem is addressed. McKelvy et al., offer a current perspective on the nursing management of the dual-diagnosis patient.[100] As part of the educational component of care, patients need to understand that even the occasional or recreational use of drugs may affect the course of their illness and treatment, eventually destabilizing their condition.[101]

Psychiatric diagnosis of a drug disorder provides valuable information for the nurse caring for the patient. First of all, it establishes the presence of a PSUD, and second, it directs the health care team toward immediate treatment and/or further assessment.

Psychoactive-Substance-Induced Organic Mental Disorders and Emergency Medical Treatment

Among clients requiring immediate attention in drug-abuse treatment settings are those admitted in acute psychoactive-substance-induced withdrawal, hallucinogenic crises, or psychoactive-substance-induced delirium and delusional disorders. In the *DSM-III-R* these problems are classified as psychoactive-substance-induced organic mental disorders because of drug effect on the nervous system. It is noted that most patients with any of these diagnoses will have an additional diagnosis of a PSUD.[102] A few helpful guidelines will be offered for the assessment of these three medical emergencies.

Acute Psychoactive-Substance-Induced Withdrawal
A withdrawal syndrome is usually precipitated after the chronic drug user either abruptly stops taking the drugs or markedly lowers the dose. The cells of the central nervous system adapt to progressively increasing doses of drugs and when they are abruptly stopped the cells react, triggering a variety of symptoms. The severity of the withdrawal syndrome depends on the interaction of several factors including: The level of dosage and combination of drugs consumed

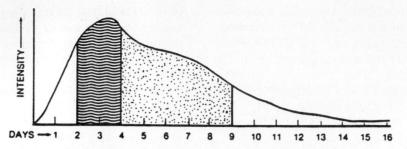

Figure 34-1. Withdrawal syndrome from the short-to-intermediate-acting CNS depressants. Peak of seizure activity is represented by wavy lines; onset of psychosis or delirium is represented by dotted area. (From Woolf, D. S., CNS depressants: Other sedative-hypnotics, in *Substance Abuse: Pharmacologic, Developmental and Clinical Perspectives*, Eds. Gerald Bennett, Christine Vourakis, and Donna S. Woolf (New York: John Wiley & Sons, Inc. 1983, p. 52, with permission.[63])

(including alcohol), length of time drug(s) abused, individual differences, and previous history of withdrawal. Intervention in withdrawal is discussed in the section on detoxification. The discussion of the withdrawal syndromes in this section offer helpful guidelines for the nurse working in any clinical setting, as well as the psychiatric and drug-abuse setting. The syndromes to be covered include general depressant withdrawal, withdrawal from opioids, and withdrawal from stimulants (e.g., cocaine, amphetamines, and related substances). Nicotine withdrawal will also be mentioned.

The general depressant withdrawal syndrome is the most dangerous of the drug withdrawal syndromes. It is characterized by symptoms ranging from mild anxiety to seizures and delirium and requires close medical and nursing attention. The drug history will give the information needed to begin immediate treatment. Determining the drugs in the current abuse

cycle is important because some short-to-intermediate-acting depressants such as meprobamate and ethchlorvynol are rapidly eliminated from the body, producing symptoms within 6 to 12 hours after cessation of the drug. Figure 34-1 identifies the course of the withdrawal syndrome for short-to-intermediate-acting drugs. Drugs such as chlordiazepoxide and diazepam are eliminated at a slower rate, creating a prolonged abstinence syndrome. It is particularly important to have specific drug information, in addition to information on alcohol (a short-acting CNS depressant), since withdrawal from alcohol may be followed a few days later by another life-threatening withdrawal syndrome. See Figure 34-2 for the course of the long-acting drug withdrawal syndrome. Along with a drug history, the assessment includes monitoring vital signs. A gradual increase in vital signs and a heightening of anxiety and tremors are important indications for immediate medical intervention.

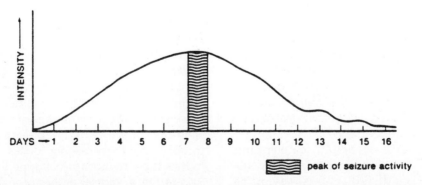

Figure 34-2. Withdrawal syndrome from the long-acting CNS depressants. (From Woolf, D. S., "CNS depressants: Other sedative–hypnotics, in *Substance Abuse: Pharmacologic, Developmental and Clinical Perspectives*, Eds. Gerald Bennett, Christine Vourakis, and Donna S. Woolf (New York: John Wiley & Sons, Inc. 1983, p. 53, with permission.[63])

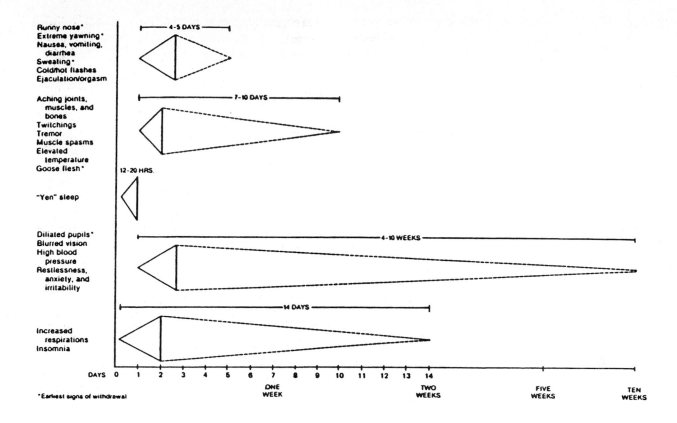

Figure 34-3. Signs and symptoms of morphine withdrawal. (From Woolf, D. S., "Opioids," in *Substance Abuse: Pharmacologic, Developmental and Clinical Perspectives*, Eds. Gerald Bennett, Christine Vourakis, and Donna S. Woolf (New York, John Wiley & Sons, Inc. 1983, p. 76, with permission.[63])

Opioid withdrawal is rarely life-threatening but causes considerable discomfort. Some addicts describe the symptoms as similar to having a severe case of the flu. Figure 34-3 identifies the course of morphine (an opioid) withdrawal, in addition to its characteristic symptoms. See the detoxification section for the nurse's role with opioid addicts. Cocaine withdrawal is characterized by fatigue, depression, irritability, and psychomotor agitation. These symptoms may last for more than 24 hours after cessation of use. Some patients also experience paranoid and suicidal ideation. The withdrawal syndrome associated with amphetamines and related substances is similar to the cocaine withdrawal syndrome. Nicotine withdrawal is generally distinguished by irritability, anxiety, restlessness, decreased heart rate, increased appetite, and weight gain.[103] Stimulant and nicotine withdrawal do not usually require emergency medical intervention.[104] Nursing assessment in patients withdrawing from stimulants and nicotine includes a drug history and the need for support and referral.

Hallucinogenic Crises

Hallucinogenic crises are characterized by flashbacks and acute fear reactions after the ingestion of drugs such as LSD and PCP. Flashbacks are spontaneous reoccurrences of drug-induced experiences. They are relatively infrequent and last for a few seconds or minutes and often precede fatigue or stress. They may appear days, weeks, or months after the last intake of a drug. The establishment of prior use of a hallucinogen is important in assessing for flashback episodes. In addition, the patient's description of the flashback(s) should be similar to the physical and psychological sensations recalled during the hallucinogenic experience. The patient should be assessed for anxiety and depression as a result of flashback episodes. Reassurance that these episodes will diminish and eventually cease is important. Patients are often afraid that flashbacks are a precursor to a psychotic break. Again, dispelling this myth is important, as is discouraging continued drug abuse. Helpful suggestions include adequate rest, good nutrition, and tension-reducing activities.

Acute fear or panic reactions may occur in the experienced as well as the novice drug abuser. The perception of the drug-induced alterations in the user's environment determines the course of the drug experience. Occasionally, the user may lose sense of the drug-induced context of the experience and panic. A gentle reassuring and supportive environment is indicated for this patient. The patient in crisis from LSD may be "talked down" in a quiet environment. Sometimes it is necessary to administer a minor tranquilizer in conjunction with support.[105]

Patients acutely intoxicated from PCP may arrive at the treatment facility in a variety of states. Some may be quiet and motionless with a blank stare, others agitated and combative, and still others may be stuporous or comatose. Immediate treatment depends on the status of the patient on admission. A complete discussion will follow in the next section on nursing intervention.

Psychoactive-Substance-Induced Delirium and Delusional Disorders

Delirium is sometimes manifested in the patient intoxicated from cocaine, amphetamines, or phencyclidine. Cocaine and amphetamine delirium are similar in that onset is usually within 1 hour of drug intake (depending on route of administration) and is over in about 6 hours. Patients exhibit labile affect, tactile and olfactory hallucinations, and may have to be restrained if they exhibit violent or aggressive behavior. Because of the erratic nature of phencyclidine (related to its absorption), symptoms may appear within 24 hours after use or may even emerge up to a week after recovery from an overdose. Symptoms are similar to delirium in cocaine and amphetamine intoxication and are often heightened. Some of the additional features these patients display are impaired judgment, belligerence, assaultiveness, and unpredictability.[106]

Psychoactive-drug-induced delusional disorders develop most commonly after stimulant use (e.g., amphetamines and cocaine). They may also occur after cannabis, hallucinogen, or phencyclidine use.[107] The features of these disorders are similar to the manifestations of paranoid schizophrenia. A drug history is very important in these patients because of the difficulty in differentiating between the two conditions. Events leading up to the emergence of symptoms are additional data for assessment. Common symptoms include paranoia, delusions,

hallucinations (visual, auditory, olfactory, and tactile), compulsive behavior characterized by simple repetitive activities, and an increased interest in sex.

There are certain symptoms of amphetamine delusional disorder not observed in schizophrenia that are helpful in a differential diagnosis. Tactile and olfactory hallucinations are rarely found in schizophrenia. Unlike the schizophrenic, the patient with an amphetamine delusional disorder is oriented to his environment and retains a clear consciousness. The amphetamine patient is also able to recall the events leading up to the psychotic episode, whereas the schizophrenic patient has no memory of the events preceding the symptoms. The amphetamine delusional patient appears anxious and does not have a flat affect. Finally, this patient does not have a distinct thought disorder typical of the schizophrenic patient.[108]

Nursing Diagnosis in Patients with Chronic Psychoactive Substance Use Disorders

The nursing process serves as a helpful organizing framework for nursing assessment and management. After assessing the pattern of drug abuse and the need for immediate medical treatment, the next requirement is nursing diagnosis of the patient.

A popular method for patient assessment leading to nursing diagnosis has been developed by Gordon. She describes a typology of 11 functional health patterns (client strengths) that are useful guidelines for a holistic assessment of the patient with a chronic PSUD. In addition to assessment of physiological patterns (such as sleep–rest, activity–exercise, elimination, and nutrition), role relationships, stress-coping, and self-concept patterns are assessed. The nature of PSUDs is complex and as the severity of the PSUD increases, greater disruption can be expected in the functional health patterns of: activity–exercise, cognitive–perceptual, sleep–rest, self-perception, self-concept, role relationships, and stress-coping tolerance. These functional health patterns are the ones most commonly disrupted, but any of the 11 patterns may be dysfunctional in the patient. The reader is referred to Gordon's textbook for a complete discussion of the functional health patterns.[109] Case examples in the nursing intervention section will demonstrate the form of dysfunctional patterns (nursing diagnoses) based on assessment.

NURSING INTERVENTION FOR PSYCHOACTIVE SUBSTANCE USE DISORDERS

Nursing intervention with the drug-abusing patient requires a variety of skills. The acutely ill patient in barbiturate withdrawal depends on the nurse to assume primary responsibility for his care. However, the chronically ill patient shares some of the responsibility for his care with the nurse. The aim is to have the patient move toward assessing his own needs and seeking appropriate assistance from a variety of resources. Although some of these resources may be professional, most will be self-help.

A conceptual framework such as Orem's self-care model serves as an appropriate theoretical basis for nurses working with patients who have PSUDs.[110] Dysfunctional patterns are viewed as self-care deficits, and nursing intervention is determined by the assessed degree of the patient's self-care deficit.

Orem identifies three general levels of nursing systems for intervention. Generally, the three levels span a continuum of nurse–patient involvement in self-care. In the supportive–educative system, the patients perform their own self-care. The nurse's role primarily involves facilitating patient goals. Collaboration and information sharing are common helping techniques nurses employ with patients. The second level is the partly compensatory system. The nurse assumes more responsibility for performing some self-care measures for the patient in this system. The last nursing system is the wholly compensatory system. In this case, the nurse assumes primary responsibility for the care of the patient. Generally, patients with PSUDs do not require this degree of nursing involvement unless they are in severe drug withdrawal or are dysfunctional from drug intoxification. At this level, patients are unable to actively participate in meeting their own self-care requirements. However, as the patient's condition improves and as he is able to assume increasing responsibility for self-care, the nursing system shifts toward the supportive–educative system.[111]

The previous section on psychiatric diagnosis of PSUDs provides useful information to incorporate into the planning of nursing care for patients. The case examples of patients with PSUDs presented later in this section will demonstrate how this information is integrated into the nursing management. For a comprehensive review of substance-abuse nursing, including chapters on the client, family, and community, the reader is referred to Bennett, Vourakis, and Woolf's *Substance Abuse*.[112]

Psychoactive-Drug-Induced Delirium and Delusions

Drug-induced delirium and delusions are generally treated symptomatically in mental health settings. As with any psychotic patient, a supportive, relaxed environment is maintained. The patient is oriented to reality by staff in the context of developing therapeutic interpersonal relationships. Tranquilizers may be given for agitation and anxiety unrelieved by interpersonal contact. If necessary, the patient may be put in seclusion to decrease environmental stimulation. If absolutely necessary, restraints are used for an extremely agitated patient. Overall, the goal is to provide a protective environment and to facilitate the patient's return to normal functioning. Some patients may require psychotherapy as part of extended care.[113]

The patient admitted with a PCP-induced delirium or delusional disorder presents additional difficulties. The erratic behavior produced in individuals is a challenge to the skills of the mental health team. The symptoms of toxic psychosis may be treated with haloperidol or sedative–hypnotics to make the patient more controllable; however, the psychosis will continue its course. In long-term PCP-precipitated psychosis chlorpromazine is recommended.[114]

Patients admitted in low-dose intoxication who are awake but with retarded speech, immobility, and blank stare should be placed in a quiet environment. The typical "talking down" technique used with other psychedelic crises should be avoided. These patients are highly sensitive to auditory and visual stimulation and may suddenly become agitated and combative. The nurse is encouraged to empathize with this patient and to utilize a gentle approach directed toward the affective level. This is accomplished by acknowledging the patient's feelings and making sure a staff member stays with him.[115,116]

PCP may alter blood pressure; therefore careful attention to this and other vital signs is important. The urine and blood should be screened for drugs as soon as possible. These procedures will assist in making a definitive diagnosis and in determining if there are other drugs present.

Additional treatment approaches vary and depend on the patient's progress. Observation may be all that is indicated. However, if symptoms persist for more than a few hours or tend to escalate, more vigorous measures are necessary. One treatment approach is based on the theory that PCP is a weak electrolyte (base) and is attracted to the acid environment of the stomach. Gastric lavage is recommended, especially if the drug is injected. Administration of cranberry juice and ascorbic acid orally may aid in the elimination of any remaining PCP because these substances acidify the urine.

The more severely intoxicated patient who is admitted in a stupor or coma needs immediate medical treatment. In addition, acidifying the urine is indicated. One way to accomplish this is to instill ammonium chloride via a nasogastric tube and administer ascorbic acid intravenously. A diuretic is suggested to promote excretion of the residual PCP. Another recommended treatment is to insert activated charcoal into the stomach via a nasogastric tube. The charcoal absorbs the PCP and is later removed by lavage. Seizures may occur, and cautious intravenous administration of 5-mg doses of diazepam per minute is recommended. As the patient regains consciousness, treatment for low-dose intoxication is indicated.[117]

Detoxification

Detoxification is a medical procedure whereby a drug similar in action to the abused drug(s) is substituted and withdrawn gradually. The withdrawal syndrome is therefore controlled, reducing the discomfort and risk associated with this condition. Including alcohol, cessation of chronic abuse of the general depressants and opioids may precipitate a physical withdrawal syndrome requiring detoxification. The severity of the withdrawal from general-depressant abuse will determine whether the patient can be safely treated in an outpatient program. A drug history (including a history of withdrawal) and an assessment of current drug use (i.e., amounts currently consumed as well as date and time of last intake), in addition to an assessment of the patient's physical and behavioral status are the parameters to consider for determination of which setting is appropriate for detoxification. Generally, detoxification from drugs other than the general depressants may be conducted on an outpatient basis.

The nurse's role in detoxification includes patient assessment for the most appropriate treatment setting and collaboration with the physician as to patient need for detoxification. In addition, the nurse usually coordinates the detoxification regimen and administers the medications. For many patients, detoxification is their initial contact with the health care system. It may also be their only contact. The nurse who is able to establish a rapport with a patient in this crisis situation may be able to counsel him into further treatment for his chronic PSUD. Some extended treatment programs offer detoxification to patients willing to commit to additional treatment.

Mild withdrawal from the general depressants does not necessitate detoxification. Severe withdrawal, however, may be life-threatening and requires treatment. The drug treatment for this condition is the same regardless of the depressant abused. Detoxification involves substituting a long-acting depressant drug for the depressant(s) abused. Phenobarbital and diazepam are frequently the detoxification drugs used because of their documented safety.[118]

First, the patient is stabilized with the substitute drug, reducing or eliminating the withdrawal symptoms. Over the next several days, the patient is given gradually decreasing amounts of the drug until the regimen is completed. At this point, withdrawal symptoms should be markedly diminished and the patient out of danger. The nurse's role is similar to that previously discussed and includes observing the patient for signs of toxicity from the effects of the substitute drug. The most prominent signs of toxicity are nystagmus, ataxia, and slurred speech. Signs of toxicity dictate withholding a couple of doses of the drug, recalculating the dosage, and then resuming the procedure. In addition, the nurse observes the patient for signs of withdrawal indicating too rapid detoxification or insufficient dosage level. Changes in the patient's physical or behavioral status may indicate withdrawal symptoms.[119]

Patients with chronic opioid substance use disorders are frequently detoxified with methadone substitution. Methadone does not alter mental functions and is the only approved opioid drug for narcotic detoxification. Detoxification can be completed in 7 to 10 days through the use of methadone.[120] The procedure is similar to general depressant detoxification. Clonidine (a nonopioid adrenergic receptor agonist) has recently emerged as a popular drug in opioid detoxification. It appears to be most useful for abrupt withdrawal from low dose methadone maintenance dose by reducing the acute opioid abstinence syndrome.

Some patients may need further pharmacological assistance after detoxification with methadone or clonidine, based on the theory that conditioned drug-seeking behavior is difficult to alter in the brief detoxification period. This is particularly important in patients who remain in environments where opioid abuse was initiated and maintained. To this end, opioid antagonists, pharmacological agents designed to block the effects of opioids without producing physical dependence, are administered. Detoxified patients maintained on antagonists who become involved in situations precipitating opioid use may avoid succumbing to regular opioid use because of the absence of the euphoric reenforcements. Naltrexone is one of the more popular potent opioid antagonists for a number of reasons, including its long action and oral effectiveness. Patients must be highly motivated to achieve success with the use of opioid antagonists.[121]

Chronic abuse of some drugs does not appear to produce a physical withdrawal syndrome. However, the psychological withdrawal symptoms, such as depression, anxiety, and despair, may be severe. Included in this category are the hallucinogens, phencyclidine, and the stimulant cocaine. There is some controversy over the ability of these drugs to cause physical dependency, especially in chronic cocaine use. At this time, however, there are no definitive answers. Marijuana and stimulants other than cocaine are known to produce a physical withdrawal syndrome. The physical and behavioral withdrawal symptoms are treated with supportive interpersonal contact and tranquilizers.

The detoxification procedure previously described in this section is not necessary for patients withdrawing from drugs other than the opioids and general depressants. In fact, mild withdrawal from the opioids and from the general depressants is treated similarly to physical and psychological withdrawal from other drugs of abuse. Nonchemical measures are primarily employed to promote comfort in these patients. Sedatives and tranquilizers may be prescribed on a temporary basis to help the patient cope with insomnia, anxiety, and depression. Other measures include psychotherapy, physical exercise, improved nutrition, meditation, and relaxation procedures.

Methadone Maintenance

Methadone maintenance programs are for people addicted to opioids. The majority of patients are heroin addicts who have repeatedly failed to remain drug-free after detoxification. Generally, a minimum of 2 years of opioid abuse is a prerequisite for admission to the program. Patients may participate in treatment indefinitely. The main purpose of methadone maintenance is to remove the addict from the criminal lifestyle established to maintain the high cost of his addiction. Maintenance on methadone allows the addict to change his life-style and to pursue resocialization. The program usually provides counseling, access to vocational rehabilitation, health care, and referrals for other kinds of services.[122]

The role of the nurse in methadone maintenance programs, in addition to dispensing methadone, health teaching, and providing health care assessments, is assisting the patient toward self-care. Orem's self-care concepts serve as guidelines for the nurse working with the chronic opioid abuser.[123]

The general goal of nursing is to promote an optimum level of functioning in patients and to enhance their integration back into the general community. Betts offers a continuum of care beginning with the acceptance of patient dependency during the early phases of treatment. During this period the nurse and patient collaborate on goals and options for goal achievement.[124] As time goes on, the patient assumes more leadership in these areas with the nurse acting more as a consultant, as proposed in Orem's supportive–educative system.[125]

The nurse has many opportunities to develop supportive relationships with patients in methadone treatment programs. The relaxed social setting established in most programs promotes casual interaction among staff and patients. The nurse may use these opportunities for health teaching and to assist clients toward resocialization. Although brief, nurse–patient interactions during the dispensing of methadone are excellent opportunities for psychotherapeutic interactions. Nurses working in methadone programs frequently participate in group counseling and may also see some clients for individual counseling.

Residential Self-Help

Therapeutic communities are the primary residential self-help programs for drug addicts. The goals of most programs are aimed at eliminating unacceptable behavior patterns and substituting patterns that allow for more effective coping in the social environment. The structure of therapeutic communities is generally regimented. Leaders of these programs argue that this structure is necessary for promoting a lifetime of abstinence and constructive use of time.[126]

The rigid structure of programs and the peer pressure of change behavior and conform to the norms of the community are not appealing to the majority of addicts. There are some addicts, though, who are able to remain drug-free and reenter society after living in a therapeutic community. Most addicts who wish to enter programs are given an opportunity to explore their ability to adapt to this type of treatment.

Synanon was the first therapeutic community in the United States, established in 1958. It is operated and controlled by the residents without professional help. Programs established since Synanon are still generally controlled by the residents; however, a few professionals are employed in these programs. Also, in contrast to Synanon, the newer programs encourage eventual reentry into society. Synanon encourages the ex-addict to live and work within the therapeutic community indefinitely.[127]

The nurse's role in relation to therapeutic communities is generally as a referral source. Familiarity with the programs in the area and their structure will assist the nurse in making appropriate referrals. Nurses may also serve as consultants to programs.

Nonresidential Self-Help

Alcoholics Anonymous (AA) is the forerunner and the model of nonresidential self-help groups. Narcotics Anonymous (NA) is the major drug-oriented self-help group. The client population in NA groups tends to be younger than in AA groups. Older drug-dependent people who fit more into middle-class society may be more compatible with members of AA groups. More recently, Potsmokers Anonymous, Pills Anonymous, and Cocaine Anonymous groups have formed. The formation of these additional drug-specific groups may be in response to members' needs to relate to people similar to themselves in values and life-style.

Drug-oriented self-help groups are open to all drug abusers and offer the support necessary to abstain from drugs. Unfortunately, the self-help group does not appeal to every drug-dependent person. Those patients willing to explore self-help groups as an option for long-term self-care should be encouraged to visit a variety of groups. The composition of self-help groups varies among groups, and a patient may feel more comfortable in particular groups. Familiarity with the types of drug-specific groups in the area will assist the nurse in making appropriate referrals.

Examples of Nursing Intervention

Nursing students are not often assigned to drug treatment programs for part of their psychiatric clinical experience. In addition to programs for opioid addicts, there are professionally run programs for alcoholics and polydrug abusers. These programs are generally 1 month in length and offer either inpatient or outpatient treatment. The majority of these programs are primarily geared to employed patients (and their families), with health insurance. Some outpatient programs may be several months in length and expect patients to participate up to 8 hours each day during the week. They are often called *day treatment programs*.

One of the challenges to a nursing student working in drug treatment programs is adapting to the variety of communication techniques used by the staff to work with the drug abuser. One problem the staff is often presented with is the patient's denial of problems. The nurse must be prepared to deal with the patient's denial of psychological problems. Therapeutic communication skills, as taught to students of nursing, primarily focus on supporting the patient by using a patient-centered approach. These techniques are important in understanding and in developing a positive relationship with the patient. However, when working with drug-abuse patients, additional techniques are necessary. After the patient is anchored to the treatment program, confrontation of his denial is the next step. The following case illustration demonstrates the use of denial and gentle but firm confrontation used by the nurse.

CASE EXAMPLE OF MRS. GRAHAM

- Psychoactive Substance Use Disorder
- Sedative–Hypnotic or Anxiolytic Dependence

Mrs. Graham, a 46-year-old housewife, was admitted to the neurology service for diagnostic tests because of complaints of persistent migraine headaches. All tests were negative. The nursing staff reported that the patient complained of nervousness and insomnia and demanded medication for both. A psychiatric consultation revealed a 2-year history of barbiturate and diazepam (Valium) abuse. She was transferred to the drug treatment unit. The patient is now in her second week of treatment and is attending various groups daily. During one group therapy session the following confrontation occurred:

PATIENT: [angrily] I can't get any help here. I need something for my headache!

NURSE: [gently but firmly] I believe your headaches are real for you. You also have a serious problem with misuse of Valium and Seconal and you are avoiding this by focusing on your headaches and other physical symptoms.

PATIENT: [angrily] Nobody around here cares about me because you won't give me anything for my headaches!

NURSE: [gently but firmly] Giving you more drugs would not be caring about you. How have the drugs made any significant changes in your headaches over the past 2 years?

PATIENT: [low voice] I don't know. . . . Well, I guess they haven't helped.

NURSE: [gently] I realize that talking about your drug taking is new to you. As you continue to attend the afternoon alcohol and drug education group, you will begin to understand what drug abuse is and what has been happening in your lfie.

A complete assessment of Mrs. Graham's functional health patterns is not feasible here. However, dysfunction in at least one pattern is readily apparent from the data given. Gordon identifies coping–stress tolerance as one pattern in her typology.[128] Mrs. Graham is ineffectively coping with stress (manifested as chronic headaches) by abusing drugs. The nursing systems in operation include the partly compensatory and supportive–educative.[129] Mrs. Graham's denial of her problem with drugs and her lack of insight preclude total participation in self-care

planning at this time. As her self-awareness increases and as she begins to assume responsibility for her health care, the supportive–educative system will suffice.

One diagnostic nursing hypothesis based on the available data on Mrs. Graham is: Coping, ineffective: drug abuse. Other tentative diagnoses applicable to Mrs. Graham include knowledge deficit: drug-abuse education and grieving, anticipatory.[130] The latter diagnosis is anticipated since drug abusers often experience a grief reaction when they have decided to give up a drug substance that they have been closely associated with for a number of years. The intervention techniques employed by the nurse working with Mrs. Graham in a group setting are appropriate strategies based on the tentative diagnosis of ineffective coping. A beginning attempt is being made to assist Mrs. Graham in recognizing how drugs are not meeting her needs. More than one group session and confrontation by several of the members, particularly other clients, may be necessary to penetrate and prevent the reemergence of the client's denial. The client's anger, somatic complaints, and other manipulative coping behaviors should be considered part of the disorder. The nurse's observation of these symptoms provides data for using the nursing process in the planning of ongoing care. The next nursing care situation exemplifies the collaborative role of the nurse as she works with a patient.

CASE EXAMPLE OF LARRY

- Psychoactive Substance Use Disorder
- Polysubstance Dependence

Larry, a 22-year-old Caucasian multidrug abuser, was referred to day treatment by the court. Participation in treatment was an alternative to incarceration for possession of cocaine and PCP. He describes himself as shy and socially inadequate except when he is on "speed," cocaine, or PCP. Larry has an 8-year-history of drug abuse, with a heavy daily pattern over the last year and a half. His mother died from complications related to chronic alcoholism when he was 16 years old. He claims they were close. He never knew his father. After his mother's death he found a job cleaning up a parking lot. He met a drug dealer who introduced Larry to using and selling drugs. He quit school and wandered from job to job. He has never had a steady girl friend, and his only friends are drug dealers and users. His regular daily pattern of heavy abuse commenced after being fired from his last job. His entire income since that time has been from selling drugs. While participating in the day treatment program, he is living at a halfway house where his meals are provided. He has been drug-free and consistent in attendance during the first 2 weeks of treatment. He only participates in the group when called on and sits alone during informal social gatherings at the treatment center.

During the first 2 weeks of treatment, Larry attended drug education groups and has acknowledged an identification with the drug problems discussed by other clients. He wants to alter his life-style and to remain drug-free. The supportive–educative nursing system in Orem's framework is the most appropriate system for Larry's care at this time.[131] The nurse's role entails supporting Larry in his life-style changes and collaborating with him on goal setting and implementation.

The assessment of Larry's functional health patterns reveals dysfunction in his self-perception–self-concept pattern and his role-relationship pattern. Larry's perception of himself as powerless in social situations, except when on drugs, indicates a self-concept and self-esteem problem. The nursing diagnostic hypothesis from the data available may be tentatively expressed as self-concept disturbance in self-esteem–social skill deficit. In collaboration with his nurse–counselor, the goal of spontaneous participation in group situations was established. Over the next week he plans to make at least one unsolicited contribution to each group session he attends. At the end of the week, Larry and his nurse–counselor will evaluate the implementation of this plan and its contribution to his goal. In addition he plans to organize an evening activity (e.g., attending a movie) following the afternoon NA meeting. He and his nurse–counselor have carefully planned each step in organizing the event to promote a positive outcome.

Larry has identified an interest in developing an occupational skill. However, he needs assistance in exploring the options and the various educational and training requirements for each. Earlier, dysfunction was noted in Larry's role-relationship pattern. There is obvious dysfunction in his work role as well as his social role. An appointment with a vocational rehabilitation counselor was discussed with Larry as a beginning step in determining his educational and vocational abilities and interests. There is a close relationship between dysfunction in Larry's social role and in his self-concept. His participation in groups at the center and his long-term attachment to self-help groups is expected to positively influence his role as a drug-free young adult.

Careful assessment of Larry's other health patterns may reveal dysfunction. People with drug problems often experience dysfunction in their sleep–rest pattern, nutritional–metabolic pattern, activity–exercise pattern, sexual–reproductive pattern, and coping–stress-tolerance pattern. Intervention in one or two of these patterns may positively affect some of the others. For example, the development of a regular schedule of exercise often improves the sleep–rest pattern in people who are recovering from drug abuse.

The final case example is of Tom, who had a chronic cocaine substance abuse disorder. A junior nursing student had the opportunity to work with Tom during her mental health clinical experience. The care plan she developed during the month she cared for him will be exhibited after presentation of Tom's history.

CASE EXAMPLE OF TOM

- Psychoactive Substance Use Disorder
- Cocaine Dependence

I. PATIENT SUMMARY

A. Personal/Family History

Tom is a 35-year-old Caucasian single male and the youngest of three children. Currently he lives by himself in a one-bedroom apartment. He describes his family as "close" and himself as the "baby" of the family. His parents are well, living together, both in their sixties and overly concerned about Tom's welfare. His father owns an auto parts company and is well off financially. Whenever Tom has been out of work the family has supported him by paying his bills and the apartment rent. He has two older sisters (both married), one 40 and the other 43 years old, who have along with Tom's parents frequently rescued Tom with money or other support when he has not met his responsibilities. He had a back problem as a child which has since resolved. He is single. He attended school through 2 years of college and has worked as an auto salesman in the past and most recently as an auto parts salesman for his father's company. The staff describe Tom as narcissistic, not listening to others when they are talking but expecting to be heard when he speaks, needing to be in control, and not willing to compromise. On admission he had pressured speech, appeared nervous, restless, and distractible. On psychological testing he indicated a high proclivity for impulsivity, moderate depression, social and interpersonal alienation, immaturity, frequent feelings of helplessness, and ruminative introspective tendencies.

B. History and Present Hospitalization

This is Tom's first admission to a psychiatric inpatient program. His admission diagnosis is cocaine dependence. He states he has been using approximately ⅛ ounce of cocaine per week by nasal inhalation. He has been using cocaine three or four times per week for the past 8 or 9 years. He denies free-basing or smoking "crack." He does drink alcohol once or twice a week. He reports no prior psychiatric or psychoactive-substance-abuse treatment. He reports occasional blood-tinged mucus after snorting cocaine; however, reports no profuse nosebleeds; otherwise, unremarkable history. He snorts cocaine three times a week and has had a $300 a week habit for the past 7 years. He first used cocaine when he came to the East Coast between the ages of 24 or 25. He does not know what he wants to do with his life; says he is depressed. He notes that working in sales is too stressful for him, says he cannot deal with people.

He is currently unemployed. He says he is unhappy with his life and wants to change. His girl friend (Sally) of the last 2 years and her brother (Jeff) recently moved out because Tom and Jeff were continually arguing about Jeff's sloppy housekeeping. Sally was free-basing cocaine and stealing from Tom to finance her habit. Neither she nor her brother were working. According to Tom, the trouble started when Jeff moved in 4 months ago. He created a mess around the apartment and would not participate in housecleaning. This led to many arguments between Tom and Jeff with the outcome of Sally and Jeff moving out. Tom had difficulty facing his life alone in the apartment. He describes himself as a fastidious person who likes to maintain a clean, orderly environment. He admitted that he was depressed and that maybe his snorting cocaine was not helping his life. He grew alarmed when he became aware he had ceased to care for his personal hygiene and the garbage was piling up in the apartment. His admission was precipitated by his brother-in-law (a physician) who talked Tom into going into the hospital for treatment.

NURSING CARE PLAN
Psychoactive Substance Use Disorder, Cocaine Dependency

ASSESSMENT

A. Problem #1

S "I couldn't believe it that I let my apartment become such a mess. I was really feeling down after Sally left." "I thought I could handle it when I went out on pass. If I could just get out of here and go back to work I know I'll be fine—I just have to avoid spending so much time at home alone."

O Patient is denying how much of his life has been revolving around cocaine abuse. He tends to talk about other issues in his life and assumes that Sally leaving, being out of work, and staying home alone are the only problems causing his depression and subsequent admission to the hospital. On the unit he spends most of his time with a 44-year-old divorced patient admitted for dependency on barbiturates. She wakes him up in the mornings and reminds him to attend the scheduled groups each day. He tends to monopolize group discussion with sad stories about how difficult life is and how things are not going his way. On a 4-hour pass the patient bought cocaine and snorted it.

NURSING DIAGNOSIS

Cognitive–perceptual pattern, knowledge deficit: denial of cocaine dependency.

GOALS

Long-Term
1. Patient will accept his dependency on cocaine and understand its effect on his life.
2. Patient will assume responsibility for his own life, pursuing activities to enhance his well-being.

Short-Term
1. With assistance, Tom will begin to connect events and relationships in his life to his pursuit and involvement with cocaine.
2. With assistance from staff, Tom will participate in social activities on the unit and begin to develop interpersonal relationships with other patients.
3. In group, encourage patient to share the meaning cocaine assumes in his life.
4. By October 24th (1 week) patient will monitor time of group meetings and be responsible for his own attendance.
5. By October 31st (2 weeks) patient will begin to admit his primary problem with cocaine dependency.

INTERVENTIONS

1. During group, staff and other patients will confront Tom with facts when he is blaming his plight in life on events other than his cocaine dependency.
2. Encourage patient to participate with other patients in social functions and recreational activities on the unit.
3. Encourage patient to request that other patients refrain from waking him up in the morning or reminding him of scheduled groups during the day.
4. Participate in the viewing of educational films and lectures on cocaine dependency.
5. Schedule informal meetings with patient to assess his understanding of films and lectures and answer any questions he has.

ASSESSMENT

A. Problem #2

S   "I can't deal with people. I can't take the pressure. It got pretty awful when Sally left. So much is expected of you in life. I only feel better when I am high; it made everything easier to deal with. Nothing else works and now that is not even working anymore."

O   During individual sessions and in group Tom is beginning to share how he used to be very active playing volleyball and tennis at least four or five times a week. Before using cocaine regularly, he also attended church, which he enjoyed. He has noticed that he has become more and more isolated in the last few years, depending more and more on his family for emotional and financial support. He wants to develop other friendships and not be so dependent on his family. He tends to head toward his room during break from group and sits by himself or with one other patient during mealtimes.

NURSING DIAGNOSIS

Coping–stress-tolerance pattern, ineffective coping (individual).

GOALS

Long-Term
1. Patient will have a variety of behaviors and resources available for coping with short- and long-term stress.
2. Patient will actively pursue a life-style to reduce excessive stress.

Short-Term
1. With assistance, Tom will begin to identify some of the major stressors in his life (including his drug use).
2. With assistance, Tom will begin to identify his role in creating and maintaining behaviors leading to excessive stress.
3. With assistance, Tom will begin to explore alternative behaviors to reduce stress and to more effectively cope with daily life.
4. By November 7th (3 weeks) patient will discuss in group the relationship between his ongoing behavior and coping patterns and his current life situation.
5. By November 7th (3 weeks) patient will identify four personal and community resources available for him to use to reduce and cope with stress in his life.

INTERVENTIONS

1. Encourage patient to keep a diary and to write down his personal history including his current situation.
2. Encourage patient to compare and contrast his personal history with his current life situation.
3. During group, encourage patient to solicit feedback from patients and staff as to his progress in the program.
4. Encourage patient to respond in group to other patients' stated goals for maintenance of a drug-free life-style after discharge.
5. Facilitate patient's exploration of personal resources preferred for use in coping with stress.
6. Schedule a meeting with patient to review mental health and recreational resources available to him in his community.

ASSESSMENT

A. Problem #3

S   "I wish I knew where I was going in life. I do not like the work I have been doing. I don't like being a salesman. It feels like too much pressure to sell something. My father keeps telling me I am good at it and I keep feeling like I should please him—yet I feel like a failure."

O   Patient is beginning to recognize that he would prefer another kind of work. He is also able to associate, in part, the work he has been doing with the additional pressure and stress he feels in his life. He exhibits conflict with doing what he perceives his father wants him to do and exploring his own occupational inclinations and interests.

NURSING DIAGNOSIS

Role-relationship pattern, unresolved independence–dependence conflict.

GOALS

Long-Term

1. Patient will pursue a career or occupation that he chooses.

Short-Term

1. With assistance, Tom will begin to explore his relationship with his father including conflicts and associated feelings.
2. With assistance, Tom will explore his assets and interests.
3. Discuss with patient the possibility of meeting with the vocational rehabilitation counselor.
4. By November 14th (4 weeks) patient will identify at least two areas of occupational interest.
5. By November 14th (4 weeks) patient will identify the beginning steps necessary for him to pursue his occupational interests.

INTERVENTIONS

1. Encourage patient to share his thoughts and feelings related to his father in group and individual therapy.
2. Encourage patient participation in activities therapy.
3. Explore with patient his interests and past accomplishments.
4. Schedule an appointment for patient with the vocational rehabilitation counselor.

This is a beginning care plan for Tom, which will need ongoing evaluation and revision. Other possible nursing diagnoses for Tom include: (1) self-perception–self-concept pattern, self-esteem disturbance, and (2) role-relationship pattern, social isolation.

The client situations discussed in this section are fairly common examples of some of the issues faced by patients with PSUDs. It is important to keep in mind that the emphasis in drug treatment often depends on the client's stage of recovery. Early in treatment, a great deal of importance is placed on detoxification and monitoring the physiological aspects of withdrawal. In conjunction with this is an attempt to assist patients in recognizing the central role that drugs have occupied in their lives and the resultant dysfunctional consequences. The reader is again referred to Bennett et al. for additional nursing care guidelines related to such special populations as youth, women, the elderly, and the culturally diverse.[132]

PSYCHOTHERAPEUTIC APPROACHES IN DRUG ABUSE

Treatment

Sociologists have noted that drug abusers, like all people, have a life pattern that over time can be viewed as a *career*.[133] Although drug addiction is a deviant career by conventional standards, it is nonetheless a way of life that has certain predictable features. Detoxification and other care measures are an effective means of moving the client from a state of physical dependency to relative physical normalcy. However, if a strong psychological dependency exists or if environmental reinforcers promote drug use, the patient may soon begin the next round in the pattern of abuse. Psychotherapeutic approaches deal directly or indirectly with the problem of psychological dependence and the changes in behavior required to effectively launch a new life career without drugs.

The principles of therapeutic interaction covered in the earlier sections of this book apply to people regardless of diagnosis, and the drug abuser is no exception. However, the nurse without some understanding of substance use disorders faces several pitfalls in counseling the drug abuser.

A common mistake made by well-intentioned counselors when working with drug abusers is to let the problem of drug abuse become a secondary concern in therapy. That is, the substance-abuse problem may only be referred to indirectly or in vague terms to minimize anxiety for the therapist and the patient.

Or drug abuse may be relegated to minimal consideration because the therapist believes it to be only a symptom of more basic psychopathology. A variation of this pitfall is to consider drug abuse "secondary" to another problem such as depression or as "reactive" to an event such as divorce. Although it may be accurate to view drug abuse as secondary or reactive in some cases, this assessment should not be an indication to ignore the drug-abuse problem or to treat it casually.

Unfortunately, the tendency of mental health professionals to overlook drug-abuse behavior as a consideration in therapy is not uncommon. One study estimated that although 23 percent of psychotherapy patients had a significant alcohol or drug-abuse problem, only 3.5 percent of these cases were identified by therapists.[134] In a study of young alcoholics in recovery, most of whom were polydrug abusers, it was common for subjects to report that mental health professionals had not responded to evidence of drug abuse.[135] One subject recalled that her psychiatrist encouraged her to continue taking Valium despite evidence that it was being abused. Another subject described what she felt to be very helpful counseling; but in the long run, the therapy failed to deal significantly with her progressive alcoholism. Effective counselors in the drug-abuse field typically consider drug abuse to be an "independent" or primary problem.[136] This is not to say that the patient does not have other problems or that drug abuse is not related to these problems.

Another pitfall that awaits the nurse-therapist working with drug abusers is unwittingly taking on the role of punisher. Although the illicit drug abuser may face punishment by the criminal justice system, the nurse should not in any way attempt to punish a patient. This is simply not the role of nursing in society. There are of course times when the nurse must present the patient with unpleasant consequences. For example, if the patient comes to therapy "high," it is often appropriate to tell him that the session cannot be productive under such circumstances and therefore must be canceled. Or if a patient brings drugs into a drug-free community or hospital program, the rule may be enforced that such behavior leads to immediate discharge. However, these actions should be conceived and administered as necessary protections for therapeutic process, not as punishment.

Punishment of the substance abuser can take subtle forms, and usually begins with a "rescue" transaction initiated by the therapist. The rescue posture implies, "I am OK, you are not OK; therefore I must save you."[137] Rescue attempts inevitably fail, leaving the therapist angry and the patient defeated. The rescue transaction can quickly lead to a "persecutor" role for the therapist.

Henry Berger, who served as a supervisor for therapists doing family therapy with families having a heroin-dependent member, described the "rescue–persecutor" pitfall quite well:

I have to use the word "countertransference." These families create enormous fantasies of rescue and enormous feelings of frustration in the therapist. I think it has something to do with the horrible nature of what is going on, the sort of slow suicide that these men get themselves into, as well as the horrible things that the addicts end up doing to their families. It is easy to become enraged at them for being so incredibly destructive, either to themselves or of their families, and try to save them. It can overwhelm you. My most crucial experience happened when I was talking about a case of David Heard's [a therapist]. We talked for a while, but I just could not understand why David was spending so much time with this guy, hours and hours, it seemed. He even went to a bar once and had some drinks with the patient, and I kept asking, "What the hell's going on?"

At David's request, I stayed late a couple of evenings for live supervision. Possibly as a coincidence, or possibly as a reaction of the family to my presence as an unknown observer, the latent violence of the family exploded to the point where the patient pulled out a knife as he argued with his father. Fortunately, no one was injured, but it was obvious that the presence of that degree of danger and rage must be felt by the therapist. It naturally tends to draw him in as a needed guardian and a safeguard against overt expression.

After that, we learned something strategically, but I also developed a lot more respect for what these therapists were up against. In addition, I stopped being so grandiose about the goals, so that my expectations were not as great anymore, and we began to sit back and say, "Let's see what we can do in 10 weeks with these families," since that was the setup for the research design of the project. I became much more relaxed, and the clinical work became much more productive during the final half of the year that we were working. Then we had a couple of families that seemed to go fairly well. I started enjoying the supervision a lot more because I also felt less pressure on me; that case was a crucial turning point.[138]

Berger's description can provide helpful direction to the nurse therapist beginning to work with substance abusers. The therapist must give up control of drug use to the patient and attempt to work on meaningful but realistic goals, given the time and resources available. A therapist should be evaluated by others and herself based on therapeutic results from an entire caseload not one or two dramatic "cures" or "failures." This kind of balanced perspective is, of course, difficult to achieve when one is a student working with a first substance-abuse patient. Working closely with an instructor or clinical supervisor is the best way for the neophyte to deal with the rescue–persecution problem.

Another problem most students in a drug treatment center face is "testing":

During the second week of a clinical experience in an outpatient drug addiction facility, three nursing students were sitting with a group of patients awaiting a scheduled group meeting. The staff leader was late in arriving to begin the group. After a few minutes, one of the more verbal patients began rapidly quizzing the nursing students about their knowledge of the etiology of addiction. Another patient joined in by asking what the students thought they could learn "in a nuthouse like this." Any responses given by the students were immediately challenged, and further questions were posed.

In situations when one is being hostilely chal-

TABLE 34-1. EGAN'S PROBLEM-SOLVING BEHAVIORS FOR EFFECTIVE THERAPISTS

1. Establish decent, nondependent relationships with clients.
2. Help clients explore problems, needs, wants, conflicts, and developmental tasks.
3. Help clients see which issues are most critical and set priorities.
4. Challenge clients to develop a new perspective through discussion and action.
5. Help clients set up realistic behavioral goals related to presenting needs.
6. Help clients take a census of possible programs for achieving each goal.
7. Help clients choose programs best fitted to their own style and needs.
8. Support and challenge clients to invest themselves in chosen programs.
9. Help clients find resources "out there" to do all the above.
10. Help clients in an ongoing way deal with the three principal evaluation questions:
    a. Are you investing yourself realistically in goal-related programs?
    b. Are the programs helping you achieve the goals you set?
    c. Does achieving the goal or goals take care of the presenting needs or problems?

From Brady, J. P., 1982, pp. 184–185, with permission.[140]

lenged, the therapeutic skill of autognosis is necessary to avoid a defensive response. Students should examine their own feelings and should look for the covert meaning behind the overt confrontation. In this example, the hostile patients felt "stood up" by the staff leader and displaced their angry feelings onto the nursing students. The covert message had little to do with the overt hostile questions. The message could be stated as, "They (the staff) don't care. Do you?" In this situation, patients should be helped to discuss their angry feelings and their fears about being rejected.

As with any patient, it is important to have a theoretical approach to psychotherapeutic intervention with substance abusers. This textbook provides a broad orientation to the major schools of psychotherapy as well as individual, group, and family approaches. The clinician with a broad background is in a good position to use an eclectic theoretical approach, calling on theories that might aid in the understanding of a particular problem and applying techniques that appear to be suitable to the therapeutic goals set in a particular case. A review of the clinical and research literature in the drug-abuse field would convince most that there is no "one" approach to treatment that can be recommended for all patients.[139]

Psychotherapist Gerald Egan identified 10 problem-solving behaviors that effective therapists exhibit regardless of their theoretical orientation. These behaviors are listed in Table 34-1. They may serve as a guide to the eclectic therapist to assist the substance abuser to engage in a full program of recovery.[140] Notice that these therapeutic behaviors focus on the patient's responsibility to be involved in self-care activities. A therapist working from this perspective views the drug-abuse self-help movement as an alternative in therapy rather than as competition. In many cases, helping an addict enter a self-help community will be the professional therapist's only action. In other cases, patients will wish to maintain an ongoing relationship with a professional therapist.

Summary

Modern society continues to cope with the growing problem of drug abuse. In response to society's need, the nursing profession continues to expand its commitment to address this problem. The nursing literature provides evidence that nurses in all specialty areas are being alerted to models of assessment and intervention. A professional nursing journal oriented specifically to problems related to addiction will soon be available.

The assignment of students to substance-abuse programs while in nursing school not only prepares them to assess these problems in other settings but it encourages some students to pursue a career in addictions nursing.

As nurse researchers, educators, and clinicians continue to give drug abuse more attention, including preventive aspects, nursing contributions in this field will grow.

Questions

1. Autognose your feelings about working with drug abusers.
2. What drugs are being abused in your geographic areas by adolescents, by women, and by chronic drug users?
3. How can nurses work with self-help drug programs?
4. How can you learn what drugs look like and smell like in order to be familiar with drugs that are abused?
5. What resources does your community have for drug abusers?

REFERENCES AND SUGGESTED READINGS

1. American Nurses' Association. *The Care of Clients with Addictions: Dimensions of Nursing Practice.* Kansas City, Mo.: American Nurses' Association, 1987.
2. Orem, D. E. *Nursing: Concepts of Practice.* New York: McGraw-Hill, 1980.
3. Harwood, H. J., Napolitano, D. M., Kristianson, P. L., & Collins, J. J. *Economic Costs to Society of Alcohol and Drug Abuse and Mental Illness* (Publication No. RTI–2374–00–01–FR). Durham, N.C.: Research Triangle Institute, 1984, pp. 9–10.
4. Washton, A. M., & Gold, M. S. Recent trends in cocaine abuse as seen from the "800-Cocaine" hotline. In A. M. Washton & M. S. Gold (Eds.), *Cocaine: A Clinician's Handbook.* New York: Guilford Press. 1987.
5. Korcok, M. U.S. aims to cut supply and demand in war on illicit drugs. *Canadian Medical Association Journal*, 1987, *136*, 428–429.
6. Dupont, R. The drug abuse decade. *Journal of Drug Issues*, 1978, *8*(Spring), 173–187.
7. Trebach, A. S. *The Heroin Solution.* New Haven: Yale University Press, 1982, pp. 240–242.
8. Washton & Gold, op. cit.
9. The debate: Drug testing. *USA Today*, March 7, 1986, p. 2.
10. Lundberg, G. Mandatory unindicated urine drug screening: Still chemical McCarthyism. *Journal of the American Medical Association*, 1967, *256*, 3003.
11. Ingles, B. *The Forbidden Game: A Social History of Drugs.* New York: Scribner's, 1975, p. 155.
12. Ibid, pp. 154–155.
13. Simmons, L. R. S., & Said, A. A. (Eds.), *Drugs, Politics, and Diplomacy.* Beverly Hills, Calif.: Sage Publications, 1974.
14. Ingles, op. cit., p. 157.
15. Ibid., pp. 156–157.
16. Inciardi, J. A. *The War on Drugs: Heroin, Cocaine, Crime and Public Policy.* Palo Alto, Calif.: Mayfield, 1986, pp. 51–86.
17. General Accounting Office. *Drug Control: International Narcotics Control Activities of the United States.* Washington, D.C.: U.S. General Accounting Office, 1987.
18. Ling, G. M., & Gomez del Prado, J. International challenge of drug abuse: A perspective from the United Nations. In R. C. Peterson (Ed.), *The International Challenge of Drug Abuse*, National Institute of Drug Abuse Research Monograph 19 (DHEW Publication No. ADM 78–654). Washington, D.C.: U.S. Government Printing Office, 1978, pp. 64–65.
19. Gregg, R. W. The international control system for narcotic drugs. In L. R. S. Simmons & A. A. Said (Eds.), *Drugs, Politics, and Diplomacy.* Beverly Hills, Calif.: Sage Publications, 1974, pp. 288–289.
20. General Accounting Office, op. cit., p. 10.
21. MacLennon, A. Drugs move up on world agenda. *Addiction Research Foundation Journal*, 1987, *16*(8), p. 16.
22. General Accounting Office, op. cit., p. 13.
23. Ibid., p. 15.
24. Hamowy, R. (Ed.). *Dealing with Drugs: Consequences of Government Control.* Lexington, Mass.: D. C. Heath, 1987.
25. Brown, P. M. A history of drug and alcohol block grant funding and its effects on Pennsylvania's prevention services system. *Journal of Drug Education*, 1986, *16*(1), 13–25.
26. Bukoski, W. J. Drug abuse prevention funding resulting from omnibus Budget Reconciliation Act of 1981. *Journal of Drug Education*, 1986, *16*(1), 51–55.
27. American Nurses' Association. *Standards of Psychiatric-Mental Health Nursing Practice.* Kansas City, Mo.: American Nurses' Association, 1982, p. 8.
28. Swisher, J. D., & Hoffman, A. Information: The irrelevant variable in drug education. In B. W. Corder, R. A. Smith, & J. D. Swisher (Eds.), *Drug Abuse Prevention: Perspectives and Approaches for Educators.* Dubuque, Iowa: Wm. C. Brown, 1975, p. 49.
29. National Institute on Drug Abuse. *Drug Abuse Prevention* (DHEW Publication No. ADM 78–588). Washington, D.C.: U.S. Government Printing Office, 1977.
30. Sheppard, M. A., Goodstadt, M. S., & Willett, M. M. Peers or parents: Who has the most influence on cannabis use? *Journal of Drug Education*, 1987, *17*(2), 123–128.
31. Hanson, D. J. Drug education: Does it work? In F. R. Scarpitti & S. K. Datesman (Eds.), *Drugs and the Youth Culture.* Beverly Hills, Calif.: Sage Publications, 1980, p. 274.
32. National Commission on Marijuana and Drug Abuse. *Drug Use in America: Problem in Perspective.* Washington, D.C.: U.S. Government Printing Office, 1973.
33. Milgram, G. G. Alcohol and drug education programs. *Journal of Drug Education*, 1987, *17*(1), 43–57.
34. Kim, S. How do we know whether a primary prevention program on drug abuse works or does not work? *International Journal of the Addictions*, 1981, *16*(2), 359–365.
35. Blizard, R. A., & Teague, R. W. Alternatives to drug use: An alternative approach to drug education. *International Journal of the Addictions*, 1981, *16*(2), 371–375.
36. Room, R. The case for a problem of prevention

approach to alcohol, drug, and mental problems. *Public Health Reports,* 1981, *96*(1), 26–33.

37. McKay, S. R. Substance abuse during the childbearing year. In G. Bennett, C. Vourakis, & D. S. Woolf (Eds.), *Substance Abuse: Pharmacologic, Developmental and Clinical Perspectives.* New York: Wiley, 1983.

38. Bakdash, D. Psychiatric/mental health nursing. In G. Bennett, C. Vourakis, & D. S. Woolf (Eds.), *Substance Abuse: Pharmacologic, Developmental and Clinical Perspectives.* New York: Wiley, 1983.

39. Church, O. M. Sairey Gamp revisited: A historical inquiry into alcoholism and drug dependency. *Nursing Administration Quarterly,* 1985, *9*(2), 10–21.

40. Naegle, M. A. Creative management of impaired nursing practice. *Nursing Administration Quarterly,* 1985, *9*(3), 22.

41. Jefferson, L. V., & Ensor, B. E. Help for the helper: Confronting a chemically impaired colleague. *American Journal of Nursing,* 1982, *82,* 575–576.

42. Estes, N. J. Group treatment of nurses with substance abuse disorders. In N. J. Estes & M. E. Heinemann (Eds.), *Alcoholism: Development, Consequences, and Interventions.* St. Louis: Mosby, 1986, pp. 283–302.

43. Ausubel, D. P. An interactional approach to narcotic addiction. In D. J. Lettieri, M. Sayers, & H. W. Pearson (Eds.), *Theories on Drug Abuse.* Washington, D.C.: U.S. Government Printing Office, 1980.

44. Greaves, G. B. An existential theory of drug dependence. In D. J. Lettieri, M. Sayers, & H. W. Pearson (Eds.), *Theories on Drug Abuse.* Washington, D.C.: U.S. Government Printing Office, 1980.

45. Khantzian, E. J. An ego/self theory of substance dependence: A contemporary psychoanalytic perspective. In D. J. Lettieri, M. Sayers, & H. W. Pearson (Eds.), *Theories on Drug Abuse.* Washington, D.C.: U.S. Government Printing Office, 1980, p. 32.

46. Frederick, C. J. Drug abuse as a learned behavior. In D. J. Lettieri, M. Sayers, & H. W. Pearson (Eds.), *Theories on Drug Abuse.* Washington, D.C.: U.S. Government Printing Office, 1980, pp. 191–194.

47. Ibid., pp. 192–193.

48. Stanton, D. A family theory of drug abuse. In D. J. Lettieri, M. Sayers, & H. W. Pearson (Eds.), *Theories on Drug Abuse.* Washington, D.C.: U.S. Government Printing Office, 1980.

49. Ibid., p. 150.

50. Ibid., pp. 150–151.

51. Johnson, B. D. Toward a theory of drug subcultures. In D. J. Lettieri, M. Sayers, & H. W. Pearson (Eds.), *Theories on Drug Abuse.* Washington, D.C.: U.S. Government Printing Office, 1980, p. 111.

52. Ibid., p. 112.

53. Winick, C. A theory of drug dependence based on role, access, and attitudes toward drugs. In D. J. Lettieri, M. Sayers, & H. W. Pearson (Eds.), *Theories on Drug Abuse.* Washington, D.C.: U.S. Government Printing Office, 1980, p. 225.

54. Ibid., p. 226.

55. Ibid., p. 227.

56. Braude, M. C., & Chao, H. M. Recommendations for future research on genetic and biological markers in drug abuse and alcoholism. In M. C. Braude & H. M. Chao (Eds.), *Genetic and Biological Markers in Drug Abuse and Alcoholism.* Washington, D.C.: U.S. Government Printing Office, 1986, pp. 109–111.

57. Simon, E. J. Opiate receptors and their implications for drug addiction. In D. J. Lettieri, M. Sayers, & H. W. Pearson (Eds.), *Theories on Drug Abuse.* Washington, D.C.: U.S. Government Printing Office, 1980.

58. Ibid.

59. American Psychiatric Association. *Diagnostic and Statistical Manual of Mental Disorders,* 3rd ed. (Rev.). Washington, D.C.: American Psychiatric Association, 1987.

60. Rounsaville, B. J., Kosten, T. R., Williams, J. B. W., & Spitzer, R. A field trial of *DSM-III-R* psychoactive substance dependence disorders. *American Journal of Psychiatry,* 1987, *144,* 351–355.

61. *DSM-III-R,* p. 166.

62. Ibid., p. 169.

63. Bennett, G., Vourakis, C., & Woolf, D. S. *Substance Abuse: Pharmacologic, Developmental and Clinical Perspective.* New York: Wiley, 1983.

64. McKelvy, M. J., Kane, J. S., & Kellison, K. Substance abuse and mental illness: Double trouble. *Journal of Psychosocial Nursing,* 1987, *25*(1), 22.

65. Ibid., pp. 20–25.

66. National Institute on Drug Abuse. *Justice-Treatment Interface:* Across-Discipline Training Course: Participant Manual, Publ. No. 79-JIC-162 P. Washington, D.C.: National Institute on Drug Abuse, GPO 1978, 9–103.

67. Holbrook, J. M. Hallucinogens. In G. Bennett, C. Vourakis, & D. S. Woolf (Eds.), *Substance Abuse: Pharmacologic, Developmental and Clinical Perspectives.* New York: Wiley, 1983.

68. Goldman, A. *Grass Roots.* New York: Harper & Row, 1979, p. 3.

69. Johnson, B. D., & Uppal, G. S. Marijuana and youth: A generation gone to pot. In F. R. Scarpitti & S. K. Datesman (Eds.), *Drugs and the Youth Culture.* Beverly Hills, Calif.: Sage Publications, 1980.

70. Ibid.

71. Milman, D. H. Effect on children and adolescents of mind-altering drugs with special reference to cannabis. In G. G. Nabas & H. C. Frick (Eds.), *Drug Abuse in the Modern World.* New York: Pergamon Press, 1980.

72. Brynner, E. D. New parental push against marijuana. *The New York Times Magazine*, February 10, 1980, pp. 36–38, 51–53.

73. National Federation of Parents convenes in D. C. *PRIDE (Parent Resources and Information on Drug Education)*, 1980, 2(4), 1.

74. Hendin, H., Pollinger, A., Ulman, R., Carr, A. *Adolescent Marijuana Abusers and Their Families* (DHHS Publication No. ADM 81–1168). Washington, D.C.: U.S. Government Printing Office, 1981, p. 46.

75. Johnson, L. D., O'Malley, P. M., & Bachman, J. G. *Use of Licit and Illicit Drugs by America's High School Students 1975–1984* (National Institute on Drugs and Drug Abuse Publication No. ADM 85–1394). Washington, D.C.: U.S. Government Printing Office, p. 12.

76. Cohen, S. Causes of the cocaine outbreak. In A. M. Washton & M. S. Gold (Eds.), *Cocaine: A Clinician's Handbook*. New York: Guilford Press, 1987, pp. 3–9.

77. Hofman, A. *LSD: My Problem Child*. New York: McGraw-Hill, 1980.

78. Jacobs, B. L. How hallucinogenic drugs work. *The American Scientist*, 1987, 75, 386.

79. Senay, E. C. *Substance Abuse Disorders in Clinical Practice*. Boston: John Wright, 1983.

80. Frosch, W. A., Robbins, E. S., & Stern, M. Untoward reactions to lysergic acid diethylamide (LSD) resulting in hospitalization. *New England Journal of Medicine*, 1965, 273, 1236.

81. Mitic, W. R., & McGuire, D. P. Adolescent inhalant use and perceived stress. *Journal of Drug Education*, 1987, 17(2), 113–121.

82. Trebach, op. cit.

83. AIDS declared Public Enemy No. 1. *American Journal of Nursing*, 1983, 83, 988.

84. Green, A. I., Meyer, R. E., & Shader, R. I. Heroin and methadone abuse: Acute and chronic management. In R. I. Shader (Ed.), *Manual of Psychiatric Therapeutics*. Boston: Little, Brown, 1975, pp. 203–210.

85. Burns, R. S., & Lerner, S. E. Phencyclidine: An emerging drug problem. *Chemical Toxicology*, 1976, 9, 435–475.

86. National Institute on Drug Abuse. *Phencyclidine Use Among Youths in Drug Abuse Treatment* (Publication No. ADM 78–635). Washington, D.C.: U.S. Government Printing Office, 1978, p. 5.

87. Lerner, S. E., & Burns, R. S. Phencyclidine use among youth: History, epidemiology, and acute and chronic intoxication. In R. C. Petersen & R. C. Stillman (Eds.), *Phencyclidine (PCP) Abuse: An Appraisal* (NIDA Publication No. ADM 78–728). Washington, D.C.: U.S. Government Printing Office, 1978, p. 92.

88. National Commission on Marijuana and Drug Abuse, op. cit., p. 145.

89. U.S. Surgeon General. *Healthy People: Report on Health Promotion and Disease Prevention*. Washington, D.C.: U.S. Government Printing Office, 1979.

90. Wolper, B., & Scheiner, Z. Family therapy approaches and drug-dependent women. In G. M. Beschner, B. G. Reed, & J. Mondanaro (Eds.), *Treatment Services for Drug-Dependent Women* (DHHS Publication No. ADM 81–1177). Washington, D.C.: U.S. Government Printing Office, 1981, p. 344.

91. Bleck, J., & Morgan, P. A. Designer drug confusion: A focus on MDMA. *Journal of Drug Education*, 1986, 16(3), 287–302.

92. American Nurses' Association. *Nursing: A Social Policy Statement*. Kansas City, Mo.: American Nurses' Association, 1980, p. 9.

93. Chychula, N. M. Screening for substance abuse in a primary care setting. *Nurse Practitioner*, 1984, 9(7), 15–24.

94. Ciske, S. J. Assessment and management of physical consequences. In G. Bennett, C. Vourakis, & D. S. Woolf (Eds.), *Substance Abuse: Pharmacologic, Developmental and Clinical Perspectives*. New York: Wiley, 1983, pp. 313–327.

95. Williams, A. Primary care of parenteral substance abusers. *Nurse Practitioner*, 1986, 11(6), 13–37.

96. Centers for Disease Control. Update: AIDS—United States. *Morbidity and Mortality Weekly Report*, 1986, 35, 17–22.

97. Ibid.

98. McKelvy, Kane, & Kellison, op. cit., pp. 20–25.

99. Ibid.

100. Ibid.

101. Bachrach, L. L. The context of care for the chronic mental patient with substance abuse problems. *Psychiatric Quarterly*, 1987, 58(1), 3–14.

102. *DSM-III-R*, p. 123.

103. Ibid., pp. 123–163.

104. Moore, D. F. Detoxification. In G. Bennett, C. Vourakis, & D. S. Woolf (Eds.), *Substance Abuse: Pharmacological, Developmental and Clinical Perspectives*. New York: Wiley, 1983.

105. Cohen, S. *The Diagnosis and Treatment of Drug and Alcohol Abuse*. New York: Haworth Press, 1986, pp. 129–131.

106. *DSM-III-R*, pp. 100–103.

107. Ibid.

108. Holbrook, J. CNS stimulants. In G. Bennett, C. Vourakis, & D. S. Woolf (Eds.), *Substance Abuse: Pharmacologic, Developmental and Clinical Perspectives*. New York: Wiley, 1983, p. 63.

109. Gordon, M. *Nursing Diagnosis Process and Application*. New York: McGraw-Hill, 1987.

110. Orem, op. cit.

111. Ibid.

112. Bennett, Vourakis, & Woolf, op. cit.

113. Cohen, op. cit. (1986), pp. 128–134.

114. Young, T., Larson, C. W., & Gacono, C. B. Chemical aspects of phencyclidine (PCP). *Inter-*

national Journal of the Addictions, 1987, 22(1), 1–15.

115. McCoy, S., Rice, M. J., & McFadden, K. PCP intoxication: Psychiatric issues of nursing care. *Journal of Psychiatric Nursing and Mental Health Services,* 1981, *19*(7), 17–23.

116. Woolf, D. S., Vourakis, C., & Bennett, G. Guidelines for management of acute phencyclidine intoxication. *Critical Care Update,* 1980, *1*(6), 16–24.

117. Ibid.

118. Moore, op. cit., pp. 333–334.

119. Ibid., p. 334.

120. Ibid., pp. 337–338.

121. Ginzburg, H. M. Naltrexone: Its clinical utility. In B. Stimmell (Ed.), *Controversies in Alcoholism and Substance Abuse.* New York: Haworth Press, 1986, pp. 83–101.

122. Bennett, G., Graves, J. E., Kavanaugh, M., & Vourakis, C. An overview of substance abuse treatment. In G. Bennett, C. Vourakis, & D. S. Woolf (Eds.), *Substance Abuse: Pharmacologic, Developmental and Clinical Perspectives.* New York: Wiley, 1983, pp. 295–297.

123. Orem, op. cit.

124. Betts, V. T. Psychotherapeutic intervention with the addict client. *Nursing Clinics of North America,* 1976, *11*, 551–558.

125. Orem, op. cit.

126. Brook, R. C., & Whitehead, P. C. *Drug-Free Therapeutic Community.* New York: Human Services Press, 1980, pp. 28–29.

127. Ibid.

128. Gordon, op. cit., pp. 135–161.

129. Orem, op. cit.

130. Gordon, op. cit., pp. 135–161.

131. Orem, op. cit.

132. Bennett, Vourakis, & Woolf, op. cit.

133. Rubington, E. Drug addiction as a deviant career. *International Journal of the Addictions,* 1967, *2*(1), 3–20.

134. Cummings, N. A. Turning bread into stones: Our modern antimiracle. *American Psychologist,* 1979, *34*, 119–129.

135. Bennett, G. Stress, social integration, and self-concept: A study of young alcoholics in recovery. *Dissertation Abstracts International.* (Ann Arbor: University of Michigan, 1983.) *44*(4) 1059B.

136. Senay, op. cit.

137. Steiner, C. M. *Healing Alcoholism.* New York: Grove Press, 1979.

138. Todd, T. C., Berger, H., & Lande, G. Supervisors' view on the special requirements of family therapy with drug-abusers. In M. D. Stanton & T. C. Todd (Eds.), *The Family Therapy of Drug Abuse and Addiction.* New York: Guilford Press, 1982, pp. 359–360.

139. Bennett, G., & Woolf, D. S. Current approaches to substance-abuse therapy. In G. Bennett, C. Vourakis, & D. S. Woolf (Eds.), *Substance Abuse: Pharmacologic, Developmental and Clinical Perspectives.* New York: Wiley, 1983.

140. Brady, J., Davison, G., Dewald, P., Eagen, G., Fadiman, J., Frank, J., Gill, M., Hoffman, I., Kempler, W., Lazarus, A., Raimy, V., Rotter, J. & Strupp, H. Some views on effective principles of psychotherapy. In M. R. Goldfried (Ed.), *Converging Themes in Psychotherapy.* New York: Springer, 1982, pp. 184–185.

Chapter 35

Alcoholism: A Treatable Disease

Mary H. Hennessey

Chapter Objectives

The students successfully attaining the goals of this chapter will be able to:

- Define alcoholism and describe the incidence and etiology.
- Conduct a nursing assessment of a person with an alcohol-abuse problem.
- Identify stalls in the therapeutic process with an alcoholic.
- Plan and negotiate a treatment plan with the alcoholic patient.
- Identify alcoholics with special problems.
- Discuss common medical and psychiatric complications of alcohol abuse.
- Discuss personal opinions and attitudes toward alcoholism and the effect of these on patient care.

Man has had a long and ambivalent history with alcohol. The first laws governing its use were in effect as early as 225 B.C. In the United States, the abuse of alcohol was recognized as a public health problem in 1775 by Dr. Benjamin Rush, a signer of the Declaration of Independence and Surgeon General in the Revolutionary War. Temperance movements and prohibition are prominent parts of this country's history. Drunk driving laws and warning labels on alcoholic beverage containers are issues of current concern.

Alcoholism is perhaps the leading public health problem in the United States today, di-rectly affecting some 10 million people. The past few years have seen significant progress in this field, and we now have fairly accurate statistics on patterns of alcohol consumption and on the prevalence of alcohol problems. The medical, psychosocial, and economic consequences of al-cohol abuse are well understood, and innovative treatment programs are reporting encouraging success rates. Progress in the laboratory is also promoting an improved understanding of the nature of alcoholism.

Unfortunately, there has been a lag in the application of this new knowledge. Concern over alcoholism as a community health problem has been a relatively recent phenomenon. Many health professionals have received minimal education regarding the use and abuse of alcohol. It is still all too common to see assessments based on inadequate data and care plans rooted in myths and stereotypes. The following situation illustrates this problem:

A 34-year-old registered nurse was admitted to a medical unit with symptoms of abdominal pain, nausea, and vomiting. Although initially anxious and frightened, she soon became a favorite of the nursing staff, who enjoyed her sense of humor and appreciated her help with the other patients. A week after admission she was discharged with a diagnosis of gastritis. The cause was not determined. A year and a half later she was dead of alcoholic cirrhosis.

THE NATURE OF ALCOHOL

Alcohol is absorbed directly from the small intestine into the bloodstream and from there is distributed to all body tissues. Approximately 10 percent of the alcohol is excreted unchanged through the lungs, kidneys, and skin; the rest is broken down by the liver. Some alcohol does enter the brain, which can oxidize and degrade it. The biochemical changes that occur in the brain during alcohol metabolism are not as yet fully understood but are the subject of widespread study.

Researchers have found that alcohol in the brain forms various kinds of isoquinolines, which act much the same as natural endorphins or narcotics, binding with the opiate receptor site. Alcohol and opiate-seeking behavior appear to be related to the body's ability to produce endorphins.[1] This research points to a possible hereditary factor as one explanation of alcoholism and moves toward establishing alcoholism as a biological entity.

The type of alcohol found in alcoholic beverages is ethyl alcohol or ethanol. An average serving of most drinks contains $\frac{1}{2}$ oz of ethanol. In other words, 12 oz of beer, 4 oz of wine, and a shot of whiskey each delivers approximately $\frac{1}{2}$ oz of alcohol.

An individual can metabolize approximately 1 oz of alcohol every 2 hours. When alcohol is ingested, a measurable blood level is attained within 15 to 20 minutes, reaching a peak after $1\frac{1}{2}$ hours and starting back down after 2 hours. If a person drinks alcohol faster than his liver can break it down, his blood alcohol concentration increases. The higher the blood alcohol concentration, the greater the drug effect on the person.

Blood alcohol concentrations (BACs) are reported as percentages and represent the amount of alcohol diluted in each 100 ml of blood. The legal limit for operating a motor vehicle in most states is 0.10 percent. This is equal to 100 mg of alcohol in 100 ml of blood. It would take the average 150-lb man four drinks to attain this level. Because women have less total body fluid, they and lighter individuals reach higher BACs with less alcohol.

Alcohol is an irregular depressant of the central nervous system. At lower concentrations there is a release of inhibitions, feelings of relaxation, diminished tension and anxiety, and impaired judgment. With increasing levels, motor function becomes impaired, speech becomes slurred, and gait staggered. At levels of 0.30 percent the person is stuporous, and at 0.35 percent surgical anesthesia is achieved. With enough alcohol, the vital centers can become involved and the person will die.

Alcohol is an addicting drug, and tolerance to its effects is experienced by the excessive drinker. A heavy drinker will find that increasingly higher amounts of alcohol are required to achieve a desired effect. Whereas an occasional drinker would be obviously drunk with a BAC of 0.25 percent, the alcoholic might show only slight signs of intoxication. There are many theories to explain this, but as yet the mechanism of tolerance is not fully understood. In the later stages of alcoholism there is a reversal of this tolerance phenomenon, and it takes less and less alcohol to affect the individual.

A person who has developed a tolerance to alcohol will also require larger amounts of other sedative drugs to achieve a desired effect. This cross-tolerance to other sedative drugs is often misunderstood in the hospital setting. It is not uncommon for nurses to look with suspicion at the alcoholic client who is still wide awake after two sleeping pills. "Perhaps," they say, "the patient is also abusing barbiturates." The fact is that since the action of drugs in the body is the same as that of alcohol, tolerance to one sedative drug means tolerance to the others. Anesthetists have long been aware of the difficulties in adjusting anesthesia for the alcoholic patient.

Although tolerance to the effects of alcohol and other sedative drugs is common, it must be remembered that the lethal limits of these drugs do not appreciably change. It is especially dangerous when alcohol is used in combination with other sedative drugs.

WITHDRAWAL

Alcohol is a physically addicting drug. When the body is deprived of alcohol after a drinking period, there is measurable sickness, which is relieved by further drinking. Consider the following example:

An alcoholic postal worker went to work on a Monday morning after a weekend of heavy drinking. He felt terrible. He had a splitting headache. His hands were trembling and he had difficulty focusing and concentrating. It was virtually impossible for him to sort mail. At 9 o'clock he stole out the back door and went through the parking lot to a liquor store across the street. He bought a bottle of vodka and returned to the parking lot. There he drank some vodka, which he promptly vomited. After repeating this three for four times, he was finally able to hold some down. He took one further drink and was able to work effectively for the remainder of the morning.

This man was experiencing withdrawal symptoms, which he self-medicated with alcohol. Along with its sedative effect, alcohol delivers a less pronounced but longer-acting effect of psychomotor agitation, which is responsible for many of the withdrawal symptoms. This is true not only for alcoholics but also anyone imbibing alcoholic beverages. Most nonalcoholics are familiar with the symptoms of a hangover.

It is critical that nurses know the symptoms of the withdrawal state and understand the criteria for anticipating withdrawal reactions (Tables 35-1 and 35-2). Untreated alcohol withdrawal can proceed to life-threatening delirium tremens. Proper treatment at an earlier stage of withdrawal can prevent the onset of delirium tremens. Alcohol detoxification centers rarely see a person suffering from "DTs." Workers in this setting appear to be more cognizant of the signs of withdrawal and realize that even an apparently resting patient could be in need of further sedation as evidenced by an increasing heart rate or rising blood pressure.

The manifestations of withdrawal reactions at the time of admission may not appear severe

TABLE 35-1. CRITERIA FOR ANTICIPATING WITHDRAWAL REACTIONS

Mild *DTs Unlikely to Develop*	Moderate *DTs Possible*	Severe *DTs Probable if Untreated*
Drinks only after work or only on weekends.	Drinks during workday and evenings.	Drinks around clock.
	Bouts last 3–6 days.	Bouts last week or more.
Daily consumption less than 1 pint in 24 hr.	Daily consumption 1 pint to 1 fifth.	Daily consumption 1 fifth or more.
Age under 35.	Age 35–40.	Age over 40.
Excessive drinking less than 5 yr.	Excessive drinking for 5–10 yr.	Excessive drinking over 10 yr.
Minimal or moderate "felt" or visible shakiness with previous withdrawal.	Visible tremulousness with previous withdrawal.	Extreme tremulousness and anxiety occurred previously.
Insomnia and nightmares on previous occasions possible.	Nightmares, illusions, or transient hallucinations previously.	Hallucinations, delusions, and disorientation occurred previously.
Regular living and eating habits.	Irregular eating habits and anorexia.	Obvious poor nutritional state.
No recent use of sedatives.	Use of sedatives.	Recent abuse of sedatives, especially barbiturates.
No recent or current major medical illness.	No current major medical illness, especially febrile.	Recent or present major medical illness, especially febrile.
No "rum fits" in past.	No "rum fits" in past.	Convulsions occurred previously.
10 to 12 hr since last drink.	6 to 8 hr since last drink.	2 to 4 hr since last drink.
Recovery from overt symptoms—few hours.	Recovery with treatment from overt symptoms—2 to 5 days.	Recovery with treatment from overt symptoms—5 to 10 days.

Modified after Williams, H., *Manual for Alcoholism Receiving Centers*, Alcoholic Rehabilitation Program State of Florida. Tallahassee, Fla.: Department of Health and Rehabilitative Services, 1976.

TABLE 35-2. SYMPTOMS OF THE WITHDRAWAL STATE

Manifestation[a]	Mild	Moderate	Severe (Delirium Tremens)
Motor control	Inner "shaky" feelings with hand tremors.	Visible tremulousness.	Gross uncontrollable bodily shaking.
Anxiety	Mild restlessness and anxiety.	Obvious motor restlessness and obviously painful anxiety.	Extreme restlessness and agitation with appearance of intense fear common.
Sleep	Restless sleep or insomnia.	Marked insomnia and nightmares.	Total wakefulness.
Appetite	Impaired appetite.	Marked anorexia.	Often rejects all food and fluid except alcohol.
Nausea	Nausea.	Nausea and vomiting.	Dry heaves and vomiting.
Confusion	Oriented, no confusion.	Variable confusion.	Marked confusion and disorientation.
Hallucinations	No hallucinations.	Often vague, transient, visual, and auditory hallucinations and illusions. Often with insight; often occurring only at night.	Visual and occasional auditory hallucinations, usually of fearful or threatening content. Misidentification of persons and frightening delusions related to hallucinatory experiences.
Pulse	Tachycardia.	Pulse, 100–120.	Pulse, 120–140.
Blood pressure	Normal or slightly elevated systolic.	Usually elevated systolic.	Elevated systolic and diastolic.
Sweating	Slight.	Usually obvious.	Marked hyperhydrosis common.
Convulsion	No.	May occur—precursor to "severe."	Convulsions common.

Modified after Williams, H., *Manual for Alcoholism Receiving Centers*, Alcoholic Rehabilitation Program State of Florida. Tallahassee, Fla.: Department of Health and Rehabilitative Services, 1976.
[a] Other manifestations: headaches; slightly elevated temperature; hyperacusis; painful calves; nystagmus.

and may subside with minimal attention; or, on the other hand, they may progress into a florid psychophysical disturbance. Table 35-1 is a guideline for anticipating withdrawal reactions based on certain historical and observational data.

Withdrawal syndromes are usually easily recognized, although confusion sometimes occurs when psychotic manifestations predominate and physiological manifestations are not prominent. Typical alcohol withdrawal manifestations may be separated into stages that simply reflect degrees of severity. Not all signs and symptoms listed for each state in Table 35-2 are invariably present. Progression from "mild" to "moderate" to "severe" can occur, but onset of "severe" (delirium tremens) can also be abrupt.

DEFINITION OF ALCOHOLISM

The difficulty in defining alcoholism is evident in the fact that there is no single, widely accepted definition. Its complexity is demonstrated in the *Criteria for the Diagnosis of Alcoholism* published by the National Council on Alcoholism.[2] This article consists of two tables, one for major and the other for minor criteria. The criteria are then weighted for diagnostic significance and divided according to types: Track I. Physiological and Clinical; and Track II. Behavioral, Psychological, and Attitudinal. The nurse can learn a great deal about alcoholism by studying these criteria.

In the *DSM-III-R* alcoholism is included

under Psychoactive Substance Use Disorders.[3] The criteria for diagnosis are as follows:

Diagnostic Criteria for Psychoactive Substance Dependence

A. At least three of the following:
1. Substance often taken in larger amounts or over a longer period than the person intended.
2. Persistent desire or one or more unsuccessful efforts to cut down or control substance use.
3. A great deal of time spent in activities necessary to get the substance (e.g., theft), taking the substance (e.g., chain smoking), or recovering from its effects.
4. Frequent intoxication or withdrawal symptoms when expected to fulfill major role obligations at work, school, or home (e.g., does not go to work because hung over, goes to school or work "high," intoxicated while taking care of his or her children), or when substance use is physically hazardous (e.g., drives when intoxicated).
5. Important social, occupational, or recreational activities given up or reduced because of substance use.
6. Continued substance use despite knowledge of having a persistent or recurrent social, psychological, or physical problem that is caused or exacerbated by the use of the substance (e.g., keeps using heroin despite family arguments about it, cocaine-induced depression, or having an ulcer made worse by drinking).
7. Marked tolerance: need for markedly increased amounts of the substance (i.e., at least a 50 percent increase) in order to achieve intoxication or desired effect, or markedly diminished effect with continued use of the same amount.
   Note: The following items may not apply to cannabis, hallucinogens, or phencyclidine (PCP):
8. Characteristic withdrawal symptoms (see specific withdrawal syndromes under Psychoactive Substance-induced Organic Mental Disorders).
9. Substance often taken to relieve or avoid withdrawal symptoms.
B. Some symptoms of the disturbance have persisted for at least 1 month, or have oc-

curred repeatedly over a longer period of time.

Criteria for Severity of Psychoactive Substance Dependence:
- **Mild:** Few, if any, symptoms in excess of those required to make the diagnosis, and the symptoms result in no more than mild impairment in occupational functioning or in usual social activities or relationships with others.
- **Moderate:** Symptoms or functional impairment between "mild" and "severe."
- **Severe:** Many symptoms in excess of those required to make the diagnosis, and the symptoms markedly interfere with occupational functioning or with usual social activities or relationships with others.
- **In Partial Remission:** During the past 6 months, some use of the substance and some symptoms of dependence.
- **In Full Remission:** During the past 6 months, either no use of the substance, or use of the substance and no symptoms of dependence.

Phases of Alcoholism

E. M. Jellinek, a well-known alcoholism researcher, viewed alcoholism as a progressive disease and described the following four phases of alcoholism[4]:

The Prealcoholic Phase
In the first, or prealcoholic phase, the person experiences greater relief from drinking than others in his social group. He moves from occasional drinking to relieve tension to daily drinking. This may occur over a time span of 6 months to 2 years. The drinker notices a change in his tolerance: it is now taking more alcohol than previously to achieve a desired effect. This phase ends when he experiences his first blackout. A blackout is a period of amnesia during or immediately following a drinking bout. During a blackout, a person is able to converse, perform tasks, and generally appear aware of his surroundings but has no memory of these events the following day.

The Premonitory Phase

In the second, or premonitory phase, alcohol has ceased to be a beverage. The person usually has a vague realization that he drinks differently from others. He begins to sneak drinks, becomes preoccupied with alcohol, and starts gulping drinks. At this stage he feels guilty about his drinking and avoids references to alcohol. Throughout this phase there are an increasing number of blackouts.

During these two phases, rationalizations of the drinking behavior are not strong, and there is some insight as well as a fear of the consequences.

The Crucial Phase

In the third, or crucial phase, the person loses control. Any drinking starts a chain reaction, which is felt as a physical demand for more alcohol. The person begins to make alibis. He feels a loss of self-esteem and compensates for this with grandiose behavior. There is an increase in aggressive behavior, followed by remorse and periods of total abstinence. The drinker tries to change the pattern of his drinking. For example, perhaps if he drank whiskey instead of gin, or drank at home instead of at the bar, he would have more control over the drinking. At this time the person's life is alcohol-centered; he becomes isolated with marked self-pity and may try a geographic escape. There are often unreasonable resentments on the part of the drinker, and a breakdown in the family may be seen. At the end of this phase, the drinker may need medical care for an alcohol-related complaint, and he begins regular morning drinking.

The Chronic Phase

In the fourth, or chronic phase, the person goes on benders, drinking for several days at a time. He carefully protects his supply. There is a marked ethical deterioration and an impairment in thinking, and the person drinks with persons below his social level. During this phase there is a loss of alcohol tolerance. It now takes only half the amount to bring on a stuporous state. Vague religious desires may then develop, and the rationalization system fails.

Formerly it was thought that an individual must reach this state in order to be amenable to receiving help. Reaching the chronic phase was seen as "hitting bottom." It is now known that successful intervention can be started at any point in the disease process. Early intervention

is stressed along with approaching the problem from the preventive angle.

These symptoms outlined by Jellinek do not necessarily appear in chronological order, and all the symptoms are not experienced by every alcoholic. Most of them are experienced, however, and this sequence can be a successful tool in identifying the progression of an individual's illness. Reviewing this sequence in a nonthreatening way with a client can be a helpful exercise in reducing denial. Upon seeing the symptoms in black and white, the alcoholic often does not feel so isolated and may find it easier to discuss his symptoms.

NURSING CARE OF THE ALCOHOLIC CLIENT

Assessment

The nurse is often in the position to detect the signs of alcoholism in a patient. During the assessment process she should collect data using effective interviewing skills, observation, history, and physical and psychological examination. The data are then used to formulate a problem statement or nursing diagnosis.

In the interview, all efforts should be made to enhance and develop the self-esteem of the patient. The patient is often frightened and defensive, desperately wanting understanding but afraid of rejection. The nurse's acceptance, concern, and attempts to understand are sources of strength to the patient. It is especially important that the patient be able to talk to the nurse without being rejected. The nurse should first pay close attention to the patient's complaints and requests for help. Points of agreement and patient's strengths should be emphasized while power struggles are avoided.

Alcoholism is a widespread problem, and questions regarding alcohol use should be included in the total assessment of any patient. These questions might best be included with those regarding dietary intake, smoking, and the use of prescribed or other drugs. Often the guarded or hostile reply to these questions will give the nurse the first clue to an alcohol problem. The nurse must also make an effort to be aware of her own biases and how these effect the interview. A nurse's attitude toward alcoholism and the alcoholic client may affect her manner of asking questions, and this could be a critical factor in determining the patient's response.

The diagnosis of alcoholism is often missed because the patient does not label the problem when seeking help and does not fit the stereotype of an alcoholic client. It must be recognized that anyone can have a serious alcohol-related problem. Research has yet to identify a specific personality type that is unique to the alcoholic. Each patient is an individual with his special needs and must be identified on that basis.

Observations made by the nurse during the interview should include the patient's manner of answering questions about alcohol, odor of alcohol or of mouthwash on the breath, tremors, and ecchymotic areas on the extremities.

While collecting the patient's history the nurse should keep in mind the high-risk factors for the development of alcoholism. These include coming from an Irish or Scandinavian background, coming from a broken home or a home with an absent or rejecting father, or having female relatives of more than one generation with a history of recurrent depression. Other high-risk factors are a family history of alcoholism or teetotalism. An individual who comes from a family where drinking is considered morally bad and later is in a situation where drinking is highly encouraged is at a particular high risk.

The nurse should also look for signs of the progression of alcoholism. A history of tolerance, blackouts, and treatment for alcohol-related medical diseases should be sought. Does the patient (or family) report gulping drinks, drinking more than the peer group, surreptitious drinking, repeated conscious attempts at abstinence, shifting from one alcoholic beverage to another, loss of interest in activities not directly associated with drinking, frequent unexplained changes in residence, absences from work, frequent job changes, or a change of jobs to one that facilitates drinking.

Other clues the nurse might pick up are decreased socialization with family or friends, family quarrels, reluctance of children to bring home friends from school, behavioral problems in children, sensitivity to comments from others about drinking, inappropriate telephone calls, and failing grades, or absences from school.

Physical Assessment

There is hardly a tissue in the body that is not harmfully affected by the heavy intake of alcohol. Many medical diagnoses are alcohol-related. Such damage is due to the direct, irritating effects of alcohol on the body, changes that take place in the body during the metabolism of alcohol, aggravation of existing disease, accidents while intoxicated, or the irregular taking of medically prescribed drugs while drinking.

In the presence of physiological withdrawal symptoms such as delirium tremens or major alcohol-related illnesses such as cirrhosis, pancreatitis, or Wernicke's encephalopathy, the diagnosis of alcoholism is usually made. The nurse doing an assessment must also be alert to clues of less diagnostic significance. These might include malaise, complaints of heartburn, an increased incidence of infection, cigarette burns on the fingers, accidents, fractures, and bruises or injuries for which treatment was delayed for at least 24 hours.

The more common alcohol-related medical and psychiatric diagnoses are illustrated in Figure 35-1.

Psychological Assessment

Alcoholism is a psychologically painful illness. The experience of being alcoholic can be compared with experiences in other life-threatening events such as prison camps, natural disasters, and nuclear war.[5] Rarely does the individual have any awareness that he is developing alcoholism. So devastating is the realization of this diagnosis that strong ego defenses are brought into play. Although the term "alcoholic personality" is widely used, no common, preexisting personality traits have been identified. Instead, commonalities are attributed to the defenses most often used when faced with the frustrating, complicated, and frightening process of slowly losing control of one's drinking and one's life.

Defense Mechanisms. It has been stated earlier in this book that ego defense mechanisms are the mind's way of defending itself. The alcoholic often feels trapped, isolated, depressed, beyond help, and stigmatized. The defense mechanisms most commonly employed by the alcoholic are denial, projection, and rationalization.

Denial is the defense mechanism most closely associated with alcoholism and is indeed characteristic of the disease. The patient can deny the presence of a problem long after family members, friends, and employers recognize its existence.

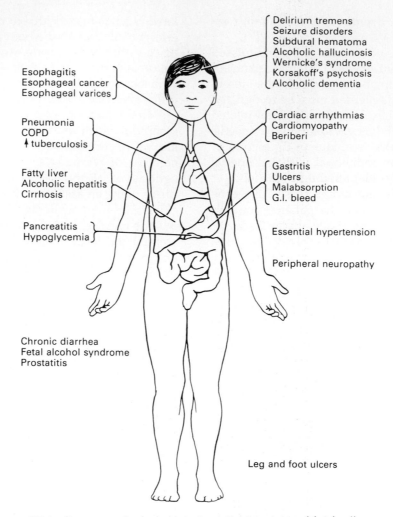

Delirium tremens
Seizure disorders
Subdural hematoma
Alcoholic hallucinosis
Wernicke's syndrome
Korsakoff's psychosis
Alcoholic dementia

Esophagitis
Esophageal cancer
Esophageal varices

Pneumonia
COPD
↑ tuberculosis

Cardiac arrhythmias
Cardiomyopathy
Beriberi

Gastritis
Ulcers
Malabsorption
G.I. bleed

Fatty liver
Alcoholic hepatitis
Cirrhosis

Pancreatitis
Hypoglycemia

Essential hypertension

Peripheral neuropathy

Chronic diarrhea
Fetal alcohol syndrome
Prostatitis

Leg and foot ulcers

Figure 35-1. Common alcohol-related medical and psychiatric diagnoses.

It is painful for an alcoholic to come to terms with the fact that his drinking is out of control and is causing harm. It is terrifying if not impossible to think of life without alcohol. Denial therefore serves a protective function. It spares the self-esteem by not acknowledging the stigmatizing diagnosis while at the same time takes away the need to curb the drinking. The professional encountering this defense mechanism often misinterprets it as willful lying on the part of the patient. The nurse who recognizes that this is not lying but a defense against painful reality will be more sensitive to the needs of the patient and therefore more effective in dealing with the denial.

The alcoholic patient often *projects* his painful feelings of guilt, inadequacy, and low self-esteem onto the nurse and then feels that the nurse regards him or her as unworthy. The pa-

tient then responds to the nurse with anger and hostility. The nurse who doesn't understand this defense mechanism may feel hurt or bewildered and in turn may respond to the patient in an angry manner. The patient receiving this response then has his original false belief reinforced.

Rationalization is another common defense mechanism and the alcoholic can find numerous ways to rationalize the drinking behavior. The reasons can vary from one drinking bout to another and may appear quite contradictory. The person may drink to celebrate a daughter's wedding or to mourn a friend's death, because of sickness or good health, because it's rainy or it's sunny, etc. It is important that the nurse understand that the patient is not merely making excuses but is using the defense mechanism of rationalization.

Psychiatric Diagnosis of Alcohol-Related Disorders

Alcoholic clients present with a wide range of psychopathology, as alcoholism can mimic almost any psychiatric disorder. If the primary problem is alcoholism, these symptoms will abate after a period of abstinence. On the other hand, the abuse of alcohol can exacerbate any preexisting psychiatric problems and should be assessed as part of the differential diagnosis of all psychiatric clients.[6]

Psychiatric disorders that are directly related to the use of alcohol include idiosyncratic intoxication, alcohol withdrawal delirium, alcoholic hallucinosis, Wernicke-Korsakoff syndrome, and alcoholic dementia.

Idiosyncratic Intoxication

In idiosyncratic intoxication an individual experiences abrupt behavioral changes after imbibing a small amount of alcohol, an amount that would be insufficient to cause intoxication in most people. The behavioral changes are generally of an aggressive nature and are atypical of this person when not drinking. The duration is quite brief, usually lasting only a few hours. The individual returns to his nondrinking state as the blood alcohol level falls, usually with amnesia for the period of intoxication. During the period of intoxication, care must be taken to protect the patient and others from injury. Treatment is abstinence and education.

Alcohol Withdrawal Delirium

Alcohol withdrawal delirium or delirium tremens usually occurs within one week of a cessation of or reduction in heavy alcohol intake. It is important to note that delirium tremens can begin while the patient is still actively drinking and should not be ruled out simply because of the odor of alcohol on the patient's breath. On the other hand, alcohol withdrawal is only one cause of delirium, and this cause should not be assumed simply on the basis of history. Many causes of delirium are life-threatening if the underlying condition is not treated. The nurse should always be concerned about the cause of the delirium.

While working with a patient in delirium, the nurse should employ the same principles used in working with other patients suffering from an acute brain syndrome. Her manner should be calm, concerned, and understanding. All procedures should be carefully explained each time they are to be performed, and new information should be introduced slowly, using face-to-face communication. It is important to reinforce reality and to keep the patient oriented. The room should be kept well lit and as familiar as possible.

Alcoholic Hallucinosis

Alcoholic hallucinosis presents with symptoms similar to acute schizophrenia, paranoid type. Typically its onset is shortly after a cessation of or reduction in heavy drinking. The symptoms include delusions of persecution and grandeur and vivid auditory hallucinations often accusatory in nature, which may engender panic and violent behavior. In the majority of cases, symptoms subside after a few hours to a week, but in some patients a chronic form develops. The treatment usually consists of hospitalization, abstinence, phenothiazines, and support.

Wernicke-Korsakoff's Syndrome

Wernicke-Korsakoff's syndrome is due to a thiamine deficiency associated with heavy alcohol intake. This is felt to be the result of both poor dietary intake and malabsorption of vitamins ingested while drinking. Once felt to be two separate entities, these two diagnoses are now generally accepted as two manifestations of the same process. Wernicke's encephalopathy is an acute neurological disease characterized by ataxia, ocular abnormalities, and confusion. This condition can lead to fatal midbrain hemorrhage if not treated with large doses of thiamine.

Korsakoff's psychosis is characterized by a severe impairment in memory and learning. The patient often appears apathetic and uninterested in his surroundings and has little insight into his memory defect. Confabulation may be used to compensate for memory gaps. Some patients do recover from Korsakoff's psychosis, but others have long-term residual damage requiring custodial care.

Alcoholic Dementia

Alcoholic dementia is diagnosed when dementia presents after prolonged, heavy use of alcohol, persists for at least 3 weeks, and all other causes of dementia are ruled out. This has long been felt to be the result of irreversible brain atrophy commonly found in heavy drinkers at autopsy. More recently, computer-assisted tomography (CT scan) has been used to study this problem. CT scans have confirmed the presence of brain atrophy in heavy drinkers but have cast doubt on the irreversibility of the process. These scans have shown a decrease in cerebral atrophy after as little as 2 weeks of abstinence.

After completing the assessment phase, the nurse should be able to recognize the presence of an alcohol problem or potential problem and to identify the stage of progression of the illness. Once the data are collected, a list of the patient's actual and potential problems should be drawn up. Some sample nursing diagnoses are as follows:

- Confusion: disorientation to time and place secondary to alcohol withdrawal.
- Nutritional alteration due to poor dietary intake and malabsorption while drinking.
- Alteration in sleep pattern related to alcohol intake or withdrawal.
- Aggressive, assaultive behavior related to drinking alcohol.
- Low self-esteem related to inability to control alcohol intake.

Assessment should not be limited to finding evidence of pathology. Efforts should also be made to identify the patient's areas of strength and accomplishments.

Planning

In planning for the care of the alcoholic patient, it is once again well to remember that the patient's self-esteem is at a low ebb. Treatment should begin by addressing the patient's immediate request for help even when other problems are far more obvious to the nurse. Successful results depend on a program that can begin at a point that is acceptable to the patient. This should include accepting the patient as a worthwhile person, recognizing and using the patient's strengths, and paying attention to his initial request for help.

The following case illustrates a not uncommon occurrence:

An alcoholic male, sober for several months, had a syncopal episode and fell on some stairs. The following morning he experienced severe back pain and pro-

ceeded to medicate himself with alcohol. A week later, due to continued back pain, he went to a walk-in clinic. The nurse observed his intoxicated state and gave him a lecture on alcohol abuse. She then discovered that he had not been taking his prescribed heart medication while drinking. An ECG was taken and the patient was sent home with a new prescription for the heart medication and a reiteration of the advice to stop drinking. On the way home the patient stopped at the nearest bar to obtain relief for the back pain, which was by then severe.

In this case the patient's immediate problem was the back pain, and this was never addressed. Furthermore, he was made to feel like an unworthy person. He left feeling worse than when he entered and further drinking was inevitable.

During the planning phase, priorities should be established, expected outcomes identified, and a timetable set up. Goals should be kept reasonable and attainable. Setting unrealistic treatment goals is a major cause of stalls in working with the alcoholic patient. Because of a failure to develop appropriate treatment goals, many nurses become easily frustrated while working with the alcoholic and subvert what might otherwise be a successful treatment approach.

Nurses may become demoralized because of recidivism and an allegedly high failure rate. This often produces hostility, which is inappropriately directed toward the patient. If nurses can appreciate that they are dealing with a chronic, relapsing illness and can learn to expect a prolonged treatment course that is sometimes interrupted by recurrences of drinking, they are better able to sustain an optimistic attitude toward the patient. Rather than entertain fantasies of "cure" dependent on total abstinence, the nurse should concentrate on lengthening the periods of sobriety while decreasing the periods of drinking. Evidence of improvement in relation to these goals is usually sufficient to maintain an optimistic attitude in both the patient and the nurse.

Effective treatment planning for the alcoholic often involves use of a variety of treatment agencies. Any one patient may require a combination of services including emergency services, crisis intervention centers, detoxification, inpatient hospitalization, outpatient treatment, after-care services, Alcoholics Anonymous (AA), and halfway houses. The patient may enter care at any point, but he is often not referred to other appropriate services and care becomes fragmented. For example, the patient who is seen on the emergency ward for treatment of a head laceration may not be referred for detoxification. An AA sponsor may neglect to refer a physically ill patient to a physician. The detoxification center may not make the effort to contact the patient's after-care coordinator. Alcoholics Anonymous is not suggested to the patient on the medical ward suffering from alcoholic hepatitis. The nurse should familiarize herself with the referral sources in her area and may find that her most important contribution is in referral and coordination of care rather than as a provider of direct service.

AGENCIES AND SERVICES FOR ALCOHOLICS

Alcohol Information Centers

Many metropolitan areas have set up telephone referral centers accessible to either patients or health care workers. These centers are equipped with the necessary information to match patients to services. Many of the centers also offer educational programs, pamphlets, films, etc., to patients, family, and health professionals.

Detoxification Centers

Some communities have established free-standing detoxification centers, and in others, detoxification is carried out in the general hospital. Detoxification is for the treatment of the acute alcohol withdrawal symptoms and should be seen as only a first step in the treatment process.

Withdrawal from alcohol is more severe and more likely to cause death than withdrawal from narcotics. In untreated advanced cases, as many as 14 percent might die. The aim of detoxification is to assist the patient through the withdrawal period with the fewest number of symptoms. Early treatment can prevent the onset of more severe and life-threatening symptoms such as delirium tremens.

Halfway Houses

Upon leaving a detoxification center, many alcoholics no longer have a stable home environment to which they can return. It may be virtually impossible for them to maintain sobriety in the environment from which they came. In this situation a halfway house can be invaluable, offering the patient a stable alcohol-free environment. Rules vary from halfway house to halfway house. Many are strongly AA oriented with required meetings on the premises. Others have few rules other than sobriety. Clients should be advised not to judge all halfway houses based on their experience in one.

Alcoholics Anonymous

Perhaps the single most effective group in the treatment of alcoholism is Alcoholics Anonymous, a self-help group founded in the 1930s whose fellowship is now worldwide. Since this is a prime resource for most alcoholics, all nurses should be familiar with how it works. The basic aim of AA is for members to help each other through a basic 12-step program. By attending meetings, patients are able to identify with other alcoholics, which is comforting and offers hope. The person is helped not to feel alone. Since there is a variation in membership from one group to another, it is wise to tell a patient not to make a decision about AA based on attendance at one meeting but to go to several meetings and continue to go to any that he feels most comfortable with. Part of the success of AA is also attributed to sponsors who are available to new members on a 24-hour basis. Nurses in any field will benefit from attending at least three AA meetings. This firsthand experience will facilitate the referral process.

Employee Assistance Programs

One of the most successful approaches to alcoholism in recent years has been the Employee Assistance Programs (EAPs). According to figures from the National Institute of Alcohol Abuse and Alcoholism, the abuse of alcohol has presented a major problem to industry. Its cost has been put at $28 billion in lost production and $18.1 billion in health and medical services. Alcoholic employees have absenteeism rates that are three to four times the norm, and accident rates that are four to five times the norm. Each problem-drinking employee loses an average of 22 workdays a year as a result of drinking and related health problems.[7]

EAPs, first introduced in the 1930s, fully came into their own in the 1970s. From a total of 300 established programs in 1972, the number increased to five and one-half thousand by 1981. EAPs report success rates as low as 40 percent and as high as 90 percent, with most programs reporting in the 70 percent to 85 percent range. Criteria for success vary between programs, but most include increased productivity, decreased absenteeism, and a decrease in other alcohol-related problems on the job. From an economic standpoint alone, EAPs are a sound investment for a company as treatment has been estimated to be 2.2 times cheaper than replacement. From a morale point of view, the EAP also makes sense because after treatment the company is left with a skilled and loyal employee rather than a succession of new trainees.[8]

ALCOHOL COUNSELING AND NURSING IMPLEMENTATION

Nurses in all settings, whether or not they plan to work with a patient over time, need a basic level of knowledge and skill to provide some alcoholism counseling. In many cases all that is needed is helping a patient accept that some of his problems may be alcohol-related, providing education regarding alcohol and alcoholism, and initiating appropriate referrals.

Stall Situations

In implementing nursing care with the alcoholic client, the nurse will encounter many situations that could lead to a stall in the therapeutic process. Some of the more common stall situations are discussed below.

Judgmental Feelings

Since the nurse's attitude toward drinking and alcoholism has a direct relationship to the response made to the patient with a drinking problem, it is necessary that the nurse be aware of her personal attitude, the reasons for it, and how it can be modified. Insensitive attitudes can cause a stall.

Attitudes may be described as the statement of one's stand or position on an issue. Attitudes are usually shaped over time by personal experiences and education and are reflected in a person's behavior. It is a rare nurse who will not have had some personal experience with an al-

coholic before meeting one in a nursing role, so she will come to that role with a preconceived attitude.

The attitude of a nurse whose prior experience included the inability to bring playmates home from school for fear of embarrassment by a drunken mother will be different from that of a nurse whose major contact with an alcoholic was Uncle Joe, who was drunk every weekend, bought ice cream, and gave out $5 bills. Different from both of these will be that of a nurse whose parents never drank and viewed drinking as sinful.

Since attitudes are the result of such prior experiences, they should not be labeled as good or bad, but they should be examined and understood and perhaps modified in the light of new knowledge and new experiences. The nurse must be aware of and accepting of her personal attitude in order to work effectively with the alcoholic patient.

Attitudes prevalent in U.S. society regarding drinking and alcoholism tend to be inconsistent and conflicting. For example, drinking and intoxication are usually seen within the realm of social drinking, whereas the alcoholic is viewed as a weak-willed moral degenerate. The disease concept of alcoholism is generally accepted on an intellectual level, but yet the sober alcoholic is often referred to as a "reformed" alcoholic. The stigma placed on the alcoholic in our society results in the development of attitudes that are moralistic and judgmental.

The National Center for Alcohol Education has identified 10 helpful attitudes to assist nurses in shaping their own attitudes toward drinking, alcoholism, and the alcoholic patient[9]:

1. Drinking alcohol has no moral implication attached to it; those who do drink alcohol are not necessarily bad or good.
2. Drunkenness is neither comical nor disgusting but rather a serious effect of an overdose of a drug.
3. Alcoholism is a disease; although complex and not completely understood, it is a disease as legitimate as any other.
4. Health care providers have professional responsibilities in treating patients and families who are the victims of alcoholism to the best of their skill, knowledge, and capabilities. If the professional is lacking in the educational preparation to do so, such education should be sought out and obtained.

5. Early recognition, diagnosis, and prevention have the same value and benefits for alcoholism as for other illnesses.

6. The alcoholic patient is a worthwhile individual who deserves the same value and benefits for alcoholism as for other illnesses.

7. Alcoholism is a treatable disease from which recovery is possible with enlightened, professional help.

8. It is the professional's ethical and human responsibility to work with the alcoholic patient, openly and without subterfuge or prejudice, to attempt to assist the patient in exploring his own drinking problems, to break through denial, and to offer appropriate treatment for alcoholism. Further, neither blame nor credit is associated with the treatment outcome if the professional has honestly and skillfully treated the patient in accordance with a sound knowledge of the disease.

9. The health professional must strive to understand the influence of his or her own background on personal attitudes toward alcoholism and alcoholic patients, to appreciate the natural tendency of most health professionals to be ambivalent and negative in regard to these issues, and to work for the development of more positive personal, professional, and community understanding of the disease.

10. No one is immune to alcoholism. It should be a concern for health professionals in all areas of practice, as well as in relationships with family, friends, and peers.

Before and during the process of caring for an alcoholic patient, the nurse should autognose her attitude about drinking and alcoholism, attempting to work out the many conflicting messages on the subject. Knowledge about the disease of alcoholism has been correlated with positive attitudes toward the care of the alcoholic patient, which can prevent a stall situation. Since alcoholism is a widespread disease encountered in all fields of nursing, the student will do well to take advantage of educational opportunities in this area.

Ambivalent Feelings

Ambivalent feelings can arise when the nurse does not accept the disease concept of alcoholism and loses sight of the defense mechanisms characteristic of the disease. Consider the following case example:

A student is caring for a 38-year-old woman with pancreatitis secondary to alcoholism. The student feels warmly toward the woman who reminds her of a favorite aunt. As she enters the room one day the student observes the patient quickly hiding a liquor bottle under some belongings. The student becomes angry at what she sees as willful self-destructive behavior. When she speaks to the patient regarding her observation, the patient says, "That little drop won't hurt me. It takes the edge off the pain. You won't tell the doctor will you?"

The student might stall the situation by responding only to her angry feelings, give a lecture on the evils of alcohol, and march out of the room with the bottle. Or she might respond to her warm feelings and tell the patient that it will be their little secret if the patient promises not to do it again. This reaction can also cause a stall.

In order to avoid a stall in this situation, the student must realize that the use of alcohol is this patient's characteristic way of dealing with pain. The student should help the patient to realize that although the alcohol is providing some temporary relief, it is in the long run compounding the problem. She should tell the patient that she will report her observation and that perhaps the staff will be able to find other, less harmful ways of dealing with the pain she is experiencing.

Overidentification with the Problem

The nurse might find herself as involved with rationalization about drinking as the patient is and feel that it is reasonable that the patient is drinking in view of the many problems he is facing. "I'd drink too if I had just lost my job with all those financial responsibilities." "A husband like hers would drive anybody to drink." Reactions like these can cause a stall situation.

It is important for the nurse to realize that the underlying problems might indeed be overwhelming and painful to the patient, but although drinking may be the way the patient has chosen to cope with these feelings, there are other choices available that should be considered.

Fear of Being Manipulated

People do not like to be manipulated. It makes them feel stupid, frustrated, and angry. Fear of being manipulated might cause the nurse to avoid working with patients who have been labeled as manipulators or to be extremely careful and unnatural in their relationship with such a patient. This can result in a stall.

The following case example and subsequent discussion show how one nurse-therapist dealt with a situation in which she had been manipulated:

On his third day in a detoxification facility, a patient called the nurse-therapist he had been seeing for a year, saying that he wanted to be discharged that day and was sure it would be possible if the nurse indicated her approval to his doctor. The nurse explained that she had no connection with the facility, that the decision was not hers to make but was one that would have to be negotiated there, and that her understanding was that the facility expected a minimum 5-day stay.

She next received a call from the patient's doctor, informing her that he was meeting with the patient and would discharge him or keep him in hospital according to her wishes.

The patient had somehow manipulated the situation so that the nurse was in a position she felt she had no right to be in. Furthermore, she felt that either decision she made would be detrimental to the patient. Her prior knowledge of this patient told her that he could not be successfully detoxified in less than 5 days. If she told the patient that he must stay, she felt that he would most likely sign out against medical advice and be lost to treatment for a time. If, on the other hand, she told him he could leave, she would expect to see him in her office for his next visit intoxicated and saying, "You were right. I should have stayed the five days."

It is important to notice that either choice the nurse made would most likely lead to a situation that was not in the best interests of the patient. This is what makes dealing with manipulation so difficult. The nurse feels forced to make a decision she is not comfortable with and resents being put in this position.

In the above situation, the nurse asked to speak with the patient. She told him that she didn't understand how he had managed it, but indeed it did appear that she had the power to make the decision. She shared with him why she was reluctant to make either choice and told him she was going to put the decision back into his hands. She asked him first to listen to why she would like him to choose to stay but made it clear that she would abide by whichever decision he made. After listening to her reasons, the patient chose to be discharged. The nurse

passed this decision on to the doctor and asked the patient to drop by her office on the way home.

In this way a stall situation was avoided. The nurse kept communication open with the patient and left the decision with the patient where it belonged. By asking him to stop by her office, she made it clear that she did not reject him for making a decision contrary to her advice.

It is important for the student to realize that there is nothing wrong with having been manipulated. It should not be seen as a conscious attempt by the patient to "con" the nurse but used as a tool that can be explained to the patient to understand his own behavior patterns.

Dependency Issues
Many nurses express concern that the alcoholic patient might demand more time and energy than the nurse thinks reasonable and that the nurse will leave the relationship feeling drained, having spent too much time with the patient. In dealing with this stall, the nurse must first consider dependency issues. It is true that alcoholic patients tend to be excessively dependent, especially during the early stages of recovery, but this is not necessarily negative. In fact, the dependency tends to be functional and adaptive as it is apt to keep the patient in treatment. Organizations such as AA have long been aware that the treatment needs of the alcoholic do not adapt to a 9 to 5 schedule and for this reason are available on a 24-hour basis. As the patient gains longer periods of sobriety, his dependency needs will decrease.

In addition to dependency issues, nurses must ask themselves whether they are acting or reacting to the issue of "too much time." Nurses are responsible for their own time. It is their responsibility to define what is reasonable and to set limits accordingly. When the nurse's limited time is not sufficient to meet all the patient's needs, other agencies should be involved. For example, a nurse seeing a patient once a week in a primary care clinic might suggest that the patient attend a daily discussion group in the hospital's alcohol clinic or attend AA meetings, and have the number of an AA sponsor or a crisis center for a possible 3 A.M. crisis.

Failure to Do Grief Work
Many nurses, seeing total abstinence as the goal, view alcohol as bad, and they feel that pa-

tient and nurse should cheer when the decision is made to stop drinking. These nurses lose sight of the fact that alcohol has been the patient's long-time companion, through good times and bad. There is a failure to appreciate the extent of the patient's loss. In many ways a commitment to sobriety has much the same impact as deciding to get a divorce. Although at this point the situation may be intolerable and separation voluntary, there are inevitably memories of the good times and a wish to have them back. The good times must be mourned if a successful adjustment is to be made. All too often, in doing alcoholism counseling, the nurse is reluctant to allow the patient to discuss the good times as well as the bad. Perhaps there is a fear that discussing the good times might lead to a relapse. It must be remembered that the patient's loss is a significant one. To ignore this loss is to hinder recovery.

Feelings of Pessimism

The word *alcoholic* to many implies a negative prognosis. Most nurses are surprised when confronted with the positive results of alcoholism treatment programs. A high value is placed on a patient's motivation for recovery; and even industrial programs, where motivation is an outside factor, report success rates as high as 85 percent. And programs dealing with "skid row" alcoholics, thought by many to be hopeless, report success rates of 15 percent.

Feelings of pessimism can reinforce the already low self-esteem of the patient. A stall situation can develop when the nurse feels that nothing can be done until the patient admits to being an alcoholic and the patient is not yet ready to take that step. However, a therapist can avoid arguments about whether or not the patient is an alcoholic without denying that the patient has problems with alcohol. Many alcoholics will accept this as the initial step to treatment, whereas they will avoid treatment altogether if it is demanded that they begin by accepting the diagnosis of alcoholism.

Another stall situation develops when the nurse, hearing that the patient must "reach bottom" before being amenable to help, interprets this to mean that the patient must have lost everything before he can begin treatment. The nurse might then feel that it is a waste of time and energy to invest in a patient who is still employed and living with this family. It is important to clear up this misunderstanding and

to realize that a patient can be helped at any stage of the illness.

Instilling the feeling of hope in the alcoholic is the cornerstone of successful treatment. Acceptance and optimism are necessary for successful treatment because the patient usually begins at a point where he feels hopeless and perceives himself in a very negative fashion. Strong support is needed from the nurse if the alcoholic is to continue in treatment.

The Scare Approach

When a patient is put on a salt-free diet because of congestive heart failure or a restricted diet for diabetes, every effort is usually made to explain to the patient in an understandable manner the reasons for this limitation. The patient is helped in a nonthreatening way to understand the physiological effects of failure to comply with the diet.

In contrast, more times than not the alcoholic is simply told to stop drinking, and this is done in a threatening manner. For example, "You're going to die if you don't stop drinking!" The alcoholic individual deserves the same consideration as other patients.

The assumption is often made that the alcoholic knows all there is to know about alcoholism and what is needed is a method to enforce compliance. Because of the reluctance of professionals to discuss alcoholism with patients, the alcoholic often knows very little about his disease. Education is an appropriate treatment strategy at any stage of treatment and can prevent a stall situation.

Disulfiram Therapy

Disulfiram (Antabuse) is an enzyme inhibitor that has been used successfully as an adjunct to treatment in alcoholism therapy. The breakdown of alcohol in the liver involves two enzymes. The first reacts with the alcohol to produce acetaldehyde, a substance toxic to the body. This is quickly broken down to acetic acid by the action of a second enzyme called aldehyde dehydrogenase. Disulfiram inhibits the action of this second enzyme, causing acetaldehyde levels to rise, resulting in palpitations, flushing, nausea, and vomiting. This is a potentially dangerous reaction, and this drug should never be given without the full knowledge and consent of the patient. It is given in daily doses and remains effective for up to 3 days after the last dose. A patient is faced with many drinking occasions throughout the course of a day and is constantly faced with the decision of whether or not to drink. When disulfiram is being taken, the decision need be made only once a day rather than at every drinking opportunity.

A drinking bout usually begins long before the first drink is taken and in most alcoholics there are recognizable signs and symptoms leading to a return to drinking. Disulfiram therapy can be useful to the patient in helping him to recognize these signs. The patient is told that no excuse for not taking the disulfiram will be considered valid and that stopping the disulfiram will be viewed as planning to drink. Since most people are relatively stereotyped in the manner in which they return to drinking, recognizing the signs can be helpful in intercepting a drinking bout.

The nurse should be alert to the number of over-the-counter and prescribed medications that contain alcohol. Medications containing alcohol percentages as low as 3.8 percent can evoke behavioral responses such as irritability, restlessness, indifference, anxiety, depression, and active avoidance of interpersonal contacts. The innocent use of an over-the-counter cough medicine has precipitated many a drinking bout. Prescribing medications containing alcohol to alcoholics reinforces denial and rationalization and implies that the person has control over alcohol intake. In persons taking disulfiram these medications will precipitate a disulfiram reaction.

Working with the Alcoholic's Family

During the implementation phase, the nurse will also want to concern herself with the patient's family. Alcoholism is often referred to as a family disease. Members of the alcoholic's family, confused by the inconsistent and erratic behavior of the drinking member, are subject to the same feelings of guilt, depression, loneliness, and low self-esteem as the alcoholic and often employ the same defense mechanisms. Ambivalent feelings are common and place a great strain on family relationships. Not understanding the illness, the family often acts in ways that sustain rather than change the drinking behavior. Alcohol and drinking become the focus of all problems. The alcoholic might cite the behavior of family members as the cause of

the drinking, whereas family members feel that if the drinking would stop, all family problems would disappear with the alcohol. There is an increased amount of fighting, battering, and child abuse in alcoholic families, perpetrated not necessarily by the drinker but by other members as well. Children of alcoholics have a higher rate of delinquency and school difficulties and are themselves at risk for developing alcoholism. Many times resentments are raised during drinking episodes that are never adequately worked out.

With so much focus on the drinking behavior, family members are often not prepared for the new set of tensions and problems brought on by the recovery process. For example, the wife of an alcoholic might have been receiving a great deal of secondary gain as friends and relatives remark on how admirably she has handled the home and family with that "no-good husband of hers." However, as the husband recovers, the admiration may be shifted to him and how well he is doing. The recovering member may also want to reassume previous roles that have been taken over by other family members. This could cause resentment and loss of status for the members who have been performing these roles. Where the family members had expected all problems to go away with the alcohol, they are now faced with a new set of problems and find that some of the old ones are intensified. If the family is unprepared and unsupported during this time of stress, there might be an unconscious attempt to return to the status quo. Although the drinking times were bad, at least each family member was familiar with his role. The stress that sobriety places on family members is too often unexpected by the family and overlooked by professionals.

Alanon, Alateen, and ACOAs

Alanon for adult family and friends of alcoholics and Alateen for children of alcoholics are excellent resources for helping a family to cope. These meetings help the family to realize that they too have needs and feelings that should be addressed. Family members are welcome to attend these meetings whether or not the drinking member is attending AA meetings. Often a family's involvement in one of these groups is an important first step because it is known that change in the behavior of one family member is bound to have an effect on the other members.

Gaining a great deal of momentum in this

country at present are concerns about the adult children of alcoholics, and there are a growing number of Alanon meetings geared specifically to the needs of this group. This movement recognizes that growing up in an alcoholic home is a traumatic experience and is made even more so by the code of silence that rules most of these families. Children develop certain roles to deal with a family environment that is unstructured and inconsistent. These responses become entrenched and maladaptive in later life. Specific characteristics seen in adult children of alcoholics include a need to be in control, difficulty with intimate relationships, difficulty in trusting, and a need for constant affirmation. For further readings in this area students are referred to the works of Black, Wegscheider-Cruse, and Brown.[10–12]

Referrals

Since nurses are often in the position of referring patients to other community agencies and coordinating their care among several facilities, they should develop an awareness of what each of these agencies offers. The optimum time to build a referral network is before a crisis arises. Nurses should take the time to visit other agencies and keep files on the components of care they offer; which clients they have the most success with; who tends to drop out; their treatment philosophy, goals, fees, and other requirements; and the name and phone number of a contact person. The files should be updated after each contact. The success of a referral often depends on the manner in which it was handled. The following six rules should facilitate the referral process.

1. Do not make the referral prematurely. Time is needed both to collect enough data to determine what kind of help is needed and to prepare the patient emotionally for the idea of referral. With a premature referral, a patient often feels that he is being "dumped."
2. Include the patient in the referral process. Discuss the idea of referral with the patient. Using behavioral descriptions rather than labels, explain to the patient why you are considering referral. This will not only increase compliance but may also uncover resources that have been helpful or unsatisfactory in the past.
3. Recognize the patient's feelings. Allowing a patient to ventilate feelings or fears increases compliance.
4. Provide realistic expectations. Overselling a resource can lead to disappointment and early dropout.
5. Provide complete and accurate information. Tell the client what to expect, using as much detail as possible. For example, Does the agency work on a first-come, first-served basis? Is there apt to be a long wait, etc.?
6. Follow through. Continued interest in the patient and his experience with the referral assures the patient of the nurse's concern. The patient's feedback is also useful data for the nurse in planning future referrals.

ALCOHOLICS WITH SPECIAL PROBLEMS

Polydrug Abuse

An ongoing difficulty in the management of many alcoholics is the problem of polydrug abuse. Particularly with younger patients, the custom of mixing alcohol with barbiturates, other sedatives, and marijuana is widespread. Current patterns in adolescent drinking suggest that, in the future, alcoholism as an isolated entity may disappear and be replaced by polydrug abuse.

It is important for nurses to recognize that all alcoholics have a high potential for abuse of other sedative drugs, especially sleeping tablets and antianxiety agents. Whenever possible, an alcoholic should be treated without medication, and all drugs should be withdrawn as soon as the individual can function without them. Whenever medications are prescribed, they should be given in relatively small quantities with nonrefillable prescriptions. If an individual does require medication, it is important that he be seen on a weekly or biweekly basis for adequate medical management.

Alcohol intoxication and alcoholism may affect the dosage requirements and safety limits of medically indicated drugs. For example, heavy drinkers metabolize warfarin sodium (Coumadin) much faster than nondrinkers. Alcohol itself has a variable effect on some of the clotting factors in the blood. Chronic alcohol ingestion increases the metabolism of tolbutamide (Orinase). A disulfiram-type reaction has been reported by 10 to 20 percent of patients who drink while taking Orinase. The depressant properties of antihistamines are enhanced by the depressant properties of alcohol. Aspirin taken with alcohol can be responsible for irri-tation of the stomach lining and hemorrhage. As previously stated, barbiturates taken with al-cohol produce an effect on the central nervous system that is much greater than the sum of the two drugs taken alone.

——— CASE EXAMPLE* ———————————————————————————

Mr. Tate, a 26-year-old, single, unemployed, black male was admitted to the rehabilitation unit, September 22, 1987, after spending 4 days on the detoxification unit in this same hospital. He was referred for addictions treatment by his mother. His chief complaint was the inability to stop using mood-altering substances, namely, alcohol and drugs. Mr. Tate was willing to participate in the 30-day inpatient addictions program. The client consumed his first drink at age 15, at which time he became drunk only on the weekends. At age 16 he began to have problems with alcohol and started drinking daily. He reports a 10-year history of alcohol dependency and he drinks 30 to 40 ounces of beer daily. Mr. Tate also has a history of cocaine dependency. He free-bases $50-worth daily.

He reports one previous detox admission in August, after which he resumed drinking and using cocaine 24 hours following discharge. He admits being noncompliant with the af-tercare plan following his last admission. Mr. Tate states that life really did not become unmanageable until he started using cocaine. He believes he can handle the alcohol but not the cocaine. He has not had previous treatment or medications for emotional problems or physical illness. There are no current legal problems.

Mr. Tate lived with his mother up until 1 week prior to his detox admission. She put him out of the home because of his addictive behavior, which included stealing things out of the house. Since that time, he has been staying with friends who also share the goal of getting "high" and "drunk."

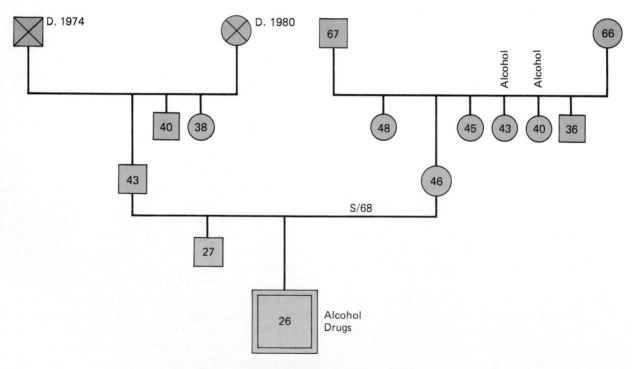

Figure 35-2. Mr. Tate's family genogram.

———————————————————————————————————

* This case is contributed by Theresa A. Catlett.

He has education to the ninth grade. However, he did receive further training in the Job Corps in the area of auto mechanics. His last job was as a dishwasher. Prior to that time, he worked as a loader in a store. He has been unable to hold a job for more than 2 months because of his addictive behavior. At present, he states he has no motivation to look for a job and that his main source of income is welfare.

Mr. Tate is the youngest of two children. His older brother is single and lives in his own apartment. Mr. Tate was raised by his mother and states he does not see his father because his parents are separated. He decribes the relationship between mother as close, until he started stealing. He states the relationship with his father is distant and poor. He considers his mother his main support system. There is no history of chemical dependency among the rest of the nuclear family. However, he reports that there are two aunts on his mother's side who are alcoholics. Figure 35-2 shows the patient's family genogram. Mr. Tate expresses feelings of loneliness and isolation. He states he feels detached and alienated from his family. He sees more attention being given to his older brother, who he describes as a "workaholic." Since childhood, he remembers his brother achieving more than him. His mother just recently received her Master's Degree and he describes her as a "work freak" and "goal-directed." Mr. Tate sees himself as being incapable of keeping up with the expectations of his family. He becomes depressed and anxious when he tries. He states he drinks and uses cocaine to prevent from "worrying" and "caring."

The client reports a history of blackouts and tremors upon withdrawal from chemical substances. He denies all other signs of withdrawal, including seizures. He currently complains of weight loss and difficulty falling asleep. He denies allergies to food and drugs.

At present, he appears alert and oriented. He is able to answer questions with good vocabulary and thought. He seems reliable. Affects appear flat and his mood depressed. No signs of withdrawal. He seems motivated and willing to participate in addiction treatment.

DSM-III-R: DRUG DEPENDENCY CONTINUOUS
Alcohol & Cocaine

NURSING DIAGNOSES

- Potential for injury due to chemical withdrawal.
- Alterations in Nutrition: Less than body requirements related to chemical dependence, manifested by weight loss.
- Sleep pattern disturbance related to difficulty in falling asleep, secondary to poor sleep–rest pattern.
- Disturbance in self-concept manifested by feelings of worthlessness and failure.
- Impaired family relationship manifested by feelings of alienation and loneliness.

GOALS

Long-Term
By the time of discharge the patient:

1. Will not have suffered from physical injury related to withdrawal.
2. Will have adequate sleep–rest pattern.
3. Will have normal eating habits with weight gain.
4. Will have a better understanding of the disease concept and AA and NA philosophy.
5. Will accept responsibility for addiction treatment and recovery process, including following aftercare plan.
6. Will have better coping stretegies.

The family will have experienced less anxiety. Each member will have developed a better sense of identity in relationship to each other and the larger family system.

Short-Term
1. The patient will be safe on the unit from physical stress at all times.
2. The patient will eat and tolerate three meals daily plus snack by day 7.
3. The patient will verbalize ability to fall asleep without difficulty by day 7.
4. The patient will verbalize and demonstrate an increase in knowledge of the addiction process by day 5.
5. The patient will attend and participate in groups and individual sessions by day 2.
6. The patient will verbalize and demonstrate a more positive self-concept by day 4.
7. The patient will verbalize and demonstrate more effective ways of coping.
8. To start family therapy sessions by end of first week.

INTERVENTIONS

1. Monitor vital signs continuously and observe for signs of withdrawal (tremors, increased BP and pulse, increased anxiety and diaphoresis). Monitor for signs indicating possible seizure activity. Maintain seizure precautions as necessary.
2. Assist patient in selection of meals (high in calories, proteins, and fibers). Use audiovisual equipment to teach the effects of chemical substances on human physiology. Assist patient in understanding the need for good nutrition. Administer vitamins daily as ordered.
3. Provide rest periods to facilitate sleep and relaxation. Maintain a quiet environment to promote sleep. Provide L-tryptophan 500 mg p.o. prn.
4. Encourage participation in all groups and lectures, including AA and NA meetings on unit. Provide reading material on AA and NA philosophy and relapse prevention. Teach importance of abstinence from alcohol and drugs. Encourage questions, provide for return demonstration of material learned, and reinforce teaching as necessary. Encourage verbalization of feelings and provide support.
5. Schedule a family session weekly. Meet with patient and his mother for 1 hour for a total of 5 sessions. Share information with family on the disease concept of addiction. Conceptualize the part each member plays in relationship to the nuclear family and family origin. Construct a family genogram and use it during sessions to help members understand their relationship to one another and their extended family. Assist family in identifying reflexive processes operating in the system. Monitor the level of anxiety during each session. Start working very early on aftercare plans with the family.

EVALUATION

Review short- and long-term goals with patient to determine positive changes and identify goals for aftercare.

The Elderly Alcoholic

A problem of growing concern is that of alcoholism among the elderly. Some long-term alcoholics, despite the high mortality, accident, and suicide rates found in this group, survive to old age. Other elderly individuals find that their usual moderate intake becomes excessive because of declining health. Still others turn to alcohol when faced with major life crises associated with aging such as retirement, loss of a loved one, new living arrangements, reduced income, and increasing social isolation.

Identification of the problem is of major concern because both family and professionals are reluctant to do so, especially in regard to individuals who develop the problem in later years.

Early treatment results of comprehensive programs that provide socialization and treatment of depression have shown optimistic results for most elderly alcoholics, including those who have had alcohol problems for some time.[13] At present, however, too many alcohol treatment programs exclude the elderly, while services for the elderly exclude the alcoholic.

Adolescent Problem Drinkers

An area of increasing concern is the number of teen-agers who drink heavily. According to a 1978 national survey conducted by the Research Triangle Institute, over 14 percent of American youth are problem drinkers, reporting drunkenness at least six times during the past year or other adverse consequences of drinking such as trouble with teachers or friends, driving while intoxicated, or trouble with the police.[14]

One of the biggest concerns over youthful drinking is the large number of teen-agers who drink and drive. Traffic accidents are the leading cause of death among young people, and from 45 to 60 percent of all fatal crashes involving teen-agers are alcohol-related. It has been found that adolescents become involved in fatal automobile crashes at blood alcohol concentrations significantly lower than those found in adults involved in similar accidents.[15] Trends to lower the drinking age, which were prevalent in the early 1970s, are now being reversed. Preliminary studies have indicated that this reversal has resulted in decreasing the number of alcohol-related traffic accidents in the 18-to 20-year-old group.[16]

Women with Alcohol Problems

In the 1950s, it was estimated that there were 5.5 male alcoholics for every female, but this difference is rapidly disappearing. Many experts predict that by the year 2000, women will make up half of all American drinkers; others feel that they already do.

Traditional studies on the progression of alcoholism, the signs and symptoms of abuse, etc., have almost exclusively been done using males as subjects. From these studies, case finding, management, and aftercare strategies have been devised. In other words, the experience of the female has not been considered in program planning.

There appear to be some real differences in the alcoholism experience for women. For example, on an emotional level it is generally more stigmatizing for a woman to suffer from alcohol problems than a male. In addition to a lack of self-esteem, female alcoholics also appear to lack a consistent self-image. And alcoholic women are much more apt to be left by their spouses than are alcoholic men.

Women are also at a much greater risk than men from socially acceptable amounts of alcohol. Since they have less body fluid, they reach higher blood alcohol concentrations with less alcohol. A woman will develop cirrhosis of the liver on half the amount of alcohol necessary to bring this about in a man, and it develops more rapidly, taking an average of 13 years to develop as compared to 22 years for a man.[17]

Women who are pregnant need to be especially cautious about their use of alcohol. The Fetal Alcohol Syndrome (FAS) resulting from heavy drinking during pregnancy can cause a range of defects including growth deficiency, mental retardation, learning disabilities, organic problems, and distinct facial characteristics. Safe levels of drinking are not known at this time, but the problem appears to be dose-related. In June of 1982, the American Medical Association joined a growing number of organizations in recommending total abstinence during pregnancy.

Alcoholism treatment facilities need to become more cognizant of the special needs of women. Women for Sobriety (WFS) is one self-help group that is aimed at the specific needs of the female alcoholic. Founded 9 years ago by a sociologist, Jean Kirkpatrick, it now has approximately 500 groups in the United States and Canada. In comparison to AA, the emphasis of Women for Sobriety is on the lives, problems, and concerns of women rather than on alcoholism. The majority of WFS members also attend AA meetings.

The Homeless Alcoholic

If the instillation of hope is indeed the cornerstone of successful treatment, then it is no wonder that the homeless or skid row alcoholic is viewed as having the poorest prognosis. The majority of homeless alcoholics first entered the treatment system at a time when the prevailing thought was that a person had to "reach bottom" before being amenable to help. "Reaching bottom" was seen as losing everything. By the time these people had lost everything—their health, employment, family, friends and self-esteem—the prevailing thought had changed. They were now seen as having lost too much to be amenable to help. In essence, they have been given a consistent picture of hopelessness and are now viewed as the most stigmatized and least worthy candidates for treatment.

Those who work with the homeless have

observed the lack of respect and inconsistent care often afforded these individuals in the health care system. In contrast, clinics set up specifically for the homeless offer their clients dignity, respect, and care. When allowed the hope that life can be better, many homeless people are able to involve themselves in the work of getting well. Because of poor health, inconsistent work history, and lack of family support this can be a long and difficult road. The client who receives consistent care and support will be the most successful.

EVALUATION

Evaluation should be continuous throughout the nursing process. The nurse might ask herself questions such as: Have the expected outcomes been achieved? Were the original goals realistic? Are the outcomes measurable? Have nursing interventions been helpful in reaching the outcomes? Have referral sources played the expected role? The answers to these questions will assist the nurse in planning the future course, which could range from reassessment to discharge.

All too often alcoholism is viewed as a dynamic process only while the patient is actively drinking or immediately thereafter. Once the drinking stops the illness is no longer addressed except in a historical fashion. Like the family member, the nurse might unrealistically expect all the problems to go away with the drinking. It must be remembered that recovery is also a dynamic process. As one alcoholic client put it, "Well, I stopped drinking and I've never felt so bad in my whole life." Continued therapeutic support is needed for some time as, paradoxically, the alcoholic learns that control of one's life is gained by acknowledging lack of control and independence is gained by acknowledging dependence.

CASE STUDY

Bill Krause is a 28-year-old airplane mechanic admitted to the orthopedic unit with a fractured femur sustained in a skiing accident.

Family History

Bill was the third of four children. His father, a truck driver, died several years ago from complications of alcoholism. Two of his father's five siblings were also alcoholic. His paternal grandparents were strict teetotalers. There was no history of alcoholism in his mother's immediate family, although his mother had an aunt and a cousin who were thought to be alcoholic. Bill has never married.

Bill gives a history of growing up in an environment that was often turbulent because of his father's drinking. He states that he vowed that he would never be like his father. He denies any problems with alcohol. He can take it or leave it; he never touches the "hard stuff" and has rarely felt drunk.

Social History

Bill has worked for the same employer for the past 12 years and is considered a good worker. He states that he has several good friends.

Drugs

Bill smokes two packs of cigarettes per day. He takes antacids for heartburn and usually has "a few beers" after work.

Drinking Pattern

Drinks daily on the way home from work, "a few beers with the guys" and perhaps a six-pack on weekends while watching football. He says that he remembers when he would feel high on a couple of beers but it takes well over a six-pack for him to feel anything now. Because of this he sometimes finds himself drinking more than he intended. He was involved in a minor automobile accident after drinking and decided to quit entirely. He managed to stay off for 3 weeks. On another occasion he was stopped for driving while intoxicated. He admits to sometimes drinking more than he had intended.

Hospital Course

On his first few days in the hospital Bill appeared anxious and restless. His appetite was poor and his sleep was disturbed. He wondered if there was anything he could take for his nerves. He was sober on admission but says he was drinking wine the day of the accident. Physical examination and laboratory findings were unremarkable. Bill is a pleasant, cooperative patient presenting no problems to the treatment personnel.

Discussion

Bill is representative of a group of underdiagnosed alcoholic patients. His admission to the ward was not overtly alcohol-related. His medical history reveals no alcohol-related problems. He has an excellent employment history and an active social life.

On closer scrutiny, however, we see that Bill's family history puts him at high risk for developing alcoholism. He in fact meets enough of the *DSM-III-R* criteria to receive the diagnosis of psychoactive substance dependence.

Bill presented as a pleasant, cooperative, well-spoken patient. He does not fit the stereotype of the alcoholic client. Although he has exhibited some denial, his defensive system doesn't appear to be particularly entrenched. How easy it would be to overlook the data regarding alcohol abuse. How sad it would be. If this opportunity is missed it may be a number of years before another presents itself.

Summary

Alcoholism is a major problem for the patient, the family, and the community. This chapter discusses the problem of alcohol in terms of its impact on the human body and behavior, historical perspectives of the problem, and the neglect of the alcoholic because of social attitudes and biases.

Common physical and psychiatric diagnoses related to alcohol abuse are presented and nursing assessment and management strategies are discussed. Program planning for the alcoholic includes a discussion of treatment needs and types of available services. Stalls of the therapeutic process include judgmental and ambivalent feelings, overidentification, labeling, dependency needs, pessimism, unrealistic treatment goals, scare approach, and failure to do grief work. The identification of alcoholics with special problems includes polydrug use, women, the elderly and adolescents. Also, the nurse's role in terms of developing linkages with the family and community of the alcoholic are discussed.

Questions

1. What are some of the common misconceptions about alcoholism?
2. How do you autognose your feelings when working with an alcoholic patient?
3. What do you find most difficult about working with an alcoholic patient?
4. What nursing interventions have you found effective in working with alcoholics?
5. What resources are available for alcoholics in your community and within hospital settings?

REFERENCES AND SUGGESTED READINGS

1. Tilton, J. E., & Worden, M. Of mice, men, and martinis. *Alcoholism, The National Magazine*, 1982, 2(3), 32.
2. Criteria Committee of the National Council on Alcoholism. Criteria for the diagnosis of alcoholism. *American Journal of Psychiatry*, 1972, 129(2), 127–135.
3. *DSM-III-R*, pp. 167–168.
4. Jellinek, E. M. Phases of alcohol addiction. *Quarterly Journal of Studies on Alcohol*, 1952, 13, 673–684.
5. Bean-Bayog, M. Psychopathology produced by alcoholism. In R. E. Meyer (Ed.), *Psychopathology and Addictive Disorders*. New York: Guilford Press, 1986.
6. Schuckit, M. A. Alcoholism and other psychiatric disorders. *Hospital and Community Psychiatry*, 1983, 34(11), 1022–1027.

7. Roth, R., The EAP works: A profitable tool for the private sector. *Alcoholism, The National Magazine*, 1981, March/April *1*(4), p. 24.
8. Ibid.
9. Kendal, E. M. Effect of attitudes on delivery of health care, *The Community Health Nurse and Alcohol-Related Problems*. Arlington, Va.: The National Center for Alcohol Education, 1978, pp. 44–45.
10. Black, C. *It Will Never Happen to Me*. Denver, Colo.: M. A. C. Printing Co., 1982.
11. Wegscheider-Cruse, S. *Another Chance*. Palo Alto, Calif.: Science and Behavior Books, 1981.
12. Brown, S. *Treating Adult Children of Alcoholics: A Developmental Perspective*. New York: John Wiley & Sons, 1988.
13. Zimberg, S. The elderly alcoholic. *The Gerontologist*, 1974, *14*, 221–224.
14. Williams, M., & Vejnoska, J. Alcohol and Youth: State prevention approaches. *Alcohol, Health and Research World*, 1981, *16*(1), 3.
15. Department of Health, Education and Welfare. *Fourth Special Report to the U. S. Congress on Alcohol and Health*. Washington, D.C.: U. S. Government Printing Office, January 1981.
16. Wagenaar, A. C. Legal minimum drinking age changes in the United States: 1970–1981. *Alcohol, Health and Research World*, 1981–82, *6*(2), 21–26.
17. Research by Dr. John Saunders, King's College Hospital, London, and reported on in *The Journal*, 1982, *11*(2). *Journal of the Addiction Research Foundation*, Toronto, Canada.

Chapter 36

Organic Dysfunctional Patterns

Ann Wolbert Burgess

Chapter Objectives

The students successfully attaining the goals of this chapter will be able to:

- Suspect organic mental dysfunctional patterns from certain patient behaviors.
- Explain the differences between acute confusional states and dementias.
- Explain why there are medical, surgical, pharmacological, and neurological causes of acute confusional states.
- Describe the different types of epilepsy.
- Assess, diagnose, and plan for patients experiencing organic dysfunctional patterns.

There has been increasing attention to and awareness of differentiating patients' symptomatology in the area of organic mental patterns. Such patterns are generally used to describe psychological and behavioral patterns associated with transient or permanent dysfunction of the brain. The term organic may be used as an adjective in three ways:

1. to describe those syndromes of psychological or behavioral change that can be attributed directly to abnormalities of brain structure or of brain chemical or electrical function;
2. to be applied to specific, identified brain diseases and dysfunctions;
3. to refer to specific changes in brain structure or function that can be detected by neuropathological, neurochemical, or neurophysiologic methods and that give rise to organic syndromes.[1]

There have been major strides in separating patients' symptomatology into manifestations of *organic* pathology and *functional* psychiatric disorders. Organic etiology includes cerebral lesions such as brain tumors (which may cause depressive and psychotic symptoms) as well as noncerebral physical illness such as thyroid disease (which may cause symptoms of depression, anxiety, or psychosis). Functional psychiatric illness, on the other hand, refers to disturbances such as unipolar depression, schizophrenia, and neurosis, for which cerebral pathology or somatic diseases have not been demonstrated to be totally causative. Although it is tempting to think of the organic syndromes and disorders as distinctly different from the functional syndromes, it would be inaccurate to conceptualize the two dysfunctional patterns as separate entities having clear lines demarcating one from the other. More appropriately, organic and functional disorders might be regarded as a continuum. The organic end of the continuum is occupied by those disorders in which the relationship between clinical symptomatoloy and underlying brain dysfunction in its literal sense is most clearly established, as would be true of the dementia caused by Alzheimer's disease. The functional end is occupied by those disorders in which this relationship is less clear in terms of identified neurochemical or neurophysiologic aberrations.[2]

The increase in interest in organic mental disorders occurs for several reasons. First, there is the growing realization that organic brain syndromes constitute a major public health, social, and economic problem because of their high prevalence and incidence among the elderly, whose numbers are steadily increasing. Second, advances in the neurosciences have provided new methodologic approaches and technical tools for the study of metabolic, vascular, electrophysiologic, biochemical, and structural cellular changes in the brain associated with psychopathological states such as disorders of cognition. Third, the current focus on chronic diseases and on critical care nursing has highlighted the problem of psychiatric manifestations of cerebral disorders resulting from cardiovascular, neoplastic, traumatic, and other diseases affecting the brain either directly or indirectly as a result of systemic metabolic disturbances.

Liaison psychiatric nursing has become increasingly involved in issues of diagnosis, management, and investigation of mental disorders caused by cerebral damage and dysfunction, some of which result from medical and surgical therapies. Psychiatric and mental health problems that complicate open-heart surgery, chronic renal dialysis, and the use of anti-Parkinson drugs illustrate the concern for the nursing care of people with organic brain impairment.

To provide some perspective on how psychiatric appearing symptoms may be found to exist in persons with an organic condition, a review of the records of a walk-in clinic revealed the following clinical conditions[3]:

- Catatonic behavior caused by pancreatic tumor.
- Depressive symptoms caused by cryptococcal meningitis.
- Manic symptoms caused by L-dopa.
- Anxiety symptoms caused by hyperthyroidism.
- "Hysterical" symptoms caused by spinal cord tumor.
- Impotence caused by prescribed medications.
- Abdominal pain caused by porphyria.
- Psychosis caused by brain tumor.
- Depression with movement disorder caused by cerebrovascular accident.
- Violent behavior caused by encephalitis.

This chapter will discuss organic mental syndromes in terms of (1) delirium; and (2) dementia.

DELIRIUM AND DEMENTIA

The two major organic brain syndromes are delirium and dementia. Delirium has traditionally been defined as an *acute* and *reversible* organic brain syndrome, in contrast to dementia, which has been defined as a slowly *progressive* and *irreversible* organic brain syndrome. Psychiatrists Keller and Manschreck argue that these definitions should be rethought because acute organic brain syndromes are often irreversible (such as are seen in carbon monoxide poisoning, encephalitis, or cerebrovascular accidents) and slowly progressive organic brain syndromes may be reversible (such as are seen in myxedema, normal pressure hydrocephalus, and vitamin B_{12} deficiency).[4] They suggest the rate of onset should not be equated with whether neuronal loss and permanent brain damage have occurred.

This departure from traditional ways of viewing organic mental disorders is seen in the *DSM-III-R.*[5] The new classification of organic mental disorders departs in several important respects from previous medical diagnoses. First, it acknowledges that prior classification systems did not do justice to the full range of psychopathological manifestations of cerebral disease and dysfunction. Thus, the new classification contains many new organic brain syndrome descriptions. Second, the new classification does away with the vague terms of *psychotic* and *nonpsychotic*. And third, the new classification breaks down the boundaries between functional and organic mental disorders; now there is an overlap between the two. There is also the option to classify some cases of paranoid, affective, and schizophrenic syndromes as organic with the hope that such reports will provide data leading to hypotheses about causative and pathogenetic relationships. Finally, the new classification stipulates that the diagnosis of an organic mental disorder requires neurological or laboratory evidence of a concurrent brain disorder or at least the history of an antecedent exposure to an identified organic factor such as head trauma or poison.

Delirium and dementia represent global disorders of cognition. They both feature impairment of acquisition, processing, storage, and retrieval of information as well as impairment of its use for problem solving, decision-making, and planning of purposeful action. Deficits in memory result from relatively widespread or diffuse dysfunction of or damage to the brain. The two syndromes overlap but are not identical.

Comparison of Delirium and Dementia

Delirium may be viewed as a disorder of wakefulness, one in which mental phenomena of both waking and sleeping states tend to intermingle. The sleep–waking cycle is disorganized, and the person often has difficulty distinguishing perceptions and images from dreams and hallucinations. Delirium features, in addition to cognitive impairment and disturbances of wakefulness, attention, alertness, and vigilance, tend to fluctuate irregularly and unpredictably over the period of a day and to be most severe at night. These disturbances probably result from a derangement of the cerebral structures subserving activation, arousal, and the sleep–wakefulness cycle. This cycle is invariably disorganized in delirium as observed through insomnia, drowsiness, and irregular succession of episodes of sleep and wakefulness.

By contrast, dementia features relatively sustained and often progressive intellectual impairment that is not accompanied by fluctuations in the level of awareness and wakefulness

or by concurrent disturbances of attention, perception, and orientation. Dementia is a chronic disorder in the sense that it has a lingering and often, though by no means always, progressive course; it may be static or remitting. Although delirium usually clears up in a matter of days or weeks, dementia has a prolonged duration and extends over months or years. The degree of reversibility, if any, depends partly on the availability and timely application of appropriate treatment. Delirium and dementia appear to reflect different phases of relatively widespread brain pathology. Delirium may be viewed as a psychopathological manifestation of acute brain failure to disruption in cerebral metabolism and neurotransmission. Dementia may be seen as a consequence either of relatively enduring pathological changes in cerebral neurons or of their death.

DELIRIUM

Delirium is an organic psychiatric syndrome commonly encountered by nurses in adult health, geriatric, and psychiatric nursing populations. The word *delirium* is derived from the Latin *de* ("from" or "out of") plus *lira* ("furrow" or "track"). The term describes an abrupt deviation from the individual's usual state in terms of level of consciousness or awareness. The syndrome of delirium is usually characterized by the following features:

- Acute or subacute onset.
- Marked variability in clinical manifestations from patient to patient and from one time to another in the same patient.
- Evidence of widespread nervous tissue dysfunction, usually involving the cerebral hemispheres, reticular activating system, and autonomic nervous system.
- Potential reversibility of the nervous tissue dysfunction, if the cause can be treated successfully.
- Absence both of pathognomonic cerebral pathological changes during the delirium and of residual pathological changes after effective treatment of the cause of the delirium.

Delirium is defined as a transient organic mental syndrome, usually of relatively acute onset, characterized by wide impairment of cognitive functions and major disturbance of cerebral metabolism. This syndrome has various synonyms such as toxic psychosis, acute brain syndrome, metabolic encephalopathy, and syndrome of cerebral insufficiency. The common denominator in all these diagnostic labels is a distortion of cerebral cellular metabolism resulting from an insult to the brain. The *DSM-III-R* psychiatric diagnostic criteria for delirium follow.

Diagnostic Criteria for Delirium

A. Reduced ability to maintain attention to external stimuli (e.g., questions must be repeated because attention wanders) and to appropriately shift attention to new external stimuli (e.g., perseverates answer to a previous question).
B. Disorganized thinking, as indicated by rambling, irrelevant, or incoherent speech.
C. At least two of the following:
  1. Reduced level of consciousness, e.g., difficulty keeping awake during examination
  2. Perceptual disturbances: misinterpretations, illusions, or hallucinations
  3. Disturbance of sleep–wake cycle with insomnia or daytime sleepiness
  4. Increased or decreased psychomotor activity
  5. Disorientation to time, place, or person
  6. Memory impairment, e.g., inability to learn new material, such as the names of several unrelated objects after 5 minutes, or to remember past events, such as history of current episode of illness
D. Clinical features develop over a short period of time (usually hours to days) and tend to fluctuate over the course of a day.
E. Either (1) or (2):
  1. Evidence from the history, physical examination, or laboratory tests of a specific organic factor (or factors) judged to be etiologically related to the disturbance
  2. In the absence of such evidence, an etiologic organic factor can be presumed if the disturbance cannot be accounted for by any nonorganic mental disorder, e.g., manic episode accounting for agitation and sleep disturbance

Epidemiology

Data with regard to the epidemiology of delirium are scarce. However, some sources estimate delirium of some degree of severity may be observed in 5 percent to 15 percent of all patients on general medical and surgical units.[6] The incidence may be higher on intensive care units (up to 40 percent), after open-heart surgery and coronary bypass surgery (30 percent to 60 percent), and in burn patients.[7-9] The incidence and prevalence of delirium are especially high in patients age 60 years or more (46 percent to 80 percent).[10]

Etiology

Delirium may result from any one of a number of factors, acting singly or in combination, that produce widespread derangement of cerebral metabolism. A necessary condition for delirium to occur is the presence of one or more organic factors (see Table 36-1). Among the factors that may predispose a person to delirium are age (60 years or older), drug addiction, and brain damage. Psychological stress, sleep and sensory deprivation, severe fatigue, and prolonged immobilization may facilitate and onset or increase the severity of delirium.[11]

A cardinal sign in patients is a disorder of attention. The patient cannot focus on incoming stimuli. He is easily distracted, unable to concentrate, is sluggish in thinking, may show mental rambling, and is confused.

There are four major causes for these mental changes. Although we acknowledge that many conditions and illnesses can cause these symptoms, we will focus only on the categories of: medical conditions, surgical conditions, pharmacological conditions, and neurological conditions. An acute confusional state is almost always secondary to a pathological process outside the nervous system. Of course, there are some confused states caused by a primary disease of the brain. A derangement of normal body metabolism is the most common feature of the acute confused state. If the metabolic imbalance can be corrected, the confused state is usually reversed and there is no permanent damage to the brain. In such a situation, an acute confusional state can be viewed as a clinical manifestation of a temporary, reversible alteration of brain chemistry and physiology.[12]

Medical Conditions

A frequent cause of acute confusional states is medical conditions that include nutritional deficiencies, internal diseases, endocrine disease, and infections.

TABLE 36-1. CAUSES OF DELIRIUM

Medical Conditions
1. Nutritional Deficiencies
   A. Avitaminosis: nicotinic acid, thiamine, cyanocobalamin (vitamin B_{12}), folate, pyridoxine
   B. Hypervitaminosis: intoxication by vitamins A and D
   C. Disorders of fluid and electrolyte metabolism: dehydration, water intoxication; alkalosis, acidosis; hypernatremia, hyponatremia, hyperkalemia, hypokalemia, hypercalcemia, hypocalcemia, hypermagnesemia, hypomagnesemia
2. Metabolic (Internal) Diseases
   A. Hypoxia
   B. Hypoglycemia
   C. Hepatic, renal, pancreatic, pulmonary insufficiency (encephalopathy)
   D. Errors of metabolism: porphyria, carcinoid syndrome, hepatolenticular degeneration (Wilson's disease)
3. Endocrine Disease
   Hormonal disorders: hyperinsulinism, hyperthyroidism, hypothyroidism, hypopituitarism, Addison's disease, Cushing's syndrome, hypoparathyroidism, hyperparathyroidism
4. Infections
   A. Systemic: pneumonia, typhoid, typhus, acute rheumatic fever, malaria, influenza, mumps, diphtheria, brucellosis, infectious mononucleosis, infectious hepatitis, subacute bacterial endocarditis, bacteremia, septicemia, Rocky Mountain spotted fever, Legionnaires' disease
   B. Intracranial (acute, subacute, and chronic): viral encephalitis, aseptic meningitis, rabies, herpes; bacterial meningitis—meningococcal, pneumococcal, etc.

Surgical Conditions
   A. Cerebral trauma occurring during surgery
   B. Surgery producing extreme anxiety

Pharmacological or Intoxication Condition
1. Intoxication
   A. Alcohol: ethyl and methyl
   B. Drugs: anticholinergic agents, sedative–hypnotics, digitalis derivatives, opiates, corticosteroids, salicylates, antibiotics, anticonvulsants, antiarrhythmic and antihypertensive drugs, antineoplastic agents, cimetidine, lithium, anti-Parkinson agents, disulfiram, indomethacin
   C. Inhalants: gasoline, glue, ether, nitrous oxide, nitrates
   D. Poisons
      (1) Industrial: carbon disulfide, organic solvents, methylchloride and bromide, heavy metals, organophosphorous insecticides, carbon monoxide
      (2) Plants and mushrooms
      (3) Toxins (e.g., snakebite)
2. Withdrawal Syndromes
   A. Alcohol (delirium tremens)
   B. Sedatives and hypnotics: barbiturates, chloral hydrate, chlordiazepoxide, diazepam, ethchlorvynol, glutethimide, meprobamate, methyprylon, paraldehyde
   C. Amphetamines

Neurological Conditions
   A. Trauma or head injuries: concussion, contusion, subdural hematoma
   B. The epilepsies: grand mal seizures and petit mal seizures
   C. Congenital brain dysfunction
   D. Intracranial neoplasms
   E. Cerebral anoxia

Adapted from Massey, E. W. & Coffey, C. E. Delirium: Diagnosis and treatment. *Southern Medical Journal*, 1983, *76*, 1147.

Nutritional Deficiencies. The relationship of general malnutrition to psychotic reactions is difficult to assess. These states usually occur under extreme conditions, for example, in economically deprived areas, prisons, and war environments in which both psychological and biologic stresses are great.

A niacin deficiency, associated with the clinical entity pellagra, was responsible for 10 percent of the admissions to state hospitals in southern United States before preventive dietary measures were taken. This deficiency is characterized by erythematous and pigmented skin, stomatitis, diarrhea, and mental symptoms ranging from anxiety and depression to severe delirium. Hallucinations and schizophrenia-like symptoms have also been reported. Treatment consists of therapeutic doses of 500 mg of nicotinic acid per day orally and vitamin B complex, thiamine, and tryptophan combined with a high-caloric balanced diet. A prompt and positive response to this regimen is generally seen.

The thiamine (B_1) deficiency (beriberi) is still endemic in Southeast Asia. Symptoms of a mild disorder are irritability, fatigability, anorexia, and insomnia. Severe cases develop neurological manifestations of numbness of the toes, calf tenderness, and muscular atrophy. Encephalopathy may follow. This disorder is seen in alcoholic patients who have a vitamin deficiency and in patients with gastric carcinoma and pernicious anemia in which poor intestinal absorption is present.

Vitamin C deficiencies, as seen in scurvy, may show depression as an early symptom. Depression is also a symptom of kwashiorkor, a tropical protein deficiency disease in young children. Children suffering from this disease die unless they are treated with a high-protein, high-vitamin diet. Even if the metabolic deficiency is corrected, the children are prone to mental retardation.

A number of metabolic diseases associated with mental deficiency and disease have been described. Although they do not constitute a clinical problem in the usual psychiatric nursing practice, they point up important areas for prevention and education that community health nurses should be aware of. If prevention cannot be accomplished, early case findings can be instrumental in early treatment.

Internal Diseases. Symptomatic psychosis can occur in severe cardiac, hepatic, pancreatic, renal, and metabolic diseases. Hypoglycemia in diabetes is usually caused by an overdose of insulin. It is important to differentiate the confusion, agitation, or lethargy caused by acidosis from that caused by hypoglycemia so that convulsions, coma, irreversible brain damage, and even death can be prevented. In an emergency situation in which there is question of hypoglycemia and a blood sugar determination cannot be done, 10 to 50 ml of 50 percent dextrose solution is generally administered intravenously.

Hepatic failure is thought to be caused by such factors as hypoxia and fluid, electrolyte, and pH changes within the brain. The signs and symptoms range from emotional lability, intellectual deficits, and psychotic ideation in impending hepatic coma to stupor and coma.

Characteristics of impending hepatic failure are a decrease in consciousness, in psychomotor activity, in speech, and in muscle strength; pres-ence of a slow tremor and perhaps jaundice; absence of anxiety; hallucinations; autonomic imbalance; or disturbance of sleep and appetite. Treatment consists of protein-free diet and purgation.

Characteristics of delirium tremens are an increase in consciousness, in psychomotor activity, in anxiety, and in muscle strength; presence of a fine tremor; rapid speech; hallucinations; autonomic imbalance; absence of jaundice; and disturbance of normal sleep and appetite. Treatment consists of high-protein diet, hydration, and sedation.

Renal insufficiency may produce apathy, depression, confusion, agitation, convulsions, stupor, and coma. Facial paralysis, nystagmus, and lower cranial nerve dysfunction are common. Symptoms may be noted in dialysis treatment because of the rapid alteration of fluid and electrolyte balance.

In certain decompensated cardiac diseases, particularly aortic stenosis and mitral insufficiency, psychotic reactions are noted. Hypoxia, along with the psychosocial factors, is undoubtedly an important factor. The stressful stimuli that produce general anxiety, or specific fear of death or feelings of being incapacitated, humiliated, provoked, or deserted contribute to delirious episodes for patients. Behavior disorders of circulatory disturbances, as in arteriosclerosis and hypertensive disease, are included in this list of potential psychotic reactions.

Endocrine Disease. Endocrine dysfunction can be a hypo- or hyperfunctional condition and can be a dysfunction of the thyroid, parathyroid, adrenal, pancreas, or pituitary glands. The characteristic symptoms of hyperthyroidism are high anxiety, oversensitivity, irritability, emotional lability, and suspicious and paranoid feelings. Some hyperthyroid patients may develop psychoses. The psychotic symptoms include manic excitement with delusions and hallucinations.

Hypothyroidism or thyroid hormone deficiency in small children causes cretinism, which is characterized by dwarfism and severe mental and physical retardation. Early detection and prompt regular administration of thyroid hormone can prevent the progression of the disease.

The thyroid deficiency in adults may produce myxedema. Paranoid and depressive symptoms are common. Mental changes progress from mild mental dullness, poor emotional control, apathy, drowsiness, anxiety, irritability, and memory defects to overt psychosis. Generally, the premorbid personality is a major factor in the psychotic symptomatology. Corrective hormonal therapy will produce a return to normal balance.

Behavior disorders in pituitary diseases range from mild to severe syndromes. Patients with Simmonds' disease or pituitary cachexia usually show depressive symptoms and apathy.

Diseases of the adrenal cortex often produce marked personality changes in patients. They become irritable and moody, and they alternate between being lethargic and impulsive.

Infections. Intercranial infections such as encephalitis and viral meningitis have symptoms of fever, headache, vomiting, stiff neck, and backache. The coma that may follow is most frequently seen in children.

Behavior disturbances may be produced by infections, the most common of which are pneumonia, pyelitis, malaria, septicemia, typhoid fever, and acute rheumatic fever.

The toxins of diphtheria and gas gangrene can cause confusion. High fever with dehydration and electrolyte imbalance can also cause a state of confusion.

Surgical Conditions

Many surgical illnesses and procedures produce delirium, hallucinations, and paranoid reactions. Two basic reactions are noted: (1) symptomatic psychosis associated with cerebral dysfunction, e.g., cerebral damage occurring during surgery; and (2) surgery that produces extreme anxiety.

Symptomatic psychosis may be more frequent after brain surgery, cardiac surgery, surgery of male and female reproductive organs, and ophthalmic surgery. In cerebral operations the direct trauma to the brain produces edema, swelling, hemorrhages, and thromboses.

Other factors that contribute to the psychological stress are surgery with prolonged anesthesia, which may cause possible brain damage, loss of blood, and infection. Postoperative psychosis is higher in children and elderly patients than in other patients.

The psychological stress of surgery is often intensified because the patient has not been properly prepared for surgery. The nurse is a key person in helping the patient deal with his fears about surgery. Some hospitals send the operating room nurses to the patient's room prior to surgery to ensure adequate teaching and preparation for the procedure. These nurses work closely with the ward staff on the floor to which the patient will return. Since the meaning of organ dysfunction, fantasies of death, mutilation, and dependency may be worrying the patient, it is essential for him to have the opportunity to express his thoughts.

Pharmacological Conditions

It would take too long to list all the various pharmacological agents that can cause psychiatric side effects. For example, the nurse needs to know that hallucinogens can cause thought disorders; psychiatric medications taken in wrong doses can cause psychiatric disturbances; and amphetamines can cause a paranoid psychosis. There are also many medical drugs that can cause side effects; for example, steroids can cause a psychosis.

Drug ingestion is a prevalent cause of behavior disturbance. Common drugs include: barbiturates, bromides, meprobamate, benzodiazepines, and other sedative–hypnotic drugs; opium derivatives and marijuana; and the psychedelic drugs.

Delirium, convulsions, and death may occur following rapid withdrawal from the alcohol-barbiturate group of sedative–hypnotic agents.

Many of the drugs are toxic to the brain and are capable of producing a clinical picture similar to schizophrenia. Alcohol is also toxic to brain tissue and can cause delirium and acute alcoholic hallucinosis.

Neurological Conditions

There are several neurological conditions that may produce behavioral disturbances, such as trauma or head injuries, epilepsies, congenital brain dysfunctions, intracranial neoplasms, cerebral anoxia, and senile and presenile brain diseases.

Trauma or Head Injuries. Cranial injuries are generally divided into closed and open injuries. Closed injuries indicate no fracture or only a linear fracture of the skull. Open injuries indicate compound and depressed fractures.

In both open and closed injuries the brain and its covering membranes may be damaged. Three divisions of acute cerebral injuries are: (1) concussion; (2) contusion and laceration; and (3) subdural and epidural hematoma.

CONCUSSION. A blow or fall, or both, usually causes a concussion. A short loss of consciousness follows. Car accidents and sports activities are common situations for such trauma.

The next symptom the patient complains of is a diffuse headache that is generally very severe. Patients will be dizzy and often feel nauseated, after which they will vomit. With a simple concussion, patients are stunned, confused, and disoriented when they wake up. They cannot tell where they are or how they arrived there, and they are confused about the time and sequence of events. They respond slowly and have great difficulty identifying persons they see.

Retrograde amnesia is usually present. The patient suffers amnesia for the immediate period preceding the blow and the accident itself.

Anterograde amnesia also is present. The patient has memory lapses during the time he is awakening from the coma. During this period of awakening the patient often seems upset, anxious, and suspicious. He is likely to cry or to try to defend himself. These symptoms generally persist for a period of from a few days to a week. If they do increase in severity, a post-traumatic psychosis may develop.

Nursing management consists of careful observation of the patient for possible development of neurological and psychiatric complications. A calm attitude is important in order not to increase the anxiety of the patient.

Medication for the headache, anxiety, or insomnia should be as mild as possible, with aspirin being the safest choice. Heavy medication is contraindicated because it will mask symptoms.

The patient should be encouraged to talk about the accident and to express his feelings about it.

CONTUSIONS AND LACERATIONS. Contusions or lacerations of the brain are usually associated with compound or depressed fractures of the skull, with bleeding from skull openings, especially ears and nose. Tearing and crushing of tissue are usually the results of local injury to the brain.

Coma following these injuries and the periods of anterograde and retrograde amnesia are more prolonged than in simple concussions. The length of the coma is significant for the prognosis. Prolonged coma produces longer-lasting symptoms. Convulsions and signs of cranial nerve injury are generally present.

Nursing management is accomplished by nurses who have had neurological training. The use of opiates for sedation is contraindicated. Strict attention must be paid to the possibility of a serious rise of the intracranial pressure. Signs of this are increased dullness, apathy, and somnolence.

An acute post-traumatic psychosis that may follow contusions and lacerations is very similar to the clinical picture of other symptomatic psychoses.

The symptoms of confusion and delirium predominate. Catatonic or manic–depressive symptoms are frequent. Intellectual and characterological changes are common.

Nursing management follows the principles of the symptomatic psychoses. Careful supervision is necessary for the confused or agitated patient who is likely to hurt himself or wander off the ward.

SUBDURAL AND EPIDURAL HEMATOMA. Venous bleeding into the subdural space generally occurs when fractures of the skull are found. However, subdural hematoma may occur in very ill senile patients who have no history of trauma.

The typical pattern in acute subdural hematoma is head injury, coma, and anterograde and retrograde amnesia. There may be a temporary return of consciousness, after which the patient lapses into deepening coma.

This course is also characteristic for epidural hematoma that is caused by arterial bleeding from the middle meningeal artery. Upon awakening, the patient usually shows unresponsiveness, dullness, apathy, irritability, and antagonism. Delirium and confused states similar to other acute traumatic psychoses occur. The patient complains of headache, and the most frequent signs are hemiplegia, hemianesthesia, and hemianopsia. Aphasic symptoms develop if the lesion is on the dormant side.

Treatment consists of operative removal of the clot. Patients in good general health have the best chance for successful surgery and recovery.

The Epilepsies. GRAND MAL SEIZURES. Grand mal seizures are a tonic–clonic attack with a loss of consciousness. Many grand mal seizures have warning symptoms of vague, uncomfortable, and anxious feelings, mood changes such as depression, elation, or lability of mood, headaches, minor gastrointestinal difficulties, sweating, and hot and cold sensations.

These symptoms are different from the aura that is part of the seizure. The most frequent kinds of aura are epigastric discomfort, dizziness, fainting, sensory phenomena such as seeing bright dots and lines, hearing sounds, and experiencing strange and unusually disagreeable odors and tastes.

The tonic phase consists of extreme rigidity of the muscles of the head, neck, trunk, and extremities. The extremities are in maximal extension, the trunk is opisthotonus, and the head and neck are thrown back. Respirations may stop for as long as a minute. Contraction of the respiratory muscle usually causes cyanosis. When the patient loses consciousness and falls in a rigid position, he is likely to hurt himself. The tonic phase ends with general trembling of the muscles, which initiates the violent contraction of the clonic phase.

During the clonic phase the patient may bite his tongue and lose control of sphincter muscles. At the end of the clonic phase the patient is in deep coma, the eyes are turned upward, and the pupils are dilated and do not react to light. Often the patient sweats profusely. Almost all patients wake up dazed and are slow to recognize their environment. They complain about sleepiness, haziness, headaches, and amnesia. Recovery may take from 1 to 4 hours.

PETIT MAL ATTACKS. The petit mal attacks may be one of three types: (1) a slight lapse of consciousness for 15 to 30 seconds with minimal twitching of facial muscles, a vacant stare, and subsequent amnesia for the attack; (2) a similar lapse of consciousness with myoclonic twitches; and (3) an episode of sudden loss of muscular tone and consciousness.

These seizures often begin in childhood and persist into adult years. It is unusual for them to begin in adult years.

PSYCHOMOTOR EPILEPSY. The term *psychomotor epilepsy* is used broadly and includes (1) increased tonicity of muscles with adversive movements of head and swallowing movements; and (2) autonomic behavior such as unbuttoning of clothing, walking, or running with complete amnesia, although consciousness may be preserved.

PSYCHIC SEIZURES. The diagnosis of psychic seizures is made with clinical and electroencephalogram confirmation of abnormal waves. Often the experiences are vague and bizarre, and the patient reports them as trance-like and dream-like. The unreal character of the experience is marked. Some patients are unable to distinguish between fantasy and reality and suffer from hallucinations, illusions, and delusions.

Another type of psychic seizure is a feeling of depersonalization with extreme anxiety and intense feelings of displeasure. These patients are not completely amnesic but show partial memory defect. The aggressive and antisocial nature of the episode can be marked.

FOCAL DISCHARGE. Focal or partial discharges are classified according to the localization of the seizure focus. The focal motor seizure begins with a twitching of a muscle, such as in the face or lips, and then spreads to the extremities. When skin sensations are involved in focal seizures, they are referred to as *sensory seizures*. Patients report tingling in a localized region of the body.

Congenital Brain Dysfunction. Prenatal factors may cause congenital brain damage. Syphilis during pregnancy was formerly a major cause of mental retardation and progressive mental deterioration (juvenile general paresis). Laboratory blood testing has assisted in preventive measures for this problem.

The virus rubella in German measles has been identified as a major cause of congenital malformation. Pregnant women contracting this disease in the first four months of pregnancy are in the high-risk category of delivering infants who may have cataracts, congenital heart disease, deafness, mental retardation, and other neurological problems. Prevention in the form of immunization three months before any conception is advised for all women.

Other prenatal sources such as hepatitis, pneumonia, influenza, cold virus, and urinary tract infection are currently being researched in the etiology of mental retardation.

Brain damage resulting in cerebral palsy may be caused by prenatal, natal, and postnatal factors. Characteristics of this disorder are weakness, incoordination, ataxia, dystonia, paralysis, visual and hearing defects, mental retardation, and emotional disturbances.

Birth traumas include all forms of brain damage resulting from complications of labor or delivery. Brain damage may result from mechanical trauma, for example, the use of forceps, breech delivery, cephalopelvic disproportion, and prolonged labor or hypoxia due to Caesarean section, bradycardia, respiratory difficulties, and anesthesia. Mechanical damage may also produce subarachnoid and intraventricular hemorrhage.

Intracranial Neoplasms. Brain tumors are found in 22 percent of all autopsied cases regardless of the primary cause of death. Brain neoplasms that cause signs and symptoms are most frequently (40 percent of all tumors) gliomas. Metastatic brain tumors account for 15 to 20 percent of brain tumors, and they commonly arise from carcinoma of the lungs and breast.

The most important neurological symptoms are convulsions, visual disturbances such as double or blurred vision, headaches, nausea, and vomiting. Convulsions occur in 50 to 80 percent of patients and are of the grand mal type. Headaches are severe though intermittent and are usually frontal or occipital.

The person with a brain tumor may be referred to a mental health facility because of psychiatric disturbances that may be the only presenting symptoms. The nurse can be alert to this possibility if she knows the signs and symptoms. If a brain tumor is in question, the patient should be referred for a complete neurological examination. The general symptoms of a brain tumor caused by increased intracranial pressure are: intellectual deterioration; defects of memory, recall, and attention; sleepiness and stupor; coarsening of personality; appearance of asocial and antisocial traits; and apathetic or euphoric reactions. Delirious and confused episodes and disturbances of consciousness are usually the result of rapid changes leading to cerebral edema or swelling, hemorrhages in the tumor, or sudden rises of intracranial pressure.

In many patients the symptoms are not that pronounced. Misinterpretation of symptoms, such as headaches and dizziness and the presence of severe anxiety, may lead to the diagnosis of hysterical or hypochondriacal reactions.

Cerebral Anoxia. The cells of the central nervous system are exceedingly sensitive to even brief periods of decreased oxygen supply. Cerebral anoxia, caused by a sudden decrease in blood flow as in some cardiac and vascular diseases, by the labor and delivery process, or by a decrease of oxygen in the atmosphere, rapidly produce a necrosis of cerebral tissue.

Situations (other than described above) in which this disturbance may occur are excessive bleeding, prolonged anesthesia, carbon monoxide poisoning, attempts at hanging or strangulation, altitude sickness, and decompensation illness. Lack of oxygen while flying at certain altitudes without pressurized equipment or in scuba diving accounts for a certain percentage of accidental fatalities.

The complex hazards of the space projects have become the subject of the specialty of space medicine. Symptoms patients complain of are dyspnea, headache, fatigue, sleepiness, anxiety, and irritability. A coma that may result in intellectual deficit may develop.

DEMENTIA

While delirium is the organic syndrome that occurs with greatest frequency, dementia is the organic syndrome with greatest prevalence, and it is dementia that creates greater problems in terms of chronicity. The term *dementia* is derived from the Latin *de* ("from" or "out of") and *mens* ("mind"). In translation, *dementia* means to be out of one's mind. Dementia refers to a clinical syndrome that is manifested most strikingly by impairment in orientation, memory, and cognition and by behavioral changes that are a result of these defects. Other essential elements in the definition of the syndrome include:

- A protracted course, often extending over many years.
- Evidence of nervous tissue dysfunction limited largely to the cerebral hemispheres.
- Ultimately, if not initially, pathological changes in the affected cerebral hemispheres that are detectable by both light and electron microscopy.

Epidemiology

Dementia creates major social problems in terms of chronicity, human distress, and the cost of economic resources and mortality. It is estimated that at least one half of the 1.2 million persons in nursing homes in the United States are confined there primarily because of dementia.

Etiology

There are various etiological factors identified for dementia.

Neurological Disease

Neurological causes of dementia include Alzheimer's disease, Huntington's chorea, multiple sclerosis, Pick's disease, cerebellar degeneration, progressive supranuclear palsy, and Parkinson's disease.

Vascular Disease

Vascular disease may result in multi-infarct dementia.

Central Nervous System Infections

Infections of the central nervous system that cause dementia include tertiary neurosyphilis, tuberculosis and fungal meningitis, viral encephalitis, human immunodeficiency virus and HIV-related disorders (AIDS), and Creutzfeldt-Jakob disease.

Brain Trauma

Brain trauma, especially chronic subdural hematoma, may produce dementia.

Toxic–Metabolic Disturbances

Such conditions include pernicious anemia, folic-acid deficiency, hypothyroidism, and bromide intoxication.

Other Brain Conditions

Two additional brain states of normal-pressure hydrocephalus and postanoxic or posthypoglycemic states are etiological factors for dementia.

Diagnostic Criteria for Dementia

A. Demonstrable evidence of impairment in short- and long-term memory. Impairment in short-term memory (inability to learn new information) may be indicated by inability to remember three objects after 5 minutes. Long-term memory impairment (inability to remember information that was known in the past) may be indicated by inability to remember past personal information (e.g., what happened yesterday, birthplace, occupation) or facts of common knowledge (e.g., past presidents, well-known dates).

B. At least one of the following:
1. Impairment in abstract thinking, as indicated by inability to find similarities and differences between related words, difficulty in defining words and concepts, and other similar tasks

2. Impaired judgment, as indicated by inability to make reasonable plans to deal with interpersonal, family, and job-related problems and issues

3. Other disturbances of higher cortical function, such as aphasia (disorder of language), apraxia (inability to carry out motor activities despite intact comprehension and motor function), agnosia (failure to recognize or identify objects despite intact sensory function), and "constructional difficulty" (e.g., inability to copy three-dimensional figures, assemble blocks, or arrange sticks in specific designs)

4. Personality change, i.e., alteration or accentuation of premorbid traits

C. The disturbance in A and B significantly interferes with work or usual social activities or relationships with others.

D. Not occurring exclusively during the course of Delirium.

E. Either (1) or (2)
1. There is evidence from the history, physical examination, or laboratory tests of a specific organic factor (or factors) judged to be etiologically related to the disturbance

2. In the absence of such evidence, an etiologic organic factor can be presumed if the disturbance cannot be accounted for by any nonorganic mental disorder, e.g., major depression, accounting for cognitive impairment

Criteria for Severity of Dementia

• *Mild*: Although work or social activities are significantly impaired, the capacity for independent living remains, with adequate personal hygiene and relatively intact judgment.

• *Moderate*: Independent living is hazardous, and some degree of supervision is necessary.

• *Severe*: Activities of daily living are so impaired that continual supervision is required, e.g., unable to maintain minimal personal hygiene; largely incoherent or mute

Senile Brain Diseases

In senile dementia, also referred to as *senile brain disease*, the symptomatology may vary from mild to severe. It is characterized by a chronic and progressive organic deficit (mental deterioration), usually occurring between 60 to 90 years of age. There is no sufficiently supported scientific evidence to explain this disease. Factors believed to strongly influence the development of this condition are metabolic, endocrine, vascular, and genetic determinants.

Senile dementia is generally accompanied by other evidence of progressive aging affecting the entire body. There is a general wasting of muscles, loss of elasticity of the skin, shrinkage of the soft tissue, unsteady gait, speech disturbances, and easy fatigability. Because of the body's aging process, the person is apt to fall and complicate his difficulties by a fracture, especially of the femur.

Dysmnesia

The cardinal symptoms of senile dementia are dysmnesia, disorientation, and difficulty with abstract reasoning. The most prominent symptom, **dysmnesia**, is an impairment in the ability to retain and recall information. The mildest kind of memory disturbance consists of lowered ability to absorb and retain new information. Initially, this symptom may appear to be absent-mindedness. In more severe cases, the person will have difficulty remembering events of the *recent* past. Incidents experienced or things learned before this period of memory failure began may still be recalled at this stage, but as the dysmnesia becomes more severe, it invades the person's memory of the time period before he was ill. This symptom progressively extends further into the person's *remote* past until it is finally global in the sense that the person neither understands the present nor remembers any part of the past.

Disorientation

The symptom of disorientation is closely related to the symptom of dysmnesia. Orientation means knowing what time it is, being able to tell where one is, and identifying the person one is dealing with. This ability is closely related to a person's memory. Thus, disorientation is rare without an appreciable memory impairment. This symptom also becomes progressively more intense. The mildest impairment usually consists of an impaired *time* sense. Initially, the person will be unable to recall when or in what order the current or previous day's events occurred, although he will still be able to describe

the events. Thereafter, he may be unable to tell the day of the month, month of the year, day of the week, or year. He will also become disoriented as to *place*. For example, in the beginning of this symptom, he will have difficulty identifying a particular place, and in more severe deterioration, he will be unable to remember his own address or where he is currently. As the deterioration continues, he will have difficulty identifying *persons* around him, forgetting their names and thereafter their relationship to him. It is not until almost every other intellectual function is impaired that the person will have difficulty identifying himself or remembering his own name. This fact can be important when distinguishing between amnesia or dissociative state.[13]

Difficulty in Abstract Reasoning

The third symptom, difficulty in abstract reasoning, is determined through asking the person to explain or rephrase a proverb (mental status exam) or by asking him to repeat five numbers in reverse order.

Persons with organic dementia suffer not only the cognitive impairment but emotional and motivational impairment as well. There tends to be a general disorganization, desocialization, and regression of behavior. People functioning at a lower neurobiological level find it more difficult to control their emotions. Aggressive behavior may be marked in some people; clinging dependent behavior is evident in others.

Syndromes of Dementia

Dementia is the major psychiatric disorder of aging. The fear of a decline in intellectual capacity is widespread among middle-aged persons as well as among the elderly. Many people state they would like to live a long life but only if they retain their mental facilities. And it is true that the functioning of a senior citizen's mind will often determine whether he lives out his life in the community or in a nursing facility.

Historically, dementia was sometimes described as the result of an indwelling spirit. However, by the nineteenth century, it was recognized as an illness. As early as 1838, a French psychiatrist Esquirol used the term *demence senile*.[14] In the 1890s, Kraepelin noted that among the group of insanities, insanity in the aged was one of the few psychiatric syndromes accompanied by gross brain changes.[15] He noted in one study of brains that half had cerebral infarcts, which he attributed to arteriosclerosis. In 1899, Alzheimer suggested that noninfarct dementia was due to a vascular disease that involved the arterioles. A few years later he reported the presence of senile plaques in cases of senile dementia. In 1906, Alzheimer described a type of presenile dementia that was accompanied by similar symptoms but occurred in persons under the age of 65.[16] It was this presenile dementia that was termed Alzheimer's disease. Together with Pick's disease, an uncommon form of dementia that was described by Arnold Pick in 1902 and primarily affects the frontal lobes, a new category of presenile dementia was established.[17]

For the next 50 years the dominant view was that arteriosclerotic disease caused senile dementia. The evidence for this belief was based on the following observations:

- Arteriosclerotic changes in the walls of blood vessels and in the diameter of blood vessels.
- That these changes occurred with advancing age.
- That arteriosclerotic changes caused narrowing of the coronary arteries, which is believed to cause a decrease of blood supply to the brain.

This viewpoint remained dominant until the mid-1960s when two English pathologists, Corsellis and Evans, studied the brains of demented and nondemented old people and found approximately the same extent of arteriosclerotic changes in both groups.[18] Subsequently, Tomlinson and associates confirmed Corsellis and Evans's findings and established the actual pathological picture of senile dementia as it is known today.[19]

The types of dementia syndromes include Wernicke-Korsakoff syndrome, Huntington's chorea, Pick's disease, Creutzfeldt-Jacob disease and Alzheimer's disease.

Wernicke-Korsakoff Syndrome
Korsakoff's syndrome, a dysmnesic syndrome, usually follows an acute delirium, twilight state, or stupor. In its classical sense, the syndrome is associated with chronic alcoholism, polyneuritis due to thiamine (vitamin B_1) deficiency, and oc-

casionally, pellagra-like skin lesions. Frequently, the person shows conspicuous memory loss. At the same time, the mechanism of **confabulation**—the making up of stories—is used to compensate for this memory loss. It has been hypothesized that this memory failure is not due to the defective storage of information but rather to a lack of access to information in storage and to the lack of new input. A major defect is the person's inability to form new associations. The answers given in the mental status examination will usually show marked defects. In contrast, this condition may or may not be observed in patients with acute brain disorders resulting from surgery or immediately following electroconvulsive treatments.

Korsakoff's syndrome may follow untreated Wernicke's encephalopathy and is characterized by alert attentiveness with a specific deficit in short-term memory. The person typically undergoes an abrupt personality change, appearing with flat affect, indifferent to his conditions, confabulatory about recent history, and free of alcohol craving. The person may be misdiagnosed as having an acute psychotic episode; however, accompanying deficits in comprehension of spoken and written language and the inability to repeat syntactically complex phrases are indicators of damage, usually vascular, to Wernicke's area in the dominant temporal lobe.

Huntington's Chorea
Huntington's chorea is a genetically inherited disease and has a progressive degenerative process involving the cerebrum, with onset usually in middle age. It is characterized by involuntary movements in the limbs and face and ultimately of the whole body. Dementia is the most notable psychiatric change, but personality variations can be noted 1 to 2 years before the overt signs. A person who has seemed fairly even-tempered may become unexplainably irritable and given to episodes of rage. A mild apathy with loss of interest in work, family, and friends comes on early. The patient complains that he is unable to concentrate. Judgment and insight gradually fail and the patient reaches a very regressed state. The suicide rate tends to be high with this group and the complication of alcoholism is common.

Pick's Disease
Pick's disease was first described by Arnold Pick in 1892.[20] Pick's disease is much rarer than Alz-

heimer's disease, and there is considerable evidence in the literature that this disease is a specific heredodegenerative process that is not associated with rapid progression in the normal aging process. In the early stages, the memory is not significantly involved, but the attention span is progressively affected, and this, in turn, is followed by a decline in memory. As deterioration continues, restlessness, aimless activity, and increased talkativeness can develop. Speech is difficult to understand. There is intellectual deterioration with early loss of abstract thinking. In the final stages of deterioration, paralysis, contractures, and epileptic seizures are often present.

Creutzfeldt-Jakob Disease

This is a subacute progressive neurological disease that usually begins in the fifth or sixth decade of life. In some cases, symptoms such as anxiety, nervousness, easy fatigability, depression, loss of appetite, affective lability, delusions, hallucinations, or behavioral changes suggest a functional psychiatric disorder. In other cases, onset of symptoms is similar to the classical picture of dementia. And in still other cases, onset of symptoms includes disturbances in speech and coordination, visual abnormalities, involuntary movements, or episodic loss of consciousness suggesting a different type of neurological disorder. Usually, however, the disorder is manifested by a dementing process, to which may be added a variety of both upper and lower motor neuron signs. The illness is rather rapidly progressive; patients usually become severely demented in less than 6 months and survive less than a year. The disease has been demonstrated to be caused by a transmissible agent. The disorder can be transmitted from humans to experimental animals with brain tissue taken from patients dying of the disease. The period between innoculation and the onset of clinical signs of the disease in the experimental animal is long, often many months, and for this reason its transmissibility was for long unrecognized.

The transmissible agent that causes Creutzfeldt-Jakob disease is a replicable, filterable particle, but one that differs from conventional viruses in several respects. It is considerably resistant to inactivation by heat, ultraviolet and ionizing radiation, proteases, nucleases, and formalin. The disease is uniformly fatal, and no means of treatment is known. Because of uncertainty as to modes of transmission and morbidity, extreme caution is advised in handling biologic substances, such as cerebrospinal fluid, from patients suspected to suffer from the disease.[21]

Alzheimer's Disease

Alzheimer's disease is a progressive, age-related, chronic cognitive dysfunction. This type of mental deterioration was first described by Alois Alzheimer in 1906.[22] The current belief is that cognitive dysfunction is not an inevitable concomitant of old age because most elderly people apparently do not experience clinically significant memory impairment. Alzheimer's disease is generally accompanied by cognitive and behavioral symptoms, the precise nature of which depends on the stage of the disease, as described below.

Phase 1. In the first phase of the disease (the forgetfulness phase) there is only subjective cognitive deficit. The individual, and occasionally people close to the patient, notice that the individual has a tendency to forget where things are placed, has more difficulty remembering names and appointments, and may have to write things down in order to remember them.

Kral described the difference between an entity he called "benign senescent forgetfulness" and a malignant form of the amnestic syndrome.[23] He noted that the malignant form was characterized by shortened retention time, the inability of the person to recall events of the recent past, and the inability to recall important as well as unimportant facts associated with an experience. By contrast, he described the benign senescent form as characterized by the inability of the subject to recall relatively unimportant data and parts of an experience, whereas the experience itself, of which the forgotten data form a part, can be recalled. Those with benign memory impairment had the same mortality rate as age-matched non-memory-impaired control subjects, while those with the malignant type of memory impairment had a much higher mortality rate.

Those patients who do not demonstrate progression of their cognitive impairment can be given the presumptive diagnosis of benign senescent forgetfulness. Those persons whose symptoms become worse and who proceed to manifest the symptoms and signs of the next stage may be presumed to have Alzheimer's disease.

Phase 2. Phase 2 is called the confusional phase and is characterized by a definite impairment of congnitive functioning in which the deficit becomes obvious. The cognitive deficit is classically particularly severe for memory of recent events. Orientation and concentration may be similarly affected. Memory for past events remains relatively intact. Vocabulary is largely spared; however, the individual may experience difficulty recalling appropriate words. During this stage, denial often replaces the earlier anxiety. There are often few symptoms apart from the cognitive deficit.

Phase 3. Phase 3, called the dementia phase, is where the person becomes severely disoriented and may, for example, confuse a spouse with a parent. Behavioral problems may now become apparent. The patient may exhibit marked anxiety despite the continuing denial. The person may not be able to carry a thought long enough to remember what to do next. In addition, psychotic symptoms such as delusions, hallucinations, paranoid ideation, and severe agitation may become manifest. These symptoms may be an extension of the cognitive deficit.[24]

DSM-III-R DIAGNOSIS

The organic mental disorders can be grouped into three categories. Since, by tradition, disorders that are related either to aging of the brain or to the ingestion of a substance are classified as mental disorders, the first two categories describe Dementias Arising in the Senium and the Presenium (Primary Degenerative Dementia of the Alzheimer Type and Multi-Infarct Dementia) and are included in this chapter. The third type, Psychoactive Substance-Induced Organic Mental Disorders, is discussed in Chapter 34.

Dementias Arising in the Senium and Presenium

Certain degenerative dementias have traditionally been referred to as senile and presenile dementias, the distinction being arbitrarily based on an age at onset over 65. Nearly all of these cases are associated with the histopathologic changes of Alzheimer's disease. Although the definitive diagnosis of Alzheimer's disease is dependent on histopathologic data, there is growing consensus that there is a high correlation between this pathology and a particular clinical picture. For this reason, the *DSM-III-R* includes a single category to encompass the progressive course of the disease. Alzheimer's disease itself is a physical disorder and is recorded as an Axis III diagnosis while the psychiatric disorder is recorded on Axis I as Primary Degenerative Dementia of the Alzheimer Type and subtyped according to age of onset.

Primary Degenerative Dementia of the Alzheimer Type

The essential feature of this condition is the presence of dementia of insidious onset and a generally progressive, deteriorating course for which all other specific causes have been excluded by the history, physical examination, and laboratory tests. The dementia involves a multifaceted loss of intellectual abilities, such as memory, judgment, abstract thought, and other higher cortical functions, and changes in personality and behavior.

Diagnostic Criteria for Primary Degenerative Dementia of the Alzheimer Type

A. Dementia.
B. Insidious onset with a generally progressive deteriorating course.
C. Exclusion of all other specific causes of Dementia by history, physical examination, and laboratory tests.

Multi-Infarct Dementia

The essential feature of this disorder is a dementia due to significant cerebrovascular disease. A single stroke may cause a relatively circumscribed change in mental state. As a general rule, a single stroke does not cause dementia; multi-infarct dementia results from the occurrence of multiple strokes at different times.

There is a stepwise deterioration in intellectual functioning that, early in the course, leaves some intellectual functions relatively intact ("patchy" deterioration). Focal neurological signs and symptoms are also present.

The onset is typically abrupt. The course is stepwise and fluctuating, with rapid changes, rather than uniformly progressive. The pattern of deficits is "patchy," depending on which regions of the brain have been destroyed. Certain cognitive functions may be affected early, whereas others remain relatively unimpaired. The dementia typically involves disturbances in memory, abstract thinking, judgment, impulse control, and personality. The focal neurological signs commonly seen include weaknesses in the limbs, reflex asymmetries, extensor plantar responses, dysarthria, and small-stepped gait. Vascular disease is always presumed to be present and responsible for both the dementia and the focal neurological signs.

Diagnostic Criteria for Multi-Infarct Dementia

A. Dementia.
B. Stepwise deteriorating course with "patchy" distribution of deficits (i.e., affecting some functions, but not others) early in the course.
C. Focal neurological signs and symptoms (e.g., exaggeration of deep tendon reflexes, extensor plantar response, pseudobulbar palsy, gait abnormalities, weakness of an extremity, etc.)
D. Evidence from history, physical examination, or laboratory tests of significant cerebrovascular disease (recorded on Axis III) that is judged to be etiologically related to the disturbance.

NURSING MANAGEMENT IN ORGANIC MENTAL DISORDERS

Nurses whose daily work involves caring for psychiatric patients with neurotic, depressive, and schizophrenic conditions must be ever alert to abnormal behavior caused by organic conditions. This awareness is extremely important since organic conditions may appear like the functional disorders.

There are particular settings in which the nurse is likely to encounter abnormal behavior resulting from organic conditions. Some of these settings include the following:

- In community work in which the patient may not have had previous medical evaluation.
- In working with people who are part of the drug culture.
- In geriatric work in which the nurse is likely to encounter patients with senile changes.

- In emergency room settings in which symptoms need to be differentially assessed.
- In intensive care settings where there may be trauma to the brain as a result of disease.
- In surgical areas where conditions may have induced cerebral symptoms.

Communicating with the Organically Impaired

Working with the organically impaired patient is recommended for nurses who wish to increase their sensitivity to overt behavior and its relationship to the organization and structure of the brain. The challenge is understanding and intervening in the social interaction of such people.

Autognosis
Students working with an organically impaired patient can ask themselves: what are my feelings and concerns regarding any type of organic mental impairment? A checklist of questions to pursue this understanding includes: Whom have I known with this disorder in my family? What kind of fears do I have regarding the loss of mental functioning? What have I learned or observed from other people that influences me positively or negatively? What are the values I place on the quality of life and the experiences of this other person?

Nurses need to say to themselves: Careful observation and patience are needed for me to be able to relate to this person in a meaningful manner. Communication consists of more than verbal response. Eye blinks, muscle tension, tonal qualities, and others forms of body language become the key areas for assessment.

Stalls
The stall warnings that the nurse–patient interaction is not functioning are twofold. In the first place, the nurse must acknowledge to herself that in working with people who suffer from organic mental disorders there is a powerful personal sense of futility that accompanies working with someone whose brain tissue is changing for some reason. If the underlying assumption is that this person cannot understand because of organic changes, that this person cannot communicate in any recognizable manner for organic reasons, the nurse will respond in a stereotypical and unhelpful manner. The reality is

that we do not know how much or how little brain tissue is necessary for processing stimuli in a meaningful manner. There are medical cases of children born with very inadequately sized brains who function at an average or normal level of intelligence. There are dramatic writings by people who were institutionalized for years because they were thought to be so brain-damaged that they were incapable of understanding or having a world of meaning. In these situations fellow patients established a relationship with these isolated people and began to understand a method of communicating with them. Through this painstaking effort they were able to elicit their lifelong story of isolation and misunderstanding by others.

Nurses need to operate on the presupposition that all forms of life communicate, no matter how differently they may be structured. Operating on this premise the nurse can now ask: What are the patient's patterns of human responding to consistent stimuli?

The second stall area to assess is: To what extent do you as a nurse believe the patient experience has to result in your being acknowledged, recognized, and satisfied? If nurses believe that their positive motivations and intentions in working with a patient are dependent upon immediate recognition of their efforts, this will stall nurses in being open and creative in making use of the best that the patient is able to do at any particular point in time.

If there is a blaming, criticizing presumption of limitation, such as this person does not know anymore or any better and cannot do whatever is being asked, there will be a breakdown in the therapeutic transaction with the patient.

The stall recovery is the challenge and pleasure of increasing one's own sensitivity to the nuances and subtleties of another human being who struggles to live. Learning how to communicate in spite of the obstacles is a primary motivator in the nursing care of organically impaired clients.

Communication Strategies

The first aspect of communicating with someone who is organically impaired is to pay careful attention to what you say and do as a nurse and to the response it elicits in the patient. Frequently nurses are frustrated and confused that their presence or touching of the patient triggers a startle reflex. The patient may talk loudly or scream. This is particularly true of older people who are confined to bed. Attempts often are made to override the screaming by short, clear, and strong vocal commands to the patient. It is important to ascertain whether the increased tonal quality of the nurse stops the screaming and focuses the attention of the patient. A combination of tonal quality and touch may be necessary to get the patient's attention and from that point attempt to relax the patient. When the patient has relaxed, the nurse continues the activity, e.g., moving the patient in or out of the bed, explaining the procedure as it is carried out. The principle is that the nurse continually evaluates the effects of communication with the patient, noting that that communication includes the tonal quality, rate of speech, the tactile interaction, the pressure, intensity, and smoothness of the interaction.

Another important principle to bear in mind in working with people with organic impairment relates to alterations in memory and sequencing of information. The nurse needs to be aware of the nature of the questions asked in relationship to time. Is the question asking the patient to go back in time, is the question based on asking the patient to respond to an immediate situation, is the question asking the patient to respond to an anticipated event time in the future? In organic conditions that impair memory, patients—for a variety of reasons—will attempt to make up for what they cannot remember or be aware of in a process referred to as confabulation. This can be checked simply by the nurse's asking questions of the patient about events that the nurse in fact knows the patient was not a part of. If the patient says yes and goes on to elaborate, the nurse can be assured that the memory concern is being dealt with by confabulation. For example, a nurse said to a patient, "Did you go to the dining hall this morning?" The patient responds, "Oh, yes. I was eating with my friends." The confabulation is established by the fact that the patient was not out of her room that morning. This example is in stark contrast to the patient who is confused and claims not to remember when asked, "When did you go to dinner with your family last week?" The patient cannot remember the day or the date or the family member. However, if the patient is given a context to remember, such as, "Remember sitting at the restaurant table with John, Julie, and Sam and there was food left over? Who agreed to take the food home?" The patient might readily respond,

"Oh, Julie took the food home." This is reminiscent of the memory development of a child where the abstract reasoning for remembering something like the day before yesterday is undeveloped but the capacity to relate and recall the details of an event are intact. The underlying implication of this principle is that the nurse must not summarily assume that a person's memory is "gone" but rather has to search for what aspects of memory are functional for the patient.

A third important principle deals with the motor-coordination and retrieval-of-language constructs. There are a variety of aphasias, that is, a variety of problems in either the retrieval of language or the production of language. Not infrequently in people with a dementia or with strokes, there is incapacity to form and retreive words. The patient may respond with one word, such as "yes," and answer "yes" to just about any comments that are made to him. If the nurse observes carefully, she will understand that at times, the "yes" tone is a "no." And eventually a pattern of interaction can be set up in which the patient's attempts to communicate are understood through this limited yes-and-no signal arrangement. For some people who lose speech altogether, eye blinks may be used for yes and no. The point is that the assumption that a person does not understand or does not remember because his expression of language is impaired is incorrect.

Nursing Assessment

Suspecting Organic Illness

The psychiatric nurse need not *diagnose* organic illness because this is a medical function that may require neurological consultation and a series of special tests such as electroencephalograms, skull x-rays, blood chemistries, and the like. The nurse should, however, learn to *suspect* organic illness.

A great deal can be learned from observing the behavior itself. There are certain behaviors that are so commonly associated with organic brain disease that their observation should lead to the diagnosis of suspected organic illness.

These behaviors include:

1. The inability to retain and recall information.
2. Disorientation as to time, place, and person. (The patient does not know the date,

where he is, or who he is.) These aspects of disorientation do not necessarily occur together.
3. Difficulty in the ability to abstract.
4. Intellectual deterioration.
5. Fluctuating state of consciousness.
6. Visual hallucinations.
7. Episodic behavioral disturbance (seizure disorders).

In a patient suffering from an organic condition, the above symptoms and behaviors do not occur alone but are likely to be accompanied by other behaviors such as paranoid delusions and depressed mood state, which also occur in functional psychiatric disorders.

The nurse must also be aware that none of the seven behaviors listed above may be apparent in a patient with a behavioral disorder resulting from an organic condition. For example, cancer of the pancreas, brain tumor, and hypothyroidism can all present as a functional depression. For any behavioral disorder, therefore, the nurse should consider the possibility of organic syndromes as well as the functional psychiatric disorders.

Assessment of Delirium

A nursing assessment of symptoms of delirium includes evaluation of wakefulness, cognition, psychomotor activity, and additional features.

Wakefulness. Some degree of disordered wakefulness and sensorium is a sine qua non in suspecting delirium. In addition, a disordered sensorium may be noted through a disturbed attention or reduced awareness of self and the environment. In delirium, the patient's level of awareness may range from minimal neglect of detail to lethargy to stupor, but it is always reduced. The patient's level of arousal and alertness (readiness to respond) may be increased or decreased, but sustained attention is invariably reduced.

Cognition. There is global impairment of cognitive functions essential to the processing of information. Some degree of impaired perception is usually present with resulting spatial–temporal disorientation, illusions, and hallucinations. Often these symptoms are most obvious at night. Thinking is disorganized to some degree as well as purposive problem solving, reasoning, and abstraction. Delusions may be present, and memory is invariably impaired.

Psychomotor Activity. Psychomotor activity may show symptoms through lethargy, catatonic stupor, or purposeless hyperactivity, often with rapid, unpredictable shifts.

Additional Features. Additional features include a wide range of emotional disturbances such as anxiety, fear, depression, nightmares, or apathy. Autonomic arousal may be noted by tachycardia, facial flushing, and hypertension.

Assessment of Dementia

Three stages of dementia may be noted. In the first stage, mood swings, feelings of general inadequacy, and fatigue are felt by the individual. Failures are most conspicuous when the person is under pressure or is faced with multiple tasks and he cannot fall back on the routine of performance. A decrease of interests, especially cultured interests, and a coarsening of interpersonal relationships are noted. In organic deficit states, in contrast to behavior disorders of old age in which the family is often overalerted for signs of impairment, this stage often goes unnoticed.

During the second stage, the patient's inefficiency is obvious to everyone but himself. When confronted with his shortcomings, he tends to make excuses or else denies them. Gross impairment in social and intellectual functioning appears, for example, crude, tactless, and impulsive behavior. A decrease in reality testing, suspicious and paranoid attitudes, and misinterpretation of relationships are common. Memory, attention, and concentration may be impaired.

In the third stage of dementia the patient is very helpless and is unable to care for himself. Intellectual deterioration is so far advanced that even the routine tasks of everyday living cannot be accomplished. The patient has great difficulty communicating and requires constant nursing care for prevention of infection, safety measures, and hygienic measures.

Assessment Tools

An important assessment tool in working with patients who have an acute or chronic organic disorder is the mental status examination (see Chapter 12). It is recommended that the mental status exam be modified to describe what a patient can or cannot do, stated in behavioral terms, when assessing for orientation, disorientation, confusion, and delirium.[25] For example, rather than noting that "the patient is confused," a more useful documentation would read:

The patient has no deficits in recent memory, as demonstrated by his ability to repeat digits in reverse order and to remember three objects. He does have deficits in memory beyond the last 4 hours, as demonstrated by his inability to subtract 8 from 45 and to count backwards by 3s from 31.[26]

One such assessment tool, designed by Marylin J. Dodd, identified six areas for behavioral observation as follows[27]:

1. Patient knows he is in a hospital, the name of the hospital, the unit or area of hospital, who is president of the United States, the month of the year, the name of the city, and the capital of the state he is in.
2. The patient knows he has pain, can communicate where the pain is, can describe the pain, and can demonstrate behavior to minimize the pain.
3. Patient can recognize visual stimuli of social network, can respond to people, can respond to number of fingers displayed, can respond to immediate environment.
4. Patient can recognize tactile stimuli.
5. Patient's memory is intact in terms of recent memory and intermediate and long-term memory.
6. Patient performs tasks on request such as coughing, turning, deep breathing, touching nose with index finger, and stretching out arms with palms up.

The Dodd assessment tool has a rating scale to diagnose the patient's mental status and is very useful in a variety of settings.[28]

Nursing Diagnosis of Self-Care Deficit

Observational data as well as a mental status diagnosis are essential for determining if the patient is experiencing a delirium or acute confusional state or if the patient's condition is part of a deteriorating dementia stage.

A nursing diagnosis of self-care deficit as applicable to delirium and dementia is provided in the following nursing care plans, showing both short-term and long-term objectives.

Management of the Patient with Delirium

If the patient is suffering from an acute confusional state, there are suggested interventions to implement until the confusion clears. These interventions are as follows[29]:

1. *Support existing sensory reception.* The nurse can ensure adequate sensory reception through the use of eyeglasses, hearing aids, radio, or television for the patient. More stimuli at nighttime is recommended for the confusion that occurs in the evening when the stimulation input is lowered. The term *sundowning* is used for this condition in older patients who have less cerebral reserve for adapting to reduced stimuli. A night light or radio is helpful for this situation.

2. *Maintain familiar environment.* Consistent and individual personal contact with the patient is strongly recommended to maintain known surroundings for the patient.

3. *Use face-to-face communication.* Talk directly to the patient using simple, direct, descriptive statements. Do not use complex explanations or questions.

4. *Provide explanations.* When giving physical care, give the patient an explanation of what you intend to do and what you are doing. Let the patient do as much for himself as possible.

5. *Assess carefully the anxiety level in the patient.* Try to keep the amount of anxiety within moderate levels. Encourage realistic optimism.

6. *Focus initially on competently functioning areas.* In order to aid internal reorientation, focus on areas the patient is already competent in.

7. *Introduce new information slowly.* Do not overwhelm the patient with a large amount of information. Providing new information slowly will help the patient to think logically.

8. *Reinforce reality* rather than responding to any delusional material presented by the patient. Always check out the content of the delusion to be sure there is not some rational explanation for the concern.

9. *Protect the severely agitated patient.* Constant staff attendance, mittens, or restraints may be necessary. Medication should be considered for patients who are agitated, delusional, or very frightened.

10. *Present a calm, concerned, understanding demeanor with patients.* It is important to remember that the confusional state may be viewed as a partially adaptive one, by which some people cope with devastating insults to their psychological and physical integrity.

Management of Excitement and Delirium

Calmness, firmness, and patience are essential nursing skills to being therapeutic with a person who is disoriented, excited, and frightened. Speaking and moving slowly, softly, and deliberately will help convey to the patient that the nurse is there to help him.

Constant observation and supervision of the patient are necessary to prevent his falling out of bed or wandering away from the ward. The suicidal intent of many of these patients should not be ignored.

It is essential to leave a light on at night because the patient becomes more confused and frightened in the dark. The nurse can decrease the patient's agitation if she can be readily available to him or within sight.

Exposure to stressful procedures, such as x-rays and diagnostic tests, may precipitate delirious patients into a panic. Team consultation is most important in the planning and carrying out of procedures.

Medical Control

Opinion on the use of medication in controlling excitement and delirium is divided. Sedation or tranquilizing drugs may be ordered. If they are, there is always a danger of giving too much on top of an unknown cause for the delirium. The patient's vital signs must be carefully noted at least 1 hour before and 1 hour after administration of any medication. The possibility of helping the patient to ventilate should be kept in mind in case of respiratory depression or cessation.

Drugs should not be given to the patient who is in shock or coma or who shows a decrease in vital signs. Patients who are in a stupor because of other drugs, narcotics, or alcohol should sleep off the effects before additional medication is administered. And wherever possible, the oral route of administration is preferred.

NURSING CARE PLAN
Patient With Delirium

HUMAN RESPONSE

1. Reduced attention span
2. Disorganized thinking
3. At least two of the following: Clouding of consciousness; Perceptual disturbances, disturbance in sleep–wakefulness cycle, increased or decreased psychomotor activity, disorientation and memory impairment

NURSING DIAGNOSIS

Sensory perceptual alteration
Alteration in thought processes
Deficit in self-care

GOALS

1. Causative agent will be identified.
2. Patient will experience relief of symptoms and a reverse of the delirium.
3. Patient will experience sensory stimulation.
4. Patient will regain sense of familiarity with surroundings.

INTERVENTIONS

1. Schedule laboratory tests. Take careful history of use of drugs, medication, and alcohol use.
2. Conduct careful nursing assessment of mental status and motor behavior. Monitor airway and breathing; vital signs; and IV. Provide adequate nutrition, fluid intake, electrolytes, and vitamin supply.
3. Provide sensory stimulation; monitor mental status and behavior. Decrease extraneous confusing noises. Schedule observation ranging from one-to-one to decreased as necessary.
4. Encourage social support.

Management of the Patient with Dementia

The primary objective in the nursing care of a person with a diagnosed dementia is to minimize the loss of self-care capacity. Working with the patient and family, the nurse can help set reasonable goals and expectations and can develop strategies for coping with the disabilities.

Community health nurses are excellent resource people in helping families to keep the person at home as long as possible. This will prevent the increase in dependency that institutions and nursing homes cannot help but foster. The nursing assessment of the different phases of dementia and teaching the family various psychological approaches that aim to maintain the person's highest level of adaptive functioning are most helpful.

Nursing procedures that the family cannot carry out can be performed by the Visiting Nurse Association, which will also facilitate the person's remaining in his familiar environment.

The following case example illustrates the progressive phases of dementia. The referral form on Mrs. Round states that the husband has been told that nothing could be done for his wife and that the husband may be expected to be depressed, for he had come to the psychiatrist "hoping for a miracle." The only other information is that the onset of her symptoms was 7 years ago and also that a son was killed in an automobile accident seven years ago.

CASE EXAMPLE

Mrs. Round, age 59, was referred to the psychiatric clinic for a consultation and evaluation interview. Her problem dated back several years to when she became "depressed and slowed down." Four years prior to this interview the patient was operated on for a strangulated bowel and was quite ill. She was transferred postoperatively to the neurology service for evaluation of "dementia" that had become precipitously apparent after surgery. She was medically discharged home following her recovery.

Mrs. Round functioned fairly well at home, but there was a gradual decline in her ability to remember, make judgments, and solve problems. For example, she had a car accident 4 months after returning home because she mistook the accelerator for the brake and crashed into a tree.

Her progressive difficulties had worsened over the previous 6 months to the point that she had become unintelligibly aphasic, confused, and disoriented. She had to be asked simple requests several times. She could not be left alone. She could feed and dress herself with directional assistance. She was not incontinent. A right hemiplegia, a leaning to the left while walking, and dropping objects from her right hand had been noted. She cried in apparent frustration every two or three days.

A diagnosis of presenile dementia caused by bilateral vascular disease was made. The results of the neurological examination showed that Mrs. Round was profoundly dysphasic with nearly unintelligible stammering, stuttering, and confusion. She could follow one-part commands but nothing more complex. An abnormal EEG with diffusely slow readings was confirmed.

NURSING CARE PLAN
Patient With Dementia

HUMAN RESPONSE

1. Impairment in short- and long-term memory
2. Impaired abstract thinking, impaired judgment, disturbances of higher cortical function, personality change

NURSING DIAGNOSIS

Alteration in thought processes
Alteration in intellectual capacity
Self-care deficit
Impaired coping and interpersonal relationships

GOALS

1. Patient will express thoughts, feelings, and behaviors regarding limitations.
2. Patient will maximize adaptive functioning to intellectual deficits, be able to accept full impact of deficit, and have correct perspective about future impact.
3. Patient and family will prioritize needs.

INTERVENTIONS

1. Schedule daily meetings with patient.
2. Teach through simple diagrams and drawings. Assist patient to mourn loss of physical part of self.
3. Monitor the administration of medications and self-care activities; acknowledge small gains and progress in self-care area.
4. Anticipate common patient–family concerns. Listen carefully to patient–family concerns. Use of peer therapy groups. Provide family support on outpatient basis.

Summary

Nurses need to constantly consider the presence of an organic condition when assessing any type of mental distress symptom. This chapter discusses four conditions of pharmacological, medical, surgical, and neurological situations related to behavior disturbance. The two major categories of delirium and dementia are described within the psychiatric diagnostic criteria and in planning nursing care.

The nurse is in an evaluative position in working in the hospital and in the community. For instance, when a nurse is seeing a patient in the community who says she is feeling poorly, the nurse should ask about medications, illnesses, and recent hospitalizations. The nurse should include in the history taking of the patient any head injuries, seizures, or loss of memory. It is helpful to use the mental status examination with the patient. The areas of orientation, memory, intellect, judgment, insight, thought content, and mood can be useful in testing for either something organically wrong with the patient or something functionally wrong.

The increased visibility of Alzheimer's disease has provided nurses with the opportunity to conduct research into ways to help patients and their families compensate for the organic impairment. The information and judgments made by the nurse in the assessment process have direct input to the treatment of referral then decided for the patient.

Questions

1. What symptoms would make you suspect an acute confusional state in a patient recovering from open-heart surgery?
2. How can infection cause a person to develop symptoms of mental distress?
3. Describe your nursing intervention with a patient with a confused mental state in a medical setting.
4. How do you assess if a patient has a progressive dementia or is "just confused?"

REFERENCES AND SUGGESTED READINGS

1. Wells, C. B. Organic mental disorders. In H. I. Kaplan and B. J. Sadock (Eds.), *Comprehensive Textbook of Psychiatry* 4th ed., Baltimore: Williams & Wilkins, 1985, p. 834.
2. Ibid.
3. Lazare, A., & Anderson, W. H. Organic differential diagnosis of psychiatric symptoms. In A. Lazare (Ed.), *Outpatient Psychiatry*. Baltimore: Williams & Wilkins, 1979, p. 249.
4. Keller, M. B., & Manschreck, T. C. Disorders of higher intellectual functioning. In A. Lazare (Ed.), *Outpatient Psychiatry*. Baltimore: Williams & Wilkins, 1979, p. 280.
5. American Psychiatric Association, *DSM-III-R*, Washington, D.C., p. 97.
6. Turner, G. O. *The Cardiovascular Care Unit*. New York: Wiley, 1978.
7. Wilson, L. U. Intensive care in delirium. *Archives of International Medicine,* 1972, *130,* 225–226.
8. Coffey, C. E., Massey, S. W., & Roberts, K. R. Natural history of neurological complications following coronary artery by-pass surgery. *Neurology,* 1982, *32,* 85–86.
9. Andreasen, N. J. C., et al., Management of emotional reactions in seriously burned adults. *New England Journal of Medicine,* 1972, *286,* 65–69.
10. Bedford, P. D. Central medical aspects of confusional stages in elderly people. *British Medical Journal,* 1959, *2,* 185–188.
11. Lipowski, Z. I. Organic mental disorder: Introduction and review of syndromes. In H. I. Kaplan, A. W. Freedman, & B. J. Sadock (Eds.), *Comprehensive Textbook of Psychiatry* (Vol. 1). Baltimore: Williams & Wilkins, 1980.
12. Seltzer, B., & Frazier, S. H. Organic mental disorders. In A. M. Nicholi, Jr. (Ed.), *The Harvard Guide to Modern Psychiatry*. Cambridge, Mass.: Harvard University Press, 1978, p. 301.

13. Detre, T. P., & Jarecki, H. G. *Modern Psychiatric Treatment*. Philadelphia: Lippincott, 1971, pp. 396–404.
14. Cited in Zilboorg, G., & Henry, W. G. *A History of Medical Psychology*. New York: Norton, 1941, p. 552.
15. Cited in Torack, R. M. *The Pathologic Physiology of Dementia*. New York: Springer-Verlag, 1978, p. 9.
16. Ibid.
17. Ibid.
18. Corsellis, J. A. N., & Evans, P. H. The relation of stenosis of the extracranial cerebral arteries to mental disorders and cerebral degeneration in old age. In *Proceedings of the Fifth International Congress of Neuropathology*. The Hague: Moulton & Co., 1965, p. 546.
19. Tomlinson, B. E., Blessed, G., & Roth, M. Observation on the brains of demented old people. *Journal of Neurological Sciences*, 1970, *11*, 205–242.
20. Torack, R. M., op. cit.
21. Wells, op. cit., pp. 864–865.
22. Torack, R. M., op. cit.
23. Kral, V. A. Senescent forgetfulness: Benign and malignant. *Canadian Medical Association Journal*, 1962, *86*, 257–260.
24. Schneck, M. K., Reisberg, B., & Ferris, S. H. An overview of current concepts of Alzheimer's disease. *American Journal of Psychiatry*, 1982, *139*, 165–173.
25. Dodd, M. J. Assessing mental status. *American Journal of Nursing*, 1978, *78*, 501.
26. Ibid.
27. Ibid.
28. Ibid.
29. Trockman, G. Caring for the confused or delirious patient. *American Journal of Nursing*, 1978, *78*, 1499.

Chapter 37

Schizophrenic Disorders

Ann Wolbert Burgess

Chapter Objectives

The students successfully attaining the goals of this chapter will be able to:

- Describe the biochemical and psychosocial theories of the causes of schizophrenia.
- Describe the schizophrenic syndromes in behavioral terms with corresponding nursing diagnoses.
- Describe the major types of schizophrenia.
- Describe the typical behaviors of persons with schizophrenia.
- Use the nursing process in caring for the schizophrenic patient.
- Plan individual care depending on the behaviors each patient displays.

The descriptive picture of what is currently termed *schizophrenia* has historical roots in Sanskrit writings as early as 1400 B.C. In the fifth century B.C., the Greek physicians distinguished dementia from mania and melancholia. In the second century, and for a thousand years following, the cause of schizophrenia was believed to be a form of possession by the devil. The schizophrenic was dealt with in jails, religious courts, and asylums. Not until the nineteenth century did classification of the signs and symptoms of the clinical picture emerge. The German psychiatrist Emil Kraeplin, in the late 1890s, classified symptoms into two broad categories based on outcome: (1) dementia praecox result-ing in deterioration; and (2) manic–depressive psychosis resulting in exacerbations and remissions.[1]

Eugene Bleuler recognized in 1911 that dementia praecox does not always lead to deterioration and that onset is not always associated with adolescence. A contemporary of Kraeplin and Freud, he attempted to apply Freud's dynamic understanding of the unconscious meaning of symptom content to the psychotic patients he observed. Adolf Meyer's belief that mental illness is the patient's reaction to environmental experiences was also integrated into Bleuler's thinking, but Bleuler never abandoned the basically organic approach advanced by Kraeplin.

The major point of departure for Bleuler was the conceptualization of dementia praecox as a syndrome, rather than as a disease entity. He argued that dementia praecox consists of a group of disorders in the same sense as the organic psychoses. He meant that the disorders differed sharply as to cause, presenting picture, and outcome.

The twentieth century has seen numerous theories proposed to explain the cause of schizophrenia. It is important to realize that each theory is incomplete separately and that few linkages occur between the various theories. Thus, schizophrenia continues to be a controversial and baffling subject not only to the clinical professions but also to society. In spite of increasing research interest and newer therapeutic drugs, many questions still remain unanswered in the etiology, diagnosis, and treatment of the disease.

ETIOLOGY OF SCHIZOPHRENIA

We will discuss the etiology of schizophrenia within two basic subject area: (1) the biologic, including genetic, biochemical, and physiological theories; and (2) the psychosocial, including behavioral, psychoanalytic, and socioepidemiologic theories.

Neurobiological Theories of Schizophrenia

A neurobiological theory of schizophrenia is proposed on the basis that genetic and biochemical factors play a part in the etiologic role.

Genetic Hypothesis

The studies on which genetic theories rest fall into two groups: (1) studies of relatives; and (2) the studies of twins. Studies of relatives from hospital records suggest that the risk for schizophrenia is higher in families with relatives with schizophrenia than in the general population. However, the incidence or prevalence of schizophrenia in relatives of patients does not necessarily mean that genetic factors play the exclusive or even the preponderant role in transmitting the predisposition. Much more transpires in families than the vertical passing on of genes.

The preferred method for testing genetic theories is the study of concordance rates for schizophrenia in monozygotic and dizygotic twins. The studies have provided strong support to the contention that genetic factors play a role in schizophrenia; however, most schizophrenic patients do not have psychotic parents.

Several hypotheses have been proposed based on a genetic theory; for example, the two-gene theory has been proposed which states that each gene is distinct, is inherited independently, and has a mutant counterpart. It is important to realize a great deal of research is under way in this area. Some interesting research of the incidence of schizophrenia in monozygotic and dizygotic twins has been and is currently in progress. Seymour Kety's research on the incidence of schizophrenia in twins and adopted children is producing some compelling evidence in support of such a theory. Although many of his findings are compatible with a genetic transmission in schizophrenia, Kety warns that other factors need careful study, such as in utero influence, birth trauma, and early parenting experiences.[2]

Genetics can only operate through biochemical mechanisms. Thus, if genes are thought to be significant, biochemical theories would also be significant. The idea of biochemical influence on schizophrenia is not new. Greek physicians speculated that insanity resided in the brain and was the result of chemical imbalances.

Currently, there are two hypotheses relating to the biologic factors of schizophrenia: (1) the transmethylation hypothesis, and (2) the dopamine hypothesis. The transmethylation hypothesis resulted from recent findings of a significantly diminished level of monoamine oxidase in the platelets of schizophrenics.[3] The dopamine hypothesis resulted from pharmacological studies that investigated the mechanism of the action of drugs that reduced the disorder and examined actions of drugs that produced or mimicked the disorder. S. Matthysse and S. S. Kety identified several types of agents that converge on dopamine synapses in the brain.[4] For example, amphetamine is a drug that produces a psychosis that is similar to schizophrenia and appears to act by potentiating dopamine at its synapses in the brain. The finding suggests that an overactivity of dopamine synapses may play an etiologic role. Other biochemical findings in schizophrenia include serotonin, histamine, and acetycholine.[5] Any cause-and-effect relationship between these agents and the disorder has yet to be determined.

In summary, Kety clearly states that a biochemical and genetic theory of schizophrenia fails to explain other schizophrenic symptoms of behavior, mood, and cognition. However, the effectiveness of certain drugs in controlling psychotic episodes, the research on the chemical nature of the synapse, and indicators of the significant role that genetic factors play in the genesis of schizophrenia, argues Kety, offer persuasive evidence of the existence of biochemical disturbances within schizophrenia.[6]

Since the schizophrenic syndrome was originally identified by Kraeplin many years ago, investigators have speculated that schizophrenic symptoms could be the result of specific brain abnormalities.[7] The search for specific structural brain abnormalities has led to inconclusive results.[8] As a result, during recent years the search for brain abnormalities has focused principally on the neurochemical level, especially the dopamine hypothesis.

The development of computerized tomography (CT) has, however, introduced a new and powerful method for measuring brain structure, thereby permitting investigators to explore again the possibility of structural brain abnormalities in schizophrenia. Johnstone and associates were the first to use this new noninvasive technique to examine the possibility of brain atrophy in chronic schizophrenia.[9] In particular, they reported on a group of 18 chronic schizophrenic patients with a significant increase in ventricular size compared with an age- and sex-matched control group. Andreasen and colleagues in a sample of 52 schizophrenic patients and 47 control nonschizophrenic patients provided additional support for the structural brain abnormality theory in schizophrenia.[10]

When Kraeplin first identified the disorder that he named "dementia praecox," he was referring to a syndrome similar to the dementias of later life but beginning at a relatively early age.[11] Since that time, several changes have occurred in the concept of schizphrenia. In stressing the importance of "fundamental symptoms" and minimizing the importance of a deteriorating course, Bleuler broadened the concept of schizophrenia to include milder cases.[12] Some investigators have added a requirement of "clear consciousness" usually defined as intact orientation and memory. A distinction between organic and functional psychoses has succeeded in precluding conceptualizing schizophrenia as

organic in origin. Another new line of study has been to investigate the importance of positive symptoms such as delusions and hallucinations in the definition of schizophrenia because they are easy to identify and define reliably. The increased interest in positive symptoms has led to a deemphasis on the importance of more "negative" symptoms, such as affective flattening or impoverished thinking, which are somewhat similar to those occurring in dementias.

There has been a continuing search for both structural and functional brain abnormalities in schizophrenia. A series of pneumoencephalographic studies have suggested that some chronic schizophrenic patients may have cerebral atrophy, while neurohistological studies of the brains of schizophrenic patients have identified quantitative changes in cortical functioning similar to viral encephalitis changes. And a marked increase in ventricular size in a subset of schizophrenic patients has been reported and replicated in at least three different studies.

These recent investigations, indicating that both ventricular enlargement and sulcal enlargement may occur in some schizophrenic patients, have reawakened interest in the Kraeplinian notions that a subset of schizophrenic patients may have a disorder similar to the dementias. This evidence has led T. J. Crow to propose that the disorder currently called "schizophrenia" may in fact represent at least two overlapping syndromes.[13] One group of patients representing what he calls "Type 1 schizophrenia" has a more acute course and a good response to neuroleptics, no evidence of intellectual impairment, and prominent delusions and hallucinations during the acute phase. Crow suggests that the underlying pathological process for Type 1 schizophrenia is a disturbance in dopaminergic transmission. On the other hand, "Type 2 schizophrenia," a disorder more closely related to the dementias, is characterized by negative symptoms such as affective flattening and poverty of speech, a greater chronicity with a poor response to treatment, and impairment in intellectual functioning. Crow speculates that the underlying pathological process in Type 2 schizophrenia is cell loss and structural changes in the brain, as evidenced by ventricular enlargement and cortical atrophy seen by CT.

The distinction between positive and negative symptoms was first introduced by Hughlings-Jackson. He defined the positive symptoms as illusions, hallucinations, delusions, and extravagant conduct and believed they were the product of activity of nervous elements without any pathological process. Negative mental symptoms, on the other hand, were believed to be products of disease.[14]

Thus, within the context of the schizophrenic syndrome, negative symptoms are those that represent a generalized loss of functioning such as occurs in the dementias: they include impoverished speech and thinking (alogia), diminished emotional spontaneity and expression (affective flattening), loss of drive (avolition), loss of ability to experience pleasure (anhedonia), and impaired attention. These symptoms, reminiscent of the "four A's" described by Bleuler, might be considered the "five A's" characteristic of "negative" or "defect" schizophrenia.[15] On the other hand, positive symptoms, reflecting a release from the higher cortical inhibitors, include such typical symptoms as hallucinations, delusions, bizarre behavior, positive formal thought disorder such as fluent derailment and incoherence, and perhaps catatonic motor behavior.

A study conducted by Nancy C. Andreasen and colleagues explored the clinical correlates of ventricular enlargement in schizophrenia by comparing 16 patients with "large" ventricles with 16 patients with the smallest ventricles from a sample of 52 schizophrenic patients.[16] Patients with ventricular enlargement showed some impairment in the sensorium and had a preponderance of "negative" symptoms (e.g., alogia, affective flattening, avolition, anhedonia), whereas those with small ventricles were characterized by "positive" symptoms (e.g., bizarre behavior, delusions, hallucinations, positive formal thought disorder). These findings, according to the researchers, offer a new model for conceptualizing and classifying schizophrenia in facilitating the search for etiology.

Negative symptoms or defect schizophrenia represents a syndrome similar in some respects to the dementias. Factors to study for etiology might include an inherited predisposition, infectious processes such as a slow virus, or other environmental insults such as poor nutrition or poor hygiene, to mention only a few. Positive schizophrenia is hypothesized to be a "release" phenomenon due to more focal brain dysfunction, possibly primarily neurochemical, and is characterized by a normal sensorium and a preponderance of positive symptoms. These two types of schizophrenia may also differ in terms of outcome and response to treatment, with neg-

ative schizophrenia leading to more severe illness with a more chronic and deteriorating course and a poorer response to treatment.

Psychosocial Theories of Schizophrenia

In contrast to the biologic factors just discussed, the psychological and social theories attempt to formulate a nonorganic basis for schizophrenia. The behavioral theorists tend to view schizophrenia as a chronic condition of nonadaptive responses. These theorists believe that early patterns of disturbed behavior are reinforced, which in turn interferes with perceptual and cognitive behavior.

Considerable focus has been placed over the years on psychoanalytic theories of schizophrenia. Melanie Klein emphasized the importance of early mother–child relationships and the development of defense mechanisms.[17] Harry Stack Sullivan stressed deeply disturbed interpersonal relationships as the basis for schizophrenia in contrast to the intrapsychic mechanisms.[18]

Psychosocial Theories of Families

It is instructive to review theories that have been misapplied at erroneous times and places in the lives of schizophrenic patients and their families. In her edited book on *Family Involvement in the Treatment of Schizophrenia*, Marion Zucker Goldstein reviews the role of psychiatric studies on the view of the family.[19] She reported that the much-maligned schizophrenogenic mother of Frieda Fromm-Reichmann's era contributed unwittingly to the development of the parent-blaming approach in subsequent years. When Lidz and Lidz began their studies, they considered that the patient's dependency and symbiotic needs followed upon the mother's inability to establish boundaries between herself and her child.[20] They also hypothesized that the father might be the prime source for schizophrenia, particularly with daughters or with sons when father has strong homosexual tendencies.[21]

By 1967, Lidz described the schizophrenic patient as seeing the world according to the parent's feelings, needs, and defenses.[22] The theories of Lidz and Lidz had a great influence on the practice of mental health professionals and implied parental responsibilities for schizophrenia.

Gregory Bateson and his colleagues studied another form of family bonding and developed the concept of the "double bind," which is a form of family ambivalence.[23] Lyman Wynne and his associates focused on the style of interpersonal relations in the family and the cognitive developments that lead to a sense of purposelessness in the schizophrenic child.[24] Wynne continues along the lines of theories of separation–individuation where unstable stretching of family boundaries of one member could lead to psychosis in another. The mode of communication in these families came to be called pseudomutuality, the unstable boundaries "the rubber fence."[25]

The recommendations of psychoanalysis or intensive psychotherapy for the mother and long-term institutionalization for the schizophrenic child were made with great frequency, primarily on the basis of the theory that this would bring about the much desired separation–individuation and independence of the schizophrenic individual and his mother. The doctor–patient alignment prevailed with the assumption that the patient's improvement was facilitated by both the patient's and the therapist's rejecting the intrusive, over- or understimulating, over- or underprotective, critical, and engulfing family (that is, mother). The concept that the therapist was at the service of the patient and was his advocate against the destructive influence of the family became entrenched in the practice of psychiatry. Gradually, this evolved into studies of patterns prevailing in the families of schizophrenic patients.

Social and epidemiologic theories look at incidence facts. Not only is schizophrenia one of the most complex problems in psychiatry, but statistically, one half of the population in many mental hospitals has the psychiatric diagnosis of schizophrenia. The prevalence of persons who have had or are likely to have schizophrenia in the United States is 1 percent, which yields a total of about 2,150,000.[26]

The factors affecting the development of schizophrenia seem to be age, sex, and marital status. The mid-teens is a frequent age of onset; more women than men are diagnosed schizophrenic; men tend to be single, and women married and then divorced.[27]

Parental Influence
There have been many research studies on the characteristics of children of psychotic parents.

One of the major research studies in the area of mentally ill mothers and their children has been led by a psychiatric nurse, Carol Hartman.[28] Her findings are based on the joint admission of the child and mother to the hospital, and they show that the early development of children of psychotic mothers did not deviate uniformly with children of conjoint admission normal mothers. However, concern remains high for these children identified as high risk, and intervention programs have been proposed.

PSYCHIATRIC DIAGNOSIS OF SCHIZOPHRENIA

There has been an increased focus on developing more precise diagnostic techniques for schizophrenia in order to more accurately predict outcome and to formulate treatment plans. One method is to develop and use standardized structured interview guides, symptom checklists or a scoring system, and computer programs for psychiatric diagnosis. The psychiatric diagnosis of schizophrenia assists in epidemiologic analysis and research interests as well as serving clinical purposes.

Attempts at Classification

There have been many attempts made to isolate the primary deficit in schizophrenia by linking performance deficits on a large number of seemingly unrelated experimental tasks to a single underlying process or deficit. A. J. Yates proposed viewing the person with schizophrenic thinking in terms of information processing models.[29] However, one major problem in disordered thinking with regard to information processing is to locate the earliest stage of information processing deficit, because once a breakdown occurs, any subsequent stage may be adversely affected.

D. L. Braft and D. P. Saccuzzo's research suggests at least two levels of deficit in paranoid thinking disorders: (1) an input deficit in the critical stimulus duration data; and (2) an independent deficit in the speed of processing. This two-factor deficit suggests that paranoid-thinking persons are impaired at both the input and more central processing stages. Normal human cognitive functioning depends on a smooth sequential flow of stimulus processing. Braft and

Saccuzzo suggest that when this normal flow is disrupted, cognitive fragmentation may occur, which is expressed as thought blocking and loose associations.[30]

Psychiatric disorders are multifaceted disorders of function, and the classification of patients is usually based on distinctive symptom patterns. These patterns can be extremely complex, with a large number of variables needing to be considered. The *International Pilot Study of Schizophrenia (IPSS)* was a project in which centers from nine countries were involved in developing patient evaluation methods that could be used for cross-cultural comparison in research with patients with schizophrenia.[31] The patients were divided into two groups—one group of 405 patients diagnosed with schizophrenia and another group of 155 nonschizophrenic patients. The first step in the process was to reduce the 443 overlapping symptoms to a more manageable number of 150 individually discriminating signs and symptoms. The next step was to reduce the overlapping symptoms to 69, and the final step was to reduce this number to a final 12 signs and symptoms. Thus, the 12 most discriminating signs and symptoms were: presence of restricted affect, poor insight, thinking aloud, poor rapport, widespread delusions, incoherent speech, unreliable information, bizarre delusions, nihilistic delusions, absence of waking early, depressed facies, and elation.

This study demonstrated a statistical method for considering patient diagnosis and an interactive approach between clinician and statistician. The *IPSS*, sponsored by the World Health Organization, is a transcultural psychiatric investigation of 1202 patients in nine countries: Republic of China, Columbia, Czechoslovakia, Denmark, India, Nigeria, the Union of Soviet Socialist Republics, the United Kingdom, and the United States. It was designed to lay scientific groundwork for future international epidemiological studies of schizophrenia and other psychiatric disorders.[32]

A Symptom Picture of Schizophrenia

The following is a portrayal of the general description that a patient or family gives of the clinical symptoms of schizophrenia:

The patient often becomes ill for the first time between the ages of 17 and 27. Personality difficulties prior to this early onset tend to go unnoticed, although a careful investigation of the patient's history may indicate early problem areas such as withdrawal behavior, the inability to mix with groups, and angry and unpredictable behavior.

Gradually the person becomes less involved with his daily life in general and becomes obsessed with ideas in particular. At this point he usually expresses verbally some ideas that seem unusual and illogical to his family and community. He thinks that these ideas have special meaning and are related specifically to him (ideas of reference). For example, an uncle may come to visit the family and the patient thinks he is there solely to spy on him. He might also feel that the static or interference one occasionally hears on the telephone is someone listening in or wiretapping the conversation. More and more frequently this kind of behavior is in evidence. The patient may then feel that the whole house is bugged, the television is speaking directly to him, and the FBI is pursuing him. These are false beliefs and delusions that tend to be negative in the beginning, with the feeling that people or some outside forces are intending to hurt him. Later on these delusions may become positive to the person and acquire a grandiose content. The person feels that he is Christ or the Virgin Mary. For example, one woman watched David Brinkley on television and felt that he was in love with her and could not proclaim this publicly but would send messages to her through the medium of television. Every gesture the newscaster made had special meaning to her. Another patient, a young boy, said, "Did you watch the TV press conference? The President said, 'We need the kid here in Washington.'"

The person experiences difficulty in perception. He may develop hallucinations, which means he can see, hear, smell, taste, or feel things in a distorted way. For example, one patient said, "Before I came here, I went to a fire and felt I was going crazy. The voices told me I was."

Another patient said, "I can't eat the food here because it is poisoned." Another patient said, "The air in here is polluted. You are trying to kill us with the gas that comes in through the ventilating system."

At times the schizophrenic patient misidentifies things that are illusions. The patient says, "I was watching TV and everyone turned white." Another patient said, "The headlines of the newspaper said, 'This boy will die. The ship will sink off the Florida Keys.'"

Frequently the behavior may be seen as normal. The only abnormality is connected with the thoughts and ideas, but closer scrutiny of the behavior often disloses gestures, stereotyped mannerisms, or actions that seem odd. This behavior is often in response to the hallucinations and delusional thoughts.

The mood and affect are usually altered. The person is withdrawn and suspicious, or he might be showing a blunting of affect. He may seem more involved with something personal that no one is aware of. His physical appearance and dress may be affected, or he may have lost interest in his personal grooming. Regressive behavior might be observed.

All the above manifestations are part of the general symptom picture of schizophrenia. A specific example of how a patient is perceived follows. The admission interview between the nurse and a 22-year-old patient shows the loosening of thoughts and feelings of the young man.

NURSE: Can you tell me how things have been going for you?

PATIENT: Trying to get my mind off myself. I'd like to get going. I'd like to play some softball. I asked my mother to bring in my low-cut sneakers and she brought in my high-cut sneakers. . . . Aren't I getting better? [Pause] . . . can't sit in the chair. [Moves to a chair behind the nurse.] Where do we go from here? I feel I have lived 50 years already. Maybe I have. What should we talk about? Seems like a lifetime. But when I see my mother, it's okay. Why talk to other people? They are not involved in it. [Silence]

NURSE: What are you doing? [Turns chair to face him.]

PATIENT: Watching you and what you are doing. It means something and not good. You are rubbing your face [nurse was not]. I've got to start somewhere. Feel like crying sometimes.

NURSE: What have you been thinking?

PATIENT: I'm ashamed of myself. I'm sick. It's hereditary. I'm trying to comfort you but you are still scared. You have the cards. I'm scared. I want to get straightened out and I can't get going. It's been two years.

NURSE: I want to hear how you are feeling.

PATIENT: This is the silent crisis. I was swimming in the pool and I cut my knee. The police took me to the hospital. Walking by the police station I was limping and my knee hurt and I wanted a ride. I'm nine years old now. I think I am riding in a truck. Can I tell you this too? He was driving a truck. There was a newspaper between us. I got scared when I saw the headlines. Another time I got lost in the zoo. I'm lost now but I'm in state hospital trying to get myself straightened out. I'm just a kid . . . fifteen years old and I'm scared of myself and what's going to happen. I'm living a farce. I wish I were thirty years old when this happened. It's pathetic and very evil. Do you mind if I stand up and walk around? You turn colors when I look at you.

In this admission conference the patient talks very freely, and it is difficult to ask any of the usual admission questions. The nurse's role is to spend time with him helping to adjust to the unit and feel more comfortable. As his discomfort decreases, he is in a better position to talk about what really hurts him.

DSM-III-R *Diagnostic Criteria for Schizophrenia*

A. Presence of characteristic psychotic symptoms in the active phase: either (1), (2), or (3) for at least 1 week (unless the symptoms are successfully treated):
   1. Two of the following:
      a. Delusions
      b. Prominent hallucinations (throughout the day for several days or several times a week for several weeks, each hallucinatory experience not being limited to a few brief moments)
      c. Incoherence or marked loosening of associations
      d. Catatonic behavior
      e. Flat or grossly inappropriate affect
   2. Bizarre delusions (i.e., involving a phenomenon that the person's culture would regard as totally implausible, e.g., thought broadcasting, being controlled by a dead person)
   3. Prominent hallucinations (as defined in 1b above) of a voice with content having no apparent relation to depression or elation, or a voice keeping up a running commentary on the person's behavior or thoughts, or two or more voices conversing with each other

B. During the course of the disturbance, functioning in such areas as work, social relations, and self-care is markedly below the highest level achieved before onset of the disturbance (or, when the onset is in childhood or adolescence, failure to achieve expected level of social development).

C. Schizoaffective Disorder and Mood Disorder with Psychotic Features have been ruled out, i.e., if a Major Depressive or Manic Syndrome has ever been present during an active phase of the disturbance, the total duration of all episodes of a mood syndrome has been brief relative to the total duration of the active and residual phases of the disturbance.

D. Continuous signs of the disturbance for at least 6 months.

TYPES OF SCHIZOPHRENIA

The *DSM-III-R* groups schizophrenia into the five types described in the following pages: the disorganized type, the catatonic type, the paranoid type, the undifferentiated type, and the residual type (see Appendix).

Disorganized Type

The essential features of the disorganized type of schizophrenic disorder are marked incoherence and flat, incongruous, or silly affect. There are no systematized delusions, although fragmentary delusions or hallucinations in which the content is not organized into a coherent theme are common. Associated features include odd mannerisms, grimaces, hypochondriacal complaints, extreme social withdrawal, and other unusual and bizarre behaviors.

Typical behaviors include giggling, unrelated smiling, and laughter. These behaviors tend to predominate and are undoubtedly responsible for the adjective "silly" being given to this behavior. If there are hallucinations, they tend to be pleasant ones (the smiling and laughing attest to this fact).

The prognosis is poor because regression is generally present. One is struck with the rapid deterioration of the personality. The person often has complete disregard for social restrictions. He eats as he chooses, urinates and defecates at will and wherever he chooses, and masturbates openly. Personal grooming, especially in the female, denotes excessive emphasis. The female may wear odd clothing, for example, blouses buttoned wrong side out and heavy the-

atrical makeup. Hairstyles tend to be representative of the years prior to the illness.

The following case illustrates this clinical type in which the patient has been hospitalized over a 20-year period in a state hospital. The following dialogue was recorded by a nursing student in her first interview with this 54-year-old woman:

I approached this woman and observed her to be slightly unkempt with a state hospital dress that was too short and ankle socks with two unmatched shoes. Her face was marked with a skin disorder, and she sounded as though she had a speech impediment until I realized she had no teeth. I introduced myself and then asked how she felt about being here in the hospital.

She said, "Could you please write to my mother?"

I repeated my question, and she started dictating, "Dear Mother. I had to go back this morning. God will take care of you. He is the power."

I asked how she felt about her mother.

She said, "I feel wonderful. God takes care of the good ones and the bad ones."

I decided to try once again and I asked her why she lived here at the hospital.

She said, "I have to live here because I didn't eat my supper."

The questions and answers continued:

STUDENT: What supper was that?
PATIENT: Yesterday, I tear up my clothes too, you know, yes I do.
STUDENT: Why do you do that?
PATIENT: They tie me up you know, but I am not going to do that anymore.
STUDENT: Why do you tear your clothes?
PATIENT: Because I am not going to lunch. I threw my hot dogs down the hopper, I did. I'm always yelling and screaming. Then they tie me up. Yes, I have to be tied up.
STUDENT: Do you like being tied up?
PATIENT: Yes, yes, I do. But I won't do it anymore.
STUDENT: Do you really like being tied up?
PATIENT: I'm not hungry. I'm not going to lunch. I feel terrible.
STUDENT: Is there anything I can get for you?
PATIENT: No, I have freckles. [Points to her arm and then abruptly gets up and leaves.]

This interaction between student and patient illustrates a stall situation. The student stalled the dialogue by continuing direct questioning of the patient's behavior rather than focusing on the feelings of the patient about either being in the hospital (original question) or about her mother (patient request to student). This example also illustrates some of the difficulties in establishing dialogue with the chronically ill schizophrenic patient.

There has been a marked decline in the number of patients suffering from this disorder, in terms of either new cases being diagnosed or schizophrenics deteriorating to this level within the hospital setting. The explanation may be that early intervention and comprehensive treatment prevent regression to the deteriorated stage.

Catatonic Type

The essential feature of the catatonic type of schizophrenic disorder is marked psychomotor disturbance, which may involve stupor, negativism, excitement, rigidity, or posturing. At times, there is rapid alternation between extremes of stupor and excitement. Associated features include odd mannerisms, stereotypic posture, and waxy flexibility. Mutism is particularly common.

Typical behaviors include abnormal and postural movements. At one end of the spectrum of behavior, the patient becomes so inactive that he cannot move, take care of himself, talk, or eat. He looks paralyzed and acts as if he is in a stupor. When the behavior reaches this point, some treatment approaches suggest tube feeding as a life-saving device to ensure adequate fluid balance; other treatment approaches suggest electroconvulsive treatments. Currently, because of early intervention, many patients do not reach this stage of deterioration and regression.

At the other end of the behavior spectrum, the patient may become extremely agitated and show excessive motor activity. This is called *catatonic excitement* and is characterized by stereotyped motion, impulsivity, and unpredictable purpose. The patient may neither eat nor sleep and thus may become dehydrated and exhausted. Negativistic behavior, or doing the opposite of what is requested, may present itself. When asking a question, the patient may keep repeating the question. Mannerisms, grimaces, and bizarre acts may be part of the symptom picture.

The more classical textbook symptoms of the stupor and waxy flexibility of the musculature, in which the patient stays in statuesque positions for hours, has become a rarity. A possible explanation is that people seek treatment earlier and therefore chemotherapy is effective in preventing the regression to this phase. The following case describes this clinical type:

Mary, a 27-year-old single woman, was admitted to the psychiatric unit from the emergency ward. She posed her hands and arms at times for brief periods during the admission interview. She could be brought back from periods of staring and standing motionless by short questions such as, "How old are you?" She volunteered that her 18-month-old baby was being cared for by her mother.

In her room she had to be directed how to put clothes away in the bureau drawer. She would stop talking in the middle of a sentence but would continue when a question was asked of her. She laughed inappropriately and said things out of context such as, "I'm a bastard." She could give no further explanation for the comment.

She said she was at the hospital because her brother was killed in a fire 4 months previously. She kept asking for cigarettes and then would say, "I'm not supposed to smoke." When asked if she had upsetting thoughts, she answered, "Yes, of burning myself with matches and going out a window."

Paranoid Type

The essential features of the paranoid type of schizophrenia are obvious persecutory or grandiose delusions, or hallucinations with a grandiose or persecutory theme. Delusional jealousies may also be present.

Associated features include anger, unfocused anxiety, argumentativeness, and violence. There may be expressed doubts about gender identity or fear of being thought of as a homosexual, or being approached by homosexuals. The impairment in functioning may be minimal if the delusional material is not acted upon. Also a formal, stilted quality or extreme intensity in interpersonal interactions is noted.

The typical behaviors include extreme suspiciousness and delusions. These behaviors may be seen in the patient's relationships with others. For example, the patient may feel that people are against him and do not like him or that they are plotting against him. Auditory hallucinations may be frequent, and the voices heard may be very threatening and may command him to do specific acts. Ideas may be bizarre. The person may believe that he is God or an important political figure.

The following case illustrates this clinical type:

The patient was brought to the hospital by police, who had received a complaint that the man was disruptive and making a scene in a public place. On interview, the man said that he believed he was telepathically in contact with several political leaders. He said he was being locked up because of the cosmic knowledge that he had, that because he knew the truth about the conspiracy against those political leaders, the conspirators had to keep him locked up in order to protect themselves.

Several weeks later the patient was able to say that he no longer believed he was psychic. He said that he had also thought he could control the world in a good way and not the bad way in which it was going. The nurse asked him when he had first started noticing this kind of thinking. The patient said that he believed he changed when he was 13. Exploration of this issue revealed that when he was 13 he was happy and enjoying being 13. During the fall he was at a football game with his grandfather, and his grandfather fell over dead with a heart attack right in front of him. He said, "All of a sudden I had to be a man." He said no one expressed his feelings about the grandfather's death—that even his grandmother controlled her feelings. The patient said, "Since then I get very frightened when my thoughts begin to drift and I cannot control them."

This case illustrates not only psychotic symptoms but also an unresolved grief reaction that lasted 11 years. Part of the therapy was to help the patient resolve his feelings about the grandfather's death instead of keeping them so tightly controlled.

Undifferentiated Type

The essential features of the undifferentiated type of schizophrenic disorder are prominent psychotic symptoms that cannot be classified in any other type of schizophrenia.

The typical behaviors include incoherence, grossly disorganized actions, prominent delusions, and hallucinations. There are many and varying behaviors noted. This is seen in the following example:

Dick, a 23-year-old college graduate and an analysis engineer, was admitted directly to the psychiatric unit. He sat slumped in the chair with his coat completely covering his face and head. His mother sat next to him looking quite upset and anxious. Dick was reluctant to walk to the ward but when encouraged with, "Would you like to get better?" he came in the door.

During the initial interview Dick said that he had been hearing voices for a long time. He said his eyes seemed funny to him, expressed fear that he was bald, and worried because he was sallow, pale, and his eyes were too red.

Later that day Dick was observed dancing around the ward humming and whistling. He would wave his hand and foot in the air in a spiral motion that ended with his falling on the floor. He replied to questions with grunts and groans. His actions were infantile; he made strange noises with his lips and mouth.

At one point in the afternoon Dick was observed crawling down the hall on his hands and knees. When asked what he was doing, he said he was smelling the flowers.

Residual Type

The essential feature of the residual type of schizophrenic disorder is a history of at least one previous episode of schizophrenia with prominent psychotic symptoms followed by an episode without prominent psychotic symptoms that required evaluation. There is continuing evidence of the illness, such as blunted or inappropriate affect, social withdrawal, loosening of associations, and eccentric behavior with illogical thinking.

NURSING ASSESSMENT IN SCHIZOPHRENIC DISORDERS

Schizophrenia is described in varying ways by clinicians. Some see it as a disease in the classical medical sense. Others see it as a maladjustment in living or an aberrant style of life. For our purposes, schizophrenia represents a complex clinical syndrome consisting of various symptoms described in behavioral terms in the *DSM-III-R* (see Appendix).

Schizophrenia is one of a group of psychotic reactions characterized by basic disturbances in the individual's relationships with people and an inability to communicate and think clearly. The person's thoughts, feelings, and behavior are often evidenced by a withdrawal behavior pattern, fluctuating moods, disordered thinking, and regressive tendencies.

Psychological assessment of an individual who is described as psychotic or diagnosed as schizophrenic requires careful nursing inquiry and observation of the person's thinking, perceiving, symbolizing, communicating, and decision-making skills and abilities. Assessment is made in each of the following areas: alterations in thought content and process, in perception, in affect, and in psychomotor behavior; changes in personality and coping style and in sense of self; lack of self-motivation; psychosocial stressors; and degeneration of adaptive functioning.

Researchers are attempting to develop more objective, reliable methods of classifying patients and are testing standardized, structured interview schedules. Roy Grinker and Philip Holzman, for example, used the Schizophrenia State Inventory (SSI) and identified the following five qualities that distinguish the young schizophrenic from the nonschizophrenic: the presence of a disorder of thinking; a diminished capacity to experience pleasure, particularly in interpersonal relationships; a strong tendency to be dependent on others; a noteworthy impairment in social competence; and an exquisitely vulnerable sense of self-regard.[33]

A symptom classification system has been devised by Dr. Schneider and is widely accepted and used throughout Europe and is gaining popularity in the United States.[34] Schneider's system is based on the presumption that there is a group of easily and reliably observed symptoms that are found only in schizophrenia. These symptoms are grouped into (1) first-rank symptoms (FRS), which are considered characteristic of schizophrenia in the absence of organic brain disease; (2) second-rank symptoms that may be used as evidence for the presence of schizophrenia but are less diagnostic than FRSs; and (3) symptoms that may be present but are not diagnostic. Schneider's first-rank symptoms are noted in the list that follows.

Schneider's First-Rank Symptoms

1. Hallucinated voices speaking the patient's thoughts aloud.
2. Hallucinated voices talking or arguing among themselves about the patient.
3. Hallucinated voices describing the patient's activity as it takes place.
4. Delusional percepts—A two-stage phenomenon consisting of a normal perception followed by a delusional interpretation of it as having a special and highly personalized significance.
5. Somatic passivity—The patient believes he is the passive recipient of bodily sensations imposed from the outside.
6. Thought insertion—The patient believes thoughts are put into his mind by an external force.
7. Thought withdrawal—The patient believes his thoughts are being removed from his mind by an outside force.
8. Thought broadcast—The patient believes his thoughts are somehow transmitted to others.
9. The patient believes that his affect is controlled by an outside force.
10. The patient believes that his impulses are controlled by an outside force.
11. The patient believes that his motor activity is controlled by an outside force.

The person who experiences these symptoms shifts his interest and attention from other people to himself. This change in his relationships with others generally results in the loss of social encounters, friendships, and goal-directed behavior. The person becomes totally absorbed in himself, his thoughts, and experiences; he withdraws from people; he loses his grasp of communication with the world or with what we experience as reality. Because of this impairment, nurse and patient have difficulty talking with each other; neither understands the other when the patient is hearing or experiencing the voices or thoughts. However, there are times in the conversation when the patient does make sense and responds to the nurse. For example, the patient says, "I can't go out for a walk today. . . . The television is broadcasting my thoughts." In another example, the patient says, "I can't go to group therapy. Dr. Karl is sending nerve gas to my brain and killing my brain cells." In each case, the patient responds rationally to the question in part of the dialogue, but he then gives an example of a psychotic symptom as the reason he cannot meet the request of going for a walk or going to group therapy.

The following is an example of how a person can slip in and out of levels of communication between psychotic statements and rational statements. This dialogue was between a nurse and an 18-year-old man on his admission to a psychiatric unit of a general hospital.

The nurse sits down to talk with the patient who is working on a model airplane. The patient says, "I know what I'd like to be doing."

The nurse says, "What is that?"

The patient replies, "Just enough to keep them happy. I can keep on an even balance. I know what I want."

The nurse says, "You are the only person who knows?"

The patient says, "A few other people; only the ones I want to know."

The nurse replies, "Certain people you trust?"

The patient says, "You are going around in circles."

The nurse begins to feel confused and says, "I am going around in circles."

The patient continues, "They all have complexes; keeps them mixed up and gets them crazy. We give them complexes. I am going from jazz to bop to bebop. Does all this sound crazy? I don't know. Sometimes I get carried away. You know what I mean?"

The nurse says, "You are trying to tell me your thoughts confuse you and send you in circles."

During this conversation the nurse could sense the times when the patient himself knew he was going off the subject. He slipped in and out of the levels considered normal, reality-oriented, understandable conversation. The nurse defined the times she felt confused in an attempt to get the patient back to the subject.

The phenomenon of multiple levels of communication can be readily witnessed in ourselves when we become distracted. This experience may have some similarity to that of the schizophrenic patient. For example, as we are listening to a lecture, we can feel our minds wander as we become preoccupied with other thoughts or daydreams. A word or question can often bring us sharply back to the level of the lecture, but sometimes the wanderings into our fantasies become so complex that we are unable to get back to the precise level of the subject of the conversation. Then we may say, "You have lost me," or "I missed the point." By having a point reclarified we can find our way back to the lecture. Similarly, it is helpful to the schizophrenic patient to reclarify reality points and situations. In the example cited above the nurse could say, "I do feel as though I am going in circles. Could we go back over your first statement in which you said that you knew what you would like to be doing?"

Alterations in Thought Content

The nursing assessment of the person's thinking can provide significant information regarding nursing intervention. This method of assessment is based on the assumption that language is the vehicle of thought; that is, language mirrors the process of thinking—what we say is what we think. Obviously, language reflects only a part of thinking; there is a great deal of thinking that is not expressed verbally. However, a careful assessment of thinking requires that we first listen closely to the patient, and then that we question the patient to determine the subjective experience associated with his language to complete our impressions of the "underlying processes."

Delusions

Delusions constitute the major disturbance in the content of thought. The delusions are most frequently bizarre, fragmented, and multiple in nature. For example, a person may hold the belief that people are spying on him or spreading false rumors about him; delusions of reference may derive from the patient watching a television program; or the person experiences thought insertion and feels unable to control his thoughts.

A **delusion** is a false, unshakable belief that cannot be influenced by reason or experience. Delusions are classified in several ways including systematic qualities and the type of delusion. In assessing systematic qualities, it is often noted that the person will build a more or less logical and consistent understanding of a particular situation based on one fundamental error.

The major assessment area regarding content of thinking is the presence of delusions. Patients may report delusions spontaneously, but usually specific questioning is required. Clues suggesting the presence of delusions include evasiveness, suspicion, or other indications or sensitivity regarding aspects of the interview. Generally, a subtle, increasingly specific use of questions is the most appropriate interview strategy. Some questions that may help in eliciting delusional trends in the patient's thinking are:

- Have you felt that something was extremely wrong and that you could not put your finger on it? Did it bother you? How did you explain it?
- Do you feel that others might be responsible for your problems or the situation you are in?

- Has anyone treated you badly or criticized you unfairly, annoyed you, or bothered you in any way that was unusual?
- Has anyone been paying particular attention to you, watching you, or talking about you?
- Have you felt that people on radio or TV were talking about you in their reports? What is the basis for these unpleasant experiences? Why are they happening to you?
- Have you felt unusually well or in very good spirits? Has this resulted in any activities on your part?
- Have you felt responsible for or blamed yourself for your illness or difficulties? Have you felt others blamed you?

Delusions often develop as a defense against intolerable feelings, impulses, or ideas that cause anxiety. The belief, although false in nature, becomes very real to the patient and nothing can challenge the belief. For example, a 17-year-old boy developed the delusion that he was wanted by a national baseball team as a bat boy. He would say:

I was going to be bat boy for the Red Sox. I've let everyone down because I didn't go with them. When the Red Sox took off for spring training, everyone was at the airport waiting for me. I know they were all there. I told Father Murphy about wanting to be a bat boy and he said he would help me. That was two months ago. Everyone is laughing at me. If I go with the Red Sox, everything will be OK. I'll get straightened out; not here in the hospital.

This delusion started out as his natural wish, and it was a subject that people naturally responded to with a 17-year-old boy. Since he was never able to follow through or to test out the idea, the unreal wish that the Red Sox wanted him in Florida for spring training increased. When a topic of conversation that would make him uncomfortable came up, he would revert to the Red Sox bat boy talk.

When he was under stress, the delusional material reappeared in the dialogue. This was the clue for the nurse to back off from the issue and to understand how uncomfortable the patient was feeling.

One could speculate that the meaning of the delusion could be that the Red Sox, who symbolize authority and idealized males, would give him strength and care for him, a boy who never had a father or any male figure in his home. Another aspect is that the status of being bat boy might mean that people would like him better as a bat boy than as a boy in a mental hospital.

It is a favorable prognostic sign when the delusional material begins to lose its solid detail and firmness of conviction.

Rating the Delusional Experience

Delusions are important symptoms of behavior to measure accurately because they often provide the basis for diagnosing severe psychiatric illness. The *DSM-III-R* emphasizes the dominant theme of the delusion, e.g., persecutory, grandiose, etc. Other theories focus on a possible etiology of the delusion, e.g., primary versus secondary, or the diagnostic significance of specific forms of delusions, e.g., delusions of passivity. Kendler and colleagues, in their study of the dimensions of delusional experience, view delusions as a multidimensional clinical phenomenon and suggest a rating scale to measure five dimensions of delusional experience, as follows[35]:

1. *Conviction*—The degree to which the patient is convinced of the reality of the delusional beliefs. An example of high conviction would be a 35-year-old woman who stated she had been in communication with God for the past 8 years. When asked if this could possibly be her imagination, she replied, "Absolutely not." An example of low conviction would be a 45-year-old man who was concerned that he might be infecting people with a dreaded disease. During the interview he stated he thought these ideas were probably his imagination; however, during the week before the interview he would occasionally become convinced of the reality of his fears and then he had to reassure himself that these were just "my sick thoughts coming back."
2. *Extension*—The degree to which the delusional belief involves various areas of the patient's life. The question concerns what persons are involved in the delusion, i.e., family, friends, coworkers, hospital personnel, other patients, or strangers. An example of high extension is a 21-year-old woman who was convinced that everyone, including her family, friends, nurses, even strangers on the street, knew that she was having an affair and were planning to persecute her. After several job changes she continued to be unsuccessful at evading her persecutors. An example of low exten-

sion is a 40-year-old man who believed he was being wiretapped. He believed his supervisor was plotting to get rid of him. When he was not at work, he noticed nothing unusual and no one tried to bother him.

3. *Bizarreness*—The degree to which the delusional belief departs from culturally determined consensual reality. An example of high bizarreness is a 29-year-old man who believed that when the space shuttle Discovery went into orbit, his picture was broadcast throughout all of space and he was declared Lord of the galaxy. An example of low bizarreness is a 38-year-old woman who believed that ever since she telephoned a local talk show to show support for the Soviets destroying the Korean airliner, she had been harassed by the State Department. When asked how she knew this, she replied that her telephone had been tapped because when she picked it up, she could hear a certain noise.

4. *Disorganization*—The degree to which the delusional beliefs are internally consistent, logical, and systematized. An example of high disorganization is a 23-year-old man who reported his beliefs during an interview as follows: His parents were dying; he was being turned into a homosexual; people were being tortured in a gas chamber and being ground up into the drinking water; and he was being poisoned at work by radioactive particles emitted from the lights in the ceiling. He made no attempt to relate these delusional beliefs to one another spontaneously or to do so when he was questioned. An example of low disorganization is a 53-year-old woman who was able to describe in detail the work of the group that had been persecuting her for over 20 years. The group was composed of persons from her graduating class who were "jealous of her great accomplishments." Upon questioning about the "group," she was able to say that only certain persons were really persecuting her and when she really thought about it, she was not sure they were really jealous of her.

5. *Pressure*—The degree to which the patient is preoccupied and concerned with the expressed delusional belief. An example of high pressure is a 54-year-old woman who was convinced the FBI had been using her as an undercover agent to give false information to the Communists about nuclear secrets. In the weeks before the interview, she had spent an enormous amount of time talking to family and friends and poring over her scrapbook for details on how the FBI recruited her. An example of low pressure is a 29-year-old man who was convinced that for the past 5 years he had been Christ. When asked how often he thought of himself as Christ, he replied, "Oh, it comes to me now and then." He denied being impressed about being Christ.

Alterations in Thought Processes

The major features of alterations in thought processes include flow of thought, control of thought, and form of thought.

Flow of Thought

Slowed or inhibited thinking may be due to a variety of conditions, including anxiety or preoccupation as well as depression or organic brain disorders or schizophrenia. *Mutism* is a condition in which the patient is unable to speak. Mutism is present in severely depressed individuals and in persons with organic brain dysfunction, as well as in persons suffering from a catatonic disturbance. *Rapid thinking* may evidence itself through pressured speech or flight of ideas. The individual may be difficult to understand because of the disturbance in the flow of thought.

In disturbances of flow of thought, there may be changes in the train of continuity of thinking. *Circumstantiality* is noted in persons who are unable to come to the point of their conversation. Such a condition may be noted in elderly patients and in obsessional patients as well as in those with formal thought disorder. The person digresses into unnecessary detail.

Tangentiality is classically observed in schizophrenia as well as in persons with organic conditions or chronic alcoholism. This flow of thought is directed toward an incidental aspect of the conversation, and the content of the statement is avoided. *Thought blocking* is another striking sign of schizophrenia and is observed when the patient suddenly stops the flow of thought in the middle of a conversation. *Perseveration* in thinking is the persistent repetition of words, ideas, or subjects so that once an individual begins to speak about a particular subject or uses a particular word, it continually appears.

Control of Thought

Although *obsessional thinking* may occur normally in children and adults, it may be aggravated and sustained by intense anxiety. The individual experiences recurrent or persistent ideas, thoughts, images, or impulses that invade the consciousness. *Thought alienation*, on the other hand, is where the individual describes his thoughts being under the control of an outside source, i.e., he no longer personally possesses his own thoughts. The person may describe *thought insertion* in which he believes thoughts are being forced into his mind from outside; *thought withdrawal* in which the person experiences single thoughts or a train of thoughts suddenly disappearing from mind with the attribution being to another source; and *thought broadcasting* in which the person feels that his thoughts are escaping from his mind and being heard by others.

Questions that may be helpful in eliciting disturbances of thought control include:

- Have you felt forced to think, say, or do certain things?
- Have your thoughts, feelings, or actions been controlled by other people? How?
- Have you felt that your thoughts were not your own, that they were being broadcast or put inside or removed from your head?
- What is the meaning of these experiences?

The following case illustrates thought control experiences of a person with schizophrenic disorder:

Ms. Hague, a 43-year-old single secretary, was brought to the emergency room by the police, who had found her sitting in the middle of a parking lot talking incoherently to herself. She had been well until 2 weeks prior to admission when her employer reported a sudden deterioration in her work performance. She had been forgetful, preoccupied, sullen, and unable to complete her work. She had been absent 2 days from work when the police picked her up.

On admission, Ms. Hague assumed bizarre postures and whispered nonsense syllables to herself. She was disheveled and exhibited poor personal hygiene. Her face was emotionless. She could not respond to questions and was unable to describe her feelings; her speech was comprehensible only for short periods. The volume and rate of her speech changed in crescendo–decrescendo manner. Her thoughts were dominated by delusions of being controlled by God; she thought God was inserting thoughts in her mind and forcing her to speak these thoughts; she claimed she could hear God speaking.

She exhibited no tearfulness. Her sleep and appetite were normal. There were no symptoms of hyperactivity, pressured speech, or grandiosity.

Form of Thought

The most common example of a disturbance in form of thought is the loosening of associations in which ideas shift from one subject to another without the person being aware of the shift. Speech may be incomprehensible; there is little if any information communicated.

Form of thinking traditionally refers to several features. First, there is the *logical character* of thinking. When there is an alteration in logic, the person's thoughts do not lead to conclusions in a manner that obeys the laws of deductive and inductive arguments. However, the logic that people employ in thinking may be difficult to evaluate because normal individuals often make logical errors. If the patient is illogical, the nurse should provide documentation for comparison with other data elicited by the patient.

Second, there is the feature of abstractness. Abstractness lies on the opposite end of a continuum with concreteness. *Concreteness* is the inability to formulate an abstract general principle from a particular group of items or to recognize common characteristics that can be grouped together under the same general category.

The third feature relating to form of thought is *coherence* or *connectedness* of clauses, phrases, and sentences that the person expresses, which allows him to be understood. The person's train of thought must be intact for him to be understood.

Fourth and closely related to coherence is the quality of *association*. The combination of thoughts, when looked at for tightness or looseness of associations, often depends on the person's word choices, the accepted uses of idioms, and the ability to keep to a theme. *Association* is the term used to identify the progression of thoughts a person has as he talks. Normally, one thought logically leads to another. When this logical association progression does not occur, the listener feels lost or confused. The person's thinking comes through to the listener as illogical, chaotic, and bizarre. For example:

I'm not in the hospital. It is the White House; a college campus. I'm trying to tell you the situation. I was shaving and getting my father's hairs. I was relaxed. Didn't jump or anything. A few hairs under the razor every day. I saw six nuns having breakfast at the automat; dinner at Joe and Nemo's.

These associations are not logical. The listener cannot make adequate sense out of one thought before the patient is speaking the next one. Generally, the illogical thoughts increase as the patient's anxiety increases. The listener has difficulty understanding the talk because the associations do not follow any logical progression. Below is another example of illogical speech:

I was standing by the window with my arms folded and a flash of blue hit my side. We're sneaking in just like the Commies. Let's get down to brass tacks. Feel off and on again. Going to throw another curve.

Alterations in Perception: Hallucinations

The assessment for perceptual changes includes evaluating for the presence of illusions and hallucinations. The following quotation is from a psychiatric admission interview with a 21-year-old man and illustrates his illusionary experiences of misinterpretation of reality-based stimuli in the environment.

I remember seeing the doctor in the emergency ward. He smiled when I shook his hand. I didn't know what was so funny, but I went along with him and smiled back. I didn't know this was a mental hospital when I first came here. I thought it was a place for abnormal males. That is what they all looked like—rather feminine. My doctor asked me if I was scared of this place—didn't know what he meant by that. He used to stare at me. He never blinked and he stared at my hands too. I had them down and he kept looking at them.

I could feel the membranes slithering across and back in my head. The doctor didn't say anything when he examined me. When he put the light to my eye, I felt the electricity go through me. He burned my eyeballs.

The head doctor talked to me; he had a curlicue. I thought he was a Communist.

When I went near someone, I would hear the voices saying, "It's time to put the number away and hang up the cleats."

The doctor told me to look at the wall. It was yellow—must have been China. . . .

Hallucinations are the major disturbance in perception, with the most common forms being auditory and visual. The voices may be families, and they often make derogatory or insulting remarks. Command hallucinations may be obeyed, thus having the capacity to create danger for the individual or others.

Useful questions that elicit or augment the description of hallucinatory experiences that are visual include:

- Do you dream vividly?
- Do you see visions in the daytime?
- Do you see flashes of light, patterns, figures, objects that others cannot see?

Questions that help to elicit auditory hallucinations include the following:

- Do noises in your head, ears, or from the outside bother you?
- Do you even hear your own thinking, your own thoughts, as if they were being spoken aloud?
- Do you hear voices when there is no one else around who could be speaking?
- If so, whose voice? Is it clear? Abusive? Accusatory?
- Can you stop the voices from occurring?

Impairment of Affect

Affect refers to feelings and emotions. In the normal state, feelings and emotions generally synchronize with the content of thoughts. When there is impairment of affect, this synchronization does not occur. The emotional response to what the person is saying is inappropriate and it does not match. The mood of the person may appear exaggerated, inconsistent, inappropriate, indifferent, flat, or blunt. In blunted affect, there is severe reduction in the intensity of affective expression; in flat affect, there is no sign of facial expression and the voice is usually monotonous.

Alterations in Psychomotor Behavior

There may be various disturbances in psychomotor behavior such as a marked decrease in reactions to the environment. Or the person may make purposeless and stereotyped, excited motor movements not influenced by external stimuli. In addition, bizarre grimacing and mannerisms may be observed along with pacing and rocking motions.

Changes in Personality and Coping Style

Another major assessment area is to determine the major mechanisms of defense used by the patient as an indication of level of personality organization. The predominant defenses used by persons with schizophrenic disorders include: ambivalence, depersonalization, projection, and negativistic behavior. Also discussed here are changes in sense of self, degeneration of adaptive functioning, lack of self-motivation, and ideas of reference.

Ambivalence

Ambivalent feelings are present in all relationships. The normal person has to constantly deal with the contradictory feelings he has within himself. The schizophrenic person also experiences ambivalence, but it is greatly exaggerated and has a special unrealistic nature toward a given object, person, or situation. For instance, the person may make glaringly opposing statements such as, "I wish my mother would drop dead. I love her so much."

In an interview when a patient asked, "Mind if I open the window?" the nurse replied, "No." The patient then said, "I opened it because I was going to jump. I want to live my life." This patient was psychotically ambivalent about his wish to live.

Knowledge of this ambivalence provides the nurse with clues to the kind of thoughts the patient is having. This patient was having self-destructive thoughts, and the nurse had to carefully evaluate and make a judgment about whether or not the patient was also hearing voices that might command him to jump out the window. The nurse applied external controls when the patient was unable to control his actions. For this patient, control by constant observation by a member of the nursing staff was indicated.

Depersonalization

Depersonalization is feeling not quite real. This state is not necessarily psychotic. In depersonalization the person feels alienated from himself. He finds it hard to distinguish himself from others, and often his own body has a strange and unreal quality to it. Psychotic examples of depersonalization are seen in the first example in this section when the patient says, "I could feel the membranes slithering across and back in my head." This statement indicates the unreal feeling the patient had in his head.

Another example is a patient who says, "My head felt like it took off on a pigeon." This statement describes the unreal quality of the patient's feeling about his head.

Projection

Projection is a defense mechanism and is used at times by everyone. In psychosis the patient is unable to distinguish between what is real and what is projected. For example, the patient says, "My mother said I had to come to the hospital. She is the nutty one. She started crying." This example would not necessarily indicate projection unless the nurse had witnessed the situation or had verification from the mother that it was the patient who had been crying.

Later this patient said to the nurse, "Have you been crying? There are tears in your eyes." The nurse, realizing that the patient was projecting, tried to encourage the patient to express his feelings by saying, "When people are upset, they can cry. Have you known people to cry?" To directly state reality would probably make the patient feel that he had to deny the fact that he was crying. If the nurse were to say to the patient, "No, I am not crying. Why do you ask?" this might cause the patient to feel that he had to defend himself and to say he was not crying.

Expressing the awareness that people do cry, which supports the feelings of the patient, and then asking if he has known someone to cry allows him to make the decision on whom he can select to talk about, his mother or even himself.

Negativistic Behavior

The person with a schizophrenic disorder often shows negativistic behavior. The negativistic defense is generally used to cover feelings of inadequacy and unworthiness. A patient behaving in a negativistic way usually will speak to no one, will go about his business, and will answer no one. Because of this behavior, he is often ignored or left alone.

Disturbances in Sense of Self

The person experiences disturbance in feeling unique, individual, and possessing a sense of his own identity. Lack of self-direction or impairment of motivation is noted. The term describing this phenomenon is *loss of ego boundaries*. There is often confusion over identity and the meaning of existence.

Degeneration of Adaptive Functioning: Autism

There is frequently the tendency to withdraw from involvement with the external world and to become preoccupied with the self and self-thoughts and delusions. This state is called *autism*. Family members and friends report the individual retreating into his world, becoming increasingly emotionally detached from others.

Autism is the extreme retreat into fantasy. The person is continually preoccupied with daydreams, fantasies, or psychotic thoughts such as are experienced in delusions and hallucinations.

Sometimes the patient coins his own words (neologisms). For example, one patient coined the word *atmospherets* and when he was angry, he would say, "Those atmospherets are doing it." He felt these little things called atmospherets were making him do the things that he did not want to do.

The symbolism of the schizophrenic can be seen in his autistic thinking. To understand what the patient is trying to communicate through his symbolic thought is one of the nurse's goals in talking with the patient. The following is an example:

I am a ball bearing; just need to get some oil and get rolling. Get down to a low level and build up slowly to go up the hill. . . . Cut out the malarky. You give me some answers. When do I go to the slave camp? I should have gone last year at this time. How long does a congressional term go? Eight years? What are you waiting for? Me to cry? They can put it on tape. I had a dream. Who runs Washington? They are going to shoot me. Those pigs. [Bangs head against wall.] They're pushing me. I'm the class clown in school except in one class. The only school around a monument. White onyx rings. Let's go by Air Force One. They're making a lot of noise. Bomb shaft open. You're beginning to dislike me. I'm getting discouraged. [Bangs chair.] I woke you up [screaming]. All my new clothes. Don't interrupt me so I can get my story straight.

A ball bearing, slave camp, congress, president, white onyx ring, and airplane are symbols for the schizophrenic patient's feelings of inadequacy and isolation. The symbols all have meanings.

Lack of Self-Motivation

Self-initiated, goal-directed activity, which often impacts on work and other role functioning, is lacking. Pronounced ambivalence regarding decisions can lead to a cessation of work–activity.

Other Behavioral Patterns Associated with Schizophrenia

Associated features include a disheveled appearance or eccentric dress. There is also ritualistic or stereotyped behavior, which may take the form of depression, anxiety, anger, or a mixture of these. There can be depersonalization, derealization, ideas of reference, and illusions. The individual may be disoriented, confused, or have memory impairment.

Ideas of reference occur when the person has the impression that he is the subject of a conversation. In general, the patient interprets cues in the environment as having reference to him. For example:

"At the dance I felt everyone was staring at me."

"There was a new group of nursing students walking down the hall and I heard one say, 'There are lots of young kids in the hospital.' I knew she was talking about me."

These ideas may symbolize the feelings of guilt, insecurity, and alienation. The nurse can deal more realistically with these feelings by helping the patient feel secure within the ward or community setting.

The following are ideas of reference that later developed into a psychotic episode and delusional ideation.

The patient, a 19-year-old college student and ice hockey player, had begun to withdraw from people and school in a subtle way. His parents, not aware of this, began nagging him about his falling school grades, the coach began pushing him for his laziness on the ice, his roommate began picking at him for not keeping the room cleaned up, and his girl friend said she was interested in another boy. Following an unsuccessful hockey game in which his performance was poor, the team lost, and the coach yelled at all the players, Charlie had many paranoid thoughts about the team members. He thought they were talking about him on the bus ride home and that they were either going to throw him in the shower or kill him.

Case Illustration of Assessment Interview

A 24-year-old white man is interviewed by the nursing instructor for the nursing students and the ward staff. The goal of the conference is to design a nursing care plan for this young man. The following is taken from one of the nursing student's reports on the conference:

Target Complaint

"I feel a lot of energy in me." This young man has been brought to the hospital by the police, who had been called to investigate a call that a man was "wandering around by the stores." The police found out that the man was confused and resistive and that he lived in the Halfway House apartment connected with the state hospital. Thus, they brought him to the hospital.

Goal

"I want to return to my job at the battery factory—the job is waiting for me when I get out."

Request

"My mind races and I go up and down." "Help me control my mind."

Fears

"I feel I'll be here forever."

Biological Data

No reported previous or present medical problems. He appears in good physical condition. Played tackle for a semiprofessional football team and looks in good shape. He has taken LSD and describes his trips as "going in circles, bouncing off things."

Psychological Data

"I hear myself think—get backup thoughts. I take waves and thoughts and they go into a laser beam and become alpha rays. Also hear other voices such as Abbie Hoffman." Feels that people watch him—like at work—and that he gets too involved with his work. When this happens, he "blows a fuse." Talked about ITT and IBM and industrial spying and business could not be trusted. Said he was in the hospital because Nixon was also. Believes he can project his thoughts: "Like I can take a pyramid and function at various points."

Social Data

The father is a football coach and has tried to encourage his son in sports, but his son really likes music and wants to play the flute but knows this would not please his father. He has a younger brother and sister. States that his mother is overbearing as are all mothers. Talks of one special friend who has not visited him in the hospital. Was doing well at the Halfway House apartment, but it was noticed he had not been taking his medications.

Cognitive and Behavioral Data

Brought a pencil and tablet to interview and frequently would draw electronic-related figures. He said he felt vibrations from his environment and drew them as oscillating lines being recorded on a machine. At another point he said he was receiving a message and had to write it down. The message was political in nature and referred to Kissinger, the USSR, and the USA.

Adaptive Strengths

Completed high school. Played football for 2 years. Has a responsible job and the employer wants him back. His parents would be available for family therapy. Has done well at the co-op apartments. Has some friends—talks of a previous girl friend. Staff responds positively to this young man.

Psychosocial Stressors

None.

Case Formulation

This 24-year-old young man presents in good physical condition and a semi-unkempt appearance, is currently socially isolated from family and friends, but was working at a nearby factory until admission; demonstrates auditory hallucinations during the interview and is suspicious that all students present are really not nursing students; writes frequently on his pad of paper and laughs inappropriately as he does this; described previous drug involvement. Has been diagnosed as a schizophrenic, paranoid type.

PSYCHIATRIC AND NURSING DIAGNOSIS FORMULATION

The assessment interview resulted in the diagnoses that are listed below:

Psychiatric Diagnoses by Axis

Axis I	295.3X Schizophrenic Disorder, paranoid
Axis II	No diagnosis
Axis III	No physical condition

Axis IV   5, serious illness in self
           (schizophrenic disorder)
Axis V   Current GAF   30
           Highest GAF this year   80

Nursing Diagnoses by Problem

- Alteration in thought content
- Alteration in thought process
- Alteration in perception
- Alteration in affect
- Alteration in psychomotor activity
- Alteration in self-care and usual work and social activities
- Alteration in sense of self; impaired coping
- Alteration in volition

NURSING INTERVENTIONS AND SCHIZOPHRENIC DISORDERS

The person suffering from schizophrenic disorder needs attention, skilled judgment, and respect. Schizophrenia is a mental illness that demonstrates more disturbance in interpersonal relationships and intrapsychic functions than in patients diagnosed with any other mental illness. The nurse feels that she is seeing mental illness in its most profound state when talking with the acutely psychotic person with schizophrenic disorder. One essentially witnesses the person with schizophrenia relinquishing control in key areas of the self. This loss of self-concept is difficult for people to understand and is horrifying to some as an example of the lack of humanness. It is important that each student master her own reaction toward the patient in order to study and treat schizophrenic disorder objectively.

There are some aspects of human behavior within normal limits in which the person does have a sense of losing contact with reality. These examples may give the student a subjective experience of what some of the unreality states that the person with changes in perceptual–cognitive functioning is experiencing may in fact be like. They are the feelings of unrealness or dreamy states, as in adolescent experiences, or even the state of being in love. In these phases we are experiencing the uncanny, sometimes frightening and sometimes idyllic feelings of dissociation and of being completely removed from the situation. To be awakened suddenly from a sound sleep can be an unreal experience; having to deal with unpleasant realities, for example, taking exams, studying, or working, can tempt us to dreamy states in which we prefer the pleasures of our fantasies to the immediate reality scene.

Watch a child play in his make-believe world. Although the people in his world are not real, the child treats them as if they are real. Observe a brother and sister playing the roles of mother and father. In the "game" their wishes of how they would like to be treated, as well as how they are treated, come through. The use of thought in the child tends to be partly creative and partly a testing process. The games help the child learn to deal with the reality of living.

The state of being in love may be likened, in a sense, to the "psychotic" state. When one is completely preoccupied with the thoughts of the beloved person, daydreaming is chronic and the perception of the loved person may be distorted. Unlike the psychotic state, however, the perfunctory reality details of living, such as eating, working, and sleeping, are usually managed. From the thought standpoint, there is a focus and a preoccupation with one theme. The creative, expressive aspect of the thoughts is usually documented through letters, poems, and other signs of endearments.

These examples point out that a thought alteration is not a sufficient condition for a diagnosis of schizophrenia. Other signs and symptoms (as discussed below) will be necessary in order to establish this diagnosis.

Traditionally, the schizophrenias and depressions were viewed as functional disorders. The emphasis was on meaning systems creating aroused or inhibited affective states. In contemporary investigations of etiology, the subtleties of the processing of information in the nervous system and brain are being understood in terms of their biochemical components. This seems at present to be the important manner of understanding the psychotic disorders and some of the major affective disorders. Here we see that the interaction of the meaning systems and the perceptual system of the individual is mediated by biochemistry as well as learning. This understanding creates the necessity for multidimensional assessments and a multimodal therapeutic approach.

Working with people who have developed secondary patterns of reasoning and communicating to deal with the underlying thought process disorders associated with the large category of schizophrenic disorders is for the nurse who welcomes a challenge. It requires courage and skill to suspend one's own personal sense of reality and to step into the beliefs and meaning structures of another who is attempting to make sense out of a very disruptive process that impacts on perception and affective expression.

Autognosis

Perhaps the most important evaluation nurses need to make is of the parameters of their sense of anxiety and fear in communicating with someone who thinks and expresses himself in a seemingly different and unpredictable manner. Perhaps the notion of unpredictableness is the most frightening aspect for new nurses working with people who have psychotic disorders.

Basic factual information is a first step in helping with this fear. First of all, most people with psychotic disorders are usually more frightened than you are. Second, any impulsive yelling or rejecting or pushing or running away is an expression of that underlying fear. Third, there is a deep sense of humiliation and inadequacy felt by people whose thinking and communication do not facilitate their participation in the world and their ability to affect the behavior of other people.

The first question that nurses have to ask themselves is: To what extent is my fear based on my own imagination of what can or might happen and to what extent is it based on solid observations of threatening behavior by the patient? The second question is: To what extent can the nurse recognize and make contact with the human, caring dimension of the patient? This latter question is based on the fact that no one is ever totally psychotic. For example, somebody may hear voices and be deluded but may also be able alert the nurse to some reality aspect occurring on the ward.

The other aspect of dealing with fear is to be familiar with the signs and characteristics of individuals, with or without psychotic disorders, who are violent. Violence is not a function of psychoses. Violent behavior has its roots in two major domains: (1) specific, organic dysfunctions within the brain; and (2) learned patterns of violence.

Another autodiagnostic tool is to question to what extent the nurse has to have sense made out of an immediate experience with people. Can the nurse tolerate the anxiety of not understanding and not knowing? Patients who are fearful often like to present obscure communications as a way of protecting themselves from being equally confused in the environment of thought disorders.

Some of the symbolism and experiential meaning level of psychotic patients can provoke extreme anxiety because it is so immature. The nurse has to be prepared to develop a sense of understanding and comfort with hearing information or witnessing certain kinds of behaviors that are developmentally inappropriate but do take on comprehensible meaning when translated in terms of the prelogical framework of the client. For example, a 32-year-old woman was admitted to a psychiatric unit because she attempted to jump out a second-story window. The sequence of her behavior was as follows: She was out shopping for the household of 17 people who lived in a seven-room flat. While in the supermarket, she had the experience that everyone was staring at her and thinking about her. Her body began to feel heavy and she began to feel as if the weight of the world was on her. Perplexed by this physical feeling, she presumed she must be God to have such a weight on her. She returned home to the apartment with all the members there and it became warm. She responded to the warmth with the thought that a fire was starting in the apartment and she had to escape. She made a dash to go out the second-floor window when she was stopped by the family members. The logic employed to cope with the feeling and emotions connected to a complex family system and life was primitive. Her sense of being overwhelmed was cast into a fable of omnipotent power counterpointed of a fear of being destroyed by fire from the outside. This example is of an acute psychotic break in a very dutiful, religious, caring woman. She was somewhat embarrassed by her thinking process and was in particular embarrassed by believing she was God. With sensitivity and some humor, the nurse was able to convey to the woman how these events were a metaphor and made immeasureable sense in a nonsensical way to a very complex life and living situation. The nurse emphasized that there were other ways of getting help than her elaborate symbolic method.

Stalls

A stall can occur when the nurse feels overwhelmed by the altered thinking of the client. When you feel you do not know what you are doing or what is going on, it is an indication that you are being challenged to step into some new territory for a period of time. Stalls really mean that rather than being resistant, the patient is offering perceptions and information that are foreign to the nurse. This is where nurse and patient learn. The nurse needs to openly discuss the fact that somehow they are not communicating and are going around in circles. This openness shares the responsibility for the relationship and for efforts in communicating between the client and the nurse. It does not place the relationship in a superordinate power struggle. If this approach is not successful, it is useful to have consultation or supervision on the matter.

Communication Strategies

Given the fact that patients are having difficulty with basic information processing in many of the psychotic disorders, it is important that patients be comfortable presenting their perceptions and reasoning without feeling they are going to be criticized or humiliated. An approach to this is to work with patients and their families in a group structure, explaining to the best of the nurse's ability some of the information that documents the alterations in thinking and feeling patterns of people who have psychotic disorders. This allows the patient and others to keep both interpersonal and personal operations at a level and scope that can be handled by the patient without inducing disruptive anxiety. At times, this is a difficult task because patients have good intelligence and are aware that they are not putting experiences together in a manner that leads to successful planning or communication with others.

Nursing Intervention for Three Types of Behaviors

In planning patient care, the nurse assesses each patient thoroughly, diagnoses nursing prob-

lems, establishes long- and short-term goals, determines appropriate approaches of care for the particular patient, and then carries through with the specific nursing intervention.*

The role of the psychiatric nurse in the care of a person with a thought disorder or who behaves in an autistic, withdrawn, or regressed way must be flexible. Because the person communicates at various levels and is in control of himself at various times, the nurse, by necessity, has to be able to adjust the nursing care as the situation demands. The care of these three types of patient behavior, presented as first-order problems, will be discussed in terms of typical behaviors, goals, and nursing intervention. It is important to observe each patient individually to determine the best nursing care. Even though a patient is diagnosed as "schizophrenic," there is no set approach for the nurse to use. The nurse must observe the behavior the patient exhibits and how it is a problem for him.

Nursing Care of the Patient with Altered Thought Processes

The following treatment plan for the patient with an alteration in thought processes related to a schizophrenic disorder is presented in Figure 37-1. The typical behaviors and nursing interventions are described.

Typical Behaviors. The patient maintains false beliefs despite experience to the contrary; he experiences distortions of reality and magical thinking; he often misinterprets the speech and actions of others; he tends to be very lonely; he experiences hallucinations; he often appears unaware of what is going on around him; he has a low frustration tolerance; he uses impersonal pronouns, e.g., "they," "them," "everyone," etc., and may talk out of context with the conversation.

Nursing Intervention. The nurse should be consistent. The autistic patient is often frightened and bewildered. He needs to realize that the staff is not frightened by his behavior and that they can be counted on for help.

The nurse should provide supervision so that the patient will not injure himself or others. The patient may experience "visions" or "voices" directing him to cause harm to himself

---

* This section through pp. 748 is written by Linda Muh Spink.

Hanna Pavilion Interdisciplinary
Treatment Plan

Specific Discipline: _____ Personnel Responsible: _____

Date Entr/ Updte	Prob. Num.	Problem Description in Behavioral Terms	Measurable Outcome Objectives	Specific Treatment Approach	Targ. Date	Date Reslvd
		Alterations in Thought Processes Related to ___	Long-Term: By discharge patient will maintain basic level of functioning, with or without assistance despite presence of disorganized or otherwise disturbed thinking.	A. Assist patient to obtain optimal levels of functioning and provide assistance where functioning is impaired, as with activities of daily living, to maintain basic level of functioning (see also Self-Care Deficit). B. Establish and maintain trusting relationship with patient. C. Communicate with patient in clear simple manner, avoiding abstractions, double meanings, and subtle wit.		
			By discharge patient will identify symptoms of illness and will discuss feelings generated by unrealistic thoughts and the consequences these have for life-style.	D. Assist patient to focus on feelings which are associated with unrealistic thought content and the effect these have on life-style. E. Teach relationship between medication effects and symptoms of illness (see Knowledge Deficit or Noncompliance). F. Help patient organize thoughts and actions by providing step-by-step directions and structured activities if patient is unable to organize self.		
			By discharge patient will identify community resources to support reality testing.	G. Inform patient of appropriate support resources in the community (e.g., mental health clinics, hotlines, support groups, etc.)		
			Short-Term: Will not harm self or others by ___ (date).	H. Reassure patient of his safety in the hospital. Institute suicide precautions if thoughts (e.g., command hallucinations) are destructive in nature (see also Potential for Violence).		
			Will not act on command hallucinations, or other unrealistic thoughts by _____ (date).	I. Instruct patient to not act on hallucinations. Reassure patient that such thoughts will not harm him.		
			Will report hallucinations to nurse as they occur by _____ (date).	J. Instruct patient to report hallucinations (e.g., voices) to nurse as they occur.		
			Will seek assistance from nurse and others to distinguish between realistic and unrealistic thoughts by _____ (date).	K. Assist patient to distinguish unrealistic thoughts from reality. Encourage patient to validate his perceptions with nursing staff and others. L. Cast doubt on unrealistic thoughts, i.e., let patient know that you do not share patient's thoughts or perceptions.		

From Novikoff, L., Tolbert, M., & Mauders, C., University Hospitals of Cleveland, Hanna Pavilion.

Figure 37-1.

or to other patients or staff. He needs the security of knowing that the nursing staff will not allow him to carry through with these dangerous impulses. A firm, directive, but gentle approach is best with the patient. One 10-year-old chronic schizophrenic girl often experienced auditory hallucinations telling her to cut herself.

A typical situation follows:

The patient runs into the kitchen, grabs a glass and breaks it, then takes broken glass and begins to cut her wrists. The nurse, running into the room, firmly grabs hold of the patient's arm. She says, "Sally, give me the glass. I will not allow you to hurt yourself.

We will wash your arm, and then you will sit by me until you feel more under control." The nurse then proceeds to carry through with the stated actions.

Often there are prn medications ordered for the schizophrenic patient, usually major tranquilizers. These medications help the patient to have more self-control and fewer confusing thoughts. The nurse can use these as an adjunct to her care to calm the agitated, impulsive patient. The patient needs to learn to accept responsibility for his actions and to ask for medications when he is feeling out of control. He should be encouraged to come to the nursing staff during these difficult times. The nurse must be careful never to use medication as a form of punishment but rather as just one method of helping the patient recover.

The nurse should increase social interaction for the patient gradually. As with the patient who is suspicious, this person also needs his activities to be increased in a gradual, nonthreatening way.

The nurse should accept the patient as a worthwhile individual without passing judgment. A person's self-image will improve when others see him as a worthwhile person. The nurse should be sensitive to the patient's feelings and should understand his need for his fantasy world. When the patient realizes that he is accepted, even with his bizarre behavior, he will find it easier to give up his autistic existence.

The nurse should never attempt to talk or argue the patient out of his delusions. The patient will give up his false beliefs when he is ready and not before.

Milton Rokeach reports in his book, *The Three Christs of Ypsilanti*, on three patients who all thought themselves God.[36] He got them together in a group, hoping that they could be talked out of their delusions because "obviously" there cannot be three Gods. By the end of the group meetings, instead of seeing reality, the three had "realized" that one was Jesus, one was God, and one was Mary. Needless to say, the patient cannot be talked out of his delusion!

The nurse should present reality. She should try to divert the patient from his delusional expression to a reality-centered situation. It is important to focus on the present, on issues that are reality-based, e.g., the weather, sports, occupational therapy activities, etc. The nurse should give reinforcement when the patient talks of reality-based things.

She should provide an opportunity for the patient to express his feelings, being careful not to perpetuate his autistic thinking.

The nurse should seek out the patient for short intervals of time. The very autistic patient cannot tolerate interactions for long periods. When spending time with the patient, the nurse should note how long he can tolerate her presence before he becomes more agitated, more delusional, etc. She can then shorten her time with the patient to less than what he can tolerate. In this way, the patient learns to associate the nurse with a positive experience, rather than as a negative, threatening situation.

The nurse should understand that even if the patient does not acknowledge her presence or seems unaware of events surrounding him, she and others do have an effect on him; it often takes time for the patient to feel secure with the nurse before he can invest in the relationship.

Nursing Care of the Withdrawn Patient

Some schizophrenic patients have negativistic behavior; they withdraw from their environment. The person who withdraws is unable to invest emotional energy outside of himself. Each person responds to stress in different ways—many schizophrenic patients choose to withdraw from their environment because the world around them is too threatening.

Typical Behaviors. The withdrawn schizophrenic is shy, aloof, lonely, apathetic, isolated, inadequate, inappropriate, autistic, and often very resistant to any form of suggestion from the environment.

Goals. In setting goals for this patient, the nurse must assess what is behind the withdrawn behavior. Usually, the patient is so afraid of others and of himself that he withdraws. Therefore, the nurse's long-term goal would be to increase the patient's self-esteem and help him to feel secure with other people. As a short-term goal, the aim would be to establish a therapeutic rapport with the patient in a one-to-one relationship.

Nursing Intervention. The nurse should limit the environment for the patient. There is security in sameness, and so this patient does best on a small unit. He should not be taken off the unit to occupational therapy or other activities until he has had an opportunity to feel comfortable with the environment and himself.

The nurse should recognize that the patient tends to isolate himself from other patients and from the staff. It is important to remember that in order for a patient to achieve psychological homeostasis, he must have interactions with other human beings. Thus, it is the nurse's responsibility to seek the patient out frequently. He has had many painful experiences with people and so has found it easier to reject others than to risk being rejected. The nurse must adopt a nonjudgmental, accepting manner with this patient. It may be necessary to sit in silence with him. It is important to understand that even if the patient gives no acknowledgment of the nurse's presence for a long period of time, consistent reaching out by the nurse will have an effect on the patient.

The nurse must make consistent, steady attempts to draw the patient into some response *without* demanding a response. The following is an example:

NURSE: Hello, John, I'm Susan, a nursing student.
PATIENT: [No response.]
NURSE: I thought I'd sit with you awhile and we could talk.
PATIENT: I have nothing to say. [Gets up and walks away.]

In this case the student stalled the therapeutic process by requiring the patient to talk. Had she only said, "I thought I'd sit with you awhile," the patient might not have felt threatened by her presence and might have been able to stay sitting with her.

As with the autistic patient, the nurse should take note of how long the patient can tolerate her presence. She should be certain that the patient does not associate her with unpleasant feelings. Gradually, the time of the visits can be lengthened. The patient has to feel secure before he can invest any energy beyond himself in another individual or group.

Again, the nurse should initiate conversation that is reality-oriented and concrete, conversation in which the patient can participate, such as the weather, sports events, a magazine—any topic that is nonthreatening. The nurse should accept that initially the conversation may be very one-sided and limited.

She should also attempt to stimulate his interest in an activity or recreation and should try to find activities that he will be able to succeed at, so as to increase his feeling of self-worth.

One very withdrawn patient indicated that years ago she had done needlepoint. The occupational therapist was notified and brought several simple needlepoint kits for her to work on. This craft served as the foundation for establishing a relationship with the patient.

As the patient is provided positive experiences, he will begin to feel better about himself, and, in turn, will have more energy to invest in his surrounding environment. As the withdrawn patient begins to socialize more on the unit, the activities he is involved in should be gradually increased. After the nurse has established a one-to-one relationship with the patient, she should, as with the suspicious patient, slowly increase his involvement with other staff and patients. The patient can be encouraged to attend occupational therapy and other activities without having to interact with many patients until he is ready. As he begins to feel good about his success, he will feel good about himself.

Nursing Care of the Regressed Patient
Some schizophrenic patients demonstrate very regressed behaviors. This is a return to a more infantile pattern of behavior.

Typical Behaviors. The regressed patient may be helpless, have temper tantrums, maintain a fetal position, withdraw from responsibility, be enuretic or encopretic, or rebel against authority in other ways.

Goals. The nurse's goals for the regressed patient center on preventing further regression and avoiding fostering dependency. Eventually, the aim is to achieve the appropriate level of functioning.

Nursing Intervention. The patient should be encouraged to participate in ward activities and the daily routine as much as possible. He should be allowed to proceed at his own pace and be gently encouraged to increase his level of functioning.

The nurse must encourage the patient to make his own decisions—making them as simple as needed for the individual patient. Positive reinforcement is very important for the regressed patient. Compliments and attention should be given when he does something well and assumes more responsibility for himself. It is important to avoid punishing the patient for periods of regression. Often these patients need protection from other patients on the unit because of their socially unacceptable behavior.

Operant conditioning, or behavior modification, is often successful with the regressed patient. It is a program set up with rewards for positive behavior, as shown in the following example:

A 23-year-old graduate student was admitted to the hospital very withdrawn and regressed. She remained in her room all of the time and was enuretic and encopretic. Two things she liked to do were to eat cookies and smoke cigarettes. A program of behavior modification was set up to reinforce her positive behavior. The patient was allowed to have one cigarette every hour routinely. If she was to have more cigarettes, she had to behave in an acceptable manner. As the days progressed, the patient was expected to assume more responsibility for herself. Within 2 weeks of admission, the patient was assuming care for herself, was no longer enuretic or encopretic, and no longer needed to be on the behavior modification program.

The schizophrenic patient may react to the nurse with hostility, regression, anger, or rejection. It is important to remember that this is not directed at the nurse as a person. The patient's need for deviant behavior will decrease as his needs are met—in other words, when he feels more secure, he will not need to communicate in a distorted manner.

BIOLOGIC MODEL OF NURSING CARE

The prominent medical treatment of schizophrenia is prescribing phenothiazine medication. Delusions, hallucinations, and bizarre behavior are often partially controlled by adequate doses of phenothiazines. Medical research is focused on determining the proper dosage schedule (e.g., rapidly increasing dosage until side effects become bothersome versus gradually increasing dosage), the pros and cons of prophylactic or maintenance antiparkinsonian drugs, and at what point, if ever, maintenance doses of phenothiazines should be discontinued.

The nurse's role is to dispense the prescribed medication and to be responsible for knowing the reactions and the side effects of the drug dosage. The nurse much watch for parkinsonian symptoms, skin rashes, bone marrow toxicity, photosensitivity, and all other reactions described in Chapter 21.

Patients must know the drugs they are receiving and they must know how to report the side effects. This should be part of the negotiations for the nursing care plan. Teaching patients and family members about their medications is an important service that the nurse provides during inpatient treatment as well as when the patient is an outpatient.[37]

PSYCHOLOGICAL MODEL OF NURSING CARE

There are two main talking therapies that the nurse may select for intervention with the schizophrenic patient: the primary therapist role and the one-to-one therapy relationship.

Primary Therapist

The role of primary therapist does not differ from that used in clinical diagnostic situations. The nurse uses the skills and techniques appropriate to the specific therapy of crisis or issue-oriented therapy, psychotherapy, or other models for which the nurse has been educated. Training to practice psychotherapy generally requires additional clinical and academic experience at the master's level and is equivalent to other professional training in psychological therapies.

One-to-One Relationship

The one-to-one relationship is indicated for patients who are acutely psychotic or who have been hospitalized for a long period of time. They need a one-to-one relationship as a prelude to other psychological interventions. Many of these people do not begin to mix in and socialize until they experience a one-to-one relationship with a reliable professional. It helps to integrate the patients into the ward or group through the experience of being able to relate to one person. They begin to reach out to another human being and do not feel so threatened. They gain some support and positive experiences that make them less likely to be frightened of other people. Many schizophrenic people are hospitalized because they cannot get along with people and most of their significant relationships outside have deteriorated. If the therapeutic relationship is continued long enough, many of the problems the patient has in dealing with people will eventually come out in the treatment situation. Learning that they are being treated differently from before can serve as a corrective emotional experience. These patients come expecting to be rejected or to be hurt or to hurt someone emotionally. The therapeutic relationship should teach a new, healthier way of interacting with another human being.

Below are the steps that are usually followed in initiating, developing, and terminating a one-to-one relationship. A case illustration follows this outline of steps.

Step One: Establishing an Alliance
- Explain to the patient who you are, why you want to talk, and for how long (weeks or months, see Chapter 15).
- Negotiate a therapeutic contract: patient request and nurse's services.
- Diagnose needs that you can meet and that won't frighten the patient.
- Collaborate with psychiatrist or staff to ensure this therapy is compatible with the overall treatment plans.
- Go slowly in the beginning, both in time spent with the patient and in content of sessions, especially in terms of talking about patient problems because nobody talks to you until they know you.
- Keep detailed notes for supervision. Take down details on what you say and what the patient says and then what you do. By reviewing this with your supervisor you both can get a picture of the dynamics of the therapy.

Step Two: Developing the Relationship
- Watch for things that might drive the patient away, for example, certain topics or issues. You are dealing with a person whose biggest problem is people, and he is easily frightened and threatened.
- Listen to what the patient wants to talk about.
- Listen for themes. As the patient feels more comfortable, he will talk about more meaningful issues. The nurse's role is to help the patient see an issue clearly enough so that he can make up his own mind. A stall can occur during this phase if you give advice because you will be controlling someone who is agreeing in order to please you.
- Use the therapeutic relationship to support looking at issues in depth. This is an indication of the patient's ability to respond to psychotherapy. If the patient moves to this point, psychotherapy might be a treatment model of choice.

Step Three: Termination
- Allow adequate time to talk about your separation and termination of the relationship. At least 3 weeks are necessary for a 3-month relationship. New symptoms and regression may occur, as well as the painful memory of previous losses. The patient and nurse need to talk about this as a reality issue.

The following case illustrates the one-to-one relationship with a severely withdrawn chronic schizophrenic patient.

CASE EXAMPLE

Lorraine Syke is a 29-year-old woman who physically looks about 16 years old. She is a shy, withdrawn young woman who has been hospitalized at a large state hospital for the past 5 years. Very few data have been gathered on her family, although one part of the history cites examples of her bearing the brunt of a foster mother's anger. She was abused both physically and verbally. The history was obtained from an older sister who stated that "Lorraine was always the scapegoat—the littlest and youngest in our family who was always picked on."

Lorraine's retreat to isolation and her feelings of unworthiness were so deep-rooted that it took a 2-week period for her to accept any kind of communication from the nurse. The following is taken from the nurse's supervision notes on the one-to-one relationship:

Before my entry on the ward, Lorraine spoke to no one, answered no one spontaneously, but was able to respond to commands of the ward staff and to function as they requested. She never answered back or displayed any anger, but she unquestioningly performed whatever was asked of her.

During my first three meetings with Lorraine, I repeated each time that I would be with her for a specific time period, and all three times Lorraine shook her head "no" and then proceeded to go through a series of nonverbal communications telling me to go away and leave her alone. She would seek all available places to keep me away, such as going into the bathroom, lying on her bed with her eyes closed, selecting a chair in the middle of the room with nothing near it for me to sit on, and walking very fast between beds and chairs of the ward, making it impossible for me to follow next to her.

On the fourth visit, Lorraine spoke her first words to me. I asked her if she had gone out with the patients the day previous. Lorraine looked at me and shook her head "no." She did, however, look as though she wanted me to continue talking because she did not make her usual movements to get away from me. She then said, "I don't go out for walks. I can't go." I asked why not. She said, "No, I get lost. I don't go anywhere."

The fifth visit proved to be the initial breakthrough in establishing an alliance for communicating. This day as I went up to her, she was able to stand in front of me and pace in step. Her feet kept moving the whole time and she began an inspection of me. She looked at me very carefully, first at my face and told me I had pretty lipstick. Then she pointed to a pin and asked me what is was. Then she asked me what time it was and took hold of my wrist to see my watch and put the watch to her ear. I took my watch off, handed it to her, and said she could listen to it tick. Lorraine did exactly as I requested and then gave the watch back to me. She paced a little faster and then asked me my name. I had repeated my name each time I went to visit her, and this time she repeated my name back after I told her once more. She then wanted to know where I came from—what town. I asked where she came from and she told me "no place." At this point Lorraine began to walk and I walked with her. It was a leisurely pace and I could keep up with her.

At this point in the relationship, the patient is reaching out to the nurse and is able to ask questions of the nurse, but she is not able to cope with the questions she is asked. The next 2 weeks were characterized by this kind of dialogue. Lorraine asked the nurse questions, but in return she was negative to each of the nurse's questions. She said there was nowhere to go, that she never went anywhere, that she didn't do anything, that she didn't like television, that she didn't like to walk, that she didn't know anyone. One day during the third week the nurse said that it was a nice day and asked Lorraine to walk outside with her. Lorraine said that she didn't go outside. Then suddenly she grabbed the nurse's hand and started down the stairs. The relationship continued with many walks outside. Lorraine was now able to verbalize freely, but her talk was so jumbled and symbolic that the nurse could not easily understand the content. Lorraine, however, just wanted to talk and did not want the nurse to say anything. During one of the early walks outside, Lorraine indicated her need to be listened

to and to be accepted. Lorraine said that she did not have a boyfriend but she did have a sister. She said that she never hears from her husband and that she has two daughters, ages 7 and 2.

The next week Lorraine presented more material that seemed to be testing whether or not the nurse would be able to accept her and her past. She repeatedly had been asking the nurse if she was a "bad girl." Finally, she mumbled something about "not a virgin—a prostitute—oh, I don't know." She continued to mumble something about the law and then she started to cry. This was the first time that human emotion appropriate to the content of the interview was expressed. It seemed that Lorraine felt very distressed that she had had a baby when she was not married, that the law defined the child as illegitimate, and that people called her bad names.

Lorraine was able to continue to talk about the sadness and loss in her life. She told of her parents' deaths and her husband's loss of desire for her. She worried about her daughters being in a foster home. She said that neither her brother nor her sister wanted her to live with them and that "no one wants me." Lorraine was able to cry at length when she talked of this part of her life, and the nurse helped to bear the feelings of loneliness and rejection. Gradually, she was able to talk more about doing something. Again, the initial presentation was a negative one. In the third month of the relationship, Lorraine said, "I don't know what to do. I don't want a job. I don't have anyone to talk with." At this point the nurse and Lorraine were sitting on a bench in the day hall of the hospital ward where another patient came along and sat down, but first she gave Lorraine a little push. Lorraine became overtly angry for the first time and said loudly, "Quit pushing me around." She then turned to the nurse and said, "Let's go." As she walked past the other patient, she said very distinctly, "Go to hell." Lorraine was beginning to feel secure in expressing both negative and positive feelings and was able to take a stand for herself. She also was able to say she had been thinking about work.

It became an appropriate time for the nurse to begin to set limits on some of Lorraine's behavior, for she was becoming very demanding of the nurse's attention and time. This example of holding firm and being consistent can be seen in the following example in which Lorraine tried several different ways to maneuver the nurse into taking her out for a walk. The patient had a bad cold, the weather was cool and rainy, and therefore the decision was made that the patient would be seen for the therapy interview inside.

PATIENT: Take me outside, please take me outside today.

NURSE: We can't go outside because of your cold. We will be able to go outside when your cold is better. Today we will stay inside.

PATIENT: I don't have any cold. [Pauses for about 4 minutes.] Come on, let's go outside.

NURSE: I have told you we can't go outside.

PATIENT: [Loudly] I don't have any cold. Oh, what's the use of talking [very disgusted tone of voice].

NURSE: You don't feel like talking if we can't go outside?

PATIENT: [Walks away angrily.] Everything is useless.

NURSE: Useless?

PATIENT: [Silence.]

NURSE: I can't take you for a walk; what can we do today?

PATIENT: [Relief is shown.] What are you supposed to do?

NURSE: Let's talk about it.

PATIENT: [Mumbles softly and then bursts out] Help me.

NURSE: Yes, I want to help you.

PATIENT: Please take me out [takes nurse's hand and pulls her toward the door].

NURSE: We can walk up and down the ward and we can talk, but I can't take you out.

PATIENT: Why can't you?

NURSE: I like being able to see you and talk to you.

PATIENT: There is nothing to talk about. Why can't you take me out? [Becomes increasingly angry and loud.]

NURSE: Seems like I can do nothing.

PATIENT: [Outburst of anger with arms thrashing and aimed at the nurse.] This is all useless. [Patient starts away from the nurse.]

NURSE: [Nurse catches up with the patient.] You are angry with me.

PATIENT: [Patient starts to cry.] I want a cigarette.

NURSE: I don't have any.

PATIENT: [Patient stops still and looks at the nurse.] I haven't heard one word you have said today. [Stamps away.]

In this situation there are at least seven different ways in which the patient dealt with the limit set by the nurse: (1) by persistently requesting to go out; (2) denying the rational reason; (3) crying; (4) indirectly asking with the request for a cigarette; (5) acting stubborn and saying, "Why talk?"; (6) using physical force; and (7) withdrawing.

Helping the patient to learn to accept the denial of wishes is not easy for the nurse. If the nurse can remain consistent and accepting through all the patient's testing maneuvers, therapeutic gains can be made.

It was shortly after this session that the nurse brought up the issue of separation and termination of the relationship. The last 3 weeks of the 4-month relationship were spent working on the problem of separation that had created an upsurge of feelings of rejection and unworthiness. However, Lorraine had shown positive growth, and the hospital staff had started noticing her more and commenting on her in a positive manner. She was seeking out staff and making requests of them. Lorraine was presented at a staff conference and plans were made to help her become involved in an activities group and to encourage her to take a hospital job. One of the hospital nurses said that she would continue to meet with Lorraine to talk about her work, her leaving the hospital, and her living in a co-op apartment.

SOCIAL MODEL OF CARE: FAMILY INVOLVEMENT IN TREATMENT

The extreme stress and disruptive life-style that families of a schizophrenic person experience because of the patient's often irrational and bizarre behavior is not well understood by many people, including mental health professionals. Also the extent of stress that a person with a psychosis causes for close family members has not been documented until recently. According to these recent studies, the symptomatology and patient outcome adversely affects many aspects of family life.[38,39]

The study of the interactions between a schizophrenic individual and his family, and how these communication patterns change over time, has achieved even greater significance for mental health staff who attempt to care for these individuals. The common goal of caretakers of schizophrenic individuals is to prevent or delay the occurrence of a relapse while enhancing the patient's optimal functioning in settings suitable to his individual needs. The achievement of this goal has now been shown by researchers working in a number of settings to be related to a combination of psychotherapy, chemotherapy, and social-skills training for patients; psychoeducation of families; and availability of community support programs for both patients and families.

The following case example illustrates the importance of including the family in the assessment and treatment of a person with a schizophrenic disorder.

CASE STUDY*

My initial interview with Shirley Bradley took place October 9, 1987. Shirley Bradley is a 46-year-old, twice-divorced, obese, neat, clean, white female who appears younger than her stated age. She is an inpatient in a state hospital who articulates concerns about her 17-year-old and 18-year-old daughters. They work full-time and live with the client's mother. Shirley states "they need a mother, they need a mother's hugs and kisses." Patient requests discharge to low-income housing, which would enable the daughters to live with her. Future discharge plans are to a Community Residential Rehabilitation (CRR) home as Shirley Bradley's mother will not take her back into the home.

A mental status examination reveals some psychomotor retardation. Angry outbursts during the session are precipitated by delusions of persecution by "demons and devils." Affect is labile, dependent on content, and is appropriate to ideation. Shirley Bradley admits to auditory and visual hallucinations related to "demons and devils." Speech ranges from normal to pressured, depending on content. Delusional material is well circumscribed, with the client exhibiting hypervigilence and blocking during delusional interference. At other

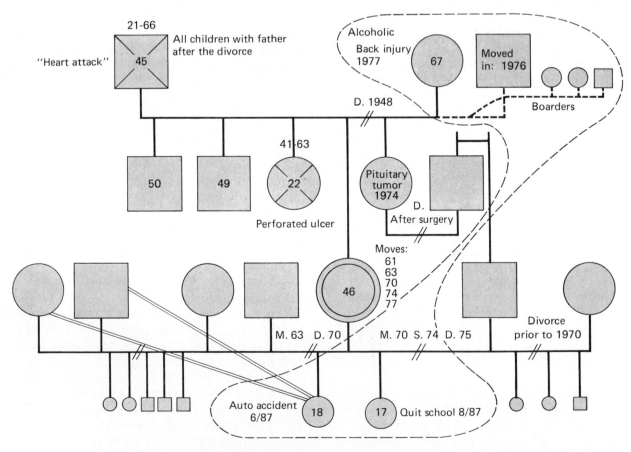

Figure 37-2. Genogram for Shirley Bradley.

---

* Case contributed by Barbara J. Rementer

times during the session the client is goal-directed, articulate and oriented ×3 spheres without apparent memory impairment. She is sad when discussing her chief complaint. She voices anger at the staffs' requirement for postdischarge supervision stating "I don't need supervision, I can do it alone." Insight and judgment are poor.

Social History. Shirley Bradley is the fourth of five children (Figure 37-2). After her parents divorced in 1948, the children lived with her father. Shirley graduated from high school in 1960. She was married in 1963. Work history is as a nurse's aid until her first pregnancy in 1967. Shirley was divorced and remarried in 1970. This second family included three step-children, who reportedly caused much stress. Shirley reports physical abuse from both husbands. Shirley left the marriage in 1974, divorced in 1975, and moved in with an ill sister "to nurse her." In 1977 Shirley and her daughters moved in with her mother, who is reportedly an alcoholic. Her mother stopped drinking in 1985 after an auto accident. Shirley is convinced that her mother is drinking. Shirley describes a "meanness" in her mother's personality over the last 4 months that had vanished after the auto accident.

Shirley describes a lifelong ability to "see spirits" that others could not see. She recalls discussing this phenomenon with her father at about 10 years of age and states he told her that "I can see them too, it's nothing to worry about." Shirley denies any interference in functioning until July 1980 when "the devil suddenly came at me with a butcher knife and sliced my belly open." Her functioning has been poor since that time. She has had multiple psychiatric hospitalizations and poor adjustment to community living.

Shirley Bradley's family is connected and supportive. She goes home every other weekend; however she sometimes returns early "because the demons threaten to hurt my girls if I don't come back." This has occurred with increased frequency in the last 2 months and would seem to correlate with a decreased level of functioning.

Medical History. There have been three episodes of self-mutilation in response to delusional material since 1980. Shirley had a hysterectomy in 1974. The remainder of her medical history is unremarkable.

NURSING CARE PLAN

DSM-III-R
Axis I   Schizophrenia Paranoid Type, Chronic 295.32
Axis II   Schizotypal Personality Disorder 301.22
Axis III None
Axis IV   Psychosocial Stressors: 17-year-old daughter quit school August 1987, 18-year-old daughter in minor auto accident June 1987. Shirley Bradley suspects mother to have resumed misuse of alcohol Severity 3
Axis V   Current G.A.F. 25
          Highest G.A.F. past year 30

ASSESSMENT

Shirley Bradley has issues surrounding family structure and family transactional patterns. Minuchin's theory will be used in formulating Shirley's care plan in hopes of improving transactional patterns by restructuring the family and clarifying boundaries. Shirley's relatively low level of functioning signifies a need to use an action-based as opposed to a cognitive-based theoretical framework in planning her care.

NURSING DIAGNOSIS

1. Alteration in communication
2. Alteration in impulse control
3. Alteration in perception
4. Alteration in role performance related to long-term hospitalization
5. Alteration of cognition related to inability to evaluate reality

GOALS

Long-Term

The ability to function in the CRR home with frequent family contact and clear family boundaries.

Short-Term

1. Anxiety reduction to allow Shirley to remain at home throughout her weekend visits.
2. Familial recognition of family state of development to allow and encourage daughters to separate.
3. Develop a more realistic attitude about future discharge plans (number 2 must be addressed first).

TREATMENT PLAN

Nursing diagnoses 1, 2, and 3 are related to sensory perceptual alterations and defined by delusions and hallucinations, causing behavior that is unacceptable to family.

Objectives	Interventions	Outcome Criteria
Clarify mystifying forms of communication to family	1. Meet with family on 10/31 to discuss anxiety-based verbalizations. 2. Encourage family not to feed into Shirley's system. 3. Encourage family not to react in an overtly negative manner.	Family will verbalize an understanding of this in 2 weeks.
Client will reduce frequency of verbalizing delusional material and responding to hallucinations. At onset 15-minute interaction without mention of delusional material; increasing by 15 minutes every 2 weeks up to 45 minutes.	1. Establish therapeutic nurse–client relationship. 2. Stay defocused from delusions during weekly sessions. 3. Encourage to verbalize anxiety in a nonpsychotic manner. 4. Develop insight into difference between internal and external stimuli. 5. Help her to identify situations that increase anxiety. 6. Identify skills in dealing with difficult situations. 7. Allow ventilation of anger in appropriate ways. 8. Substitute activities for behavior in physical and art therapies.	Shirley will control psychotic behavior enough to resume consistent every-other-weekend visits with her family in 2 months. Shirley swims four times weekly; art five times weekly.

Nursing Diagnosis 4 is related to hospitalization for most of last 7 years and characterized by a desire to "mother" 17- and 18-year-old daughters.

Objectives	Interventions	Outcome Criteria
Restructuring family to clarify boundaries. Elimination of Shirley's perceived need to nurture daughters.	Structural family therapy for 5 to 6 months after remission of Nursing Diagnoses 1 and 2. To meet with the family once weekly.	1. Shirley will be aware of age-appropriate behaviors for herself and her daughters in 4 months. 2. Daughters will be able to separate from grandmother and mother in a mature manner and without guilt when each is ready. 3. Grandmother will gradually reduce nurturance of granddaughters. 4. Shirley will verbalize acceptance of living in CRR in 5 months.

Nursing Diagnosis 5 is related to inability to evaluate reality and characterized by inability to solve problems and inappropriate responses.

Objectives	Interventions	Outcome Criteria
Shirley will gain some insight regarding the effect of her behavior on interpersonal relationships. Shirley will become aware of the purpose her behavior serves for her.	In weekly hour-long one-to-one sessions and later in the prescribed family therapy reality orientation at Shirley's level of perception, therapist should engage when anxiety levels cause agitation and reengage when anxiety level is acceptable.	Verbalizes understanding about family's inability to tolerate behavior. Ability to explain anxiety increase coinciding with aberrant behavior increase.

EVALUATION AND FOLLOW-UP

Two important components of nursing care of patients with schizophrenic reactions include the course of schizophrenia and follow-up efforts.

The Course of Schizophrenia

The course of schizophrenia is as difficult to define as is its diagnosis, its symptoms, or its etiology. Some courses progress rapidly, others slowly, and others are static. Some may run the entire gamut and are called *chronic syndromes*. People with chronic syndromes tend to spend their days on the wards of state hospitals. Others may have their psychosis arrested at earlier stages, and only under heavy stress will the symptoms become manifest again.

The clinical picture of the patient long hospitalized in a mental hospital is often thought to be a result of schizophrenia. It is currently believed, however, to be a result of a social breakdown rather than the disease of schizophrenia, a view that is engendered by the fact that these patients can be rehabilitated. That is, what is seen in the continued care wards of state hospitals is not a phenomenon of the disease schizophrenia but is what happens when someone is put in a situation in which sensory deprivation exists.

Prolonged Schizophrenia

Clinical experience has appeared to support the view that persons with repeated episodes of schizophrenia can expect to have a chronic course with residual symptoms and lasting deficits in such areas as work, social relations, and self-care. A group of researchers carefully reviewed prior studies of schizophrenic patients' outcomes and, together with findings from the recent long-term follow-up studies, have corrected the negative perception that schizophrenia has a poor outcome. Their research suggests that there is considerable heterogeneity in the long-term outcome of schizophrenia, with marginal or deteriorated states more the exception than the rule. Among the contributors to the misperception of chronicity are biased sampling, both past and present, as well as a multitude of environmental and psychosocial factors that affect patient outcomes.

The study suggests that the term *prolonged schizophrenia* be substituted for the term *chronic schizophrenia*. The term *prolonged schizophrenia* does not have the implications of relentless progressive deterioration, residual symptoms, deficits in functioning, and hopelessness that are commonly associated with the term *chronic*.[40]

Follow-up Care

Work with chronically mentally ill people requires careful follow-up care. Patients who have received hospitalized care need some type of aftercare planning. Various aftercare programs have been developed to help the patient during the transition from the hospital back into the community. Following are some of the programs in which nurses have been most involved.

Group Therapy

Patients come back for supportive group sessions on a weekly, biweekly, or monthly basis. One of the goals is the enhancement of social functioning and participation. Patients are able to discuss the problems they encounter in their adjustment to normal social responsibilities.

Cooperative Apartments

For patients who have been hospitalized for a long period of time and are homeless, a program to move long-term patients into apartments that are supervised by a landlord–supervisor is proving successful. Initially, the landlord–supervisor oversees the everyday tasks of the person, and gradually the person is encouraged to gain autonomy. Studies have shown that this kind of aftercare has a positive effect on expatients. The programs cost considerably less than alternative community aftercare facilities such as halfway houses, family-care homes, and nursing homes.

Indigenous Community Workers

In another project, indigenous members of the community were trained to help discharged patients deal with the daily activities of living in the community. Some workers took patients into their own homes; other workers regularly visited the patients in their apartments.

All these methods are ways to strengthen community resources to enable the discharged patient to move out of the hospital and back into the community. Inherent in this progressive movement is the importance of safeguarding that all this is not done in order to transfer the problem of caring for the mentally ill to the community. It is hoped that all community planning considers the person's wishes; that is, the person with schizophrenia should be free to live alone when he wishes, live with his family when he wishes and can, or live with similar persons in a communal social setting that is cohesive enough to give support yet casual enough not to be too demanding. It is also essential that supervised care be given when it is necessary.

Community Assessment

The community mental health nurse has an important role in working with the previously hospitalized or disturbed person in the community. When a person presents himself to the clinic, one of the first things to do is to differentiate the chronic state from the acute state of emotional disturbance. The chronic patient who has increased psychotic symptoms because of a loss of an important member in his social network is different from the patient who is experiencing schizophrenic symptoms for the first time. For example, in the chronic patient's situation, the treatment might be the social model to help restructure his social milieu. If the patient's brother, for instance, left home because he was drafted or because he was going away to college, or if this brother who was the only one to understand him died, then the question to ask is, "What does this person need to best manage at the level he was accustomed to?" There must be a substitute available to the patient for him to readjust to the missing brother.

The stable level of social adjustment is important to look at when assessing the patient in the community. Is he working or fitting into some kind of social matrix by his living arrangements? Where is he psychologically in general? Is he going to hurt himself or someone else? What is his ability to function outside a hospital?

It is important to know whether or not the behavior takes antisocial forms and whether or not it bothers other people. How ill is the patient considered by the people around him in the community? The nurse can use the group process in initiating group activities for discussions about living and adjusting to the community.

NURSING CARE PLAN*
Schizophrenic Disorders

HUMAN RESPONSE

1. Bizarre delusions, e.g., delusions of being controlled, thought broadcasting, thought insertion, or thought withdrawal.
2. Incoherence, marked loosening of associations, illogical thinking, or poverty of content of speech.
3. Auditory hallucinations; delusions with persecutory or jealous content.
4. Blunted, flat, or inappropriate affect.
5 Catatonic or other grossly disorganized behavior.
6. Deterioration from a previous level of functioning, e.g., work, social relations, and self-care.
7. Social isolation or withdrawal; markedly peculiar behavior (e.g., talking to self in public, hoarding items).
8. Digressive, vague, overelaborate, circumstantial, metaphorical speech; nonarticulated life goals.

NURSING DIAGNOSIS

- Alteration in thought content.
- Alteration in thought process.
- Alteration in perception.
- Alteration in affect.
- Alteration in psychomotor activity.
- Alteration in self-care and in usual work and social activities.
- Alteration in sense of self; impaired coping.
- Alteration in volition.

GOALS

1. Patient will demonstrate a decrease in delusions as well as improvement in reality testing.
2. Patient will demonstrate an increased ability to form thoughts in a logical, goal-directed manner.
3. Patient will demonstrate a decrease in delusions and hallucinations, and an improvement in reality testing.
4. Patient will demonstrate an increased ability to recognize and express his emotions in an appropriate manner.
5. Patient will demonstrate an increased ability to control disorganized behavior.
6. Patient will demonstrate skills to participate in therapeutic unit activities or structured community social activities.
7. Patient will demonstrate an increased level of functioning.
8. Patient will demonstrate an increase in self-esteem and autonomy.
9. Patient will demonstrate an increase in motivation and goal-directed behaviors.

INTERVENTIONS

1. Approach the patient in a calm and reassuring manner. Establish a trust relationship with the patient by:
   a. Setting limits on his behavior and establishing a consistent approach to nursing care.
   b. Controlling environmental stimuli according to the patient's needs and emotional status.
   c. Listening to the patient in a nonjudgmental manner. Validate reality and reassure the patient when perceptual distortions occur. Protect the patient from any external danger arising from distortions in perception. Limit discussion of delusional material, and redirect the patient as necessary. Administer appropriate psychotropic medications and evaluate their effect. Refer to Nursing Care Plan in Chapter 47 for suicidal behavior in the presence of command delusional thoughts to hurt self.
2. Allow time daily to listen to the patient's communication. Provide an atmosphere conducive to communication (i.e., free from distractions). Seek clarification from the patient and acknowledge when communications are not understood. Assist the patient in focusing on the topics being discussed.
3. Continue interventions for alterations in thought content and in thought processes. Avoid touching the patient without first telling him. Explain all procedures and treatments prior to administering. Assist patient in determining what is real and unreal.
4. Assist the patient in recognizing and expressing his emotions. Provide an acceptable outlet for the appropriate expression of emotion. Validate appropriate emotional responses for the patient. Provide feedback for the patient when emotional responses do not match reality.
5. Discuss behavior with the patient (e.g., withdrawal, agitation) when observed. Provide an acceptable outlet for the appropriate expression of feelings. Control environmental stimuli according to the patient's needs and emotional state. Set limits verbally on disorganized behavior. Administer psychotropic medications as ordered and evaluate their effects. Use seclusion or restraints as ordered and as necessary to control disorganized behavior.
6. Spend time with the patient to facilitate trust and communication. Include the patient in the plans for his care. Encourage the patient to assume responsibility for activities of daily living and to become independent in self-care.
7. Reassure the patient of his individuality and uniqueness through the use of individual and group activities. Assist the patient in developing increased self-esteem through reinforcement of positive behavior and participation in the unit's program of activities. Encourage the patient to accept responsibility for his own care and behavior, to the fullest extent possible.
8. Encourage the patient's participation in goal-directed activities (i.e., care of self, and therapeutic unit or community programs). Encourage the patient to consider alternatives for future life plans, and to set appropriate goals. Consult appropriate resources for discharge planning.

This nursing care plan was prepared by Eileen E. Rinear and Janice Kleinschmidt.

Summary

Not only are there many theories on the causes of schizophrenia, but there are insufficient data to decide which of these theories, if any, are correct. One probable reason for this situation is that schizophrenia is not a unitary disease with an invariant etiology. In fact, most diseases are not homogeneous entities with distinctive etiologies. For example, several different forms of pneumonia exist.

In this chapter the psychiatric diagnosis of schizophrenia was discussed as a complex clinical syndrome consisting of various symptoms. The manifest symptomatology was described in terms of the fundamental symptoms of ambivalence, associative disturbance, autism, and affective impairment. Other symptoms described were ideas of reference, delusions, hallucinations, depersonalization, projection, and negativistic behavior. The clinical types of schizophrenia (paranoid, catatonic, disorganized, residual, and undifferentiated) were discussed.

The prognosis, etiology, prevention studies, and course of schizophrenia were covered. The psychiatric and nursing diagnoses for the schizophrenic person were identified according to the *DSM-III-R* categories, and specific nursing approaches were described, including defining reality, responding to the thought disturbance, handling patient control, strengthening the self-image of the patient, and strengthening interpersonal relationships of the patient. The psychological model, which included the nurse as primary therapist and the one-to-one relationship, the biological model, and community assessment by the community health nurse were described.

Nursing care plans for schizophrenic disorders were provided.

Questions

1. Describe how the schizophrenic views the world.
2. Differentiate schizophrenic disorders from paranoid disorders.
3. What implications are there for nursing research in schizophrenic disorders?
4. How do schizophrenic persons manage on an outpatient basis?
5. What medications are patients receiving for schizophrenia in your clinical setting?

REFERENCES AND SUGGESTED READINGS

1. Kraeplin, E. [*Dementia Praecox and Paraphrenia*] (R. M. Barclay & G. M. Robertson, trans.). New York: R. E. Krieger, 1971. (Originally published in 1919.)
2. Kety, S. S. Genetic and biochemical aspects of schizophrenia. In A. M. Nicholi, Jr. (Ed.), *The Harvard Guide to Modern Psychiatry*. Cambridge, Mass.: Harvard University Press, 1978, pp. 94–98.
3. Ibid., pp. 98–99.
4. Matthysse, S., & Kety, S. S. (Eds.). *Catecholamines and Schizophrenia*. Elmsford, N. Y.: Pergamon Press, 1975.
5. Ibid., p. 101.
6. Ibid.
7. Kraeplin, op. cit.
8. Fisman, M. The brain stem in psychosis. *British Journal of Psychiatry*, 1975, 126, 414, 422.
9. Johnstone, E. C., et al., Cerebral ventricular size and cognitive impairment in chronic schizophrenia. *Lancet*, 1976, 2, 924–926.
10. Andreasen, N. C., et al., Ventricular enlargement in schizophrenia: Definition and prevalence. *American Journal of Psychiatry*, 1982, 139, 292–296.
11. Kraeplin, op. cit.
12. Bleuler, E. *Dementia Praecox*. New York: International Universities Press, 1950.
13. Crow, T. J. Molecular pathology of schizophrenia: More than one disease process? *British Medical Journal*, 1980, 280, 1–9.
14. Hughlings-Jackson, J. *Selected Writings* (H. Taylor, Ed.). London: Hodder & Stoughton, 1931.
15. Bleuler, op. cit.
16. Andreasen, N. C., op. cit. Ventricular enlargement in schizophrenia: Relationship to positive and negative symptoms. *American Journal of Psychiatry*, 1982, 139, 297–302.
17. Klein, M. *The Psychoanalysis of Children*. London: Hogarth Press, 1932.
18. Sullivan, H. S. *Schizophrenia as a Human Process*. New York: Norton, 1962.

19. Goldstein, M. Z. (Ed.). *Family Involvement in the Treatment of Schizophrenia.* Washington, D. C.: American Psychiatric Press, 1986.

20. Lidz, R. W., & Lidz, T. The therapeutic considerations arising from the intense symbiotic needs of schizophrenic patients. In B. Brody & F. C. Redlich (Eds.), *Psychotherapy with Schizophrenics.* New York: International Universities Press, 1952.

21. Fleck, S., Lidz, T., Cornelison, A. R., et al., Incestuous and homosexual problems. In T. Lidz, S. Fleck, & A. R. Cornelison (Eds.), *Schizophrenia and the Family.* New York: International Universities Press, 1965.

22. Lidz, T. The family, personality development, and schizophrenia. In Y. Romano (Ed.), *The Origins of Schizophrenia.* The Hague: Excerpta Medica Foundation, 1967.

23. Bateson, G., et al., Toward a theory of schizophrenia. *Behavioral Science*, 1956, *1*, 251.

24. Wynne, L., et al., Pseudomutuality in the family relations of schizophrenics. *Psychiatry*, 1958, *21*, 205–220.

25. Green, J. R., & Framo, J. *Family Therapy: Major Contributions.* New York: International Universities Press, 1984.

26. Day, M., & Semrad, E. V. Schizophrenic reactions. In A. M. Nicholi, Jr. (Ed.), *The Harvard Guide to Modern Psychiatry.* Cambridge, Mass.: Harvard University Press, 1978, p. 207.

27. Ibid., pp. 206–207.

28. Hartman, C. Psychiatric nursing perspectives, In H. Grunebaum, J. Weiss, B. Cohler, C. Hartman, & D. Gallant (Eds.), *Mentally Ill Mothers and Their Children.* Chicago: University of Chicago Press, 1974, pp. 83–211.

29. Yates, A. J. Psychological deficits. *Annual Review of Psychology*, 1966, *17*, 453–461.

30. Braft, D. L., & Saccuzzo, D. P. Information processing dysfunction in paranoid schizophrenia: A two-factor deficit. *American Journal of Psychiatry*, 1981, *138*, 1051–1056.

31. World Health Organization. *International Pilot Study of Schizophrenia* (Vol. 1). Geneva: World Health Organization, 1973.

32. Ibid.

33. Grinker, R. R., & Holzman, P. S. Schizophrenic pathology in young adults. *Archives of General Psychiatry*, 1973, *28*, 169–175.

34. Schneider, J. [*Clinical Psychopathology*] (M. W. Hamilton, trans.). New York: Grune & Stratton, 1959.

35. Kendler, K. S., Glazer, W. M., & Morganstern, J. H. Dimensions of delusional experience. *American Journal of Psychiatry*, 1983, *140*, 466–469.

36. Rokeach, M. *The Three Christs of Ypsilanti.* New York: Random House, 1967.

37. Greenberg, L., Fine, S., Cohen, C., Larson, K., Baily, A., Rubinton, P., & Glick, I. An interdisciplinary psychoeducation program for schizophrenic patients and their families in an acute care setting, *Hospital & Community Psychiatry*, 1988, *39*(3), 277–282.

38. Falloon, I., Boyd, J., McGill, C., et al., Family management in the prevention of exacerbations of schizophrenia: A controlled study. *New England Journal of Medicine*, 1982, *306*, 1437–1440.

39. Goldstein, op. cit.

Chapter *38*

Delusional (Paranoid) Disorders

Ann Wolbert Burgess

Chapter Objectives

The students successfully attaining the goals of this chapter will be able to:

- Describe delusional disorders.
- Identify five major themes of delusional disorders.
- Plan nursing care for patients with suspicious behavior.

Paranoia is the term used to describe a syndrome in which the logical nature of the system of belief concerning persecution or threat is tight and coherent and there is no evidence of other disturbances. *Paranoia* is derived from two Greek roots, *para*, meaning beside, and *nous*, meaning mind; thus, the term implies a mind beside itself.

The essential features of delusional paranoid disorders are extreme suspiciousness, persistent persecutory delusions, or delusional jealousy. The delusions may be simple or elaborate and may involve a single theme or a series of connected themes. These themes include being spied upon, conspired against, cheated, followed, drugged, poisoned, harassed, or obstructed in the pursuit of goals. Minor incidents such as small slights may be exaggerated and can become the focus of a delusional system. In

order to give a psychiatric diagnosis of delusional paranoid disorder, the presence of delusions must not be due to any other mental disorder, such as a schizophrenic, schizophreniform, affective, or organic mental disorder.

THEMES IN DELUSIONAL PARANOID DISORDERS

There are five major themes commonly seen in delusional disorder: erotomaniac, grandiose, jealous, persecutory, and somatic. Determination of the type of delusional disorder is based on the predominant delusional theme. Cases having more than one delusional theme are frequent (see Table 38-1).

761

TABLE 38-1. COMMON TYPES OF DELUSIONS

Type	Symptoms
Delusions of persecution	The person believes that he is the victim of persecution. The delusion may have a self-reference ("People are talking about me"); a self-harm quality ("I am being poisoned"); or an influence ("The FBI are after me").
Delusions of jealousy	Delusions of marital or sexual infidelity. ("My wife is having an affair.")
Delusions of love	The person believes another person to be in love with him, though they may not have even met. ("David Brinkley loves me; he sends me a special message through the television set.")
Delusions of grandeur	The person assigns self-importance and uniqueness. ("I am a good friend of the President.")
Somatic delusions	The person believes he has some incurable illness. ("I believe I have AIDS.")
Delusions of guilt	The person demonstrates self-reproach. ("I am a sinner.")
Delusions of nihilism	The person denies the existence of friends, family, the world, and himself. He may even assert that he is dead.
Delusions of poverty	The person believes that he is impoverished. ("I have no money or belongings.")

Erotomaniac Type

The central theme of an erotic delusion is that one is loved by another. The delusion concerns spiritual union and idealized romantic love rather than sexual attraction. The person toward whom the delusion is directed is usually of higher status, such as a famous person, a superior at work, or even a stranger. Efforts are usually made to contact the object of the delusion, through telephone, letters, calls, gifts, visits, and even surveillance and stalking. The prevalence of erotic delusions is such as to be a significant source of harassment to public figures.

Grandiose Type

Grandiose delusions commonly take the form of the person's being convinced that he possesses something great but unrecognized, such as talent or knowledge, or has made an important discovery, which may be taken to the government or FBI. Grandiose delusions may have a religious content, and people with these delusions can become leaders of religious cults.

Jealous Type

When delusions of jealousy are present, a person is convinced, without due cause, that his spouse or lover is unfaithful. Usually the person confronts the partner with some type of evi-

dence (e.g., disarrayed clothing) to justify the delusion. The person with the delusion may physically attack the partner.

Persecutory Type

The persecutory delusion, the most common type, may be simple or elaborate, and usually involves a single theme or series of connected themes, such as being conspired against. People with persecutory delusions are often resentful and angry and may resort to violence against those they believe are hurting them.

Somatic Type

Somatic delusions occur in various forms. Most common are convictions that the person emits a foul odor from his skin, mouth, rectum, or vagina; that he has an infestation of insects in the skin; or that certain parts of the body are not functioning. People with somatic delusions usually consult nonpsychiatric physicians for treatment of their perceived somatic condition.

PSYCHIATRIC DIAGNOSIS

The diagnosis of paranoid disorder is made when an individual exhibits dominant persecutory delusions or delusions of jealousy that are unexplained by other psychiatric disorders. Generally the delusions are developed logically and are well systematized. The emotional responses to these delusions appear appropriate; the personality remains intact or deteriorates minimally over a prolonged time period.

The diagnostic criteria for delusion disorder includes the following[1]:

A. Nonbizarre delusion(s) (i.e., involving situations that occur in real life, such as being followed, poisoned, infected, loved at a distance, having a disease, being deceived by one's spouse or lover) of at least 1 month's duration.
B. Auditory or visual hallucinations, if present, are not prominent [as defined in Schizophrenia].
C. Apart from the delusion(s) or its ramifications, behavior is not obviously odd or bizarre.
D. If a major depressive or manic syndrome has been present during the delusional disturbance, the total duration of all episodes of the mood syndrome has been brief relative to the total duration of the delusional disturbance.
E. Has never met criterion A for Schizophrenia, and it cannot be established that an organic factor initiated and maintained the disturbance.

THE EGO DEFENSE OF PROJECTION

Paranoid people rely heavily on the ego defense of projection. Essentially other people are blamed for their actions. One of the patterns of communication of people who are paranoid is a theme of victim ("Things are always happening to me") and a theme of suspicion ("That person is after me"). The person tends to focus on what other people are doing, and the language pattern deals with other people.

Because of this focus on other people, paranoid individuals think they are mind readers. For example, a patient said to a nurse: "Here they are, out after me again and you are not listening to one thing I am saying!" The nurse, who had been listening to the patient but was patiently waiting for an opportunity to speak, gently asked, "How do you know this?" The patient then proceeded to talk about people in

his life who had not listened to him, which assisted the nurse to focus the interview on the feeling of disappointment when the patient was not listened to. At a later point in the interview, the nurse reaffirmed to the patient that she had been listening to him.

The use of projection is to defend the person against painful feelings. This defense is used when people are distressed and depressed and experiencing a great deal of internal pain. Projecting is a way of relieving the pain and the way it is being caused. Paranoid people see their feelings state as externally caused. They tend to feel victimized and impinged upon by others, and the "counterfeeling" is for power and control that they attempt to gain through the use of language.

Analysis of Speech

Research is now underway on the speech and language of people with varying diagnostic categories. Advances have been made in the use of computers to analyze content of speech. Through this use of computer content analysis, Oxman, Rosenberg, and Tucker have been able to discriminate schizophrenic from nonschizophrenic patients on the basis of the semantic content of their speech.[2] In their study, paranoid people distinguished themselves primarily by the avoidance of word classes common to the nonparanoid groups (i.e., family, low status, etc.).

The language of paranoia tends to dehumanize others and situations. There is a nonorientation or narrowing of interest from reality. The speech conveys no interest in connecting with others; the defense is an introversion or an avoidance of human-oriented themes. Rather, the paranoid person tends to manifest, through his use of the ideal value category, a sense that he wishes to be judged as normal or indeed superior and beyond reproach. Paranoid patients who are hospitalized work hard to refute the implication that their hospitalization reflects any stigma or failing ("I just feel I am coming into my own identity. . . . I've done pretty well with the adversities I have faced.").

The language of paranoia implies a double emphasis: first, on the patient's current difficulties, and then on his innate superiority. The patient's troubles are seen as external and transitory, things that he will come through to achieve such ideals as fame, success, and identity.

VARIABILITY OF DEFINITION

The presentation of paranoid delusions in a variety of situations and diagnostic categories is consistent with the model of paranoia as a protective psychological response to different types of stress or etiologic factors—factors such as fear of the unknown, homosexual panic, psychotropic drugs, depression, mania, organic brain syndromes, or schizophrenia. Each of these stresses can represent a profound threat to the self and to self-esteem. The paranoid response to threat is usually withdrawal from intimate ties and an intense effort to retain the appearance of normalcy.

In certain susceptible individuals, this paranoid defense escalates to an independent, maladaptive state, which fails in its aim to reduce anxiety and further disrupts the patient's capacity to function. Patients manifesting the maladaptive paranoid stance (whether the patient is simply paranoid, schizophrenic, or suffering organic impairment) relate to their world in an isolating and abstract way. Content analysis shows their primary concerns, generally presented indirectly, as self-protection through distancing and an exaggerated assertion of their normalcy. This latter behavior seems to represent an attempt to shore up a damaged sense of self. The projective mode we associate with paranoia is thematically expressed in a refusal to represent the self as an agent of action but rather to represent the self as an object of external, impersonal forces. This dynamic is semantically tied to an effort to turn the attention of others away from the self, an effort that also arises from the paranoid's sense of himself as shamefully defective. The paranoid's sense of transparency is responded to by efforts to become opaque and by an escalating vigilance and suspiciousness, which entails delusions.

The difficulty of defining the boundaries of paranoia as a clinical entity is highlighted by a study by Freedman and Schwab, who found a 40 percent prevalence of paranoia in 264 patients with mixed diagnoses.[3] Their study, as well as other studies on paranoia, illustrate the variability in the definition of paranoia. Four different definitions of paranoia include: suspiciousness, ideas of reference, paranoid delusions with psychosis, and systemized delusions without any other signs of psychosis. When paranoid thinking is broadly defined, it is as common a term as depression. When paranoia is defined as a disorder, the major clinical distinction remains between paranoia as a separate delusional disorder and paranoia as a subtype of schizophrenia.

With regard to schizophrenia, one of the diagnostic tools that continues to stand out as a means of differentiating between types of schizophrenic patients is the paranoid versus nonparanoid distinction. Paranoid schizophrenia, in addition to being equated with suspiciousness or bizarreness, is also characterized by delusions of control, reference, persecution, grandeur, or jealousy, but it is not characterized by requirements of specificity or fixity.

When paranoia is described on a continuum, the assumption is that a universal mental mechanism can result in a normal development and adaptation, or in an abnormal personality style, or, for particularly vulnerable individuals, in a psychosis. Genetic predisposition, superimposed organic illness, family dynamics, and environmental stress are factors that can determine the degree of pathology, but a paranoid orientation is regarded as a universal possibility.

POTENTIAL FOR VIOLENCE

The potential for violence is present in persons with this pattern of thinking. Often society fails to detect the potential for violence in time for intervention. In one mass murder, a father killed 14 of his family members, two known associates, and wounded four additional persons. A news report cited the following information:

No one in town really knew the 47-year-old Simmons, a former Air Force officer who went through a string of low-paying jobs during the 4 years he lived in the area. He was described as a recluse who sometimes answered a friendly inquiry with a glare.

He did not let his wife out of the house without him, except to do the laundry; she apparently knew how to drive but was not allowed to do so.

The five children living at home were sentenced in effect to internal exile. They were not permitted to go to church or to socialize, though they sometimes did by deceiving him.

The four who were of school age were not allowed to walk to the bus; he drove them. When they returned in the late afternoon, he had them do chores

until dark—mostly carrying piles of firewood or rocks or earth from the road at the bottom of the driveway. He worked them like a general.

Simmons' obsession with privacy seemed almost absolute. His home was his fortress. Visitors said he would lie on the couch and drink beer, watch the news, and not say a word.

He was known to beat his wife and he hit his children when they tried to keep him from striking his wife. He had been charged with three counts of incest after his daughter testified before a grand jury that he had impregnated her. She was 17 at the time, and the child she bore was 6 when both of them were murdered. The incest charges were dismissed after police found that Simmons had fled the state in the middle of the night.

Apparently, Simmons' wife was saving her money and gathering up nerve to file for a divorce when he found out and killed all 14 of them.

After killing his family, Simmons then sought out and killed two additional people, a young woman who had spurned his advances the year before when they worked on a truck farm and her supervisor, who had admonished him for his actions. He had sent the young woman notes, small gifts, flowers. He had showed up at her door and may have been following her, even after she told him she had married since they had last known each other.

His statement after the murders was to the effect that he had killed everyone who had hurt him.

NURSING MANAGEMENT

Nursing Care of the Suspicious Patient

The suspicious person tends to be distrustful of people and subjectively feels an uneasiness around people. The suspicious patient often projects onto others his own unhappiness and mistrust.

Typical Behaviors

This patient can be expected to remain aloof from others, be extremely sensitive, resentful, hostile, irritable, or quarrelsome. He often believes others are "out to get him" and fears persecution. This patient will see the environment, no matter how therapeutic, as hostile and threatening, especially if he has been hospitalized against his wishes. He may refuse all forms of medical and nursing intervention. Delusions of persecution and of grandeur and ideas of reference are common.

One such patient, on being brought to the hospital, tried to take control of the steering wheel from her husband because she thought he was taking her to a hospital run by Communists.

Goals

One nursing goal for the suspicious patient would be to establish a trusting relationship with first one member of the nursing staff, and then with other staff and patients. Whether this will be a long- or short-term goal will depend on the chronicity of the patient's illness. The nurse must be flexible when determining appropriate goals for the patient.

Another goal would be to increase the patient's self-esteem by providing for successful experiences for the patient. The more positive experiences a patient has, the sooner he will be able to feel good about himself and learn to trust others.

Nursing Intervention

Initially, contact between the patient and the staff and other patients should be kept at a minimum. The patient who is highly suspicious of others can be intimidated by an overbearing, friendly attitude of the staff or other patients. The patient must have "room to breathe." This patient does better in a smaller unit, preferably in a private room. He should be allowed to set his own pace in closeness with others.

The nurse should give concise explanations of routine and necessary procedures. Long verbal accounts will only serve to anger this patient. At the same time, a lack of explanation of procedures will decrease the patient's sense of trust in the staff. A clear explanation of the daily routine of the ward will diminish the patient's anxiety.

The nurse should not whisper or act secretively in the patient's presence. Common courtesy expects this, but it is especially important when caring for the suspicious patient. The nurse must be careful not to give the patient any reason to be suspicious. For example, a nurse may know she's just telling a coworker about her date Saturday night, but the patient does not know this. He may experience an illusion with this behavior and will develop it into his delusional system. Obviously, this will greatly hamper the therapeutic relationship the nurse may be developing with this patient.

The nurse should avoid laughing or talking in front of the patient when he can see but not hear what is being said. Again, the patient with many suspicions will assume the nurse is talking about him. This could provoke impulsive destructive behavior if the patient is still highly agitated.

Social participation should be limited until the patient can tolerate a larger group. This patient should not be expected to attend community meetings, group activities, ward parties, etc. He must be allowed to establish a degree of trust in the staff and therapeutic community before he is expected to socialize in large groups. The nurse can act as a role model for the patient initially within a small group. Once the nurse has established a rapport with her patient, she may begin to initiate social activities for the patient, perhaps a simple card game, or Ping Pong, or pool. When the patient can tolerate this activity, the nurse should slowly bring in more people to the setting, perhaps including another patient or trusted staff member, in the social activity. The intent is that the patient will, at his own pace, begin to socialize with others in a nonthreatening environment. The patient can also gradually be encouraged to participate in activities in the occupational therapy department, also at a slow pace.

The nurse should avoid involving the patient in competitive, aggressive activities. A game of touch football would be threatening as well as frightening for the suspicious person. Initially, he cannot tolerate this type of activity. A nature walk with a small group of other patients would be far less threatening to him than a touch football game. The activity should be planned so that, although the patient is involved with others, he can still be alone when necessary until he is ready to handle more interaction.

The nurse should allow the patient a choice of activities. Whenever possible, the patient should be able to choose among several acceptable activities. This allows him the chance to assume responsibility for his actions and to feel that he does, in fact, have some control over what goes on in his environment. It is helpful to let him know the schedule ahead of time. If changes in some activity are necessary, the nurse should let the patient know in advance with a simple, concise explanation.

The nurse should not argue with the patient. She cannot talk him out of his suspicions. This will only serve to increase his agitation. If limits must be set, the nurse should not get into arguments over them. She should be certain that the patient understands the limits before it is necessary to invoke them.

The nurse should be honest and keep any promises made. This is extremely important for helping the patient to reestablish trust in people. If the nurse says she will spend time in an hour with him, and then finds herself unable to do so, it is important to go to him to explain that she will be unable to be there as promised, and agree on another time for the meeting.

The nurse should be consistent. The patient must know what is expected from him and what to expect from the staff. There is security with sameness, and the staff must see that this environment is secure for the individual.

The nurse must assess the physical needs of the patient. She must be certain that adequate hygiene and nutrition are provided. If the patient does not eat because of suspiciousness, he may be allowed the opportunity to prepare his own meals. His physiological needs must be met before he can regain psychological homeostasis.

All behavior has meaning to the individual. Even though the nurse may not fully understand the meaning of a behavior, it is important to realize that to the patient the behavior has great significance. The nurse should try to understand the patient's behavior so that she can have greater empathy for the mental pain he is experiencing.

Communicating With Paranoid Patients

The defining characteristics of paranoid people are suspiciousness and jealousy. To be able to think this way, the most important belief is that you know what other people think, that you can read their minds and that you know exactly what they think and feel, based on your sense and perception of the other. There is no verification or checking it out: the basic premise is that a person knows the inner world and experiences of another person.

This works in the following manner. The person says to himself: I know that nurse doesn't like me because this morning she didn't say hello. She thinks that I am a wimp; well, I'll show her. With that, the person picks up the ashtray on the ward and throws it into the fireplace, smashing it and making a loud noise when the nurse asked him to turn his radio down. The excessive display of anger in the face of the simple request alerts the nurse the misperception and incongruence of the patient's response to external reality. However, the nurse has to accept that no matter what her original intentions were, the response of the patient is the meaning of her communication. This means that the personal thoughts and constructs of the patient have to be elicited for an understanding of how the simple request to turn down the radio justified the violent outburst in the patient's mind.

The strategies here would be to establish rapport with the client and ask the client what was it in the nurse's behavior that elicited such a strong reaction in the patient. This question may not be responded to directly, and the nurse must also be aware that the patient can assume that the nurse believes herself responsible for the patient's behavior because she has requested that he identify aspects of her behavior that were either annoying or upsetting to him. The important step, though, is to make it perfectly clear to the patient that you are confused because your intentions were not to be pushy or commanding or critical. It is important for you to know how you come across so that your behavior isn't misleading. This is the beginning of separating inner world from overt behavior. At this point the nurse is using herself to outline a different set of premises. In addition, she makes it clear that she can't possibly know what the patient is thinking. He will have to tell her. It is even useful to reiterate that one really does not know what is going on in the mind of another person, and one only makes inferences about that from people's behavior, but one does have to check out whether those inferences are correct.

The most characteristic reaction and response to someone who tends to project and be suspicious is to be frightened. Other reactions to projections are to be angry and defensive, often feeling blamed or guilty. These two emotional reactions can often be the basis for establishing rapport and trust between the nurse and the patient. If the nurse states, "I am frightened of you because I really do not know what is on your mind and what you are thinking or how you are interpreting what I am doing," this often disarms the paranoid person, who is convinced of his personal perceptions. However, there is the person who will say, "This is not true. The voices tell me you know and that you are just lying to me." The nurse is then alerted to the delusional state of the patient and the defensive position being taken. It usually means that in some way the nurse is too close to the patient, either spatially or affectively. There are a couple of important strategies to use at this time.

1. Acknowledge that you feel uncomfortable and that maybe each of you needs to clarify the situation because it isn't the way you understand things, though you understand it is the way the patient sees it. When the patient feels like talking, you will come back at a later point.
2. Ask the patient to consider his point of view with you and another person, thus providing more people and a sense of protection and safety.

In this example the revelation that the voices are telling the patient what is going on alerts the nurse to the fact that either she or other people working with the patient will need to talk with the patient when he is less frightened and angry about the voices. This discussion is carried in a manner that is respectful of the experiences of the patient, but it does inform the patient that the nurse's beliefs about the origins of the voices are different from his.

CASE EXAMPLE OF A PARANOID PATIENT

Ms. Kraft was a 63-year-old divorced mother of four children. She had a past history of psychiatric illness, stating to the nursing student that she had been "in and out of state hospitals fourteen times."

On a home visit, the student observed Ms. Kraft to be very talkative and providing a great deal of detail on her two daughters, daughter-in-law, and older sister in terms of their actions and behavior, specifically against her (Ms. Kraft). Upon discussing these women and their negative actions and attitudes, Ms. Kraft would occasionally grit her teeth and rub her nose. She maintained eye contact with the student and would also frequently brush back her hair with her hand.

Ms. Kraft's main theme was that both her daughters and sister were against her and trying to put her back into the state hospital. She became very anxious as she described feeling persecuted and plotted against.

Ms. Kraft was noted to have adequate family interaction, living with her youngest son and seeing two of her children quite frequently. Even though she believed her daughters to be against her, she remained in contact with them.

The following excerpt from a nursing process recording illustrates the use of projection, mind-reading trait, and persecutory beliefs:

MS. KRAFT: I know my two daughters want me out of this house so they can get my money.
STUDENT: How do you know that?
MS. KRAFT: I can tell by watching them talk to each other. They really want my money. Don't you think so?
STUDENT: I really don't know what they think. I have not talked to them.
MS. KRAFT: Well, I think if they can get my son out

of here, then they will send me back to the hospital. You think they are right, don't you?

STUDENT: What makes you think that?

MS. KRAFT: The way you looked when I said that.

STUDENT: I really didn't think that. You seem to be drawing conclusions about my thoughts without checking them out. I'll be glad to tell you if such a thought passed through my mind. Do you sometimes think you know what other people are thinking?

MS. KRAFT: Yes—I do that a lot.

STUDENT: That is something we can talk about more.

In this interaction, the student gently challenged the patient's paranoid position of thinking that she knew what other people were thinking by focusing the conversation on herself and her own thoughts. This intervention for reality testing will help to build a sense of trust in the patient (see Nursing Care Plan on Paranoid Disorders).

Psychiatric and Nursing Diagnosis Formulation

The assessment interview resulted in the diagnoses that are listed below.

Psychiatric Diagnoses by Axis

Axis I: 297.100 Delusional Disorder
Axis II: No diagnosis
Axis III: No physical condition noted
Axis IV: 4, moderate
Axis V: Fair

NURSING CARE PLAN
Paranoid Disorders

HUMAN RESPONSE

1. Persistent persecutory delusion or delusional jealousy.
   Patient example: Daughters wanted her money and to put her in state hospital.
2. Emotion and behavior appropriate to the content of the delusional system.
3. Chronic and stable persecutory delusional system of at least 6 months duration.
   Patient example: Previous hospital admissions.

NURSING DIAGNOSES

- Alteration in thought content.
- Appropriate affect and behavior when talking of delusional thoughts.
- Alteration in thought process.

INTERVENTIONS

1. Analyze thought content and persecutory theme. Listen carefully to patient. Develop trust with patient by sharing thoughts regarding content. Really test where possible, specific to use of projection and mind-reading trait.
2. Validate the feeling generated by patient when talking of thoughts.
3. Verify prior hospitalization and review each admission to determine positive or negative outcome.

GOALS

1. Patient will experience trusting therapeutic relationship. Patient will analyze own thoughts and will identify them when projecting and drawing conclusions.
2. Patient will agree that feeling and behavior matches thought content.
3. Patient will speak with objectivity regarding hospitalizations and results.

Summary

The delusional (paranoid) disorders were discussed in this chapter and case examples were provided to illustrate the language use of the paranoid person. Nursing care plans describe the challenge of working with this type of patient.

Questions

1. Differentiate schizophrenic disorders from delusional paranoid disorders.
2. How do schizophrenic and paranoid persons manage on an outpatient basis?
3. What is the relationship of aggressive and/or violent behavior in the paranoid patient?

REFERENCES AND SUGGESTED READINGS

1. American Psychiatric Association. *DSM-III-R.* Washington, D.C.: American Psychiatric Association, 1987, p. 202.

2. Oxman, T. E., Rosenberg, S. D., & Tucker, G. J. The language of paranoia. *American Journal of Psychiatry*, 1982, *139*, 275–282.

3. Freedman, R., & Schwab, P. J. Paranoid symptoms in patients on a general psychiatric unit. *Archives of General Psychiatry*, 1978, *35*, 387–390.

Chapter 39

Mood Disorders

Ann Wolbert Burgess

Chapter Objectives

The students successfully attaining the goals of this chapter will be able to:

- Identify major approaches in understanding the affective dysfunctional patterns.
- Explain the process of autognosis in working with a depressed client.
- Design a nursing care plan for a depressed patient integrating psychiatric and nursing diagnoses.
- Describe the nursing management of a manic patient.
- State typical behaviors of a manic patient.
- Describe unresolved grief.
- Identify the reasons people fail to grieve.
- Describe the nursing management for unresolved grief.

There are a variety of psychiatric states and syndromes that are classified under the rubric of mood disorders. Primary mood disorders, also referred to as bipolar and unipolar, manic–depressive illness, and affective disorders are recurrent illnesses that include episodes of depression and may include mania or hypomania.

Mood disorders are common and serious conditions. It is estimated that, at any given time, 10 to 15 million Americans (5 to 7 percent) suffer from some form of depression or bipolar illness.[1] The epidemiology for mental disorders in the general population ranges between 17 to 23 percent of adults. The prevalence of major depression (unipolar illness) is 7 percent, extending to 20 to 25 percent with minor depression and 1 to 2 percent with bipolar illness. The median age of onset is 24, with the range between 10 and 60 years of age. The bipolar patterns show an earlier age of onset, beginning in the late teens or early twenties (median age 25); they are generally more recurrent and the frequency of episodes is generally greater. Bipolar illness represents about 25 to 35 percent of major mood disorders.[2]

The unipolar age of onset is more diffuse because of the various subgroup distributions. The average age of onset does not indicate how early or late the illness can start. Consideration must be given to lifetime behavior patterns, family history, medical problems, and sociocultural patterns.[3] A National Institute of Mental Health collaborative study found that 15 percent of the patients who met the criteria for major depressive illness experienced a phenomenon termed "double depression," described as a major depression superimposed on a chronic minor depression.[4]

The pattern of sex distribution in the unipolar and bipolar subgroups differs. Bipolar illness is distributed between males and females, although females have a tendency to have a higher depression:mania ratio than do males.[5] The majority of rapid cycles (more than four episodes of mood disruption in a year) are women. Many of the studies suggest that females distribute 2:1 among unipolar patients, but this is not a consistent finding.[6]

Mood disorders are by their nature recurrent and cyclic. Several studies have confirmed the classic observation that depression is a recurrent illness. In a study of 101 patients suffering from primary unipolar depression who were followed up for at least 1 year after recovery from the index episode, 51 relapsed into a new depressive episode within the year of recovery. Only those variables related to the period immediately after discharge distinguished nonrelapsers from relapsers. Relapsers showed more symptoms from the original depressive episode, poor social adaptation, a more pathological personality profile, and lower tricyclic plasma levels, despite similar medication dosages. The data are consistent with the hypothesis of an incomplete recovery from the index episode as a risk factor for relapse within one year.[7]

MOOD STATES

The dominant features that link the affective disorders together are disturbances in the patient's mood. Mood refers to a prolonged emotion that colors the whole psychological life. The mood generally involves either elation or depression. The manic and depressive syndromes each consist of characteristic symptoms that tend to occur together. These disturbances, to be discussed in this chapter, are most often a form of manic or depressive behavior, but they may also include unresolved grief.

In the majority of mood states—depressions and manic conditions—the etiology is uncertain, and researchers speculate that varying combinations of stress, personality, central nervous system changes, and other factors contribute to the behavioral state. A description of the two major behavioral states, the manic episode and the depressive episode, will be offered first.

Manic Episode Viewed as a Mood State

In a manic episode, the predominant mood is usually elevated, expansive, or irritable and there are associate symptoms of the manic syndrome. These symptoms include pressure of speech, hyperactivity, inflated self-esteem, flight of ideas, distractibility, a decreased need for sleep, and an excessive involvement with activities that have the potential for painful consequences.

The elevated mood is more often described as cheerful, euphoric, or high. The mood is judged excessive by those who know the individual well. The expansive quality of the mood disturbance is characterized by unselective enthusiasm and unceasing enthusiasm for interacting with people and for seeking involvement with the environment. If the individual is frustrated or thwarted in his attempts, the mood disturbance may change to that of irritability.

The hyperactive behavior often involves excessive planning of and participation in multiple activities (e.g., occupational, political, religious, and sexual). There are efforts to renew old acquaintances which may include telephoning friends at all hours of the night. The domineering, intrusive, and demanding nature of these interactions is not recognized by the individual. Often, the expansiveness, optimism, grandiosity, and lack of judgment lead to activities of reckless driving, buying sprees, questionable business investments, and sexual behavior unusual for the individual. The activities may have a bizarre quality to them such as dressing in colorful or strange garments, wearing excessive makeup, or giving advice to passing strangers.

The speech of the person is typically loud, rapid, and difficult to interrupt. It may be filled with jokes, puns, and amusing irrelevancies. It may become theatrical, with dramatic manner-isms and singing. If the mood is irritable, there may be hostile comments, complaints, and angry tirades.

Flight of ideas is usually present. The accelerated speech may contain frequently changed topics. The individual is easily distracted and is observed through rapid changes in speech or activity in response to external stimuli, such as background noise or signs or pictures on the wall.

Characteristically, there is an inflated self-esteem, ranging from uncritical self-confidence to marked grandiosity, which may be delusional. The individual does not hesitate to start projects for which he has little aptitude, such as composing music, writing a novel, or seeking publicity for an impractical invention. Grandiose beliefs involving a special relationship to God or some well-known figure from the political, religious, or entertainment world are common.

The individual has great amounts of energy and has a decreased need for sleep. When the sleep disturbance is severe, the individual may go for days without sleep and yet not feel tired.

The term "hypomania" is used to describe a clinical syndrome that is similar to, but not so severe as to cause marked impairment in social or occupational functioning or to require hospitalization.[8]

Depression Viewed as a Mood State

Depression covers a broad spectrum of moods and behaviors. Depression is a common complaint, not only among psychiatric patients but also among large numbers of people who are not psychiatrically ill and may never seek psychiatric help.[9]

The mood state of depression may occur in a normal person, in a patient with a psychiatric syndrome, or in a medical patient. Anyone can experience depression.

The mood of depression may be described as one of despair, gloom, a sense of foreboding, a feeling of emptiness, or a feeling of numbness. This mood state may be qualitatively and quantitatively different from other mood states. Whether or not the mood of depression in normal people differs from the mood of depression in people who have clinical depression is a matter that has not yet been decided. The same word is used, but it is not clear whether or not

there is a clinical differentiation between the two.

When patients who have recovered from a severe depression are asked to compare the everyday kind of depression with this kind of clinical depression, they reply that the two kinds of depression are very different. Patients say that the severe depression comes over them like a very dark cloud, but the depression of everyday life is more transitory.

Depression Versus Sadness

It is clinically important to distinguish between the mood of depression and the mood of sadness.[10] The emotion of sadness may so resemble pathological depression that mental health professionals sometimes fail to note the distinction between the two. Consequently, the normal emotion of sadness may be improperly treated by antidepressant medications or by a referral for psychotherapy. This distinction between sadness and depression may be as relevant to the management of the depressed patient as the distinction between the murmur of mitral insufficiency and the functional heart murmur is to the medical management of the cardiac patient. The two murmurs may sound the same, but the conditions are very different from the medical treatment aspect. Similarly, two people can look sad and depressed, but the etiology and nursing interventions for each one may be very different.

NEUROBIOLOGICAL THEORIES

Although the etiology of mood disorders remains unclear, one of the current approaches to study of mental illness is through neurobiological exploration of the brain. There is ongoing research into the biologic factors of mood disorders, including studying the amine and other neurotransmitter systems, circadian biologic rhythms, neuroendocrine regulation, genetic transmission, and limbic system defect. Included in the major neurotransmitter systems are norepinephrine, serotonin, dopamine, and acetylcholine. It is suggested that depression might be the result of an imbalance among one or more of these neurotransmitters.[11]

The circadian rhythm research investigates the hypothesis that mood disorder involves disturbance in the regulation of biologic rhythms that synchronize body functions. It is well reported that affective illness is recurrent and that episodes of depression and mania recur and remit spontaneously. Two specific types of circular forms of the illness are the rapid-cycling and the seasonal affective disorder.[12]

The research strategies designed to understand the neuroendocrine regulation in mood disorders involve the manipulation of neurohormones. The feedback between messenger hormones and the target organs may suggest many types of defective neuroendocrine secretion. Extensive investigation has suggested an overactive hypothalamus-pituitary-adrenal axis in depressive illness.[13]

The current interest in the possible relationship of female depression with sex hormones comes from observations that clinical depression tends to occur in association with events in the reproductive cycle such as menstruation, use of contraceptive drugs, postpartum, and the menopause. However, to date, the research data on a pattern of relationship of endocrine to clinical affective states are inconsistent and should be considered merely speculative because there are reported studies correlating depression with female endocrines.[14]

Genetic Studies

The majority of genetic studies in depression are concerned with evidence that suggests:

1. There is an increased risk of depression in the first-generation relatives of diagnosed depressives as compared to the general population.
2. There is a higher concordance rate in monozygotic twins than is found in dizygotic twins.

Summarizing all the studies, there is reasonable evidence for a genetic factor operating in some types of depressive disorders. But the samples studied are still small, and the most common subtypes of depression have not been reported on yet.[15]

Dexamethasone Suppression Test

There have been major advances in the diagnosing of depression through biochemical means. The dexamethasone suppression test (DST) has gained considerable attention in the mental health field as a possible diagnostic marker for endogenous depression as well as for its implications for treatment and prognostic factors. Studies have found that 40 to 50 percent of patients suffering from endogenous depression or from major depressive disorder with melancholia show early escape from cortisol suppression after the administration of dexamethasone.

A 1987 report by the American Psychiatric Association's Task Force on Laboratory Tests in Psychiatry on the DST was made as follows:

In the past decade, the search for a clinically useful marker for major depression had led the dexamethasone suppression test (DST) to become the single most extensively studied biological test in psychiatry. The DST is one of the first laboratory tests in psychiatry and, as such, represents a significant advancement. However, like many laboratory tests in clinical medicine, the DST does less than one might hope. Due to the limited sensitivity of the DST, the APA task force concludes that the usefulness of the test is not high when a patient is either very likely or very unlikely to have a major mood disorder. When a patient's clinical condition strongly suggests a major mood disorder, a positive DST result is reassuring and confirmatory. It may not alter the choice of treatment, but it may encourage some patients to accept recommended somatic treatments. A negative test outcome should not discourage a trial of somatic treatment if other clinical findings support a decision to treat. In summary, the task force urges the psychiatric community neither to accept the DST uncritically for clinical application nor to discard it. The DST is a promising beginning but it is hoped that better tests will eventually replace it.[16]

PSYCHOSOCIAL THEORIES

Various theories have been developed specific to the mood state of depression. The following discussion includes psychodynamic, cognitive, and social.

Psychodynamic Theory

The psychodynamic theories regarding the dynamic structure of the depressions had their beginnings in Freud's paper, "Mourning and Melancholia," in which the gaps between grief and depression are described.[17] Normal grief, observed Freud, shades into the abnormal, and a complex of mechanisms such as oral dependency, identification with the lost object, inhibition, anger turned inward, and specific issues regarding loss are observed.[18]

Extending Freud's studies, Edward Bibring looked at depression as a state of helplessness and powerlessness after experiences of illness, failure, and loneliness.[19] Bibring continued his research in psychoanalytic theory and defined depression as an ego state in which the individual's emotional expression of helplessness and powerlessness occurs. The depression, as an ego state, is characterized by loss of self-esteem in reaction to three dynamic issues: (1) the wish to be worthy, loved, and appreciated; (2) the wish to be good, loving, and unaggressive; and (3) the wish to be strong, superior, and secure. When these three aspirations are threatened, they lower the person's self-esteem and bring on a depression.

The following summary is based on Edward Bibring's "The Mechanism of Depression."[20]

1. The wish to be worthy, to be loved, to be appreciated, and not to be inferior or unworthy. People who have these aspirations struggle with strong needs to be loved and cared for. These aspirations are viewed as oral issues, which means these people have the potential to become depressed when the fear of not being loved or cared for occurs. They receive their "ego supplies" of being given to and cared for from people who are important to them. The depression may occur when someone who has cared about them leaves or dies.

2. The wish to be good, to be loving and not to be aggressive, hateful, or destructive. These people struggle with issues relevant to being in control and being good versus not being in control or being bad. When these people feel that they are bad or out of control, they may be prone to depression. Sometimes when aggressive or angry feelings within the self become too painful to acknowledge, depression may occur. For example, when someone important to the patient dies, the patient may feel that he might have done something to prevent the death or that he might have contributed to the death. These feelings could precipitate a depression.

3. The wish to be strong, superior, great, se-

cure and not to be weak and insecure. Some people, often men, become depressed when they lose in competition. They are concerned about being strong and winning and not losing. For example, a business failure or poor choice in the stock market may depress this kind of person. The person does not talk about not being loved or about whether he is good or bad in the moral sense, but he feels defeated and this is the issue with which he struggles.

Cognitive Theory

Moods and affects differ in complexity, and Arieti notes that depression appears to require a state of maturation and cognitive constructs that aid in structuring one's ideas of one's self and of others.[21] These cognitive structures may not be fully conscious.

Depression is related to sadness, but it also implies a deviation from the normal way of thinking about and experiencing sadness. Sadness, as defined by Arieti and Bemporad, is the normal response of the human being when he apprehends a situation that he would have preferred had not happened and that he considers adverse to his well-being.[22] Sadness, however, does have positive values. It becomes a motivational source that induces the individual to remedy the effect of the adverse event. When a remedy is found, when the grief work is completed, sadness diminishes or disappears. For example, sadness caused by the death of a loved person will eventually disappear when the survivor feels that the person has left important parts (effects) of himself on earth; or when the survivor comes to think that the person is still alive in some place (alive spiritually); or, on the contrary, when he comes to think that the deceased is not so indispensable as he once thought but can be replaced by another relationship. In other words, the normal person is able, to a large extent, to metabolize sorrow and sadness. The person prone to depression may lack this cognitive capacity.

Depression starts as something positive. A complex situation that was totally unconscious or not yet clarified begins to emerge either as a sudden realization or as a process of slow maturation and progressive understanding. It frequently takes the form of the recognition that a long commitment to a person or to a goal, or to a combination of both, will end in failure. In some cases, the person is unable to do the sorrow work. This marks the beginning of the negative construct. Together with personal impoverishment, the person has the conviction that the unhappy state will continue forever. He feels trapped and in a state of helplessness because the feeling of no power in the situation is overwhelming; he feels he cannot relieve the painful affect and sees no compensatory avenues. The reasons why a realization that at first may have positive values ends up by being destructive and leads either to a temporary or prolonged feeling of helplessness are to be found in the patient's history.

Arieti and Bemporad view the depressive adult as an individual who, as a result of child-rearing practices as well as other experiences, has narrowed his sources of meaning and gratification to a dangerous extent.[23] Furthermore, this person suffers from a paucity of cognitive alternatives that would ordinarily keep him from progressing into further despair following a loss of meaning from the environment. Becker has compared the depressive person's mood to the despair of the actor who knows only one set of lines and who loses the one audience who wants to hear it.[24] This limitation to new ways of thinking and this self-inhibition from new experiences may best characterize depression.

Sociological Theory

There is a sociological explanation for depression. Pauline Bart, a sociologist, has suggested that depression is usually defined as a response to loss, making us aware of the differences between psychological and sociological views.[25] In psychological theory, the problem is viewed as intrapsychic in origin, whereas in sociological theory, the problem is located at the interface of the individual and society. It is important to keep in mind, however, that these differences refer only to presumed etiology, and that the overt symptoms of depressive states, e.g., negative alteration of mood, self-depreciation, paralysis of will, vegetative manifestations, and so on, are seen as similar from both points of view.

The sociological point of view has been cogently expressed by Bart.[26] In a deliberate effort to go beyond the usual case-centered approach to the study of mental illness, she has undertaken three methodologically diverse studies of depression in middle-aged women. The results of the first study, a cross-cultural survey of 30 societies, indicated that, contrary to the American experience, women usually gain, not lose, status in middle age, and that, furthermore, this period is not generally considered to be a stressful one. Bart felt that these findings served to reject a biologic, or hormonal, explanation for depressive reactions of menopause, and suggested instead the importance of sociocultural factors. In her later two studies, involving epidemiologic and interview data, respectively, Bart expanded this thesis, eventually concluding that the depression seen in middle-aged women is due to their lack of important social roles and subsequent loss of self-esteem and that, furthermore, the greater the previous investment in their now declining roles, the greater the chance of depression.[27]

Social scientists and clinical practitioners have become increasingly occupied with explaining why so many women become depressed. Myrna Weissman, a research psychologist, offers two views derived from the sociocultural perspective:

1. The *social status hypothesis* is based on social discrimination against women in which women find their situation depressing because the discrimination makes it difficult for them to achieve mastery by direct action and self-assertion, further contributing to their psychological distress. Applied to depression, the hypothesis is that the inequities felt lead to legal and economic helplessness, dependency on others, chronic low self-esteem, low aspirations, and, ultimately, clinical depression.[28]
2. The *learned helplessness hypothesis* proposes that socially conditioned, stereotypical images produce in women a cognitive set against assertion, which is reinforced by social expectations. Applied to depression, the classic "femininity" values are redefined as learned helplessness.[29]

Weissman further states:

The most convincing evidence that social role plays a part in the vulnerability of women to depression is the data that suggest that marriage has a protective effect for men but a detrimental effect for women. This supports the view that elements of the traditional female role may contribute to depression.[30]

MOOD STATES AND THE *DSM-III-R*

The view of mood states as clinical syndromes includes identifying a number of specific symptoms of certain severity and persistence that produce impairment or disorders. Psychiatric diagnoses are derived from such syndromes.

The major mood disorders include the following *DSM-III-R* categories[31]:

- Manic episode
- Major depressive episode
- Bipolar disorder (mixed; manic; depressed)
- Other specific affective disorders (cyclothymia, major depression, dysthymia)

Manic Episode

The essential feature of a manic episode is a distinct period during which the predominant mood is elevated. The disturbance is severe enough to cause impairment in occupational functioning or in usual social relationships. The person may require hospitalization to prevent harm to himself or others.

Diagnostic Criteria for Manic Episode

A. A distinct period of abnormally and persistently elevated, expansive, or irritable mood.
B. During the period of mood disturbance, at least three of the following symptoms have persisted (four if the mood is only irritable) and have been present to a significant degree.
   1. Inflated self-esteem or grandiosity
   2. Decreased need for sleep, e.g., feels rested after only 3 hours of sleep
   3. More talkative than usual or pressure to keep talking
   4. Flight of ideas or subjective experience that thoughts are racing
   5. Distractibility, i.e., attention too easily drawn to unimportant or irrelevant external stimuli
   6. Increase in goal-directed activity (either socially, at work or school, or sexually) or psychomotor agitation
   7. Excessive involvement in pleasurable activities that have a high potential for painful consequences, e.g., the person engages in unrestrained buying sprees, sexual indiscretions, or foolish business investments

CASE EXAMPLE OF A PATIENT WITH A MANIC EPISODE

Dr. Paul called his cousin early one morning from a distant seashore town. He had been up for the last $3\frac{1}{2}$ days and nights extremely involved in his work and community projects. He was finding himself unable to stop talking to his wife. She was exhausted and realized that her husband had moved into a manic state. It had been 10 years since the last episode and Dr. Paul had maintained himself primarily on psychotherapy. He had discontinued taking drugs for some time because of increased kidney problems from the lithium medication.

The telephone call facilitated Dr. Paul's admission to the emergency room of the hospital. When he arrived, his face was flushed, his eyes were darting and racing around, his rate of speech was rapid, and his thought content was loosely associated. His mouth was dry, and even though he was thirsty and would make a move to get water from the drinking fountain, he would stop as he was distracted by a flow of ideas not connected with the original intention of going to the drinking fountain to get water. Dr. Paul was told that he was doing well in terms of hanging on; that if he could, he should rest and either think about his wife's cool hand on his brow or his wife holding his hand to block the racing thoughts. He was frightened but was reassured that he was doing the right thing by being at the emergency room. He knew he had responded to previous drug therapy and medications would be instituted to help him.

His flow of ideas were as follows: He explained that his thoughts were pouring out and to make sense of them he invoked his law of magic. This allowed him to put meaning around meaningless association of thoughts. He would think to himself: I am a little boy climbing an apple tree. I hate the boss at work who told me that my report wasn't in on time. The car needs fixing. He further explained at one point, he was getting frightened because his memory was going and he couldn't keep all of the thoughts together.

This example graphically illustrates how in a manic episode the wiring and communication within various areas of the brain is violently disrupted by a chemical imbalance and what appears to occur, in part, is that all information stored in the brain pops up without any rhyme or reason. This can be likened to a computer that fails when information stored in the computer appears in an existing file, though no effort was made to link or collect this information from the other files.

The example of Dr. Paul indicates the human need to make sense regardless of another level of awareness that things don't make sense. Being an intelligent man, Dr. Paul found the best way to deal with the unrelatedness of ideas and memories was to use magic where everything could be assumed to be related and make sense. But his fear increased as fatigue set in and he could no longer use memory, thus demonstrating the importance of memory as an ego-integrative phenomenon both of the brain and the personal sense of self.

Major Depressive Episode

Diagnostic Criteria for Major Depressive Episode

A. At least five of the following symptoms have been present during the same 2-week period and represent a change from previous functioning; at least one of the symptoms is either (1) depressed mood; or (2) loss of interest or pleasure.
   1. Depressed mood (or can be irritable mood in children and adolescents) most of the day, nearly every day, as indicated either by subjective account or observations of others
   2. Markedly diminished interest or pleasure in activities
   3. Significant weight or appetite loss or gain
   4. Insomnia or hypersomnia nearly every day
   5. Psychomotor agitation or retardation
   6. Fatigue or loss of energy nearly every day
   7. Feelings of worthlessness or excessive guilt
   8. Diminished ability to think or concentrate
   9. Recurrent thoughts of death or suicide ideation

CASE HISTORY OF A MAJOR DEPRESSION

A 68-year-old widow presents at a psychiatric hospital admission conference as a highly anxious, trembling, teary woman with alternate statements of complaints and sentimentalism regarding her family. She states her depression began 1 year previously when she was hospitalized for a cholecystectomy and bowel resection.

Following a 3-month period in the hospital, she went to live with her eldest son in a relatively small house where she had to sleep in the living room. The son was from her first marriage. She had had little contact with either him or his brother since they left home for the service 25 years earlier. The sons felt they had been on their own since adolescence when the mother had remarried after her first husband died.

The sons felt that their "mother didn't bother them too much until she found herself a widow again." The second husband died from a heart attack 2 years prior to her psychiatric admission. Since this loss, the mother had been trying to make arrangements to live with the eldest son in spite of the fact that she had her own apartment in an apartment building for people over 50. She felt she was quite isolated there and did not join in the activities of the project. The sons said they were willing to do their share but felt she was capable of helping herself.

The sons described the mother as being a difficult person to get along with and one who pushed people away from her by being too demanding.

The patient did well until a year ago when she began to have physical complaints. She said that she had felt "depressed" after her second husband died. Since her surgery she has been extremely depressed, feeling that life was not worth living and was also unable to drive her car because she "felt so badly." Her previously neat obsessive personality changed, and she did not pay attention to her dress or keep her apartment clean. There was a 4-lb weight loss and difficulty falling asleep. In the hospital she eagerly took her medications and was continually asking for more medicine. She created conflict between herself and the other patients by passing along gossip that the other patients resented. She was very reactive to the interpersonal stimuli on the ward. The diagnostic impression was reactive depression caused by her surgery as the precipitating event, with the additional stress factors of the loss of her husband who was the important person in her life; isolation in an apartment building where little contact was made with others and in which others were relatively intolerant of depressive behavior, and her sons' lack of involvement in her life.

During the hospitalization, the patient was constantly pleading to have staff intercede with her sons to have her live with them. She became physically shaky whenever she was with staff and patients on the ward.

She was quite hopeful that after the wedding of her grandchild, the granchild's room would become available to her to live in. When she realized that her son was not going to invite her to live with his family, she began to regress for about a 4-week period. This behavior took the form of her not getting out of bed in the morning, constantly demanding extra time from staff, demanding her meals on the unit, and refusing to do her ward work or to become involved in ward activities, ward meetings, or group therapy. The therapeutic task for the staff was to help her verbalize and resolve her disappointment over not being able to have what she wanted (to live with the son) and to help her reinvest in new activities such as interacting with patients, staff, and the ward activities.

Within the 4-week period she was able to deal with the feelings of loss and disappointment and did become sociable with the staff and patients. She decided not to live in a nursing home as she had previously thought was her only alternative, and was able to make plans to return to her own apartment. She went from full hospitalization to weekends in her apartment until she had made new friends in the apartment building, and with the new interest was discharged from the hospital.

The nursing management focused on helping her to bear the feelings of her sadness and to deal realistically with the alternatives of living in her own apartment, making new friends, and accepting the relationship that her sons could offer her at this time.

Severity Rating

The rating of a major depressive episode is by the following: (1) mild (minor impairment); (2) moderate (some functional impairment); (3) severe without psychotic features (major impairment); (4) with psychotic features; (5) in partial remission; (6) in full remission; and (0) unspecified.

The following case of Mrs. Frank is an example of a patient with a major depression with mood-congruent psychotic features and illustrates a nursing management plan with recommendation for family theory.

--- CASE EXAMPLE* ---

Mrs. Frank is a 59-year-old Caucasian married woman whose initial complaints of confusion and depression precipitated her admission to a private psychiatric hospital for 16 days. She had three prior psychiatric hospitalizations at other facilities, the first occuring approximately 20 years ago and the most recent 10 years ago. Her husband, who served as informant, said that "she'd get into these depressions."

Mrs. Frank left her husband of 35 years 1 year ago following an "argument over twenty dollars." During this separation, Mrs. Frank lived in an apartment several hundred yards from the family home. She wanted to keep in touch with her husband but he refused because he was angry that she had left. One and one half weeks prior to admission she asked her husband if she could return, and although they got into another argument over why she had left, he told her "You do what you want to do." With that minimal permission, she moved back into their home.

Following her return home, Mrs. Frank became increasingly confused, began pacing, was restless and experienced numerous crying spells. The patient complained that her husband never allowed her to make decisions. The husband responded that "she drives herself to depression, taking arguments and carrying it on and on."

Background Information. Mrs. Frank was the youngest of nine children. Her childhood was described as stable, though her father died when she was 12 and this experience was described as "very hard" for her. The family then lived on income from the father's social security as well as earnings from older siblings. Her mother did not work outside the home. Mrs. Frank attended Catholic schools through the eighth grade and did not like school very much. She considered herself a fair student though indicated that she could not get on the cheerleading squad because her grades were not good enough. She was not involved in other extracurricular activities. She began casually dating her husband when she was around 15 years of age and reported receiving "lickings" from her mother for coming home late, reportedly around nine o'clock in the evening.

---

* Case contributed by Elizabeth G. Nissley.

Mrs. Frank's one brother committed suicide at home when she was 21. An explanation of "problems following service in World War II" was given for this. Another sister had been psychiatrically hospitalized after the death of a child.

Mrs. Frank married her husband when she was 22. She worked full time until the birth of their first child and part time thereafter, usually in a shirt factory. They have five children, ranging in age from 25 to 35. The fourth child, who is 27, is still living at home. Mrs. Frank spoke of being caught in the middle of her family. She said that she frequently baby-sits for her daughters and that they argue over who gets to use her the most. There had been one previous separation in the marriage approximately 25 years before, when Mrs. Frank lived with the children in another town for 3 months. She would threaten to leave whenever they had an argument, with these arguments usually focusing on money issues.

Assessment. Mrs. Frank presented as a thin, unkempt, distraught woman looking older than her stated age. Her responses to numerous questions did not in any way reflect the questions that were asked. Her general body movements were restless. Her facial expression was tearful and affect was irritable, angry, and fearful. There appeared to be an underlying depression in her mood. She spoke in a rapid manner.

The patient said that she had no appetite and was not sleeping well. The husband indicated that she had not eaten a "decent meal" in the past 10 days since her return home. She denied any allergies or medical problems. She stated that she smokes one to two packs of cigarettes per day and drinks only when the family goes out to eat. The patient denied drug use.

Mrs. Frank was not active in her Catholic faith nor did she have other outside involvements. She had not worked but was receiving Social Security disability since her last psychiatric hospitalization. She was able to identify that she was having difficulty with her family but showed little insight into the current problems. She was not able to state any goals for the hospitalization other than a desire to return home. The husband indicated that she might return home but also stated that "if it were not for seeing the condition that she was in 2 weeks ago, I would not have let her come back."

Mrs. Frank denied any hallucinations or suicidal ideation. Ideas of reference and delusions of persecution were noted. Speech was loosely associated. The patient was oriented to time, place, and person. Her memory was poor and judgment appeared impaired.

The *DSM-III-R* diagnosis given to Mrs. Frank was major depression, recurrent episode with mood-congruent psychotic features. Criteria substantiating this diagnosis were restlessness, insomnia, poor appetite with significant weight loss, diminished ability to concentrate, psychomotor retardation, and loss of energy. The interdisciplinary treatment team goal was to decrease confusion and depression. Interventions of individual psychotherapy, antidepressant and antipsychotic medication, and a variety of success-oriented activities such as music, horticulture, recreation, and art communication were initiated.

Two nursing diagnoses were given: depressive behavior and coping, ineffective individual. In consultation with the patient, the following goals were established: (1) will meet basic needs for adequate nutrition, sleep during nighttime hours, and personal hygiene while reducing feelings of worthlessness; (2) will demonstrate awareness of reality; (3) will be able to redefine ideas about self in relation to the family situation; and (4) will understand causes and responses to depression through health education.

Nursing interventions focused on obtaining a diet history and, in consultation with the dietary department, encouraging preferred high-calorie foods. Weight was monitored and supplements given as ordered. Mrs. Frank's sleep patterns were observed. A quiet nighttime environment, warm drinks, and sleeping medication as prescribed were all used as needed to promote sleep.

The patient was encouraged to assume responsibility for her grooming. As her confusion decreased, she was also encouraged to participate in activities on the unit. A one-to-one relationship with her primary nursing therapist gave opportunity to assess her belief patterns and to discuss the impact of lowered energy levels on feelings of depression and the control she may have over the depressed state.

Mrs. Frank's changing status was observed and evaluated as she showed decreased confusion and made positive statements and plans for discharge to her home. Her performance of the activities of daily living and return to a normal mood pattern indicated that the goals for decreased depressive behavior were being met.

Application of Model to Case

In addition to the *DSM-III-R* and nursing diagnoses and the interventions needed for the brief inpatient stay and stabilization of Mrs. Frank, Mrs. Frank and her family need a family therapist to work on trust issues that have precipitated dysfunctional family interactions in the past.

The therapist would initiate therapy with Mrs. Frank and her husband and would consider the interests of these two primary family members who have expressed concern for each other and have maintained a marriage relationship for most of 35 years. The therapist would explore what entitlement Mrs. Frank might have as the youngest child in her extended family and one who lost her father in what was perceived as a very significant unresolved loss. With the multidirectional approach, the therapist would include all possible other family members, siding with them whether they can be physically present or not. Family work would be planned. The family legacy of both husband and wife and their loyalties to preceding generations and to their own children would be explored. This would bring into session the issues of one adult son still living at home, the feelings that Mrs. Frank has of being caught in the middle, and the dissension over her baby-sitting obligations.

The goal would be to unlink the invisible loyalties that bind Mrs. Frank to her symptomatic depressive behavior and enable her and her husband to increase trust within the family system.[32]

Through demonstration of multilateral listening concern for the content of each person, the therapist would also be modeling new resources for the family. The intent would enable them to continue building trust even after therapy is completed.

Bipolar Disorder

A bipolar disorder may be classified as depressed, manic, or mixed (e.g., features of both depressed and manic episodes). The essential feature of a manic episode is a distinct period of time where the predominant mood is elevated,

expansive, or irritable and when there are accompanying symptoms of the manic syndrome. A cursory observation of the patient reveals that he looks happy, is totally unconcerned, cheerful, high. The expansive quality of the mood is noted by unceasing and unselective enthusiasms for interacting with people and for searching out involvement with the environment. Manic or hypomanic people tend to have quick wits and possess a good sense of humor. In the manic state the verbal and physical exertion of the person is greatly increased, and he can easily exhaust himself to the point where he does not eat or take care of himself. Just as the depressed patient neglects himself in a self-harmful manner, the manic person neglects himself by overactivity in that he does not have time for the reality details of eating, dressing, and organizing his time. Similarly, the depressed person does not have the energy or interest to do these things.

The person with a depression may go into a manic phase from the depressed phase; this then accounts for a cyclic diagnosis such as bipolar depression.

The following case illustrates the cyclic aspect of bipolar depression.

CASE HISTORY OF A BIPOLAR DEPRESSION

Mr. Land stated that his problem was "recurring depression." He first began having "emotional problems" at 11 years of age. He described becoming dizzy in the library and running home to his grandmother (who lived with the family) in a "panic." His family physician referred him to a psychiatrist at that time. He described himself as a shy and an introverted child but extremely overactive. He always felt "five years ahead" of his peers both in maturity and physical skills. He felt that he was better than his friends except in the really important things like work. He also felt inferior because his friends never had "depressive attacks."

Mr. Land said that his attacks come every year and usually last about 3 months. They used to come in the winter but more recently have been coming in the spring or early summer. He describes himself as a "night owl" who constantly goes out with his friends (when not depressed) and is always the life of the party. He says that he goes from one extreme to another and that there is no "in between." When "up," he is always rushed, has a very poor appetite, constantly going, and doing things on impulse without thinking them through. When he is "down" and depressed, he constantly thinks about all the catastrophic things that could happen to him or his family. He wakes up "shaky" at night in "anxiety attacks" and cannot carry out the activities of normal living such as attending to his appearance. He withdraws from people, cannot concentrate, and everything "appears as if he were looking out from a walled-off vacuum." He becomes afraid to travel and usually has to leave his job.

He knows he does not rest when he should and is like a "machine driving himself even when the fuel is low." He said that his depressive states usually follow some precipitating event such as being transferred to a new position in his work.

He said that no doctor has given him an answer to "why it happens." Each time the depressions occur, they "have to run their course." Once they are started, he cannot prevent himself from going into them and they "engulf" him totally. He can usually see the symptoms coming on. He stated that depression is like "being dead; that everyone seems far away, and although he usually loved people, he did not care about anyone at all." He has not felt suicidal during these periods.

Mr. Land describes his father as a "great guy" but someone he cannot talk with. He has an older (middle-aged) cousin whom he greatly respects. He frequently goes to him for talks in which the cousin "sets him straight" and gives him support and encouragement. He describes his mother as an "overprotective Italian" woman who spoiled him when he was a child; she gave him everything materially. She has always compared him to his older brother (who is 30), who is the "golden son" who can do no wrong. His mother still brings Mr. Land clothing and food whenever she goes shopping. His wife does not get along with his mother because she (the mother) tries to interfere with the raising of their two children. Mr. Land said that his mother has always given money to "smooth things over."

Mr. Land was married 5 years ago and experienced a depression 2 months after the marriage. He said his relationship with his wife is at present "going very well." His wife does become upset when he is depressed and tells him to "try and fight it." He describes his wife as a sensitive woman. He said he does not want any sympathy from his family when he has these depressive periods because it only makes him feel worse.

Other Specific Affective Disorders

Cyclothymic Disorder

A cyclothymic disorder is a chronic mood disturbance of at least 2-years duration, involving periods of depression and hypomania, but not of sufficient severity and duration to qualify as a major affective disorder.

The symptoms in both the depressive periods and the hypomanic periods are seen in the major affective disorders and include: insomnia, feelings of inadequacy, decreased productivity, social withdrawal, loss of libido, restriction in pleasurable activities, guilt over past activities, hypomotor activity, depressed speech, and tearfulness or crying. In the hypomanic period, symptoms include: less need for sleep, hyperactivity, inflated self-esteem, increased productivity, sharpened and creative thinking, hypersexuality, excessive involvement in pleasurable activities, physical restlessness, hyperspeech, and exaggeration.

Dysthymic Disorder

Dysthymic disorder is a chronic disturbance of mood. The term *dysthymia* means "ill-humored" and refers to an inclination to melancholy. Although it has been used for all distressing affective states with anxious, depressive, and obsessional qualities, as well as being a synonym for the entire domain of depressive disorders, the more common use tends to limit it to mild and protracted depressions. The classic picture of the person with dysthymia is that of an individual who is habitually introverted, gloomy, overconscientious, brooding, incapable of fun, and preoccupied with personal inadequacy. These same characteristics have been used to describe the depressive personality.

The defining characteristics of dysthymic disorder include:

A. Depressed mood. Persistent or intermittent depressive manifestations of at least 2 years duration. Presence, while depressed, of at least two of the following:
   1. Poor appetite or overeating
   2. Insomnia or hypersomnia
   3. Low energy or fatigue
   4. Low self-esteem
   5. Poor concentration or difficulty making decisions
   6. Feelings of hopelessness

Onset is insidious or may follow a major depressive episode.

The characteristic of long duration may be discussed in terms of chronicity. The subsyndromal aspect of this disorder suggests a characterological depression. Symptoms of severe depression are not present. The disorder also often has a late onset. Prior diagnostic terms of "involutional depression or melancholia" have been noted. The personality of the person before illness is often stated to be rigid, overconscientious, and emotionally constricted. The illness may be viewed as a regression of the obsessive-defensive life style of the individual.

The onset of the illness is slow with an increase of hypochondriasis, pessimism, and irritability. The main symptoms are motor agitation and restlessness, a pervading anxiety and apprehension, and occasionally delusions associated with an exaggerated hypochondriasis and paranoid ideation.

The following is a case example of a primary depression with residual chronicity:

CASE EXAMPLE

Ms. Lupo, a 50-year-old woman, developed chronic depression following three melancholic episodes—the first at age 40—that had not been resolved completely. During the second episode she was involved in a divorce, her father died of a heart attack, and her son was in an accident that left him seriously disfigured. Ms. Lupo had very little in the way of social support; her mother had committed suicide when Ms. Lupo was in her late teens, and her only sister also suffered from recurrent depressions. While in the midst of the third episode of melancholy, Ms. Lupo underwent a knee operation for a painful benign tumor; this led to narcotic and sedative-hypnotic dependence. Despite vigorous trials with various classes of antidepressants and two courses of ECT, Ms. Lupo has continued to experience intermittent crying spells, insomnia, and periodic death wishes, and she has developed fears of going out of her home. During psychiatric visits she exhibits a pattern of clinging helplessness, pessimism, and resignation.

NURSING ASSESSMENT AND DIAGNOSIS OF MOOD DISORDERS

The dominant features that link the mood disorders together are disturbances in self-care behavior, in motor behavior, and in affect and mood. These disturbances, to be discussed in terms of nursing management, are most often a form of depressive or manic behavior.

Psychological assessment of the individual who is described as being manic or depressed requires careful nursing inquiry in observing, listening, and speaking to the patient, to the family, and to the other health care profession-

als. When gathering data, nurses must carefully assess the following areas: self-care behavior, alterations in psychomotor behavior, alterations of mood and affect, personality coping style, psychosocial stressors, and level of adaptive functioning.

Self-Care Behavior

A crucial assessment area is the capacity of the patient to care for himself. We suggest a simple three-point evaluation scale: (1) patient needs constant assistance with self-care activities of daily living; (2) patient needs some assistance with self-care activities; and (3) patient manages self-care activities on his own. Assessment is made of the patient's ability in the following self-care activities.

- Able to maintain adequate food and fluid intake.
- Able to maintain personal hygiene with minimal assistance.
- Demonstrates the ability to maintain appropriate self-control.
- Is able to interact socially in an appropriate manner for short periods of time.
- Is able to discuss the events leading up to the need for psychiatric care.
- Participates in the evaluation of progress made toward the achievement of formulated goals.

Alterations in Psychomotor Behavior

Psychomotor malfunctioning has long been recognized as a central feature of depression and mania. Clinical portrayals of depressive psychomotor retardation and of main psychomotor acceleration have remained consistent over many years. Patients with psychomotor deceleration have been described as unable to respond quickly or spontaneously, either in thought or in action. Features closely related to this defect are: slowed speech; fixed expression; reluctance to answer questions; difficulty in establishing contact; slowed, deliberate, labored movements; apathy, indifference, or unresponsiveness; low, weak, or whispered voice; and stupor.

This description can be readily compared with that compiled by writers in the nineteenth century. Depressed patients were described as individuals who no longer wished for action but remained motionless and passive or occasionally rocked themselves to and fro. It was observed that the patient's circulation became languid; the face pale; the muscles flaccid; the eyelids drooped; the head hung on the contracted chest; the lips, cheeks, and lower jaw all sank downward from their own weight. Hence all the features lengthened, as the face of a person who hears bad news falls.

Historical descriptions of hypomania and mania have also emphasized psychomotor malfunctioning. Current publications still emphasize psychomotor aspects. The typical behaviors of the person include: talking easily, winningly, and humorously; "he talks and talks and talks"; and he is constantly on the go and never seems to tire.

Neuroanatomic Substrate of Psychomotor Regulation

Neuroanatomic networks that integrate "psychic" and "motor" functions in humans have not yet been completely mapped. During the past several decades, however, substantial progress has been made in identifying certain substrates of psychomotor activities. Although a comprehensive neuroanatomic review is beyond the scope of this chapter, it is fundamental to note that pathways have been identified between components of the limbic system, with its well-documented affective, autonomic, and neuroendocrine functions. These connections provide at least a partial explanation for the long-established clinical observation that the motor disturbance of patients with Parkinson's disease, Huntington's chorea, and other extrapyramidal conditions are exacerbated by stress of affective arousal. These connections might also provide the anatomic basis for understanding why psychomotor features are so prominent in the "functional" psychoses.

Alterations of Mood and Affect

Because of the major disruption in mood and psychomotor activity of the depressed patient, the feelings communicated by the patient are very important to assess.

Feelings frequently observed in individuals who are depressed are feelings of loneliness, worthlessness, hopelessness, powerlessness, and anger. But how does the nurse know if these feelings are actually present?

Feelings of *loneliness* may be verbalized by the individual who is depressed, by comments like: "I always am alone on holidays; no one cares about me." Many people are sometimes lonely, but they have the inner strength to reach out to others to alleviate their needs to be close to others. When an individual experiences pathological loneliness, the feeling is much more intense than being lonely, and the person is not able to reach out to others for fear of being turned away or emotionally hurt. Thus the nurse must assess the degree of loneliness felt by the individual.

Worthlessness is another feeling that may be expressed by individuals who are depressed. Feelings of worthlessness are frequently verbalized by comments like: "No one needs me anymore." "Everything I do is no good and no one even cares what I do." This individual feels that he is not valued as a person, and his low self-concept is reinforced.

Hopelessness is frequently felt by individuals who are depressed. Hopelessness is expressed either verbally or behaviorally as the lack of goals or reasons for being alive. The individual feels all is useless and may withdraw. The nurse may hear, "I just don't care anymore," or "I don't have anything to live for."

Powerlessness is a feeling that can be described as the lack of needed resources to make decisions about one's own life. The individual who feels powerless may express himself by saying, "They make all the decisions here anyway, so who cares about what I think?"

Anger also may be an expressed feeling. There are a large number of depressed patients who seem to be angry and who seem willing to express their anger. The expression of negative feelings may be observed directly by the nurse. Many times the nurse may be the recipient of these negative feelings. An example would be as the nurse enters the patient's room, the patient shouts, "Get out of here; I don't want to see you!"

Many times individuals who are depressed are not able to verbalize their feelings. When a patient cannot verbalize his feelings, the nurse must be cognizant of the nonverbal messages of the individual. Nonverbal messages communicated by a depressed individual may be interpreted as a need to be cared for by the nurse. Frequently the feelings again are loneliness, worthlessness, and hopelessness. These feelings are related to the patient's need for dependency, which may be demonstrated by a demanding and clinging type of behavior.

Other nonverbal messages are communicated by lack of eye contact, slowed body movements, poor posture, lack of interest in personal appearance, sleep disturbances, and eating disturbances. Frequently somatic complaints are expressed, and the individual appears uninterested in all activities of life.

The six major affective or mood states are: happiness, sadness, anger, fear, surprise, and disgust. Although people have been observing facial expressions for centuries, the specific ways to describe a particular set of facial wrin-

kles into a judgment that a person is angry or sad, etc., is difficult. Part of the difficulty is that few objective measurements of facial musculature have been attempted.

Family Assessment

A family assessment is important for all patients. The following case describes a college student experiencing a bipolar depression and the implications for family work.

─── CASE HISTORY* ───────────────────────────────

Mr. Corso is a 20-year-old, single, Caucasian male at present residing with his parents. He is a junior in college, and he is of the Roman Catholic faith. He was referred for after-care after a brief psychiatric hospitalization.

The client's chief complaint is, "I'm a failure. I've let everybody in my family down and I can't deal with it."

This well-groomed, casually dressed man, who appeared younger than his stated age, arrived for his appointment accompanied by his parents. Mr. Corso relates that until February 7, 1987, he was attending college and did well both academically and socially for two years. This 1986–87 school year, however, he began having increased difficulty in his school environment. He explained this by saying that he was spending a great deal of his time studying in order to maintain "a straight A average." He began experiencing insomnia, fatigue, and a decreased interest in activities going on around him. He failed to shave or shower for several days at a time and often "forgot" to eat. A weight loss of 23 pounds over the past month was experienced. He denies having dated over the past 3 or 4 months and had little social contact with others. He experienced marked inability to concentrate, which prompted him to withdraw from college in February of this year.

He returned to his parents' home, but as his symptoms persisted, he sought voluntary admission to the Psychiatric Center. This was his first psychiatric hospitalization.

According to the discharge summary from the hospital, his admission physical and laboratory studies, which included a CBC, urinalysis, biochemical profile II, T_3 and T_4, serology, chest x-ray, and cardiogram, were unremarkable. The patient also had psychological testing, which showed no evidence of psychosis but a clear severe depressive disorder with problems surrounding dependency needs. He was seen in daily individual reality-oriented psychotherapy and was placed on Nortriptyline 20 mg BID.

His hospitalization lasted 11 days, during which time he experienced a rapid clinical improvement, with his affect normalizing in a matter of days. He was given a provisional and final diagnosis of 296.52 Bipolar Disorder, Depressed. Discharge plans included referral to a community mental health center for medication monitoring and supportive therapy.

Mr. Corso denied any present health problems. He had chicken pox and measles during childhood but reported no other history of medical or surgical problems. He denied the present use of tobacco or alcohol, admitting to smoking marijuana at college parties on occasion, "maybe 5 or 6 times altogether." His last use of marijuana was in the spring of 1986. He experimented with alcohol a few times in high school but did not like it. He has not used alcohol since that time.

Mr. Corso described his home life as happy. He is the youngest of three children, having a brother 27 years old and a sister 25 years old. He relates a close relationship with his

───────────────────────────

* This case is contributed by Charlotte McDowell.

parents, especially his mother. He verbalized concern about the pressure he feels regarding living up to the success of his father and siblings, all of whom are successful lawyers. His sister is married to a lawyer as well.

The patient did quite well both academically and socially throughout elementary and high school. He played on the football team, was president of his senior class and student council, and had a leading role in the school play. He was a member of the National Honor Society and had a steady girl friend during the last 2 years of high school. He stated that he did not feel confident around girls, however. He attended Mass with his family on a regular basis.

He related first noticing difficulty during his sophomore year at college when he began worrying more and more about his career choice. He had planned to attend law school when he first went away to college but had a growing desire to be a history major with the hopes of someday teaching American History. Upon discussing this with his family during a weekend visit from college, he reports being met with angry disapproval and resistance from his father. He "felt" his mother would be supportive, in time, although she did not verbalize this to him.

Mr. Corso was cooperative, oriented in all three spheres, and his speech was coherent, logical, and goal-directed. His memory was intact. His affect was flat and his mood depressed. He was rigid and unsmiling and spoke slowly and quite softly after long delays. When he talked about the events leading up to his recent psychiatric hospitalization, he seemed puzzled and distressed. He described himself as feeling guilty about recent events and hopeless about the future. He denied homicidal or suicidal ideation. He denied hallucinations and exhibited no evidence of thought disturbances. His cognitive functioning appeared quite good and he expressed motivation to change. His insight about what happened to him was limited. His judgment was good. He stated he wanted to get help in being able to stand up to his parents, especially his father, in making decisions about his future.

Mr. Corso and his parents expressed a willingness to attend family therapy once a week. All three have expressed a desire to improve communication within the family. Mr. Corso's mother expressed a willingness to "do anything I can to help my son get well again."

In applying Bowen's family model in working with Mr. Corso's family, a specific care plan would be formulated with the purpose of shifting the focus of therapy away from Mr. Corso and redirecting it toward the dysfunctional family patterns.[33]

Plan of Treatment

A working nursing diagnosis of impaired family roles related to lack of differentiation as evidenced by unsatisfactory communication among family members would be applied.[34]

The goals of therapy would be to:

1. Decrease the anxiety within the system
2. Decrease the amount of fusion among the individuals
3. Increase the level of differentiation among members
4. Improve communication among family members

Therapy would begin by obtaining a complete and detailed family history over at least three generations. This would be done to enable each member to see how the family system has functioned in the past and how it is now functioning, and the interrelationship of functional behavior patterns over time. A genogram, a diagramatic representation of the multigenerational family, would be an important part of the history-taking process. By mapping out significant life events for each family member, an analysis of the presence of repetitive family patterns across generations could be examined.

During each phase of therapy it is of paramount importance for the therapist to remain emotionally disengaged but at the same time actively involved in guiding the family members in their work. Recognition of the many interfamily triangles is a central component of therapy.

Early recognition by the therapist of the strengths and weaknesses within the family system will prove invaluable to her. By working with the strength of the system, the therapist will elicit changes, however small, which will have a ripple effect within the system. By pointing out positive changes that have occurred in therapy, the practitioner hopes to keep each of the family members motivated to work toward the stated and unstated goals of therapy. This increase in differentiation-of-self among the family members will enable the system to function in a more positive way during times of increased anxiety. That is the ultimate goal in using a family therapy model.

In the early phases of therapy, the focus would be toward decreasing anxiety and reactivity among the members of the family system. Focusing on thinking through issues rather than on emotions evoked would be a basic method of accomplishing these short-term goals.

Evaluation of effectiveness of therapy would be accomplished through observation of the family systems, as well as feedback from its members in terms of being able to discuss important issues with each member while respecting input from the others. Inability to take a stand on an important issue, e.g., Mr. Corso's feelings regarding his desire for autonomy in career choice, would be an indication that therapy was not progressing toward attaining the desired outcome.

Encouraging dialogue that would focus on family-desired changes would not only focus away from Mr. Corso as the symptom-bearer of family dysfunction but would also encourage the family to work toward making these changes occur within the system.

Discussion of how each member saw himself in terms of family roles would allow the issue of overfunctioning and underfunctioning to be explored. This would be a natural way to talk about fusion among family members and explore ways in which to disengage toward a more differentiated self.

The above steps would have occurred over many weekly family sessions, depending upon the motivation of the family members, the skill of the therapist in remaining outside the family triangles, and a multitude of other factors. As Mr. Corso's presenting symptoms centered around his depression subsided, the therapist could feel confident that this family had responded positively to treatment. Anxiety and fusion would have begun to abate and effective communication would be taking place. Differentiation among family members would be taking place in a slow but steady manner.

NURSING MANAGEMENT OF MANIC EPISODES

Nursing the patient with manic behavior disorder, as with the other clinical syndromes, requires application of the nursing process. Because there is no "standard" way to treat any patient, each individual must be assessed to determine the care based on the behaviors and particular problems the patient experiences. A nursing care plan for patients experiencing a manic episode is provided.

Defining Characteristics

The manic patient tends to be very extroverted and euphoric. He demonstrates a flight of ideas, accelerated speech, and motor activity (occasionally to the point of physical exhaustion), clang or rhyming associations, and a domineering, sarcastic, ridiculing manner. The manic patient makes many requests, demands much time, and becomes irritable and arrogant if ignored. He has overbearing manners, a short concentration span, and seeks to control others. He has delusions of grandeur, leading to the devising of bold schemes that collapse easily. Typically the patient spends money wildly and indulges in alcohol. Defenses seen are often regression, denial, reaction-formation, and identification. In short, the manic patient can be a very exhausting, difficult patient, and thus a very challenging one for the nurse.

One young man was convinced that he was a talented musician and spent many hours composing music. When he wasn't composing, he was on the telephone to publishing houses in Boston and New York. In actual fact, he had little talent in this field. It was a task to get him to rest even 4 hours per night.

Goals

A long-term nursing goal for the manic patient would involve helping him to increase his feelings of security and self-esteem because it is possible that the mania is covering a severe depression. Short-term goals will vary, depending on how the mania is manifested. It is of prime importance that all physical needs of the patient are met because physiological homeostasis must be met before psychological homeostasis can be achieved. Other short-term goals may include helping the patient learn to vent his anger appropriately, learning to get along with others in a group, and learning acceptable behaviors.

Nursing Intervention and Social Model of Care

A therapeutic milieu is very important in treating manic behavior. A calm, quiet environment is best for the manic patient. Bright lights and disco music will only serve to increase his manic behavior. This patient does best on a small unit, in a private room if possible—more for the other patients' sake than his. His room is best located at the end of the hall, away from the noise of the living room or nurses' station. The more subdued the environment, in color, lights, music, etc., the more calming an effect the environment will have on the patient.

Consistency among the staff is very important for this patient. Limits must be set on demanding behavior. It is very important that the nursing care plan be updated and complete. The patient will feel more secure if he knows that all the staff are in agreement as to what he is or is not allowed to do. If the staff are inconsistent, they will find the patient's mania escalating. If the patient is unhappy with restrictions, he should be allowed an opportunity to express his annoyance in an appropriate manner. Be certain to give short concise explanations of limits, rules, etc. Lengthy discussion tends to increase manic behavior.

The nurse should encourage the manic patient to participate in activities that require large-muscle activity rather than in something requiring precision work. The gross motor activity allows the patient an opportunity to release some of his excess energy in a socially acceptable way and to achieve success. A game of volleyball is far more effective an outlet for this patient than a game of Scrabble. This patient does not have the attention span to concentrate on small tasks. Be careful to avoid highly competitive games, for this will also tend to increase manic behavior.

In occupational therapy the patient should be given relatively simple tasks to complete. Of course this will depend on the patient's past experiences. However, it must be remembered that it is important not to frustrate the patient or the manic behavior will increase.

It is important that the nurse be careful to avoid punishing the patient or withdrawing from him because of his very demanding behavior. At times these patients can be very trying, and they bring out the "worst" in the nurse. As stated earlier, limits must be firmly established, but the nurse will find it much more effective to reinforce the positive behaviors the patient demonstrates than to punish the negative behaviors. She should make a concerted effort to spend time with the patient when he is not demanding. It is important to remember that although the patient's manic behavior is often geared toward the nursing staff, the nurse should not take any lavish praise or insults personally. The nurse, representing security and consistency, is often one of the "safest" people the patient can "attack."

The nurse may well have to protect other patients from being recipients of the manic patient's hostility. Again, setting firm limits will aid in implementing this. In addition, the manic patient may have to be protected from the other patients. Other patients on the unit will tire of the loud, often obnoxious behavior of the manic patient and will tend to "dump on him." Many a community meeting has been spent with patients upset over late TV hours, noise at 3:00 A.M., and so forth. Again, firm limit setting can be helpful in solving this problem.

The nurse must understand that some manic patients can be very witty, charming, and enjoyable at times. At these times the nurse must be careful not to encourage the patient too much or he will typically carry the behavior to an extreme and become very "high."

Because the manic patient often resists sleeping regularly or eating properly, the nurse must see that all needs for rest, nutrition, sleep, and elimination are met. These patients often ignore their hygiene because they feel so "pressed" for time. Thus, the nurse must protect the patient from the possibility of actual physical exhaustion.

Often manic patients are placed on lithium carbonate to help control the mania. The nurse must be alert to signs of toxicity and must see that frequent lithium levels are taken as ordered. Many times a major tranquilizer will be ordered to help the patient become calmer. The medication can be used appropriately as one approach to helping the patient learn to deal with his hyperactivity, but it should never be used as punishment.

Occasionally it is necessary to use seclusion as a means of calming down the hyperactive patient. The limited stimuli can serve as a calming influence on him. However, it is very important not to use seclusion as punishment but rather as another form of external control for the patient. Seclusion should be used judiciously—only when absolutely necessary.

The manic hyperactive patient can be a frustrating patient because he so often sets the tone of the entire unit. The nurse may find herself "up," tense, and jumpy after spending time with this patient. However, if the plan of care is implemented consistently, the patient will find that his needs can be met without his behaving in a deviant manner.

Communication Strategies in Working with Hyperexcited Patients

Manic patients have racing thoughts, are engaging and humorous. When they are excited, they feel very humiliated in being confronted, so their way of dealing with it is to project and to try to humiliate you and put you on the spot. They have some thought disorder.

Confrontation of manics with their behavior needs to be done gently and in a warm and consistent way. They have tight prejudicial beliefs. They have an immature character structure and difficulty in intimacy. The nurse can encourage

NURSING CARE PLAN
Manic Episode

HUMAN RESPONSE

1. Increase in activity or physical restlessness.
2. More talkative than usual or pressure to keep talking.
3. Flight of ideas or subjective experience that thoughts are racing.
4. Inflated self-esteem (grandiosity that may be delusional).
5. Decreased need for sleep.
6. Distractibility.
7. Excessive involvement in activities that have a high potential for painful consequences that are not recognized.

NURSING DIAGNOSES[39]

- Ineffective individual coping.
- Impaired verbal communication.
- Alteration in thought processes.
- Disturbance in self-concept.
- Sleep pattern disturbance.
- Alterations in thought processes.
- Sensory perceptual alteration.
- Alteration in self-care.

GOALS*

1. Patient will gain external control by validation of stressors. Patient is maintained on an activity level within physiologically healthy limits.
2. Patient's hyperverbal behavior will decrease.
3. Disordered thinking will decrease. Patient verbalizes medication doses and physiological impact of drugs to body.
4. Self-representation is within reality limits.
5. Patient will be able to sleep during nighttime hours.
6. Patient controls attention given to irrelevant stimuli.
7. Patient will regain ability to discriminate excessive involvement in activities.
8. Patient will regain ability to perform hygienic needs.

INTERVENTIONS*

1. Document psychosocial stressors and major ego defenses; validate with patient. Observe patient and set appropriate controls on activity.
2. Assist patient to listen to himself rather than projecting.
3. Assist patient to note the changes in his thoughts and to gain external control. Monitor psychotropic medications, e.g., lithium reactions. Administer prn medications before behavior escalates and at the first sign of agitation.
4. Review with patient feelings and thoughts about self, self-image, and self-esteem. Reality test with patient self-representation. Frequently reorient to surroundings. Redirect patient away from delusions or hallucinations.
5. Observe sleep pattern for latency, early morning awakening, hypersomnia, interrupted sleep. Medicate prn as per order; evaluate effect, observe for side effects, provide safety measures when necessary with sedatives, side rails, etc. Discourage stimulating activities. Discourage stimulating environment. Discourage caffeine products before sleep. Offer warm decaffeinated beverages before sleep. Assess need for communication prior to sleep. Discourage daytime sleeping.
6. Discourage potentially stimulating environment for patient. Establish set time for talking with patient. Encourage patient to verbalize thought alterations. Limit number of staff contacts during distractibility phase. Conversation should be direct and concise. Avoid arguing and setting up power struggles with patient. Introduce reality in a nonthreatening, nonchallenging manner.
7. Review activities in weeks prior to manic episode in terms of thoughts, feelings, and behavior. Assist patient to gain control over painful affects relevant to activities.
8. Assist patient with personal hygiene as necessary. Routine should be as consistent as possible. Encourage independence.

---

* Sections contributed by Eileen E. Rinear and Janice Trichtinger.

---

the patient to listen to himself by saying, "Are you hearing what you are saying?"

NURSING MANAGEMENT OF DEPRESSION

As indicated in the earlier discussion of depression, there are many different types of depression and many different treatment methods used for depression. The nurse must use knowledge and skill to plan nursing interventions, implement these interventions, and evaluate the care that has been provided to the individual. A nursing care plan for major depressive episodes is provided.

Autognosis

Before nurses begin to assess the behavior of an individual, they should autognose their own feelings about depression in order to be most

effective in working with the patient. Frequently nurses experience feelings of helplessness. Some other feelings nurses may anticipate in working with the depressed individual are as follows:

1. At times the nurse feels frustrated because she wants to help but cannot when the patient is not responding. Often motor retardation is evident during severe depressions, and this lack of physical or emotional response by the patient may make the nurse feel helpless and frustrated.
2. Bad-tempered hostility and hypercritical attitude are often found in certain kinds of depressions. This patient will try to get the nurse to conclude that his whole family is utterly disagreeable. He will try to have the nurse sympathize with his view of the situation.
3. Some depressed patients display a self-berating quality. The nurse simply cannot talk them out of it because they enjoy playing the role of a martyr. In effect, the patient

is saying, "I am the worst person in the world and there is no one as bad as me." Instead of trying to convince him otherwise, it is more helpful to be supportive and wait it out. Bearing the feeling the patient is expressing will aid in the resolution of the feeling.

Behavioral Model and Interventions

In planning care for depressed patients, the nurse must determine the behavioral problems and must implement plans of care that will meet individual needs. The nursing interventions are suggested as follows:

Encouraging Self-Care
In planning care for depressed, withdrawn, or regressed patients, the nurse must determine with the patient the level of self-care capacity. Ideally, the patient, using short-term goals, advances from requiring complete assistance with self-care, to requiring supervision, and then to being completely able to care for self. Self-care consists of adequate food and fluid intake, maintenance of personal hygiene, adequate sleep, and normal physical activity. The activities of daily living provide a basis for the monitoring of the self-care deficits.

Providing Observation
The person who is depressed often needs constant observation to ensure that he does not attempt to harm himself. Most nursing units have specific protocol regarding patient observation patterns. For example, a patient may be on constant observation—which means 10-minute checks or longer-spaced time periods.

Providing Controls
A major behavioral intervention is to provide controls for the patient. Often patients with a depression feel so low and have so little self-esteem and hope regarding their situation that they may lose control of their self-protective impulses. Loss of control may result in the patient's attempting to hurt himself through a self-destructive act.

When a patient cannot control his own impulses, the nurse assumes responsibility for the safety of the patient. The regressive behavior of the patient is severe, and this may be one of the reasons for the hospitalization of the patient. The nursing interventions for providing controls for the patient in the hospital setting are implemented in the following ways:

- Close observation of the patient and restriction of the patient to observable areas on the ward.
- Implementation of the one-to-one relationship.
- Determining when the patient may leave the unit with staff or visitors or alone.
- Removal of potentially injurious items such as razor blades and scissors. This procedure is usually part of the routine admission procedure for patients who have self-destructive impulses. Although it is documented that the removal of all potentially injurious items will not necessarily ensure that a person will not hurt himself, removal of the items does help to decrease such impulsive gestures of the patient as wrist slashing and swallowing of pills from hidden medications.

Using Communication Strategies
The primary communication pattern in the withdrawn and depressed person is *internal reference*. The internal questions include:

- Why is this happening to me?
- Why do things always happen to me?

There are clues in communicating with people who use repetitive, ruminating processes. At an operational level, the person is carrying on an internal dialogue of self-recrimination, and this is revealed in the individual's communication. The question is rhetorical, and a strategy for response by the nurse is, "What in fact happened to you? How is it you believe this should not have happened to you?" You are dealing with a whole theory of how the person cares about "being perfect." You can also learn how this person derives his expectations and disappointments in himself and others.

There is the causal belief: "I am so bad; I am causing all this problem," rather than believing that life events have a way of happening and it is a matter of how to cope with them.

The communication strategy includes the following:

1. Work on the patient's belief system and patterns (presuppositions).

2. Work on the state of withdrawal and depression with the patient and demonstrate how much control he has over that state. If the person feels depressed, the nurse can say, "Can you imagine yourself feeling even more depressed?" If he says yes, the nurse can ask how he did that; i.e., what did he say, think, what came to mind? The nurse then says: "Now, make it less than that." This strategy is based on control. If the patient can increase feeling depressed, he can also decrease the feeling and that means he has self-control. The purpose is to assist the patient to be aware of how his own cognitions play a part in maintaining the depressive position. Once the patient understands his thinking patterns, this knowledge has a great bearing on his internal state. Once this position is achieved, another goal is established. This next goal may be to assist the patient in working on his pattern of expectation of self and others.

3. Help the patient recognize the control he has over his affective state.

4. Help the patient to progress into dealing with presuppositions, beliefs, and expectations.

Psychological Model and Interventions

The nursing interventions related to (1) developing a good nurse–patient relationship; (2) helping the patient bear and resolve painful feelings; (3) responding to the dynamic issue of the patient; (4) helping the patient feel cared for; (5) helping the patient gain self control; and (6) helping the patient adjust his goals are important psychological aspects in the nursing care of the depressed patient.

Developing the Nurse–Patient Relationship

In developing a nurse–patient relationship, the nurse must remember that the initial contact with the patient is the beginning of their relationship. Since trust and care are important components of the nurse–patient relationship, the nurse must begin to establish trust and demonstrate care during the initial interview. One nursing approach that demonstrates caring and begins to develop trust is the nurse's ability to bear the feelings expressed by the patient.

Resolving the Feeling

It may be very difficult and painful to sit with a depressed patient, but the situation and the patient require it. Being able to bear sadness and grief is made possible for many people by the presence of a caring person who listens, talks, and shares the discomfort. A lonely person, whether because of circumstances or his own personality difficulties, may not be able to deal with the sadness in his life. The nurse helps the person to bear the feelings he does not want to bear alone. What is said to the patient is not as important as the fact that the nurse is present. The depressed patient is often desperately lonely and unable to cope effectively.

It is helpful to remember that depression is usually a time-limited condition. Eventually the depression will lift, but much patience will be needed before it does. If it is difficult to allocate an extra amount of time listening to the sadness of the patient, the nurse should try to allot a specific amount of time she knows she can remain with the patient. Sitting and bearing the feelings are therapeutic for the patient, even though the results of this approach are not immediately evident.

Bearing a painful feeling is the first step in the total process of resolution and mastery of the feeling, but not everyone knows how to do this. In the course of their personality development, some people have never learned to cope directly with the experience and to discriminate between various feelings. Instead, they handle internal discomfort and distress by impulsive actions. Some people have never allowed themselves to experience feelings because they have been taught that demonstrating feelings or any similar emotion is a sign of weakness.

To successfully deal with one's feelings means that a resolution of the feeling has occurred. That is, the person must make peace with the situation and its ensuing conflicts, feelings, and problems. For example, in the situation in which the feeling of sadness caused by a loss must be resolved and peace made, the nurse can be of significant support to the patient during the process. For sadness to be resolved, the feeling must be acknowledged cognitively and viscerally, that is, in the head and the heart.[35] The meaning of the loss must be thought about and talked about. The feeling, which may be accompanied by tears and by physical distress in the head, chest, stomach, and other portions of the anatomy, must be experienced. Only then can the person give up and part with that which has been lost.

The nurse helps the patient express his feeling, and she can specifically go over the reality details of his physical symptoms as he works to resolve his sadness so that the patient's pain is lessened by knowing that he is making peace within himself, that he is making therapeutic progress, that someone does care about him and his distress, that he is not alone in his sadness, that he is sharing it in a human way with another person.

When the resolution of sadness is optimal, people can move on to new obligations and opportunities.[36] For example, they can say: "I have lost someone whom I love, but I am able to love again." "I have not lost a son; I have gained a daughter." "I may have lost my uterus, but I am still a woman." "I may be older, but I am wiser and freer." "My dream has collapsed, but I am free of its tyranny." "My children no longer need me in the old ways, but I have something different and vital to offer them." Even the patient with a terminal illness must come to terms with his sadness if the remaining hours, days, or weeks are to have any human meaning.

Responding to the Dynamic Issue

An understanding of the concept of the intrapsychic issue is the basis for the therapeutic skill of determining and responding to the issue. If the assumption is that depression may be viewed as patients struggling with different dynamic issues specific to them, each patient must be looked at separately.

For example, there are some patients who are demanding and clinging and want everything possible done for them. The nurse feels compelled to give the patient something. Other patients feel they are so without merit and worthless that they are not entitled to anything. Some patients say they hate themselves, but when the nurse contradicts them and says that they are fine people, they will become angry with the nurse.

Helping the Patient Feel Cared For

There are several things the nurse can do when a patient is depressed because he feels unloved and uncared for. The patient can be taught how to get those ego supplies he wants. He can be taught some of the social skills of how people develop important relationships. The nurse can help the patient look at situations in which he emotionally pushes away people with whom he could become close. For example, when a wife tells of how critical she is of her husband and says that nothing he does seems to please her, the nurse might say, "What I hear you saying is that your inclination is to push your husband away. It might be more helpful to listen to him more instead of constantly criticizing him." Helping the person who has a strict and hypercritical attitude to soften his approach is often a useful way to help teach more fruitful ways of interacting with people.

If the person is depressed because someone who cared about him is gone, the nurse can help the person grieve. By this process the patient can be helped to give up unrealistic aspirations. For example, if the patient says, "I wish I had my mother back even though she has died," the nurse can say, "You may not be able to have her back, but I can help you grieve so that your wishes will be more realistic." The nurse is often the replacement for the lost person during the grieving process.

When there is a longing for the external supplies that are now gone or have been cut off, the nurse can diminish the need for those supplies by helping the person to resocialize and not to be so demanding of others.

Helping the Patient Gain Self-Control

The nurse can help the patient to get his life back under control by helping him to reorganize his life. This involves the nurse's listening to the person describe in detail his usual style of life and then working with the person to restructure the disorganized parts of his life. Or the nurse can help to ease the patient's superego that demanded that everything be so orderly that his life became disorganized.

Helping the Patient Adjust Goals

When some people feel they have failed and have not accomplished their goals, they may become depressed. The nurse can help these patients to reevaluate what they really want to accomplish and help them to readjust their goals. This might involve helping a patient to grieve for a lost goal or a goal he had to give up. The problem may be seen in medical situations, for example, among paraplegics. The athletic person whose dynamic issue is to achieve may have a great deal of difficulty when he is injured because he has to give up his goals for athletic achievement. In contrast, the paraplegic who has the dynamic issue of being cared for may not become depressed in this situation because he may well thrive on the nurses' caring for him.

Determining the dynamic issue is very important in the nursing approach to the patient who is depressed.

Social Model and Interventions

The social model of care includes the therapeutic milieu of the ward environment. An important nursing intervention with depressed patients is facilitating their expression and mastery of feelings and strengthening their performance level with activities. The following nursing interventions related to feelings include milieu activities.

Loneliness
As the nurse assists the patient to bear the pain of loneliness, the nurse recognizes the emptiness felt by the patient. The nurse assists the patient gradually to move toward social interactions. Opportunities for socialization and interpersonal contact are carefully selected, so that the patient will be able to receive positive feelings about himself from the experience. The patient can be taught the social skills useful in developing work and personal relationships.

Worthlessness
Feelings of worthlessness are related to the patient's low self-concept. Any activity that the nurse and patient may engage in together that will produce a positive outcome will assist in increasing the patient's feeling of worth. The importance of providing respect for the individual's self-esteem is essential. The patient's dignity must be maintained.

Powerlessness
When an individual feels powerless, the nurse needs to provide opportunities for the patient to participate in the formulation of plans for care. The nurse should allow the patient to make decisions that are appropriate to his functioning ability. When possible, the patient should assume responsibility for his care on the unit or in a selected work environment. The nurse may also assist the patient to get his life back under control. This involves the nurse's listening to the person describe in detail his life-style and then assisting him to restructure his life.

Anger
There are some patients for whom anger turned upon the self in the classical Freudian way seems to cause depression. This phenomenon, however, is not a universal cause for depression as was previously supposed. On the contrary, there are many depressed patients who seem to be angry and who seem willing to express their anger. It is most helpful to patients who wish to express anger that they have an opportunity to participate in an adjunct therapy such as occupational therapy in order that their anger be channeled appropriately.

Biologic Model and Interventions

Frequently the nurse assists in the implementation of the biologic model. Somatic treatments are often prescribed by the psychiatrist in the medical management of depression. Antidepressant medicines may be used before electroconvulsive therapy.

Medications
Whenever nurses administer medications, they must be knowledgeable about the dosage, the route of administration, the side effects, and the expected effect. Chapter 21 describes in detail the information needed to adminster antidepressant medications.

The nurse must monitor the physiological state of the patient as well as the emotional state. Total care for the patient is essential. Therefore the nurse must observe the eating, sleeping, and activity patterns for a depressed patient and must record the data on the patient's record. Frequently eating and sleeping present problems for the depressed patient. The nurse has the responsibility to ensure that the patient has time to eat and sleep.

Evaluating the Symptom Cluster in the Community Setting

The nurse in the community setting (in home visiting, in industry, in schools) needs to know what symptoms to evaluate in the depressed person. Because somatic therapies can be helpful, especially in the endogenous depressions and the manic episodes, the nurse, by evaluating the symptom cluster; may be able to refer the patient for somatic treatment or medication.

The assessment of the symptom cluster enables the nurse to determine if the patient is suffering from a depression of the endogenous type or the reactive type. When the nurse discovers an endogenous cluster of symptoms, she should give serious thought to referral for medical treatment. The symptoms of severe weight loss, psychomotor retardation, diurnal variation, hopelessness, worthlessness, and inhibition of feelings are all of the endogenous type of depression. These people usually respond well to antidepressants or electroconvulsive therapy.

In the endogenous depressed patient, the premorbid personality is quite good, and the person tends to describe the depression as "coming out of the blue." He feels enveloped in the depression, but then it may suddenly lift. Medication can work well as a biochemical factor in reversing the symptomatology. When the nurse assesses this kind of depression, she might immediately think, "Here is a penicillin type of depression and the patient should see a physician." The medical model of treatment is indicated.

NURSING CARE PLAN
Major Depressive Episode

HUMAN RESPONSE

1. Poor appetite and significant weight loss or increased appetite and significant weight gain.
2. Insomnia or hypersomnia.
3. Psychomotor agitation or retardation.
4. Loss of interest or pleasure in usual activities or decrease in sex drive.
5. Loss of energy; fatigue.
6. Feelings of worthlessness, self-reproach, or excessive or inappropriate guilt.
7. Diminished ability to think or concentrate.
8. Recurrent thoughts of death, suicidal ideation, wishes to be dead; suicidal attempt.

NURSING DIAGNOSES[37]

- Alterations in nutrition; more or less than body requirements.
- Sleep pattern disturbance.
- Disturbance in psychomotor activity.
- Alteration in self-care and interests.
- Alteration in energy level.
- Disturbance in self-concept.
- Alteration in thought processes.
- Potential for self-endangering behaviors.

GOALS

1. Adequate nutritional status will be achieved and maintained.
2. Patient will be able to sleep during nighttime hours.
3. Patient verbalizes level of adaptive functioning.
4. Patient will regain self-care behaviors. Patient can acknowledge alterations in usual activities. Patient has control over energy level to participate in social activities. Patient expresses awareness and control over changes in partner and sexual relationships.
5. Patient will have data on possible organic or functional etiology for decreased energy level. Patient can verbalize relationship between low energy level and affective state.
6. The patient verbalizes the presuppositions he holds regarding depression. The patient acknowledges control over affect. The patient can form a working relationship.
7. The patient will demonstrate reality awareness.
8. The patient will regain control over self-care and commitment to living.

NURSING INTERVENTIONS*

1. a. *Decreased appetite:* Obtain diet history to determine food preferences and eating habits. Consult dietary department. Encourage high-calorie foods. Monitor patient's intake. Give supplements whenever possible. Monitor weight. Encourage participation in exercise program. If dehydrated: IVs as ordered; monitor intake and output; encourage fluids by mouth.

   b. *Increased appetite:* Obtain diet history to determine food preferences and eating habits. Consult dietary department. Encourage low-calorie meals and snacks. Discourage high-calorie snacking. Encourage small-fragment feeding. Have patient set goals for weight reduction. Assist patient to monitor calorie intake. Monitor patient's intake and weight. Encourage participation in exercise program and group activities such as Weight Watchers. Explore patient's cognition relative to eating and dieting and depression.

2. Observe sleep pattern for: insomnia, early morning awakening, hypersomnia, interrupted sleep. Medicate prn as per order: evaluate effect, observe for side effects, provide safety measures when necessary with sedatives (side rails, etc.). Discourage stimulating activities and environment. Discourage caffeine products before sleep. Offer warm decaffeinated beverages before sleep. Assess need to communicate before sleep. Discourage daytime sleeping.

3. Assess adaptive functioning over the year with the patient acknowledging accomplishments as well as disappointments.

4. Encourage patient to assume responsibility for hygiene and grooming, dressing, and care of living environment. Assist patient in noting change in interest level with usual activities. Encourage patient to assure responsibility for participating in ward or social activities. Explore with patient changes in sexual interests and libido. Assess biochemical changes and psychosocial stressors.

5. Review results of physical and system examination for organic causes. Establish one-to-one relationship to discuss impact of lowered energy level on feelings of depression.

6. Assess with patient causal belief patterns and affective state. Demonstrate to patient that he has control over depressed state. Establish communication through nurse–patient relationship.

7. Assess reality perception. Provide controls for patient if psychotic depression present. Observe for self-harm.

8. Observe for self-harm: Determine observation pattern (i.e., constant, 10-minute checks, etc.). Establish one-to-one relationship. Dispense medications as ordered; observe patient compliance; monitor for side effects. Provide controls for patient who is acutely suicidal (see Chapter 47).

---

* Eileen E. Rinear and Janice Trichtinger contributed sections of this nursing intervention.

When the nurse assesses a reactive cluster of symptoms in a person in the community, and if the depressive symptoms are not too severe and are related to an environmental stress, the patient can most likely be treated by interpersonal intervention. The community mental health nurse may decide to treat the depression with a social or psychological model, or may refer the person to a local mental health center.

Stalls in Treatment

Refusing Medications
As Chapter 18 reports, recent court decisions permit a patient the right to refuse treatment.

Although the patient may have such a right, it does not remove the patient from the care of psychiatric staff. Such a stall in treatment has the potential to trigger a general withdrawal on the part of staff and patient. One case example follows that summarizes a clinical situation described by psychiatrist Jeffrey L. Geller:

CASE EXAMPLE
Ms. Albert, a 34-year-old divorced mother of one daughter, was involuntarily admitted to a state hospital under a physician-authorized 10-day emergency condition. This was her third psychiatric and first

state hospitalization. Ms. Albert had a recent 25-lb weight loss, was unable to care for her daughter, and had refused all efforts to provide food and care for 3 weeks. On admission, Ms. Albert was depressed, guarded, and unkempt. She denied having hallucinations or delusions, exhibited poor judgment and insight, and claimed a poor memory.

Although Ms. Albert became a voluntary patient on day 8 following admission, she remained isolated, depressed, and taciturn throughout the first 5 months of inpatient care. Although she showed no evidence of thought disorder, she began to regress, exhibiting bizarre mannerisms, refusing to change her clothes, and lying motionless on the floor. A variety of medications were administered including trifluoperazine, haloperidol, amitriptylene, imipramine, and perphenazine. On hospital day 204, Ms. Albert refused all treatments. This refusal behavior continued for 472 days. Shortly after she refused all treatment, her behavior improved in that she became more alert, more coherent, and more conscientious about her hygiene. But she remained unable to care for herself. She could not be discharged because of the concern that she might harm herself and that she could not complete self-care activities. After 3 months of refusing treatment, her behavior again deteriorated. She was described as regressed, delusional, vulgar, assaultive, and incontinent. She established a pattern wherein she claimed a corner of the ward as her own and lay there except for meals and occasional outbursts. This period lasted 13 months, with the only medication being seven injections of chlorpromazine. There were 7 accident reports and 20 episodes of mechanical restraint. After hospital day 454, Dr. Geller began daily visits to Ms. Albert's corner, where initially she would shout obscenities or make delusional proclamations.

On hospital day 718, Dr. Geller ordered 10 mg TID of haloperidol, after discussing his plan with her for 2 weeks. Ms. Albert refused to take the medication the first time it was offered by the nurse but agreed on the second day. Following an intermittent pattern of taking the medication, Ms. Albert began coming on her own to the nursing station at medication time and began to participate in the ward routine. Self-care improved: she started to use her own bed, dressed more appropriately, and carried on conversations with staff and patients. Nursing evaluation of her 30 days after accepting medication noted that she had achieved her highest level of functioning since admission.

When asked why she refused medication, Ms. Albert stated that she did not take the medicines because she was afraid they would hurt her. She reported taking the medications as she began to trust people and after finding out the medicines made her less confused.[38]

In this example, when the patient refused medication, the staff turned their efforts from therapeutic support to trying to obtain legal intervention. They admitted feeling helpless and frustrated. They clearly viewed the case as a legal problem rather than indicative of the patient's disorder and staff countertransference. The psychiatrist, working with the nursing staff, was able to treat the patient rather than continuing to be caught in the confusing interface of psychiatry and the law.

WORKING WITH PATIENTS WITH MOOD DISORDERS

Nurses who wish to work with people who have mood disorders have to be prepared to deal with sadness, guilt, rage, passivity, helplessness, and hopelessness. Depression is familiar to everyone. Nurses can stall their therapeutic interventions by either becoming overly involved with the depressive state or becoming fearful or annoyed and minimizing or ignoring the depressed state.

Nurses working with mood disorders are challenged to examine how the patient's thinking creates unhappy, helpless, depressed emotional experiences. Taking sides, blaming, making comparisons, feeling gypped, believing oneself imperfect, unable to meet expectations, being subject to demands in the face of feeling helpless and overwhelmed all form the superstructure of the cognitive and perceptual orientation of somebody who has depressed affect and feels in his body a lack of energy, power, effectiveness. The depressed person can actually feel physically ill, as the gastrointestinal tract is often upset when people are depressed. In addition the nurse may react more to the excessive sleeping of a depressed person than to the lack of sleep or disrupted sleep of a depressed person.

Autognosis

People with severe mood disorders stir strong reactions in others. When the state of depression is hidden from others, it can only be discerned through themes of the individual that tend to be morose or sad, avoidance of usual pleasurable activities, or in some situations, a contrary state of being jovial, making fun of or laughing about oneself or one's situation when it is not congruent or appropriate to the conflict or predicament of the individual. In the mood disorders in which there is a shift from depression to excessive activity, the nurse is challenged to gather observations and information about the client to discern whether he has moved from a state of deep depression to one of relative integration and normal affective range or to an increasing state of hyperactivity. There is often a tendency for people, when they move from the depressed state, to avoid contact with the health services because of their shift in mood and their desire to involve themselves in the more energetic state. Consequently, the mood shift is not always a well-documented course of events, either observed or established through careful interviewing.

Communication Strategies

The communication strategies for people with mood disorders focuses on some of the following patterns characteristic of people who are depressed. One pattern is self-blame and feeling lack of qualification. This is picked up with the appraisal that the person should have done something or been something or accomplished something. The "should" is the key. It is a command and often punitive in tone. One will observe the patient is unwittingly carrying on an internal dialogue, mumbling in his head, I should have done this. Closely connected to the "shoulds" are the beliefs and premises regarding expectations. These premises can involve unreasonable expectations of the person that lead to a sense of failure and inadequacy, or the expectations of what others should do build for intense disappointment. Paralleling the "shoulds" and the expectations are patterns of communication in which the person constantly makes comparisons. He compares himself to another person in a negative light or he compares the treatment of other people to his own and thinks they are treated better or more favorably. This evolves into ascertaining the person's premises about what is just and right or wrong. It is within the structure of obligation, commands, expectations, and what is right, wrong, just, or unjust that the individual's sense of self is highlighted in a negative depriving or disqualifying construct that diminishes the sense of self. This diminished state can be one of worthlessness, helplessness, or ineffectualness. Communication strategies aim at assisting patients in becoming aware of their beliefs and

premises, the conclusions they arrive at, and their connection to their dysphoric state. Altering these beliefs and structures requires that the patient begin to identify broader and additional relevant criteria, by which he judges himself and others as well as events and their outcomes.

Stalls that occur in working with depressed clients usually come for the nurse who confronts in the client a repeated belief structure that has not been addressed or challenged by the nurse. What usually occurs is that the nurse and client will repeat the difficulty over and over. For example, the patient explains: "My mother always yells at me." The nurse responds, "That must make you unhappy." The patient continues: "Yes, it makes me very unhappy. I don't believe she loves me." The nurse responds: "It must be difficult to not be loved and yelled at by your mother." As this scenario goes on and develops over a 5- to 10-minute period, both will feel an intense state of dysphoria. There is no challenge to the belief that mother "always yells" at her. A suggested correction could be: "Are there times she doesn't yell?" There is no challenge to her conclusion that because she yells, she doesn't love her daughter. There is no sorting for other experiences of the daughter with mother.

UNRESOLVED GRIEF

Virtually everyone must deal with grief at some time in his life. Grief situations follow the loss or death of significant persons as well as less overt examples of separation.

A person who is unable to experience sadness often presents himself for psychiatric care with this depressive mood state as an important clinical feature. He may be reacting with functional complaints to some loss in his personal life, or he may be reacting to a loss resulting from a medical diagnosis or procedure. This patient then presents himself with symptoms of gloom, despair, and feelings of emptiness.

Depression may occur because the person is unable to bear his sadness. Instead of acknowledging and facing the loss, he feels numb or detached. He denies the loss by saying, "It couldn't have happened. It is beyond belief." The denial may even take the form of a psychosis. If the patient is depressed over something he has done, he may project the blame onto someone else or criticize himself in a totally unreal or highly exaggerated way. His agitation relieves his tension. His motor retardation keeps his mind from active thinking. In other words, the person avoids his sadness by depressive symptoms: he feels nothing, denies the loss, avoids responsibility by projecting the blame, and uses motor activity. Depression, then, may be viewed as a defense against sadness and grief.

There are a number of psychomotor behaviors that people may use to avoid feelings of sadness or grief. Persons may drink, eat, or sleep excessively, or behave impulsively. They may also use pain as a depressive equivalent to avoid sadness and other painful affects.

This section deals with unresolved grief, a condition that has a major bearing on the dysfunctional affective states.

The most common reaction to unresolved grief is a mild, chronic depression. In most instances this reaction is hardly noticeable. The patient may withdraw from friends, stop going to church, feel guilty in various situations, and suffer various aches and pains. More severe reactions to failure to grieve include severe depressions, schizophrenic reactions, psychosomatic disorders, or "acting-out" behavior. Under the stress of unresolved grief, the patient will regress according to his individual vulnerability.

Why People Fail to Grieve

We find it useful for the purpose of therapy to classify the causes of failure to grieve (or pathological grief) into social and psychological factors.

Social Factors

Social Negation of a Loss. Pathological grief may result from situations in which the loss is not socially defined as a loss. This may occur following an abortion. The expectation is either that the woman will keep the event a secret or that she should be grateful that the procedure is completed. The situation may be further complicated by the anger directed toward the woman for being "careless" and for inconveniencing others. Similar dynamics occur when a woman gives up an infant for adoption. With both adoption and abortion, there is a grief process to be done, but social support necessary for the process is often inadequate.

Because of the number of patients who present for help following an abortion or giving up a child, we routinely inquire about these possibilities in all women of childbearing age. The diagnosis is more certain when the presentation for help occurs, as it often does, on the anniversary of the loss.

A Socially Unspeakable Loss. Pathological grief may result when the loss is so "unspeakable" that members of the social system of the bereaved cannot be of any help. As an example, a 24-year-old, bright, attractive young woman was found dead from an overdose of morphine. There was no prior history of drug abuse. It was never determined if the death resulted from foul play, accident, or suicide. Because of the uncertainty, no one would ask the bereaved mother the usual questions that facilitate the grieving process; for example, When did it happen? Where did it happen? How did it happen? The mother failed to grieve and made a suicide attempt a month after the funeral in an attempt to "join my daughter." Following the suicide attempt, the patient was referred to a psychiatrist with whom the loss could be discussed. The patient was able to grieve successfully in ten weekly visits.

Geographic Distance from Social Support. Unresolved grief may occur if the person is away from his social supports at the time of mourning. In one situation, a mother decided not to tell her 20-year-old daughter of the father's death until college examinations were completed. By the time the daughter returned home, the family had completed their grieving. They were perplexed over the daughter's tears and provided little in the way of support for her grief. She sought psychiatric help the following year.

Sometimes the bereaved is socially isolated from his family because of geographic distance or psychological alienation. This person has neither family nor close friends. It is to be hoped that he will seek help from clinics or mental health personnel.

Assuming the Social Role of the "Strong One." Some people are designated to be the "strong ones" by those around them. In family situations they are expected to make the arrangements for the funeral and be supportive to everyone else. Needless to say, these people miss the opportunity to deal with their own grief.

The "strong one" impasse also occurs outside the family setting. For example, an operating room nurse was seen crying by the physician and nurse colleagues. They insisted that she go to the psychiatric clinic for "therapy" even though they knew her best friend had been killed in an auto accident just 2 days before. Her social support system believed that operating room nurses—like Marines—are not supposed to cry.

Uncertainty over the Loss. When the loss is uncertain, for example, a husband who is missing in action, both the wife and the social support system are unable to deal with the possible loss.

Psychological Factors

Guilt. The bereaved may be unable to grieve because of the enormous guilt he anticipates experiencing should the mourning process proceed. This concern over guilt occurs most frequently in patients with harsh superegos (often having many obsessional personality features) whose feeling toward the deceased are markedly ambivalent. Alongside their positive feelings for the deceased is an intense hate coupled with the superego injunction "Thou shalt not hate." Guilt may result not only from ambivalent feelings but from a responsibility the patient felt he ignored—not driving carefully, failing to anticipate a suicide, or not watching a child go into the road or the ocean.

The Loss as an Extension of Self (Narcissistic Loss). There may be difficulty in mourning when the person who is lost is perceived as an extension of the patient. One woman referred to her dead mother as "half of myself." Another young woman who lost a daughter, who promised to be everything the patient was not, felt the death left "a gaping hole, as if something was torn out by the roots." She later explained why she had to suppress the grief response: "If I believe that she is dead, then I am dead." Patients who suffer such a loss of self may feel they can never be the same again. "I will get over this, but I will be a different person."

Inadequate Ego Development. There is a group of patients who have not achieved an adequate integration of basic ego functions necessary to experience the process of mourning. Such patients may respond to the loss of a significant other or any separation with serious ego regression. They may experience depression, anxiety, explosive rage, despair, and hopelessness, which is defended by primitive mechanisms often leading to psychotic behavior.

Idiosyncratic Resistances to Mourning. There are other resistances to mourning that may ultimately lead to the syndrome of unresolved grief. This is often more a fear of the mourning process itself than a fear of acknowledging the loss.

1. Some people fear seeing themselves as weak or being seen by others as weak. The yearning and the sadness of mourning are a surrender, an injury to their self-esteem.
2. Others are concerned that their mourning will hurt those who are available and want to help. "I don't want to upset her."
3. Another common resistance stems from the fear of the patient that he will lose control and never regain it, specifically as it relates to the outpouring of tears. One patient related, "I am afraid I will cry and cry and never stop. I will cry in the streets. I will cry over the entire world. And then I will drown in my tears." In this situation, there is the fear of damaging and being damaged by his mourning.
4. Some people feel guilty as a result of the satisfying feeling of crying.
5. One patient suffering from unresolved grief had an anxiety attack whenever she lost anything, even a button. As a child, she watched her father physically attack her mother whenever anything was misplaced or lost. She perceived these attacks as threats on her mother's life and on her own life as she came to her mother's defense. As an adult, to mourn the death of her child would be to acknowledge something was lost and to reexperience the anxiety associated with father's attacks upon her mother and herself.

Overwhelmed by Multiple Loss. Some people who experience multiple losses, such as the death of an entire family, have difficulty grieving on two counts. First, the loss is too overwhelming to contemplate. Second, the family who supports the grief is no longer available.

One patient experienced a multiple loss as a result of five miscarriages caused by a uterine defect. In therapy, the patient grieved the loss of each fetus one at a time. The patient had a name and a set of hopes and dreams for each fetus.

Reawakening an Old Loss. Some people are reluctant to grieve because the current loss reawakens a more painful loss that has not yet been dealt with. The death of a distant aunt, for instance, may reawaken the death of a mother many years ago.

The Diagnosis of Unresolved Grief

The diagnosis of unresolved grief may be inferred from the following historical data and interview observations:

1. If a patient fails to grieve after the death of a loved one, the diagnosis of unresolved grief should be considered. The patient may not have cried, may have absented himself from the funeral, and may have put thoughts of the deceased out of his mind.

2. Unresolved grief should be considered when the patient becomes symptomatic on the anniversary of a loss, when the symptoms recur the same time each year, or when symptoms occur during the holidays (especially Thanksgiving and Christmas).

3. Unresolved grief should be considered when the patient avoids visiting the grave and refuses to participate in religious memorial services of loved ones when these practices are a part of the patient's culture.

4. Unresolved grief should be considered when the patient develops a chronicity of normal grief symptoms, especially persistent guilt and lowered self-esteem.

5. Unresolved grief should be considered when the patient continues to search for the lost person after a prolonged period of time. Some patients make the search while they are in fugue states. Others may wander from town to town or act as if they are expecting the dead one to return. They may even consider suicide to effect a reunion.

6. Unresolved grief should be considered when a relatively minor event triggers symptoms of grief. This event is psychodynamically connected to the original loss.

7. Unresolved grief should be considered whenever a patient is unable to discuss the deceased with relative equanimity. When the voice cracks and quivers and the eyes become moist, unresolved grief is likely.

8. Unresolved grief should be considered when an interview is characterized by themes of loss.

9. Unresolved grief should be considered when the patient experiences bodily symptoms similar to those of the dead person after the normal period of grief.

10. Unresolved grief should be considered when the patient's relationships with friends and relatives shift for the worse following the death. This may represent a displacement of feelings from the dead person. For example, one patient, angry at a stillbirth "that almost killed me," found it difficult to love the next infant until the grief was resolved.

The Treatment of Unresolved Grief

In order for a delayed or incomplete grief reaction to be successfully dealt with, the person has to experience the feelings and thoughts that were initially avoided. He is likely to cry, to have detailed recollections of the dead person, to dream more actively of the dead person, to reminisce. This process is often completed in 6 to 10 weeks. With a successful outcome, we have seen patients who no longer have bodily aches that plagued them from the time of the loss. They experience positive and warm feelings toward the deceased, remembering them not as they were during their dying days and in the coffin but as they were in happier times. They experience a "sweet sadness" over the deceased, not a bitterness. One patient described feeling, after completing the delayed grief, that the "ax was now out of her heart." There is sometimes a feeling that time has resumed after "standing still ever since the loss occurred." Two patients commented that the New Year's Eve after the grief work was very special. "I said good-bye 1974 and good-bye 1964 (the year of the loss)." After successful grief work, people feel increased self-esteem, less guilt, and may resume church affiliation if that was their pattern prior to the loss. They begin to visit the cemetery. Relationships that had been compromised because of a displacement of feelings from the dead person are changed in a healthier direction. One patient who failed to grieve over a miscarriage of an 8-month female fetus had extraordinary difficulty relating to her next-born daughter. After successfully dealing with the grief, the patient commented on how appealing and responsive her daughter had become.

How can one assist with the regrief process? Who can provide this assistance?

For the large numbers of people who fail to grieve because of the absence of an available and supportive social matrix, help can be easily provided. The therapeutic person needs only to gently encourage the patient to discuss the loss and then to bear with the bereaved during the grief process. The therapeutic person will be carefully but subtly scrutinized by the grieving person to see whether or not there is strength, respect, and kindness. It may be helpful to educate and reassure the person as to what is expected, what is all right. We reassure the bereaved, if necessary, that they will not cry forever, or permanently lose control, or go crazy if they grieve. We have never seen these untoward consequences. On the contrary, these things may occur where there is a failure to grieve. If the person complains that the past is the past and should remain buried, we reply that the past is very much in the present because it has not really been buried. Grieving is necessary in order to put the past in its proper perspective.

For those people who experience considerable difficulty in grieving, especially those for whom there are psychological causes for failure to grieve, more active measures may be necessary. Special therapeutic skills may be necessary here. The clinician may help the bereaved reconstruct memories in order to elicit the feelings. "What did she look like?" "What happened the last time you talked with her?" "Where were you standing when you visited the hospital?" "Who else was in the room?"

When failure to grieve results from strongly ambivalent feelings toward the deceased, it is useful and necessary for the person to express the negative feelings. This must be done, however, not by confrontation but by a gentle and supportive approach. For instance, the bereaved may be reassured by the clinician of the strength of the positive feelings that he knows exist. Only then may the patient be willing to verbalize the negative feelings. Sometimes it is easier to assist the bereaved to discuss "disappointments with" rather than "anger toward" the dead person. In discussing negative feelings, it is often easier for the bereaved to use words such as "irritation," "annoyance," or "aggravation" rather than "anger."

With multiple losses, the bereaved will need to deal with them one at a time.

When there is an overcathexis toward the dead person, a firm therapeutic relationship may have to be established before the bereaved dares "give up" the dead person.

The overall response to regrief work is difficult to predict. We have seen no one get worse. We have seen most people improve to varying degrees. In the most dramatic cases we have seen people improve to their level of functioning before the death occurred, even if the event occurred 25 years before. In other situations, improvement is limited by pathological personalities, which are not clearly apparent until the grief work is done.

In general helping a person with regrief work can be a most gratifying experience for the therapeutic person.

Subjective Reactions

Several conditions may develop that would interfere with the nurse's ability to deal adequately with the patient's grief. These are:

1. If the nurse has not successfully grieved for her own losses, listening to the patient's grief may reawaken and revive the nurse's pains.
2. When the deceased resembled one of the nurse's loved ones in age, sex, or other conditions, the nurse may be too pained in contemplating and fearing a similar disaster to support the patient's grief.

The following is a case history of unresolved grief:

CASE ILLUSTRATION

Pam, a 21-year-old student, was presented at a psychiatric community clinic following referral from the Student Health Service. As she talked during the interview, she would periodically dig her fingernails into her palms, and she acknowledged having deliberately cut her arm on several occasions.

Pam talked of having had feelings of "falling apart" and of not being able to control herself, but that she currently felt more in control of her behavior. She felt that her difficulties were caused by her being away from home for the first time. However, she would become upset when she went home because "mother is so sad and father so old."

Pam almost immediately began talking about her sister's death 6 years previously. She did this with a great deal of intense emotion, explaining that it was very difficult for her to talk about it because they had been very close, with her sister being a "mother" to her.

Historically, Pam's mother did not notice her childhood problems, but her sister did and tried to help her. Pam views herself as having been a tomboy (because father had wanted a boy and Pam had tried to please him), fat, very self-conscious, shy, and ugly because of a severe acne problem. The sister began helping Pam by getting her to lose weight and was about to take her to a dermatologist when she was murdered.

The nurse asked Pam to describe the events relevant to the murder, which she did, as follows: The sister went to work as usual the morning after a holiday. The employer called the home around 10 A.M. to find out where she was. The family became concerned and called the police, who felt it was not that serious a concern for alarm at 11 A.M. but stated they would begin a search. The father went to retrace the daughter's usual path to work. The father found his daughter strangled with her stocking in an isolated field that was part of a shortcut she often took to go to work.

Pam wept at this point and said that the feelings she had were of hatred and these feelings were difficult for her to think about as they upset her so much. The resentful feelings she had were toward the police department who wouldn't respond quickly to go to look for her sister, and then when the father did find the body, they sent their rookies to "mess up the clues so that the murderer was never found."

The hatred feelings were also for the townspeople who made the family feel like "freaks" and forced them to withdraw, as a family, into their house "like strange animals in a cage." The family did receive a lot of crank calls and weird letters at the time, and people continually talked about the incident in the town.

Pam saw this as the reason for her subsequent withdrawal from social contacts (she had one girl friend) and for not dating in high school. Pam could recall feeling "numb" at the funeral and remembered looking at people to see their reaction. She then recalled her grandfather's funeral when she was 7 when she did the same thing and they had to take her out of the church. She did not cry at the time of her sister's death, but about 2 years later when a person whom she liked very much died, she cried with great feeling, realizing then that she was also weeping for her sister.

After the sister's death, Pam slept in her sister's bed (Pam's had been the lower part of a trundle bed), and she wore her sister's clothes. Her sister had been 2 years older than Pam.

Pam frequently had nightmares about a man coming in the window with a knife to stab her and had to receive medication from a local physician. These nightmares developed into a fear that she has continued to have so that she would not allow anyone to walk behind her. (She would not even allow her boyfriend to walk behind her.) She had been to her sister's grave only twice in the 6-year period.

Case Analysis of Unresolved Grief

One can readily make the diagnosis that the patient in the above example is suffering from unresolved grief for two reasons:

1. The patient is unable to discuss with equanimity a death that occurred 6 years previously. With a supportive listener, she immediately began to discuss the death with intense emotion.
2. There was a history of failure to grieve at the time of death.

As to the reasons for her inability to grieve, the patient suggests that it was because she and her sister had been very close, with the sister being a "mother" to her. This closeness is further illustrated by the patient sleeping in the sister's bed and wearing her clothes. In addition, the patient has nightmares that she too is being murdered. It becomes clear that the failure to grieve is related to some quality regarding the relationship between the patient and her sister. The data suggest two hypotheses. First, although the patient verbalizes positive feelings toward the sister, she must have harbored many negative feelings toward someone who got from her mother what the patient could not get. In effect, besides loving the sister, the patient hated her. The death consequently evoked too much guilt to let the patient grieve. Digging her fingernails into her palms and cutting her arm on several occasions were a means of relieving guilt. As an alternative hypothesis, it may be postulated that the patient was so attached to the sister, as the only one who cared, that to grieve would be to acknowledge that the sister really died. By not grieving, the sister is somehow still alive.

Whichever hypothesis is correct, the nurse

must provide a supportive relationship that will allow the patient to mourn her sister. In the process, the nurse will discover and help the patient realize and understand the nature of the relationship to the sister that made the grief process so difficult.

Summary

This chapter showed that there are two major mood disorders: (1) manic episode viewed as a mood state; and (2) depression viewed as a mood state. The various explanations of affective disorders included the psychodynamic, cognitive, sociological, and biologic theories.

When providing nursing care for individuals who are depressed or manic, the nurse uses knowledge and skills to implement the nursing process. The nurse assesses the behavior and feelings of the patient, plans nursing interventions based on her assessments, intervenes with the patient, and evaluates the outcome of the plan with the patient and other health care professionals.

Providing care for individuals who are depressed or in a manic state is best accomplished after the nurse autognoses her own feelings. In order to assist other individuals deal with their feelings, nurses must understand their own feelings.

Unresolved grief is an important clinical condition that nurses must assess and diagnose in their work. This chapter reviewed the normal grief process, why people fail to grieve, how one can make the diagnosis of unresolved grief, and the nursing management of unresolved grief.

Questions

1. When should a depressed person seek mental health evaluation?
2. Spend an hour with a person who is depressed, and then identify the feelings you experienced and the feelings expressed by the patient.
3. What are three nursing concerns in providing care for a manic patient?
4. Describe a case in which you made the diagnosis of unresolved grief.
5. What is the relationship between unresolved grief and depression?

REFERENCES AND SUGGESTED READINGS

1. Freedman, D. X. Psychiatric epidemiology counts. *Archives of General Psychiatry*, 1984, *41*, 931–938.
2. Goodwin, F. K., & Jamison, K. R. The natural course of manic–depressive illness. In R. M. Post & J. C. Ballenger (Eds.), *Neurobiology of Mood Disorders*. Baltimore: Williams & Wilkins, 1984, p. 20.
3. Simmons-Alling, S. New approaches to managing affective disorders. *Archives of Psychiatric Nursing*, 1987, *1*(4), 219–220.
4. Keller, M. B., Klerman, G. L., Lavori, P. W., Coryell, W., Endicott, J., & Taylor, J. Long-term outcome of episodes of major depression. *Journal of the American Medical Association*, 1984, *252*, 788–792.
5. Roy–Byrne, P., Post, R. M., Uhde, T. W., Porcu, T., & Davis, D. The longitudinal course of recurrent affective illness: Life chart data from research patients at the NIMH. *Acta Psychiatrica Scandinavica (Copenhagen)*, 1985, *317*, 23–24.
6. Simmons-Alling, op. cit., p. 220.
7. Faravelli, C., Ambonetti, A., Pallanti, S., & Pazzagli, A. Depressive relapses and incomplete recovery from index episodes. *American Journal of Psychiatry*, 1986, *143*, 888–891.

8. American Psychiatric Association. *DSM-III-R*. Washington, D.C.: American Psychiatric Association, 1987, p. 217.
9. Weissman, M., et. al. Symptom patterns in primary and secondary depression: A comparison of primary depressives with depressed opiate addicts, alcoholics, and schizophrenics. *Archives of General Psychiatry*, 1977, 34, 854–862.
10. Lazare, A. The difference between sadness and depression. *Medical Insight*, 1970, 2(23), 23–26.
11. Simmons-Alling, S., op. cit., p. 221.
12. Ibid.
13. Ibid.
14. Kidd, K. K., & Weissman, M. M. Why we do not yet understand the genetics of affective disorders. In J. Cole, A. F. Schatzberg, & S. H. Frazier, (Eds.), *Depression: Biology, Dynamics, Treatment*. New York: Plenum, 1978.
15. Ibid.
16. APA Task Force on Laboratory Tests in Psychiatry. *American Journal of Psychiatry*, 1987, 144, 1253–1262.
17. Freud, S. [Mourning and melancholia]. In *Standard Edition*. London: Hogarth Press, 1955, p. 14. (First published in 1917.)
18. Ibid.
19. Bibring, E. The mechanism of depression. In P. Greenacre (Ed.), *Affective Disorders*. New York: International Universities Press, 1953.
20. Ibid., pp. 13–48.
21. Arieti, S. The structural and psycodynamic role of cognition in the human psyche. In S. Arieti (Ed.), *The World Biennial of Psychiatry and Psychotherapy* (Vol. 1). New York: Basic Books, 1970, p. 3.
22. Arieti, S., & Bemporad, J. Psychological organization of depression. *American Journal of Psychiatry*, 1980, 137, 1360–1365.
23. Ibid., pp. 1363–1364.
24. Becker, E. *Revolution in Psychiatry*. New York: Free Press, 1964.
25. Bart, P. Depression in middle-aged women. In Bardwick, J. M. (Ed.), *Readings on the Psychology of Women*. New York: Harper & Row, 1972.
26. Ibid.
27. Ibid.
28. Weissman, M. M. Depression in women: Progress and gaps in understanding and treatment. Paper presented at the American Psychological Association Project, *Women and Psychotherapy*, Washington, D.C., March 22–24, 1979.
29. Ibid.
30. Ibid.
31. *DSM-III-R*, pp. 213–233.
32. Boszormenyi-Nagy, I., & Spark, G. *Invisible Loyalties*. New York: Harper & Row, 1973.
33. Bowen, M. *Family Therapy in Clinical Practice*. Northvale, N.J.: Jason Aronson, 1986.
34. Loomis, M., O'Toole, A., Brown, M., Pothier, P., West, P., & Wilson, H. Development of a classification system for psychiatric/mental health nursing: Individual response class. *Archives of Psychiatric Nursing*, 1987, 1(1) 16–24.
35. Lazare, op. cit., p. 27.
36. Ibid., p. 30.
37. Loomis, op. cit., p. 21.
38. Geller, J. L. Sustaining treatment with hospitalized patient who refuses treatment. *American Journal of Psychiatry*, 1982, 139, 112–113.

Chapter **40**

Anxiety Disorders

Ann Wolbert Burgess

Chapter Objectives

The students successfully attaining the goals of this chapter will be able to:

- Define a dysfunctional pattern caused by tension.
- Identify the symptoms of anxiety.
- Define four types of anxiety reactions.
- Devise a nursing care plan integrating psychiatric and nursing diagnoses.

One of the diagnostic tasks for psychiatric nurses is to identify actual or potential emotional problems related to anxiety, physical symptoms, dissociative responses, and sexual dysfunction. This task requires some background and knowledge of an individual's capacity for coping with the everyday stresses of life, the ego defenses, and personality traits and styles. Prior to the development of the *DSM-III-R*, the inability to cope with life demands, on a minor scale, merited a diagnosis of "neurotic behavior." And although the term *neurotic* used to have status—to the point of almost being a household word—its usefulness has waned, and in the *DSM-III-R*, "neurosis" is no longer used as a classification. This deletion is due to the change from theoretical to descriptive formulation as the basis for classification. It is be-

lieved that conflict exists in people with psychiatric disorders as well as in people without psychiatric disorders, and therefore the theoretical formulation is not used as a basis for class formation in the *DSM-III-R*.

CONCEPT OF ANXIETY

Anxiety is a universal experience. However, people vary significantly in their ability to tolerate feelings of anxiety and in their ability to cope with anxiety-producing situations. Anxiety is both a psychological and physical experience; thus, an individual will report both psychological and somatic symptoms when he complains of anxiety. The symptoms are similar to fear, but they are triggered by internal states and are out of proportion to any reality of external stimuli or danger.

Typical subjective psychological experiences of anxiety include descriptions of apprehension, dread, edginess, fear, fright, inability to concentrate, irritability, nervousness, panic, restlessness, scared feeling, tension, terror, and uneasiness. Typical physical signs and symptoms of anxiety include anorexia, butterflies in the stomach, tightness in the chest, diarrhea, dizziness, dyspnea, dry mouth, faintness, flushing, headache, hyperventilation, light-headedness, muscle tension, nausea, pallor, palpitations, sexual dysfunction, shortness of breath, stomach pain, tachycardia, tremulousness, urinary frequency, and vomiting.

As the symptoms of anxiety range from psychological to somatic, the understanding of anxiety in a theoretical sense has included both psychological and physical explanations.

Psychodynamic Theory

Sigmund Freud reported that anxiety was a signal of threats that could potentially overwhelm the ego; if the threat was actual, the response would be "traumatic" anxiety. Most anxiety, however, reflects unconscious signals of early dangers; for example, separation may trigger a mild form of anxiety. Freud believed that neurotic behavior was the result of unconscious conflict, and this premise was the key to his formulations. He explained that neurotic symptoms are constructed by the ego.[1] Conflict develops between the forbidden, unconscious impulses of the id and the reality strivings of the ego; the superego can side with one or the other.[2]

The ego, which represents the integrity and liaison between the id, superego, and reality of the environment, must control the impulses of the id by satisfying them or by manipulating the environment. When this is not possible, the anxiety becomes too much for the ego to tolerate, and defense or coping mechanisms must be used to restore equilibrium. Repression and suppression are the primary coping mechanisms. These processes are unconscious. Such conflicts generate anxiety and threaten psychological stability. Conflicts that cannot be resolved are repressed by the ego, or, as Robert Waelder states, are ignored by being swept under the rug.[3] Symptoms frequently reported

by patients are increased anxiety, increased guilt, and depression. Figure 40-1 diagrams this conflict.

Interpersonal Theory

Anxiety as experienced in neurosis has been explained by Harry Stack Sullivan as "anticipated unfavorable appraisal of one's current activity by someone whose opinion is significant."[4] This view of interpersonal theory stresses the importance of interaction or communication. His theory has been based on the assumption that human behavior is positively directed toward goals of collaboration and of mutual satisfaction and security, unless interfered with by anxiety. Therefore, the need for relief of anxiety is the need for interpersonal security.

Sullivan believes that anxiety is the chief disruptive force in interpersonal relations and the main factor in the development of serious difficulties in living. In terms of development, Sullivan sees that anxiety is created in the infant by the mother. When the mother experiences tension, possibly because of her own insecurities about mothering, this creates anxiety in the infant. This is also called "malevolent transformation" in which the need for tenderness has, under the impact of anxiety, been replaced by malevolent behavior. This "malevolent transformation" causes decreased self-esteem and self-respect in the infant.[5]

An example of this interaction between mother and infant can best be illustrated by a case example from a community nurse:

An 18-year-old married woman came to the Community Mental Health Center shortly after delivering her first child, a girl. The woman lived in a two-family

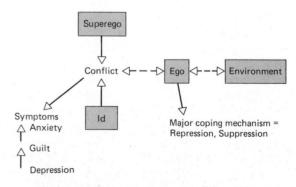

Figure 40-1. Internal psychic processes.

house on the second floor with her husband and baby. Her own mother and father lived downstairs. Ever since the new mother had returned home, she had not been able to care sufficiently for the infant as she had done while in the hospital. She had severe doubts about her ability and competency. Her husband had been staying home from work to care for the infant. While in the hospital the mother had been adequately able to bathe, change, and feed the infant. The change in the young mother's behavior seemed to have been precipitated by her return home. Upon discussion with the community nurse, the woman began to realize that her own mother had had severe reservations about her having a child because she was so young. The woman began to understand that her fears were generated by her own mother's words and concern about her capability. When the young mother became aware of this, she was able to have more freedom and choice of action to assess her own capabilities in caring for her infant. When her own anxiety decreased, the tension in the infant also decreased. This early intervention by the nurse in the mother–child relationship is an important aspect of prevention.

Hildegard Peplau believes anxiety is one of the key concepts in psychiatric work. Nurses use this concept to help explain and understand behaviors observed not only in patients but also in themselves. Peplau defines anxiety as "energy; a secondary behavior following an experience, a subjective experience; an emotion without a specific object; anxiety is reaction and fear is expression in objectivated form; inability to achieve self-realization; threat to some value; and danger to self-respect."[6]

Anxiety is experienced by the individual in such physiological functions as increased heart rate and respiration, increased urinary urgency, dryness of mouth, cold sweat, and fluctuation in blood pressure. It can also be experienced as a "vague discomfort" and feelings of "helplessness" or "impotence." Anxiety is experienced as an apprehension that jeopardizes one's whole existence. This feeling is to be distinguished from fear, which can be perceived as coming from a specific object.

Peplau agrees with Sullivan that anxiety is a threat to the security of an individual. This threat can be biologic; anxiety is also always communicated interpersonally.[7]

It is important that nurses know what effect anxiety has upon observable behavior. These effects—biopsychosocial, cognitive, and perceptual—can be incorporated into the nursing assessment for planning nursing intervention. Nurses also need to remember that anxiety is communicated interpersonally, and they should be aware of their own level of anxiety during patient interaction.

CLINICAL TYPES OF ANXIETY DISORDERS

In the clinical types of disorders to be discussed, anxiety is either the *dominant problem*, as in generalized anxiety disorder and panic disorder; or is experienced if the individual attempts to *confront* the threatened situation, as in phobic disorders; or is experienced if the individual tries to *resist* the thoughts and feelings, as in obsessive–compulsive disorders; or is *reexperienced* after an unusual traumatic event as in post-traumatic stress disorder.

Symptomatic Anxiety

Anxiety states occur in varying degrees of intensity, from a vague, constant or intermittent feeling of unpleasantness and preoccupation to extreme panic, and also as a constant state of tension. The anxiety state may include sadness, anger, and guilt. Persons experiencing the anxiety reaction report physical symptoms of dry mouth, rapid heartbeat, diarrhea, frequent urination, sweating, nausea, hyperventilation, dizziness, faintness, headache, fatigue, insomnia, various aches, and sexual dysfunction. Patients also experience chronic irritability and tension, feel insecure, and lack confidence.

The following excerpt from an interview with a patient suffering from symptoms of anxiety neurosis illustrates the mental anguish these patients experience.

NURSE: How are you feeling tonight?
PATIENT: The day has been awful. All I do is worry.
NURSE: What are some of your worries?
PATIENT: I have pains in my chest and a burning in my stomach and chest. Everyone tells me these symptoms are my "nerves," but I'm worried that it might be cancer or heart disease or an ulcer. I have to be well to care for my sick kids and husband. He can't help me because he's a man and has his job all day.

Then I think about my responsibility at home. I hate the housework part and the kids being sick all the time.

I saw my sister at the doctor's office. She

used to take care of me when I was little, and I'm afraid I'll be a chronic mentally ill case like her.

Then I worry about the noise, the crowds, and riding in a car. Maybe I should just forget about my kids and the responsibilities. Maybe I'll never be better. Or maybe I should just go home. I'll just have to force myself to do the things I hate to do.

Almost all patients with a psychiatric diagnosis of neurosis have symptomatic anxiety. Depressed patients may be so agitated that they cannot sit down, and they may experience a pervasive sense of dread. The anxiety of compulsive patients may trigger ritual diversions, and their anxiety increases if the ritual is disturbed. The somaticizing person is no less anxious about fears of having cancer with the fifth physician than with the first. Anxieties can sometimes be differentiated from fears in that the term *anxiety* is applied to states that are diffuse and are without clearly focused targets.

Anxiety disorders are classified by their major presenting symptomatology and defense systems. The essential features of each disorder are discussed below.

Generalized Anxiety Disorder

Persistent anxiety of at least 6 months duration is the essential feature of generalized anxiety disorder. There are also signs of motor tension (shakiness, jumpiness, trembling, tension, fatigue, twitching eyelids, furrowed brow, sighing respirations, etc.); autonomic hyperactivity (sweating, heart pounding, cold hands, dry mouth, upset stomach, etc.); apprehensive expectation (feels anxious, worries, ruminates, anticipates dread); and vigilance and scanning (feels impatient, on edge, easily distractible, interrupted sleep, fatigue on awakening).

The criteria for psychiatric diagnosis follow.[8]

Diagnostic Criteria for Generalized Anxiety Disorder

A. Unrealistic or excessive anxiety and worry (apprehensive expectation) about two or more life circumstances, e.g., worry about possible misfortune to one's child (who is in no danger) and worry about finances (for no good reason), for a period of 6 months or longer, during which the person has been bothered more days than not by these con-

cerns. In children and adolescents, this may take the form of anxiety and worry about academic, athletic, and social performance.

B. If another Axis I disorder is present, the focus of the anxiety and worry in A is unrelated to it, e.g., the anxiety or worry is not about having a panic attack (as in panic disorder), being embarrassed in public (as in social phobia), being contaminated (as in obsessive–compulsive disorder), or gaining weight (as in anorexia nervosa).

C. The disturbance does not occur only during the course of a mood disorder or a psychotic disorder.

D. At least 6 of the following 18 symptoms are often present when anxious (do not include symptoms present only during panic attacks):
Motor Tension
1. Trembling, twitching, or feeling shaky
2. Muscle tension, aches, or soreness
3. Restlessness
4. Easy fatigability
Autonomic Hyperactivity
5. Shortness of breath or smothering sensations
6. Palpitations or accelerated heart rate (tachycardia)
7. Sweating, or cold clammy hands
8. Dry mouth
9. Dizziness or light-headedness
10. Nausea, diarrhea, or other abdominal distress
11. Flushes (hot flashes) or chills
12. Frequent urination
13. Trouble swallowing or "lump in throat"
Vigilance and Scanning
14. Feeling keyed up or on edge
15. Exaggerated startle response
16. Difficulty concentrating or "mind going blank" because of anxiety
17. Trouble falling or staying asleep
18. Irritability

E. It cannot be established that an organic factor initiated and maintained the disturbance, e.g., hyperthyroidism, caffeine intoxication.

CASE EXAMPLE

A 21-year-old college student, just before final examinations began, experienced a severe anxiety attack accompanied by feelings of panic and impending doom. The day prior to the attack was her birthday and the fourth anniversary of her favorite aunt's death. The symptoms described by the student included fatigue, tension, sweating, cold palms, worrying, feeling of dread, racing heart, feeling edgy and nervous, and an inability to sleep. The nurse learned that the mourning for the aunt had been incomplete and that the student at the time had felt a sense of responsibility to care for her mother, who was very upset over the death of her sister. The student recalled having been anxious and depressed for several weeks just prior to her birthdays for the past several years. She never connected the anniversary of the aunt's death with her anxiety attacks.

Nursing Intervention

The nursing care plan for generalized anxiety disorder includes the nursing interventions of identifying the precipitant, educating the patient, and cognitive reframing. (See the nursing care plan on generalized anxiety disorder.)

Identify the Precipitant. Look for antecedents within a few hours prior to the acute onset of the disorder or at the maximum, within a few weeks. These events need not be the original traumatic incidents but may be related to them. The types of events precipitating severe anxiety are an extension of those precipitating normal

anxiety, such as separation, fears of being hurt or injured, and fear of facing new tasks or new ventures.

Educating the Patient. The patient is in need of ego mastery. The experienced anxiety overwhelms his ability to be in psychological and physiological control; thus, most patients will wish to be assisted in strengthening their control over anxiety. One strategy is to provide a diagnosis to the patient. Understanding the attack as one of anxiety reduces the uncertainty of what was experienced. A second strategy is to inform the patient that the anxiety attacks will pass without any specific action on the part of the patient. Anxiety attacks are self-limiting. This information can be anxiety-reducing for the patient.

Cognitive Reframing. Together with the nurse, the patient can review and rehearse the thoughts that led to the anxiety attack. Speaking the thoughts out loud and in the presence of the nurse helps the patient to gain control over the thoughts. The patient can be asked to pace the

---

NURSING CARE PLAN
Generalized Anxiety Disorder

HUMAN RESPONSE

1. Generalized, persistent anxiety with multiple physical symptoms (see symptom list).
2. The anxious mood has been continuous for at least 1 month.

NURSING DIAGNOSES

- Ineffective individual coping.
- Disturbance in self-concept.

GOALS

1. The patient will demonstrate increased insight into stressors precipitating the anxiety attacks.
2. The patient will demonstrate increased ability to control and master the anxious mood state.

INTERVENTIONS

1. Observe stressors that precipitate the patient's symptoms of anxiety.
2. Provide education by explaining the anxiety attack.
3. Use cognitive reframing to move the patient from an internal to an external frame of reference.

attack and actually time the symptoms as a method to shorten the time frame. This strategy assists in putting the patient's mind on another task (timing the symptoms) and concurrently shifts the thinking to a positive action.

The rehearsal of the anxiety-laden thoughts and images may also open up previously suppressed or repressed material, which can be discussed with the nurse. This technique will also reduce the intensity of the anxiety.

Panic Disorder

The essential features of panic disorder include recurrent panic attacks at unpredictable times as well as in certain situations such as carrying out a specific task. The person describes a sudden onset of intense apprehension, terror, and fear, accompanied by physiological symptoms of dyspnea, palpitations, chest discomfort, cold and hot flashes, sweating, etc. These attack periods generally last minutes; more rarely, hours. The psychiatric diagnostic criteria for panic disorder care plan follow.[9]

Diagnostic Criteria for Panic Disorder

A. One or more panic attacks have occurred that were (1) unexpected, i.e., did not occur immediately before or on exposure to a situation that almost always caused anxiety, and (2) not triggered by situations in which the person was the focus of others' attention.
B. Either four attacks, as defined in criterion A, have occurred within a 4-week period, or one or more attacks have been followed by a period of at least a month of persistent fear of having another attack.
C. At least four of the following symptoms developed during at least one of the attacks:
  1. Shortness of breath (dyspnea) or smothering sensations
  2. Dizziness, unsteady feelings, or faintness
  3. Palpitations or accelerated heart rate (tachycardia)
  4. Trembling or shaking
  5. Sweating
  6. Choking
  7. Nausea or abdominal distress
  8. Depersonalization or derealization
  9. Numbness or tingling sensations (paresthesias)
  10. Flushes (hot flashes) or chills
  11. Chest pain or discomfort
  12. Fear of dying
  13. Fear of going crazy or of doing something uncontrolled
  Note: Attacks involving four or more symptoms are panic attacks; attacks involving fewer than four symptoms are limited symptom attacks (see Agoraphobia without History of Panic Disorder).
D. During at least some of the attacks, at least four of the C symptoms developed suddenly and increased in intensity within 10 minutes of the beginning of the first C symptom noticed in the attack.
E. It cannot be established that an organic factor initiated and maintained the disturbance, e.g., amphetamine or caffeine intoxication, hyperthyroidism.
  Note: Mitral valve prolapse may be an associated condition, but does not preclude a diagnosis of panic disorder.

Diagnostic Criteria for Panic Disorder with Agoraphobia

A. Meets the criteria for panic disorder.
B. Agoraphobia: Fear of being in places or situations from which escape might be difficult (or embarrassing) or in which help might not be available in the event of a panic attack. (Include cases in which persistent avoidance behavior originated during an active phase of panic disorder, even if the person does not attribute the avoidance behavior to fear of having a panic attack.) As a result of this fear, the person either restricts travel or needs a companion when away from home, or else endures agoraphobic situations despite intense anxiety. Common agoraphobic situations include being outside the home alone, being in a crowd or standing in a line, being on a bridge, and traveling in a bus, train, or car.

Diagnostic Criteria for Panic Disorder Without Agoraphobia

A. Meets the criteria for panic disorder.
B. Absence of agoraphobia, as defined above.

The types of panic disorders include panic disorder with and without agoraphobia. In agoraphobia, the patient has a marked fear of being alone, or of being in public places from which escape would be difficult in the face of sudden danger. This individual fears crowds, bridges, tunnels, and public transportation—where escape is limited without assistance. The individual either avoids public places or travels in the company of a family member or friend. There is usually a progressive constriction of normal activities until the avoidance behavior dominates the individual's life. The patient will describe physiological symptoms of breath holding or difficulty in breathing, nausea, sweating, weakness, palpitations, and various epigastric sensations when confronted with the feared activity (e.g., flying).

The following case illustrates panic disorder with agoraphobia.

CASE EXAMPLE

A 21-year-old woman, the eldest of ten children, had a prior history of good socialization skills as well as

dating. She had a strong interest in auto mechanics as an occupation and attended a school, where she excelled. However, she soon developed a fear of being around people, which impacted on her socializing with friends and she sought counseling. Her presenting request was her distress over not being able to leave the house.

The story unfolded that she was having increasing difficulty in getting a job as an auto mechanic although she was the top student in her class. She was being discriminated against as a female seeking employment in a male-dominated area. Also, she was receiving major criticism from family and friends for her vocational pursuit.

In the first interview it became apparent that she was very depressed over social response to her. Therapy focused on her sense of low self-esteem, failure, and rejection. As the depressive symptoms were dealt with, the phobia began to subside. She felt stronger as a woman and was able to pursue her vocation as an auto mechanic.

NURSING CARE PLAN
Panic Disorder

HUMAN RESPONSE

1. One or more panic attacks occurred that were unexpected and not triggered by situations in which person was the focus of others' attention.
2. Panic attacks have periods of apprehension or fear and at least four symptoms of respiratory or circulatory origin.

NURSING DIAGNOSES

- Ineffective individual coping.
- Alteration in breathing and other physiological patterns.

GOALS

1. The patient will demonstrate increased insight into stressors precipitating the panic attacks.
2. The patient will demonstrate increased ability to control and master the panic state.

INTERVENTIONS

1. Observe stressors that precipitate the patient's symptoms of anxiety.
2. Develop and maintain a calm and confident nurse–patient relationship: relax the patient, move the patient from an internal to an external state. Encourage the patient to verbalize his feelings as well as the perceived stressors, and offer appropriate encouragement and reassurance. Encourage the patient to seek staff support when symptoms of anxiety are first recognized. Control environmental stimuli according to the patient's needs and emotional status (e.g., seclusion). Administer appropriate psychotropic medications and evaluate effects of same. Protect the patient from himself during episodes of panic (e.g., seclusion or restraint).

Nursing Intervention

In severe panic attacks, the person is flooded with anxiety and he cannot close off the anxiety. He begins to respond to the panic and the affect escalates. The intervention is as follows:

1. Relax the patient and break the cognitive pattern, particularly the internal dialogue. The dialogue usually proceeds as follows:

PERSON: I feel my heart racing, my palms sweating. What is the matter with me? I know I am going to have another attack. I know it is going to come. (The result is that the anxiety increases.)

One difficulty for the person experiencing the anxiety is that he is not sure when the attack is going to end. If this were known, the person would be able to calm down.

2. Have the person put his mind on another issue. Suggest taking deep breaths, which changes the physiological pattern.
3. Move the person from an internal to an external source. This technique draws the person out of himself rather than going into the anxiety. Do not ask about the attack or the anxiety because that will only increase the feeling. In essence, it is a "talking the person down" type of experience and moving him away from a focused concentration.

─── CASE EXAMPLE* ───

Dora Stone is a 27-year-old divorced white female who presents with a chief complaint of panic attacks and anxiety. Dora first started with the attacks after her marriage at age 17. She describes this marriage as abusive, both mentally and physically. She had one daughter and one miscarriage. This marriage lasted five years with multiple separations and reconciliations. Dora did not seek treatment following the marriage. She is in contact with her exhusband because of her daughter; however, she feels that she is raising her daughter alone.

Dora describes herself as "spoiled" by her parents. During her marriage, she had her parents come to get her in the middle of the night on multiple occasions. After her divorce, she lived with her parents. She now lives with her boyfriend of 5 years who "treats her like a queen." Dora has always lived with family or a significant other.

The reason for seeking treatment at this time is due to her concern and that of her physician for her health. Also, another precipitating feature was a heart attack that her father had within the past 2 months. She was away for the weekend when her father became ill and her mother was unable to get in touch with her. She became very upset at the thought of her father dying and this was further compounded by her mother's statement, "We have always been there for you and when we needed you, you weren't there."

During the same time frame as her father's illness, her ex-husband moved around the corner from her. This caused conflict within Dora's relationship with her boyfriend. Her boyfriend felt that her exhusband wanted her back. He had one episode of intoxication during which he had an accident. This precipitated him losing his driver's license and subsequently his job. She states no problems since with his drinking.

She now presents with a complaint of insomnia. This has become a major problem in the past week. She has been unable to sleep for two nights.

Diet history includes caffeine and a love for chocolate. She consumes a liter of soda, minimum, daily. She has also increased her weight by increased munching throughout the day.

Past medical history includes asthma, and frequent upper respiratory tract infections. No cardiac history stated.

Gyn. Para 2 Gravida 1

Social history includes social drinking, and denies smoking.

Medications— Birth control pills
              Xanax 0.5 mg QID

* This case is contributed by Colleen O'Brien.

DSM-III-R 300.01
Panic Disorder, Severe

NURSING DIAGNOSIS

Ineffective individual coping related to anxiety.

LONG-TERM GOAL

The patient will be able to cope effectively with anxiety and use it for motivation to institute change in life.

SHORT-TERM GOAL

Patient will be able to cope with anxiety and reduce it from severe to moderate.

ASSESSMENT

Patient is unable to work outside the home. Patient complains of "panic attacks" and this includes hyperventilation.

PLAN

1. Be clear and concise in communication with patient.
2. Discuss panic attacks timing to determine any factors that may precipitate event.
3. Encourage coping mechanisms: (a) verbalization, (b) physical activity.
4. Teach relaxation exercises to patient and formulate with patient ways to incorporate into her day and when stressed.
5. Teach deep-breathing exercises and have patient demonstrate back to nurse.

EVALUATION

1. Patient states decrease level of anxiety to a more tolerable level.
2. Patient channels energy into activity, relaxation, or deep-breathing exercises.

NURSING DIAGNOSIS

Sleep pattern disturbance related to anxiety.

ASSESSMENT

Patient has been unable to sleep for two nights.

PLAN

1. Discuss with patient perception of cause.
2. Allow patient to verbalize about anxiety.
3. Prepare optimum restful environment.
4. Provide relaxation tape at hour of sleep.
5. Refrain from daytime naps.
6. Establish regular daily activity.

EVALUATION

1. Identified factors that affected sleeping patterns.
2. Used environment and relaxation tape to achieve a night's sleep.
3. Established routine of daily walks.

NURSING DIAGNOSIS

Knowledge deficit regarding recognition and effective management of anxiety.

LONG-TERM GOAL

Patient will be able to identify sources of anxiety and to use coping mechanisms to manage own anxiety.

PLAN

1. Identify sources of anxiety.
2. Encourage verbalization about concerns.
3. Allow for anxiety level in ability to learn.
4. Encourage patient responsibility in decision process.
5. Establish activity routine.
6. Involve family in care and process.

EVALUATION

1. Listed anxiety factors.
2. Demonstrated increased self-knowledge about factors that cause anxiety.
3. Patient stated that increased activity decreased level of anxiety.
4. Patient expressed improved sense of responsibility for her own life.

Phobic Disorders

A persistent and irrational fear of a specific object, activity, or situation that results in a compelling desire to avoid the dreaded object is the essential feature of phobic disorders. The individual recognizes that the fear is excessive or unreasonable in proportion to the actual dangerousness of the object, activity, or situation.

The phobic person is characterized as having an intense fear of objects or places, or even of particular groups of people. The phobia defends against conscious as well as unconscious anxiety generated from a variety of situations. Phobias include the chief defense mechanisms of regression, projection, and displacement. In becoming phobic, the person fears an external object rather than an internal and unknown source of distress. Phobias are common experiences in childhood, such as a fear of animals, darkness, lightning, and strangers. In adulthood, a phobia can become a crippling experience.

There are many times in which an individual will experience an irrational avoidance of such things as certain insects or modes of transportation, but this usually has no major effect on his life. In fact, certain phobic behaviors derive from childhood and from observing the statements or behavior of one's parents (e.g., hiding under the bed during a thunderstorm). A diagnosis of phobic disorder is made when the avoidant behavior interferes with the individual's social or role functioning. The phobic disorders are subdivided into social phobia and simple phobia.

Simple Phobia

The person with a simple phobia has a persistent fear or compelling desire to avoid an object or a situation. The person may fear a specific animal (zoophobia), confined places (claustrophobia), heights (acrophobia), and air travel.

Social Phobia

The individual suffering from a social phobia avoids situations in which he may be exposed to scrutiny by others. There is a companion fear that he will behave in a manner that will be embarrassing or humiliating. Examples of social phobias include fears of speaking in public, writing in the presence of others, eating in public, and using public rest rooms. The person is usually aware that the fear will be observed by others, e.g., a hand tremor being noticed while writing.

In one case, a 60-year-old woman sought counseling because her husband was offered a new job in another state. She feared moving. Her history revealed the onset of anxiety symptoms 2 years after her marriage at age 25. She became panicked in a bus, requiring her getting off at the next bus stop. Over the years her phobias expanded, and in the past 15 years she had been unable to travel by public transportation, in tunnels, or over bridges. She was unable to shop in markets, eat in restaurants, ride in elevators, cross wide highways, use any public facility. She feared worms and live animals. She had few social friends and avoided social gatherings.

Nursing Intervention

The overall goals of intervention are:

1. The reduction of anxiety.
2. The mastery of the feared experience, usually by actual exposure.
3. The understanding and integration of conflicted areas when these feared experiences are symbolically charged.

Behavior Modification. Behavior modification is sometimes used in conjunction with, or to the exclusion of, psychotherapy. Relaxation exercises can help control anxiety. Desensitization is a technique used to gradually help the patient execute the action that he most fears, like riding in an elevator. The patient would begin with relaxation exercises, such as breathing exercises, to control his anxiety. Next, he would step in front of an elevator, and then leave. After this he would step in front of the elevator and push the button, and then leave. The final steps would include the addition of stepping into the elevator, and so on, until the patient could successfully ride in the elevator without anxiety.

The following example illustrates a situation where behavior modification was required:

Matt Douglas was a 21-year-old single man who lived with his parents and worked in a machine shop. He was referred by his physician to the inpatient unit after no physical cause had been found for severe chest pains. The patient had been going out with a woman to whom he wanted to become engaged, when these symptoms occurred. The patient also experienced a fear of crowds and riding in cars or buses, which interfered with his social life and work performance.

The patient was the youngest son of four children and was the only child still living at home with his parents. His father was a working alcoholic who

would come home from work and argue and often beat his wife. The patient was always his mother's "protector." He would intervene in these fights and beatings and would soothe his mother at night, talking to her or rubbing her back. The patient had never desired to move away from home until he wished to marry, which is when the symptoms of anxiety and phobias appeared.

These symptoms were caused by the conflict over the dependency needs and sexual fantasies the patient had toward his mother. The patient was gradually able to decrease his anxiety, using behavior modification techniques, and he increased his understanding of the reasons for his difficulty in leaving home. The patient was able to return to work in a short time, moved out of his home into his own apartment, and married shortly afterward.

Obsessive–Compulsive Disorder

Recurrent obsessions or compulsions are essential features of obsessive–compulsive disorders. Obsessions are repeated persistent *thoughts* that are seen as intrusive and, at least in part, as ego alien. These thoughts are highly charged with emotional significance. Compulsions are the *action* components, i.e., repetitive, intrusive, and largely ego alien acts.

Obsessive–compulsive disorder is classified under anxiety disorders in the *DSM-III-R* because of the prominence of anxiety.[10] This disorder is viewed as a defense against anxiety. Additional ego defenses used by the individual include: repression, isolation, reaction formation, and undoing.

Examples of commonly described obsessions include:

1. Thoughts of violence, e.g., ideas of stabbing, shooting, maiming, hitting.
2. Thoughts of contamination, e.g., images of germs, dirt, feces.
3. Repetitive doubt and concern that something is not right or that a tragic event may occur or that perfection was not achieved.
4. Repeating or counting images or words or objects in the environment.

Examples of commonly described compulsions include:

1. Touching—usually repetitively, often combined with counting.
2. Washing, especially hands, which seem to come in contact with contaminants.

3. Doing and undoing, opening and closing doors, walking backwards and forwards, changing the order or organization of things.
4. Checking, especially to make sure that no disaster has occurred and that someone has not been injured.

The obsessional person, although under the burden of defenses intended to minimize and deflect anxiety and anger, is nonetheless anxious and angry. Not only do the rituals fail to provide him with the sense of security, it burdens him further with the symptoms.

The psychiatric criteria follow.

Diagnostic Criteria for Obsessive–Compulsive Disorder

A. Either obsessions or compulsions:
   Obsessions: (1), (2), (3), and (4):
   1. Recurrent and persistent ideas, thoughts, impulses, or images that are experienced, at least initially, as intrusive and senseless, e.g., a parent's having repeated impulses to kill a loved child, a religious person's having recurrent blasphemous thoughts
   2. The person attempts to ignore or suppress such thoughts or impulses or to neutralize them with some other thought or action
   3. The person recognizes that the obsessions are the product of his own mind, not imposed from without (as in thought insertion)
   4. If another Axis I disorder is present, the content of the obsession is unrelated to it, e.g., the ideas, thoughts, impulses, or images are not about food in the presence of an eating disorder, about drugs in the presence of a psychoactive substance use disorder, or guilty thoughts in the presence of a major depression
   Compulsions: (1), (2), and (3):
   1. Repetitive, purposeful, and intentional behaviors that are performed in response to an obsession, or according to certain rules or in a stereotyped fashion
   2. The behavior is designed to neutralize or to prevent discomfort or some dreaded event or situation; however, either the activity is not connected in a realistic way with what it is designed to neutralize or prevent, or it is clearly excessive
   3. The person recognizes that his behavior

is excessive or unreasonable (this may not be true for young children; it may no longer be true for people whose obsessions have evolved into overvalued ideas)
B. The obsessions or compulsions cause marked distress, are time-consuming (take more than an hour a day), or significantly interfere with the person's normal routine, occupational functioning, or usual social activities or relationships with others.

CASE EXAMPLE ONE

Sister Patricia, a 40-year-old nun, was admitted to the psychiatric unit after her community was unable to manage her behavior. The patient was a teacher who had not worked for about 6 months because of an increase in her obsessive-compulsive behavior of washing. The patient washed her arms, hands, clothes, walls, and furniture. This behavior increased until finally she was unable to sleep because she was washing her clothes throughout the night and early morning hours.

The patient's ritualistic behavior was a long-standing problem. She had been behaving this way for many years with an increase in severity as she got older. The patient had no recent stressful events that caused her behavior to worsen, the symptoms persisted and increased as the patient matured. The accumulated anxiety caused an increase of her depression and low self-esteem. The chronicity of her behaviors made resolution and nursing management more difficult.

The patient felt she must wash the unit, especially the bathroom, herself, and her clothes constantly. This behavior interfered with her attendance at therapy and activity groups and private sessions. Taking away all the behaviors would have been ineffective and would have increased her anxiety, so the patient might have failed at her treatment. The approach was to give the patient a schedule to follow, so that she had to limit her ritualistic behavior but not extinguish it entirely. Gradually the patient was able to attend more milieu and therapy groups and decrease her ritualistic behavior.

CASE EXAMPLE TWO

A 23-year-old married woman came to the mental health clinic because "life is gray." The story unfolded that there were various secrets in her life, especially that she practiced rituals. For example, she was compelled to read everything three times and tap three times before opening anything. She also felt compelled to read the obituaries every day. The rituals were done in the service of protecting the people around her. The patient felt the rituals were a part of her. They frightened her, and she wondered if she was crazy. On the other hand, to explore them in therapy would increase her anxiety. Part of her ambivalence in exploring them was that she believed that they separated her from her two sisters and gave her a "specialness."

The nursing intervention was first to identify the rituals; next the task was to determine the purpose of the rituals; and third was to identify what she would need in order to give up the rituals. Under stress, she was able to note that the rituals increased in intensity. She was able to remember that the rituals started when she was age 7 or 8 and that she was always the "good girl" in the family. Thus, one could speculate that the rituals were a defense against assertiveness, impulses, and instincts that were opposed to her being a "good girl."

CASE EXAMPLE THREE

In another example of an obsessive–compulsive person, the symptoms accelerated. A fire chief was at a major fire when a wall collapsed and killed some of his men as well as endangering himself. After recovering from the trauma suffered during the fire, he returned to work, but he began to doubt his ability. Concurrently there were cuts in the city budget and his anxieties began to build. He began to worry constantly about fire. He was unable to leave his house without feeling the walls, and he soon began to run back to his house during the day to check the walls. These symptoms forced him into early retirement on disability.

Nursing Intervention

The nursing care plan includes the psychiatric diagnoses as well as interventions and expected outcome and evaluation. The interventions include close observation, reality testing, symptom substitution, and goal-oriented interviews.

Close Observation.

Acute and pervasive obsessive–compulsive symptoms are often rapidly evolving states that need careful monitoring. The patient needs to be observed for the intensity and severity of symptoms and for the possible emergence of both depression and psychosis.

Reality Testing.

The nurse can provide reality-testing methods for the patient who has exaggerated or grandiose thoughts connected to performance of rituals. Reality limits may be unclear, and the nurse may assist as in the following dialogue:

PATIENT: I am doing this for my salvation and my family's—and maybe for yours also.

NURSE: Tell me again why you think your ritual is for my salvation?

PATIENT: Well, when I said that, it may not sound right, but that's what I think when I'm doing it.

NURSE: Do I understand you to mean that while you do the ritual you think it is for your salvation, your family's as well as mine?

PATIENT: I did. But when I hear you say it, it doesn't sound right. I had better think about that again.

Symptom Substitution.

At times, it may be helpful for the nurse to suggest a symptom substitution. For example, when a patient has the compulsion to check and recheck something, the nurse can ask him to sit and think about what he is going to talk over with his therapist at the next appointment. This technique introduces a delay in the performance of a compulsion and should be followed with a verbal acknowledgement that the compulsion was not acted on.

J. G. Taylor has devised a technique known as "thought stopping" to interrupt obsessive patterns.[11] The patient is instructed to yell as loudly as possible the word *stop* in the middle of his obsessions. Behavioral techniques used without other therapeutic approaches are successful with patients for whom the obsessive–compulsive symptoms affect only a narrow range of their functioning and whose personality is relatively healthy.

Goal-Oriented Interviews.

The nurse works with the patient, through the contract, on goal-oriented issues. Although one should not ignore the obsessive–compulsive symptoms, neither should the nurse allow the interview to progress in an endless discussion of symptoms. The nurse needs to establish goals beyond the reduction of symptoms in the area of strengthening interpersonal relationships.

Post-Traumatic Stress Disorder (PTSD)

The *DSM-III-R* category Post-Traumatic Stress Disorder provides a conceptual bridge linking a wide variety of traumatic events, such as war, terrorism, natural disasters, and rape, to a specific set of symptoms. The psychiatric diagnostic criteria for post-traumatic stress disorder follow.[12]

NURSING CARE PLAN
Obsessive–Compulsive Disorder

HUMAN RESPONSE

1. Recurrent, persistent ideas, thoughts, images, or impulses that are ego-dystonic.
2. Repetitive and seemingly purposeful behaviors performed according to certain rules.
3. The obsessions or compulsions interfere with social or role functioning.

NURSING DIAGNOSES

- Alteration in thinking.
- Ineffective individual coping.
- Ineffective coping with others.

GOALS

1. The patient will become aware of thoughts as senseless and purposeless.
2. The patient will verbally acknowledge that the compulsion was not acted on.
3. The patient will master the anxiety that triggers the obsession or compulsion.

NURSING INTERVENTIONS

1. Develop and maintain a confident and calm nurse–patient relationship. Maintain close observation and monitoring of symptoms. Provide reality testing regarding thoughts.
2. Symptom substitution to delay the performance of a compulsion.
3. Identify the precipitant. Educate the patient for mastering control of anxiety. Cognitive reframing.

Diagnostic Criteria for Post-traumatic Stress Disorder

A. The person has experienced an event that is outside the range of usual human experience and that would be markedly distressing to almost anyone, e.g., serious threat to one's life or physical integrity; serious threat or harm to one's children, spouse, or other close relatives and friends; sudden destruction of one's home or community; or seeing another person who has recently been, or is being, seriously injured or killed as the result of an accident or physical violence.

B. The traumatic event is persistently reexperienced in at least one of the following ways:
1. Recurrent and intrusive distressing recollections of the event (in young children, repetitive play in which themes or aspects of the trauma are expressed)
2. Recurrent distressing dreams of the event
3. Sudden acting or feeling as if the trau-

matic event were recurring (includes a sense of reliving the experience, illusions, hallucinations, and dissociative [flashback] episodes, even those that occur upon awakening or when intoxicated)
4. Intense psychological distress at exposure to events that symbolize or resemble an aspect of the traumatic event, including anniversaries of the trauma

C. Persistent avoidance of stimuli associated with the trauma or numbing of general responsiveness (not present before the trauma), as indicated by at least three of the following:
1. Efforts to avoid thoughts or feelings associated with the trauma
2. Efforts to avoid activities or situations that arouse recollections of the trauma
3. Inability to recall an important aspect of the trauma (psychogenic amnesia)
4. Markedly diminished interest in signifi-

cant activities (in young children, loss of recently acquired developmental skills such as toilet training or language skills)
  5. Feeling of detachment or estrangement from others
  6. Restricted range of affect, e.g., unable to have loving feelings
  7. Sense of a foreshortened future, e.g., does not expect to have a career, marriage, or children, or a long life
D. Persistent symptoms of increased arousal (not present before the trauma), as indicated by at least two of the following:
  1. Difficulty falling or staying asleep
  2. Irritability or outbursts of anger
  3. Difficulty concentrating
  4. Hypervigilance
  5. Exaggerated startle response
  6. Physiological reactivity upon exposure to events that symbolize or resemble an aspect of the traumatic event (e.g., a woman who was raped in an elevator breaks out in a sweat when entering any elevator)
E. Duration of the disturbance (symptoms in B, C, and D) of at least 1 month. Specify delayed onset of symptoms was at least 6 months after trauma.

Over the past decade there has emerged a growing scientific literature on the effects of massive psychic trauma on human mental functioning and on the psychosocial development of the survivor. The results of studies conducted with survivors of the atomic bomb at Hiroshima; the 1972 flood at Buffalo Creek, West Virginia; the Nazi persecution in World War II; the veterans of the Vietnam War; and studies of rape and incest victims have shown that PTSD often develops after the catastrophic stressors have terminated. It is now recognized by clinicians, scholars, and others that immersion in the death experience and exposure to profound life–death threats may lead to survivor syndromes in which there persists a lasting psychic residue of the traumatic event. Perhaps for this reason the *DSM-III-R* identifies PTSD as a valid clinical entity that characterizes behavioral adaptation following profoundly stressful life events.[13]

The core feature of PTSD is that the survivor reexperiences elements of the trauma in dreams, with uncontrollable and emotionally distressing intrusive images, dissociative states of consciousness, and unconscious behavioral reenactments of the traumatic situation. Many survivors also report psychic numbing, a loss of normal affect, depression, a loss of interest in work and significant activities, survivor and moral guilt, loss of intimacy, sleep disturbances, anger, rage, mistrust, helplessness, and approach or avoidance tendencies of stimuli with trauma-related associational value.

The following case reports a situation in which a clinical situation reactivated a stress disorder and illustrates the complex and intricate interplay between present events. It also describes therapeutic interventions to assist in the resolution of the traumatic conflicts.

Mr. Ormsby, a 55-year-old divorced man, was admitted with severe anxiety, multiple somatic complaints, feelings of hopelessness, self-care deficits, depression, and suicidal ideation. He had required psychiatric hospitalization for "nerves" shortly after his discharge from the service at the end of World War II. He subsequently had a good adjustment and stable marriage and work history. Three years before this admission, Mr. Ormsby left his job as an emergency room technician and began drinking heavily. Eventually his wife left him, and the actual signing of the divorce papers precipitated the symptoms that led to this hospitalization.

It was only after another patient on the ward began talking of his difficulties during World War II that Mr. Ormsby revealed the following history. He had been stationed in the South Pacific and had survived two battles in which his ship had been destroyed and many people around him had been violently killed. Shortly after these events his unit was instructed that island children were being wired as human bombs, and an order was issued to shoot all children approaching the camp. When Mr. Ormsby was on duty, he had been forced to shoot a 10-year-old boy. After this incident Mr. Ormsby began having nightmares of exploding shells, violent scenes of people being killed, and scenes of himself killing the boy. These nightmares cleared over a period of a few years.

Mr. Ormsby's onset of symptoms 3 years previously came after an episode at work in the emergency room when he was told to clean up a child in one of the rooms. He was unaware that the child (a 9-year-old boy) was already dead when he was brought to the emergency room. When Mr. Ormsby discovered that the boy was dead, he was horrified, left work, and never returned. His nightmares resumed, but he felt unable to discuss these war episodes with his wife. At times he would wake up screaming and throw his wife to the floor to "cover" her from exploding shells. It was this unexplained behavior that forced their separation.

During the hospitalization, Mr. Ormsby was able to talk about the war episodes for the first time in over three decades. He participated in a group of

NURSING CARE PLAN
Post-Traumatic Stress Disorder

HUMAN RESPONSE

1. Stressor outside the range of usual human experience, i.e., rape, combat, flood.
2. Reexperiencing of the trauma through recollection, dreams; feeling the event was again occurring.
3. Numbing of responsiveness to external world.
4. Development of new symptoms including hyperalertness, sleep disturbance, guilt, memory impairment, as well as avoidance of activities and symbolic events resembling the trauma.

NURSING DIAGNOSES

- Rape trauma syndrome.
- Alteration in perception.
- Alteration in mood and affect.
- Ineffective individual coping. Alteration in sleep pattern.

GOALS

1. The patient understands that other people validate the traumatic nature of the event.
2. The patient will regain control of thoughts, feelings, and behaviors.
3. The patient will psychologically separate from the event and move into the future.

INTERVENTIONS

1. Validate to the patient that the event is classified in the traumatic stress category.
2. Review with patient distress related to intrusive imagery: teach patient self-relaxation, reduce anxiety and symptoms. Encourage verbalization of feelings.
3. Assist patient in dealing with fears and phobias. Assist patient to use own resources of social support.
4. Cognitive reframing in helping patient move from negative label to positive use of crisis: identify belief system of patient to event. Densensitize patient to traumatic images.

World War II veterans who focused on the expression of feelings about traumatic war experiences. Gradually, Mr. Ormsby's depression cleared and he reported being less anxious than at any time since the war. He was able to sleep through the night without nightmares and resumed working.[14]

Despite advances in our understanding of anxiety disorders, the psychiatric diagnostic nomenclature is still imprecise. Studies have shown, for example, that both panic and generalized forms of anxiety occur in most of the anxiety disorders.[15] Certain anxiety-disorder diagnoses are more easily separable, for example, social and simple phobia, because of the discrete nature of the cues precipitating anxiety, obsessive–compulsive disorder because of the unique phenomenology and clinical presentation, and post-traumatic stress disorder because of the presence of past trauma and recurrent traumatic memories. However, the categories of panic, agoraphobia, and generalized anxiety still seem to merge into one another, occasionally along with depression.[16]

The researchers on treatment of anxiety disorders have looked at both pharmacological and psychotherapeutic approaches. For example, Gitlin and colleagues noted that 14 weeks of behavior therapy consisting of education, relaxation, breathing, cognitive anxiety management, and exposure was effective for 10 of 11 patients with minimal panic behavior.[17] While other studies are reporting success in using this model of care, to date there are no studies of short-term dynamic therapy, either alone or in combination with medications, in treating panic disorder. As with behavior therapy, however, when psycho-dynamic treatment is effective in increasing coping, it may decrease the tendency toward relapse as well as decrease the morbidity if acute panic attacks should recur.[18] Nursing research is vitally needed in this area, especially since nurses are treating many victims of rape, battering, and child molestation.

Summary

This chapter discusses the psychiatric diagnostic criteria and nursing diagnoses related to the anxiety disorders of generalized anxiety disorder, panic disorder, phobic disorder, obsessive–compulsive disorder, and post-traumatic stress disorder. These clinical states and conditions are presented in terms of thoughts, feelings, and behaviors that interfere with daily living. The resultant actions that reflect a subjective and objective discrepancy between the person's potential and actual performance are addressed in terms of assisting the patient to achieve the highest adaptive functioning level. Nursing care plans are provided to illustrate the development of nursing interventions.

Questions

1. What role does anxiety play in the anxiety disorders?
2. Develop a nursing care plan for a patient diagnosed with an anxiety disorder.
3. Give an example of a post-traumatic stress disorder.

REFERENCES AND SUGGESTED READINGS

1. Freud, S. The ego and the id. In S. Freud, *Standard Edition*. London, Hogarth Press, 1961, p. 19. (First published in 1923.)
2. Freud, S. *A General Introduction to Psychoanalysis*. Garden City, N. Y.: Garden City Publishing, 1943, p. 217.
3. Waelder, R. *Basic Theory of Psychoanalysis*. New York: International Universities Press, 1960.
4. Sullivan, H. S. *Interpersonal Theory of Psychiatry*. New York: Norton, 1953, p. 113.
5. Ibid., pp. 213–216.
6. Peplau, H. A working definition of anxiety. In S. Burd & M. Marshall (Eds.), *Some Clinical Approaches to Psychiatric Nursing*. New York: Macmillan, 1963, pp. 323–324.
7. Ibid., p. 325.
8. American Psychiatric Association. *Diagnostic and Statistical Manual*, 3rd ed. (Rev.). Washington, D.C.: American Psychiatric Association, 1987, pp. 252–253.
9. Ibid., pp. 238–239.
10. Ibid., p. 247.
11. Taylor, J. G. Behavioral interpretation of obsessive–compulsive neurosis. *Behavior Research Therapy*, 1963, *1*, 237–244.
12. *DSM-III-R*, p. 250.
13. Ibid.
14. Christiansen, R. M., et al., Reactivation of traumatic conflicts. *American Journal of Psychiatry*, 1981, *138*, 984.
15. Barlow, D. H. The dimensions of anxiety disorders. In A. H. Tuma & J. D. Maser (Eds.), *Anxiety and the Anxiety Disorders*. Hillsdale, N. J.: Erlbaum, 1985.
16. Tyrer, P. Neurosis divisible. *Lancet*, 1984, *1*, 685–688.
17. Gitlin, B., Martin, J., & Shears, M. K., et al., Behavior therapy for panic disorders. *Journal of Nervous and Mental Disease*, 1985, *173*, 742–743.
18. Roy-Byrne, P. P., & Katon, W. An update on treatment of anxiety disorders. *Hospital and Community Psychiatry*, 1987, *38*, 835–843.

Chapter 41

Somatoform Disorders

Ann Wolbert Burgess

Chapter Objectives

The students successfully attaining the goals of this chapter will be able to:

- Describe the somatoform disorders.
- Identify the dynamics of conversion reaction.
- Integrate psychiatric and nursing diagnoses in planning patient care.

The somatoform disorders consist of a group of conditions in which somatic symptoms are due to psychological rather than biologic factors. Unlike factitious disorder or malingering, the symptom production in somatoform disorder is not intentional, i.e., the person does not experience the sense of controlling the production of the symptoms. Although the symptoms are physical, the specific pathophysiological processes involved are not demonstrable or understandable by existing laboratory procedures and are conceptualized most clearly by means of psychological constructs. For that reason, they are classified as mental disorders.

Patients who have persistent and troubling somatic symptoms without identifiable organic causes may be expressing psychological distress in bodily terms. This somatization is more likely among those with a recent decline in self-es-

teem, those undergoing serious life stresses, and those whose characteristic coping patterns and defense mechanisms are failing.

Several different types of psychological disturbance present themselves in this section. The first disorder, body dysmorphic disorder, is characterized by preoccupation with some imagined defect in physical appearance. Conversion disorder refers to a condition in which psychological factors are judged to be causally related to a loss or alteration of physical functioning that suggests a physical disorder. Hypochondriasis involves a preoccupation with the fear of having, or the belief that one has, a serious disease. Somatization disorder is a chronic, polysymptomatic disorder that begins early in life and that was previously referred to as either hysteria or Briquet's syndrome. Somatoform pain disorder is characterized by preoccupation with pain that is not attributable to any other mental or physical disorder.

BODY DYSMORPHIC DISORDER

The essential feature of this disorder is preoccupation with some imagined defect in appearance in a normal-appearing person. The most common complaints include facial flaws, such as spots on the skin, wrinkles, shape of facial feature, or excessive facial hair. The defining characteristics include the following[1]:

- Preoccupation with some imagined defect in appearance in a normal-appearing person. If a slight physical anomaly is present, the person's concern is grossly excessive.
- The belief in the defect is not of delusional intensity.
- Occurrence not exclusively during the course of anorexia nervosa or transsexualism.

CONVERSION DISORDER

The predominant feature of conversion disorder is a loss of or alteration in physical functioning that appears to be a physical disorder but which instead is apparently an expression of a psychological conflict or need. The problem is not under voluntary control and after careful study, the problem cannot be explained by any physical disorder or known pathophysiological mechanism.

There are two mechanisms that are used to explain why a person may have a conversion symptom. In one mechanism, the individual achieves a "primary gain" by keeping the psychological conflict out of conscious awareness. For example, after an upsetting confrontation and argument, an individual develops a physical symptom rather than dealing with the inner conflict. Thus, the symptom of blindness might result from viewing a very traumatic event, or the paralysis of an arm might result after an argument where physical violence was witnessed. In the second mechanism, the individual achieves "secondary gain" from the symptom by avoiding a particular activity that is traumatic. For example, a "paralyzed" hand can prevent a soldier from entering into combat.

The psychiatric criteria for conversion disorder follow.[2]

Diagnostic Criteria for Conversion Disorder

A. A loss of, or alteration in, physical functioning suggesting a physical disorder.
B. Psychological factors are judged to be etiologically related to the symptom because of a temporal relationship between a psychosocial stressor that is apparently related to a psychological conflict or need and initiation or exacerbation of the symptom.
C. The person is not conscious of intentionally producing the symptom.
D. The symptom is not a culturally sanctioned response pattern and cannot, after appropriate investigation, be explained by a known physical disorder.
E. The symptom is not limited to pain or to a disturbance in sexual functioning.

The conversion reactions are named for the major intrapsychic mechanisms. Conversion is an unconscious process by which intrapsychic conflicts find symbolic expression through a variety of body symptoms. Only the voluntary nervous system is affected, resulting in such temporary symptoms as paralysis, blindness, and deafness. Such symptoms may have a particular significance for the patient such as enuresis or encopresis occurring in a child who has been sexually traumatized by an adult. The patients may show a lack of concern about their symptoms because these symptoms may provide secondary gains by winning the person sympathy or by relieving him of unpleasant responsibilities. The primary coping mechanism is repression.

The conversion reactions were the first illness of psychogenic origin to be so recognized and the first neurotic reactions to receive intense psychological study. In the early 1900s, conversion symptoms were familiar to physicians. The term *hysteria* was often attached to these symptoms.

It is important to distinguish this kind of hysterical neurosis from psychophysiological disorders in which the autonomic nervous system is affected, from neurological lesions, and from malingering, which is a conscious act. The nursing care plan for conversion disorder is provided.

NURSING CARE PLAN*
Conversion Disorder

HUMAN RESPONSE

Loss or alteration in physical functioning suggesting a physical disorder.

NURSING DIAGNOSIS

Impaired reality testing.

GOALS

1. The patient will demonstrate improved reality testing and a decrease in somatic symptoms.
2. The patient will demonstrate increased insight into stressors associated with physical symptoms, as well as an increased repertoire of coping behaviors to deal with them.

INTERVENTIONS

1. Allow the patient to verbalize his fears, anxieties, and needs.
2. Redirect the patient's conversation away from focusing on his symptoms, when appropriate.
3. Reinforce reality to the patient in a nonthreatening manner, whenever possible.
4. Observe and record behavioral antecedents to the patient's symptoms.
5. Offer and teach the patient alternatives for coping with stress.
6. Encourage the patient to assume responsibility for own care and to participate in therapeutic activities whenever possible.
7. Administer appropriate psychotropic medications and evaluate effects.

* Data from Eileen E. Rinear and Janice Trichtinger.

CASE EXAMPLE

Mrs. Hall, a 38-year-old married mother of four, was in her usual state of mental health until the 25th anniversary of her mother's suicide. Mr. Hall described a specific event that heralded the onset of psychiatric symptoms. They were attending a party at which most of the guests had many alcoholic drinks. Mrs. Hall walked into a bedroom and found her husband and another man in physical contact with another woman. Mrs. Hall screamed, called the other woman a "slut," and went "absolutely wild, hysterical" according to the husband. Shortly thereafter, Mrs. Hall felt depressed and experienced frequent episodes of crying. She noted a decrease in energy and was unable to complete her household chores or care for herself. There was a decrease in appetite and an 18-lb weight loss, difficulty falling asleep, and pains throughout her body. These symptoms continued for about 4 months before she sought medical attention. She initially saw an internist for arm pains. She was

then referred to a psychiatrist who hospitalized her and administered thirteen electroconvulsive treatments. There was no clinical improvement. Six months later, there still had been no improvement, and she was admitted to another psychiatric hospital during which time the following life events were uncovered:

1. Mrs. Hall was the eldest of four children. Her mother, described as "mentally ill," committed suicide at age 38 when the patient was age 13. Mrs. Hall held the father responsible because of his "cruelty." Mrs. Hall claimed she felt distant from her mother, who usually left the care of the children to domestic help. The mother's suicide was from an overdose of sleeping pills. At her mother's funeral, a friend stopped the patient from jumping into the grave.
2. The father was an insurance broker, and the patient recalled him as always being drunk and

chasing the maid, his wife, or the children about the house. He opposed the patient's marriage because he desired both her physical presence and her wages. She secretly married at age 19 in an attempt to get away from her father, who 3 years after the marriage, died of gastrointestinal hemorrhage secondary to alcoholism. Mrs. Hall found it difficult to understand why she was unable to remember where her father is buried.

3. Mrs. Hall described her marriage as unhappy, "one constant argument, one long grudge." Her husband had always left clues that he was having extramarital affairs. Mrs. Hall said she rarely enjoyed sex; orgasm was infrequent. At the time of admission there were four children: ages 19 (female), 15 (male), 12 (female), and 5 (male). The patient voiced no concern over her eldest daughter's sharing of the husband's bed during the hospitalization or the joint bathing of the two youngest children.

4. Mrs. Hall came from a family of four children. There was a 37-year-old sister and two brothers ages 33 and 30. Both brothers had had psychiatric care. The younger brother received electroconvulsive treatments when he was 25. Mrs. Hall was a high-school graduate who worked as a saleswoman prior to her marriage. The male psychiatrist treating Mrs. Hall described her personality traits in the following way: aggressive, sarcastic, demanding, clinging in her dependence, pessimistic, suggestible, emotionally labile, and sexually provocative.

During the first weeks of hospitalization there was a gradual diminution of depressive symptoms. Then suddenly there was an acute exacerbation of the depression following a quarrel with her husband. Simultaneously, the patient was experiencing uncomfortable feelings in her body, especially in the presence of the therapist: "I feel suspended . . . I feel it's absolutely choking me, whatever it is . . . I feel suspended . . . I feel like my whole body tickles, like a raw nerve, a crawling sensation." This interview material was a response to an inquiry about the sexualized transference. The patient visited home the next weekend. During the visit her husband said that he could no longer stand her complaining and that he was "fed up." On the evening of her return to the hospital the patient developed camptocormia. She walked with a flexed spine that made an 80° angle with her pelvic girdle. Her head and trunk were nearly parallel to the ground. While in bed the patient could maintain her body in a straight line without difficulty. Except for the abnormal posture,

the neurological exam was within normal limits. Just prior to the onset of symptoms, the depressive symptoms had reached their height. With the onset of camptocormia there was an abrupt change in the depressive syndrome. Sadness and anxiety were markedly diminished, and appetite and sleep pattern improved. Mrs. Hall displayed a positive demeanor. Although the depressive symptoms decreased, there was an increase in somatic concerns including the conversion symptoms of transitory blindess and paralysis of the hands.

The conversion symptoms continued for another 2 weeks but subsided when important changes occurred in the patient's relationship with her husband and male therapist. First, the husband changed his view of his wife from a malingerer to someone who was severely distressed and in need of protection and comfort. This new understanding removed the patient's fear of being abandoned. Second, the male therapist (because of a change in supervisors) reviewed his approach and became more supportive. Previously he had been overemphasizing the sexualized transference. The patient commented on the fact that he was becoming more like a mother than a father and appeared relieved with this changed therapeutic relationship.

Nursing Diagnosis of Unresolved Sexual Trauma

The above case was reported in the second edition of this text without any further nursing interpretation. The patient was treated between the years 1963 and 1968. During the interval since then, considerable information regarding hysteria, conversion, and anxiety disorders has surfaced. With these new insights, a postscript to this case is offered, specifically with the nursing diagnosis of unresolved sexual trauma. If this case were to be treated in 1985, the following hypotheses would be made:

1. The antecedent event of the patient walking into a physical scene involving two men and a woman triggered an enormous amount of anxiety with repressed roots in her own past. Several speculations might be: (1) The patient witnessing a similar event as a young child, or (2) the patient being a nonconsenting person in a sexual assault as a child. The resultant symptoms

are indicative of an unresolved symptom of post-traumatic stress disorder.

2. The abusive father's hypersexuality was known by the patient from witnessing as well as experiencing. The indicators are her running away from him, her sexual dysfunction, and her lack of concern over the overt sexual explicitness of the relationship between her own children and their father.

3. The patient describes a dissociative experience during an interview with the therapist that has strong themes of a childhood sexual abuse incident. The therapist comments on the "sexualized transference" that exacerbates the experience and triggers the camptocormia and conversion symptoms. These symptoms subside when the husband takes the patient's psychiatric condition seriously, and when the therapist is viewed less as the sexualized and threatening father and more as the supportive mother.

HYPOCHONDRIASIS

Hypochondriasis is another personality dimension in which somatic symptoms form a prominent feature. Hypochondriasis is best used to refer to an enduring manner of coping with psychological, interpersonal, and physical distress characterized by a prominent concern with bodily symptoms and their causes and implications. There is an excessive and fearful preoccupation with the body, with multiple worrisome symptoms in the absence of significant pathology. Patients generally describe their condition with great urgency, intensity, and persistence, and reassurance by the physician or other health care members is totally ineffective. These individuals respond poorly to traditional medical treatments, which only serves to frustrate the physician whose intent is to "cure" the person of his symptoms. It is important to understand that the somatic symptoms are an integral part of the person's social relationships and psychological conflict and that "cure" of the symptoms is probably an unrealistic goal. Rather, intervention needs to be aimed at recognizing the crucial function that somatic symptoms play in the individual's life and to help the person "live" with the symptoms in as adaptive a manner as possible. The psychiatric diagnostic criteria for hypochondriasis follows.[4]

Diagnostic Criteria for Hypochondriasis

A. Preoccupation with the fear of having, or the belief that one has, a serious disease, based on the person's interpretation of physical signs or sensations as evidence of physical illness.

B. Appropriate physical evaluation does not support the diagnosis of any physical disorder that can account for the physical signs or sensations or the person's unwarranted interpretations of them, *and* the symptoms in A are not just symptoms of panic attacks.

C. The fear of having, or belief that one has, a disease persists despite medical reassurance.

D. Duration of the disturbance is at least 6 months.

E. The belief in A is not of delusional intensity.[5]

Psychiatrists Barsky and Klerman have proposed that the general concept of somatic style should be used to investigate symptom formation, bodily perception, and medical illness as a psychological and social event.[6] They argue that the concept of hypochondriasis is confusing because of its many untested implications and conflicting historical connotations and because of modern medicine's emphasis on disease rather than illness. Practicing physicians focus on physical pathology and demonstrable pathophysiology (i.e., disease) while neglecting the patient's perception of, and response to, this pathology (i.e., his illness).

Hypochondriasis may be viewed in a number of ways, as discussed below.

Hypochondriasis as a Psychiatric Disorder

In the *DSM-III-R*, hypochondriasis is viewed as a psychiatric disorder, and is described as having four major characteristics: (1) physical symptoms disproportionate to demonstrable organic disease; (2) a fear of disease and the conviction that one is sick; (3) a preoccupation with one's body; and (4) the persistent and unsatisfactory pursuit of medical care.[7] The disorder may be primary and occur without any other mental disorder, or it may occur secondarily in the course of a preexisting psychiatric illness such as depression, anxiety, or schizophrenia.[8]

The physical symptoms are usually vague,

variable, and generalized, although they may at times be quite specific. Pain is the most common symptom, and bowel and cardiorespiratory complaints are also frequent. The most commonly involved regions of the body are the head and neck, abdomen, and chest. The organ systems most frequently implicated are the gastrointestinal, musculoskeletal, and central nervous systems.

Hypochondriasis as the Result of Intrapsychic and Unconscious Emotional Forces

Psychiatrist John Nemiah has pointed out that hypochondriasis can be understood in one of two ways: (1) as an alternate channel through which to deflect sexual, aggressive, or oral drives; and (2) as an ego defense against guilt or low self-esteem.[9] The conceptualization of the intrapsychic defense is closely related to the notions of primary and secondary gain. Primary gain is the reduction in intrapsychic conflict and the partial drive gratification accomplished by the defensive operation. Secondary gain refers to the acceptable and "legitimate" interpersonal advantages that one has when one has a physical disease. The physically symptomatic person gains sympathy, attention, support, and many types of concrete assistance.

Hypochondriasis as the Result of a Perceptual or Cognitive Abnormality

There are three versions of the view of hypochondriasis as a perceptual or cognitive abnormality: (1) hypochondriacal patients amplify and augment normal bodily sensations; (2) they incorrectly assess and misinterpret the somatic symptoms of emotional arousal and of normal bodily functions; and (3) hypochondriacal patients are constitutionally predisposed to thinking and perceiving in physical and concrete terms rather than in emotional and subjective terms. These three versions are not mutually exclusive.

Hypochondriasis as a Learned Social Behavior

The most salient feature of hypochondriasis as a learned social behavior is not what patients feel but what they do and say. They exhibit illness behavior as if being a patient were their sole avocation and their full-time vocation. They are perpetually visiting doctors, monitoring their health status, recording their condition, and treating themselves. These patients have learned that illness behavior is a way to obtain care and support and attention. They may have assumed the sick role initially as a result of an accident, injury, or medical illness or by modeling themselves after someone who successfully used the sick role. However, once the behaviors occur, they are positively reinforced and maintained by the supportive, nurturant, and encouraging responses of family and friends.

Barsky and Klerman suggest that rather than deliberating whether or not the label "hypochondriasis" can be accurately affixed to a particular patient, the patient might be assessed on four axes as follows[10]:

1. Does the patient have multiple functional symptoms, a fear and conviction of disease, and bodily preoccupations? If yes, then search for those psychiatric disorders that can have such features, namely, depression, anxiety, and schizophrenia.
2. Is the patient troubled by problems of anger and hostility, orality and dependency, diminished self-esteem, or guilt and masochism?
3. What does the patient believe is causing his bodily sensations?
4. How has the patient learned to use illness and patienthood to cope with interpersonal conflict and stressful life events?

SOMATIZATION DISORDER

Prior to the publication of the *DSM-III-R*, the somatization disorder was known as Briquet's syndrome or hysterical neurosis, conversion type. Patients with these symptoms are not popular with medical practitioners because of their persistent physical complaints without physical findings. The psychiatric criteria for somatization disorder follow.[11]

Diagnostic Criteria for Somatization Disorder

A. A history of many physical complaints or a belief that one is sickly, beginning before the age of 30 and persisting for several years.

B. At least 13 symptoms from the list below. To count a symptom as significant, the following criteria must be met:
1. No organic pathology or pathophysiological mechanism (e.g., a physical disorder or the effects of injury, medication, drugs, or alcohol) to account for the symptom or, when there is related organic pathology, the complaint or resulting social or occupational impairment is grossly in excess of what would be expected from the physical findings
2. Has not occurred only during a panic attack
3. Has caused the person to take medicine (other than over-the-counter pain medication), see a doctor, or alter life-style

Gastrointestinal symptoms:
1. **Vomiting (other than during pregnancy)**
2. Abdominal pain (other than when menstruating)
3. Nausea (other than motion sickness)
4. Bloating (gassy)
5. Diarrhea
6. Intolerance of (gets sick from) several different foods

Pain symptoms:
7. **Pain in extremities**
8. Back pain
9. Joint pain
10. Pain during urination
11. Other pain (excluding headaches)

Cardiopulmonary symptoms:
12. **Shortness of breath when not exerting oneself**
13. Palpitations
14. Chest pain
15. Dizziness

Conversion or pseudoneurological symptoms:
16. **Amnesia**
17. **Difficulty swallowing**
18. Loss of voice
19. Deafness
20. Double vision
21. Blurred vision
22. Blindness
23. Fainting or loss of consciousness
24. Seizure or convulsion
25. Trouble walking
26. Paralysis or muscle weakness
27. Urinary retention or difficulty urinating

Sexual symptoms for the major part of the person's life after opportunities for sexual activity:
28. **Burning sensation in sexual organs or rectum (other than during intercourse)**

29. Sexual indifference
30. Pain during intercourse
31. Impotence

Female reproductive symptoms judged by the person to occur more frequently or severely than in most women:
32. **Painful menstruation**
33. Irregular menstrual periods
34. Excessive menstrual bleeding
35. Vomiting throughout pregnancy

Note: The seven items in boldface may be used to screen for the disorder. The presence of two or more of these items suggests a high likelihood of the disorder.

CASE EXAMPLE

Mrs. Gardner, a 30-year-old widow, was admitted to the psychiatric unit with numerous physical symptoms including urinary incontinence, nausea, generalized pain, and dizziness. The patient was about to be married for the second time and experienced the severity in symptoms while writing wedding invitations. Her fiancé's brother had been killed suddenly while working at his job on the railroad several weeks prior to admission. This death was similar to that of the patient's first husband, who was also killed suddenly in an automobile accident one year after their marriage. As a child, the patient had enuresis frequently until age 7. Although the diagnosis of multiple sclerosis was ruled out at this admission, this diagnosis might still show up in later years.

Nursing intervention was focused on the milieu management of the patient. She initially showed no distress over her symptoms. She was able to give up the catheter and urine bag when the milieu exerted negative reinforcement for this behavior. After this intervention, Mrs. Gardner was able to control her own urine. She concurrently began talking to the nurse about her fear of losing her fiancé as she had lost her first husband, which was causing her to fear another marriage. The nurse helped Mrs. Gardner connect this dynamic understanding with the multiple symptoms she experienced prior to admission, especially her urinary incontinence. Mrs. Gardner was discharged with no reccurrence of the symptoms. Mrs. Gardner and her new husband continued couples therapy on an outpatient basis after their marriage.

SOMATOFORM PAIN DISORDER

Certain personality types have been noted to be particularly prone to somatization. One of these has been described by Engel as the "pain prone person."[12] This personality is described as a pessimistic, gloomy, self-deprecating individual

NURSING CARE PLAN*
Somatization Disorder

HUMAN RESPONSE

Multiple somatic symptoms (i.e., complaints of long duration, usually beginning before age 30, and with a chronic but variable course).

NURSING DIAGNOSIS

Alteration in coping style: Use of physical symptoms as defense against anxiety and depression.

GOALS

1. Patient will demonstrate a decrease in somatic complaints.
2. Patient will demonstrate increased insight into his symptoms as well as improved coping patterns.

INTERVENTIONS

1. Observe and record frequency of somatic complaints.
2. Provide patients with frequent 1:1 contact to enlist his trust and confidence.
3. Evaluate current symptoms in the context of the patient's previous medical history and level of functioning.
4. Observe and record dramatic or vague somatic complaints.
5. Recognize that the patient's distress is very real to him and validate same.
6. Listen to the patient's somatic complaints in a supportive nonjudgmental manner and redirect the patient's focus of conversation away from them, as appropriate.
7. Record vital signs as ordered by the physician or when deemed appropriate within the context of the patient's symptoms.
8. Notify the patient's attending physician or the medical resident if symptoms persist.

* Data contributed by Eileen E. Rinear and Janice Trichtinger.

burdened by guilt and unable to bear success. A review of past history reveals interpersonal relationships, psychological experiences, and physical health characterized by repeated injuries, humiliations, and defeats. Most importantly, pain has become an adjustment to life, a means of coping and a method for dealing with stress and loss.[13]

In somatoform pain disorder, the individual complains of pain, but there are no adequate physical findings or psychological factors to explain the disorder. Either the pain symptom is inconsistent with the anatomic location, or it mimics a known disease such as angina or sciatica. The psychiatric diagnostic criteria for somatoform pain disorder follow.[14]

Diagnostic Criteria for Somatoform Pain Disorder

A. Preoccupation with pain for at least 6 months.
B. Either (1) or (2):
1. Appropriate evaluation uncovers no organic pathology or pathophysiological mechanism (e.g., a physical disorder or the effects of injury) to account for the pain
2. When there is related organic pathology, the complaint of pain or resulting social or occupational impairment is grossly in excess of what would be expected from the physical findings

NURSING CARE PLAN*
Somatoform Pain Disorder

HUMAN RESPONSE

Somatoform pain, not related to any other mental or physical disorders.

NURSING DIAGNOSIS

Alteration in comfort level; pain.

GOALS

1. The patient will demonstrate a decrease in his complaints of pain.
2. The patient will demonstrate increased insight into his pain, as well as improved ability to cope with it.

INTERVENTIONS

1. Observe and record characteristics of pain (severity, duration, and precipitants) especially for: paresthesia, muscle pain, back and joint pain, and genital pain.
2. Administer prn pain medication and observe and record effects.
3. Observe the patient's ability or inability to voluntarily control his pain.
4. Use palliative nursing care techniques to promote patient comfort and facilitate a trust relationship between him and a member of the staff.
5. Encourage the patient to accept responsibility for his own physical care and to participate in therapeutic unit activities.

* Data from Eileen E. Rinear and Janice Trichtinger.

Summary

This chapter describes a group of mental health conditions in which physical symptoms are due to emotional factors rather than physiological factors. The psychiatric disorders described include somatization disorder, conversion disorder, psychogenic pain disorder, and hypochondriasis. The nursing care plans for each disorder include nursing interventions and expected outcomes. Case examples illustrate the types of situations nurses may encounter in both general and psychiatric populations.

Questions

1. Describe a nursing approach you would take in working with a patient who complains of chronic pain but for which no physical evidence has been documented.
2. How would you respond to a patient who states that everyone tells him that his "problem of chronic headaches is in his head?"
3. Describe a patient from a general hospital or community setting whom you diagnose as having a somatoform disorder.

REFERENCES AND SUGGESTED READINGS

1. American Psychiatric Association. *Diagnostic and Statistical Manual*, 3rd ed. (Rev.). Washington, D.C.: American Psychiatric Association, 1987, p. 256.
2. Ibid., p. 259.
3.
4. Ibid., p. 251.
5. *DSM-III-R*, p. 261.
6. Barsky, A. J., & Klerman, G. L. Overview: Hypochondriasis, bodily complaints, and somatic styles. *American Journal of Psychiatry*, 1983, *140*, 273–282.
7. *DSM-III-R*, p. 261.
8. Kleinman, A., Eisenberg, L., & Good, B. Culture, illness, and care: Clinical lessons from anthropologic and cross-cultural research. *Annals of Internal Medicine*, 1978, *88*, 251–258.
9. Nemiah, J. Somatization disorder. In H. I. Kaplan & B. J. Sadock (Eds.), *Comprehensive Textbook of Psychiatry*, 4th ed. Baltimore: Williams & Wilkins, 1985.
10. Barsky & Klerman, op. cit., p. 281.
11. *DSM-III-R*, pp. 263–264.
12. Engel, G. L. Psychogenic pain and the pain-prone patient. *American Journal of Psychiatry*, 1959, *26*, 899–918.
13. Ibid.
14. *DSM-III-R*, p. 266.

Chapter 42

Dissociative Disorders

Ann Wolbert Burgess

Chapter Objectives

The students successfully attaining the goals of this chapter will be able to:

- Describe the behavioral characteristics of dissociative disorders.
- Describe the relationship between the ego defense of splitting and multiple personality.
- Integrate psychiatric and nursing diagnoses in planning patient care.
- Describe relationship of multiple personality disorder and post-traumatic stress disorder.

The essential feature of dissociative disorders is a sudden, temporary alteration in the normally integrative functions of consciousness, identity, or motor behavior. Important personal events cannot be recalled if the alteration occurs in consciousness. If the alteration occurs in identity, either the individual's customary identity is temporarily forgotten and a new identity is assumed, or the customary feelings of one's own reality are lost and are replaced by a feeling of unreality. If the alteration occurs in motor behavior, there is a concurrent disturbance in consciousness or identity as in the wandering that occurs in a fugue state.

CONCEPT OF DISSOCIATION

Dissociation is the splitting off of an intolerable idea or emotion from the person's consciousness so that it is a separate identity from the person's consciousness. In essence, the idea or emotion has a life of its own. For example, drifting into a fantasy mentally when in an intolerable situation illustrates the phenomenon of splitting. Dissociation is an adaptive mechanism allowing one to "tune out" for awhile. Any person can "split" if stressed severely. This process occurs in people with dissociative disorders, where the individual has little or no control over its occurrence and no recollection of where he was during the interval. In the subtypes of dissociative disorders, (1) the person can recall nothing of the past (*psychogenic amnesia*); (2) the person goes off and suddenly comes back (*fugue states*); (3) the person continually dissociates (*multiple personality*); or (4) the person acts mechanically as though in a trance (*depersonalization*). Many dissociative states relate to early severe abuse. This cognitive coping begins as an adaptive means to defend against the trauma event, but by adulthood or adolescence, it reveals itself as a pathological trauma.

The dissociative component in acts of violence is a new area of clinical investigation, especially as it relates to the cycle of victimization. Violence, when validated as an expression of post-traumatic stress disorder, usually has a dissociative, stereotyped quality, as if a former event were being reenacted. For example, a young teen-ager, 11 months after shooting her father during a visitation meeting as part of a separation arrangement by the father's divorce attorneys, described the act as follows:

He told me everything would change after the divorce and that my sister and I would have to see him whenever he wanted. I was terrified. He always got what he wanted. He had grabbed me that evening and I pulled away. Then everything became spontaneous . . . I don't know what happened in what order. I left the room, got the gun, loaded it, and came back and shot him. I didn't want to be hurt anymore.

The girl stopped firing the gun when she saw the blood. She was shocked to learn she had fired twelve bullets. The girl, previously raped by her father, dissociated under the fear of a repeated assault and became homicidal in the service of self-defense.

There are many memory problems experienced by the individual. The memory separates the dissociative states, and the person loses periods of time. The person frequently will say, "I can't recall events from my childhood." This person experiences periodic episodic amnesia. Questions that nurses can ask if suspecting a dissociative or memory problem include the following:

- Do you ever lose time?
- Do you ever find yourself somewhere and can't recall how you got there?
- Do you ever find yourself in clothes you can't recall putting on?

The symptoms reported by such persons frequently include depressions, suicide attempts that may not be clearly remembered, and antisocial behavior. The dissociative episodes will continue from childhood through adulthood unless the person receives treatment. Some of the physical symptoms include: migraines, limb movement difficulty, intense pain, loss of voice, blindness, deafness, auditory and visual hallucinations, out of body experiences, and confused body identity.

The memory barriers are adaptive in helping the person to avoid recalling the abusive situations. Another advantage to dissociating is that the person does not feel the pain. It is much like a hypnotic amnesia. For children, it seems like this all happened to someone else and not to them. But when they grow older, dissociating is more autonomous, and they are not controlling it as they did in childhood. They enter other states of consciousness that are screened off. The danger in the dissociation as an adaptive mechanism is that it produces an encapsulation and isolation experience.

Dissociation relates to the frequency and nature of the abuse *and* to the various relationships the child has with the adult. For example, the placement of children in foster homes can set up this dissociative response. This change from natural home to foster home may be viewed as a cutting off for the child between ages 3 and 6 of a life structure. If children are carefully observed, one can note periods when the dissociative response is seen. Some of the behavioral signs include:

- The construction of imaginary playmates.
- The use of different names or ages for themselves.
- Taking on the role of an animal.
- Imagining they were adopted or came from another family.
- Separation from the past.
- Gender confusion.
- Regressive behavior.

TYPES OF DISSOCIATIVE DISORDERS

The types of dissociative disorders include: psychogenic amnesia, psychogenic fugue, multiple personality, and depersonalization disorder.

Psychogenic Amnesia

Amnesia is the inability to remember. The extent of the disturbance in psychogenic amnesia is too great to be explained by ordinary forgetfulness. The disturbance is not due to an organic mental disorder (e.g., blackouts during alcohol intoxication) and represents a sudden inability to recall important personal information.

Four types of disturbance in recall are noted. In *localized* amnesia, the most common type, there is failure to recall all events occurring during a circumscribed period of time. For example, the survivor of a serious motor accident that injured and killed other people may not be able to recall anything that happened from the time of the accident to days later. In *selective* amnesia, there is a failure to recall some, but not all, of the events occurring during a circumscribed time period. For example, after a sudden death, a family member remembers hearing of the death but cannot recall conversations with the hospital staff. In *generalized* amnesia, there is failure of recall that encompasses the individual's entire life; and in *continuous* amnesia, the individual cannot recall events subsequent to a specific time up to and including the present.

Psychogenic Fugue

The Latin root of the word *fugue* ("to flee") encompasses both the observable state of wandering and traveling and the hypothesized precipitant of flight from painful circumstances. During the fugue state, the individual usually assumes modified identities and has no recall of what happened. Fugue has been related to multiple personality and narcissistic personality, with the ego defense of splitting; it is also related to sleepwalking.

CASE EXAMPLE

Jane Norton is a 21-year-old single woman who lives with her mother and stepfather and works as a secretary. She was admitted to an inpatient unit for a 3-month period because of fugue states in which she would wander off and act as a 6-year-old child called Ellen. After hospital discharge and during outpatient treatment, her anxiety built up as a result of the discussion of events in her past. The fugue states reappeared and interfered with her work and social functioning. Therapy revealed that during the patient's adolescence she had been sexually assaulted by her father. One of the coping strategies used by the patient to deal with the traumatic event and to control her anxiety about the abuse was to return to her childhood (i.e., a dissociative strategy) and to become the 6-year-old Ellen again.

The nursing intervention was directed at assisting Jane Norton to use reality-respecting coping defenses when under stress rather than the reality-distorting defense of dissociation. The nurses helped Jane in reality testing and always responded to her using her adult name and identity. This adult reality-based expectation gave Jane a clear message that the nurses could help her with her feelings of anxiety as an adult in the context of the real situation that was stimulating the anxiety that triggered the fugue state. The patient also talked about the unresolved sexual trauma in therapy and gained control over feelings of helplessness and vulnerability. The talking therapy and the milieu therapy gradually strengthened the patient in her attempts to reintegrate the childhood trauma with her adult personality.

Multiple Personality Disorder

The essential feature of multiple personality disorder is the presence within the individual of two or more distinct subpersonalities, each of which is dominant at a particular time. Each subpersonality is a fully integrated and complex unit with unique memories, behavior patterns, and social relationships that determine the nature of the individual's acts when that subpersonality is dominant. When there are more than two subpersonalities, each is aware, to varying degrees, of the others. Over the past 80 years there has been an increasing interest in the relationship of these various subpersonalities to each other.

Multiple personality disorder may not be the presenting complaint of the individual. Rather, it is often discovered under other circumstances. Usually the dominant subpersonality presents first as a rigid, restricted, and self-punitive person who feels angry, deprived, and rejected. The second subpersonality is commonly the opposite—impulsive, flamboyant, and sexual; and may appear suddenly in relation to stress, drugs, or alcohol.

Within the last decade, multiple personality has been diagnosed, treated, and studied with increasing frequency. Multiple personality disorder is a complex, chronic dissociative psychopathy characterized by disturbances of identity and memory. Lay interest in celebrated cases of multiple personality disorder and its portrayal through television have gradually brought it to the attention of the professional community. The impact of Schreiber's description of Wilbur's treatment of "Sybil" reached a professional as well as general public audience.[1]

Interest in multiple personality disorder increases, observes Kluft, when interest in hypnosis is high; a renaissance of interest in hypnosis has been underway for more than a decade.[2] Also, the struggles of combat veterans have alerted therapists to post-traumatic stress disorder. Many clinicians working with both multiple personality disorder and post-traumatic stress disorder have remarked on the similarity of the two conditions.[3]

Etiology of the Disorder
Using a four-factor theory, Kluft suggests multiple personality occurs when (1) a child with the capacity to dissociate is (2) exposed to overwhelming stimuli that cannot be managed with less drastic defenses. Thus, the capacity to dissociate is enlisted in the service of defense. (3) Dissociated contents become linked with one of many possible substrates and shaping influences for personality organization. (4) If there are inadequate stimulus barriers and restorative experiences or an excess of double-binding messages that inhibit the child's capacity to process his experience, multiple personality disorder can result.[4] This four-factor theory is supported by findings that patients with multiple personality disorder are highly hypnotizable.

Diagnosing Multiple Personality Disorder
Kluft suggests that clinicians carefully scrutinize any of the following symptoms and suspect multiple personality disorder when noting the symptom.[5]

- A history of prior treatment failure
- Three or more prior diagnoses
- Concurrent psychiatric and somatic symptoms
- Fluctuating symptoms and an inconsistent level of functioning
- Severe headaches
- A history of time distortion or time lapses
- The patient's having been told by others of behaviors he has forgotten
- The patient's having been told by others of observable changes in his facies, voice, and behavioral style

- The patient's discovery in his domicile, vehicle, or place of work, of productions, possessions, or strange handwriting that he can neither account for nor recognize
- Auditory hallucinations, which should be assessed with special care
- The use of "we" in a collective sense
- The eliciting of what appear to be separate personalities with hypnosis or amytal

Treatment
The treatment discussion is derived from Braun and Kluft.[6,7] Because multiple personality disorder is found in a diverse group of individuals with a wide range of axis I and axis II diagnoses, treatment must be highly individualized. The tasks of therapy are the same as those in any intense, change-oriented approach with the exception that the patient does not have a unified personality. Therefore, the therapist cannot presume the presence of an observing ego but rather must anticipate that there will be disruptions in ego functioning processes. Treatment relies heavily on the strength of the therapeutic alliance, which must be cultivated globally and with each personality. The personalities are treated equally, with respect and empathetic concern. The following general steps are outlined.

1. Create an atmosphere of safety and trust.
2. The diagnosis must be made and shared with the accessible personalities.
3. Establish communication with the accessible personalities.
4. Assess the personalities' pressures toward harming self or others and contract against such activities.
5. Learn the origin, functions, and problems of each personality and the manner in which they relate to one another.
6. Work on the personalities' issues and problems.
7. Understand the traumatic events preceding development of the personalities using modalities such as art therapy, movement therapy, or hypnosis.
8. Develop communication with the personalities.
9. Help resolve the personalities' conflicts and integrate them.
10. Help patient develop new defenses and coping skills.
11. Teach patient to optimize available social supports.

12. Provide supportive therapy to solidify gains.
13. Provide long-term follow-up.

The following case example is written by a young woman in whom 11 different subpersonalities were diagnosed. An account of the treatment and the assistance of psychiatric nurses is included.

CASE EXAMPLE

Dear Ann:

I just received your letter. I've been in the hospital for the past 2 weeks, just a checkup to make sure all the personalities stayed "in." Unfortunately, four did not, but my doctor said they had overlooked some important material dealing with the gang rape when I was 11½. Needless to say, the two weeks there were very painful. Again, therapy was 5 days a week, lasting anywhere from 3 hours to 7 hours. The staff on the unit were invaluable. The nurses played an important role in my therapy. They helped to defuse potentially embarrassing situations on the unit when other personalities came out. Two or three of the "girls" were close to these two nurses; consequently, these two nurses were asked to participate in my therapy sessions. The staff were supportive, positive, and always reassured me that I was going to make it. After some of the therapy sessions, I wanted to quit. I just knew I wasn't going to make it, live through it, at least a hundred times. But I did. Summarizing all my personalities may prove difficult, but I will try.

Personality #1: Katrina, age 27, was a dominant personality with blond hair, blue eyes, slender, and was anorexic. She was a prostitute who hated men and was very street wise; she caused pain to others and tried to kill Wendy. Katrina and Wendy are sisters and have the same mother (she was an aunt and I spent some of my summers with them). Katrina loves roses, is religious, and never plays with dolls. Katrina took the longest to trust the male therapist; she never hurt the female therapist.

Personality #2: Sarah Jane and Samuel Arthur, ages 13 and both blonds (twins as I am). Sarah came when I was 4, took abuse from my brother, hid in the closet, and was very frightened. As she grew older, she became very polite and extremely loyal to Sam. Sam had an extreme fear of dogs. He also "came out" when he thought Sarah might be in danger. He was very strong in therapy (physically), but a handshake with the therapist was binding (when aged, Sam and Sarah became just Sarah).

Personality #3: Katherine Ann, age 23, blond hair and blue eyes, was a dominant personality and the protector of the "family." She was a real fighter, held anger, was an obsessive cleaner, bossy and demanding; would not cry or show any emotions except anger (she helped me when I was raped and when Mom locked me in the attic and during the gang rape). She was *very* nonsexual.

Personality #4: Wendy, age 7½, long dark hair, blue eyes, and a dominant personality. She sucked her thumb, like to cuddle with two of the doctors, spoke French, was creative (she drew well and I don't); also religious. Her nickname with the other "girls" was Chatty Wendy. She wanted to play on the hospital grounds with the doctors, was full of vitality and very humorous. She loved vanilla ice cream and peanut butter and jelly sandwiches. She took abuse from my oldest brother also, saw my father (not her father) beat my mother, and was gang-raped also. Staff and doctors liked her best and one nurse translated the French in therapy sessions. When Wendy was older, she became very suicidal.

Personality #5: Kate, age 6 years and a dominant personality. She claimed a neighbor as her mother; loved shiny things (watches, rings, etc.). She got along better with the female therapist (I had two); Kate at first only used sign language (again, I had an interpreter for therapy). She was also polite, sensitive, generous, and liked to wear make-up when aged. Kate had bits and pieces of several traumas, which is why she wouldn't speak of the "unspeakable" but would sign it.

Personality #6: Katrinka, age 5, cried a lot, saw things but couldn't speak. She used finger spelling. She was terrified of wing-tipped shoes and always untied everyone's shoes in therapy because when she got kicked (like Dad did), it wouldn't hurt so much. She was modeling herself after Katrina and looked forward to making money too.

Personality #7: Melinda, age 3 or 4. She liked women best, was deaf, and the youngest and just wanted to be held. She adopted a female therapist as her mom. She was sweet and gentle and autistic.

Personality #8: Amanda, age 29 and a dominant personality. She was afraid of mirrors and of who might be behind her. She was intelligent and knew and understood most of the others. She was the writer and published poems before me. Seemed to bring calm and order to the others.

Personality #9: Kathyann, age 3½, with red hair and green eyes. She had no trauma. She came when I was locked in the attic but remained untouched. She stayed innocent—the child in me. When she came, Katherine Ann left for a number of years (she was aged to 10 years old through therapy).

Personality #10: Shelly Eileen, age 57 years, gray hair and brown eyes, a dominant personality. She was the same age as my mom was when she died. She was called the I.S.H.—Inner Self Helper. She knew everyone and everything of the others and what needed to be done in therapy. She was grandmotherly. When the others were aged, she grew younger spontaneously until she reached my age. Wendy, Kate, Katherine Ann, and Katrina could all communicate with her when asked.

Personality #11: Cory, unknown age. Wendy created her when she realized she "hated" what other people had done to us. Unable to handle such a "sinful" emotion, she created Cory. Cory stayed a secret until the end of therapy. Cory hated everything and everybody—the opposite of Wendy totally.

All personalities looked different and had separate parents, speech patterns, mannerisms, etc. They had their likes and dislikes—from people to food to colors. All, when aged (through therapy), had to deal with family deaths, miscarriage (I was 19), abortion (age 17 by brother), my hysterectomy, and the sadness of not having babies. Much of this aging process was accomplished in therapy. The most traumatic incident (horror!) was being sold by my mother at 11½ to the Mafia, who in turn exposed me to some type of religious cult (it is being investigated by a priest now) and then on into prostitution. Fortunately, that was only a couple of times. I am having the most trouble with this now and need a lot of support to get through this difficult time.

The integration of the personalities was complicated but so exciting to meet them all and ask questions of each other. Sadness too—they'll never come around if or when I might need them. It's like saying goodbye to old friends. I do have the gift of time now and "I'm no longer outnumbered." I have a T-shirt with that on it. Anyway, days are longer; colors brighter; sounds sharper, etc. It's not easy to get used to such a dramatic change and it will take time.

The nurses kept reminding me we were all the same and how much I had survived. They pointed out all my strengths and helped to keep a perspective in an incredibly confusing time. They cried with me when I learned of the traumas and personalities; they laughed with me when Wendy stopped up the showers on the unit to give stuffed animals a bath. It took me awhile to laugh; I admit I cried when I found that out! Later they got me to relax about it. I've been "just me" for 16 days, but every day is a struggle. The longer I stay me, the better chance I have of never splitting again. I draw, write poetry, and know a spattering of French, and my marriage is a lot better.

Fondly,
Kathi

Nursing Intervention for Multiple Personality Disorder. As previously stated, the treatment of multiple personality disorder is a long-term process. The splitting mechanism between the personality configurations is initially unconscious and hidden from both the patient and others. Dealing with previously unresolved conflicts needs to occur slowly and with a willingness to travel an anxiety-laden path.

The nurse can note the progress of the various stages. First, the person becomes aware of and is able to talk about the various subpersonalities and what each means. There may be avoidance and diversionary mechanisms used, including amnesia, thought-blocking, "acting out," and obsessive–compulsive behaviors whenever there is the retelling of traumatic childhood events. As noted in the above case example, the various subpersonalities were advanced or "aged" in order to integrate into one personality. The goal is the eventual recovery of the memories and the toleration of the accompanying feelings of anger, rage, guilt, shame, and humiliation. This experience promotes mastery, a more integrated personality, and less conflicted interpersonal relationships.

Depersonalization Disorder

Depersonalization disorder is the subjective sense of detachment from self, which is frequently reported as a barrier between self and perceptions. This sense of depersonalization may relate to fragments of such things as limbs or a voice, as well as the whole self. Derealization, a closely related phenomenon, is the experience of detachment from the outside world as if it were a stage setting in which there is affective detachment.

CASE EXAMPLE

A single parent, a 17-year-old young woman, began feeling as though her hands and lower part of her body did not belong to her. This experience followed the birth of her baby. She became depressed, could not concentrate, and was unable to communicate with her parents. She was frightened by these experiences of depersonalization. She was referred for therapy, where she was able to begin to verbalize anger and resentment over a variety of situations, most importantly the circumstances surrounding her pregnancy and the birth of the baby. These situations included fears, threats, and abuses, which had never been expressed. With proper therapy, there was a reduction in symptoms of depersonalization and clearing of her cognitive functions, which significantly helped her functioning at school and her eventual recovery.

Summary

This chapter describes dissociative disorders in terms of behavioral characteristics; the ego defense of splitting; the psychiatric diagnoses of psychogenic amnesia, fugue state, multiple personality and depersonalization; and nursing intervention goals. Special attention is placed on the linkage of multiple personality to early child abuse and sexual victimization.

Questions

1. What differentiates the normal state of "splitting" with the dysfunctional state?
2. Describe a clinical case where you observed the patient dissociating.
3. What is the relationship between early childhood sexual victimization and multiple personality?

REFERENCES AND SUGGESTED READINGS

1. Schreiber, F. R. *Sybil*. Chicago: Regnery, 1973.
2. Kluft, R. P. An update on multiple personality disorder. *Hospital & Community Psychiatry*, 1987, *38*, 363–373.
3. Spiegel, D. Multiple personality as a post-traumatic stress. *Psychiatric Clinics of North America*, 1984, *7*, 101–110.
4. Kluft, R. P. Treatment of multiple personality disorder: A study of 33 cases. *Psychiatric Clinics of North America*, 1984, *7*, 9–29.
5. Kluft, op. cit.
6. Braun, B. G. (Ed.) *Treatment of Multiple Personality Disorder*. Washington, D.C.: American Psychiatric Press, 1986.
7. Kluft, R. P. The treatment of multiple personality disorder: Current concepts. In E. F. Flach (Ed.), *Directions in Psychiatry* (Vol. 5, Lesson 24). New York: Hatherleigh, 1985.

Chapter 43

Sexual Disorders

Ann Wolbert Burgess, Carol R. Hartman, and Christine A. Grant

Chapter Objectives

The students successfully attaining the goals of this chapter will be able to:

- Explain sexual growth and development and their relationship to partners.
- Describe the human sexual response cycle and the expression of sexuality.
- Identify the two major groups of sexual disorders and the residual class, other sexual disorders, as classified by the *DSM-III-R*.
- Plan nursing care with nursing diagnoses for the patient with a sexual disorder.
- Describe sexual deviations dangerous to self and dangerous to others.
- Understand treatment issues with paraphilia and incest families.

Human sexuality is a pervasive force arising from the biologic and chemical ability of a species to reproduce and refurbish its group.* The human has added to the dimension of instinct and drive such psychosocial processes as values (i.e., companionship, need for love), morality, ethics, and legality.[1] Although sexuality is often equated with sexual behavior (genitality), this constitutes but a portion of the sexual sphere. Sexuality encompasses communication, inter-personal intimacy, self-affirmation, responsibility, sensuality, mutual pleasuring, and love. It is a human potential beginning before birth and terminating with death. It involves all the biologic and experiential factors that influence an individual's relationship with members of the same and opposite sex and more importantly, the individual's self-concept as male or female. Although every individual is a sexual being, the expression of sexuality may be altered by personal choice, psychosocial factors, health status, or environment.

The nature of nursing practice is such that nurses will encounter clients from various social and cultural groups, of every age, and with var-

---

* NOTE: This chapter is adapted from Chapter 19, Psychosexual disorders, by Carol R. Hartman, Ronna Krozy, William H. Masters, and Mark F. Schwartz, in A. W. Burgess (Ed.), *Psychiatric Nursing in the Hospital and the Community*, 4th ed., (Englewood Cliffs, N.J.: Prentice-Hall, 1985).

ious conditions that may threaten their sexual well-being. Through the close interpersonal relationships that nurses have with their clients, it is safe to assume that nurses will be confronted with sexual issues that challenge their own knowledge and values. Isabel P. Robinault contends that "personhood is the threshold of sexuality."[2] Thus, in order to treat clients holistically and humanistically, sexuality must be a part of the nursing process. The nurse must not only assess, educate, and intervene (directly or indirectly) in clients' sexual issues, but should be fully aware of her own attitudinal set. It is only through conscious self-awareness that the nurse can begin to evaluate her effectiveness in assisting clients to reach the optimal level of functioning.

A great deal of research is being conducted at present, rapidly changing our body of knowledge. It is beyond the scope of this chapter to treat comprehensively the entire realm of sexuality. Nurses, in pursuing the topic more fully, should consult some of the excellent resources available as well as consider undertaking a formal sex education course.

At the same time, this chapter will facilitate the nurse's understanding of human sexual growth and development, human sexual response, variations in sexual partnerships and expressions, and conditions that affect sexual function.

Increasing nurses' sexual awareness will enable them to interact appropriately with their clients and will prevent immobilization or blocking of sexual cues. Not only will they be able to assist clients whose conditions interfere with their sexual function, but they will also be able to define parameters of nursing's responsibility to healthy sexuality.

SEXUAL GROWTH AND DEVELOPMENT

Accurate knowledge about sexual physiology and functioning is basic to understanding human sexuality. The process of sexual maturation, including reproduction, desire, and function, is generally a function of the endocrine system. Every individual becomes a male or female as a result of biopsychosocial influences.

Biologic Influence

The presence of certain hormones bring about the differentiation of the embryonic sex-cell mass into female or male genitalia. Hormonal signals initiated by the special chromosomal pattern established in the embryo at conception results in the sex of the offspring. Each ovum produced by the female carries an X chromosome, whereas each sperm produced in the male carries either one X (female) or one Y (male) chromosome. Only one of the 200 million sperm contained in one single ejaculate will penetrate and fertilize the female ovum. An X-bearing sperm fertilizing the ovum will produce an XX, or a female child. The sperm bearing the Y chromosome will produce an XY, or a male child.[3]

The complex human sexual system, under the control of hormones, begins with the differentiation of the gonads into male testes or female ovaries. The reproductive system of the embryo is simply an undifferentiated genital thickening on the posterior outer layer of the embryonic cavity. This internal sexual transformation is visible at about 6 weeks' gestation.

During this earlier embryonic phase the gonads emerge as ridges of tissue. They are not differentiated sexually and can become either testes or ovaries. At this same point in development two duct systems develop. The wolffian and müllerian duct systems are two primitive genital ducts that are the precursors of specific sexual structures.

The primitive gonads transform into testes when the chemical substance H-Y antigen starts the process. This antigen, controlled by the Y chromosome, must be present for the male to develop; otherwise the primitive gonads will always develop into ovaries.[4,5]

Once the sex of the embryo has been established by the gonadal development, the ducts of the opposite sex remain undeveloped or degenerate.[6] In the male, a chemical called müllerian duct inhibiting substance causes the müllerian ducts to shrink and virtually disappear. Testosterone, an androgen, is produced and the wolffian ducts develop into the epididymis, vas deferens, seminal vesicles, and ejaculatory ducts.[7] Testosterone is converted to dihydrotestosterone, another androgen, which in turn is responsible for the development of the penis, scrotum, and prostate gland.[8]

The female organs are not dependent on hormones. Ovaries develop around the 12th week after gestation and the müllerian duct system develops into the uterus, fallopian tubes, and the inner third of the vagina.[9] The wolffian duct system shrinks because of the absence of androgens. By the 14th week the embryo is clearly differentiated into either a male or female with visible internal sex structures.

The external genitalia are identical up until the seventh week of development. Initially the ovaries and the testes are formed in the abdomen and with the influence of androgen the male testes move into the scrotum. The lack of androgen stimulation results in the clitoris, vulva, and vagina development, and eventually the ovaries settle into the pelvis. The external genitalia are initially located between the umbilical cord and the embryo's tail. The area called the genital tubercle eventually becomes the clitoris in the female and the glans of the penis in the male. A groove that forms in front of the genital tubercle around the fourth week of life produces a separation that is known as the perineum.

Genetic sex is fixed at the time of fertilization but it is not until the fifth or sixth week of development that the genes actually influence the embryo. Normal development depends on the presence of androgen, and if the male is deprived of androgen then the müllerian system regresses, the wolffian system does not develop, and hermaphroditism results.[10] The hermaphrodite is born with both testicular and ovarian tissue. The pseuodohermaphrodites have gonads that match their sex chromosomes but their genitals represent the opposite sex.

Klinefelter's syndrome, a common chromosomal abnormality, occurs when there is an extra X chromosome in the male. This condition occurs about once in every 500 live male births but is often not discovered until the male reaches maturity. The testosterone production is reduced, the testes are abnormal, and sperm production does not occur. Low sexual desire and impotence have been noted, although the condition may improve with regular testosterone injections.[11]

Turner's syndrome is the absence of an X chromosome. The result is nonfunctioning ovaries and subsequent absence of menstruation. Infertility, shortness, and a variety of abnormalities that may involve facial appearance and internal organs occurs. Turner's syndrome occurs in about one in 2,500 live female births.[12]

Besides sex chromosome disorders and genetic conditions the exposure of the fetus to drugs taken by the mother can also influence the sexual development of the embryo. A study by Yalom, Green, and Fisk revealed that teenage boys of diabetic mothers who received estrogen and progesterone during pregnancy were rated as having lower masculine behavior and athletic prowess than other boys of the same age.[13] Zussman, Zussman, and Dalton found less physical activity and participation in heterosexual activity in a group of boys ages 16 to 19 who had been exposed to high levels of progesterone in utero.[14,15] Although inconclusive, the studies do suggest that prenatal hormonal exposure may influence later life-styles.

Our sexuality is influenced by both biology and learning. This interaction throughout our lives affects our sexual behavior and emotions. The separation of these two influences is impossible. Highlighting the unique inter-relatedness of the biologic and learning influences are the following examples as presented in Masters, Johnson, and Kolodny.[16]

The first is one of the most famous cases in the annals of modern sexology, which was reported by John Money.[17,18] When identical twin brothers underwent circumcision at 7 months of age, an operating error led to the loss of the penis of one twin. After considerable anguish and consultation with various medical experts, the parents were finally referred to Johns Hopkins University, and a joint decision was made that the twin missing a penis would be raised as a girl. At 17 months, the child's name, clothing, and hair-style were changed, and four months later the first of a series of surgical procedures designed to reconstruct the genitals as female was started. Family members were provided with the best available advice about ways of coping with this gender reassignment.

The parents took great care to treat their twins as son and daughter even while knowing that both were biologically male. As a result, the daughter quickly began to prefer dresses to slacks and showed other "typical" signs of femininity, such as a desire for neatness. When the twins were 4½, the mother remarked: "One thing that really amazes me is that she is so feminine . . . She just loves to have her hair set; she could sit under the drier all day long to have her hair set."[19] The twins were encouraged to develop play patterns and interests in toys along traditional lines—dolls for the girl, cars and tools for the boy. The mother also reported that her son and daughter imitated their parents' behavior differentially, the son following his father's example and the daughter imitating what the mother did. According to Money, these two children achieved normal (and different) gender identities and gender roles although they both had identical chromosomal, anatomic, and hormonal sex during prenatal development and for the first 7 months of life.

The case has now taken a new twist, however, and the "girl" twin's adjustment to a female gender identity may not be as straightforward as Money previously suggested. According to interviews with the girl's psychiatrist conducted by the British Broadcasting System, she is having many problems as a teen-ager and is so unfeminine in appearance and behavior that classmates taunt her by calling her "cavewoman."[20] While a final picture of her psychosexual development may not emerge for another decade and while the current problem may reflect a need to adjust her estrogen dose properly, it is now difficult to use this case to support the position that gender development depends primarily on learning.

Another research study claims to support just the opposite conclusion. In 1974, 38 male pseudohermaphrodites were discovered in four rural villages of the Dominican Republic. Although these subjects have normal sex chromosomes, an inherited enzyme defect causes improper formation of the external genitals, even though prenatal testosterone production is normal. The testes and internal sex organs are completely male. But at birth, the affected babies have an incompletely formed scrotum that looks like labia, a very small penis that looks like a clitoris, and a partially formed vagina. As a result, many of them are raised as female. Then, during puberty, normal male testosterone production starts, and definite masculine changes occur. The voice deepens, male-pattern muscles develop, the "clitoris" grows into a penis, and the testes descend into the scrotum. Normal erections occur and intercourse is possible.

Of the 18 genetically male children with this condition who were raised as girls, 17 changed to a male gender-identity and 16 of 18 shifted to a male gender-role during or after puberty.[21] The authors of this report believe that these findings show that when sex of rearing is contrary to the biological sex, the biological sex will prevail if normal hormone production occurs during puberty.[22]

The biologic influences of one's sexuality interact with the psychological and social factors that are in operation from birth forward. The psychosocial development in human sexuality is concerned with sex identity (a biologically assigned classification), gender identity (the personal perception of being male or female), and gender role (the outward expression of socially accepted masculine or feminine traits).

The sexual classification assigned at birth generally guides the roles, relationships, and behaviors that an individual will assume throughout life. Gender identity formation occurs during early childhood, beginning somewhere between 18 months and 3 years of age. The development of gender identity and gender role is shrouded with controversy and there are several theories postulated to explain the sequence and interrelationships.

The social learning model suggests that gender development is learned from the personal role models and cultural influences that the child experiences during growth. The child imitates and models the parents' behavior and is rewarded for this imitation. A "child learns sex-typed behavior the same way he or she learns any other type of behavior, through a combination of reward, punishment, and observation of what other people are doing."[23] Rewards are apt to be seen in the form of praise: "He's built just like his father," or, "little girls don't climb trees and get dirty," or, "that's women's work." The child thus learns which behaviors will be sanctioned through specific direction and imitation of the same-sex parent or surrogate role model. This process, known as "differential socialization" influences the child's gender identity and gender role.[24,25]

The cognitive-development theory posits that children form a firm gender identity around ages five or six when they understand that gender is constant, i.e., that dressing up in Mommy's shoes does not change a boy into a girl. This theory suggests that children learn by observation and imitation, not for parental reward as the learning theory suggests but rather simply to obtain self-identity.[26]

The biosocial interaction theory stresses critical periods in sexual development that influence gender development. This comprehensive manner of encompassing all sexual development phases includes prenatal programming, psychology, and society's norms and their interactions with the biologic factors.[27]

Sexual development is a pervasive process that occurs throughout the life cycle. This takes place within the context of one's culture and religion, guided by "a mixture of ethical beliefs, social assumptions and personal experiences."[28] Typical patterns of sexual development have been observed and researched during childhood and offer insight into the development of gender identity and role assumption.

Infantile sexuality is closely related to the sensuous closeness of parent and child.[29] The cuddling, holding, caressing, and physical interactions between child and parent are the precursors for forming intimate relationships and being comfortable with one's own sexuality.

Freud theorized that the libido existed from infancy and that sexual development occurred within five stages; oral, anal, phallic, latency, and genital. Modern sexology has been profoundly influenced by Freud's work, although criticism has centered around his disregard for cultural influences and his biases concerning female sexuality.

Modern research has revealed that babies "express joy when their genitals are stimulated" and demonstrate irritability when they are interrupted while masturbating.[30,31] The responses of parents to this genital play influences the child's sexual behavior and has many implications to the child's gender identity formation.

SEXUAL PARTNERSHIPS AND RELATIONSHIPS

The human enters numerous relationships to satisfy personal and social needs. In our society adults have many pressures triggering a strong need for intimacy.[32] Among these pressures are maintenance of economic order through the efforts of family units rather than single individuals, and the maintenance of social order through the division of labor. The search for love, security, intimacy, affiliation, and gratification also form the bases for establishing interpersonal liaisons. Thus, sexual partnerships or relationships may be viewed by their legal status, social status, gender status, or activity status.

Legal Relationships

Marriage in the United States is a legal heterosexual union governed by state regulation (i.e., age of majority). One exception is common-law marriage whereby participants after a designated number of years together may be entitled to some of the rights engendered by legal marriage.

The married heterosexual couple is the preferred legal relationship in most cultures. However, those who wish to form other relationships are able to do so, though with more difficulty.[33] Sexual relations outside of marriage, though often considered unlawful or immoral, arise from personal choice.

Social Partnerships

Various social partnerships exist. These range from premarital relationships (casual dating to engagement) to those occurring within or after marriage.

The incidence of premarital sexual behavior has steadily risen since Alfred Kinsey's studies in the late 1940s and early 1950s.[34] One interesting phenomenon is the growing incidence of "living together" or "lewd and lascivious cohabitation" as it is legally classified in many states. Proponents argue that living together allows individuals to learn about each other intimately on a day-to-day basis, in order to decide whether marriage is justified. Opponents feel that a spiritual commitment is not possible without legal sanction. In fact, one study showed that contrary to their female partners, males in a living-together situation tended not to be committed toward marriage.[35] One might assume that incongruent expectations between these couples could lead to future problems.

Extramarital relationships, or adultery, may be defined as "nonmarital sexual intercourse between a man and woman, at least one of whom is married at the time to someone else."[36] R. A. Harper notes that extramarital intercourse among males decreases with age and, conversely, increases with age among women.[37]

Adultery is generally nonconsensual. Great pains are usually taken to hide it, although there may be realistic suspicions on the part of the spouse. Various reasons (e.g., illness, boredom, aging) exist for engaging in extramarital affairs, and recently some differentiation has been made between healthy and disturbed reasons.[38]

Another phenomenon is consensual adultery or "extramarital relationships of which the spouse knows and approves. Open marriage allows each spouse to establish closer or transitory relationships outside of marriage. Although discretion is usually practiced, inclusion of sexual partners in family activities may occur, resulting in confusion and trauma for children.[39]

Mate-swapping, as defined by R. R. Bell, is the "sexual exchange of partners among two or more married couples."[40] Another type of extramarital relationship is group sex, which

sometimes involves many people. Men and women may participate in equal or unequal numbers of whom none, some, or all may be married. Heterosexual or homosexual relations, or both, may occur at the same time within the same group. The significant aspect of group sex is that the experience is shared by all the participants, physically or visually.[41]

The rationale for entry into group sexual relationships differs widely. It has been shown that extramarital relationships frequently create jealousy, disharmony, and strain within a marriage, with unhappiness exceeding the worth of the experiences.[42]

Postmarital relationships created by divorce or widowhood are social partnerships worthy of discussion. Loss is sustained in both instances, and in addition, a feeling of failure and stigma often accompanies divorce. Divorced men and women tend to be younger than widowed ones, and entry into singlehood creates uncertainty. The trauma of divorce may hamper emotional commitment, and sexual relationships may be entered into for physical intimacy rather than emotional fulfillment.

Widowhood differs in that hostility does not usually exist toward the deceased spouse. However, the survivor may be subtly or openly chastized for seeking a new partner, seen as a lack of fidelity to the lost mate.

For both the widowed and the divorced, celibacy is decreasingly practiced. Many remarry, although the older woman may encounter greater difficulty because of the smaller number of males and the social acceptance of males initiating contact and dating younger women.[43]

Partnerships Based on Gender

Homosexuality is believed to have existed since the evolution of man. The causes of homosexuality—sexual relations between members of the same sex—have been diversely proposed: (1) social learning or conditioning; (2) heredity or genetic disorders; (3) family pathology; or (4) trauma-induced. Although some similarities are found in the backgrounds of homosexuals, these backgrounds do not necessarily differ from those of many heterosexuals.[44]

The category homosexuality has sociopolitical roots as the rationale for the removal from an official psychiatric category list. The activist movement called the Gay Rights Movement directly affected the mental health field as follows.

Gay Rights Movement

The 1970s witnessed a new social group gather in strength—the Gay Rights or Homophile movement. The first public outcry of the movement followed a riot by homosexuals in late June 1969, at a gay bar called the Stonewall in Greenwich Village, New York. This riot was precipi-

tated by a police encounter with the management of the bar. The time was ripe. The message from the homosexuals involved in the riot was their anger and retaliation at being discriminated against and their request to be treated as human beings. This historic riot provided the basis for organizing the first Gay Liberation Front group in New York, and it served as a model for many more groups forming throughout the country.

The underlying theme of the Gay Liberation approach to homosexuality is outlined by Franklin Kameny as follows: (1) homosexuals are fully the equal of heterosexuals; and (2) homosexuality is fully the equal of heterosexuality.[45] With the first precept goes the full bid by homosexuals for equality in employment, civil rights, and decent treatment; and with the second precept goes the acceptance of the sexual life-style. It is the second issue that presents the greatest problems for professionals. Kameny continues to outline those areas that need active work for people to see homosexuals as equals:

1. To dispel in the popular mind the sickness myth that has been created.
2. To change society's attitudes toward homosexuals and homosexuality.
3. To temper and ultimately to eliminate the prejudice felt and the discrimination, contempt, disdain, and dislike shown toward homosexuals.
4. To create and implement new, effective methods, applicable to large numbers of people, of supporting and reinforcing the homosexual in his homosexuality, in order to repair the psychic damage done by society.[46]

The Gay Rights movement has pressured the mental health professions to reevaluate their position on the subject. Increasingly, articles and research on the issue have appeared in journals. After reviewing the current materials on the topic, Eli Coleman states:

The main difference between homosexuals and heterosexuals is their choice of affectional and sexual preference. In addition, treatment modalities based upon the illness model have not reported very convincing evidence of success in "curing" homosexuals.[47]

All the mental health disciplines have taken positive steps to correct their traditional views on homosexuality. The most significant result of the early debates over the issue was the decision made in 1973 by the American Psychiatric Association to remove homosexuality from the standard official nomenclature. The American Psychological Association no longer lists "Homosexuality and Sexual Deviations" in its nomenclature. In addition, "Sexual Life-Styles" has been added to the study of social psychology.[48] The National Association of Social Workers at its national conference went on record to state that homosexuality was not a disorder, and it approved a set of resolutions to encourage homosexuals to enter the social work profession. And at the 1978 American Nurses' Association's Biannual Meeting in Hawaii, Resolution 51 was adopted by the 1978 House of Delegates on "Sexual Life-Style Minorities and Human Rights." It was resolved that the ANA would support the enactment of civil rights laws at the local, state, and federal levels that would provide the same protection to persons regardless of sexual and affectional preference as is currently guaranteed to others on the basis of sex, age, ethnicity, and color. Thus, persons not dissatisfied with their gender preference, ego-syntonic, were not to be labeled psychiatrically ill.

Homosexual partnerships among males are generally depicted as frequent, transient, and casual. Because of the difference in social conventions, extended dating or love commitments are unnecessary. At the same time, homosexuals often act with moral and ethical considerations, and there is a movement to consider homosexual "marriages" legal and binding.[49]

Among female homosexuals, relationships are often long-term, stable, and monogamous. They are based on the need for love, personal intimacy, and sex.[50]

Although bisexuality was an increasing alternative life-style and identity in the 1970s, the AIDS epidemic has had an influence on the sexual activity of people. Bisexuality may be defined as simultaneous sexual interaction with males and females. This phenomenon is believed to have arisen as a result of modern sexual permissiveness.

Activity

The last approach to sexual partnerships may be based on activity and includes prostitution and celibacy.

Prostitution refers to engaging in sexual ac-

tivity for profit and may be homosexual, bisexual, or heterosexual. Although the reasons that males and females enter into prostitution are various and complex, it is important to note the increasingly clear linkage between early sexual trauma within the family and early entry into prostitution in the life histories of many adolescent male and female prostitutes. Another interesting speculation regarding motivation is made by Charles Winick and Paul M. Kinsie who suggest that people who do not have power in our society may use their sex to achieve some of their goals.[51]

Gigolos are males who sell sexual services to women. They are usually young, attractive, and cater to older women who fear loss of appeal. It is not unusual to find gigolos in resorts serving the rich, in massage parlors, and in escort services.[52]

Male homosexual prostitutes often find their clientele through advertising or pickups. H. Benjamin and R. E. L. Masters interestingly note that many of these men are motivated by money, ultimately giving up their activities for marriage and child rearing.[53]

E. H. Erikson states that humans should have the potential for mutual orgasm but should also be capable of sustaining "a certain amount of frustration in the matter without undue regression wherever emotional preference or considerations of duty or loyalty call for it."[54] Celibacy is the conscious choice of adults to abstain from various degrees of sexual activity. Several forms of celibacy exist.

Complete celibacy excludes all willful sexual activity. Partial celibacy allows masturbation but excludes sexual exchange between persons. Experiential celibacy is a chosen life-style or value with or without having experienced other sexual modes and without a particular celibate ideology. Religious celibacy is an ideological practice related to beliefs in chastity. Roman Catholic celibacy is derived from "a negative evaluation of sexuality in the Christian heritage as well as a duty to love all equally."[55] Feminist celibacy derives from sociopolitical factors that hold that sexual activity uses the energy that could be "channeled into the struggle for female equality." Finally, celibacy for health may be practiced for medical purposes or, as proclaimed in yoga, to maximize energy and level of consciousness.[56]

Nurses need to be aware of the various types of relationships that their clients may have and autognose their feelings about their clients'

846 CLINICAL SYNDROMES AND HUMAN RESPONSES

sexual life-style in order to ensure a positive response to the following questions: Will the nurse be able to intervene effectively with the homosexual couple, the prostitute, the unmarried parent, the client who chooses nonparenting? Will the nurse offer sensitive counseling to the divorced or widowed with sexual needs? Understanding the acceptance of the client's chosen life-style is important in facilitating the nurse–client relationship.

HUMAN SEXUAL RESPONSE AND EXPRESSION

Human Sexual Response

According to W. H. Masters and V. E. Johnson, the sexual response pattern for males and females consists of four phases: excitement, plateau, climax, and resolution.[57] (For males, immediately after orgasm and prior to resolution, there is a refractory period where no response is possible.).

Each phase brings with it specific sex organ response as well as generalized body response (for example, lubrication, erection, perspiration, tachycardia). The length of each phase varies greatly, with the longest phases being excitement and resolution.

The orgasmic response in males often differs from females. Generally, the male experiences one orgasm following ejaculatory demand and requires a period of time before erection and orgasm are again possible. Three patterns of orgasmic response have, however, been reported in women. The first is similar to the male. The second shows a rippling effect of multiorgasms at the plateau level, and the third shows mounting excitement levels, bypassing the plateau, to orgasm and resolution. Figure 43-1 depicts such patterns.

Sexual Expression

Sexual arousal in humans is expressed in a variety of ways that may or may not include orgasmic discharge and does not preclude abstinence and conscious suppression of sexually charged stimuli.

Heterosexual Modes of Sexual Expression

Petting may be defined as the continuum from simple kissing with clothes on to mutual genital stimulation and complete nudity without engaging in intercourse. *Intercourse* (copulation, coitus) refers to the insertion of the penis into the vagina.

Oral genital contact includes *fellatio* (taking the penis into the mouth), *cunnilingus* (mouth and tongue stimulation of the female genitalia), *analingus* (anal stimulation with the tongue), and *mutual fellatio/cunnilingus* (or "69" based on the similarity of the body configuration).

Anal sex usually connotes penile insertion into the anus. This is the least practiced sexual expression among heterosexuals but is practiced by some male homosexuals.

Autoeroticism or self-stimulation may occur by manipulation of the genitals with a hand or mechanical device such as a vibrator, stream of water, or artificial phallus or vagina. *Masturbation* may take place in the presence of another partner—for example, during intercourse to effect orgasm, or by oneself. *Autoeroticism* often involves fantasy or sexually explicit materials to enhance the experience.

Abstinence may refer either to the total withdrawal of an individual from any sexual activity including masturbation or to varying degrees of activity without intercourse.

Homosexual Modes of Sexual Expression

Freedman, in his study of homosexuals, describes the sexual practices of gay males and females in an attempt to clarify the "considerable confusion about what homosexually oriented men and women actually do in bed."[58] Males engage in differentiated and preferential sexual practices as their experience increases. Among these practices are massage, mutual masturbation, fellatio, body rubbing, and anal intercourse. Body rubbing may cause painful friction if lubricant is not used. Anal intercourse may be intolerable to some males because of physical irritation or the feeling that it is depersonalizing. Multiple sex, sadomasochism (with dominance and bondage), sexual devices, and pornographic materials are also utilized. Freedman also mentions the use of "poppers" (isoamyl nitrate) or marijuana to heighten the experience.[59] Males often engage in a homosexual encounter before identifying themselves as gay; the converse is true of women. Sexual conquest is often the intent of males. For the gay woman, emphasis is often placed on tenderness and love. The sexual practices of gay women usually in-

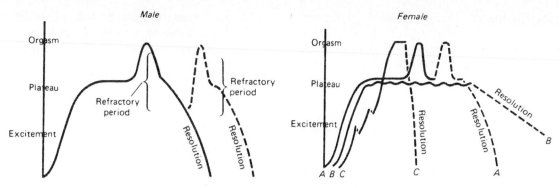

Figure 43-1. Male and female phases of sexual response.

volve cunnilingus and mutual masturbation. Tribadism (body-rubbing in the face-to-face position resulting in orgasm) is less frequently practiced. A dildo may be used in instances where partners wish to assume heterosexual roles. Gay women do not generally engage in group sex or sadomasochism, or use sexually arousing photos, but some do use marijuana.[60]

Sexual Devices

The purpose of sexual devices is to stimulate and heighten an individual's sexual response.

Vibrators
Vibratory sensations of the clitoris, vagina, anus, and penis are known to stimulate the sensitive nerve endings creating orgasm. Vibrators may be shaped like a penis, in length up to 10 or 12 inches, with or without various speeds. They are often recommended for nonorgasmic women in an attempt to teach them about their sexual potential.

Dildos and Artificial Vaginas
A dildo is a penis-shaped rod for vaginal insertion. It is often made of latex and replicates a real penis in terms of texture, color, size, shape, and flexibility. Artificial vaginas correspond to dildos in that they replicate vaginal structure. They are often semiflexible to provide penile friction and are ridged to simulate rugae.

Ticklers
Ticklers are rods or penile attachments of soft rubber fingerlike projections believed to provide additional vaginal stimulation.

Penile Rings
Penile rings are often used by male homosexuals to maintain erection and provide greater exposure of the penis while clothed. The rings are made of metal or plastic and encircle the base of the penis.

Penis Extenders
Penis extenders are another form of dildo. They are strapped onto the male and may be used in erectile dysfunction, spinal cord injury, or in cases of traumatic amputation of the penis. The psychological effect of using this device must be considered in a counseling situation.[61]

Love Dolls
A love doll may be male or female, solid or inflatable, and equipped with simulated genitalia for the purpose of intercourse or masturbatory fantasy.

Special Clothing
Extremely provocative clothes are sold as sexual enticements. Examples are see-through underwear, frontless brassieres, split crotch underpants, and pouch underpants for men. Black leather outfits are often sold for their effect in sadomasochistic and bondage practice.

Bondage Materials
Whips, chains, handcuffs, and leather straps are used for the purpose of enhancing sexual excitement by simulating bondage or rape, or inflicting pain.

Additional Devices
Fur, feathers, and other soft materials are used to caress various body parts for pleasurable and sensual effects.

848 CLINICAL SYNDROMES AND HUMAN RESPONSES

Pornography

As sexual violence is increasing in our society, people are asking for reasons and if there is a link between pornography and sexual violence. Cited as a common defining characteristic of the paraphilias, which are indicative of various sexual deviations, is the presence of sexually arousing fantasies or imagery. Many of these images are found explicitly in pornography.

The questions most often asked are: Is pornography harmful or harmless? What is "obscene"? Does restricting pornography transgress rights to free speech? Does pornography provide healthy outlets for impulses that would result in sexual deviance, or does it cause sexual acting out? Finally, how does it affect children?

Pornography and obscenity are illegal in all states, with numerous laws governing display, transportation, mailing, and distribution of "erotica." Diverse interpretation, however, left to the individual communities, has created problems in enforcement of such laws, resulting in a lack of protection for individuals who are unwittingly exposed to pornographic material. One area of general agreement is the need to eliminate "kiddie porn." Strict laws prevent the use of children depicted in sexual acts and punish offenders who solicit children for child abuse.

How is pornography defined? J. S. Delora and C. A. B. Warren define *pornography* as the "written, visual, or spoken presentation of sexual interaction or genitals . . . [whose purpose is most often] . . . a blend of entrepreneurial economics and sexuality; the making of money by the production and distribution of depictions of sexuality that will sexually arouse the consumers."[62] Pornography may include *obscenity*, "which can be defined as utterances, gestures, sketches . . . judged repugnant according to the mores of our society."[63]

A feminist definition of pornography was proposed by Dworkin and Mackinnon as the sexually explicit subordination of women, graphically depicted, whether in pictures or words, that also includes the presentation of women in one or more of the following ways:

1. As dehumanized sexual objects, things, or commodities
2. As sexual objects who enjoy pain or humiliation
3. As sexual objects who experience sexual pleasure in being raped

4. As sexual objects tied up, cut up, mutilated, bruised, or physically hurt
5. In postures of sexual submission or sexual servility, including inviting penetration
6. With body parts—including but not limited to vaginas, breasts, and buttocks—exhibited, such that women are reduced to those parts
7. As whores by nature
8. As being penetrated by objects or animals
9. In scenarios of degradation, injury, or torture and shown as filthy or inferior, bleeding, bruised, or hurt in a context that makes these conditions sexual.[64]

Federal Reports

In 1970, the U.S. Presidential Commission on Obscenity and Pornography stated that "the commission cannot conclude that exposure to erotic materials is a factor in the causation of crime or sex delinquency."[65] Sixteen years later, however, the Attorney General's Commission on Pornography came out with a different conclusion: "We are satisfied that the vast majority of depictions of violence in a sexually explicit manner are likely to increase the incidence of sexual violence in this country."[66] These two contradictory statements seem to indicate that crucial changes have taken place in the sixteen years since the first report.[67]

Probably the greatest change regarding public views on pornography has occurred in the nature of the materials under consideration. Although both commissions discussed sexually explicit materials, the later investigation tended to concentrate more on sexually violent depictions, which the commission found to be not only increasingly available, but also more frequently used in the publications that featured them. A second major change has been in the quantity and quality of academic research examining the effects of pornography. Academic interest in pornography increased with the publication of studies. Moreover, such studies, which contain reviews of earlier studies, were able to use methodological advances in the social sciences, such as more sophisticated techniques of statistical analysis. In addition, use of the penile plethysmograph meant that researchers need no longer rely on self-reports of sexual arousal, a method found to be relatively unreliable.[68]

The 1986 commission, in keeping with its specific mandate to study the "available empirical evidence on the relationship between exposure to pornographic materials and antisocial behavior," presents a thorough and scientific analysis of the major research findings in this field. These findings are summarized as follows.

In evaluating the results for sexually violent material, it appears that exposure to such materials (1) leads to a greater acceptance of rape myths and violence against women; (2) has more pronounced effects when the victim is shown enjoying the use of force or violence; (3) is arousing for rapists and for some males in the general population; and (4) has resulted in sexual aggression against women in the laboratory.[69]

PSYCHIATRIC DIAGNOSES

The sexual disorders are divided into two groups.[70] The paraphilias are characterized by arousal in response to sexual objects or situations that are not part of normative arousal-activity patterns and that in varying degrees may interfere with the capacity for reciprocal, affectionate sexual activity. The sexual dysfunctions are characterized by inhibitions in sexual desire or the psychophysiological changes that characterize the sexual response cycle. Finally, there is a residual class, other sexual disorders, for disorders in sexual functioning that are not classifiable in any of the specific categories.

PARAPHILIAS

The essential feature of disorders in this subclass is recurrent intense sexual urges and sexually arousing fantasies generally involving either (1) nonhuman objects; (2) the suffering or humiliation of oneself or one's partner (not merely simulated); or (3) children or other nonconsenting persons. The diagnosis is made only if the person has acted on these urges or is markedly distressed by them. In other classifications these disorders are referred to as sexual deviations. The term *paraphilia* is preferred because it correctly emphasizes that the deviation (*para*) lies in that to which the person is attracted (*philia*).

The specific paraphilias include: (1) exhibitionism; (2) fetishism; (3) frotteurism; (4) pedophilia; (5) sexual masochism; (6) sexual sadism; (7) transvestic fetishism; and (8) voyeurism.

People with paraphilia commonly suffer from several varieties and may have additional mental disorders. The paraphilia has criteria for severity as follows:

Mild	The person is markedly distressed by the recurrent paraphilic urges but has never acted on them.
Moderate	The person has occasionally acted on the paraphilic urge.
Severe	The person has repeatedly acted on the paraphilic urge.

Diagnostic Criteria for Voyeurism

The essential features of this disorder are recurrent, intense, sexual urges and sexually arousing fantasies, of at least 6 months duration, involving acts of observing unsuspecting people, usually strangers, who are either naked, in the process of disrobing, or engaging in sexual activity. The act of looking (peeping) is for the purpose of achieving sexual excitement, and no sexual activity with the person is sought. Orgasm, usually produced by masturbation, may occur during this voyeuristic activity, or later in response to the memory of what the person has witnessed. Often these people enjoy the fantasy of having a sexual experience with the observed person, but in reality this does not occur.

Diagnostic Criteria for Transvestic Fetishism

The essential features of this disorder are recurrent, intense, sexual urges and sexually arousing fantasies, of at least 6 months duration, involving cross-dressing. The person usually keeps a collection of women's clothes that he intermittently uses to cross-dress when alone. While cross-dressed he usually masturbates and imagines other males being attracted to him as a woman in his female attire.

CASE EXAMPLE

Syd was 12 years old when he first ran away from home because of his difficulty in concentrating at school and because of his mother and stepfather's inability to accept his fetishism and cross-dressing. From the age of 5, Syd said he had wanted to dress and be a girl. He thought about being a girl, preferred playing with dolls, and frequently would use his mother's makeup. This latter behavior upset his father to the point that he would tear the boy's mattress apart looking for the cosmetics. Until age 5 Syd was raised by his mother, an aunt, and his grandmother. His aunt encouraged his feminine interests and often made up his face with her makeup. Syd had strong, positive memories of his female caretakers. His mother's remarriage when he was 5 was very upsetting to Syd.

Syd's first sexual experience was at age 11 when he was approached by an adult male for oral sex while in a public bathroom. When he ran away, he was given refuge by the manager of a men's clothing department. This man talked openly of the gay clubs and the "queens" who cross-dressed. This man bought Syd his first woman's wardrobe and makeup in exchange for sex. After the man tired of him, Syd earned money hustling at gay bars and on the street. At age 14, Syd had tried all the street drugs and had been treated for sexually transmitted diseases. His hope is to be able to afford a sex-change operation.

Diagnostic Criteria for Exhibitionism

Over a period of at least 6 months, recurrent intense sexual urges and sexually arousing fantasies involving the exposure of one's genitals to an unsuspecting stranger characterize this disorder. The person has acted on these urges or is markedly distressed by them. Sometimes the person masturbates while exposing himself (or fantasizes exposing himself).

Diagnostic Criteria for Frotteurism

The essential features of this disorder are recurrent, intense, sexual urges and sexually arousing fantasies, of at least 6 months duration, involving touching and rubbing against a nonconsenting person. It is the touching, not the coercive nature of the act that is sexually exciting. Both rubbing and fondling are included within this category.

The person with this paraphilia usually commits frottage in crowded places, such as on public transportation or a busy sidewalk, from which he can easily move to escape arrest. The person rubs his genitals against the victim's thighs and buttocks or fondles her genitalia or breasts with his hands. While doing this he usually fantasizes an exclusive, caring relationship with his victim. The victim may not initially protest the frottage because she cannot imagine that such a provocative sexual act would be committed in such a public place.

Diagnostic Criteria for Fetishism

This disorder is characterized by recurrent intense sexual urges and sexually arousing fantasies involving the use of nonliving objects by themselves (e.g., female undergarments) over a period of at least 6 months. The person may at other times use the nonliving object with a sexual partner. Among the common fetish items are bras, women's underpants, stockings, shoes, boots, or other wearing apparel. The person may masturbate while holding, rubbing, or smelling the fetish object or may ask his sexual partner to wear the object during their sexual encounters. Usually the fetish is required or strongly preferred for sexual excitement, and in its absence there may be erectile failure in males.

Diagnostic Criteria for Sexual Masochism

The essential features of this disorder are recurrent, intense, sexual urges and sexually arousing fantasies of at least 6 months duration, involving the act (real, not simulated) of being humiliated, beaten, bound, or otherwise made to suffer.

Masochistic acts may be fantasized, such as being raped while being held or bound by others so that there is no possibility of escape. Others act on the masochistic sexual urges themselves through binding themselves, sticking themselves with pins, shocking themselves electrically; or self-mutilation or masochistic acts may be sought with a partner. Such acts include restraint (physical bondage), blindfolding (sensory bondage), paddling, spanking, whipping (flagellation), pinning and piercing (infibulation), and humiliation (such as being urinated or defecated on, being forced to crawl and bark like a dog, or being subjected to verbal abuse). Forced cross-dressing may be sought out for its humiliating associations. The term *infantilism* is sometimes used to describe a desire to be treated as a helpless infant and clothed in diapers.

One particularly dangerous form of sexual masochism is called hypoxyphilia and involves sexual arousal by oxygen deprivation. In this form, the person produces oxygen deprivation by means of a noose, ligature, plastic bag, mask, chemical (often a volatile nitrate that produces a temporary decrease in brain oxygenation by peripheral vasodilation), or chest compression, but allows himself the opportunity to escape asphyxiation before consciousness is lost. People engaging in such behavior report that the activity is accompanied by sexual fantasies in which they asphyxiate or harm others, others asphyxiate or harm them, or they escape near brushes with death. Oxygen-depriving activities may be engaged in alone or with a partner.

Sexual Deviations Dangerous to the Self: Autoerotic Practices

There are a wide variety of autoerotic practices known to humans. The motivation is primarily self-stimulation by sexual means. In the vast majority of these cases, the goal is achieved with no untoward effects on the individual. However, this is not true of autoerotic asphyxia.

Hypoxyphilia, solo sexual practice that seeks to induce hypoxia for a sexual euphoria through the use of an injurious agent, is strongly emphasized in the professional, scholarly, and commercial literature as a dangerous activity.[71-73] When cases are correctly identified, conservative estimates now suggest that between 500 to 1000 deaths occur annually, with the majority in the adolescent and young adult age range.[74]

Although the forensic and law enforcement literature describes the investigative and medical components of autoerotic asphyxial deaths, little exists in the behavioral or social science literature that describes this form of fatality or the response of the family members or associates to this type of death.[75] Several factors are responsible for this deficiency: (1) there is often a misdiagnosis of suicide or homicide rather than a diagnosis of accidental death, and thus an underreporting of the manner of death[76]; (2) there also is now a general acceptance and encouragement of all types of consenting sexual activity and a concomitant reluctance to acknowledge or emphasize the dangerous component in certain sexual activities (e.g., sexual bondage); and (3) there is social stigma surrounding a sexually motivated death.

Need for Case Finding: Statistical Evidence

Clearly there is a need for case finding for young people who use this type of sexual practice and

a need for mental health clinicians to understand the activity for the counseling of families. One of the major encouragements we found for bringing this problem to the attention of professionals came from the parents of young victims who had been shocked at the sudden death of their child and who had known nothing about the manner in which their child died. If parents who have lost children to this type of death believe it is timely to talk about the subject, not only to investigators but also to the news media, the professionals whose work may bring them into contact with families need accurate information. Thus, in an attempt to correct this oversight in the psychiatric–mental health literature, data from the social network of the 132 victims who died during a dangerous autoerotic act were analyzed as to the impact of this type of death on the family, specifically as related to pathological grief reaction.[77]

Data were systematically abstracted from 157 cases received by the Behavioral Science Unit of the FBI Academy. Of the 132 cases of autoerotic asphyxial deaths, 127 were male and 5 were female, with the mean age of 26.5 years. Four victims were preadolescent, 37 were teenagers, 46 were in their twenties, 28 in their thirties, 8 in their forties, 6 in their fifties, 2 in their sixties, and 1 in his seventies. There were 124 white victims, 5 black victims, 2 were Native American, and 1 was Hispanic. Seventy-six of the victims were single, 30 were married, 3 were separated, 1 divorced, and 2 widowed, and there were no marriage data on 20.

Emotional Response to Sudden Sexual Death

The emotional response to the death of a family member is particularly traumatic when the discovery of the body is made by a family member or associate, when the death is sudden and untimely, when the decedent is young, and especially when the death is sexual in nature. These are the factors generally present in autoerotic fatalities.

In the majority of cases in this study, the victim was found dead by a family member or friend. Of the 34 cases with data from the teenage group, 25 parents discovered their son dead. Of the 17 cases with data and where the victim was married, 11 wives found their husband dead. In the nonmarried group, out of 59 cases with data, 10 parents and 9 relatives found the decedent. More frequently in this group, the victim was found dead by friends, roommates, landlords, janitors, maids, employers, colleagues, police, or search parties.

People hearing of a victim's death are stunned and shocked at the suddenness of the news. The victim is usually described as having been in good spirits, good physical health, active, and having a future orientation. There rarely is any suspicion of suicidal ideation. Thus, the feeling of shock that is experienced is often due to the fact that there has been such a short time interval between seeing the victim and the death of the victim.

The victims are young and predominantly male. The extraordinary prevalance of males practicing dangerous autoerotic acts is a fact well supported in the literature.[78,79]

A sexual death resulting from the use of an injurious agent during a masturbatory ritual is considered an unusual type of death because many people—professionals included—have never heard of it. Although many people are familiar with autoerotic practices using manual stimulation, it appears that a significantly smaller number of people are aware of techniques for reducing oxygen to the brain to achieve an altered state of consciousness and to enhance erotic sensations and fantasy.

Characteristics of Autoerotic Death

The sexually associated features of this type of death concern: (1) the position and condition of the body; (2) the injurious agent and self-rescue mechanism; (3) the attire and indications of bondage and masochism; (4) the props and sexual paraphernalia; and (5) the evidence of sexual activity. All of these features confuse and puzzle family members and associates.

Location, Position, and Condition of the Body.
Erotic imagery, an important psychodynamic feature of autoerotic practice, may be enhanced by the victim's specifically selecting a secluded location in order to act out his fantasies. In the study, although the position of the body most often was partially suspended with feet barely touching a surface, victims were also found sitting, kneeling, lying face upward or downward, and suspended by their hands. The physical condition and the appearance of the body were dependent upon (1) the length of time the victim had been dead and how much tissue decomposition had occurred, and (2) the type of injurious agent used and the physical

injury to the body. Common characteristics of asphyxial deaths that family members have observed include a protruding discolored tongue (purple or black); bleeding from the ear, nose, or mouth; and indented ligature marks to the neck or body when protective padding was not used.

Injurious Agent and Self-Rescue Mechanism.
The most common injurious agent was a ligature that compressed the neck and included ropes, cords, belts, chains, and whips. Other injurious agents identified in this study included devices for passing electrical current through the body, restrictive containers, obstruction of the breathing passages with gags, and the inhalation of toxic gases or chemicals through masks, hoses, and plastic bags. A self-rescue mechanism—necessary in this sexual activity—is any provision that the victim has made to reduce or remove the effects of the injurious agent. A slip knot is frequently used when the injurious agent is a ligature, knives may be nearby for use in cutting a rope, keys may be found to unlock a padlock, or the victim may have needed to do nothing more than extend his legs and stand up to relieve the pressure to the neck. In the study sample, in the use of the rescue device, the victim miscalculated the amount of time, substance, pressure, or current.

Attire and Medications of Bondage and Masochism.
Twenty-six of the 127 male victims were cross-dressed at the time of death, with teen-agers wearing their sisters' clothing and some husbands wearing their wives clothing. There also were fetish items found in the victim's residence that held sexual significance such as leather, rubber, nylon, and lace articles. Bondage, a major feature with these deaths, included physically restraining materials or devices. The majority of cases used a ligature around the neck, often with protective padding, and with other parts of the body also bound, including wrists, arms, legs, ankles, chest, and mouth. Less subtle forms included hoods, handcuffs, decorative chains, ace bandages, gags, and constrictive garments. The victim may also be found with evidence of masochism, specifically his having inflicted injury to his genitals, nipples, or other parts of the body.

Props and Sexual Paraphanalia.
A wide variety of fantasy aids—commercial erotica and pornography, books, records, sketches, diaries,

mirrors—were found with the victim or in his residence and are believed to be related to enhancing and expanding the fantasy scenario. Sexual paraphernalia found included dildos, vibrators, and fetish items.

Evidence of Sexual Activity. Although the victim may not have engaged in manual masturbation during the final autoerotic act, he is often found with pants unzipped or genitals exposed or the genitals wrapped to collect semen. Again, the sexual nature of the death is distressing to many family members, and so they may alter the clothing before the authorities arrive.

Problems in Dealing With the Investigation of Death

Law enforcement investigators try to determine if the victim has had prior experience with hypoxyphilia in order to establish the manner of death as accidental rather than suicidal. In talks with relatives and associates of the victim in regard to evidence of prior practice, some people reported no awareness of the victim's activity. In other cases, relatives and associates made observations but, lacking the knowledge of dangerous autoerotic activity, failed to link the observations, such as a preoccupation with tying knots, physical signs of red marks on the neck, bloodshot eyes, or confused behavior for short time periods, with this disorder. And there were a few cases in which wives were aware of their husband's preference for autoerotic activity over partner sexual activity. Rosenblum and Faber report on a case in which a 15-year-old boy was treated for this activity and in which the parents were aware of the activity but failed to bring it to the attention of anyone.[80]

There are problems for the person engaging in this type of sexual activity because the stigma and secrecy surrounding the behavior prevents him from disclosing. There also are problems for the families in dealing with this type of sexual activity because they may not know about it or how to observe for signs or what to do if they do discover the child with the sexually oriented equipment. And there are problems for clinicians, too, because there is no specific psychiatric classification or discussion of this behavior. There are a group of paraphilias and sexual deviations that are beginning to be studied but have not yet become part of the standard nomenclature in psychiatry.[81] These deviations are something of an uncharted territory, partly be-

cause professionals have shied away from studying these areas since they represent taboo topics. Also, investigators who did know about them were inhibited from study because of the concerns of colleagues that their careers would be tainted if they dealt with sexual matters. The conservatism of academic institutions has also inhibited study. And because the gathering of information in some of these areas meant dealing with unpleasant and unseemly materials, study was further delayed.

Nursing Implications

It is important for nurses to be knowledgeable about the various types of autoerotic deaths and the ways in which the death is distinguished from a suicide or homicide. The nurse may be consulted by the police investigating the case for any observations regarding the possibility that the death was autoerotic. For example, if the victim is brought into the emergency room of a hospital, the nurse can make observations, about the body; and if she hears information regarding the life-style of the victim, she can bring this to the attention of the police officials. The nurse may also be part of a crisis intervention team that provides care to the families of suicide or accidental death victims. The families of a victim of an autoerotic death will have many feelings about the nature of the death, and it is hoped that the nurse will be able to encourage the family members to talk and share their feelings. The nurse should be able to provide referrals for counseling because family members are considered at high risk for unresolved grief.

Attention is called to this type of sexual activity because we are aware of the sizable number of deaths resulting from it, such that it cannot be ignored any longer by mental health clinicians. People need to be warned of the lethality of the activity. And we are finding that families do want some basic information about the manner in which their family member died, as well as emotional support through the grieving process in order to prevent pathological grief.

Diagnostic Criteria for Sexual Sadism

The essential features of this disorder are recurrent, intense sexual urges and sexually arousing fantasies, of at least 6 months duration, involving acts (real, not simulated) in which the psychological or physical suffering (including humiliation) of the victim is sexually exciting.

Sadistic fantasies or acts may involve activities that indicate the dominance of the person over his victim (e.g., forcing the victim to crawl, or keeping the victim in a cage), or restraint, blindfolding, paddling, spanking, whipping, pinching, beating, burning, electrical shocks, rape, cutting or stabbing, strangulation, torture, mutilation, or killing. The sadistic fantasies are likely to have been present in childhood.

Paraphilias and Incest Families

The Paraphiliac

Definition. Paraphilia is predominantly a male psychiatric disorder.*

The term *paraphilia* literally means "beside-love." This suggests that there is a critical pathognomonic feature comprised of a multiplicity of cognitive, affective, and behavioral patterns that constitute this syndrome. In cases of paraphilia, there has been interference with or displacement of establishment and maintenance of intimacy between two adults. Common features among the various paraphilias are the inability to cope with closeness and attachment to other adults and the inevitable loneliness that is an integral part of social separation. Paraphiliacs usually cope with their social pathology by withdrawing into the secretly comfortable world of fantasy.

Paraphilia involves obsessive–compulsive behavioral patterns and appears to have a number of clinical similarities to addiction. The paraphiliac engages in obsessional sexual thinking and compulsively "acts out" his fantasies. The illicit compulsion may involve cross-dressing, fetishes for leather, undergarments, inanimate objects, pornography, exposing the genitals, making obscene telephone calls, peeping into windows, or fondling children. Generally unresponsive to nondeviant, affectional sexual stimuli, the paraphiliac becomes dependent on highly specific imagery or socially inappropriate, external stimulation to achieve sexual arousal.

Addictive Components. Like other addicts,

---

* This section, pp. 854–862 has been written by Mark F. Schwartz and William H. Masters from the Masters & Johnson Institute, St. Louis, Mo.

the paraphiliac experiences almost a "trance-like" sense of relaxation, relief, and homeostasis when involved in the illicit sexual activity, and conversely, exhibits social disease when not sexually "acting out." "Acting out" becomes an escape from distasteful aspects of life. The paraphiliac usually evidences adolescent-like narcissism, which results in his frequently attempting to extract unrealistic demands from his environment. Since he usually fails in this effort, he is continually frustrated and frequently angry. Other cognitional and thinking errors (discussed later) also add to his continuing frustration. Finally, chronically low self-esteem, self-depreciatory preoccupation, and poor assertiveness skills result in the paraphiliac repetitively feeling victimized. One exhibitionist, for example, became furious on a daily basis for over a year because his office mate played the radio and his wife asked his help with her college work. In another example, a male pedophile was enraged that the parking lot near the clinic was closed so that he could not participate in the therapy session. These individuals feel an overwhelming sense of inadequacy and a lack of control. The paraphiliac's "acting out" experience becomes an expression of rage or an attempt at control, giving him a temporary sense that "he is calling the shots."

Paradoxically, this illusion of control is quickly abated, leaving as a residual an overwhelming feeling of inadequacy. These sexual addicts being pushed by their "sickness" spend hours each day searching for the right situation to "act out." The paraphiliac becomes unable to make decisions based on personal morality and rarely recognizes potential harm to self or others. What follows is further internalization of "Why bother?" "I can't," "I'm sick," and other cognitions indicative of an absence of a sense of mastery and self-responsibility. Such cognitions then generalize and result in a myriad of other manifestations of self-sabotage, which in turn "fuel" the addiction. Alcohol abuse may accentuate this pattern by providing still another factor for rationalization.

Pedophilia and Incest: Description of the Syndromes

Pedophilia. For the paraphiliac uncomfortable in sociosexual interaction with adult males and females, eroticism may emerge either in response to an object (*fetishism*), through sexual interaction with an adult conducted at a safe distance (*voyeurism, exhibitionism, obscene telephone calling*), or by a sexual act with a nonthreatening child (*pedophilia*). Since the pedophile's social development has been impeded, he typically verbalizes a sense of uneasiness with other adults. Usually the only time he can feel comfortable and "be himself" is with a child. Psychosocial trauma has caused a fixation of or an impediment to his cognitive maturation, so the pedophile often thinks, feels, and acts like a child.

Incest Offenders. Incest offenders may or may not be paraphiliacs. But since many are pedophiles, and those who are not pedophiles are clinically so similar, the incest family will be included in this discussion. Many incest offenders are pedophiles who have married and continued their pedophilia with greater safety by sexually approaching their own child or stepchild. Several pedophiles in our sample have married in order to fondle their wife's daughter by a previous marriage or to impregnate their wife in order to fondle the resultant infant. Although most incest offenders deny being sexually aroused by children, plethysmography studies suggest that many of these men have greater arousal to children than they are willing to admit even to themselves.[82]

Another reason incest is included in this discussion is that in our experience, incest offenders require very similar treatment to that of the paraphiliac, with the major difference being that intervention for the incest offender also includes a family therapy component.

The husband-and-wife relationship in the incestuous family evolves into an immature, undifferentiated couple—creating confusion, conflict habituation, and other types of destructive dependent relationships. The homes of these men and women reflect any combination of the following: chaos (few rules are consistently followed), enmeshment (everyone's involved in one another's business), disengagement (no one cares what the others say or do, and rigidity (extreme authoritarianism).[83] In about 40 percent of reported cases, the incest offender or wife is alcoholic. According to recent data and our own clinical experience, the nonalcoholic offender may actually display more psychopathology than the alcoholic.[84]

Some incest offenders are extremely rigid and authoritarian, sometimes even physically abusive to other family members. The rigidity protects the offender from overwhelming feelings of inadequacy in dealing with daily transactions. The incest perpetrator is often intimidated by other men and uneasy in his work and social interactions. One perpetrator who dropped out of school at age 16 had recently been promoted to an administrative position. He stated, "I feel like I have to fake it every day." He said he felt the same way with his wife—"uneasy, inadequate, incompetent," yet without her he was unbearably lonely. At times, he was overtly acquiescent with her. At other times, particularly when drinking, his rage manifested itself with physical violence.

Treatment Program: The Masters and Johnson Model

There are three phases to the Masters and Johnson treatment program for the incestuous family. During phase one, the men participate in ten 3-hour group therapy sessions. These are counseling sessions designed to establish social, dating, and intimacy skills and to improve stress-management, problem-solving, and communication skills. The sessions are conducted in advance of phase two, intensive conjoint therapy. The perpetrators are helped to find adult female partners or to improve their relationship with their established partners.

Phase two, which entails 2 weeks of intensive conjoint therapy, uses all of the critical components of the Masters and Johnson model—social isolation, daily therapeutic intervention, dual-sex therapy team, integration of marital therapies, communication skills, experience with sensate focus, and directive eclectic psychotherapy focused on improving the state of intimacy between two adults.

Phase three is follow-up. All clients are followed actively for a minimum of 2 years. Phase four, for incest families only, is family therapy.

Immediate Intervention. If the individual has a *noxious paraphilia* (paraphiliac behavior that is harmful to self or others), it is essential to stop the "acting out" as rapidly as possible. Among the many different therapeutic approaches to the problem, contracting with the patient to stop the behavior for at least 3 months is a primary requisite. Several techniques have been employed to ensure compliance with the contract. Antiandrogen injections (depo-provera, dosage titrated according to individual's body weight) have been used by some researchers.[85] Behavioral techniques such as fantasy satiation or other forms of aversive conditioning can also be quite effective, while eliminating concern for medication side effects.[86] A third alternative is temporary institutionalization, particularly during phase one of the psychotherapy program.

Phase One: Behavioral Skills Training.

The most frequently encountered clinical presentation of paraphilia is that of a single man who describes very little interaction with adult partners. Despite the fact that the man may have significant sexual experience, or even if he is married, multiple behavioral skill deficits are still common. Therefore, the first phase of the Masters and Johnson Institute's rapid intervention program consists of ten sessions of 3-hour group therapy aimed at information giving, role playing, and social skills training. Trained female graduate students sit in on the group and role-play with the patients.

SOCIAL SKILLS. Some discussion of the techniques employed to improve or implement social skills is necessary since the techniques represent a synthesis of approaches and procedures described by others in the field.[87] The Masters and Johnson Institute's approach conceptualizes social behavior as a network of interacting components, including the individual's cognitions, his behavior, and his social environment. The individual is seen as an active organism in which all three components mutually influence social competence.[88]

This treatment model postulates a ladder approach toward modification of maladaptive behavior and the subsequent development of behavioral proficiencies (Table 43-1). Individuals in the group therapy educational experience progress through various levels of social competency at an individually tailored rate. First the patient is taught how to start conversations. Then advice is given regarding dress and hygiene and how to maintain appropriate eye contact without distracting motor gestures. The individual learns appropriate self-disclosure, how to keep a conversation flowing, how to handle silences, how to listen attentively, and how to terminate conversations.[89] The second step is for the man to learn how to ask a woman for a date and to make the date fun. Paraphiliacs need to understand the complicated sociosexual scripts of how the male typically initiates social interaction in our double-standard culture. A third step is to establish a moderate level of intimacy with a consenting female partner.

TABLE 43-1. COGNITION AND BEHAVIORAL DEFICIT CHECKLIST

Stage 1

Give and receive compliments	Active listening
Assertive talk and behavior	Receptivity to nonverbal clues
Feeling talk	Terminating conversation
Handling silence	Keeping conversations flowing
Eye contact	
Initiating conversations	Authority on certain subjects
Lengthening answers	
Focusing on positives	Dressing and grooming
Learning about others	Evaluating feedback
Relaxation skills	
Appropriate affect	
Appropriate self-disclosure	

Stage 2

Empathy skills	Appropriate physical contact
Intermediate levels of self-disclosure	Interpreting body language
Self-talk	Ending a date
Finding dates	
Making dates fun	

Stage 3

Irrational beliefs	Misinterprets feedbacks
Faulty thinking styles	Hyperresponsive
Negative self-statements	Self-deprecatory preoccupation
Unrealistic expectations	Easily threatened and defensive
Anticipated failure	

Stage 4

Touching	Problem-solving skills
Sexual skills	Using negative emotions as signals for action
Intimate self-disclosure	
Expressing and representing desires directly	Disagreement skills
Negotiating skills	Recognizing dependency and helplessness

Stage 5

Shared interests	Separate interests
Self-disclosure	Privacy
Positive regard	Dislikes self
Shared feelings	Privacy of feelings
Shared thoughts	Privacy of thoughts
Sexual needs	Lack of sexual needs
Closeness	Distance
Compassion	Dispassion
Empathy	Lack of empathy
Problem-solving	Lack of problem-solving
Doing things for each other	Doing things for self
Consideration	Inconsideration
Unselfishness	Selfishness
Touch	Lack of tough
Time together	Time alone
Trust	Distrust

Source: Masters and Johnson Institute, St. Louis, Mo., 1983.

A female facilitator is critical to effective group treatment. She provides the necessary female identity for the man to test out his irrational beliefs about women. When his misconceptions prove obviously false, the level of his social anxieties usually is reduced. Primary therapeutic emphasis in the group is placed on role modeling, which permits the client to see how others perform a specific skill to make it socially effective.[90] Through continuous rehearsal of his newfound skills, the paraphiliac develops a greater sense of self-mastery and esteem, which in turn increases his confidence to use these skills in his environment.

Some paraphiliacs may be relatively competent in their social skills initially, but most have difficulty with moderate levels of intimacy. At this stage, men are provided with suggestions regarding potential ways and means to meet partners. Once a partner is found, the men are given progressively specific, but flexibly graded instructions: starting with a coffee date,[91] or movies with a specific time to end the date, and meetings in partner's home with no physical interaction; then kissing and petting but no intercourse; and, finally, intercourse with a lot of nongenital touching. After each date, the patient is asked to detail and evaluate his social experience and is then provided with specific suggestions regarding social, dating, intimacy, or sexual skills.

ATTITUDE CHANGE. Another component of social skills is attitude change. Most sex offenders manifest uneasiness with specific aspects of adult sexual functioning. Early in therapy, definitive sex education is provided, including the use of visual materials if indicated. As an integral part of this educative process, female sexuality is discussed in depth by a female therapist, who simultaneously models the competent woman.

RESTRUCTURING THE THINKING STYLES OF THE PARAPHILIAC. Cognitive restructuring is critical to successful rehabilitation of the paraphiliac. Therefore, destructive thinking styles require continual reassessment in all phases of the therapy process. Certain cognitions are destructive to self-esteem. They include: irrational beliefs, self-depreciatory preoccupation, negative self-statements, unrealistic expectations, anticipated failures, misinterpretation of feedback, and easily elicited defensiveness.[92] Negative self-esteem is maintained by each individual's unique

cognitive filtering system. During the therapeutic process, the paraphiliac's biases in processing input from the environment are confronted and are explained by the therapist, after which reality is tested by the patient. Paraphiliacs are asked to attend to the positives rather than the negatives in their lives.

Therapists attempt to note and underscore styles of destructive thinking in context. One patient stated, "I'd rather be put in jail than have to call my wife to tell her I won't come home tonight because I have to work. In suggesting I call, you people are taking away all of my freedom." Obviously this man needed to test reality to realize that the act of calling his wife did not jeopardize his freedom. One unmarried patient stated, "I am not interested in any woman who starts a conversation with me." This man held the irrational belief that any friendly woman is a "whore." Obviously, this irrational belief needed to be exposed to therapeutic scrutiny and be tested. A married patient said, "When a woman speaks her mind, she wears the pants." This individual needed to discover that allowing his wife to represent herself was in his best interests. In group therapy, therapists and facilitators continuously need to be looking for faulty thinking styles that require reality testing.

Another common problem for the paraphiliac is the feeling of being a victim of life's circumstances, of constantly being pushed and pulled between undesirable alternatives. The socially immature offender will often respond to stress by moaning like a child, complaining, and blaming others for his problems. As previously noted, he evidences little capacity for self-responsibility or for taking positive action. Such individuals often evidence personalities that are unattractive to potential partners, or they tend to attach themselves to partners who will "mother" them but who may not be erotically stimulating. In response to even minor stresses, such as traffic jams, the paraphiliac may exhibit rage and then retreat into his fantasy world. Instead of changing the situation or finding a constructive means of stress reduction, that is, taking the "front door" by confronting and managing the stressful situation, the paraphiliac retreats through the "back door" into deviant sexual fantasy or behavior.

In group therapy sessions, clients are encouraged to set small attainable goals to facilitate confidence that "I can create and support the environment I live in." For distress that cannot be reduced, stress management techniques such as physical exercise, joining social organizations, and relaxation techniques are introduced.

Stress also results from consistent passivity instead of responsible, assertive behavior. Assertiveness skills are taught and practiced in role playing. Occasionally, paraphiliacs may cope with their helplessness and passivity with inappropriate aggression. Therefore, attention is given to mastering basic communication skills. Assertiveness skills need to be coupled with a change in self-esteem so that the paraphiliacs feel they have the "right" to express their desires to others. This is particularly true in interactions with new relational partners since the paraphiliac's initial feeling is often, "I'm lucky if she stays with a person as terrible as me, so I can't risk telling her if I'm upset or annoyed."[93]

Problem-solving skills are also rehearsed in group therapy. The individual is helped to feel a sense of mastery whatever problems arise. Group members are taught to function as a creative team to solve problems rather than attacking one another.

Yochelson and Samenow have documented "errors of thinking" common among paraphiliacs and incest perpetrators (see Table 43-2).[94] Each of these errors will be discussed briefly. The first is the "closed channel." Rarely will the paraphiliac or the incest offender tell the full truth (at least initially) to the health-care professional evaluating his problem. He typically has ambivalent motivation. These individuals despise their sexual "acting out," yet fear the loss of these experiences since "acting out" is the one high that helps them escape their distasteful lives.

Confabulation has been a way of life. Paraphiliacs and incest offenders successfully lie even to themselves; for example, some incest offenders state convincingly that they are not aroused by children—until you show them plethysmographic results of their erections in response to kids.

Total self-disclosure by the paraphiliac of his incestuous behavior is requisite to successful therapy, much like the alcoholic who must begin his treatment program by admitting his alcoholism. Lack of trust is also significant in this context. The paraphiliac will not allow himself to even hope that change in his "acting out" behavior is possible. A positive attitude is necessary for change and should be initially established as the client talks with other group members and with the therapists.

The "victim stance" is dealt with by pointing out the kinds of things done to him by society as well as the things he has done to himself as a result of his behavior. Situations in which the individual acted self-destructively are repeatedly pointed out. The therapist's style is not condemning but rather challenging. "Do you want to continue to 'act out' or try a new approach in the future?" All aspects of directive therapy are oriented to giving paraphiliacs and incest offenders a mode of handling previously unsolvable problems. By making small changes on a daily basis, the individual begins to realize that any effort to achieve short-term and long-term goals maximizes the probability of happiness.

Perhaps the most important motivating factor in eliciting behavioral change is repeatedly reminding the perpetrator of the effect of his behavior on the victim. Whenever he feels an urge to "act out," he must ask himself, "How will my behavior affect this other person?" In addition, if the behavior is potentially noxious, a second thought to be encouraged is, "What will be the possible consequences of my actions?"

Phase Two: Focus on Relationship Issues. The core of the Masters and Johnson treatment approach for sex offenders is a variation of the short-term intensive model described in their text *Human Sexual Inadequacy*.[95] Once the man has found a female partner and has completed the 10-week group therapy program, he is placed in couples therapy. Some men with advanced social skills are permitted to bypass the group therapy phase of the program.

Couples therapy comprises a 14-day period in social isolation from daily home and job responsibilities during which the paraphiliac and his female partner are asked to devote themselves to their relationship. The couple "try on" different ways of interacting socially and sensually. The experience of positive interchange on a daily basis increases motivation for continuing change.

Most paraphiliacs living in close quarters with a partner will evidence a myriad of resistances to intimacy. These resistances are diagnostic and can be utilized by the therapist. Confronting each partner with a single destructive transaction, describing how he or she perpetuates the specific distress, and then suggesting a way to do it differently (which they can try on in the next 24 hours) is the key to effective short-term therapy. Therapeutic rapport, established

TABLE 43-2. THINKING STYLES COMMON TO PARAPHILIACS

Category	Example
Closed channel	A "two-way" channel of communication with therapist and others based on self-disclosure, receptivity, and self-criticism is not established. Details of history are filled with omission, exaggeration, distortion, circumlocution. Selective listening, particularly of people believed to be dissuading him from his pursuit, is common. He commonly criticizes others but angrily rejects criticism of himself. He will deliberately mislead others by feeding them what he thinks they want to hear.
I can't	The individual states that there is nothing he cannot do if he wants to, yet is often powerless. Therefore, "I can't" becomes equivalent to "I won't," indicating his refusal to perform on someone else's terms. He dismisses effort and hard work.
Victim stance	Individual blames others on the grounds that he is a victim; he refuses to take responsibility for his role in situations.
Lack of perspective	He does not learn from experience or plan for the long term. He refuses to deter gratification; desires instant triumph instead of working slowly to obtain goal.
Failure to put oneself in another's position	He rarely stops to think about what other people think, feel, and expect. He has little regard for rules, customs, and laws or the noncriminal's way of thinking or living.
Failure to consider injury to others	He minimizes or does not view himself as injuring anyone. When held accountable, he regards himself as the injured party.
Failure to assume obligation	He feels obligation is a position of weakness and vulnerability to other's control. Family responsibilities, punctuality, and chores are not taken seriously.
Failure to assume responsible initiatives	He generates tremendous energy and initiative in a direction that is not socially acceptable. He does what is necessary to get what he wants. Ordinary social incentives have little meaning.
Ownership	Ownership represents an extreme form of control. If the individual wants something another owns, it is as good as his. Ownership extends to others' space. He invades others' privacy at will, yet insists on his own privacy. He is secretive about his life but feels entitled to know about others.
Fear of fear	Fear does not guide his behavior. It is a put-down word, destroying his self-esteem. For example, he will not allow himself to fear the possibility of his wife leaving; instead he denies and acts overly optimistic.
Lack of trust	Rarely trusts another—"It's a weakness."
Refusal to be dependent	Dependence is weakness. He is good at asking for assistance with the easiest of tasks, arguing for others to do his work for him.
Lack of interest in responsible performance	He deserves a particular status but is unwilling to achieve the status responsibility.
Pretentiousness	He thinks of himself as better than those around him. He scoffs at individuals who do things "by the book."
Failure to take an effort to endure adversity	He will endure adversity for crime but not for responsible living.
Poor decision making	He makes decisions a different way—whatever is expedient to get what he wants.
Other thinking errors	Overgeneralization, selective abstraction, arbitrary inference, magnification, minimization, dichotomous thinking, negative self-statement, personalization, unrealistic expectations, anticipated failure, misinterprets feedback, hyperresponsive, self-deprecatory preoccupation, easily threatened and defensive, and black-and-white thinking, others.

(From Yochelson, S., 1977.[94])

through insight, empathy, and support, is particularly critical in these cases. Many paraphiliacs and incest offenders are emotionally rigid and tend to respond with a childlike defensiveness and withdrawal from confrontation with authority. In addition, they typically are pessimistic and ambivalent about their potential for change. Frequently their ambivalence about losing the excitement of the addictive aspects of the paraphilia will manifest itself as therapeutic sabotage. Since sabotage is predictable, it can either be prevented with anticipatory guidance or be identified and used to help the individual or couple deal with their "fear of success."

SENSATE FOCUS. When treating sexual dysfunction, sensate focus is a most effective means of eliciting factors that interfere with "natural" sexual responsiveness. In similar fashion, when treating paraphilia, sensate focus is extremely valuable in eliciting factors that have interfered with heterosexual unfolding. Once the interfering factors are identified, directive psychotherapy can be used in an effort to neutralize the "roadblocks." Certainly, sensate focus can also be therapeutic in and of itself. These techniques are a means of gradually introducing stimuli that are potentially anxiety-provoking, while allowing the individual to maintain a sense of control.

Through sensate focus experience, a man previously oriented to paraphilia is given an opportunity to interact sexually with a woman without having to contend with culturally oriented demands for male sexual expertise or performance facility. Consequently, he has the opportunity to learn a great deal about female sexual responsivity in a nondemanding environment. In addition, he becomes more aware of his own sexuality in relation to women and of the potential for sexual pleasure without intercourse. He begins to realize that pleasurable states of sexual excitement and sexual comfort can be attained with adult partners.

Some paraphiliacs manifest aversion to the female body. For example, one pedophile in response to a suggestion to touch his partner's genital area experienced flashbacks to childhood of his mother sitting in the bathtub with him and insisting that he put his hands on her labia and into her vagina. He required several days of nondemanding genital touching with his partner before he could focus on her body exclusively. This clinical adaptation of the sensate focus experience allowed the man to respond "naturally" to tactile stimulation without paraphiliac imagery.

Partners of Paraphiliacs. The female cotherapist continually orients the female partner to be lover, friend, and companion. In turn, the woman provides an effective observer's source of continual informational feedback, not as another therapist but rather as an interested and involved party.

Obviously the female partner's appearance, personality, and sexual confidence are critical factors directly affecting the progress and ultimately the prognosis of couples therapy. When an unmarried paraphiliac searches for a female partner to bring to therapy, he usually chooses a socially nonthreatening woman. She is often physically unattractive and noncomplementary in intelligence and personality. And she frequently is also sexually unsophisticated. Yet, therapy can be benefited by her presence as long as she: (1) does not evidence significant individual psychopathology; (2) is sufficiently motivated to help; and (3) does not develop overt antipathy toward her partner. The sexually naive paraphiliac usually acquires a great deal of sociosexual information from this nonthreatening partner, which, in due course, he transfers to other potential relationships.

Treatment of Incest Families

Successful treatment of incest families requires a more sophisticated therapeutic process than the intervention techniques described for the paraphiliac offender. Intervention simultaneously focuses on the victim, the offender, the wife, and the family. Table 43-3 lists the five phases of the Masters and Johnson Treatment Program for Child Sexual Abuse Through a Schematic Diagram of the Demonstration Project. This program integrates individual, couple, group, and family therapy modalities into a rapid treatment program of 15 to 20 weeks in duration. The specific goals of the treatment program are listed in Table 43-4 and the Evaluation Criteria of the Treatment Program are listed in Table 43-5.

Unique characterological aspects of the incest offender are his extreme rigidity, authoritarianism, and defensiveness. Repeated confrontation with factors contributing to and maintaining the incest is required. For example, it may be necessary to change dramatically the family's style of living. Several men were en-

TABLE 43-3. SCHEMATIC DIAGRAM OF THE DEMONSTRATION PROJECT FOR CHILD SEXUAL ABUSE TREATMENT

Location	Activity	Time Period	Staff
Phase 1—Assessment			
Masters & Johnson Institute	Initial Screening		
	Husband	1 hour	Primary Investigator
	Partner	1 hour	Primary Investigator
Washington University Child Guidance Clinic	Individual Screening and Family Assessment Children/Parents	1 hour	Child Psychiatrist
Masters & Johnson Institute and Washington University Child Guidance Clinic	Psychologic Testing and Screening (General Psychological testing history)	2 hours / 4 hours	Primary Investigator / Psychologist
Appropriate Referral			
Phase II—Pretherapy Counseling and Individual Child Therapy			
Masters & Johnson Institute	Evaluation Pretesting (11 tests)		
	Husband	4 hours	Primary Investigator
	Partner	4 hours	Primary Investigator
Washington University Child Guidance Clinic	Individual Therapy (Children) Group Therapy	10 sessions / 10 2-hour sessions	Child Psychiatrist / 2 Group Leaders or Therapists
Masters & Johnson Institute	Group Therapy (same sex group)	10 2½-hour sessions	2 Group Leaders or Therapists
Phase III—Conjoint Sex & Marital Therapy & Dyad Therapy			
Masters & Johnson Institute	Intensive Conjoint Marital and Sexual Therapy	14 sessions	Dual Sex Cotherapy Team
Masters & Johnson Institute and Washington University Child Guidance Clinic	Mother-Victim Dyad Therapy	2 sessions	Group Therapist Family Therapist
Phase IV—Family Therapy			
Washington University Child Guidance Clinic and Masters & Johnson Institute	Family Therapy	8 sessions	Family Therapist and Masters & Johnson Cotherapists
Phase V—Follow-Up			
Masters & Johnson Institute	Evaluative Post Testing	4 hours / 1 hour	Psychologist / Child Psychiatrist
Child Guidance Clinic	Post Testing Follow-Up	1 hour 3 months 6 months 1 year 2 years	Child Psychologist / Therapist

couraged to obtain high-school equivalency degrees in an effort to reverse their hopeless, goalless, powerless existence. Others were helped to find and maintain jobs.

The wives in incestuous families are helped to recognize how they also may have had a role in maintaining the abusive sexual behavior. As a means of improving the status of the marital relationship, many wives are introduced to pleasure in sexual activity for the first time. Husband and wife are helped to feel more at ease with peers. Many wives begin to dress differently and give more attention to good grooming. Those who have resorted to adolescent, "acting out" behavior are taught to interact less self-destructively.

In family therapy the following areas are explored: (1) the nature of leadership and dis-

TABLE 43-4. THE MASTERS AND JOHNSON TREATMENT GOALS FOR CHILD SEXUAL ABUSE

GOALS OF THE CHILD SEXUAL ABUSE PROGRAM

1. Stop incest; prevent reoccurrence; minimize trauma to the victim; and alter the circumstances that promoted it in 3–4 months by focusing on relational dyad and triad (assuming only one victim).
2. Reunite the family as long as it's not harmful to the child.
3. Establish a profile of offenders' wives and victims; identify contributing factors; identify factors that are critical components for psychotherapeutic focus; and identify prognostic indicators for success and failure in meeting the above stated goals.

DEFINITION OF INCEST

1. Breast or genital contact between a child and parent with the intent of providing sexual excitement to the perpetrator.

CRITERIA OF PROGRAM ACCEPTANCE

1. Victim states that incest has occurred with a primary care giver.
2. There must be a relational dyad of perpetrator and female partner and both must be willing to participate.
3. No active psychosis in perpetrator or wife, and no chronic psychosis for victim.
4. The perpetrator has no record of using a weapon or of extreme violence.
5. If the perpetrator is alcoholic- or drug-dependent, he must complete an inpatient treatment program, plus remain in aftercare while attending the incest program. If the perpetrator has not been drug-dependent for 3 months prior to evaluation, he may not be required to participate in inpatient care. AA attendance may be required.
6. Individuals must be able and willing to complete all phases of the program. Termination with other therapists may be essential.
7. Victims over 18 are excluded from the program unless they have a younger sibling who has been victimized.
8. No mental retardation (IQ below 50) of victim or severe retardation of parents, as judged in evaluation.
9. Must be within catchment area for reimbursement or able to pay.

Based on Masters and Johnson Treatment Program for Child Sexual Abuse.

cipline; (2) pathological coalitions within the family triad (alignment and collusion for secrecy); (3) appropriate ways of being close; (4) ability to take responsibility for parenting; (5) appropriate roles for mother and daughter; (6) family problem solving; and (7) the use of therapists for preventive assistance.

Conclusions

The psychotherapy program for paraphiliacs and incest families has not had the necessary follow-up period to document its effectiveness statistically. Therefore, the concepts and principles described in this section are tentative. The initial therapy failure rate, however, has been low, and major alterations have been noted in behavior and in psychological testing profiles that have been maintained in follow-up.

Like the alcoholic, the paraphiliac offender can rarely be considered cured. Rehabilitation may be a chronic process, so long-term follow-up is required.

Mental health professionals need to encourage cooperative arrangements with the legal system to provide efficacious humane treatment of the paraphiliac. Research efforts are currently being focused on predicting which clients can and cannot benefit from brief intensive psychotherapy.

Conceptualizing incest as a pair-bonding disorder generates the components of the conjoint treatment program. There is little logic in offering extensive rehabilitation support for incest victims but not for incest offenders (the current situation in most cities). Thus, the focus on a family treatment model for symptom reversals in incestuous families and paraphilia is suggested. Intimate reciprocated pair-bonding and adult sexual functioning problems are emphasized.

Paraphilias Not Otherwise Specified

Examples of other paraphilias include the following: telephone scatologia (lewdness), necrophilia (corpses), partialism (exclusive focus on part of body), zoophilia (animals), coprophilia (feces), klismaphilia (enemas), urophilia (urine).

SEXUAL DYSFUNCTIONS

Inhibition in the sexual appetitive phase or in the psychophysiological changes that characterize the complete sexual response cycle is the essential feature of psychosexual dysfunctions. Four phases are defined in a complete sexual

TABLE 43-5. MASTERS AND JOHNSON CHILD SEXUAL ABUSE PROGRAM: EVALUATING TREATMENT SUCCESS

Criteria Desirable for Treatment Success	Source of Determination	Criteria Met
1. No reoffense occurs.	Self-report and agency contacts	_____
2. Father admits and discusses incest.	Group therapy	_____
3. Father assumes responsibility and apologizes to victim.	Family therapy	_____
4. Father verbalizes concern and empathy for victim.	Group and family therapy	_____
5. Father has minimal arousal to kids, maximal to adults.	Fantasy homework, reported relations with wife, self-report, and erection tests	_____
6. Father's rigidity and authoritarianism decrease.	Therapist, psychological tests (Budner & Rokeach tests), and sex-role measures (Bem, Spencer tests)	_____
7. Father and mother establish intimacy in and out of bedroom.	Couples therapist, self-report, and psychological tests (Locke-Wallace, Derogatis tests)	_____
8. Father and mother demonstrate increased parenting skills.	Role-playing, group exercises, family therapy, interactions with children, and self-report	_____
9. Father and mother establish communication skills.	Therapist's impressions, self-report, and written homework exercises	_____
10. Mother and father display signs of interdependence, (i.e., symbiosis; fusion and extreme dependency are less extreme).	Therapist and self-report of independent activities.	_____
11. Father and daughter establish an appropriate parent–child relationship without peerlike quarreling and inappropriate physical interaction.	Self-report and family observation	_____
12. Mother and father have clear understanding of adult cognitional patterns and how they differ from child and adolescent cognitions.	Group therapy and post testing	_____
13. Mother shows clinical signs of improved self-esteem.	Homework, self-report, therapist's observation, and psychological test scores	_____
14. Mother shows improved assertiveness skills.	Therapist's observation, role-plays, homework.	_____
15. Mother and daughter establish an appropriate parent–child relationship in which mother does not seek advice or nurturing from child. Not peerlike relationship.	Family therapy and self-report	_____
16. Mother verbalizes an understanding of the necessity and demonstrates willingness to protect the child.	Group and family therapy	_____
17. Mother believes daughter; does not blame daughter.	Group and family therapy	_____
18. Mother, father, and daughter demonstrate understanding of the dynamics within the family that contributed to the abuse and their roles in the family system.	Therapist and self-report	_____
19. Family secrecy is no longer active.	Family therapy	_____
20. Child understands the right of parents to form intimate attachment to one another and that such intimacy between adults does not preclude parents' closeness to children.	Group and family therapy, and self-report	_____

TABLE 43-5. (*continued*)

Criteria Desirable for Treatment Success	Source of Determination	Criteria Met
21. Family responsibilities are spelled out and negotiated. Child is given age-appropriate home duties.	Family therapy and follow-up self-report.	_____
22. Child does not experience psychological dysfunctions resulting from the sexual abuse.	Child psychiatrist's evaluation	_____
23. Child understands rights to protect her body.	Child and family therapy	_____
24. Child demonstrates ability to develop appropriate relationships with males.	Child and family therapy	_____
25. Child holds a legitimate and secure place in the triad.	Family therapy	_____
26. Child demonstrates ability to share concerns with mother and feels mother will protect her.	Child psychiatrist's report and family therapy	_____

response cycle: (1) *appetitive phase*, which consists of thoughts and desires to have sexual activity; (2) *excitement*, which consists of a subjective sense of sexual pleasure and accompanying physiological changes; (3) *orgasm*, which consists of the peaking of sexual pleasure with release of sexual tension and rhythmic contraction of perineal muscles and pelvic reproductive organs; and (4) *resolution*, which consists of a sense of general relaxation, well-being, and muscular relaxation.

Inhibitions in the response cycle may occur at one or more of these phases, especially at the first, second, or third phase. The specific sexual dysfunctions are described below:

Hypoactive Sexual Desire
This dysfunction involves a persistent and pervasive inhibition of sexual desire. This lack of desire is a source of distress to either the individual or his partner.

Sexual Aversion
This dysfunction is a persistent or recurrent extreme aversion to, and avoidance of, all or almost all, genital sexual contact with a sexual partner.

Female Sexual Arousal Disorder
This dysfunction includes either persistent or recurrent partial or complete failure to attain or maintain the lubrication-swelling response of sexual excitement until completion of the sexual activity or persistent or recurrent lack of a subjective sense of sexual excitement and pleasure in a female during sexual activity.

Male Erectile Disorder
This dysfunction includes either persistent or recurrent partial or complete failure in a male to attain or maintain erection until completion of the sexual activity, or persistent or recurrent lack of a subjective sense of sexual excitement and pleasure in a male during sexual activity.

Sexual Disorders Not Otherwise Specified
Sexual disorders that are not classifiable in any of the previous categories are included in this classification. In rare instances, this category may be used concurrently with one of the specific diagnoses when both are necessary to explain or describe the clinical disturbance.

Examples of this disorder include the following:

1. Marked feelings of inadequacy concerning body habitus, size and shape of sex organs, sexual performance, or other traits related to self-imposed standards of masculinity or femininity
2. Distress about a pattern of repeated sexual conquests or other forms of nonparaphilic sexual addiction, involving a succession of people who exist only as things to be used
3. Persistent and marked distress about one's sexual orientation

Sexual Dysfunctions and Nursing Diagnoses

Sexual dysfunction is a disruption or extreme variation of sexual behavior.* Sexual dysfunc-

---

* The section on "Sexual Dysfunctions and Nursing Diagnoses" (pp. 864–869) is written by Carol R. Hartman.

tion as a *disruption* is defined by an identifiable disturbance of one or more phases of the sexual response cycle (orgasm phase disorders, excitement phase disorders, or desire phase disorders), by excessive pain, or by phobic avoidance of sex (both simple and panic). Sexual dysfunction as an *extreme variation* of sexual behavior is defined by the object (human or inanimate) that is required for sexual arousal and release or by disregard for the rights of, damage to, pain, fear, and sensitivities of another person.

Sexual Dysfunctions: Biophysiological Etiology

Ill health is one of the greatest detriments to sexual expression, not only because it prioritizes energy use toward recuperation, but it often lowers an individual's sense of personal worth and attractiveness. Many conditions directly impede sexual response by interfering with endocrine levels, blood circulation, nerve transmission, and mobility, or by creating genital or generalized pain. Various surgical procedures and drugs may also affect the body. Sexual dysfunction may be a temporary concomitant of an illness or treatment, or it may be permanent. In either case, patients must be appropriately counseled so that they will know what to expect and what behavioral options they might consider.

Examples of Biophysiological Conditions Leading to Sexual Dysfunction.

DIABETES. Millions of individuals are affected by diabetes mellitus, a condition that causes gradual impotence in almost 50 percent of males and orgasmic dysfunction in 35 percent of females. Diabetically caused sexual dysfunction is often irreversible and requires sensitive couples counseling.[96]

ALCOHOLISM. Alcoholism results in impotence in 40 percent of males, decreased libido in 30 to 40 percent, and retarded ejaculation in 5 to 10 percent. In females, 30 to 40 percent experience difficulties in sexual arousal, and 15 percent experience loss or reduction of orgasmic frequency.[97]

RENAL FAILURE. Clients with chronic renal failure who receive hemodialysis have a high degree of sexual dysfunction. In males, 90 percent experience depressed libido and 80 percent erective difficulties; in females, 80 percent experience decreased libido, 70 percent difficulty in sexual arousal, and 50 percent reduced orgasmic response. Hemodialysis usually does not improve sexual function, although some improvement may be seen postimplantation. It is important to note that males with chronic renal failure have a suicide rate 200 times that of the general population.[98]

CARDIOVASCULAR DISEASE. When pain or weakness accompany cardiovascular disease, sexual expression may be inhibited. Following a heart attack, however, many clients self-restrict their sexual activity because of unnecessary fear or ignorance. Studies have shown that sexual activity may be resumed when the individual can tolerate climbing two flights of stairs without pain or can walk briskly around the block.[99] Four to 5 weeks are usually enough time to abstain from sexual activity.

Kaplan provides an excellent summary of conditions that affect sexual functioning in males and females.[100]

DRUGS. Numerous drugs, although effective in treating illness, create sexual side effects: for example, decreased libido and erectile, ejaculatory, and orgasmic dysfunction. Antihypertensive drugs also frequently affect sexual performance by interfering with nerve transmission. One example, Guanethidine, has been shown to cause impotence in 13.6 percent of males, with decreased libido in 59 percent, and retarded ejaculation in 63.6 percent.

Of the psychotropic drugs that affect sexual capacity, monoamine oxidase inhibitors cause impotence in up to 75 percent of males. Tranquilizers may create fatigue rather than decreased libido. Drug abuse with heroin and methadone results in 80 to 90 percent decreased libido, and barbiturate abuse results in impotence in 60 percent of males, sexual response difficulty in 60 percent of females. Thus, it is important to counsel clients on the possible effects of drug therapy on sexual functioning. Noncompliance, particularly with hypertension treatment, often results when clients realize their impotence is drug-induced. Patients should be aware of the ability to reverse the condition through a change of drug or dosage.[101]

Sexual Dysfunctions: Intrapsychic Etiology

Sexual dysfunctions may have immediate and specific or remote psychological causes. They reflect intrapsychic conflict creating anxiety and blockage of erotic feeling toward lovemaking.

A variety of fears play a role in sexual dysfunction[102]:

- Fear of failure or performance anxiety
- Fear of displeasing one's partner or being displeased
- Fear of being abandoned or rejected
- Fear of loss of control

A traumatic sexual experience, e.g., a hurried attempt at coitus in the backseat of a car, may create premature ejaculation. Rape may be the cause of sexual aversion and vaginismus.[103]

Cultural or religious taboos, where sex is seen as sinful and dirty, can negatively condition an individual toward nonresponsiveness.

In addition, under conditions of severe stress or depression, sexual energy may be decreased. Low self-esteem may cause sexual dysfunction by preventing the ability "to accept pleasure from another, to be aware of one's individuality, and to be able to seek the boundaries of one's sexual preference."[104] Mutilative surgery, disfigurement, or handicap may create poor body image. "When the body is considered unattractive, anxiety and increased muscle tension are the likely response to admiration from a sexual partner."[105]

Sexual Dysfunctions: Interpersonal Etiology

The interpersonal component of the relationship between sexual partners very often affects, to some degree, the quality of their sexual interaction.[106] Hostility can lead to deliberately withholding pleasure through sexual sabotage: creating tension before lovemaking, suggesting sex at an inopportune time, making oneself deliberately unattractive, or producing deliberate frustrations. On the other hand, lack of knowledge about sexual anatomy and poor communication about preferences may create years of sexual tension in even the most stable, loving relationships.[107]

Nursing Diagnosis and Care

When a behavioral matrix such as sexual functioning becomes the focus of an acute health problem, objective evidence as well as the subjective data is essential. The more closely that the objective evidence coincides with a definitive etiology, the more apt the intervention is to

be specific. Sexual dysfunction as a diagnosis provides a broad spectrum of general data with various possible etiologic factors. Collaboration with other professionals as well as the specialized expertise of the nurse will be required for both the nursing diagnosis and the particular intervention modes. Nursing diagnosis and care of sexual dysfunction will be discussed under the three subnursing subdiagnoses below.

Sexual Dysfunction Related to Anxiety Specific to Performance, Secondary, With no Disruption of Sexual Response Patterns and no Extreme Variation of Sexual Behavior. When the sexual dysfunction is organic, nursing care focuses on the educative aspects of the patient and on counseling around misconceptions regarding the dysfunction process, its treatment, and the patient's response. Since sexual functioning most often involves a partner, nursing intervention will also be directed toward the appropriate partner.

EXAMPLE

A husband is recovering from a mild heart attack. The husband and wife are hesitant to resume their sexual relationship for fear the husband will have another heart attack. Sexual desire is present as well as sexual arousal and orgasmic experiences. For these people, a causal connection has been made between the energy expended in the sexual act and a heart attack. Information and experience in monitoring exertion with concomitant signs such as pulse rate and chest pain become important for the husband. This is usually done through gradual increments in physical activity. Involvement of the wife provides experience for her as well as an opportunity for both of them to open up communication between themselves. Unrealistic expectations can be revealed and countered. In addition, the couple can become comfortable in exploring relaxing, pleasurable and less strenuous methods for enjoying their sexual relationship.

Steps in nursing care are as follows:

- Assess and establish existence of intact sexual response patterns and no extreme variation of sexual behavior.
- Establish clear definition of primary organic problem (i.e., heart attack).
- Establish information relevant to the influence of the organic problem on sexual behavior.
- Clarify the patient's and the significant oth-

er's key perceptions regarding the relationship of the organic problem to sexual functioning.

- Provide experiences necessary to enhance functioning, e.g., information, counseling, focused exercises.
- Evaluate effectiveness of intervention.

When the etiologic factor of the sexual dysfunction is psychological, education and counseling are the primary interventions. This is particularly true when the problems are minor in nature. Severity of the primary psychological and relationship problems is determined in part by assessment of the psychological makeup of the person or couple and of the critical interactional components of the relationship.

If the dysfunction is simple and minor, nursing care is as follows:

- Explain causal connection between attitudinal set and behavior and its relationship to sexual concern.
- Gain cooperation and agreement to work toward change. Clarify that change is compatible, comfortable, and acceptable to patient and partner.
- Evaluate outcome. If unsatisfactory, reassess, and if necessary refer for further evaluation or more specific psychiatric treatment of psychological or relationship problem.

Removing a sexual complaint can escalate anxiety by exposing other human demands of relating such as commitment and intimacy. Problems in these personal areas of human existence are often masked through various symptoms of dysfunction. The symptoms may be used as defenses by the individual. At times in complex relationship problems, the partner with the complaint may in fact be a foil for the more severe psychological problems of the nonsymptomatic partner. When the symptom is removed, there is an imbalance in the relationship, and the partner's underlying psychological difficulties come to the forefront.

Sexual Dysfunction Related to Disruption of Orgasm Phase, Desire Phase, Pain, or Phobic Avoidance of Sex.

ORGASM PHASE. The orgasm phase is quite susceptible to primary organic problems. This is true for both males and females. The effectiveness of nursing care is dependent on proper medical intervention and on an understanding of the impact of the medical problem and treatment regimen. Since many of the medical issues are irreversible or are necessary for the total functioning of the individual, nursing care will focus on the rehabilitative measures. If the medical problem is treatable, the nursing care is aimed at quelling the anxiety of the individual regarding sexual functioning during the treatment period as well as working with the partner. Education and counseling in conjunction with the medical regimen constitute primary nursing intervention.

Some medical interventions greatly alter bodily structure as well as impinge on the physiology of orgasm. Therefore special attention has to be paid to the process of the client gaining acceptance of the body image changes and resuming pleasure in sensuous, erotic, and interpersonal comforting experiences. Partners need support and counseling during this period.

When the etiologic conditions are the result of immediate psychological causes or of out-of-awareness cognitive patterns (such as images or internal dialogue), expectations play a large role in interfering with the sexual response pattern. Anorgasm or inhibited orgasm in the woman has of recent years been debated as to its etiology or, for that matter, as to whether orgasm is a necessary condition of female sexuality. The purpose of the nursing care proposed here is not to enter this disputed issue, but rather to present, from clinical experience, some etiologic factors that, when taken into consideration, alter the sexual response patterns in some women. In addition, it is known that certain dysfunctional response patterns, present or past, can contribute to a lack of perception of erotic sensations. This can be the result of both habit and distraction; both play an important role in the dysfunctional patterns in orgasm phase.

DESIRE PHASE. Desire phase disorders may have organic causes. One organic reason is that there is an established alteration in neural hormones that specifically mediate sexual desire. The length of time that there has been no sexual desire becomes important in planning care. If the problem is chronic in a physically healthy, functioning individual, without signs of severe mental illness, complex dynamic intrapsychic issues are usually considered. These require long-term psychotherapy with possible combined sex therapy. Nursing care would most often involve referral.

When the desire phase problem is short-term and is related to factors such as stress and depression, nursing care focuses on the reduction of stressors contributing to the mood state, making clear the causal link with low or absent sexual desire. If there is a pattern of avoidance of sexually stimulating experiences, this should be explored with the patient. This is particularly true in someone who has lost a spouse and is confused as to the meaning of sexual desire and the loss of the spouse.

PAIN. Pain associated with sex is more often than not based on organic causes. Nursing intervention is primarily directed toward making sure the patient is thoroughly evaluated for underlying organic causes.

PHOBIC AVOIDANCE OF SEX. Avoidance of sex and sexual arousal must be evaluated carefully for underlying panic disorder. In recent years, panic disorders have been hypothesized as being related to an underlying propensity to overreact physiologically to intense feeling states. Some people speculate there is a genetic precursor. At any rate, experiments with drugs have demonstrated a reduction in the panic response. When the response is down and psychotherapy and sex therapy are combined, there have been favorable results. However, severe neurotic and borderline states can underline the panic.

Simple phobic responses are usually amenable to psychotherapy or to behavior therapy combined with instruction. When panic or phobic avoidance is evident, referral is the appropriate nursing intervention.

Nursing Interventions. Nursing interventions often involve the cognitive technique of thought stopping and reeducation. These are best accomplished with the patient and the patient's partner. Special knowledge, techniques, and counseling skills are necessary for identifying and changing dysfunctional patterns. Some clinical specialists in psychiatric nursing do this type of sex therapy, as do nurse clinical specialists in the area of dysfunctional disease or neurological diseases. Sex therapy provokes anxiety and requires motivation to carry through. People with problematic psychological functioning and precarious relationships may not withstand the therapy and can decompensate under its stress. On the other hand, a patient with a known psychiatric problem who has

had periods of undisputed sexual functioning can be assisted with an approach that focuses directly on sexual functioning. In these situations, the dysfunction is not a defense against the underlying psychological problem.

Traumatic events may precipitate a psychological cause for a dysfunction. Of particular importance is understanding whether the patient has been the object of rape, incest, or a brutalizing abusive situation. Counseling on this issue of unresolved sexual trauma would be the primary intervention. Focused sex therapy may be required in conjunction with the resolution of the past event.

When counseling is addressed to underlying psychological or relationship issues, it must be remembered that pain can be a defense against pleasure and until acceptance of pleasure has been established, removing the pain may provide intense anxiety and can cause withdrawal from counseling.

In general, nursing care for the first two subdiagnoses of sexual dysfunction can be summarized as follows:

- Determine if disorder has an organic or psychogenic cause.
- If there is doubt, refer for more specialized evaluation.
- If organic and psychogenic causes are established, as well as their primary and secondary relationships, one of the following nursing interventions most appropriate to the causes and the level of sexual dysfunction should be used: education, general counseling on personal and relationship issues, and focused exercises to alter cognitive sets or physical behavior that impedes sexual and erotic behaviors. Include the partner.

Sexual Dysfunction as an Extreme Variation or Deviation of Sexual Behavior, Where There is Little or no Regard for the Welfare of Another Person. The pedophile is an example of this sort of dysfunction.

Intervention with this disorder requires efforts of a specialist. Because of the degree of deviance and often the pain and exploitation of others, there are only spotty efforts in developing consistent exploration into the management and cessation of the behaviors involved. The behavior is very compulsive and repetitive.

Nurses are in contact with these people in many settings—the prison, the home, and areas of the health care system. In addition, nurses are often involved in either providing or referring services to the *victims* of people who fall under this category of sexual dysfunction.

Where infants, children, and adolescents are the sexual object or where violence is engaged in with or without an age-appropriate partner, endocrine and genetic hypotheses have been set forth. With the pedophile, experiments are underway using hormonal therapy in conjunction with behavioral and psychotherapeutic efforts. This treatment group is a small and highly selected population. For the most part pedophiliacs are released and reside in the gen-

eral community without much being offered either for their treatment or for the treatment of their victims.

For the nurse in the community who does have contact with paraphiliacs, the following nursing care is suggested. First, attempt to get some supervision from an interested mental health professional. Second, establish a contract with the individual to work toward stopping the deviant behavior, make clear that sexual activity injurious to another person must be reported to the authorities, establish protection for potential victims (that is, children of incest offenders), and establish methods of stopping the behavior.

Summary

This chapter has described the wide area of human sexuality with which the nurse must be familiar in order to understand the client's sexual health. Information relevant to carrying out the nursing process was presented. The psychiatric diagnoses of the *DSM-III-R* were presented and focused on the essential features of the disorders. Nursing diagnoses of sexual dysfunctions included disturbances of the sexual response cycle and deviations of sexual behavior. Sexual deviation was discussed in terms of sexual practices dangerous to one's self, as in autoerotic death. The treatment model used at the Masters and Johnson Institute to treat paraphiliacs and incest families was described.

Questions

1. Why is it important to understand human sexuality in order to provide client care?
2. What types of questions are nurses asked about sex?
3. A patient starts rubbing your leg when you are giving him a bed bath. How would you respond to his behavior, and how would you understand his behavior?
4. Argue the pros and cons of prison versus hospital settings for pedophiles and incest offenders.

REFERENCES AND SUGGESTED READINGS

1. Katchadourian, H. A., & Lunde, D. T. *Fundamentals of Human Sexuality*, 2nd ed. New York: Holt, Rinehart & Winston, 1975, pp. 1–18.
2. Robinault, I. P. *Sex, Society, and the Disabled: A Developmental Inquiry into Roles, Reactions, and Responsibilities.* New York: Harper & Row, 1978, p. 11.
3. McCary, J. L., & McCary, S. P. (1982) *McCary's Human Sexuality*, 4th ed. Belmont, Calif: Wadsworth.
4. Wachtel, S. S. H-Y Antigen and sexual development. In H. Vallet & I. Porter (Eds.), *Genetic Mechanisms of Sexual Development*, pp. 271–277. New York: Academic Press, 1979.
5. Haseltine, F., & Ohno, S. Mechanisms of gonadal differentiation. *Science*, 1981, 211(4488), 1272–1278.
6. McCary & McCary, 1982.

7. Masters, W. H., Johnson, V. E., & Kolodny, R. C. *Human Sexuality*, 2nd ed. Little, Brown and Company: Boston, 1985.

8. Imperato-McGinley, J., & Peterson, R. Male pseudohermaphroditism: The complexities of male phenotypic development. *American Journal of Medicine*, 1976, *61*, 251–272.

9. Money, J., & Ehrhardt, A. E. *Man & Woman, Boy & Girl*. Baltimore: Johns Hopkins University Press, 1972.

10. Money & Ehrhardt, 1972.

11. Kolodny, R. C., Masters, W. H., & Johnson, V. E. *Textbook of Sexual Medicine*. Boston: Little, Brown, 1979.

12. Masters, Johnson, & Kolodny, 1985.

13. Yalom, I. D., Green, R., & Fisk, N. Prenatal exposure to female hormones. *Archives of General Psychiatry*, 1973, *28*, 554–561.

14. Zussman, J. U., Zussman, P. P., & Dalton, K. K. Abstract, Third Annual Meeting of the International Academy of Sex Research. Bloomington, Ind., 1977.

15. Zussman, J. U., Zussman, P. P., & Dalton, K. K. Post-pubertal effect of prenatal administration of progesterone. Paper presented at the Society for Research in Child Development. Denver, April 1975.

16. Masters, Johnson, & Kolodny, 1985.

17. Money & Ehrhardt, 1972.

18. Money, J. Ablatio penis: Normal male infant sex-reassigned as a girl. *Archives of Sexual Behavior*, 1975, *4*, 65–72.

19. Money, 1975.

20. Diamond, M. Sexual identity, monozygotic twins reared in discordant sex roles and a BBC follow-up. *Archives of Sexual Behavior*, 1982, *11*, 181–186.

21. Imperato-McGinley, J., et al. Androgens and the evolution of male-gender identity among male pseudohermaphrodites with 5 α-reductase deficiency. *New England Journal of Medicine*, 1979, *300*(22), 1233–1237.

22. Masters, Johnson, & Kolodny, 1985.

23. Skolnick, A. 1986. Early attachment and personal relations across the life course. In D. Featherman & R. Lerner (Eds.), *Life Span Development and Behavior*, vol. 7, Hillsdale, N.J.: Erlbaum, 1986.

24. Kagen, J. Psychology of sex differences. In F. Beach, (Ed.). *Human Sexuality in Four Perspectives*, pp. 87–114. Baltimore: Johns Hopkins University Press, 1976.

25. Petersen, A. Biopsychosocial processes in the development of sex-related differences. In Parsons, J. E. (Ed.), *The Psychobiology of Sex Differences and Sex Roles*, pp. 31–55. New York: Hemisphere Publishing Corp., 1980.

26. Kaplan, A., & Sedney, M. A. *Psychology and Sex Roles: An Androgynous Perspective*. Boston: Little, Brown, 1980.

27. Johnson, Masters, & Kolodny, 1985.

28. Luria, Z., Friedman, S., & Rose, M. D. (1987). *Human Sexuality*. New York: Wiley.

29. Higham, E. Sexuality in the infant and neonate: birth to two years. In Wolman, B. B., & Money, J. (Eds.), *Handbook of Human Sexuality*, pp. 16–27. Englewood Cliffs, N.J.: Prentice-Hall, 1980.

30. Kaplan, H. S. *The New Sex Therapy*. New York: Brunner/Mazel, 1974.

31. Bakwin, H. Erotic feelings in infants and young children. *Medical Aspects of Human Sexuality*, 1974, *8*(10), 200–215.

32. Stall, C. S. *Female and Male: Socialization, Social Roles, and Social Structure*. Dubuque, Iowa: Wm. C. Brown, 1974, p. 161.

33. Ibid., p. 182.

34. Kinsey, A. C., Pomeroy, W. B., Martin, C. E., & Gebhard, P. H. *Sexual Behavior in the Human Male*. Philadelphia: Saunders, 1948.

35. Lyness, J. J., Lipetz, M. E., & Davis, K. E. Living together: An alternative to marriage. *Journal of Marriage and the Family*, 1972, *34*, 305–311.

36. McCary, J. L. *Human Sexuality*, 2nd ed. New York: Van Nostrand Reinhold, 1973, p. 322.

37. Harper, R. A. Extramarital sex relations. In A. Ellis & A. Abarbanal (Eds.), *The Encyclopedia of Sexual Behavior* (Vol. 1). New York: Hawthorn, 1961.

38. Ellis, A. Healthy and disturbed reasons for having extramarital relations. In G. Neubeck (Ed.), *Extramarital Relations*. Englewood Cliffs, N.J.: Prentice-Hall, 1969.

39. DeLora, J. S., & Warren, C. A. B. *Understanding Sexual Interaction*. Boston: Hougton Mifflin, 1977, p. 253.

40. Bell, R. R. "Swinging," the sexual exchange of marriage partners. *Sexual Behavior*, 1971, May, 70.

41. McCary, op. cit., p. 393.

42. Ibid., p. 402.

43. DeLora & Warren, op. cit., pp. 223–227.

44. Freedman, M. *Homosexuality and Psychological Functioning*. Belmont, Calif.: Brooks/Cole, 1971, p. 1.

45. Kameny, F. E. Gay liberation and psychiatry. In H. M. Ruitenbeck (Ed.), *Homosexuality: A Changing Picture*. London: Souvenir Press, 1973, pp. 70–82.

46. Ibid., pp. 81–82.

47. Coleman, E. Toward a new model of treatment for homosexuality: A review. *Journal of Homosexuality*, 1978, *3*, 355.

48. Silverstein, C. Even psychiatry can profit from its past mistakes. *Journal of Homosexuality*, 1976–77, *2*, 157.

49. Freedman, op. cit., p. 87.

50. Ibid., p. 26.

51. Winick, C., & Kinsie, P. M. *The Lively Commerce*. Chicago: Quadrangle, 1971, p. 49.

52. Ibid.

53. Benjamin, H., & Masters, R. E. L. *Prostitution and Morality*. New York: Julian Press, 1964.
54. Erikson, E. H. *Childhood and Society*, 2nd ed. New York: Norton, 1963, p. 265.
55. DeLora & Warren, op. cit., pp. 299–305.
56. Ibid.
57. Masters, W. H., & Johnson, V. E. *Human Sexual Response*. Boston: Little, Brown, 1966.
58. Freedman, op. cit., p. 18.
59. Ibid., pp. 18–26.
60. Ibid.
61. Stewart, T. D., & Gerson, S. N. Penile prosthesis: Psychological factors. *Urology*, 1976, 7, 400–402.
62. DeLora & Warren, op. cit., pp. 332–333.
63. McCary, op. cit., p. 379.
64. Dworkin, A., & McKinnon, C. Antipornography laws proposed as amendment to Minneapolis, Minn., Code of Ordinances, civil rights title 7, chapters 139, 141. Hearing, December 12–13, 1984.
65. U.S. Presidential Commission on Obscenity and Pornography. *Report of the Commission on Obscenity and Pornography*. Washington, D.C.: U.S. Government Printing Office, 1970.
66. U.S. Attorney General's Commission on Pornography. *Final Report*. Washington, D.C.: U.S. Government Printing Office, 1986.
67. Dines-Levy, G. An analysis of pornography research. In A. W. Burgess (Ed.), *Rape and Sexual Assault* (Vol. 2). New York: Garland, 1988, pp. 317–323.
68. Abel, G., Barlow, D. H., Blanchard, E. B., & Guild, D. The components of rapists' sexual arousal. *Archives of General Psychiatry*, 1977, 34, 895–903.
69. U.S. Attorney General's Commission on Pornography, op. cit., p. 1005.
70. American Psychiatric Association. *Diagnostic and Statistical Manual*, 3rd ed. (Rev.). Washington, D.C.: American Psychiatric Association, 1987.
71. Litman, R., & Swearingen, C. Bondage and suicide. *Archives of General Psychiatry*, 1972, 27, 80–85.
72. Hazelwood, R. R., Dietz, P. E., & Burgess, A. W. *Autoerotic Fatalities*. Lexington, Mass.: Lexington, 1983.
73. Milner, R. Orgasm of death. *Hustler*, August 1981, pp. 33–34.
74. Hazelwood, Dietz, & Burgess, op. cit.
75. Hazelwood, R. R., Dietz, P. E., & Burgess, A. W. The investigation of autoerotic fatalities. *Journal of Police Science and Administration*, 1981, 9, 404, 411.
76. Hazelwood, R. R., Burgess, A. W., & Groth, A. N. Death during dangerous autoerotic practice. *Social Science and Medicine*, 1981, 15E, 129–133.
77. Hazelwood, Dietz, & Burgess, op. cit. (1983).
78. Ford, R. Death by hanging of adolescent and young adolescent males. *Journal of Forensic Science*, 1957, 2, 171–176.
79. Resnik, H. Eroticized repetitive hangings: A form of self-destructive behavior. *American Journal of Psychotherapy*, 1972, 26, 4–21.
80. Rosenblum, S., & Faber, M. The adolescent sexual asphyxia syndrome. *American Academy of Child Psychiatry*, 1979, 17, 546–558.
81. Hazelwood, Dietz, & Burgess, op. cit. (1983).
82. Lams, D., & O'Neill, J. Variations on masturbatory conditioning. *Behavioral Psychotherapy*, 1981, 91–98.
83. Ingerbritson, M. *Incest and Alcoholism: Dual Addictions*. Lecture given at the Masters & Johnson Institute in St. Louis, Mo., January, 1983.
84. Ibid.
85. Money, J. Use of androgen-depleting hormones in the treatment of male sex-offenders. *Journal of Sex Research*, 1970, 6, 165–172.
86. Abel, G., & Blanchard, E. The role of fantasy in the treatment of sexual deviation. *Archives of General Psychiatry*, 1974, 30, 467–475.
87. Bellach, A., & Herson, M. *Research and Practice in Social Skills Training*. New York: Plenum, 1979.
88. Bandura, A. The self-system in reciprocal determinism. *American Psychologist*, 1978, 33, 344–358.
89. Zimbardo, P. *Shyness, What It Is and What to Do About It*. Reading, Mass.: Addison-Wesley, 1977.
90. Eiseer, R., Fredericksen, L., & Peterson, G. The relationship of cognitive variables to the expression of assertiveness. *Behavior Therapy*, 1978, 9, 419–427.
91. Zilbergeld, B. *Male Sexuality*. New York: Bantam, 1978.
92. Merluzzi, T., Glass, C., & Genest, M. (Eds.). *Cognitive Assessment*. New York: Guilford, 1981.
93. Lange, A., & Jakubowski, P. *Responsible Assertive Behavior*. Champaign, Ill.: Research Press.
94. Yochelson, S., & Samenow, S. *The Criminal Personality*. New York: Bantam, 1977.
95. Masters, W., & Johnson, V. *Human Sexual Inadequacy*. Boston: Little, Brown, 1970.
96. Kolodny, R. C. Chronic illness and sex. Paper presented at *Seminar on Human Sexuality*, American Assoc. for Sex Educators, Clinicians & Therapists, Boston, November 7–8, 1978, pp. 1–3.
97. Ibid., pp. 3–5.
98. Ibid., pp. 5–6.
99. Steffl, B. M. Sexuality and aging: Implications for nurses and other helping professionals. In R. L. Solnick (Ed.), *Sexuality and Aging* (Rev. ed.). Los Angeles: University of Southern California, Ethel Percy Andrus Gerontology Center, 1978, p. 139.
100. Kaplan, H. W. *The New Sex Therapy*. New York: Brunner/Mazel, 1974, pp. 80–85.
101. Kolodny, R. C. Drugs and sex. Paper presented at *Seminar on Human Sexuality*, Am. Assoc. Sex

Educators, Clinicians & Therapists, Boston, November 7–8, 1978, pp. 1–4.

102. DeLora & Warren, op. cit., p. 460.

103. Johnson, V. E. Sexual aversion. Paper presented at *Seminar on Human Sexuality*, AASECT, Boston, November 7–8, 1978, p. 1.

104. Burchell, R. C. Self-esteem and sexuality. *Medical Aspects of Human Sexuality*, 1975, (January), 81.

105. Ibid.

106. DeLora & Warren, p. 463.

107. Ibid.

Chapter 44

Stress Response and Physical Illness

Nancy R. Starefos and Marita Prater

Chapter Objectives

The students successfully attaining the goals of this chapter will be able to:

- Define stress, stressors, and adaptation as these terms relate to human responses.
- Identify biopsychosocial components affecting individual perceptions of stress.
- Identify common effects of stress on physiological, psychological, cognitive, and perceptual systems.
- Chart the four levels of anxiety (stress response) as based on the work of Hildegard Peplau.
- Develop a plan of care for a client with a psychophysiological disorder using the assessment model.
- Discuss ways to assist the client in developing awareness of his physical illness and his role in successful adaptation.
- Identify areas of nursing research for assessment, intervention, and prevention of maladaptive stress responses.

The stress response and its possible effect on health status have assumed increasing importance in nursing and in the community at large in recent years. As research on the subject has proliferated and new understandings have been disseminated, the public has become more aware of the potential effects of stress on their lives.

Nurses in particular have taken notice of the stress response. (The number of articles on oc-cupational stress in nursing are an indication of this phenomenon.)

There is no doubt that nurses should be concerned with the stress response. All nurses are aware of the effects of stress on themselves and their patients, no matter what their age or physical or emotional condition. Even the American Nurses' Association (ANA) definition of nursing implies that nurses deal with the human stress response; "Nursing is the diagnosis and treatment of human responses to actual or potential health problems; . . . assisting sick and well people, individually and in groups, in the promotion, maintenance, and restoration of health."[1]

Nursing sees humans as biopsychosocial beings who must be viewed in totality as they interact with their environment. As such, human responses must be viewed in terms of their precipitating factors, human perceptions of themselves and the events occurring within and around them, as well as their perceptions of any consequences. Stress responses are as complex as they are common. Many factors must be considered in providing care and support to others. The development of an understanding of these considerations in the stress response will be reviewed in the following section.

THEORETICAL BACKGROUND

The interrelationship between the mind and the body has always fascinated clinicians; it has been an area of investigation by health professions for centuries. The Greeks and Romans observed that the mind (psyche) could influence dysfunction and disease in the body (soma), but the discipline we know today as psychophysiological disorders began only about 55 years ago in the Western world. Currently, there is renewed interest in understanding the role of psychophysiological factors in physical and emotional illness.

The original of the term psychosomatic was replaced in the nomenclature in 1952 by the term psychophysiological autonomic and visceral disorders. In 1987, the DSM-III-R introduced the classification of Psychological Factors Affecting Physical Condition. This classification permits acknowledgment that psychophysiological factors contribute to the initiation or exacerbation of a physical condition. Although the physical condition most often will be due to a physical disorder, there may be instances where there is only a single symptom such as vomiting. This classification is used for physical conditions where psychological factors are believed to be contributory.

Examples of physical conditions for which this classification is most appropriate, but are not limited to, include: tension headache, migraine headache, painful menstruation, obesity, angina pectoris, neurodermatitis, acne, rheumatoid arthritis, asthma, tachycardia, ulcerative colitis, urinary frequency, nausea and vomiting, regional enteritis, arrhythmia, duodenal ulcer, cardiospasm, and pylorospasm. These conditions have, in the past, been referred to as either psychosomatic or psychophysiological.

The psychiatric diagnostic criteria for this classification of Psychological Factors Affecting Physical Condition include the following[2]:

1. Psychologically meaningful environmental stimuli are temporarily related to the initiation or exacerbation of a physical condition that is recorded on axis III of the DSM-III.
2. The physical condition involves either demonstrable organic pathology (e.g., angina pectoris) or a known pathophysiological process (e.g., nausea, vomiting).
3. The condition is not due to a somatoform disorder.

A brief historical review of psychophysiological research indicates three phases, as listed below.

1. Before 1920, the emphasis in Western psychosomatic medicine was philosophical. Generalizations about mind–body inter-relationships were highly speculative.
2. Between 1920 and 1955, two directions of study developed: the psychophysiological and the psychodynamic. Psychiatrist Franz Alexander formulated many psychodynamic assumptions central to psychosomatic medicine and was the pioneer leader in this second approach.[3]
3. The third phase of investigation beginning after 1955 is characterized by stronger research methodology and more emphasis on the study of psychophysiological responses to environmental stimuli.

In the nineteenth century, the diagnostic category "functional nervous disorder" was used to describe what are known today as psychophysiological or psychosomatic disorders. Functional disorders were believed to occur in the absence of physical causes. The prevalent mechanistic view of medicine and physiology could not accommodate these conditions, so they came to be considered beyond scientific explanation.

The term psychosomatic is believed to have been coined by J. C. A. Heinroth in 1818 when he discussed insomnia.[4] Earlier roots of philosophical psychiatry dealing with mind–body issues can be traced to 1775 when French physician Franz Anton Mesmer stated that verbal suggestion could produce physiological changes through the use of magnets and the "animal magnetism" in his own person. The work of the French neurologist Jean Martin Charcot in the 1880s greatly advanced the technique of hypnotism as an accepted technique. Charcot's treatment of hysterical patients demonstrated the role of psychological factors in the origin of physical symptoms such as hysterical seizures and subsequently influenced Sigmund Freud and his work.

In 1905, Freud's formulation of the "unconscious" contributed to explaining the psychosomatic phenomenon. In his papers on the psychodynamics of anxiety and conversion hysteria, Freud related the "conversion symptom" to regressions or fixations at earlier levels of emotional development.[5] He described the symptom as a physically expressed compromise between a forbidden impulse and the defense against it. For example, the wish to kick someone would be repressed and the drive to discharge would be converted into the symptom of a paralyzed leg. The symptoms, therefore, would have a symbolic connection to the wish.

Psychosomatic illness became established as a category of pathology largely through the influence of Freudian theory. Freud recognized, however, that psychogenesis could not explain such conditions fully.[6] Paralleling Freud's psychological theories to explain physiological disturbances came the neurophysiological research of Russian physiologist Ivan P. Pavlov, as well as the work of American physiologist Walter B. Cannon and Canadian physician Hans Selye. Cannon's work provided the basic conceptual model for psychosomatic medicine. He emphasized that bodily changes caused by emotional responses to stress prepare the individual defensively for the struggle for survival. Cannon also described *homeostasis,* a mechanism by which the individual mobilizes himself to maintain a dynamic equilibrium, despite environmental stress, by means of feedback devices.[7,8]

Hans Selye further clarified the body's organized reaction to stress, which he called the *general adaptation syndrome.* He found that all types of demands on the individual produce the same biologic response. According to Selye, stress is the nonspecific response of the body to any demand made upon it.[9] Whether the stressor (demand) is physical, such as a change in room temperature, trauma, or infection, or psychological, such as the loss of a loved one, the individual is forced to adapt to the situation. Stressors may include socioeconomic, environmental, and cultural influences. Each stressor to which the individual is exposed requires him to respond and to try to return to a state of equilibrium. Stressors may be perceived as positive or negative, but in either case a person must make an adaptive response.

A stressful situation, according to Selye, occurs in three stages. The first stage is the initial reaction and period of adjustment, which he terms the "alarm reaction." In the second stage, the individual uses his resources to the fullest in the "stage of resistance." If the stressor subsides, the person returns to a state of equilibrium. If the stressor continues over a prolonged period or is of such severity that the individual's resources become exhausted, he enters a third stage, the "stage of exhaustion." The individual can no longer continue to adapt and develops a pathological state that, if unresolved, leads to death.[10]

Rene Dubos, in his theory of adaptation, also stated that man has limits to his adaptability.[11] Repeated stimulation of the adaptive response may be seriously damaging, eventually leading to irreversible wear and tear. Competitive situations, crowded environments, and continual changes affect people both psychologically and physically.

CONCEPTUAL FRAMEWORK

Stress and Illness

It has long been known that stress plays a major role in illness. Scientists are now approaching a clearer understanding of the mechanisms involved, which is a hopeful sign for the future. The links between the brain and the body involve the autonomic nervous system, the neuroendocrine system, the musculoskeletal system, and the immune system. The recent understanding of these links provides the basis for scientific research to define causal relationships. For example, alterations in the autonomic and endocrine systems can cause inhibition of the immune system, increasing susceptibility to disease. In addition, certain genetic types are particularly susceptible to immunodeficiency states. In stressful environmental conditions, a susceptible individual can readily develop a temporary acquired immunodeficiency. Some cases of immunodeficiency lead to overt disease, whereas others are merely temporary phenomena. Research on physical factors leading to immunodeficiency is extensive. Such factors include malnutrition, aging, infection, trauma, irradiation, the AIDS virus, and immunosuppressant drugs.[12]

Despite extensive research into the relationship of stress and illness during the past several decades, the specificity of the relationship remains vague. Research has shown that there are a variety of hormonal responses to various types of stress,[13] but directly applicable discoveries have not come easily. Some of the difficulty evolves from the definitions of stress and illness. Research is just beginning on the more difficult and subtle area of coping and adaptational processes, to define what is stressful, what is stress, and the relationship between them.[14]

Concept of Stress, Stressors, and Adaptation

Although there are several varying definitions of stress, for the purposes of this chapter, stress will be defined as:

1. The nonspecific response of the body to any demand made upon it, as per Hans Selye.
2. An existing state that has varying degrees of intensity, depending upon currently existing external and internal factors and human perception.
3. An existing state that on some level is necessary for life and that necessitates an adaptive response.

A stressor is thus defined as any internal or external demand made upon the human system. Consequently, a stressor could include physiological, psychological, sociocultural, or environmental influences that force an individual to respond or adapt to such demands. In this context, adaptation refers to the process in which the human system changes in response to stress. The change may be adaptive in that homeostasis or equilibrium is resumed. However, it may also be maladaptive, which results in continued stress and conceivably pathology or even death.

Psychophysiological Responses to Stress

Physiological Responses

Both Dubois and Selye recognized the extreme importance of the mechanisms by which the mind acts on the body. Both described the effect of stress on the endocrine system, causing widespread physiological changes. As can be seen from Figure 44-1, the interpretation of a stress situation in the brain leads to stimulation of the hypothalamus, which is the control center of both autonomic nervous system responses and the majority of hormone activities.

Psychophysiological disorders involve physiological changes in body systems such as the skin, gastrointestinal tract, respiratory system, or cardiovascular system. The organs involved are affected by both the autonomic nervous system and the endocrine system. Both systems function independently of conscious thought. Thus the changes that occur in these organs cannot be controlled by any effort of will.

The autonomic nervous system is composed of two main branches, the sympathetic nervous system and the parasympathetic nervous system. Both branches innervate the major body organs and have opposite effects (Fig. 44-1). For example, the sympathetic nervous system stimulates an increase in heart rate, whereas the parasympathetic nervous system slows the heart rate. The sympathetic nervous system in general prepares the body to act in an emergency situation—the "fight or flight" response. Peripheral vasoconstriction and increased heart rate cause an increase in blood pressure and thus promote optimum circulation. Activity slows in the gastrointestinal tract, which is not needed in the emergency. The parasympathetic nervous system, on the other hand, increases gastrointestinal secretion and peristalsis and generally provides activities for the general maintenance of the organism.

Both branches of the autonomic nervous system, although not consciously controlled, are greatly influenced by the emotional state of the individual.

Studies have shown that the stomach lining becomes markedly engorged and hyperemic when an individual becomes angry or anxious, producing an increased secretion of hydrochloric acid. Conversely, when an individual is depressed, the stomach lining remains pale and secretes little. Persons who are depressed are known to have changes in appetite, often being

tions created additional problems in interpersonal relationships. Even though the episodes of diarrhea continued, she did not perceive the relationship between her physical symptoms and her stressful situation but blamed it on a virus. She ignored comments about her weight loss and frequent absences. By the time of admission, she had lost 35 pounds and was pale, drawn, and anxious. She was diagnosed upon admission as having ulcerative colitis, acute exacerbation.

Nursing assessment of Barbara's response and level of stress would entail the following;

1. Adaptive capacity: From a *developmental* perspective, Barbara is a young adult, who by now has the cognitive capabilities for problem-solving skills and for seeking out a variety of support systems. Given her educational history, she appears to be bright, which further enhances such skills. However, her experience with more insight-oriented processing is limited and needs further development. *Physiologically*, Barbara has been healthy up until this point with all sensory and most other physiological systems functioning effectively. *Interpersonally*, Barbara is capable of establishing and maintaining some level of interpersonal relationships, as evidenced by her having a fiancé and continued contact with her family. However, these relationships are both a support system as well as a stressor for Barbara. In addition, she is beginning to establish stressful relationships with coworkers.

2. Stressors: Sources of stress appear to stem from a variety of areas. Developmental stressors for Barbara are establishing intimate relationships or being engaged and forming an occupation or beginning a job as an account executive. Psychological stressors entail Barbara's own need to excel or become an overachiever as a means of establishing a positive self-image. Sociocultural stressors include Barbara's family's insistence on conforming to their expectations around religious and family beliefs.

3. Individual's perception of stress: Because of Barbara's limited insight (e.g., she did not perceive the relationship between her physical symptoms and her stressful situation), Barbara would not initially be able to explore the subjective feelings that influence her perceptions of these stressors. However, her responses to stress indicate that she does view her stressful situation to be "anxiety provoking."

4. Person's response: Barbara appears to be responding at a severe level of stress or anxiety. Her perceptions are becoming more narrowed (i.e., focusing around her physiological symptoms), and she incorrectly interprets the problem as being viral or external to herself. Maladaptive responses have also already been implemented, as evidenced by her establishing extra meetings, working overtime, and demanding superhuman efforts of her staff. These maladaptive responses have further led to somatic complaints and problems such as diarrhea, weight loss of 35 pounds and pale, ashen appearance.

Nursing Diagnoses

Analysis of assessment data obtained for psychophysiological disorders should lead to one or a varying combination of the following nursing diagnoses:

1. Anxiety and the respective level of anxiety observed or
2. Ineffective individual coping or
3. Other nursing diagnoses that refer specifically to the physiological manifestations or responses to stress.

In Barbara's case, nursing diagnosis, based on the assessment data obtained, would entail (1) anxiety, severe level; (2) ineffective individual coping related to avoidance behavior; (3) alteration in bowel elimination and diarrhea; and (4) nutritional alteration related to weight loss and anxiety.

RANGE OF INTERVENTIONS: PLANNING AND IMPLEMENTATION OF NURSING CARE

Although the nursing care for psychophysiological disorders varies for each individual, certain guidelines are appropriate.

In terms of establishing care priorities, nurses must assess, early on, whether the patient exhibits any pathological symptoms that are life-threatening and establish interventions that will at least stabilize the patient's physiological status. Once this stabilization occurs or is already determined to be present, other nursing interventions can be implemented.

Reduction of stressors can be a primary nursing activity in caring for a patient with a psychophysiologic disorder. For the hospitalized patient, the lack of privacy, increased dependence, strange noises and odors, institutional food, and staff attitudes are all potential stressors that can be ameliorated through nursing intervention. It is incumbent upon the nurse to talk with the patient to determine which stressor—environmental or otherwise—is a priority problem. The nurse can act to assist the patient to deal with stressors such as uncertainty about the unknown, separation from family, or worry over finances, through her interest and concern. The nurse should not become discouraged if the stressors are such that she can do nothing about them (e.g., family illness, job situation). Her role then is to provide a setting for the patient to be able to comfortably discuss his concerns with an appropriate resource person. She should always remember the need to provide the patient with a sense of control and the need to reduce the occurrence of unpredictable events.

As much as possible, the locus of decision making should rest with the patient to increase his sense of control over his own health and care. Consider for example the individual waiting for an x-ray for 3 hours, unsure of when his test will begin. This stress, added to the physiological stress of being allowed no food and the psychological stress of fear of the test and its outcome, significantly raises his anxiety level, and he should have an explanation of what will be experienced during the test.

The issue of control depends in part upon the individual's perception of his circumstances. It should be remembered that an individual has the capacity to control his own behavior (eating, drinking, smoking, communicating). How he perceives his behavior has a direct effect on his illness. The brain does not always work logically in this regard. The nurse should assist the person to identify how his response to stress is affecting his physical health. It is vital that he see this relationship in order to promote any long-term change in his responses. The nurse must remember that the defense mechanisms that the person is using may be the best adaptation that he can make for the time being. Any attempts at breaking down denial, for example, may be counterproductive. Some people resist the idea that their emotions are affecting their physical state, since to them it is a sign of weakness or a threat to their integrity. The emotions involved may be strong and the responses deeply ingrained. A sustained, trusting relationship with a skilled professional is needed in such cases.

Nursing interventions should also focus around diminishing the clients level of anxiety or response to stress. As previously stated, individuals whose level of response is mild to moderate are often themselves capable of adapting and growing and learning within the stressful situation. Here nursing interventions primarily involve patient education and problem-solving tasks that further enhance a patient's potential to adapt or change. However, if a patient's level of stress is within the severe-to-

panic range, the nurse must first implement interventions to reduce the level of stress or anxiety before such problem-solving and educational strategies can even be effective. In addition, if the nurse can successfully help the patient to reduce the level of stress response, maladaptive responses and potential crisis states can perhaps be avoided.

To diminish the stress level, first and foremost the nurse needs a calm, organized, skillful approach. The person experiencing severe or panic levels of anxiety needs help in getting more comfortable. Oftentimes, large-muscle activities such as brisk walking can begin to help. If this is not possible, working with the patient through deep-breathing activities or specific muscle relaxation techniques may also help to make him more comfortable. Remember, patients at these levels have severe limitations in perception and interpretive powers, so the nurse needs to be the one to take direct, simple, concrete actions. Also, the nurse should always stay with this person until his level of panic has diminished.

Nurses frequently first encounter patients when pathology has already occurred, as a result of the patient's maladaptive response to the stressor(s). As previously stated, the nurse will first have to ensure that the patient's physiological status is stable. Once this has been established, the nurse should begin working toward developing a trusting, therapeutic relationship so that the patient can explore the connection between his psychological response to stress and his present physiological condition. Through understanding of the patient, the nurse can assist him to alter maladaptive coping responses and can support adaptive responses. She can provide outlets for his emotions, activities both satisfying to the patient and helpful in dissipating negative emotions. Active participation in events and a sense of responsibility are also helpful and have been shown to reduce mortality rates by 50 percent in a group of elderly patients.[28]

Promotion of a social support system is vital, especially during periods of crisis. Studies have shown that the presence of a support system is directly linked to increased coping ability.[29] In fact, the presence of a support person (friend, relative) has been shown to be more directly related to low morbidity than even the use of preventive measures such as diet and exercise. Even the continued presence of a pet can foster a positive feeling in the individual. Available personal and community resources should be explored. People important to the patient should be identified and encouraged to participate in the individual's care. The multidisciplinary team can play an important role by contributing its own expertise in determining care, often with the coordination of the nurse. Teaching and counseling are extremely important factors in control of psychophysiologic disease and require coordinated efforts of all health team members.

In developing a nursing care plan for Barbara, the following interventions should be identified for implementation:

1. In order to ensure physiological stabilization in Barbara's case, specific nursing actions may need to take priority, depending on current assessment data:
   a. Monitor fluid balance and electrolyte levels.
   b. Monitor stools (frequency, content).
   c. Maintain bed rest in nonstressful environment.
   d. Administer parenteral fluids and transfusions as needed.
   e. Monitor vital signs regularly.
2. In order to address problems specifically related to severe level of anxiety and inadequate individual coping, the nurse first has to assist Barbara in diminishing her anxiety level so that she can begin to explore alternative methods of coping.

   To assist Barbara in diminishing her level of anxiety, the nurse should, in a calm, organized manner:
   a. Provide outlets for her anxiety (e.g., helping her to engage in physical activities as tolerated, introducing simple concrete tasks to perform).
   b. Stay with the patient until her anxiety level has diminished.
   c. Allow for talking by being available and communicating that she has time to listen.
   d. Assist in performing specific relaxation techniques such as deep-breathing exercises or specific muscle relaxation exercises.
   e. Provide patient with a sense of control, as much as possible.
3. Once Barbara's level of anxiety or stress response has diminished, specific interventions for developing more adequate coping responses can be implemented by the nurse. These include:

a. Assisting the patient to identify her responses to stress, both positive and negative.
b. Helping her develop some insight as to how her somatic complaints are exacerbated by and a manifestation of her response to stress.
c. Identifying, with the patient, alternative coping mechanisms such as relaxation techniques and realistic goal setting when solving problems.
4. In conjunction with assisting Barbara in developing more adequate coping responses, the nurse should also assess whether interventions around altering specific stressors and establishing support systems are possible. In Barbara's case, the nurse could:
   a. Encourage incorporating her fiancé and family members in discussions as appropriate.
   b. Provide Barbara and her family with information about the disease condition as appropriate.
   c. Attempt to elicit concerns of the family members.
   d. Assist the family members in understanding possible sources of stress and constructive responses to stress.

CASE EXAMPLE TWO

Brian, age 6, a known asthmatic, had just arrived in the emergency room with wheezing, increased respirations, and complaining of shortness of breath. Medical history revealed no known allergies and only minor complaints of earache and common childhood infections. He had been basically healthy prior to the first hospitalization for acute bronchial asthma, which occurred at age 4. He appeared frightened and would cling tightly to his mother while in the emergency room.

In attempting to obtain a history of present illness from the mother, the nurse observed that the mother could barely focus on her questions and seemed to only address her child's physical symptoms. However, the nurse could elicit from the mother that Brian's parents had divorced when he was 3. Brian had only seen his father sporadically since then. Brian's mother then had to begin working part time to support them, and she stated that she felt "overwhelmed" by their situation. In addition, they had no close family members or friends for support, since they were new to the area.

Assessment Data

Developmentally, Brian is only 6 years old and basically must rely on adults to solve problems for him.

He has been basically healthy except for the development of acute bronchial asthma since age 4. He and his mother have minimal economic and psychosocial supports since they are new to the area. Stressors entail divorce of parents, economic difficulties, and moving to a new community.

Human Response to Stress

- Brian: Increased respirations, wheezing, shortness of breath, frightened, clinging to mother.
- Mother: Narrowed perceptual focus, unable to attend to questions, feeling "overwhelmed."

Nursing Diagnosis

- Brian: Ineffective breathing pattern related to asthma
  Anxiety
- Mother: Anxiety
  Ineffective coping, family

Goals

Long-Term
1. Patient will have decreasing episodes of dyspnea as a response to stress
2. Situational support systems will be established for the family within 6 months.

Short-term
1. Within 2 hours the patient's respiratory rate will decrease, with diminished wheezing and shortness of breath.
2. Mother's anxiety level will diminish from a severe to moderate or mild level, as evidenced by an increased ability to attend to questions and to respond directly to her child's needs.
3. Patient's anxiety level will diminish as evidenced by signs of relaxation as the acute episode subsides and less clinging behavior toward the mother.

Interventions

1. Assess adequacy of oxygenation and ensure patient airway.
2. Encourage mother to engage in simple, concrete tasks around comforting son.
3. Allow for verbalization of feelings, from both mother and son.
4. Introduce each intervention to Brian and mother in simple, concrete terms.
5. Begin to explore with Brian and mother their feelings around recent changes, as time constraints allow.

6. Refer to community support systems, such as counseling services for stress reduction, social services, and community-involved activities to increase socialization opportunities.

OTHER STRESS MANAGEMENT TECHNIQUES

Prevention

Nursing intervention may occur at any stage during the development of a psychophysiologic disorder. Probably the most important stage, and the stage on which nursing should focus greater efforts, is that of prevention. Children at an early age can be taught effective means of coping with stress—open communication, identification of stress symptoms, stress reduction techniques, and identification of individual stress level and coping style. In today's high-pressure society, such skills should be routinely taught. Adults, too, can learn to better cope with their lives. With the increasing commitment to health seen in today's society, stress reduction programs can be used to contribute significantly to better health in the future.

Biofeedback

Since it has been demonstrated that a person can control his own heart rate, blood pressure, and other physiological events, much research has been done to determine the possibilities of this power of the mind over other parts of the body. Biofeedback works by providing the individual with direct feedback to know the results of efforts to alter a physiological function. Ordinarily, we are not aware of our internal physiology, and have no idea, for example, when our blood pressure becomes dangerously high or when our brain-wave pattern changes. If given enough feedback information, a person can learn to control his blood pressure or learn to alter his brain-wave pattern, at least temporarily. The information comes from machines that are designed to detect small changes in physiological activity and convert them into flashes of light or audible tones that change in frequency. After some practice, the individual often finds that he can control his blood pressure or relieve his migraine headache even without the use of a machine. Because the promise of biofeedback is exciting, it has been occasionally promoted as a panacea. Legitimate researchers are more reserved in their projections for the future. Biofeedback research is progressing slowly and carefully.

Relaxation Techniques and Imagery

Another technique that is seeing increasing use is that of imagery. Some people use imagery to quit smoking, lose weight, or improve athletic skills. Doctors and other health professionals use it to overcome negative emotions or to assist their patients to pay attention to their bodily symptoms and their own inner wisdom. All imagery techniques begin with relaxation, which is the most important part of the process. Relaxation techniques are needed to interrupt a chain of chronic hyperalert state and to allow a change from negative to more positive images. Most people have some awareness of relaxation techniques, of which there are several. One relaxation technique has the person close his eyes and concentrate on one muscle group at a time, starting with the toes, consciously relaxing each muscle group in ascending order. Another type of relaxation technique has the individual imagine himself in a quiet, pleasant place, perhaps a favorite spot by the water, and focus on remembered sensations of sight, touch, sound, and smell. Once an individual is relaxed, he is more likely to be successful in the use of imagery.

According to psychologist Arnold Lazarus, mental imagery can change a person's negative images into positive ones. He says that humans are governed by their predictions about the future. Both our optimistic and pessimistic anticipations take the form of mental imagery. A person's actions are dependent upon the way in which he *anticipates* events. In order to change a negative reaction, according to Lazarus, it is only necessary to change the mental image, since the imaging process affects the same nerve cells as the actual action. Lazarus feels that understanding of the underlying mechanism is not necessary in order to get results. The basic rule is: "If you wish to accomplish something in reality, first picture yourself achieving it in imagination."[30]

The premise underlying the use of imagery is that it brings into play the right side of the brain, which functions in a spatial, visual way rather than in a verbal way. Incorporating the right hemisphere makes more creative use of brain potential. Some individuals can call up mental images readily, whereas for others, practice is required. Imagery can consist of visualizing yourself as your idealized self-image, visualizing in detail the accomplishment of a goal, using coping imagery to overcome fears, using negative imagery to avoid fattening foods, or using time compression to gain perspective. Lazarus also uses imagery techniques to control the symptoms of ulcerative colitis, tension headaches, peptic ulcers, and other psychosomatic disorders. Deeply comforting images from the past seem to have soothing effects on the gastrointestinal tract, for example. A young woman who suffered from ulcerative colitis showed a marked reduction in symptoms after she began to visualize herself being hugged as an infant.[31] To be effective, imagery must be practiced thoroughly and faithfully. The repetition improves the nerve cell responses and allows the desired response to occur more readily.

CURRENT RESEARCH ON STRESS AND PSYCHOPHYSIOLOGICAL DISORDERS

Research with neurotransmitters such as norepinephrine, acetylcholine, dopamine, and endorphins may lead to an entirely new view of psychophysiological disorders. As with recent research findings regarding depressive states, the problem in psychophysiological disorders may well be due to an imbalance between neurotransmitters.

Because emotions can cause illness, it has been postulated that the mind may be used to cure disease. The use of therapeutic touch is one avenue that is currently being explored as a means to positively affect the individual. Biofeedback and transcendental meditation are two popular methods now being used by the general population. By the use of such techniques, an individual can alter his own psychophysiological state. Biofeedback and therapeutic touch are also being studied for use as nursing techniques.

Recent research shows that the brain has control over many more bodily functions than previously realized. For example, the brain has been found to have a previously unknown influence over the immune system. This finding has many implications in terms of causation and treatment of the autoimmune diseases. Abnormal immune response has been connected with conditions as varied as ulcerative colitis, rheumatoid arthritis, and even cancer. The implications are very exciting, for they mean that each individual potentially has a means of presenting or at least exerting some control over conditions against which there was formerly no recourse.

Many body systems are altered by the state of mind—brain waves, oxygen consumption, blood pressure, and gastrointestinal motility, for example. One need only think of the Indian yogi who can get along without oxygen for 15 minutes in a closed container by lowering his metabolic needs through meditation. It is interesting to speculate what other bodily needs and functions may be altered by the state of mind.

Negative emotions have been proven to affect many bodily states adversely. By decreasing the immune response, for example, an individual is left susceptible to a wide variety of conditions from the common cold to a chronic crippling condition. An altered state of mind may be able to prevent such consequences. Alteration of a person's frame of mind can be accomplished by numerous techniques, including the above-mentioned meditation, hypnosis, relaxation techniques, and the use of mental imagery. Even asking the person to take a deep breath creates a temporary relaxation.

Nursing Research on Stress

The profession of nursing has increasingly begun to research the interrelationship of stress responses to the development and treatment or prevention of physiological disorders. For example, there are several studies that refer to the effectiveness of stress management programs as either primary or secondary interventions for clients with specific psychophysiological disorders. One such study by B. Milne, G. Joachim, and J. Niedhardt relates their findings of the effectiveness of a stress management program for inflammatory bowel disease patients. The program revolved around six classes on stress management, which included autogenic training (repetition of phrases describing a desired body condition), personal planning skills, and communication techniques. Their conclusion that "practicing stress management techniques decreased disease activity and was associated with improved psychosocial functioning," has direct implications for nursing practice.[32]

Other studies emerging around stress man-agement techniques include those of patients with such psychophysiological disorders as hypertension or asthma. For example, a study by Nola J. Pender found that progressive muscle relaxation was useful in increasing beliefs in personal control of health.[33] Another study of hypertensive patients found that well-controlled hypertensives had better health adjustment scores and fewer hypertension-related problems and felt that their health was under their own control.[34] Management of stress associated asthma is discussed in a research study by N. M. Clark, et al.[35]

The effect of social support and coping responses are being studied in many populations, such as the functionally disabled.[36] Studies are also being done on the effect of developmental level on perceived stress and on the effect of cultural beliefs, but many more studies need to be done in these areas.[37] More studies also need to be done on the methods that nurses use to assess their patients for stress. According to one author, it appears that nurses do not accurately assess the effects of pre-existing patient stress.[38]

There is also an increasing amount of research being done in the area of the effects of stress on the profession of nursing itself. There appears to be a consensus among nursing researchers that nursing has been identified as a high-stress profession.[39] In order to ensure continued efficacy within the profession, identifying stressors and modifiers of stress can help in leading to interventions that reduce excessive stress within nursing itself.

In conclusion, our health reflects how we live our lives. What we believe can heal us or kill us. (As an example, consider voodoo medicine.) Psychological factors have even been shown to affect tumor growth, showing that life-change events and emotional states are transmitted by neural and hormonal influences to the cellular level. On the other hand, love and humor are now being suggested to be antidotes to disease. For an interesting discussion of this topic, see Norman Cousins' book, *Anatomy of an Illness as Perceived by the Patient*.[40] We live in an exciting time because there are so many new avenues to explore and so many possibilities for improving the health of the population. The new science of psychoneuroimmunology (which is studying the ways in which thoughts and beliefs can predispose to disease and alter the course of ongoing disease) may provide a major breakthrough in understanding and perhaps preventing many of the chronic psychophysiological ailments in our society.

The health professions are becoming increasingly aware of the need for a "holistic" approach whereby the patient can be intimately involved in his own care in the prevention as well as the treatment of disease. There is a great need in our high-pressure society for a general awareness of the causes and results of stress and the means that individuals can use to reduce stress and cope with it effectively. As Hans Selye has said, "Fight for the highest attainable aim, but do not put up resistance in vain."[41]

Summary

This chapter has focused on the interrelationship of psychological factors and physiological function. Although the precise role that each factor plays on the outcome health behavior of the individual is not known, it is clear that psychological factors are important in the expression of illness. The concept of stress and adaptation is emphasized, and the nursing process is applied to case examples. Prevention issues were identified in terms of necessary nursing research, patient teaching and counseling, identification of life stressors, and biofeedback research.

Questions

1. What is the most critical factor affecting how a person will respond to a stressful situation, and why?
2. Write a patient example for each level of anxiety conceptualized by Peplau.
3. Identify two patient teaching–counseling approaches to aid a person with a psychophysiological disorder to cope with stressors in his life.
4. Cite two nursing research studies on stress and physiological response.

REFERENCES AND SUGGESTED READINGS

1. American Nurses' Association. *Nursing: A Social Policy Statement*. Kansas City, Mo.: American Nurses' Association, 1982.
2. American Psychiatric Association. *Diagnostic and Statistical Manual*, 3rd ed. (Rev.). Washington, D.C.: American Psychiatric Association, 1987, pp. 333–334.
3. Alexander, F. *Psychosomatic Medicine*. New York: Norton, 1960.
4. Sheehan, D. V., & Hackett, T. P. Psychosomatic disorders. In A. M. Nicholi, Jr. (Ed.), *The Harvard Guide to Modern Psychiatry*. Cambridge, Mass.: Harvard University Press, 1978, pp. 320–321.
5. Ibid.
6. McMahon, C. E., & Oberg, D. Functional illness and the status of psychosomatic concepts in nineteenth century medicine. *Journal of the American Society of Psychosomatic Dentistry and Medicine*, 1983, 30(4), 156–161.
7. Cannon, W. B. *The Wisdom of the Body*. New York, Norton, 1932.
8. Selye, H. The stress syndrome. *American Journal of Nursing*, 1965, 65(3), 972–999.
9. Selye, op. cit., p. 98.
10. Ibid.
11. Dubos, R. *Man Adapting*. New Haven: Yale University Press, 1965.
12. Borysenko, M., & Borysenko, J. Stress, behavior and immunity: Animal models and mediating mechanisms. *General Hospital Psychiatry*, 1982, 4, 59–67.
13. Mason, J. W. Specificity in the organization of neuroendocrine response profiles. In P. Seeman & G. Brown (Eds.), *Frontiers of Neurology and Neuroscience Research*. Toronto: University of Toronto, 1974, p. 68.

14. Kimball, C. P. Stress and psychosomatic illness. *Journal of Psychosomatic Research*, 1982, 26(1), 63–71.

15. Rubin, R. T. Life stress and illness patterns in the United States Navy, part 3: Prior life changes and illness onset on the attack carriers crew. *Archives of Environmental Health*, 1969, 19, 758.

16. Elliot, G. R., & Eisdorfer, C. *Stress and Human Health: Analysis and Implications of Research*. New York: Springer, 1982.

17. Hovanitz, C. A. Life event stress and coping style as contributors to psychopathology. *Journal of Clinical Psychology*, 1986, 42(1), 34–42.

18. Sarason, I. G., Johnson, J. H., & Siegel, J. M. Assessing the impact of life changes: Development of the Life Experiences Survey. *Journal of Consulting and Clinical Psychology*, 1978, 46, 932–946.

19. Vogel, W. Coping, stress, stressors and health consequences. *Neuropsychobiology*, 1985, 13(3), 120–135.

20. Tobin, D. J., Holroyd, K., & Reynolds, R. *The Assessment of Coping: Psychometric Development of the Coping Strategies Inventory*. Paper presented at the meeting of the Association for the Advancement of Behavior Therapy, Los Angeles, Feb. 1982.

21. Hovanitz, op. cit.

22. Felton, B. J., Revenson, T. A., & Hinrichsen, G. A. Stress and coping in the explanation of psychological adjustment among chronically ill adults. *Social Science and Medicine*, 1984, 18, 889–898.

23. McFarlane, A. H., Norman, C. R., Streiner, D. L., et al. The process of social stress. *Journal of Health and Social Behavior*, 1983, 24, 160–173.

24. Thoits, P. A. Conceptual, methodological, and theoretical problems in studying social support as a buffer against life stress. *Journal of Health and Social Behavior*, 1982, 23, 145–159.

25. Richman, J. A., & Flaherty, J. A. Stress, coping resources and psychiatric disorders: Alternative paradigms from a life cycle perspective. *Comprehensive Psychiatry*, 1985, 26, 456–466.

26. Haggerty, J. J. The psychosomatic family: An overview. *Psychosomatics*, 1983, 24, 615–623.

27. Campsey, J. R. Psychophysiologic illness. *Journal of Psychiatric Nursing and Mental Health Services*, 1979, 17(11), 27.

28. Minkler, M. People need people: Social support and health. Paper presented at *Conference on The Healing Brain*, Falmouth, Mass., August 15, 1982, sponsored by Pacific Medical Center and the Institute for the Study of Human Knowledge, San Francisco.

29. Ibid.

30. Lazarus, A. *In the Mind's Eye*. New York: Rawson Associates, 1977, p. 73.

31. Ibid., p. 154.

32. Milne, B., Joachim, G., & Niedhardt, J. A stress management programme for inflammatory bowel disease patients. *Journal of Advanced Nursing*, 1986, 11, 561–567.

33. Pender, N. J. Effects of progressive muscle relaxation training on anxiety and health locus of control among hypertensive adults. *Research in Nursing and Health*, 1985, 8(1), 67–72.

34. Powers, M. J., & Jalowiec, A. Profile of the well-controlled, well-adjusted hypertensive patient. *Nursing Research*, 1987, 36(2), 106–111.

35. Clark, N. M. Managing better: Children, parents and asthma. *Patient Education Counseling*, 1986, 8(March), 27–38.

36. McNett, S. C. Social support, threat, and coping responses and effectiveness in the functionally disabled. *Nursing Research*, 1987, 36(2), 98–103.

37. Yarcheski, A., & Mahon, N. E. Perceived stress and symptom patterns in early adolescents: The role of mediating variables. *Research in Nursing and Health*, 1986, 9, 289–297.

38. Ross, S. E. M., & MacKay, R. C. Postoperative stress: Do nurses accurately assess their patients? *Journal of Psychosocial Nursing*, 1986, 24(4), 17–21.

39. Trygstad, L. N. Stress and coping in psychiatric nursing. *Journal of Psychosocial Nursing*, 1986, 24(10), 23–27.

40. Cousins, N. *Anatomy of an Illness as Perceived by the Patient*. New York: Norton, 1979.

41. Salye, op. cit., p. 99.

Developmental Disabilities

Eunice Shishmanian

Chapter Objectives

The students successfully attaining the goals of this chapter will be able to:

- List four types of prenatal conditions that can result in mental retardation.
- Summarize the factors that can result in developmental delay during and following birth.
- Identify the prevalence of mental retardation in the United States.
- Describe the nursing assessment skills of the interview, behavior observation, physical observation, and testing tools in collecting data on developmental delay.
- Describe factors involved in negotiating a treatment plan after a diagnosis has been given to a family with a child with mental retardation.
- Identify eight nursing interventions for working with a family with a child who is developmentally disabled.
- Identify areas of nursing research in developmental disabilities.

Development is a lifelong process—one that begins at conception and proceeds in a pattern leading to maturity. It is influenced by internal factors (health, genetics, and organic functioning) and external factors (the environment and the society in which one lives). This chapter will explore the dimensions of developmental disabilities.

DEVELOPMENTAL DISABILITIES

Definition

The developmentally disabled person is one whose adaptive ability has been compromised in one or more areas of functioning by an alteration in the pattern or rate in stages of development during childhood. The current official definition in the Comprehensive Rehabilitation Services Act addresses the functional needs of the person requiring services rather than the use of a diagnostic classification.[1] According to the law, the term *developmental disability* refers to severe chronic disability that is attributable to a mental or physical impairment or a combination of mental and physical impairments; is manifested before the person attains age 22; is likely to continue indefinitely; results in substantial functional limitations in three or more of the following areas of major life activity: self-care, learning, mobility, self-direction, capacity for independent living, and economic self-sufficiency; and reflects the person's need for a combination and sequence of special interdisciplinary or generic care treatment or other services that are of lifelong or extended duration and are individually planned and coordinated.[2]

Subaverage general intellectual functioning that originates during the developmental period and is associated with impairment in adaptive behavior is termed *mental retardation* (mental deficiency). It is a social attribute consisting of at least three components: organic, functional, and social. The organic component is referred to as the *impairment*, the functional component as the *disability*, and the social component as the *handicap*. The functional disability is measured in terms of subaverage intellectual capacity, whereas the extent of the social handicap varies with age and social setting.

Etiology

The etiology of mental retardation is often unidentifiable. The known causes can be considered in two main groups of factors: genetic and acquired conditions (Table 45-1).

Approaches to Diagnosis

A diagnosis of mental retardation is warranted in individuals who demonstrate deficits in both measured intelligence, and social-adaptive behavior.

Intelligence is measured by the use of a standardized intelligence test from which the I.Q. (intelligence quotient) score is computed. The test attempts to sample a wide range of knowledge and skills and to compare the person's test

TABLE 45-1. CAUSES OF MENTAL RETARDATION

Genetic Conditions
  Chromosomal
    Down syndrome
    Klinefelter syndrome
  Errors of metabolism
    Phenylketonuria
    Hypothyroidism
    Hurler disease
    Tay-Sachs disease
Acquired Conditions
  Prenatal
    Rubella and other viruses
    Toxins
    Placental insufficiency
    Blood type incompatibility
  Perinatal
    Anoxia
    Birth injury
    Prematurity
    Kernicterus
  Postnatal
    Infections—meningitis, encephalitis
    Poison—lead, medications
    Poor nutrition
    Trauma—central nervous system insult
    Sociocultural factors—deprivation

performance to a standard established for his chronological age. The test is based on the assumption that the person being tested has had similar opportunities to learn, and shares a common language and culture with those persons on whom the test was standardized. Special assessment techniques are required in the presence of other specific handicaps such as an impairment of hearing or vision or musculoskeletal abnormalities. The person whose performance is similar to his age group is considered average (assigned a score ratio of 100), with those falling below or above being compared to persons younger or older. The I.Q. expresses the relationship of "mental age" or "test age" to chronological age, with an I.Q. of 100 being assigned to represent the average. The basic formula is:

$$\frac{\text{Mental age}}{\text{Chronological age}} \times 100 = \text{I.Q.}$$

Thus, as an example, if Joey is 8 years old and has achieved a mental age of 4 years on a standardized intelligence test, his I.Q. would be computed as follows:

$$\frac{\text{Joey's mental age} = 4}{\text{Joey's chronological age} = 8} \times 100 = \text{I.Q.} = 50$$

Difficulties are encountered in that these tests were originated to measure academic achievement, and they yield unreliable measurements in children with poor motor coordination or impaired speech development because performance on most tests requires use of motor skills and written or spoken language.

Social-adaptive behavior refers to the individual's ability to cope with the social, educational, and vocational demands of his environment. It includes the degree to which the individual satisfactorily meets the culture's demands for social and personal responsibility and is able to function independently. As with intellectual functioning, social-adaptive behavior is evaluated by comparing an individual with members of his own age group. Therefore, maturational skills, i.e., sitting, standing, and walking, would be emphasized in the early years; academic performance during school-age years; and vocational and social competency in adult years. Assessment at present must be made from data about everyday behaviors in conjunction with objective measures.

A positive correlation should exist between measured intelligence and social-adaptive behavior, but it is not uncommon to see retarded individuals whose adaptive functioning is higher than that achieved on cognitive tests. This points to the importance of the evaluation being accomplished by a team of qualified professionals, including representatives from the medical, social, and educational disciplines.

Levels of mental retardation are classified according to the intelligence quotient achieved. Although a classification is a rationale for obtaining services and experiences for the individual, it may also serve to stigmatize the person and may exclude him from opportunities and services.

Categorical definitions are used to indicate the potential to grow, to learn, and to develop, and are based on the I.Q (Table 45-2).

Mildly retarded children are often not diagnosed until they begin school attendance. They are able to learn basic academic reading and arithmetic skills with some special training. As adults most are capable of learning to do productive work and thus be self-supporting and live independently.

Moderately retarded young children may have fair motor development and can learn to talk and care for their basic needs. They will require a program of special training throughout their school years and are able to learn func-tional academic skills. As adults they can perform semiskilled work under supervised situations as in a sheltered workshop or supported work program. They may be able to achieve competitive employment and live in the community with varying degrees of assistance.

Severely retarded children experience slow development of motor and communication skills and may have physical handicaps. Special education services and use of adaptive equipment may enable them to learn to talk and communicate. They will vary in their ability to contribute to learning to care for themselves and will require supervision in work and the living situation.

Most profoundly retarded persons require ongoing medical or nursing services in order to remediate physical–medical disabilities, prevent further difficulties, and maintain life. They will need help in feeding, bathing, and general care as well as protection. They can learn to relate to others, to play, and to participate with assistance in self-care.

Within the spectrum of health services, the profession of nursing has a responsibility to provide for the handicapped population. The scope of nursing involvement encompasses preventive, interventive, and management activities. Nursing needs extend throughout the entire life-span. Techniques must be adapted on the basis of the assessment of the disabled individual's needs and capabilities.

In the past it was believed that emotional reactions were not possible for persons with compromised cognitive abilities. Retarded persons were not perceived as being aware of societal values and therefore were felt to be unaware of not meeting these values. Thus, the mentally retarded were regarded as unable to experience human emotions. As a result, the presence of emotional disorders in a severely developmentally handicapped child was frequently overlooked or even denied.

The recent attention of mental health professionals to mental retardation has increased our knowledge about the emotional development and psychopathology of retarded persons.[3] We now know that developmentally handicapped persons can experience a full range of emotions, although they may not be able to communicate these feelings in the usual ways that we are accustomed to. It is also known that they may develop the same emotional disorders as nonretarded persons and may be di-

TABLE 45-2. LEVELS OF RETARDATION BASED ON STANDARDIZED INTELLIGENCE TESTS

Level of Retardation	Standardized Intelligence Tests	
	Stanford-Binet[a]	Wechsler[b]
Mild	52–67	55–69
Moderate	36–51	40–54
Severe	20–35	25–39
Profound	Below 20	Below 35

[a] Terman, L. M., Merrill, M. A. *Stanford-Binet Intelligence Scale*. Boston: Houghton Mifflin, 1960.
[b] Wechsler, D. *Wechsler Intelligence Scale for Children*. New York: The Psychological Corporation, 1974.

agnosed and treated by the same, although modified, techniques.

Each child is a unique individual. One must not stereotype him by considering him a member of a group with a specific handicap. Mental retardation is not a specific disorder but rather a behavioral functional syndrome. Therefore, retarded persons form a more heterogeneous group than nonretarded ones. For example, a mildly retarded young adult living in a community residence and attending a workshop program has more in common with his nonretarded neighbor than with a profoundly retarded, nonverbal young adult who is totally dependent on others. Yet both are classified as "retarded."

Psychosocial adaptation depends on a complicated interaction of many biologic and environmental factors. One cannot generalize about the personality of any child. Personality patterns are not unique to retarded children, although certain patterns are more frequently encountered.

The *DSM-III-R*, introduced in 1987, is an effort to improve the reliability of diagnostic judgments by the use of specific diagnostic criteria and a multi-axial approach. This format represents the current state of knowledge about diagnosing mental disorders. It provides a more comprehensive approach toward the goal of a reliable means of common assessment, language, and definition in approach for all professionals involved in psychiatric care. The *DSM-III-R* makes available official codes and terms for all recognized mental disorders. A brief description of categories within the five axes follows:

Axis I and axis II (see Appendix) provide a listing of the clinical disorders appropriate to adults and specific developmental disorders of children and adolescents. Levels of intellectual functioning (I.Q.) are assigned categories. These categories represent the psychological or intra-personal area of functioning. Axis III denotes the physical disorder or condition that is relevant to the understanding and management of the client. Examples would be a seizure disorder, soft neurological signs, or a conductive hearing loss. Axis IV relates to the severity of psychosocial stressors that contribute to exacerbation of the mental disorder; these are rated by degree on a seven-point scale. Examples would be separation of the child's parents or abuse such as physical trauma by a caretaker. Axis V speaks to the highest level of adaptive functioning during the past year.

The following examples illustrate usage of the *DSM-III-R* categories:

EXAMPLE ONE

Ralph was a 5-year-old globally delayed little boy with a significant medical history suggestive of a combination of genetic and traumatic etiologic agents. He showed a high degree of distractability as well as attractability. He had many personal strengths and was an enjoyable child. He seemed quite needy and eager for attention both at home and at school. Piano playing provided a way for him to express himself nonverbally without frustration and afforded positive attention.

Axis I	Attention deficit disorder without hyperactivity.
Axis II	No diagnosis.
Axis III	Developmental delay. Peripheral vision impairment.
Axis IV	Five, severe. Single mother with significant depression. Loss of grandparents. Persistent harsh parental discipline.
Axis V	Five, poor. Problems getting along both at home and at school.

EXAMPLE TWO

Mia was a 3-year-old little girl with a diagnosis of Down's syndrome. She was a social child relating warmly to adults. Psychological testing placed her cognitive functioning in the range of moderate retardation. She was independent in feeding behaviors, participated in dressing herself, and was in the process of being toilet-trained. She communicated with a small repertoire of single words and the use of gestures. She participated regularly in family activities and was a well-accepted member of her family. Parents sought guidance for an appropriate educational program.

Axis I   No diagnosis.
Axis II   Mental retardation, moderate.
Axis III   Down syndrome, trisomy 21. Recurrent otitis media.
Axis IV   Two, mild. Adjustment to new school program.
Axis V   No diagnosis.

Psychiatric diagnostic techniques must be adapted for use with the retarded population. A diagnosis has to be established within a comprehensive context as there are often multiple handicaps as well as the child's dependence on and involvement with many caretakers. Medical assessment, family assessment, a developmental and behavioral history, and school information have to be integrated with information gathered from the examination of the child. Verbal and nonverbal techniques should be used, and should be adapted to the child's communication level. Information must be collected concerning the child's functioning in all important areas. Use of the *DSM-III-R* diagnostic criteria provides a framework for understanding the child. However, the clinician is urged to use the full profile obtained from comprehensive assessments to gain a well-rounded picture. Only in this way can a plan of intervention based on strengths as well as weaknesses be effective.

Studies are underway on the adaptation of the *DSM-III-R* for use with developmentally handicapped children referred for comprehensive assessment. Preliminary results indicate that in a sample of 126 retarded children, symptoms warranting formal psychiatric diagnosis were present in 70 percent of the patients. Thus, diagnostic criteria of mental disorders can be used with developmentally delayed children provided they are modified according to the development level.[4]

Learning Disabilities

The term *learning disabilities* refers primarily to the low-severity, high-prevalence disabilities of school children who are not affected by generalized cognitive impairment (mental retardation). The functional profiles of such children indicate that they are not well adapted to learning or social adjustment. Specific developmental disabilities are characterized by inadequate development of specific academic, language, speech, and motor skills. A wide range of syndromic classifications and descriptive terminology has been developed to describe these disorders, including such concepts as learning disability, dyslexia, hyperactivity, and minimal brain dysfunction, perceptual-motor impairment, and language disability. The most recent official definition proposed (Public Law 94-142) considers a learning disability to imply disorder in language usage that is manifested in imperfect listening, thinking, speaking, reading, writing, spelling, or mathematics ability. The currently accepted viewpoint is that the term *learning disability* is more useful as a concept than as a category. Areas of difficulty in learning include: skills in perception, information processing, or thinking; selective attention, memory, language, social interaction skills; and academic skills such as reading, writing, spelling, and arithmetic.

A diagnosis of mental retardation in a child does not preclude the additional diagnosis of a specific developmental disorder. Learning difficulties of children with mild degrees of mental retardation are often very similar to those of children with subtle learning problems. Educational assessment of both groups is also very similar. Both need special education and individual educational plans. Teaching and learning experiences are designed for remediation of the specific problems. The variety of techniques in teaching currently used are in accord with two major schools of thought, namely a Basic Ability Approach and the Direct Skills Approach. For children with generalized though mild mental retardation, however, the likelihood of ultimate success is reduced because of their multiplicity of delays in perceptual and cognitive areas.

Prevalence

Mental retardation is the most prevalent developmental disability in the United States, with 30 out of every 1000 persons affected. A prevalence ratio of 0.3 percent of our total population exists, which includes profound, severe, and moderate retardation. Retardation is frequently accompanied by other related disorders (physical and emotional), which may be severe enough to constitute handicaps in themselves. It is difficult to estimate the prevalence of developmental disabilities, owing to a lack of clear definitional criteria and poor data-recording procedures at all levels. The Education of All Handicapped Children Act, designed to provide equal educational opportunity for all children between ages 3 and 21, employs the term *special needs* in reference to the handicapped child.[5] National figures on the incidence of children with special needs may exceed 12.5 percent. It is estimated that there are in excess of 8 million handicapped children between the ages of 3 and 18 in the United States.[6] Estimates of handicapped individuals may range as high as 18.7 percent of the noninstitutionalized population between the ages of 18 and 64 years according to a document published in 1973 by the Urban Institute entitled *Report of the Comprehensive Needs Study.*[7]

If we include the immediate families of the developmentally disabled, the number of involved persons grows to more than 20 million. The problem touches a number of persons beyond calculation in the interactions of daily life.

HISTORICAL PERSPECTIVE

It has been said that the degree of civilization of any society may be judged by the way in which it provides for its handicapped members. Throughout history, attitudes toward the disabled populations have been reflected in the terminology employed and the services provided.

Before the nineteenth century, there is little information available about the problems of mental retardation. Hippocrates mentioned cranial malformations in his writings. The laws of Sparta and ancient Rome allowed for the extermination of severely retarded infants. Mental retardation and mental illness were viewed as similar until a clear distinction was made by John Locke in 1689.

The first humane approach to mental retardation coincided with the time of the French and the American revolutions. It was at this time that the first efforts to end inhumane treatment of both the mentally retarded and the mentally ill were made in France by Philippe Pinel, who advocated humane treatment for the mentally ill, and by J. M. G. Itard, who developed plans for the education and training of the mentally re-

tarded. Then, in the middle of the nineteenth century, J. J. Guggenbuhl of Switzerland first introduced the idea of institutional treatment for mental retardation. He made mental retardation a respectable field of medicine and educational endeavor.

In the United States in the early 1800s, the mentally ill and retarded resided with their families or, if lacking friends, were placed in poorhouses or jails. The Industrial Revolution saw an influx of immigrants into the country and a shift from rural society to urban areas. Aberrant behavior was looked upon as the result of the chaotic social, political, and economic environment of the times.

During the last half of the nineteenth century and early twentieth century, traditional social procedures were greatly stressed. Europe was heralding cures of insanity by caring for these individuals in residential institutions. Thus was developed the concept of "moral treatment," along with an increasing belief in the physical cause of deviant behaviors. Between 1850 and 1930, institutional care was defined as the most proper treatment method. Idiocy and feeble-mindedness were looked upon as societal problems created by such social errors as alcoholism and sexual perversion. Thus institutionalization was a protective mechanism for society and was assumed by professionals to be therapeutic for all inmates.

In the early 1900s, psychological testing became a mechanism by which to classify intellectual functioning. The educational system became a means of training for economic and civic roles. The educational approach was considered the appropriate treatment of social problems. However, this was not acceptable to some parents, who voiced loud disapproval on the basis of what was happening to their children in school. Schools had special classes that became classrooms for all categories of atypical children, i.e., the emotionally disturbed, the mentally retarded, delinquent children, and the physically handicapped. There was continued emphasis on the identification of individuals by labeling them with intelligence quotients. Labels conjure stereotypic pictures and do not allow for the vast range of individual differences found in the people so labeled. Thus, although the label may be necessary to allow data collection and to facilitate communication, it is dangerous in that it can lead people to interact with mentally retarded persons without any recognition of individual differences.

Crucial Discoveries

In the twentieth century, some crucial discoveries were made regarding the causes of mental retardation. A. E. Garrod's concept of the inborn errors of metabolism attracted medical curiosity and showed promise of possibilities to prevent or avoid the defective metabolic pathways. The genetic principles propounded by Gregor Mendel expanded the science of genetics. And I. A. Folling's discovery of phenylketonuria in 1935 paved the way for state legislation to perform PKU tests on all newborn infants. Other medical insights prompted improvement in obstetrical techniques, control of syphilis, and the Rh incompatibility factor.

The past 30 years have seen considerable progress in the biomedical and behavioral sciences toward new and more effective approaches in the care and education of handicapped persons. During the 1950s, groups of parents of retarded children joined forces to seek citizen rights and to create educational programs for the retarded. They organized the National Association for Retarded Citizens (the ARCs) in 1950. Through this association, advocacy is exerted at local and national levels. President John Kennedy in 1961 appointed the President's Panel on Mental Retardation, which identified a national need for services to the handicapped, for training of professionals, and for research in the field. Two years later in 1963, legislation was passed to implement many suggestions of the panel, and funds began to flow to the states for development of state and community programs and to finance demonstration service projects. In the 1980s emphasis has been placed on recognition of the handicapped as self-respecting and contributing members of the community eligible for the benefits of all citizens.

THE NURSING PROCESS

The effectiveness of the nurse requires an awareness of her attitude toward handicapped people. The psychodynamics of interaction with the patient are guided by a previously established value system that has developed through the incorporation of parental attitudes and teaching, education, life's experiences, religious beliefs, and the individual's ethnic and cultural milieu. Thus the nurse must work through her own feelings about human exceptionality. This involves an honest appraisal of personal attitudes and prejudices. This process usually requires direct involvement and personal experiences with persons with disabilities. Such insights are best achieved under the tutelage of a mentor.

As an exercise, place yourself in the following situation. How would you feel if you were assigned to care for a 14-year-old moderately retarded girl about to undergo surgical repair of scoliosis? What mental image of her appearance would come to mind? Would you be fearful of her? What mind-set would be most beneficial for this girl?

Early detection of developmental disabilities in children is essential to positive adaptation and prevention of secondary handicaps. Nurses as members of health care teams are in a position to detect difficulties early and to make referrals for more comprehensive evaluations. Identification is achieved through the mechanisms of screening and assessment.

Screening refers to a superficial assessment of a large population in regard to a specific problem area. For example, school nurses perform vision screening tests for classes of children at regular grade intervals and refer those with unsatisfactory results for ophthalmological examination. The criteria for screening are broad enough to encompass all individuals with suspected visual problems.

Assessment

The nursing assessment is the systematic collection of information to identify areas of strengths and weaknesses. It may refer to a broad general area, such as that of overall development, or to a small specific component, such as that of sleep patterns. The value of the assessment depends on the expertise of the professional in using assessment techniques and tools.

Ability to identify developmental lags and deviations is based on the nurse's having a working knowledge and understanding of normal patterns of growth and development. The sequence of growth is fairly stable and proceeds in a constant direction. However, each child has an individual velocity and pattern that must be monitored over time in order to determine if suspicion warrants concern.

Development is affected by both somatic

and environmental factors. This is represented by the concept of human ecology—the interaction of the young child with his environment.

The environment encompasses the persons interacting with the child and the area in which they (the child and relevant others) spend their time. Relationships and modes of interaction between parents and child are among the most important factors in the interactive environment. Intellectual abilities, financial status, and physical and mental health of the primary caretakers are other factors warranting assessment. This information provides a basis for conclusions regarding parent capability for meeting the developmental needs of a handicapped child.

A combination of several approaches is useful in the assessment of an individual's developmental progression and are listed below:

- Interview
- Behavioral observation
- Physical observation
- Testing tools

Skillful interviewing provides the nurse with important data about the individual and his environment. Parents are, as a rule, accurate reporters of their child's behavior. They are able to combine historical perspective with a wide variability of situational experiences. They are the ones who know their child best. Parents have usually tried a variety of solutions to the problem and have determined successes and failures. Most parents strive to sacrifice and meet their child's needs; thus in severe cases of developmental disability, their present concerns are truly beyond their coping ability.

Exploration should include information on the following areas:

Child	Sleep patterns
	Eating patterns
	Temperament
	Elimination patterns
	Play behavior
	Social-interactional behaviors
Family-Child	General health status
	Parental involvement with the child
	Sibling interactions
	Family supports
	Family stresses

Both formal and informal methods of observation yield information about relating and functional behaviors. Observation of the child and parents together provides assessment of interactions. Such observations are essential to an understanding of the parent–child relationship.

The following is an example of an informal observation:

Joey, 4 years old, and his mother are visiting for an annual health visit. Joey has one toy that he plays with but throws three times during the 20-minute visit. During the conversation he distracts his mother five times by seeking her attention. Her responses denote impatient hostility rather than guidance in acceptable behavior and a comforting acceptance of the situation.

The following is an example of a formal observation:

(This presents only a small sample of observations to be made during eating.) Observation of Joey's mealtime behaviors denotes information about the child's developmental skills. How does Joey approach the meal? What is his behavior over a 10- to 15-minute time span? How does he position himself? How does he use his body during eating? How does he use utensils for eating? What is the quality of language used?

Observation should include a systematic assessment of physical characteristics. Organic impairment will alter developmental progression in a variety of ways. The presence of physical symptoms, appearing singly or in combination with one another, requires additional assessment by the physician.

A variety of testing tools are available as aids for standardized assessment of developmental progress. These tools are useful in denoting progress or delay as well as areas of strength and weakness. They provide accurate judgments about behaviors observed. In addition, they are helpful in encouraging parents to maintain reasonable expectations for age and abilities. They act as a guide for planning strategies for an intervention or treatment plan.

The Denver Developmental Screening Tool is a standardized tool with acknowledged reliability and validity.[8] It yields a developmental profile of an infant or child in four areas: gross motor, language, fine motor, and personal-social skills. Results provide a quick visual picture of the child's strengths and weaknesses in each area. M. Erickson describes other tools in her book, *Assessment and Management of Developmental Changes in Children.*[9]

Diagnosis

A diagnosis of *mental retardation* is an event of great emotional trauma for parents. An interdisciplinary team assessment, including medical, psychological, neurological, nursing, and others, is crucial to providing the family and professionals complete information about the child as a basis for planning intervention strategies. The philosophical approach to imparting the diagnostic information will, in part, determine the parents' ability to cope with this difficult situation.

The timing of the diagnosis is important in understanding its impact. Retardation that is identified shortly after the birth of a baby comes at the culmination of the parents' psychological preparation for the arrival of a normal infant. During the course of pregnancy, the mother and father have developed an idealized mental image of their baby—one that is a composite of their creative dreams and ideals derived from past and present experiences. One of the early tasks of all parenting is to resolve the discrepancy between this idealized image of the infant and the real infant. This task is made more challenging when the baby is born with a physical or mental disability. Parents must simultaneously mourn the loss of the anticipated child and adapt to the real child.

The attachment of mother to infant begins prior to pregnancy, proceeds during the pregnancy, and continues actively during the postpartum period. Complex interactions including the events of the birth, seeing and touching the baby, and giving care help to bond this relationship. The infant is totally dependent on his care giver to meet his physical and emotional needs, and the strength and character of this relationship will influence his future attachments with other individuals and his personality structure.

Parental reactions and the degree of their difficulty in relating to their handicapped infant are dependent on the characteristics of the child's disabilities as perceived by the parent. If parents are told a diagnosis before becoming acquainted with their baby, their response may well be in terms of their stereotype of what the baby has, rather than what he is.

Emotional responses to the news of a handicapped baby progress through specific complex reactions, with each parent needing varying amounts of time to deal with the crisis. The course moves through shock, denial, sadness,

and anger, to equilibrium and reorganization. Although the process is similar among parents, it is highly individualized.

One cannot generalize about the impact a developmentally disabled child will make on his family. The variations in families, children, individual parents, and communities, and the myriad of interactions that result make generalizations invalid. Differences exist in parent's ability to accept and to care for the child. As time goes on, the acute emotional response to the diagnosis is modified to a long-lasting sorrow. This is described as "chronic sorrow" by S. Olshansky.[10] At times, repressed feelings surface that are symbolic to the individuals involved. The disabled child presents a new challenge to the family that will effect all family members. Therefore, this family group is called upon to develop strategies for coping with the variety of special issues which influence family life.

Parents seek truthful, accurate information presented in a sympathetic manner. There is no easy way to tell parents that their child has a problem, but an informed, compassionate attitude will convey the empathy one human can give another. The sensitive manner and caring atmosphere created by professionals during this period of intense anxiety will provide assistance to the family in coping with their feelings. Parents look to other significant people in their environment for support and information as well as for cues to appropriate feelings and behavior. It is important to relate something positive about the child in order to maintain hopefulness while realistically presenting the problem of what is wrong. Informing other family members is often of great concern as parents may feel inadequate or uncomfortable about sharing this information with loved ones. Professionals can assist by offering their counseling to others significantly involved with the family and child.

Nursing Plan

The art and expertise of nursing are a sound basis for interventive involvement with children with developmental disabilities and their families. The spectrum of interventions may include: the meaning of the crisis for the family, counseling regarding the diagnosis, providing parents ongoing teaching of the child's growth, development and health care needs, giving help in the planning of activities of daily care, relieving stress on the caretakers, and identifying program choices for the child.

Understanding the Nature of the Crisis for the Family

The presence of significant developmental delay in a young child has psychological implications for the parents. A crisis occurs in which feelings of loss are experienced for the child as formerly perceived and for any future expectations. A period of grief and mourning follow, during which the parents must deal with disappointment, anger, shame, and loneliness. Parents blame themselves for the child's situation. The social stigma of retardation reinforces many negative attitudes. The mystique of this handicap often causes families to experience social rejection. The parent then perceives her or himself as an unworthy person unacceptable to others. During this period of depression, the parents' relationship with the child may be strained. The parents may direct their energies inward and may withdraw, which may be demonstrated by a lack of support and warmth for the child. In this early emotional climate, it is most difficult for the child to develop a positive self-image. Children tend to integrate the early emotional climate into their permanent personality structure.

Counseling the Family Regarding the Diagnosis

Parents need acceptance of their feelings and supportive counseling toward regaining equilibrium. They also need to develop familiarity with the baby in order to foster a comfortable relationship and ability to care for their child. Their questions must be answered and information provided as they are ready to receive it. Assistance in locating suitable community resources is also necessary.

With time, families are able to focus on issues of the child's development. There will be a need for continuing evaluation of the child's developmental progress and guidance about appropriate objectives and the ways to achieve them.

For some children, the nature of a disability is not identified until after a period of apparently normal development. Mild retardation often goes unnoticed until the child enters school. Parents may have been unaware or denied subtle signs of developmental difficulties. They may have avoided situations that exposed the child's inability to behave in age-appropriate ways. Others may have denied the reality of their observations or devalued the effectiveness of their management of the child. The child may not have been exposed to opportunities to develop skills. Some parents may have placed a great deal of pressure on the child to perform. In desperation or frustration over the child's behavior, the parents will eventually seek professional consultation.

A considerable period of time will be required for most parents to adjust to the fact that their child has a severe impairment that will prevent him from assuming even limited self-care. The same responses as were described earlier are in operation with the initial reaction being a defensive mechanism of denial. This is followed by a period of confusion and frustration when the questions of why it happened and what it will mean for the future confront them. An opportunity for parents to develop a gradual awareness of the child's disability will avoid the uncomfortable situation of the professional attempting to convince the parents of their child's problem. The task is to aid the parents in becoming aware of their child's handicap. More recently, emphasis has been placed on assessment of the process of a child's development and guidance in supporting optimal patterns rather than waiting for an abnormal behavior to become established for a diagnosis. The framework of an active treatment program facilitates discussion of the individual's strengths and weaknesses.

Families whose members have learned to cope with the sorrow that came into their midst may find this to be an achievement that encourages mutual support and courage and fosters communication. Sharing and reliance on each other through many experiences can enrich members' ability to deal with all phases of life. There develops an acceptance of the quality of love for others and a belief in offering opportunity for all individuals to develop to their potential.

Providing Parents with Ongoing Teaching of the Child's Growth and Development

Parenting is a learned experience developed throughout life from observation and experiences of role models, namely, parents and friends. This interactive process is reciprocal and is based on a feedback situation of giving and responding. The parent gives to the child, who responds and thus reinforces the parent with feelings of success. Therefore, in the creation of a self-enhancing environment, parents need ongoing experiences that will give them feelings of adequacy.

For the average child, learning takes place quite spontaneously by responding to a variety of stimuli. Learning to play is a natural activity of the child, as can be noted in observing an infant enjoying movement of his arms and legs. The orderly cephalo-caudal progression of motor development, with advancement from gross skills to more refined motor ability, enables the child increasingly to explore and use his environment. Play with people and objects is the child's way of learning about the world. It offers opportunity for growth in understanding, in mastery of self, and in acquisition of skills.

The presence of impairments in areas affecting neurological, sensory, cognitive, or motor functioning causes alteration and delay of the learning process. Thus, the individual with mental retardation or multiple handicaps learns differently and at a slower rate than the average child. He requires special adaptation of developmental experiences in order to fulfill his potential for learning and achievement. The level of ultimate attainment will vary according to the type and degree of innate handicap and the suitability of learning opportunities that are provided. Much of the learning in early childhood takes place through imitation of the actions and responses of parents. For the disabled child, imitative learning takes place slowly. Tasks must be reduced to individual steps, steps that are demonstrated and practiced with as much repetition as needed. Parents and professionals may become discouraged with the slowness of achievement of major milestones, but progress is noted when focus is placed on small individual steps within the skill. As an example, consider the separate actions a child goes through when independently drinking from a cup:

- Orients to cup by looking at it.
- Reaches for cup.
- Touches cup.
- Grasps cup.
- Lifts cup.
- Delivers cup to mouth.
- Opens mouth.
- Places cup on lip.
- Opposes lip to rim of cup.
- Tips cup.
- Coordinates swallow and respiration.
- Tips cup from mouth.
- Returns cup to table.

Giving Help in Planning Activities of Daily Care

Providing daily care for the handicapped individual increases the emotional and physical burden on the caretakers. Some children will require nursing care procedures, i.e., gastrostomy feedings, adaptive equipment, ostomy care, and so forth. Parents will need to learn how to perform these special procedures. They will also need ongoing guidance in ways to handle and position children to maximize opportunities for learning from the environment, to facilitate comfort, and to promote good body movement. In addition to time required in giving care, more time is needed to make daily activities learning opportunities for the child or young adult. For example the 2-year-old who continues to require that the majority of nourishment be fed to him but developmentally is working on hand-to-mouth transfer needs experiences for encouraging this independent behavior. The retarded child will remain dependent on the care giver for protection for a long period of time. Protection must be provided from life-threatening physical problems, such as seizures or aspiration, or from dangers of the environment, such as for the mobile retarded child who is unable to perceive the dangers of traffic.

Relieving Stress on Caretakers

Caretakers are exposed to a great deal of stress with the amount of time expended and the energies required to care for the handicapped. There is little opportunity for self-actualization and relaxation. Parents attempt to meet all their children's needs and often end up with little time for themselves. Families at various stages have constraints on their mobility; for example, vacations must be planned around their "special needs" member. Sitters are often difficult to obtain, and respite programs continue to be limited. There is an increased financial burden that persists, and usually mothers do not have the freedom to work.

Parents frequently become advocates for this disabled member on all fronts. They must communicate their concerns and problems to a professional in order to learn about the service systems and to become aware of available resources. Professional responsibilities include informing parents and affording them options from which to choose what appears best for them. Individuals with handicaps are frequently bruised by public contacts, so parents comfort and shield the disabled one. Such incidents are continually used as opportunities to teach others acceptance of the disabled person. Public law mandates education for all children in the least restrictive environment, but parents are called upon to ensure that this is interpreted in the best interest of their child. Close coordination between school and home will ensure that objectives and management techniques are consistent, and parents can thus benefit from the expertise of the educator.

Progression from adolescence to adulthood includes the development of independence and gradual separation from parents. This process is far more difficult for the handicapped and requires special programming. The range of adult life-styles include independent living, marriage, or group living according to the individual's capabilities and desires. Options are continually broadening for the handicapped individual in these areas, but careful assessment, planning, and support are needed to ensure success. Parents can look to the future with anticipation that there is somewhere for their handicapped child to go where he may live and have the guidance or help needed.

Identifying Program Choices for the Child

Until the past decade, parents of children observed to have more severe disabilities at birth, i.e., Down's syndrome, hydrocephalus, etc., were counseled to place the child in an institution. Formerly, most thinking advocated avoiding becoming attached to the infant because life expectancy was limited, and the potential for the child becoming a rewarding family member was nearly impossible. Advances in medicine and research have proven this thinking incorrect. Modern trends in the approach to care are based on the premise that the disabled child will thrive best if treated as normally as possible. The former practice of placing a child in an institution has shifted to that of encouraging families to raise their child in the home environment with mainstreaming in the community. **Mainstreaming** means that services for the disabled should not be isolated from those available to normal individuals and should be provided under similar service structures as those for nonhandicapped whenever possible. The psychological and social well-being of the family is strengthened by accommodating to their child's needs. The goal is to provide the range of health, educational, and social programs available to normal individuals, but at the same time to provide supplementary assistance to alleviate the additional demands the handicapped child's care places on the family.

Although the family may successfully provide a nurturing environment for the individual, problems may arise in relation to the school and the community. Much education remains to be accomplished to effect changes in society's attitude of rejection of the handicapped. Public education is mandated for "special needs children," but difficulties continue in trying to achieve comfortable social acceptance by teachers and peers. There continues to be difficulty in gaining residences for the retarded in the community. Families are faced with recurring issues of community rejection and emotional hurts. Some parents withdraw from social relationships, and others have found much support from contacts with other parents of handicapped children or parent organizations. Such organizations have impacted on national policy as well as helped obtain local community services.

Evaluation

In the nursing approach to planning care for the handicapped child within the home, an effective conceptual framework considers the total family's needs. Focus must be on the identification of the needs of the family and the needs of the child, with intervention incorporating a feasible approach to each need. Family, parents, and child will require various supports with this life-long problem.

Children are unique, but they all have the same basic needs for physical, social, mental, and emotional growth. Like all children, the retarded child bears the traits of his parents, has an individual personality, and requires the nurturance of a loving, warm environment. Like all persons, the retarded need to experience acceptance, understanding, and love.

The evaluation component of the nursing plan continually looks at the goals jointly identified by the family and by the nurse to assess the effectiveness of the plan. Sufficient time should be allowed in counseling to carefully review the goals established and to revise them as needed. This process must be in conjunction with ongoing assessment of the child's developmental progression by a professional with expertise in developmental disabilities.

Prevention

Nurses play a vital role in primary prevention through health education, which includes sex education, family planning, prevention of gynecologic infectious diseases, and emphasis on adequate prenatal and obstetrical care. Research is continually suggesting the complex dimensions of the relationship of the prevention of developmental delay and the preconceptual, prenatal, and perinatal periods of development. Nurses take responsibility in health care programs for nutrition, immunization, and environmental modification. There is provision of nutritional information and guidance to families. Immunizations prevent disabling conditions that can result from childhood infections. Through health teaching, families are taught sound health practices and concepts of environmental stimulation.

Nurses participating in well-child care settings are in the position to discover developmental delays through systematic assessment of development and planned screening programs. Thus, by means of early identification, treatment programs can be instituted to enhance the developmental potential of the child. Children may risk developmental delay because of an environment that is not conducive to growth and development. The nurse's role is one of case finding, contributing to assessment and treatment plans, and referring for evaluation.

Summary

This chapter has presented an overview of current knowledge in the area of developmental disabilities including attention to underlying causes, prevention, diagnosis, and treatment. The chapter has emphasized understanding of the impact upon the involved individual and his family as a basis for nursing interventions.

Questions

1. Compute the I.Q. of a child age 12 who has achieved a mental age of 8.
2. What parallels and dissimilarities are there in the history of the fields of mental retardation and mental illness?
3. What feelings must families face when a child is diagnosed to have developmental delay?
4. What primary prevention interventions in mental retardation are ongoing in your community?
5. Define the term *learning disability*.

REFERENCES AND SUGGESTED READINGS

1. Rehabilitation Comprehensive Services and Developmental Disabilities Amendments of 1978, PL 95–602. Washington, D.C.: U.S. Government Printing Office, 1978.
2. Ibid.
3. Donaldson, J. Y., & Menolascino, F. J. Past, current, and future roles of child psychiatry in mental retardation. *Journal of American Academy of Child Psychiatry*, 1977, 16, 38.
4. Syzmanski, L. S. Emotional problems in a child with serious developmental handicap. In M. D. Levine, W. Carey, A. Crocker, & R. Gross (Eds.), *Developmental–Behavioral Pediatrics*. Philadelphia: Saunders, 1983.

5. Menolascino, F. *Challenge in Mental Retardation: Progressive Ideology and Services*. New York: Human Sciences Press, 1977.
6. Tarjan, G., et al. Natural history of mental retardation: Some aspects of epidemiology. *American Journal of Mental Deficiencies*, 1973, 77, 369–379.
7. Education of All Handicapped Children Act, PL 94–142. Washington, D.C.: U.S. Government Printing Office, 1975.
8. Frankenberg, W. R., & Camp, B. (Eds.), *Pediatric Screening Test*. Springfield, Ill.: Charles C. Thomas, 1975.
9. Erikson, M. *Assessment and Management of Developmental Changes in Children*. St. Louis: Mosby, 1978.
10. Olshansky, S. Chronic sorrow: A response to having a mentally defective child. *Social Casework*, 1962, 43, 190–193.

Chapter *46*

Personality Disorders

Ann Wolbert Burgess

Chapter Objectives

The students successfully attaining the goals of this chapter will be able to:

- Identify uses of the term *personality disorder* as it has been used over the decades.
- Differentiate personality traits from personality disorders.
- List behavioral characteristics of the 11 types of personality disorders.
- Explain why people with personality disorders, especially borderline personalities, have difficulty changing their behavior through psychotherapy.
- Plan nursing care, using nursing diagnoses, for the various personality disorders.

Personality traits are the well developed and relatively stable patterns of behavior, cognitive skills, and variations of mood and attitudes that define an individual. Personality traits differentiate one person from another. They determine how one appears, how one behaves, how one is liked and judged by others, and what one accomplishes in life. These traits have evolved over years of living. Their essential function is defensive. Thus, they also may be called character defenses.

Clusters of personality traits are referred to as personality styles or types. When these traits or styles repetitively limit the attempts and potential for mastery, disrupt interpersonal relationships, fail to balance independence, depen-

dence, and autonomy, or bring to bear insufficient moral parameters in human interactions a diagnosis of personality disorder is given an individual. Whereas the flexible, resourceful, and healthy person fails under conditions of severe stress (e.g., harsh adversity, major illness, significant trauma), a person with a personality disorder fails in an average environment.[1]

Historically, the psychiatric diagnosis of "personality disorder" or, alternatively, "character disorder" has been used in a variety of ways[2]:

- Descriptively (e.g., the histrionic character as overexcitable, dramatic, labile, and suggestible).

- To connote a stage of psychosexual development (e.g., oral character).
- To convey negative social qualities (e.g., delinquent personality, sociopathic personality).
- To emphasize degree of impairment (e.g., psychotic character, inadequate personality).
- To describe behavioral subtypes (e.g., addictive personality).
- To highlight the persistence of affects (e.g., depressive character).
- To imply specific patterns of object relations and ego skills or the lack of them (e.g., borderline personality, narcissistic personality).

Normal character development organizes and delimits perceptions and experience, provides mechanisms for the seeking of new experience, and integrates the new experience with past and current instinctual needs. The result is an expanding capacity for both the safety and gratification of the individual. In normal personalities, there is a balance of risk taking, searching, integrating, restricting, and consolidating elements. At different times of life and under different conditions, different elements predominate but all elements remain functional.

With nonnormative or pathological character development, both the balance and the elements are maladaptive. The result is that specific coping defenses are used to excess, and they tend to constrict or exaggerate the functioning of the individual. This distinction provides a general framework to better understand the personality disorders, which are classified on axis II of the *DSM-III-R*, and provide a basis for planning nursing care.

Traditionally, clinicians have diagnosed personality disorders in terms of a single specific disorder. The *DSM-III-R* offers a marked departure from this prior position by stating that since many individuals exhibit features that are not limited to a single disorder, more than one disorder diagnosis may be made if the individual meets the criteria for more than one.[3]

This chapter will discuss the psychiatric diagnosis classification system of personality disorders in three major clusters:

Cluster A　Paranoid, schizoid, and schizotypal.
Cluster B　Antisocial, borderline, histrionic, and narcissistic.
Cluster C　Avoidant, dependent, obsessive–compulsive, and passive–aggressive.

PARANOID PERSONALITY DISORDER

The diagnosis of paranoid personality disorder is given to the person in whom there is an unwarranted and pervasive suspiciousness and mistrust of people, hypersensitivity, and restricted affect. There is a constant search by this individual for confirmation of the idea that particular people, or all people, will betray him or otherwise do harm. Evidence to the contrary is likely to be ignored. Our society makes an attitude of suspicion justified and adaptive in certain situations; however, the flexible person is willing to abandon such suspicions when presented with convincing evidence to the contrary. The paranoid personality ignores such evidence and may even become suspicious of the person presenting the evidence and challenging the beliefs.

People with paranoid personality styles may be either shy, seclusive, furtive, and frightened of involvement, or they may be aggressive, ambitious, outwardly hostile, and arrogant. Whatever variation we see, these individuals spend a great deal of their energy searching for clues that will confirm to them that danger is forever lurking. They seem particularly prone to hurts and humiliations. They tend to avoid blame even when it is warranted. They are viewed by others as secretive, devious, guarded, and scheming. They may question the loyalty of others, always expecting trickery, and for this reason there may be pathological jealousy.

These individuals may exaggerate situations, making "mountains out of molehills." They frequently are argumentative, find it difficult to relax, are critical of others, have great difficulty accepting criticism themselves, and may be litigious. Because their affect is restrictive, they may appear cold, odd, or eccentric. They have no sense of humor and are usually serious. Their perception of themselves is that they are objective, rational, and unemotional, and indeed they usually lack warm, tender, and sentimental feelings.

There is a preoccupation with the need to be in control and to have power. Thus, any threat to this need is met with hostility and defensiveness. They are keenly aware of power and rank and who is superior and who is inferior, and they may be jealous of those in power. A major area where maladaptive patterns are noted is in the workplace. Occupational difficulties are common, especially in relating to authority figures and coworkers.

The following list of diagnostic criteria is from the *DSM-III-R*[4]:

Diagnostic Criteria for Paranoid Personality Disorder

A. A pervasive and unwarranted tendency, beginning by early adulthood and present in a variety of contexts, to interpret the actions of people as deliberately demeaning or threatening, as indicated by at least four of the following:
    1. Expects, without sufficient basis, to be exploited or harmed by others
    2. Questions, without justification, the loyalty or trustworthiness of friends or associates
    3. Reads hidden demeaning or threatening meanings into benign remarks or events, e.g., suspects that a neighbor put out trash early to annoy him
    4. Bears grudges or is unforgiving of insults or slights
    5. Is reluctant to confide in others because of unwarranted fear that the information will be used against him
    6. Is easily slighted and quick to react with anger or to counterattack
    7. Questions, without justification, fidelity of spouse or sexual partner

The above list of criteria is provided to help the nurse understand some of the paranoid behaviors that may be expected in clinical situations. Slight rejections and inadvertent oversights on the part of the nurse as well as the feeling of vulnerability that is part of being hospitalized as a patient may precipitate an array of paranoid behaviors. These may take the form of inappropriate anger, threats of revenge, threats of litigations, claims that the nurse is like "all the others," and proclamations of self-righteousness. In this way, the patient exaggerates his main ego defense—projection—and projects all of the perceived badness into the world. Pathological behaviors of paranoid patients may be minimized by avoiding situations in which the patient feels that his autonomy is threatened or in which he feels trapped. Whenever possible, the nurse should not try to control the patient's freedom of choice and movement, nor should the nurse argue or reassure the patient. Instead, the nurse should strive to be a safe person who does not take sides so that the patient may have the opportunity to begin to break out of his psychological isolation.

SCHIZOID PERSONALITY DISORDER

The schizoid personality is characterized by a tendency to withdraw from others, a chronic sense of loneliness, and a subjective sense of emptiness. These patients may be very aware of their intense need for people, and they may fear that their needs, if expressed, will overwhelm and hurt the other person. They maintain distance in order to protect themselves from rejection, to protect the other person from their own aggression, and to protect themselves from the feared aggression of others. Schizoid patients may also describe excruciating feelings of discomfort when someone attempts to be close, kind, warm, or affectionate. Many of these patients never marry. They obtain solitary jobs in which there is barely enough interpersonal contact to sustain them. They may feel comfortable dealing with other people by telephone, correspondence, or through brief and fleeting contacts. The *DSM-III-R* lists the following criteria for schizoid personality disorder[5]:

Diagnostic Criteria for Schizoid Personality Disorder

A. A pervasive pattern of indifference to social relationships and restricted range of emotional experience and expression, beginning by early adulthood and present in a variety of contexts, as indicated by at least four of the following:
    1. Neither desires nor enjoys close relationships, including being part of a family
    2. Almost always chooses solitary activities
    3. Rarely, if ever, claims or appears to experience strong emotions, such as anger and joy
    4. Indicates little if any desire to have sexual experiences with another person (age being taken into account)
    5. Is indifferent to the praise and criticism of others

6. Has no close friends or confidants (or only one) other than first-degree relatives
7. Displays constricted affect, e.g., is aloof, cold, rarely reciprocates gestures or facial expressions, such as smiles or nods

Schizoid persons may seek treatment after they have been completely isolated from their few sustaining contacts or after they have been overwhelmed by the intensity of a close relationship. They are likely to present with depressive symptoms characterized by an empty, hungry quality. Often these patients resort to drugs, alcohol, or excessive food, which may be regarded as depressive equivalents.

In the nursing intervention, the nurse needs to be ever mindful of the patient's need for human contact on one hand and his need for respectful distance on the other. A delicate balance must be maintained. Some patients respond to a one-to-one interpersonal contact in which they learn that there is more pleasure than fright in a relationship. Thus, the nurse–patient relationship may be an instructive and correctional experience for the patient. For others, group therapies or occupational therapy may be more useful. It is essential that there is interdisciplinary planning for the overall intervention with the person diagnosed with schizoid personality disorder.

SCHIZOTYPAL PERSONALITY DISORDER

The essential features of the diagnosis of schizotypal personality disorder include various oddities in thought, perception, speech, and behavior that are not severe enough to meet the criteria for schizophrenia. Rather than a single feature to this disorder, there are multiple features. The disturbance in the content of thought may be noted through magical thinking, ideas of reference, or paranoid ideation. Perceptual disturbances are noted through recurrent illusions, depersonalization, or derealization; marked peculiarities of speech; and concepts presented in odd ways. There is social isolation and constricted affect, which is noted in face-to-face encounters.

The *DSM-III-R* lists the following criteria for this disorder[6]:

Diagnostic Criteria for Schizotypal Personality Disorder

A. A pervasive pattern of deficits in interpersonal relatedness and peculiarities of ideation, appearance, and behavior, beginning by early adulthood and present in a variety of contexts, as indicated by at least five of the following:
1. Ideas of reference (excluding delusions of reference)
2. Excessive social anxiety, e.g., extreme discomfort in social situations involving unfamiliar people
3. Odd beliefs, or magical thinking, influencing behavior and inconsistent with subcultural norms, e.g., superstitiousness, belief in clairvoyance, telepathy, or "sixth sense," "others can feel my feelings" (in childhood and adolescence, bizarre fantasies or preoccupations)
4. Unusual perceptual experiences, e.g., illusions, sensing the presence of a force or person not actually present (e.g., "I felt as if my dead mother were in the room with me")
5. Odd or eccentric behavior or appearance, e.g., unkempt, unusual mannerisms, talks to self
6. No close friends or confidants (or only one) other than first-degree relatives
7. Odd speech (without loosening of associations or incoherence), e.g., speech that is impoverished, digressive, vague, or inappropriately abstract
8. Inappropriate or constricted affect, e.g., silly, aloof, rarely reciprocates gestures or facial expressions, such as smiles or nods
9. Suspiciousness or paranoid ideation

ANTISOCIAL PERSONALITY DISORDER

In the diagnosis of antisocial personality disorder, there is a history of continuous and chronic antisocial behavior in which the rights of others are violated. This behavior begins before age 15 and there frequently is failure in sustaining good job performance. Early childhood signs include lying, stealing, fighting, truancy, and resisting authority. In adolescence there is unusually early or aggressive sexual behavior, drinking, and use of drugs. The diagnostic criteria are listed below[7]:

Diagnostic Criteria for Antisocial Personality Disorder

A. Current age at least 18
B. Evidence of conduct disorder with onset before age 15, as indicated by a history of three or more of the following:
   1. Was often truant
   2. Ran away from home overnight at least twice while living with parent or in surrogate home (or once without returning)
   3. Often initiated physical fights
   4. Used a weapon in more than one fight
   5. Forced someone into sexual activity with him or her
   6. Was physically cruel to animals
   7. Was physically cruel to other people
   8. Deliberately destroyed others' property (other than by fire setting)
   9. Deliberately engaged in fire setting
   10. Often lied (other than to avoid physical or sexual abuse)
   11. Has stolen without confrontation of a victim on more than one occasion (including forgery)
   12. Has stolen with confrontation of a victim (e.g., mugging, purse snatching, extortion, armed robbery)
C. A pattern of irresponsible and antisocial behavior since the age of 15, as indicated by at least four of the following:
   1. Is unable to sustain consistent work behavior, as indicated by any of the following (including similar behavior in academic settings if the person is a student);
      a. Significant unemployment for 6 months or more within 5 years when expected to work and work was available
      b. Repeated absences from work unexplained by illness in self or family
      c. Abandonment of several jobs without realistic plans for others
   2. Fails to conform to social norms with respect to lawful behavior, as indicated by repeatedly performing antisocial acts that are grounds for arrest (whether arrested or not), e.g., destroying property, harassing others, stealing, pursuing an illegal occupation
   3. Is irritable and aggressive, as indicated by repeated physical fights or assaults (not required by one's job or to defend someone or oneself), including spouse- or child-beating
   4. Repeatedly fails to honor financial obligations, as indicated by defaulting on debts or failing to provide child support or support for other dependents on a regular basis
   5. Fails to plan ahead, or is impulsive, as indicated by one or both of the following:
      a. Traveling from place to place without a prearranged job or clear goal for the period of travel or clear idea about when the travel will terminate
      b. Lack of a fixed address for a month or more
   6. Has no regard for the truth, as indicated by repeated lying, use of aliases, or "conning" others for personal profit or pleasure
   7. Is reckless regarding his own or others' personal safety, as indicated by driving while intoxicated, or recurrent speeding
   8. If a parent or guardian, lacks ability to function as a responsible parent, as indicated by one or more of the following:
      a. Malnutrition of child
      b. Child's illness resulting from lack of minimal hygiene
      c. Failure to obtain medical care for a seriously ill child
      d. Child's dependence on neighbors or nonresident relatives for food or shelter
      e. Failure to arrange for a caretaker for young child when parent is away from home
      f. Repeated squandering, on personal items, of money required for household necessities
   9. Has never sustained a totally monogamous relationship for more than 1 year
   10. Lacks remorse (feels justified in having hurt, mistreated, or stolen from another)

BORDERLINE PERSONALITY ORGANIZATION

There is a group of patients, referred to as *borderline*, who lie on the diagnostic continuum between normal personality organization and psychotic personality organization. From one perspective they have many of the strengths of the neurotic patient, but on more careful examination they appear sicker. From another perspective these patients may appear at times to be seriously ill (like the schizophrenic patient), only to surprise the observer with their many strengths. Because of such apparent contradictions, these patients have troubled psychiatric nurses in terms of planning intervention and care.

There are several reasons why there has been attention focused on the personality disorders defined as borderline. First, the use of psychiatric medications has reduced the flagrant schizophrenic symptoms and has transferred attention to a large group of generally nonpsychotic but nonetheless severely impaired patients. Second, the conceptual expansion of personality disorders by fixation at libidinal stages to classification by ego defenses and object relations has widened the range of borderline diagnosis.

From a broad clinical perspective, borderline patients may differ from neurotic and schizophrenic patients in the following ways.

1. When there is regression to psychosis, the regression is relatively brief (a few days to a few weeks), and the patient then returns to his usual normal level of functioning.
2. There is a stability to the chaotic nature of the patient's functioning. In other words, what appears to be chaos is a part of the patient's life-style.
3. The patient is usually very demanding in interpersonal relationships and has exaggerated disappointment reactions to relatively minor frustrations.
4. The depression and anger are not usually a part of an acute depressive reaction but are a pervasive part of the patient's character.

In 1959 a research team began a study of the ego functions of borderline patients at the Illinois State Psychiatric Institute. In this study the overall characteristics of the borderline syndrome were defined as follows[8]:

1. Anger constitutes the main affect the border patient experiences. This affect is directed at a variety of targets.
2. The border patient characteristically has difficulty in his social and personal relationships.
3. There is an absence of consistent and positive self-identity. This trait is probably re-

lated to the lack of consistent and affectional relationships. Anger tends to be a defense against closeness in a relationship.
4. Depression and feelings of loneliness are present. The difficulty in achieving satisfactory interpersonal relationships makes the patient prone to loneliness.

The Ego Defense of Splitting

The major ego defense in borderline personalities is *splitting*, which is a primitive and ineffective intrapsychic mechanism. Change and ambivalence cannot be managed. The concept of splitting has a long and complex history in the field of mental health. Common themes in the clinical literature indicate that splitting has been described in various ways:

• As alternating states of dual consciousness in histrionic patients.
• As detachment from reality in psychotic patients.
• As dissociation of true and false selves in the schizoid individual.
• As defensive separation of gratifying and frustrating experiences of the self and others by the developing infant that may persist into adulthood.

Splitting leads to a division of external objects into "all bad" and "all good" categories, with a consequent inability to view objects as having mixtures of good and bad qualities. To the individual using extensive splitting, the world seems populated by devils and angels but devoid of truly human figures. Extreme devaluation and idealization of others follow from this, as do shifts from one extreme view to another. This marked use of splitting leads to chaotic interpersonal relationships, characterized by unpredictability and instability.

The division of external objects into mutually exclusive, totally good and bad categories plays havoc with cognitive processes involved in decision making. Certain options are recklessly exercised, only to be later vehemently rejected; other choices are readily abandoned with much subsequent regret. Relationships are suddenly broken, only to be mended the next day. Hospitals are left against medical advice, only to be voluntarily reentered. Plans for self-improvement are made with great enthusiasm (i.e., giving up smoking), only to be neglected.

In addition to the inability to experience ambivalence and the problem of impaired decision making, there is oscillation of self-esteem. Splitting produces mutual dissociation of the self-representations formed under loving and depriving influences in the early formative years. Individuals who use extensive splitting may feel despicably worthless when faced with a narcissistic injury or a realistic setback. Subsequent positive external events may quickly turn this negative self-appraisal into a view of the self as superior, lovable, and outstanding. These two contradictory feelings, which are experienced with comparable conviction, remain separate and are not assimilated into a more realistic and somewhat ambivalent view of the self.

Splitting may also cause a peculiar disturbance of impulse control seen in narcissistic and borderline patients. Their impulsive actions are ego-syntonic, and even pleasurable, at the time of their occurrence. Moreover, these actions produce little subsequent guilt, only a bland denial of their emotional significance. Many instances of promiscuity, kleptomania, and substance abuse represent such splitting.

The lack of fusion of libidinal and aggressive drives inherent in the mechanism of splitting leads to dissociation of their corresponding affects. Anger, for instance, is experienced only as rage; and murderous and suicidal impulses readily surface in response to frustration. Concomitantly, clinical observation of individuals in whom splitting is the central defensive mechanism has revealed the capacity of these individuals for profound exhilarating happiness under favorable circumstances. Splitting may also lead to passionate awe, infatuations, and worshipping idealization.

Splitting is a central defense seen in borderline, narcissistic, schizoid, and antisocial personality disorders. These disorders are clinically characterized by the presence of contradictory self-representations, the inability to tolerate ambivalence, chaotic interpersonal relationships, intense affects, and continued conscious involvement with childhood conflicts. Discomfort comes from erroneous basic assumptions about the self and others. Such patients are unlike those with compulsive, histrionic, dependent, and avoidant character disorders whose defenses center around repression. The latter demonstrate a cohesive identity, ambivalent but stable interpersonal relationships, muted affects, and elimination of childhood conflicts from conscious awareness by means of repression. Dis-

comfort, when present, is related to symbolically disguised derivatives of the unconscious drives and prohibitions.

Symptom Picture of Borderline Patients

The patient's *mood* is typically angry and complaining. Underlying this defensive posture is anxiety and depression. Reports by the individual of prolonged periods of happiness or gratification is lacking and even pleasant past experiences are reported in a distorted manner as unfulfilling.

Often, the behavior of the individual is impulsive and erratic, although there may be superficial efforts to be effective in social situations. The impulsive behavior, which includes drug or alcohol abuse or suicidal gestures, is often in the service of the following personality functions:

- To direct or organize part of the patient's experience that otherwise seems drifting and undirected.
- To temporarily relieve highly dysphoric affect.
- To manipulate others.

The person's *cognitive* area—both the ability to organize experience and to judge, perceive, and integrate an experience—is impaired. Those borderline-diagnosed persons who maintain consistent work usually do so under highly organized conditions. Generally, it is quite difficult for such individuals to organize themselves and follow through on their own approaches. School difficulties and short-term employment records are common.

The person may behave in bland, nondescript style. Negative and positive affect may be absent, and the person takes cues from other people in an attempt to relate by assuming a complementary role. This individual behaves as expected; the role vacillates depending on the other person to whom he adapts. He often feels no personal identity. The following case example deals with the type of personality presenting in this bland, nondescript style.

CASE EXAMPLE

A young man presented himself at a walk-in clinic with the complaint that he felt he was going to fail in his college courses. This student was the nephew of a prominent bishop and came from a famous family of clergymen. Whenever he was asked in therapy how he felt, he would say "My uncle, the bishop, said this or someone said that." The question of his feelings would never be answered because he really did not know how he felt about himself. Therapy focused on helping the student gain a positive identity.

Psychotic Symptoms

Borderline persons may also become psychotic. Psychoses in borderline patients tend to be stress-related, reversible, transient, ego-alien, without systematic or organized delusion systems, and usually do not include hallucinations. Generally, one can see the psychosis on admission or when the person is in the stressful situation (e.g., during an interview or in a family therapy session). Patients in this group show inappropriate and negative behavior toward other people. They may sleep and eat erratically and become careless about their personal grooming. Anger comes out in explosive ways and depression is present.

Self-Image

The self-image of the borderline person fluctuates between a highly exaggerated self-esteem and feelings of worthlessness, although the former is more likely to be verbalized. The feeling of entitlement is strong; that is, the person feels entitled to what he wishes, and he blames others for a lack of fulfillment. With such a view, the person may perceive himself as a "chronic victim" (e.g., "bad things always happen to me"). The person also sees himself as vulnerable, especially to being abandoned.

Interpersonal Relationships

In the interpersonal relationship area, the individual is oriented toward what others can do for him, particularly for comfort and nurturance. Frequently, there is a rapid, overidealized, clinging quality brought to new relationships, followed by an equally rapid disappointment when the needs are not met. This disappointment brings forth anger and rage. The following case example illustrates a nursing student's assessment and care plan with specific emphasis on the relationship issue.

The *DSM-III-R* lists behavioral patterns that are the product of an amalgamation of symptoms and signs reported to be key features of the disorder. The essential feature in a person-

ality disorder is instability in a variety of areas, including interpersonal behavior, mood, and self-image.[9] No single feature is invariably present. Interpersonal relations are often intense and unstable, with marked shifts of attitude over time. Frequently there is impulsive and unpredictable behavior that is potentially physically self-damaging. Mood is often unstable, with marked shifts from a normal to a dysphoric mood or with inappropriate intense anger or lack of control of anger. There is a profound identity disturbance about several issues relating to self-image, gender identity, or long-term goals or values. There may be problems tolerating being alone and chronic feelings of emptiness or boredom.

The following list of diagnostic criteria is taken from the *DSM-III-R*, as is the psychiatric diagnosis that follows the case example.[10]

Diagnostic Criteria for Borderline Personality Disorder

A. Pervasive pattern of instability of mood, interpersonal relationships, and self-image, beginning by early adulthood and present in a variety of contexts, as indicated by at least five of the following:
  1. A pattern of unstable and intense interpersonal relationships characterized by alternating between extremes of overidealization and devaluation
  2. Impulsiveness in at least two areas that are potentially self-damaging, e.g., spending, sex, substance use, shoplifting, reckless driving, binge eating. (Do not include suicidal or self-mutilating behavior covered in 5.)
  3. Affective instability: marked shifts from base-line mood to depression, irritability, or anxiety, usually lasting a few hours and only rarely more than a few days
  4. Inappropriate, intense anger or lack of control of anger, e.g., frequent displays of temper, constant anger, recurrent physical fights
  5. Recurrent suicidal threats, gestures, or behavior, or self-mutilating behavior
  6. Marked and persistent identity disturbance manifested by uncertainty about at least two of the following: self-image, sexual orientation, long-term goals or career choice, type of friends desired, preferred values

7. Chronic feelings of emptiness or boredom

8. Frantic efforts to avoid real or imagined abandonment. (Do not include suicidal or self-multilating behavior covered in 5.)

CASE EXAMPLE

Ms. Simon is a 54-year-old divorced woman who comes from an upper middle-class family. She has had an extensive past history of psychiatric difficulties, beginning when she was in her mid-teens. She also has a history of alcoholism, although she has not been drinking for the past 3 years. She is also tobacco-dependent. Her psychiatric diagnosis is borderline personality disorder. She has attempted suicide several times by overdosing on one or more of her medications, on which she is dependent. She was hospitalized for 5 weeks on a psychiatric inpatient unit of a university hospital following a suicide attempt.

The nursing student made an initial visit with Ms. Simon prior to her return home. At this visit it was learned that Ms. Simon was married briefly, less than a year, and that the divorce was initiated by the husband due to the "terrible temper tantrums" of the wife. Ms. Simon was employed for short periods of time in the health care field. For the past 20 years, she has been living with her father. Ms. Simon was verbal during the interview, initiating much of the conversation and talking of her complaints of the hospital. In a 15-minute time span she smoked five cigarettes. Two problems she identified included: (1) her not getting out of the hospital as quickly as she had anticipated, and (2) her difficulty sleeping through the night.

She wanted to have sleeping medication but was aware that her physician would not approve additional medication. She asked the student to intervene on her behalf and ask the physician for the medication. Ms. Simon also told the student of past agoraphobia panic attacks, which she described experiencing whenever she would go outside.

Psychiatric and nursing diagnoses and case formulation are listed below.

NURSING CARE PLAN
Borderline Personality Disorder

HUMAN RESPONSE

1. Impulsivity or unpredictability (spending, sex, gambling, substance use, shoplifting, overeating, self-destructive acts).
   Patient example: Suicide attempts, prior substance abuse, and tobacco dependence.
2. Unstable interpersonal relationships (i.e., marked by manipulative behavior, dependency, and fluctuation between idealization and devaluation of the other).
   Patient example: Marital conflict and divorce.
3. Inappropriate, intense anger or lack of control of anger (temper displays).
   Patient example: Ex-husband's description of temper tantrums.
4. Identity disturbance.
   Patient example: Unstable work history despite college education and health care training.
5. Affective instability (mood shifts, irritability, anxiety).
   Patient example: Reported temper outbursts.
6. Intolerance of being alone.
   Patient example: Living in parental home; unstable work history.
7. Physically self-damaging acts.
   Patient example: History of suicidal attempts.
8. Chronic feelings of emptiness or boredom.
   Patient example: Work history; complaints to nursing student.

NURSING DIAGNOSES

- Impaired reality testing.
- Impaired interpersonal relationships.
- Alteration in mood and affect.
- Alteration in self-concept.
- Potential for violence (self).
- Alteration in energy.

GOALS

1. The patient will be able to verbalize an understanding of her destructive, impulsive, or unpredictable behavior. The patient will show an increased tolerance for frustration and an improvement in impulse control. The patient will begin to behave in ways that are socially more acceptable.
2. The patient can identify development of new nonchaotic relationships. The patient can identify that she cannot manipulate staff. Staff conferences are held routinely for planning patient care.
3. The patient will demonstrate an increased ability to identify her feelings of anger. The patient will seek assistance in dealing with her anger in a constructive manner.
4. Patient will verbalize difficulties in new relationships. The patient strengthens and lengthens interpersonal relationships.
5. Positive reinforcement strengthens ego capacity.
6. The patient will express a more positive view of self, as well as begin to identify differences between herself and others.
7. The patient will demonstrate improved reality testing as well as an increased willingness to accept responsibility for her own behavior. Patient can explain unit rules and rationale. Patient can articulate the unit rules.

INTERVENTIONS

1. Observe the patient's behavior and document in summary form daily and prn. Let the patient know when her behavior is viewed inappropriate. Assist the patient in identifying alternative behaviors that are more acceptable socially. Spend time daily with the patient to facilitate verbalization of her feelings. Assist the patient with gaining control of her behavior (i.e., by removing her from stress-producing situations. Develop a mutual written contract with the patient, negotiating appropriate and inappropriate behavior. Administer appropriate psychotropic medications and observe and record the effects of same. Use seclusion (and restraints) if necessary to prevent the patient from harming self or others. Also, see standard on Care of the Suicidal Patient.
2. Assist the patient in identifying her expectation of self and others and in evaluating how realistic such expectations are. Assist the patient in examining her own behavior and in evaluating the extent to which this contributes to her relationship difficulties. Develop and implement a coordinated, consistent staff approach to the care of the patient. Schedule regular staff conferences to evaluate plan of care and to reduce the effects of attempts by the patient to split the staff and create conflict among personnel. Spend time with the patient daily to facilitate verbalization of her feelings. Staff should identify own reactions to patient. Work with the patient's family or significant others to assist them in understanding the psychopathology so that they are better able to aid in the recovery process.
3. Assist patient in identifying her feelings. Encourage verbalization of anger within reason. Assist the patient in channeling her anger in a more constructable manner (e.g., use punching bag). Set limits verbally on the patient's behavior. Provide a consistent, supportive and firm approach to the patient's care. Control environmental stimuli according to the patient's needs and emotional status. Administer appropriate psychotropic medications and note effects of same. Use seclusion and/or restraints to decrease environmental stimuli and control angry behavior.
4. Observe patterns of interaction between the patient and others in her environment. Provide realistic, positive reinforcement to the patient when behavior is deemed

appropriate. Explain and reinforce unit policies to the patient and encourage her understanding of same. Verbalizing feelings assists in mastery of self-image.

5. Provide a consistent, supportive, and firm approach to care. Explain the rules of the unit to the patient, wait for her to verbalize understanding of same, and reinforce as necessary. Reinforce reality to the patient in a nonthreatening manner. Recognize and discuss the use of impaired coping behavior and explore alternatives to same. Have the patient assume responsibility for her own physical care and self needs, to the fullest extent possible. Discuss the patient's responsibilities for her own behavior in observed interactions with others as well as in unit activities.

6. Establish a trusting nurse–patient relationship. Allow the patient to verbalize her feelings within reason. Give positive feedback to the patient for tasks accomplished and for the use of appropriate behaviors.

7. Set firm and clear limits on unacceptable behavior. Support the patient's efforts to acknowledge and accept differences between her own values and beliefs and those of others.

8. Support the patient in her attempts to accept differences between self and others with regard to values/beliefs. Encourage patient to participate in both independent and group activities to increase self-esteem, feelings of accomplishment, and positive social interaction skills.

* Written by Eileen E. Rinear and Janice Trichtinger.

Nursing Intervention with the Borderline Client

A major goal in treatment is to promote the ego capacities as they relate to the organization and processing of experience. Development of reality-based skills is essential for the client who tends to be overwhelmed at the task of mastery and competence of a skill. His lack of self-confidence triggers a drop in self-esteem and a concurrent affective response of anger or depression. The nurse needs to slowly build a therapeutic relationship that is based on trust.

The borderline personality usually displays a lack of anxiety tolerance, a lack of impulse control, and characteristics of narcissism and entitlement. The patient typically views others as distant objects with no real emotional involvement and as objects for manipulation. Primary process thinking is evident with the borderline patient. Defense mechanisms seen are splitting, projection, denial, and primitive ideation. The borderline patient is a difficult, challenging patient to work with.

Borderline patients are often more difficult to manage than either neurotic or schizophrenic patients. They may, at first, be socially engaging with the nurse, but as soon as their wishes are frustrated, they become enraged, petulant, or hurt. They may threaten to terminate the relationship, leave the hospital, or commit suicide.

The demands of these patients seem endless. And when any need is frustrated, they demonstrate their expertise in provoking guilt. For example, one patient said, "Doctor, give me a pill for my anxiety." The physician suggested that the patient wait for 10 minutes to discuss her feelings during her scheduled therapy appointment. But within 2 minutes the patient returned to the physician with bleeding wrists extended out to him, saying, "Now see! See what you have done." With maneuvers such as this, the patient first makes the staff want to help; then she makes the staff helpless; then she provokes guilt. To complete the clinical picture, the patient often tries to play one staff member off against another. The staff are angry at each other; the patient begins to act up on the ward, ensuring that she is the center of attention. She has successfully recreated her own family dynamics.

This type of situation is typical of borderline patients. Therefore, to prevent staff "splitting," the nursing management is of prime importance in the course of treatment of this patient. It is important to understand that although the borderline patient attempts to manipulate the staff, she does not do so consciously. The patient feels very inadequate and worthless and so feels she cannot get anything done for her unless she manipulates. This can be learned behavior from previously experienced family patterns. The staff must provide consistency at all times with set limits and controls. Good communications between the staff members working with this patient are essential. Care plans must be thorough and shift reports very inclusive. The borderline patient is adept at manipulating situations so that the staff will feel defensive and helpless. This patient will often play up to one staff member with such comments as, "You really are the only one here who cares about me;" "You are so helpful, no one else really understands me;" and so on. This staff member, if not aware of the patient's manipulativeness, becomes protective of the patient, defending her to other staff members and wondering why they are really not paying attention to the patient. Without realizing it, the staff, who once worked well together, are now arguing about the right approach to use, the right medication, the right anything. Many clinicians use this type of behavior diagnostically to help the staff to come to a diagnosis of borderline personality in the patient. The "splitting" of staff in this manner is very typical of the borderline patient.

One such patient who had been screaming and yelling at several other patients and stomping through the unit stormed into the nurses' station demanding her car keys. Although she had car privileges, the nurse determined that the patient was in such a "state" that she should not be allowed to leave the grounds until she calmed down. The patient began her usual tirade at the staff, leading to the staff feeling very defensive and helpless. The nurse, instead of firmly sticking to her decision, agreed to call the patient's doctor with the patient present. As it happened, the physician did not support the nurse's decision and allowed the patient to leave the grounds. This undermined the unity of the staff. The entire disciplinary team working with this patient must work together in order to help the patient learn better patterns of growth.

The female borderline patient often acts out her aggression. This behavior may be directed at the staff, at other patients, or at self with self-destructive impulses. Often the borderline patient will cut her wrists or take an overdose of medication. It is therefore important that a safe environment be provided while the patient is being assessed for suicidal impulses. "Acting out" will usually be a continual part of the hos-

pital stay. It is therefore important for the nurse to help the patient explore her feelings and ways of dealing with people. A direct, honest approach is the most successful method for the nurse to use with this patient. The nurse should be sure to reinforce positive behavior. When the patient is not "acting out," the staff should be certain to spend time with the patient to reinforce the appropriate behavior. When the patient handles herself appropriately, limits can be lifted.

Discharge from the hospital or termination from outpatient treatment is a very stressful time to the borderline patient who may "act out" in various ways. Sometimes the "acting out" is an attempt to get the physician or nurse to postpone the discharge.

At other times, the "acting out" is designed to force the staff to terminate the hospitalization. One example was a young female with rheumatoid arthritis who knew the time for her discharge had arrived, but she continued to stall. One day she swung her cane at several windows and at a nurse's back. She screamed, "Now I'll bet I'll be discharged!" The physician was persuaded by the staff to give this girl another chance, especially since she had not yet found a place to live. One week later, the incident was repeated. She said, "Now I'm sure I'll be discharged." She was.

Many of these patients consciously realize that their place is out of the hospital and that they must be discharged. Nevertheless, they do not want to take responsibility for their discharge from a ward that has been warm and comforting. The part of the ambivalent person that wants to stay and be dependent can express anger and righteous indignation at being discharged. The anger they insist on creating in their termination is also a part of an attempt to sever the therapeutic relationship completely. In effect, they are saying, "If you will not care for me completely, I want nothing to do with you."

The angry parting often recapitulates both the patient's family history and previous therapeutic efforts. To allow this kind of parting to occur is to miss the opportunity to deal therapeutically with a major therapeutic problem. The general management principles in the discharge from treatment of these patients is as follows.

1. Nurses must first deal with their own omnipotent fantasies. They cannot be mother, father, or friend to the patient.

2. Nurses must set reasonable goals with the patient and be careful not to promise what they cannot give.

3. In the push and pull of the therapeutic relationship, the patient will want to deal with his anxiety by action, such as wrist cutting, sexual promiscuity, running, asking for discharge. Limits and controls must be set to prevent this discharge of anxiety by action.

4. Limits are lifted according to how the patient handles responsibility. The patient has to learn to bear the uncomfortable feelings. This is accomplished by blocking the route to action, by helping the patient to verbalize the feeling in as much detail as possible, and by the support that comes from the presence of the nurse.

5. The patient's attempts to make the nurse feel helpless, angry, and guilty must be seen as the patient's problem. It can easily be shown how this is a pattern of relating to subsequent people in his life and how this leads to a great deal of psychic pain. These issues recur every few days, but if handled successfully, they will recur with diminishing intensity. It is common to see an increase in hypochondriasis and depressive symptomatology if the nurse is successful in dealing with the patient's characterological way of dealing with anxiety. These symptoms are usually temporary as the patient progresses and as the nurse helps the patient bear the painful feelings.

When nurses are careful in setting goals, when they set limits judicially, when they can deal through transference with the patient's maladaptive way of interacting, and when they are clear as to whose problem is whose, the termination is relatively simple. When two people are neither guilty nor angry, it is always easier to say good-bye. When the pitfalls of the therapeutic relationship are avoided, nurses can show patients that they owe it to themselves and their growth as more mature persons to leave properly.

Comprehensive Behavioral Treatment

Planning a comprehensive treatment program for borderline patients is essential for helping the patient to maintain an optimum level of functioning. The following behavioral treatment program, as outlined by psychologist Ralph M. Turner, includes a focus on (1) reducing social anxiety; (2) restructuring cognitions; (3) anxiety management training; and (4) contingency management during an acute hospitalization.[11]

Social-Anxiety Reduction Procedures and Interpersonal Social Skills Building

A useful behavior therapy strategy for reducing social anxiety and increasing interpersonal skills is social skills group therapy. The essential components of this type of treatment are:

- Didactic training in interpersonal behavior.
- Role playing.
- Rehearsing appropriate interpersonal behavior.
- Feedback geared to improve the patient's interpersonal skills.
- Exposure to actual problem situations for group analysis.

Group format is the usual procedure. The group provides the opportunity for patients to share experiences and to learn from each other. Interaction with others is a key learning step. Sessions generally begin with a review of the previous week's homework assignment. Assignments are determined from a hierarchy of anxiety-arousing situations developed for each patient. The patient is helped to progress from relatively simple interpersonal tasks through increasingly difficult situations. The second section of the group meeting involves the leader teaching such behaviors as empathetic listening, skills in conversation, the use of humor, assertiveness, methods for dealing with criticism, etc. Then patients rehearse and receive feedback on their ability to carry out the skills learned during the group meeting. Finally, specific problems encountered in day-to-day life are discussed, and active attempts to resolve problems are made.

Cognitive Restructuring

The cognitive restructuring components consist of the following:

- The patient is taught to understand the role of cognitions in contributing to his behavior through a didactic mode.
- The patient is taught to discriminate and systematically observe negative self-statements and images that are disruptive.

- Training is conducted in the essentials of problem solving, including problem definition, anticipation of consequences, evaluation of alternative strategies, and comprehending feedback.
- The patient role-plays and rehearses engaging in positive self-statements, the use of coping strategies, and the applied use of problem-solving skills.

The goal of the cognitive restructuring is to assist the patient in learning how to counter: (1) his tendency to demean himself; (2) the use of an all-or-nothing philosophy; or (3) the belief that he needs complete love and approval from everyone.

Patients with borderline diagnoses have difficulties in managing adaptive strategies in their thinking. Thus, the final stage of cognitive therapy is to help the patient to apply the strategies to everyday life situations. Once a patient has substituted more reality-oriented interpretations for the maladaptive cognitions and has learned to identify and alter the dysfunctional beliefs that predisposed him to distort experiences, major strides toward adaptive behaviors have been made.

Anxiety Management Training

Since borderline patients experience high levels of anxiety, are easily stressed by various environmental stimuli, and develop multiple phobic responses, a general method of anxiety reduction is needed. Anxiety management training, a derivative of systematic desensitization, has been developed to help individuals learn to reduce anxiety in a wide variety of unpredictable stress situations. The procedure is composed of the same elements incorporated into desensitization (relaxation training, hierarchy construction, and graded imaginal exposure to the hierarchy items), but the program is performed in a different pattern.

First, the patient is taught progressive relaxation or some other relaxation procedure. Then, a hierarchy of stress-producing situations is developed through patient self-recording of stressful events with the therapist. Next, the patient is exposed to the stressful hierarchy scenes in imagination and is requested to pay attention to exactly how and where the anxiety was first registered. The patient is then trained to use the onset of anxiety as a cue, or signal, to engage in the relaxation response. To accomplish this, the patient imagines a stressful experience, signals the onset of anxiety, and simultaneously engages in relaxation. These imaginal exposures occur until the patient reports no discomfort with the situation.

Management during Hospitalization

Patients may need to be hospitalized during acute crises. Management during the hospitalization (called *contingency management*) is designed to firmly establish "If-Then" rules. This is precisely what patients with impaired ego control need. Contingency management helps to teach structure and to aid the person to gain insight into the connections between behavior and environmental responses to those behaviors.

The "token economy" is one management program in which the essential components include: (1) the target behavior; (2) the token; (3) the explicit contingency; and (4) backup reinforcers. The target behavior is the behavior that both staff and patient wish to modify. For example, aggressive "acting out" behavior might be selected for modification. The token can be anything that is durable and can be used as a medium for exchange. Next, the explicit contingencies must be developed describing what behaviors and under what specific circumstances will lead to the acquisition of how many tokens. For example, every 10-minute period with no aggressive outburst will lead to the acquisition of one token. The contingency must also define the rate of exchange of tokens for backup reinforcers. Backup reinforcers are what the tokens purchase. For example, reinforcers might be food, time to play games, extra time off the grounds, etc.

In conclusion, no single behavioral intervention can adequately modify a patient's behavior. However, the consistent and carefully planned program steps can assist the patient in taking major strides in reaching his optimum level of functioning.

HISTRIONIC PERSONALITY DISORDER

The essential feature in the histrionic personality disorder is an overly dramatic, reactive, and intensely expressed behavior coupled with characteristic disturbances in interpersonal relationships. Individuals with such exaggerated traits are lively, and they frequently draw attention to themselves. Minor stimuli trigger emotional excitability such as angry, irrational outbursts or tantrums. These people crave novelty and excitement and quickly become bored with normal routines.

The histrionic personality is characterized by a constellation of personality traits, which includes exhibitionism, egocentricity, suggestibility, and lability of emotions. In addition to these traits, these persons have difficulty in triangular situations; by this, we mean that in a situation with a male and a female, the patient becomes competitive with the person of the same sex and seductive with the person of the opposite sex. Although hysterical dynamics occur in both sexes, the literature focuses almost entirely on the "hysterical" female, probably because most of the literature is still written by male therapists.

The degree of ego strength and the use of the defense of splitting usually determine the level of adaptive versus maladaptive functioning. At the lesser-developed end of the spectrum, patients are both histrionic (flamboyant, exude a sexual demeanor lacking in subtlety, and are impulsive) and narcissistic (stormy interpersonal relationships and erratic academic and work capacity). The most common diagnosis is either borderline or narcissistic personality with hysterical features.

The healthier histrionic personalities show major areas of competence and stability, can be organized and successfully competitive, and can develop and sustain friendships. A major deficit area is in the selection of partners, or once the partner has been selected, there is difficulty in sustaining the relationship. These persons will complain of a sense of unfulfillment, a deep longing for a central gratifying relationship, and a sense of desperation that it may never come about. Thus, the person may become depressed and lose any perspective on his overall self-worth as well as on his or her adequacy of maleness or femaleness. The affect may be profound enough to trigger serious depression and self-directed anger.[12] Althought the literature usually describes female patients, Nemiah associates this disorder in men with passive, feminine, and homosexual characteristics.[13]

The diagnostic criteria for histrionic personality disorder are shown below[14]:

Diagnostic Criteria for Histrionic Personality Disorder

A. Pervasive pattern of excessive emotionality and attention-seeking behavior, beginning by early adulthood and present in a variety of contexts, as indicated by at least four of the following:
   1. Constantly seeks or demands reassurance, approval, or praise
   2. Is inappropriately sexually seductive in appearance or behavior
   3. Is overly concerned with physical attractiveness
   4. Expresses emotion with inappropriate exaggeration, e.g., embraces casual acquaintances with excessive ardor, uncontrollable sobbing on minor sentimental occasions, has temper tantrums
   5. Is uncomfortable in situations in which he is not the center of attention
   6. Displays rapidly shifting and shallow expression of emotions
   7. Is self-centered, actions being directed toward obtaining immediate satisfaction; has no tolerance for the frustration of delayed gratification
   8. Has a style of speech that is excessively impressionistic and lacking in detail, e.g., when asked to describe mother, can be no more specific than, "She was a beautiful person."

CASE EXAMPLE

A 51-year-old never-married man was observed by a nursing student in a mental health clinic to burst dramatically into the waiting room of the office area. With great swooping movements, he removed his raincoat and hat and loudly announced to all present, the secretary included, that he desperately needed help. He become impatient and angry after being told he would have to wait about 45 minutes to be seen by an intake staff member. When he did enter the intake worker's office, he immediately commented on the appearance of the therapist. He then proceeded to relate in a flamboyant manner that he was very upset over the death of his great-aunt with whom he had lived for the past 5 years. He stated he had been upset since the funeral, had trouble sleeping, felt very depressed, and decided he needed to talk to someone.

The intake worker then remarked that he would have to wait for another appointment to begin therapy. At that point, the man became quite upset and insisted he see someone right away. After a brief staff meeting, it was decided that the situation met the criteria for a crisis and he was assigned to a graduate nursing student. She came in to talk with the patient and when she suggested dates and times, he proceeded to refuse all of them. Finally after several negotiation attempts, a weekly therapy time was determined.

The nursing student saw the patient for 12 sessions. After five sessions he revealed that he also had a drinking problem. The salient issue was that of being labeled a "drunk" by several of his associates, which was contrary to his flamboyant view of himself. This issue was addressed as well as some mid-life issues regarding his valuation of his life to this point. The patient was able to gain understanding of himself; his attention to dates and details improved; and he was able to set goals and meet them.

In planning nursing care, assessment needs to be made of the predominate ego defense mechanisms. Usually, repression and denial are the major modes of intrapsychic defense. Jacobson cites three examples of presentation patterns of hysterical personalities: (1) the woman who becomes depressed after the termination of her third romantic relationship with a married man and her statement that men are "untrustworthy," yet is not aware of her own pattern of partner choice; (2) the man who suddenly veers away from prominence or success just prior to obtaining it; and (3) the person who can be sexually expressive with selected partners but not with his or her spouse.[15]

In clinical practice, the nurse is likely to see persons diagnosed with histrionic personality disorders who have considerable ego impairment. These patients usually describe severe deprivation in their early years. Female patients may display a provocative demeanor, which needs to be viewed as a masked way of asking for caring. There may be unresolved sexual trauma in the childhood history of this patient. The patient may behave in a provocative way toward male staff and in a competitive way toward female staff. The nurse can best help the patient by being supportive and caring in response to the competitive provocations as well as the seductive behaviors. Caring in a nonsexualized manner is key in the response to these patients. The treatment strategies recognize that the maladaptation in interpersonal relationships resides in the relationship that evolved between patient and parent.

NARCISSISTIC PERSONALITY DISORDER

The history of the terminology of narcissistic personality disorder derives from Greek mythology and the myth of Narcissus. There are two sources to the myth. First, and best known, is that Narcissus, noted for his beauty, rejected the love of others and drew upon himself the vengeance of the gods. He fell in love with his own reflection in the waters of a spring and either pined away or killed himself. The second version is that Narcissus, to console himself for the death of a favorite twin sister, peered into the still water at his reflection to try to recall her features. Havelock Ellis cited this myth to illustrate a psychological state in reporting a case of male autoeroticism, and Freud used the term in discussing concern about self-love and love for others.[16,17] Narcissism in early ego psychology was included in general concepts of self and identity.

Over the past decade, there has been increasing attention to the concept of narcissism as a measure of personality development. There is debate on whether narcissistic character disorder should refer to a small number of people with discrete characteristics or to a wide variety of disorders of narcissism and whether the disorder represents a distortion of normal narcissism or the development of a special pathological configuration.[18]

In the clinical literature, the adjective *narcissism* is used in at least three ways: (1) referring to self-concept or self-image; (2) referring to self-love or self-esteem; and (3) referring to pathological self-attention or self-aggrandizement. Self-esteem has been defined as a prerequisite for self-maintenance. Disorders of narcissism, broadly stated, should include, according to Jacobson, patients whose self-esteem is too low as well as inappropriately too high.[19] Usually, however, we refer to narcissistic personality disorder when:

1. The individual has an inflated sense of esteem with extreme self-centeredness.
2. The individual shows deficient empathy for others despite an assiduous wish for their admiration.

These are individuals who feel entitled to special treatment without reciprocity, who have grandiose fantasies and perceptions, and who have little capacity for warm or mutual interpersonal relationships.[20]

Kernberg describes persons with this condition as having excessive self-absorption, intense ambition, grandiose fantasies, overdependence on acclaim, and an unremitting need to search for brilliance, power, and beauty.[21] He stressed the pathological nature of their inner world, regardless of their superficially adaptive behavior. This pathology is shown in an inability to love; a lack of empathy; chronic feelings of boredom, emptiness, and uncertainty about identity; and exploitation of others. Kernberg also emphasized the presence of chronic intense envy and defenses against such envy, particularly devaluation, omnipotent control, and narcissistic withdrawal. These defenses appear in their contempt for, or anxious attachment to, secretly admired or envied others. There is also a tendency toward sexual promiscuity, homosexuality, perversions, and substance abuse and a peculiarly corruptible conscience, a readiness to shift values quickly to gain favor.

Kohut's writing on narcissism notes that these persons complain of disturbances in several areas: Sexually, they may report perverse fantasies or lack of interest in sex; socially, they may experience work inhibitions and difficulty in forming and maintaining relationships, as well as participating in delinquent activities; and personally, they may demonstrate lack of humor, little empathy for others' needs and feelings, pathological lying, or hypochondriacal preoccupations.[22] These patients also display overt grandiosity in unrealistic schemes, exaggerated self-regard, demands for attention, and inappropriate idealization of certain others. Profoundly angry reactions are noted, such as a narcissistic rage as a reaction to injury to self-esteem. The central features are the need for revenge—the undoing of hurt by whatever means—and compulsion in this pursuit with utter disregard for reasonable limitations.

A list of the diagnostic criteria for narcissistic personality disorder is given below[23]:

Diagnostic Criteria for Narcissistic Personality Disorder

A. Pervasive pattern of grandiosity (in fantasy or behavior), lack of empathy, and hypersensitivity to the evaluation of others, beginning by early adulthood and present in a variety of contexts, as indicated by at least five of the following:

1. Reacts to criticism with feelings of rage, shame, or humiliation (even if not expressed)
2. Is interpersonally exploitative: takes advantage of others to achieve his own ends
3. Has a grandiose sense of self-importance, e.g., exaggerates achievements and talents, expects to be noticed as "special" without appropriate achievement
4. Believes that his problems are unique and can be understood only by other special people
5. Is preoccupied with fantasies of unlimited success, power, brilliance, beauty, or ideal love
6. Has a sense of entitlement: unreasonable expectation of especially favorable treatment, e.g., assumes that he does not have to wait in line when others must do so
7. Requires constant attention and admiration, e.g., keeps fishing for compliments
8. Lack of empathy: inability to recognize and experience how others feel, e.g., annoyance and surprise when a friend who is seriously ill cancels a date
9. Is preoccupied with feelings of envy

In planning nursing care, important clues to working with the person with a narcissistic personality disorder are derived from autognosis. The countertransference (feelings engendered in the nurse while working with the patient) may be intense. Kohut states that the therapist may feel bored in response to the patient's state of nonrelatedness.[24] The patient may talk readily enough but may appear to be removed or unconcerned about the therapist as a person. It is also noted that these patients may become quite suicidal and depressed during treatment.

CASE EXAMPLE

A 42-year-old never-married man was seen on intake evaluation at a mental health clinic. He was immaculately dressed and worked as the director of a performing arts group that performed specifically for deaf audiences. His first question to the intake worker related to knowing the professional credentials of all the staff members. In the interview, the patient revealed that he was quite unhappy in his life and that although he was intimately involved with a 23-year-old man, he was finding it difficult to make a commitment to the relationship.

The patient was assigned to a psychiatric nursing student. Although he was guarded and defensive in the interviews, he was punctual for all his sessions. It was painful for him to speak of issues in his life. He felt great entitlement and was very disappointed and upset when things did not go his way. He had great difficulty with people in authority and did not feel the people with whom he had to interact understood the nature of his artistic talents and work. There was tremendous conflict in his interpersonal relationships and anger in his interactions. However, the patient was quite compassionate, and what held him in therapy was his desire to get along with people. He valued his work greatly and wanted to achieve major accomplishments.

As he began to trust the nurse, she could gently begin to approach why he had to always feel he was right in a situation. The patient insisted that it was not that he had to be right. With that admission, the nurse then asked what it would mean for him to be wrong. This statement opened up the issue of being wrong and what unfolded then was his review of his relationship with his mother and father. His parents had divorced and he was essentially raised by his mother. Although she cared for him, she was never really engaged with him, from his perception. Thus, as a young boy he dealt with his loneliness by taking care of himself. He did not experience comfort and warmth from his mother but rather by taking care of himself. Behind his narcissism was his fear of intimacy and any kind of feedback that anything was wrong with him.

The intervention at this point with a person with narcissistic traits is to deal with the person's response to feedback and his defensiveness about it. Essentially the strategy is to talk to the person about his need to be self-centered and the defense that it serves. The idea can be carefully introduced that when such persons talk to people, they put up a mirror that reflects themselves. As long as the mirror is there, they see what is familiar and what they know and what they can control. Such individuals are very comfortable because they know how to interpret the mirror (i.e., themselves). But if the mirror is removed and there is another human being to whom to relate, these individuals are at a loss to understand the feedback they are receiving, and this confrontation is very frightening. This situation has developed because early in life, the persons have had the world revolve around their own reflection as a kind of protection in the service of nurturance and comfort. This condition may evolve as in the case example above or from parents who overidealize their child and isolate him from the feedback of others.

The intervention is to remove the mirror in a caring and trusting manner and permit the person to experience that he does not disappear; that it is OK to be separate and to appreciate the feedback and impressions of other persons.

AVOIDANT PERSONALITY DISORDER

The individual with a diagnosis of avoidant personality disorder is hypersensitive to potential rejection, humiliation, or shame. There is also an unwillingness to develop relationships unless given strong guarantees of uncritical acceptance. The individual usually is isolated socially and evidences low self-esteem. Thus, these individuals withdraw from opportunities where they might develop social relationships and have very few close friends. These people desire affection and acceptance yet are distressed by their lack of ability to relate comfortably to others.

The diagnostic criteria for avoidant personality disorder are listed below[25]:

Diagnostic Criteria for Avoidant Personality Disorder

A. Pervasive pattern of social discomfort, fear of negative evaluation, and timidity, beginning by early adulthood and present in a variety of contexts, as indicated by at least four of the following:
1. Is easily hurt by criticism or disapproval
2. Has no close friends or confidants (or only one) other than first-degree relatives
3. Is unwilling to get involved with people unless certain of being liked
4. Avoids social or occupational activities that involve significant interpersonal contact, e.g., refuses a promotion that will increase social demands
5. Is reticent in social situations because of fear of saying something inappropriate or foolish or of being unable to answer a question
6. Fears of being embarrassed by blushing, crying, or showing signs of anxiety in front of other people
7. Exaggerates the potential difficulties, physical dangers, or risks getting involved in doing something ordinary but outside his usual routine, e.g., may cancel social plans because he anticipates

being exhausted by the effort of getting there

CASE EXAMPLE

A 20-year-old university student sought counseling at the local mental health clinic for "depression." She had the belief that people were laughing at her on the street. During an intake interview, the patient revealed that she had just completed a course with a professor that she liked very much and whom she thought was interested in her personally. Her fantasy was that at the end of the course he would invite her for a date. However, the end of the semester arrived and nothing happened with the professor. She became depressed and came to the clinic.

Further interviews revealed that the patient came from divorced parents. When she would visit her father, he would constantly criticize her. He also would invite young women to the house for casual affairs.

The patient was a shy, quiet young woman who did not know how to make friends. She had few friends in high school and felt isolated. She had a low self-image and was very sensitive to rejection.

The intervention was through the development of a nurse–patient relationship. The nurse assisted the patient in the painful task of recognizing that the criticisms by her father were not correct. The second therapeutic step was to point out that the patient was continuing the process started by her father. That is, if her father was not there to criticize her, she would criticize and demean herself. Helping the patient to stop the cycle of criticism meant confronting the issue of her loneliness and strengthening her to begin to socialize and develop her own friends. The therapeutic tasks were to help the patient separate from her father via the criticism and to explore her feelings regarding her insensitive father. As the patient became stronger in therapy, she was able to stand up to her father and tell him how she felt. She was able to get a job and thus could stop being totally financially dependent upon him. She began making her own social network.

DEPENDENT PERSONALITY DISORDER

The person diagnosed with a dependent personality disorder passively allows others to assume responsibility for major areas of his life because of a lack of self-confidence and an inability to function independently. This person subordinates his own needs to those of others on whom he is dependent. This behavior is in the service of avoiding any possibility of having to be self-reliant.

Characteristically, the individual leaves major decisions to others. He is also reluctant to make demands on others for fear of jeopardizing the relationship. This person lacks self-confidence and berates his own abilities and talents. The diagnostic criteria for this disorder are listed below[26]:

Diagnostic Criteria for Dependent Personality Disorder

A. Pervasive pattern of dependent and submissive behavior, beginning by early adulthood and present in a variety of at least five of the following:
   1. Is unable to make everyday decisions without an excessive amount of advice or reassurance from others
   2. Allows others to make most of his important decisions, e.g., where to live, what job to take
   3. Agrees with people even when he believes they are wrong, because of fear of being rejected
   4. Has difficulty initiating projects or doing things on his own
   5. Volunteers to do things that are unpleasant or demeaning in order to get other people to like him
   6. Feels uncomfortable or helpless when alone, or goes to great lengths to avoid being alone
   7. Feels devastated or helpless when close relationships end
   8. Is frequently preoccupied with fears of being abandoned
   9. Is easily hurt by criticism or disapproval

OBSESSIVE–COMPULSIVE PERSONALITY DISORDER

The individual diagnosed with an obsessive–compulsive personality disorder generally has restricted ability to express warm and tender emotions. There is a perfectionistic quality to the individual that interferes with his ability to view a total situation. There is an insistence that others submit to his way of doing things. In addition, there is excessive commitment to work and productivity to the exclusion of pleasure. There is also a tendency to indecisiveness. Interpersonal relationships have a rigid and stilted quality. These persons are perceived as serious and nonhumorous. They rarely give compliments or gifts. Their preoccupation with rules, efficiency, trivial details, and procedures interferes with their perspective on the total picture. Often, time is poorly managed and important tasks are left to the last moment, which interferes with the idealized goal of perfection and efficiency.

Diagnostic criteria for this disorder are listed below[27]:

Diagnostic Criteria for Obsessive–Compulsive Personality Disorder

A. Pervasive pattern of perfectionism and inflexibility, beginning by early adulthood and present in a variety of contexts, as indicated by at least five of the following:
1. Perfectionism that interferes with task completion, e.g., inability to complete a project because own overly strict standards are not met
2. Preoccupation with details, rules, lists, order, organization, or schedules to the extent that the major point of the activity is lost
3. Unreasonable insistence that others submit to exactly his way of doing things, or unreasonable reluctance to allow others to do things because of the conviction that they will not do them correctly
4. Excessive devotion to work and productivity to the exclusion of leisure activities and friendships (not accounted for by obvious economic necessity)
5. Indecisiveness: decision making is either avoided, postponed, or protracted, e.g., the person cannot get assignments done on time because of ruminating about priorities (do not include if indecisiveness is due to excessive need for advice or reassurance from others)
6. Overconscientiousness, scrupulousness, and inflexibility about matters of morality, ethics, or values (not accounted for by cultural or religious identification)
7. Restricted expression of affection

8. Lack of generosity in giving time, money, or gifts when no personal gain is likely to result
9. Inability to discard worn-out or worthless objects even when they have no sentimental value

PASSIVE–AGGRESSIVE PERSONALITY DISORDER

The individual with a diagnosis of passive–aggressive personality disorder resists the demands for adequate performance in both work and social situations; however, the resistance is expressed indirectly rather than directly. For example, the person who is chronically late for appointments or "forgets" to bring important papers to a meeting may be exhibiting this pattern of behavior. Diagnostic criteria for this disorder are shown below[28]:

Diagnostic Criteria for Passive–Aggressive Personality Disorder

A. Pervasive pattern of passive resistance to demands for adequate social and occupational performance, beginning by early adulthood and present in a variety of contexts, as indicated by at least five of the following:
1. Procrastinates, i.e., puts off things that need to be done so that deadlines are not met
2. Becomes sulky, irritable, or argumentative when asked to do something he does not want to do
3. Seems to work deliberately slowly or to do a bad job on tasks that he really does not want to do
4. Protests, without justification, that others make unreasonable demands on him
5. Avoids obligations by claiming to have "forgotten"
6. Believes that he is doing a much better job than others think he is doing
7. Resents useful suggestions from others concerning how he could be more productive
8. Obstructs the efforts of others by failing to do his share of the work
9. Unreasonably criticizes or scorns people in positions of authority

Summary

This chapter has described a typology of personality disorders that are classified on Axis II of the *DSM-III-R*. Persons with personality disorders generally do not seek mental health intervention unless the defensive nature of their disorder breaks down in some way, usually from a crisis situation. These persons seek assistance when they experience symptoms of anxiety, nonperformance, depression, or loss, or after a confrontation with the law.

Three major clusters of personality disorders were discussed as follows: (1) paranoid, schizoid, and schizotypal; (2) antisocial, borderline, histrionic, and narcissistic; and (3) avoidant, dependent, obsessive–compulsive, and passive–aggressive.

The nursing care of individuals with personality disorders rests heavily on the nurse's ability to autognose and deal with emotional reactions to the characteristic traits of the patient; on firm, consistent limit setting of the behavior; on communication of expectations for a change in behavior to the patient; and on a consistency of team approach in understanding the dynamics of the behavior.

Questions

1. Give an example of a patient with a personality disorder whom you have worked with from a general nursing situation.
2. Why is a client with a personality disorder more likely to be seen in nonpsychiatric settings than a person with a psychosis?
3. Why do you think so little has been done in developing treatment interventions for the sociopath?

REFERENCES AND SUGGESTED READINGS

1. Jacobson, G. Personality disorders. In A. Lazare (Ed.), *Outpatient Psychiatry*. Baltimore: Williams & Wilkins, 1979, p. 419.
2. Ibid.
3. American Psychiatric Association: *Diagnostic and Statistical Manual*, 3rd ed. (Rev.) Washington, D. C.: American Psychiatric Association, 1987, [pp. 335–358].
4. Ibid., [p. 337].
5. Ibid., [p. 339].
6. Ibid., [pp. 340–341].
7. Ibid., [pp. 342–346].
8. Grinker, R. R., Sr., Werble, B., & Drye, R. R. *The Borderline Syndrome*. New York: Basic Books, 1968, pp. 90–91.
9. *DSM-III-R*, [pp. 346–347].
10. Ibid.
11. Turner, R. M. Behavioral therapy with borderline patients. *Carrier Foundation Letter*, 1983, *88*(4), 2–3.
12. Jacobson, op. cit., pp. 432–433.
13. Nemiah, J. Conversion reaction. In A. M. Freedman & H. I. Kaplan (Eds.), *Comprehensive Textbook of Psychiatry*. Baltimore: Williams & Wilkins, 1967, p. 882.
14. *DSM-III-R*, [pp. 348–349].
15. Jacobson, op. cit., p. 433.
16. Ellis, H. Autoeroticism: A psychotic study. *Alienist and Neurologist*, 1898, *19*, 260–299.
17. Freud, S. On narcissism: An introduction. In E. Jones (Ed.), *Sigmund Freud Collected Papers* (Vol. 4). New York: Basic Books, 1959, pp. 30–49. (Originally published, 1914.)
18. Kernberg, O. *Borderline Conditions and Pathological Narcissism*. New York: Jason Aronson, 1975.
19. Jacobson, op. cit., p. 431.
20. Ibid.
21. Kernberg, op. cit., p. 264.
22. Kohut, H. *Analysis of the Self*. New York: International Universities Press, 1971.
23. *DSM-III-R*, [pp. 349–351].
24. Kohut, op. cit.
25. *DSM-III-R*, [pp. 351–353].
26. Ibid., [pp. 353–354].
27. Ibid., [pp. 354–356].
28. Ibid., [pp. 357–358].

PART VI

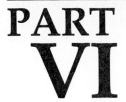

Special Populations

Nurses frequently are frontline health professionals who either "case find" or directly intervene with special population groups within various health care settings. The intervention may be direct care (secondary prevention), continued care (tertiary prevention), or primary prevention. Focus in this section is placed on the very young, the elderly, the seriously depressed or combative individual, the runaway, the chronically mentally ill, victims and perpetrators of sexual violence, and the person with an AIDS diagnosis.

CHAPTER 47: THE SUICIDAL PATIENT

Nurses need to be able to assess and diagnose the suicidal risk of patients and to plan nursing care that includes goals for self-recovery.

CHAPTER 48: THE COMBATIVE PATIENT

With the increase of violence in our society, nurses need to be able to assess and diagnose the potential for violence of patients and to plan nursing care that includes safeguards for controlling aggressive behaviors.

CHAPTER 49: CHILD ABUSE, NEGLECT AND SEXUAL VICTIMIZATION

Nurses, as mandated reporters of child abuse, need to know the various indicators of physical abuse, sexual abuse, psychological abuse, and neglect. This chapter focuses on the interview and assessment of the family and child and outlines steps for prevention of abuse.

CHAPTER 50: VICTIMS OF RAPE

With an increasing number of women reporting sexual trauma, nurses need to know the symptoms reaction and crisis response of victims of rape.

CHAPTER 51: VICTIMS OF FAMILY VIOLENCE: INCEST AND BATTERING

The physical and sexual assault of children and women by family members is being brought to the attention of health professionals. Some of the myths and issues of the violent home are discussed, including program services and shelters for women and their children.

927

CHAPTER 52: THE CHRONICALLY MENTALLY DISABLED

Nurses are noting an increase in the chronically mentally ill who are being seen in emergency rooms as well as mental health centers.

CHAPTER 53: AGING AND MENTAL HEALTH

Research has documented the way in which adults age and those stressors that place them at risk for developing maladaptive patterns. This chapter describes the role that nurses can assume in reducing stress and in increasing the coping capacity of the aging.

CHAPTER 54: THE PSYCHOSOCIAL ISSUES CONCERNING ACQUIRED IMMUNE DEFICIENCY SYNDROME

The 1980s has been witness to a major epidemic of Autoimmune Disease (AIDS). This chapter describes educational information regarding the disease as well as care of the dying AIDS patient.

Chapter 47

The Suicidal Patient

Ann Wolbert Burgess

Chapter Objectives

The students successfully attaining the goals of this chapter will be able to:

- Identify the assessment areas of suicidal behavior.
- Assess the nature of suicidal intent.
- Compare the psychiatric syndromes of depression, schizophrenia, organic mental disorders, and personality disorders to suicidal behavior.
- Describe the nursing management of suicidal behavior in outpatient settings as well as inpatient settings.
- Describe nursing care plans for the suicidal patient.

A question for consideration is whether suicidal behavior is a diagnosis or it is merely an expression of a variety of different mental states, each with its own and different determinants and prognoses? In Shaffer's literature review of suicidal children and adolescents, he concluded that suicidal children differ from others (both normals and nonsuicidal controls) only in their propensity to repeat the suicidal behavior.[1] Further support for Shaffer's thesis is noted in the literature, especially Pokorny's prospective study of 4,800 patients hospitalized for psychiatric illness.[2,3] In that study, the suicide rate for the 15 percent who had made suicide attempts or threats was triple that of the nonsuicidal hos-

pitalized population.[4] There appears to be increasing consensus on the importance of multiple suicide attempts when one is comparing a suicidal with a nonsuicidal population, even though there is no consensus on most external and intrapsychic factors in suicidal prediction.[5]

A review of studies investigating factors relating to suicidal intent suggests that hopelessness is an important psychological construct for understanding suicide. Beck observed clinically that when depressed patients believe there is no solution to serious life problems, they view suicide as a way out of an intolerable situation.[6] Hopelessness, according to Beck, is a core characteristic of depression and serves as the link between depression and suicide. Furthermore, hopelessness associated with other psychiatric disorders also predisposes the patient to suicidal behavior.[7]

Suicide continues to be a pressing biopsychosocial concern in our society. Statistics, difficult as they are to obtain and interpret, are indicating an increase in suicide rates for adolescents and children, minority populations, and women. Nurses are influential in helping a suicidal person to consider other solutions to his problems rather than death.

Suicide is not a twentieth-century phenomenon and probably dates back prior to written history. The magnitude of the problem is still unknown, along with other human acts that trigger strong emotional biases in people and may go unreported and undiagnosed. A recognition of the problem in our society began in the 1950s, and research on the subject prompted the formation of the Los Angeles Suicide Prevention Center in 1957 by psychologists Edwin S. Shneidman and Norman L. Farberow. This center has served as a model for other suicide prevention centers throughout the country.

Two important facts to be stressed regarding the field of suicidology are: (1) its pioneer multidisciplinary approach to a social issue; and (2) the tremendous progress that has been made in the field in a relatively short period of time.

PSYCHIATRIC DIAGNOSIS IN SUICIDE

A key prognostic factor in assessing the likelihood of a patient repeating suicidal behavior is the identification of underlying psychiatric illness. The most frequently encountered psychiatric illness will be described below, including depression, schizophrenia, organic brain syndrome, and certain of the personality disorders.*

Depressive Syndromes

The depressive syndromes present a common clinical picture that is distinguishable from transient mood states. The patient presents a forlorn, generally immobile countenance with varying degrees of psychomotor retardation or

---

* This section is based in part on O. S. Surman & A. Lazare, Management of the attempted suicide patient, *Medical Insight*, 1972, 4(July), 14–21. Copyright, Insight Publishing Co., Inc.

agitation, with diminished appetite, and almost invariably with insomnia. His thought content is marked by hopelessness, guilt, anger, desperation, loneliness, and feelings of worthlessness. Concomitant suicidal ideas may emerge because he feels that he deserves to be dead, that others would be better off if he were absent, or that suicide is the only escape from what appears to be an intolerable situation. Further progression of the syndrome may be accompanied by evidence of delusion and hallucinations and occasionally by an associated confusional picture and impairment of intellectual functioning.

Diagnosis is made by clinical observation and direct questioning of the patient and relatives. Often, the patient has a history of depressive episodes that may have responded to antidepressant medication or electroconvulsive therapy and that may have required hospitalization. The organic brain syndromes can generally be ruled out through the case history and through testing.

Depression is the pneumonia of psychiatry; if left untreated, it often has high morbidity and mortality. Treatment, however, often leads to complete remission. Attempted suicide in a depressed patient calls for rapid, definitive treatment by psychotherapy, antidepressant medication, or electroconvulsive treatment. When the depressive symptoms are severe with marked alteration in normal life-style functions or pronounced feelings of hopelessness and guilt, outpatient management is a high risk. The patient may be so convinced of his hopelessness that he is unable to cooperate in an outpatient program; his antidepressant medication may present the temptation of a lethal overdose. And there is often a considerable time lag before treatment takes effect. It is advisable to hospitalize the depressed patient who has attempted suicide when his depressive symptoms are severe, when he is out of contact with reality, or when he presents continuing suicidal ideation.

The Schizophrenic Syndromes

The schizophrenic syndromes are characterized by impairment of the capacity to distinguish reality from fantasy. There is a progressive tendency toward disordered communication, altered emotional responsiveness, and social isolation. The onset of the syndrome may be insidious or sudden. Classically, the patient's presentation is marked by bizarreness in dress, in deportment, and in speech. There is an air of cold indifference or inappropriate outbursts of anger, sadness, or mirth. The stream of talk is generally loosely connected, and its content is marked by bizarre somatic preoccupations, ideas of a grandiose or paranoid nature, fear of thought control or feelings of estrangement and depersonalization. Suicidal thinking may relate to any or all of these thoughts. With progressive decompensation there are frank delusions and hallucinations; suicidal behavior at this point may relate to the delusional system or be dictated by an hallucinated voice.

Diagnosis is made in the same way as in the depressive syndromes—by clinical observation, direct questioning, and a review of the client's past psychiatric history. There may also be a family history of similar illness.

Although schizophrenia is frequently managed successfully on an outpatient basis by using a combination of phenothiazines and psychotherapy, the schizophrenic patient who has attempted suicide is at extreme risk even when the attempt appears to be a minor one. Because of the client's impaired cognitive function and tendency toward isolation and disordered communication, suicidal behavior is highly unpredictable.[8] For this reason, hospitalization is almost always indicated.

Organic Brain Syndromes

Organic brain syndromes are psychotic reactions of organic etiology, which may be reversible (acute brain syndrome) or irreversible (chronic brain syndrome). The nature of the dysfunction may be toxic, metabolic, traumatic, hemorrhagic, vascular, or infectious. Attempted suicide may occur in any of the organic psychoses, but it is most common in the presence of drug and alcohol abuse and more recently in the toxic psychoses induced by hallucinogenic drugs.

The diagnosis of an organic brain syndrome, is made through the use of history, physical examination, and laboratory data.

Like all persons in psychotic states, these patients are highly unpredictable and require close observation following a suicide attempt. Once medical management has successfully reversed central nervous system impairment (when this is possible), it is necessary to perform a careful psychological reassessment, particularly when the etiology is related to substance abuse (i.e., alcohol or drug abuse). The disturbed patient who has limited adaptive resources, whose history is characterized by impulsive behavior, and who deals with stress by resorting to some form of substance use is likely to repeat the patterns that result in central nervous system impairment and suicidal behavior. In such cases, psychiatric hospitalization is often advisable.

Personality Disorders

Personality disorders consist of a broad group of characterological impairments; however, clients who have attempted suicide frequently present life styles that are characteristic of two major subgroups: (1) histrionic personality disorder, and (2) borderline personality disorder.

Histrionic Personality Disorder

The criteria for histrionic personality disorder include behaviors that are characteristic of the individual's current and long-term functioning, are not limited to episodes of illness, and cause either significant impairment in social or occupational functioning or subjective distress.

Attempted suicide in the patient with a histrionic personality disorder is often a dramatic display or acting out of an interpersonal conflict. The person's demanding dependency frequently antagonizes others (especially the medical staff) and evokes an angry response. A power struggle may then ensue in which the patient becomes increasingly willful and intransigent. This struggle is best avoided if one views the suicide attempt objectively as an inadequate or maladaptive means of dealing with life stress. The major goal in management is to support the client through the crisis and to encourage healthier and more appropriate modes of problem solving. This intervention is best initiated by mobilizing support from family and friends and by referral to a mental health professional. Although these clients require a great deal of help and careful follow-up, hospitalization can often be avoided.

Borderline Personality Disorder

The criteria for the diagnosis of borderline personality disorders include behaviors that are characteristic of the individual's current and long-term functioning, are not limited to episodes of illness, and that either cause significant impairment in social or occupational functioning or subjective distress.

The borderline patient may be highly engaging in the absence of stress, but he often meets frustration with frantic attempts to manipulate the social situation, which may take the form of suicidal threats or actions. These patients need support until the initial crisis has passed; however, the nurse must be alert to the tendency of these patients to present unrealistically high demands, to engineer staff conflicts and "splitting" of personnel, and to evoke anger within their caretakers. Management therefore requires that the nurse support and set firm limits when offering assistance, and she should clearly define the reality of the situation and the patient's responsibility. If this approach fails and the patient is unable to cooperate, hospitalization is often advisable.

ASSESSMENT OF SUICIDAL BEHAVIOR

The assessment of suicidal behavior includes two important sources of data: (1) the nature of the suicidal risk; and (2) the nature of the intent.

The Nature of the Suicidal Risk

A major problem confronting nurses is how to identify the person who is a serious suicidal risk. Although it is a fact that suicides will continue, no one has data at present as to what extent suicides are being prevented. Nurses are continually assessing patients for degrees of suicide risk. Strong emphasis is being placed on finding a reliable, quantitative measure of lethality. Although a variety of frameworks for evaluating suicidal risk have been cited in the literature, it should be recognized that none is completely reliable or all-encompassing as a predictive measure, at the present time. It is important that nurses guard against dividing people into those who carry out a "serious act" and those who make "gestures." Every suicide attempt is serious; a person must have few alternatives to solving his problems if he puts his life in jeopardy by a self-destructive act. The gesture and the serious attempt should be seen as points on the continuum of suicidal behavior. The nurse should, therefore, weigh all of the data carefully when using such a framework as a guide

in formulating appropriate intervention strategies. Since the risk of repeated suicidal behavior is an ever-present one, it is recommended that consultation with a psychiatrist be sought whenever possible when dealing with suicidal individuals.

In an excellent book on suicide, nurse–authors Hatton and Valente clearly describe assessment of suicidal risk as follows[9]:

1. Identifying the client through demographic data. Key information to collect is name, age, sex, race, education, religion, and living arrangement. Studies have shown that men between the ages of 35 and 50 are persons at greatest risk for suicide; men over 65 who feel isolated, alienated, or deprived physically or mentally are also high risk. Women make more suicidal attempts, but successful suicides are made by men. Studies are now looking at the ethnic factor and suicide rates, specifically blacks, Asians, Mexican-Americans, and American Indians. In regard to living arrangement, clients need to be asked who is the person the client is living with; what is the quality and quantity of the relationship; is the client satisfied with the relationship; and how are the arrangements in terms of economics, emotions, and social needs?
2. Clinical characteristics need to be assessed in terms of:
   a. The hazard. (Why did you come today? What has happened recently in your life that is different? When did it happen?)
   b. The crisis the client is experiencing internally. (How bad is the person feeling inside? How severe are the symptoms of depression?)
   c. Coping strategies and devices used by the client to manage his life. (How does he cope? What is the level of the client's impulse control?)
   d. Significant others. (Who does the client usually rely on? Who is available through the social network for the client?)
   e. Social and personal resources in terms of basic necessities for living, transportation, health care facilities, employment, and hobbies.
   f. Past suicidal attempts in terms of method used and time interval between attempts.
   g. History of psychiatric problems.
   h. Current psychiatric or medical status. (Any current acute or chronic problems?

Has the client consulted a physician within the last 6 months?)

  i. Life-style in terms of quality and maintenance over a period of time of that person's job, interpersonal relationships, and coping strategies.

  j. Suicidal plan in terms of: method, ability to carry out method, specificity of plan in terms of detail and access, and lethality in terms of method and success.

3. High-risk factors include:

  a. Multiple high-lethality suicide attempts in client's history.

  b. Alcohol abuse. (Alcohol abuse figures high in the behaviors of chronically suicidal persons.)

  c. Disorientation or disorganization, which implies the suicidal person is not perceiving the world in a realistic, clear way.

  d. Hostility in which the client displays rampant hostility toward the self or others, and where the hostility is of a long-standing nature.

The Nature of the Intent

A first consideration in the therapeutic approach to the person who has attempted suicide is to listen very carefully to what the person says about the suicide attempt and the nature of the intent. The intensity of the wish to die is an issue that must be directly discussed with the person. If a suicide attempt has already been made, this provides an opening for the nurse. The questions to ask may be, "What did you wish would happen when you took the pills?" or, "What did you think would happen when you cut your wrists?" or, "How do you feel now?" or, "What do you wish would happen now?" In addition to other assessment questions, the nurse can also ask if the person has had previous depressive periods and if there have been previous attempts at suicide.

The nurse may be reluctant to ask about suicide, but it has been our experience that the patient is never hurt by direct, respectful questions. The patient generally responds to the questions and understands them as part of the total interview. The patient's impulse control level and how desperate he is regarding self-destruction must be assessed promptly.

As the nurse listens to the patient describe his suicidal act, the nature of the attempt is assessed. Of course, the person who attempts suicide in a severe and self-mutilating fashion is in greater danger of being successful than the person who swallows a relatively minor dose of medication or who superficially cuts his wrist. However, nurses have seen cases where an individual uses a relatively innocuous method of self-injury with the firm conviction that he will succeed. It appears that minor attempts of suicidal behavior may also occur in psychotic or severely depressed people who lack the energy or initiative to act any more aggressively against themselves.

A second consideration is whether the person makes a suicidal attempt in an isolated setting. For example, the person who ingests medication in front of a spouse during a family argument is not considered to be at high risk. It is important, however, to remember that most suicidal behavior is ambivalent, and although the person wishes to escape what appears to be an intolerable reality, at the same time he wishes to be discovered. M. Farber refers to this aspect of suicidal behavior as a "gamble with death."[10] This feature of suicidal behavior points out the manipulative aspect. However, it is most disquieting to find that the person who commits suicide almost always leaves a warning.[11]

Estimating Suicidal Risk

A prevailing problem in the work of suicide prevention is determining the degree of suicide risk in individual patients. Very often, this task is conducted on a clinical and intuitive basis. In an attempt to advance suicidal assessment, Motto, Heilbron, and Juster developed an empirical suicide risk scale and tested it prospectively on 2,753 subjects using 101 psychosocial variables. In a two-year follow-up study, 136 (4.9 percent) of the subjects had committed suicide. Using rigorous statistical analysis, 15 variables were identified as significant predictors of suicidal outcome.[12] These variables are as follows:

1. Age: risk increases with age.
2. Occupation: executive, administrator, owner of business, professional, semi-skilled worker.
3. Financial resources: risk increases with resources.
4. Emotional disorder in family: depression, alcoholism.
5. Sexual orientation: bisexual, active; homosexual, inactive.

6. Previous psychiatric hospital admission: risk increases with number of admissions.
7. Result of previous efforts to obtain help: negative or variable.
8. Threatened financial loss: yes.
9. Special stress: severe.
10. Sleep (hours per night): risk increases with number of hours per night.
11. Weight change, present episode: gain or 1 to 9 percent loss.
12. Ideas of persecution or reference: yes.
13. Suicidal impulses: yes.
14. Seriousness of present suicide attempt or intent: unambivalent or ambivalent but weighted toward suicide.
15. Interviewer's reaction to subject: risk increases with negativity of reaction.

In view of the studies, the following high-risk factors are useful in determining the urgency and severity of cases involving potential suicide:

1. Prior attempt.
2. A detailed and refined suicide plan.
3. A lethal means for self-destruction (e.g., gun).
4. An available mechanism for self-destruction.
5. Expression of bizarre death-related fantasies.
6. Emotional status that extends beyond sadness to despair, or exhibition of almost defiant attitudes toward others.

PREVENTION AND INTERVENTION

Authorities at the Los Angeles Suicide Prevention Center have noted that the potentially suicidal person is experiencing a severe crisis, one that results in some degree of disruption in the thought process, as well as in an alteration of customary reactions and behaviors. Suicidal crises are often precipitated by life stresses that the individual perceives as so overwhelming that continued living ceases to possess meaning for him. In addition, it has been observed that among suicidal persons of all age groups, those who do not succeed at first will often try again— many with lethal success. It is also believed that for every successful suicide, some eight attempts are made; therefore, suicidal threats and gestures should be taken seriously and should be considered as sufficient reasons for intervention.[13]

Toward this end, increasing emphasis has been placed on the importance of broad-based, public education programs on suicide prevention. It is hoped that such programs will promote a greater recognition and awareness of the danger signals exhibited by most suicidal individuals before the acting out of their self-destructive thoughts, so that such individuals may be urged to seek professional assistance before it is too late. Accordingly, authorities have suggested the need for the correction of eight prevalent myths concerning suicide, which are listed below[14]:

Myth 1   Individuals who verbalize suicidal thoughts do not actually follow through with suicide attempts.
Fact   Eight out of every 10 suicides that occur have been preceded by clear, definite warnings. Suicidal threats must be taken seriously.
Myth 2   Suicide is an impulsive action on the part of an individual.
Fact   Studies indicate that many suicidal individuals give numerous clues or warning signals as to their intentions, often over an extended period of time.
Myth 3   Suicidal individuals are completely intent on dying.
Fact   Most authorities agree that the suicidal individual is undecided about living and that the wish to die is an ambivalent one. Thus, it is erroneous to assume the position of, "Why bother, we can't stop them anyway?"
Myth 4   Persons are suicidal for life.
Fact   Numerous case histories reveal that an individual who has been assisted through a suicidal crisis can go on to live a long and productive life.
Myth 5   "Improvement" of depressive states is an indication that the danger of suicide has passed.
Fact   Many suicides occur within the 3-month period that immediately follows the onset of "improvement." During this time, one must remain especially vigilant.
Myth 6   Suicides selectively affect certain economic and occupational classes.

Fact   While it is true that some population groups may be considered to be at higher risk for suicide than others, it is also true that this phenomenon is a relatively democratic one that is spread throughout all levels of society.

Myth 7   Suicidal individuals are psychiatrically ill.

Fact   While it is true that some suicidal individuals may have an underlying psychiatric disorder, it is also true that others may simply be feeling sad or unhappy as a result of some temporary emotional crisis or a sudden loss of hope.

Myth 8   Suicidal tendencies are hereditary.

Fact   Suicide is an individual matter that can be prevented but not inherited.

Emphasis has recently been placed on the roles that people in a variety of occupations can play in regard to suicide prevention and crisis intervention. Training has been suggested for groups of people such as beauticians, barbers, and bartenders because they have an opportunity to talk with their clients about matters of concern and are in a position to observe personality and behavioral differences.

Advice is often asked of nurses regarding depressed individuals. The following guidelines for people faced with a potentially suicidal individual were given by clinical psychologist Guy T. Pilato:

1. All suicidal ideations should be taken seriously.
2. Avoid debating the issue of life versus death with the individual. Often, the suicidal individual has given considerable thought, over a period of time, to his life circumstances and may have good arguments for terminating his life.
3. Show a concern for the individual as well as willingness to listen to him.
4. Adopt a position of confidence (i.e., "I can handle this conversation that we are having."). Try to avoid disclosing personal anxieties to the individual whose life situation is already upset.
5. Remember that crises are time-limited, and as such, possess both a beginning and an end. Assist the individual through the crisis period.
6. Encourage the client to seek professional assistance.
7. Personalize the referral process by offering to accompany the individual to the counselor or therapist selected.

Shneidman and Mandelkorn have suggested the following guidelines for the management of the suicidal person over the telephone[15]:

1. It is essential that the counselor establish and maintain continuing communication with the suicidal person; this may take the following form:
   a. How did you get into this trouble?
   b. What are some of the solutions you have considered?
   c. Have you thought about how you will do it?
   d. When?
2. A suicidal crisis almost always concerns two people—the suicidal individual and some sort of significant other. Telephone therapists must first determine who that significant person is—a father, mother, wife, lover, friend, or whoever; then attempt to arrange an immediate interview with the two persons. The significant other must be advised of the situation and urged, if possible, to become involved in the life-saving effort.
3. Some authorities stress how important it is for the caller to feel assured that the person who is interviewing him is a sympathetic and knowledgeable authority who can be of assistance and provide some realistic hope.
4. The primary goal of crisis intervention is to prevent the individual from terminating his life, not to restructure his personality, instantaneously, over the telephone. Thus, prescribing a cure for the caller's difficulties under such delicate and precarious circumstances is not appropriate or therapeutic.
5. It may be useful to inform the suicidal individual that you can assist him in reevaluating his life situation and in making immediate realistic changes. Sometimes minimal assistance initially is all that is necessary for preventing death, since the person who is contemplating suicide is still clinging to life.

NURSING MANAGEMENT OF SUICIDAL BEHAVIOR

The suicide crisis is a common psychiatric emergency that is seen in outpatient settings such as in emergency departments of general hospitals. Since there is an ever-present danger that the suicide attempt will be repeated with lethal consequences, psychiatric consultation is advisable. When such consultation is not available, the most important decision following treatment for the crisis is whether to hospitalize the person in a psychiatric facility or refer him for outpatient evaluation.

Behavior that Threatens the Patient's Own Life

Behavior that threatens the patient's own life includes suicide threats, actual attempts, and the potential of suicide attempts. This type of behavior is most frequently associated clinically with severe depression, various forms of psychosis, or conditions related to acute and chronic alcoholism, drug abuse, interpersonal conflicts, and acute paranoia.

EXAMPLES

1. A 20-year-old patient is brought to the emergency room by his father. The father states the patient has been acting strangely at home—collecting knives, walking around the house holding knives and waving them at family members, pointing them at himself, and talking to himself about death and dying. The patient is sitting in the waiting area getting his chart completed when the psychiatric nurse practitioner is called. Upon the arrival of the psychiatric nurse practitioner, the patient becomes increasingly frightened, says he wants to leave, and if everyone doesn't go away, he'll pull out the knife he has in his pocket and stab himself in the neck (pointing to neck).
2. A person is standing in the subway station threatening to jump in front of a train, stating he was commanded by God to end his life here on earth. He is brought to the emergency department by police who were called to the scene.
3. A 30-year-old woman is brought by ambulance, accompanied by her mother and sister who speak only Spanish. The patient is drowsy and lethargic upon arrival. She said she had ingested an unknown quantity of sleeping pills and Valium in the past 3 days since the death of her

boyfriend who had hung himself in jail. She had put him into jail following an argument and a beating. The patient stated, "I just want to sleep and sleep" and denied she was trying to kill herself.

The primary task of the nurse, whether the behavior is threatened or has been actually carried out, is to (1) evaluate the suicidal potential of the patient, i.e., establish the patient's explicit attempt to die, and (2) make a decision as to whether the patient can be treated as an outpatient or will require hospitalization.

Management is geared toward structuring a safe, comfortable, and quiet environment for the interview to take place, i.e., away from the activity of the emergency room. The nurse should check for weapons, have security backup available, and reassure the patient that he will be safe in the emergency room and that the staff will not let him do anything to hurt himself.

Outpatient Care

When there is no sign of psychosis, severe depression, or a highly disordered personality structure, and when the social situation is relatively stable and the attempt has not been of a highly lethal nature, the nurse can be further reassured if the patient regrets his recent suicidal behavior and assures that he will return for help if future events threaten to overwhelm him. Alternatively, the nurse should never disregard a patient who states that he is sorry he did not succeed or threatens to try again. This individual is clearly asking for help, however disordered the nature of his communication. The nurse should also be extremely cautious about the patient who has suffered a loss and believes that death will reunite him with a loved one.

Just as the suicide act communicates a wish for escape and at the same time a plea for rescue, so the wish for rescue is frequently associated with a tendency to alienate the helper. The suicide act is often an expression of the patient's rage against the environment turned in against himself, what Shneidman has called "murder in the 180th degree."[16,17] This is of consequence in management because the patient's anger and hopelessness may evoke similar feelings from even the most empathetic nurse and may increase the patient's tendency to see the environment as hostile and unforgiving.

During the initial interview, it is essential to listen very carefully to what the person says about the nature of the suicidal intent. After the information is evaluated, it is important to assess the patient's feelings of inadequacy in coping with the immediate and chronic stresses in his life, his level of hope, and his view of the situation as being intolerable. The nurse listens and tries to understand the client's view of his existence at that very moment.

In working with patients who are not psychotic or toxic, Allen and Allen have found it useful to follow the method of checking to see if the patient is willing to make a "no-suicide contract."[18] This is done by asking the patient if he will make a *contract with himself* not to kill himself, accidentally or on purpose, now or in the future. If the person hedges, then see whether a contract can be made for a year, a month, or even a day. This gives some measure of the person's intentions. Persons who say that they won't kill themselves this year are a much less immediate risk than those who say they might kill themselves tonight. The contract must be between the patient and himself. The therapist is only a witness to the contract, and since the contract is not between the patient and the therapist, it is more difficult for the patient to commit suicide to punish the therapist. If the patient keeps suicide as an option, will he make a contract to contact the therapist, or failing that, to go to the emergency room should he feel suicidal? The latter prevents the patient from letting the phone ring once, then hanging up. If the patient is unwilling to make such a contract, he needs to be hospitalized. Assessment of the patient's social supports and home environment includes evaluation of both the healthy support that such entities provide him as well as the support that these may lend to his pathology. The patient's supportive network needs to be actively mobilized.[19]

In our experience, people who make suicide attempts are outside of a caring system; that is, they are not being cared for by a professional or mental health worker. And people who are successful in their suicidal behavior are generally not actively engaged in treatment. They may be involved in situations in which the therapist has terminated treatment or is on vacation or is in the process of leaving, and thus the patient is in transit.

The main intervention in this situation is that someone must take responsibility to care for and to watch over the patient. A danger for nurses is that they are so busy making referrals for the suicidal person that, in essence, he is getting no care. We caution against this danger of making transfers and referrals because it gives the message that no one in the system really cares. The quality of hopelessness decreases when the patient feels that someone does care in a human way. This feeling may be a lifeline at that point in time.

—— CASE EXAMPLE* ——————

Miss Zito presented herself at the local mental health center with "depression and suicidal thoughts" on the advice of her supervisor at work. She related that she had had passing periods of "the blues" before, but her feelings at present were much more severe and began after she broke up with her boyfriend 2 months before. She related the following symptoms: frequent crying spells, inability to concentrate on the job, great difficulty in falling asleep at night, poor appetite, and weight loss. She felt it a great effort to get out of bed in the morning. Miss Zito was an attractive, neatly dressed, twenty-two-year-old woman with puffy, dark circles under her eyes. She answered questions relevantly, but slowly with a flat tone of voice. She moved very little throughout the interview.

Miss Zito stated that her breakup with her boyfriend was full of turmoil. He was demanding that she decide whether or not she would marry him. Miss Zito's mother did not seem to like this man and Miss Zito felt caught in the middle.

Miss Zito was from an Italian family. Her parents divorced when she was 11 years old after many years of fighting. Mr. Zito left on Miss Zito's 11th birthday and she has felt somehow responsible for his leaving. She describes Mrs. Zito as "the long-suffering type" who says she sacrificed her life to make her children happy and all she got in return was grief and unhappiness. She never smiled or talked much with her daughter. When Miss

* This case is contributed by Margaret Eckroth.

Zito began dating, Mrs. Zito never asked about her date, instead stating how tired she was because she had waited up for her. She made disparaging remarks about the boy Miss Zito had been with and men in general. Miss Zito related she had several friends but always found sharing her feelings with them very difficult. She relates having had the same difficulty with her boyfriend.

The *DSM-III-R* diagnosis for Miss Zito is Major Depressive Episode. This diagnosis is substantiated by the presence of depressed mood, loss of interest or pleasure, weight loss, insomnia, loss of energy, and diminished ability to concentrate for over 2 weeks.

NURSING CARE PLAN

NURSING DIAGNOSES

- Alteration in thought processes as evidenced by negative views of self and environment
- Inefficient individual coping related to situational crisis
- Potential for suicide

NURSING GOALS

1. Meet basic needs while reducing pervasive feelings of worthlessness, hopelessness, and helplessness.
2. Redefine ideas of self or the situation and help to expand coping strategies.

NURSING INTERVENTIONS

1. Prevent isolation from others.
2. Confront irrational demands.
3. Use firmness when patient hesitates to do things for self.
4. Avoid arguments or making moral judgments regarding what the patient should or should not do.
5. Help patient identify thoughts that occurred just prior to feelings of hopelessness, helplessness, and sadness.
6. Observe for indications of self-harm potential.

The effectiveness of therapy based on this nursing care plan will be evaluated by the following criteria:

1. Decrease in depressive symptoms; development of normal mood pattern.
2. Makes positive statements about self.
3. Uses problem-solving skills.
4. Reflects desire to live in making future plans.

The nursing diagnosis of alteration in thought processes might be treated according to the cognitive therapy model.

According to Beck, the thought content of the depressed patient centers on a significant loss the patient perceives to be essential to his happiness.[20] He anticipates negative outcomes from any important undertaking; he regards himself as deficient in the attributes necessary for achieving goals. This theme may be formulated in terms of the cognitive triad: a negative conception of the self; a negative interpretation of life experiences; and a nihilistic view of the future.

Beck states that early experiences with loss of a significant other may predispose the person to overreact to a similar happening later in life.[21] Miss Zito had just such an experience with the loss of her father; thus she had a tendency to make extreme judgments when other losses occur. After experiencing the loss of her boyfriend Miss Zito regarded herself as deficient, inadequate, unworthy, and attributed this loss to a deficiency in herself. Miss Zito at that time saw her future as hopeless.

The course of therapy according to Beck's model was to first identify why Miss Zito was depressed, what the rules she used to interpret and evaluate the events in her life. Miss Zito was given a homework assignment to keep a log of automatic thoughts to help her to identify the rules she lived by. Later this log was expanded to include a rational response to the automatic thoughts. Miss Zito was also asked to log her daily activities and record which ones were pleasurable and which ones were not. This activity was to penetrate the blindness depressed people develop, insisting nothing gives them pleasure.

Next, the rules that Miss Zito lived by were challenged. If they were found to be false or self-defeating, she was encouraged to drop them and substitute more realistic, adaptable ones.

The outcome of this therapy was that Miss Zito changed the self-defeating rules she lived by into more realistic ones. By changing her cognitions she changed her feelings and her behavior. She was no longer depressed and was able to work through other problems using her newly acquired problem-solving skills.

The use of cognitive therapy has become increasingly popular. This form of therapy takes into account a unique aspect of human functioning that the other major schools of psychology ignore, that being the human ability to think. This capacity allows therapists to turn responsibility for therapy back over to the patient. The therapist then coaches the patient in thinking and working through his problem, thus teaching the patient problem-solving skills for generalization to other areas of his life.

Inpatient Hospitalization

The risk of repeated suicidal behavior and the indications for hospitalization can be assessed by referring to the psychiatric diagnosis, nature of intent, social matrix, and current and past history. Hospitalization is indicated when there is high risk in any of these areas.*

* This section, thorugh page 942, on nursing care of the inpatient hospitalized suicidal patient was written, in part, by Linda Muh Spink.

Inpatient psychiatric units of hospitals are a major resource for referral of suicidal persons. These units have a dual task: First, they have an administrative obligation to prevent suicide and to protect the patient; and second, they must provide the caring aspects of the therapeutic environment.

The nursing care of the hospitalized suicidal patient includes assessment of typical behaviors, the setting of goals, and patient management in the milieu.

Typical Behaviors

The suicidal patient often has feelings of severe self-depreciation, guilt, hopelessness, helplessness, and worthlessness. There are many somatic complaints because all energy is focused on the self. These complaints include fatigue, sleep disturbances, anorexia, weight loss, constipation, and decreased muscle tone. There may be a retardation of physical behaviors as demonstrated by slowed gait, slumped shoulders, and slow motion, plus a retardation of cognitive functions as demonstrated by slowed thinking processes, reduced comprehension, and impaired verbal responses. Depressed patients can also become agitated in their behavior rather than retarded. They can pace the floors for hours on end, wringing their hands, and pulling at their hair and crying. The nurse must continuously be watchful for signs that these patients may be planning to turn their hostility onto themselves, resulting in actual physical harm and a suicidal attempt.

Setting Goals

Whichever form of behavior the patient demonstrates (agitated or retarded), the goals the nurse sets for this patient must be individualized and must be based on the patient's present behaviors and past history. The first consideration, of course, is preventing the patient from self-destructive actions. A long-term goal for this type of patient would be to help him learn to express feelings of aggression and hostility in an appropriate, socially acceptable manner. Variations of this goal would be indicated as short-term goals for the patient, depending on his behavior and past experience. This type of patient is often so overwhelmed with feelings of worthlessness that an important short-term nursing goal is to increase the patient's self-esteem. Once the patient begins to feel good about himself, he can then begin to invest energy elsewhere.

The Therapeutic Milieu

The patient who is very withdrawn and at the depth of his depression does not usually have the energy to attempt suicide. All energy is being turned inward, leaving little energy for other activities. However, as there are signs of improvement from the depression, the risk of suicide increases. Such "improvement" may not indicate clinical progress but rather the relief experienced by the patient at a decision to commit suicide. In addition, the patient whose depression is manifested by agitated behavior *always* has the energy for self-destructive behavior and so must be watched especially closely.

Potentially suicidal patients should be in a room near the nurses' station where close observation is easily accomplished. Preferably, the suicidal patient should not be in a private room but rather with at least one other patient. In a therapeutic community, the patients often support each other and help each other deal with their problems in ways that the staff cannot. Many times another patient has reported to the staff that a patient needs help. Having another patient in the room with the suicidal patient provides one more pair of eyes, should the patient be contemplating harming himself. At no time, however, should the nursing staff ever rely on another patient to be watching a patient for suicide attempts. This is too heavy a burden to place on another patient who has problems of his own.

Until such time as the patient has inner control over self-destructive wishes, he must be on suicide precautions. Exactly what these precautions entail will vary somewhat from hospital to hospital. However, obvious hazards should always be removed from the environment. Many units have a locked cupboard where patients' razors, scissors, mirrors, etc., can be placed. Some nursing units still remove everything from the suicidal patient. However, most staff members have learned that to remove everything the patient could hurt himself on is impossible and demeaning to the patient. The patient who is actively set on destructive behavior will find a way to do it. For example, one such patient, Anna, attempted to eat the tacks nailing the carpeting to the floor. A patient such as this requires frequent checks or even continual supervision. Occasionally four-point restraints are used for a very suicidal patient; however, this should be a last resort. (Laws regarding the use of restraints vary from state to state and must be carefully observed.) Anna

was placed in restraints because this was the only means of keeping her from destructive behavior. She found tremendous relief in being in the restraints—whether she viewed this as her "just" punishment or as a strong external control is uncertain. She stated she felt the need to know that no matter how she felt, while in the restraints she knew she could not hurt herself and thus found it reassuring. Thus, the use of restraints should not be viewed as punishment but rather as an additional external control.

The patient who is suicidal must be encouraged to seek out staff when feeling an urge to injure himself. Although it is important that the staff be ever-alert, the patient must learn self-control. One way to achieve this is by encouraging the patient to come to the staff when feeling a loss of this control. Anna, the patient cited above, learned to come to the staff when she needed help controlling her destructive impulses. With encouragement from the staff, Anna learned to say whether she felt that sitting and talking with a staff member would help her or whether she needed medication or even restraints for a short while. In this way, a patient can learn to assume responsibility for himself and eventually can learn to exert control over himself.

It is often helpful to make a "contract" with the hospitalized patient. This contract is usually set up between a nurse and a patient for a predetermined period of time. If the nurse has observed the patient to be having difficulty controlling his self-destructive impulses, she would first seek him out to assess how real is the danger of his harming himself. After spending time with the patient, the nurse can directly ask the patient whether he feels he can agree to come to the nurse when he feels himself losing control over the impulse to hurt himself. The contract must be dealt with directly and openly with the patient. The nurse indicates her concern to the patient and asks if he can agree that within a stated time frame, which would vary depending on the patient, he will definitely not hurt himself. Some hospitals use a verbal contract, but others will have the patient put this agreement in writing. If the nurse deals honestly with the patient, the patient will accept this responsibility and state whether or not he feels he can keep a contract. The nurse must then make a point to check often on the patient and to be certain to sit down with the patient again before the determined time limit is over. A contract is useful for both inpatient and outpatient clients. The time frame set will depend on the nurse's assessment of the patient's ability to handle the stress he is experiencing. The following example illustrates such a contract.

Anna had been able to maintain control of her self-destructive impulses and had been out of restraints for several days. However, she continued to have difficult times. The nursing staff had learned Anna's nonverbal cues at these times and would seek her out and sit with her. The past 2 days Anna was able to seek out the nurses. This conversation was the second contract the patient had made with the staff.

ANNA: I can't stand this anymore—[pacing, chewing on her clenched fists]
NURSE: I can see you are feeling uptight. Let's talk for awhile.
ANNA: Yes, OK—I'm just so scared. . . .

The nurse and patient then sat together for 15 minutes talking of scared feelings.

NURSE: Anna, I'm going to have to leave in 5 minutes. I'm wondering how you are now—do you think you need the restraints again? Or can you control your feelings of wanting to hurt yourself? How can we help you best?
ANNA: Oh . . . I don't know [chewing on knuckles]. No, I think I'm OK. . . .
NURSE: I need you to be able to promise me that you'll seek out the charge nurse if you feel you're losing control.
ANNA: [no comment]
NURSE: You have to be able to honestly tell me that in the next hour you will not hurt yourself and that you will go to the charge nurse if you are having difficulty.
ANNA: Yes. . . . I can agree to that—at least until 8:45. I'll go to her. . . .
NURSE: OK. I'm glad you feel you can handle that. I'll tell the charge nurse our agreement and she can talk with you then.
ANNA: OK. Bye now.

This method worked well for Anna. She was able to keep the contract—at least she held out for 45 minutes. About 15 minutes before the hour was up she came to the charge nurse stating she feared she was losing control. This particular evening she needed to go back into restraints for an hour. However, she had made progress because *she* had assumed responsibility for herself and had handled it as well as she

could. For Anna this was growth, and this was pointed out to her to help raise her self-esteem.

The suicidal patient needs a simple routine without many demands until he is ready for more interaction. If the unit has numerous, loud activities going on at one time, the patient who is severely depressed will tend to withdraw even more and feel worse about his depression. He should be encouraged to join other patients without too high expectations being placed on him. Because this patient tends to withdraw much of the time, the staff need to seek him out. The patient frequently needs to be provided an opportunity for outward expression of hostility, under supervision, as this provides for catharsis. The occupational therapy department (activity department) can provide the patient with activities that will help ventilate his hostility and provide for successful experiences to increase self-esteem. Some patients may find release in creative crafts; others may prefer chores such as ironing or washing the walls, tables, etc.

Suicidal patients often are so withdrawn that they need help making decisions. The patient does not have the energy to expend on decision making. The nurse must provide the patient with simple choices to encourage responsibility without being frustrated. Initially the decision may be as simple as the choice between orange juice or grapefruit juice for breakfast. The patient should not be pushed. As improvement is noted, the decisions should be more complex. The nurse must be careful to avoid the inclination to be especially gay and cheerful with the depressed patient. A smiling, bouncy nurse will make the patient even more acutely aware of his depression. Do not tell the patient how much he has to live for, or how much his family loves him and needs him, etc. This serves to deny the patient's true feelings and will stall the nurse–patient relationship. If the patient senses the nurse cannot handle talking about his depression, then he will withdraw even more inwardly.

Because the patient absorbs his energy into himself, there is little energy left to care for his personal hygiene or nutrition. Therefore is very important that the nurse see to these needs until the patient is able to do so. Nourishing fluids such as milkshakes or eggnog can be offered frequently to increase the patient's caloric intake. Constipation is a common problem for the depressed patient because of decreased food intake and lack of exercise, so stool softeners may be indicated. Patients will often need much encouragement to adequately maintain their personal hygiene. Positive reinforcement should be given when patients show an interest in good grooming.

Communication Strategies

Distraught people often do let people know both in direct and indirect ways their thoughts and feelings about suicide. There are people who do not verbally announce they are suicidal but again the situation they are in often clearly indicates that alternatives and options are not perceived by the person. There are some people who, because of their religious beliefs, are guilt-ridden by any conscious acknowledgment of suicidal thoughts yet who are at risk because their behavior indicates they are suicidal though they are not consciously aware of it. Again, the assessment here is focused on how compromised this person is from his view of himself and his life. For example, a mother who is having difficulty caring for her children and is becoming increasingly angry with them and whose husband leaves and works two jobs and is unable to understand her being upset with the children can be at high risk for suicide if at the same time she strongly believes it is wrong to be angry, in particular, that it is wrong to have angry, hateful thoughts toward one's children.

The nurse needs to step into the dominant belief system of the person who is depressed. This will usually provoke intense emotional states in the nurse. For example, if you believe that you are not loved and you are worthless, what would it be like to leave the hospital and interview for a job? If you believe you were the cause of the automobile accident that killed your aunt and has placed your sister in the intensive care unit, what might you consider doing knowing that your uncle is coming to the hospital to meet you? In this latter example, the young man was walking out of the emergency room door because the family had arrived when the nurse stopped him. The nurse had observed this young man's face, noticed the shocked state and realized no one had talked to him. She sensed that he was in an uncompromising situation, which was confirmed when she stopped him and he broke down crying and admitted that he had decided to leave and kill himself. He was able to communicate his total distress over his aunt's death and his fear that he in no way could face his uncle and his parents for what had hap-

pened. There were extensive family meetings and in this situation he agreed to a voluntary stay in the hospital.

CASE EXAMPLE*

Jerry Bauer, a 31-year-old never-married male, was admitted to the psychiatric unit following a serious suicidal attempt. The suicidal attempt was the culmination of a year marked by the death of a sister (from cancer), the loss of employment, and the loss of independence (incurred by a move back to his parents' home). One month prior to hospitalization, Jerry Bauer began to hear voices. He was frightened more by the existence of the voices than by their content. Troubled by his inability to stem the chanting of the voices, along with increasing anhedonia and shrinking self-respect, Jerry Bauer overdosed on diazepam (Valium).

Nursing Assessment

At the time of this nursing assessment, Jerry Bauer was in locked seclusion. His continuous pacing stopped with the entrance of the student. He was unshaven and emaciated, but his blank facial expression was his most distinctive feature. He made direct eye contact, although he frequently looked downward. Jerry's voice was monotone and barely audible. He volunteered little spontaneous conversation but answered all questions.

Jerry Bauer described his life over the course of the last year. He felt great sorrow over the death of his sister. After the funeral, he began to experience a sense of despair relative to his career as a teacher. He felt that his impact upon the students was negligible. He decided to quit his job. The termination of his job led to a financial crisis. He had to give up his apartment and move to his parents' home. The emotional climate at his parent's home was tense. Jerry made a fledgling attempt to escape from the home environment and search for employment. The search was short-lived as he met with rejection by potential employers. Jerry began to spend most of the day alone in his room. Initially, books were his primary diversion. He soon began to lose interest in reading. His nights and days became indistinguishable, accentuated by agonizing periods of boredom. Jerry loathed his inability to help himself. As boredom and self-loathing built to a crescendo, Jerry began to hear voices. The voices were descriptive and turned ordinary objects such as pencils into fantastic images, such as space rockets. Jerry was aware that the voices were not real and he was terrified by their increasing frequency. He needed to escape and suicide was his plan.

---

* This case was contributed by Barbara Greengold.

DSM-III-4 Diagnosis: Major Depression with Psychotic Features

The medical intervention was electroconvulsive therapy (ECT).

Nursing Diagnosis

Knowledge deficit related to ECT.

Short-Term Goal

Patient will understand what ECT is and what outcomes can be predicted by its use.

Intervention

Provision of written information about ECT followed by discussion and questions.

Evaluation

Jerry studied the ECT literature in detail. The more he read, the less convinced he was of the efficacy of ECT as a treatment modality. However, Jerry was aware of the reality that his insurance coverage was limited. His parents had told him that if he was not well when the insurance for private hospitalization ran out, they would commit him to a public mental hospital. The insurance company agreed to extend coverage if ECT was undertaken.

Jerry had 18 ECT sessions. He reported a diminution of voices, spoke of returning to his apartment, and began to consider going back to work. Jerry was released from the hospital and returned to his parents' home the day his insurance coverage expired.

Postvention: A Program for Bereaved Survivors of Suicide

Not all suicides can be prevented. Although the subject has not been extensively studied, there is some literature available on the experiences of families and individuals who have been bereaved by a suicide. One of these studies focuses on children as survivors of a parent's suicide; another study reports on widows of suicides; another on the families of adolescent suicides; and yet another on significant others as survivors.[22–25]

One author notes that:

survivors of the suicidal death of a loved one form a neglected group with individual needs and collective problems. Their vulnerability to subsequent episodes of depression with or without suicidal behavior has been suggested by follow-up studies. Their psycho-

logical situation is distinct from the bereavement following natural death in both intrapsychic and interpersonal ways.[26]

According to Schuyler, a conservative estimate reveals that on the average five survivors from the immediate family are intimately affected by each suicidal loss, constituting a special interest group to which approximately 250,000 new members are added annually. The point is made that as soon as a suicidal death occurs, the survivors lose an inalienable right—the right to live an unstigmatized life.[27]

It has been observed that suicidal death, in contrast to natural death, is invariably associated with a tendency on the part of survivors to blame themselves, especially, if their relationship with the deceased was an ambivalent and conflicting one.[28] Another common reaction exhibited by the survivors of a suicidal death is anger directed at the deceased individual.

A suicidal death raises many questions, including[29]:

1. Was the suicidal individual aware of and capable of controlling his own actions?
2. Will surviving children, when there are any, be more likely to become suicide victims because of their sibling's death? One study investigated suicide among twins and found no substantive evidence to support the belief that specific suicidal tendencies are inherited.
3. Is suicidal death a sin, and if so, is the victim relegated to eternal damnation?
4. Finally, with suicidal death, strange hypotheses often emerge. For example, was a murder committed? Was there a mysterious intruder who came in the night and took the victim away?

It has also been observed that survivors of suicidal deaths often search for scapegoats. If the deceased was undergoing therapy, the therapist is the obvious choice. If the person was in a hospital or under the care of a physician, the physician is seen as responsible for the death. If the person abused drugs or alcohol, these agents are viewed as the causative factors.[30]

Suicidal death may also be associated with identification of the survivor with the deceased. Tragically, this may take the form of imitation or adoption, of the survivor, of the suicidal behavior itself. Or during the process of adaptation to his loss, the survivor may adopt a distorted picture of himself, which in turn may precipitate clinical depression. Preoccupation with the grief process may also lead to disturbances in the survivor's relationships with others, and social isolation is common following a suicidal death. Finally, regardless of whether the underlying motivational factor is identification with the deceased, an attempt to rejoin the loved one, or a learned reaction to stress, it is these behaviors that place the survivor of a suicidal death at considerable risk for lethal behavior and suggest the advantages of a positive counseling relationship.[31]

In counseling the survivors of suicidal deaths, the following recommendations are made:

1. The survivor needs to reach an understanding of the suicidal death, which preserves his own self-worth and satisfies his search for meaning. Initially, the pattern of self-blame predominates, along with anger at having been denied the opportunity to intervene. Comments such as, "I know I could have stopped him," are not unusual at this time. Sometimes the suicidal nature of the death is denied. ("It was an accident. It must be certified as an accident. The gun was loaded because there had been prowlers.") The earlier life of the survivors may be searched for clues to explain the death. ("My husband should have spent more time with the boy.")

2. The survivor needs to express his feelings in an atmosphere of acceptance. These emotions often include sadness, anger, grief, loneliness, anxiety, and abandonment. Once the patient feels that the counselor can tolerate his expression of feelings, the therapist can move on to the task of beginning to assist the survivor in "ordering" his feelings. Irrational fear, guilt, or shame can then be openly dealt with and brought to the patient's attention.

3. In addition to dealing with the suicidal nature of the death, the patient should be encouraged to mourn his loss, and to consider his life in the absence of the deceased person. Preoccupation with the suicide may be employed by the survivor, as a defensive measure, to avoid the conscious awareness of the emotional pain associated with his loss.

4. Counselors must monitor survivors, in much the same way that they inquire into the thoughts and plans of a potentially suicidal individual believed to be at risk. The therapist's response to information concerning suicidal intent among survivors must be active and include availability of the counselor to his client, as well as encouragement of the survivor to consider the consequences of his proposed actions.

5. Since the social response to a survivor is often dominated by the stigma attached to suicide, the counselor must make a special effort to identify and encourage support from others in the patient's environment. This must be done as an adjunctive measure to the support and reassurance that he provides for the client. At this time of cognitive confusion and emotional turmoil, it is critical that the coping mechanisms of the patient be reinforced.

A program in *postvention*—Shneidman's term for the activities following the suicide of a significant other—serves to assist the survivors in coping with their emotional and psychological responses to the loss and is most frequently conducted through home visit intervention by nurses.[32] In the San Bernardino (California) Suicide Survivor Follow-Up Program, the coroner's office collaborates with the local departments of mental and public health by forwarding to them at once a copy of the death certificate of each reported suicide, so that a nurse can make a home visit to the bereaved family.[33]

Summary

Nurses have an important role in working with the suicidal client both in the outpatient setting as well as in inpatient hospitals. Careful assessment, diagnosis, and planning are necessary to negotiate a regimen useful and helpful to the client. Evaluation of the plan is essential. Nurses are also collaborating with other disciplines to provide crisis intervention to those individuals bereaved by a suicide.

Questions

1. What are the key factors to consider when someone tells you he wants to kill himself?
2. Give an example of a suicidal gesture and a suicidal attempt and discuss the factor of lethality of intent.
3. A classmate tells you that a friend of hers said she had a gun in her pocketbook and wanted to kill herself. What would you advise?
4. Design a nursing care plan using the nursing process for a suicidal patient who is hospitalized.
5. What are your thoughts and feelings regarding "postvention" programs?

REFERENCES AND SUGGESTED READINGS

1. Shaffer, D. Diagnostic considerations in suicidal behavior in children and adolescents. *Journal of the American Academy of Child Psychiatry*, 1982, 4, 414–416.
2. Stanley, E., & Barter, J. Adolescent suicidal behavior. *Journal of Orthopsychiatry*, 1970, 1, 87–96.
3. Rauenhorst, J. Follow-up of young women who attempt suicide. *Diseases of the Nervous System*, 1972, 33, 792–797.
4. Pokorny, A. Prediction of suicide in psychiatric patients. *Archives of General Psychiatry*, 1983, 40, 249–257.
5. Gispert, M., Davis, M. S., Marsh, L., & Wheeler, K. Predictive factors in repeated suicide attempts by adolescents. *Hospital and Community Psychiatry*, 1987, 38, 390–393.
6. Beck, A. T. *Depression: Clinical, Experimental, and Theoretical Aspects*. New York: Harper & Row, 1967.
7. Beck, A. T., Steer, R. A., Kovacs, M., & Garrison, B. Hopelessness and eventual suicide: A 10-year prospective study of patients hospitalized with suicidal ideation. *American Journal of Psychiatry*, 1985, 142, 559.
8. Shneidman, E. S., & Lane, D. M. Psychologic and social work clues to suicide in a schizophrenic. In E. S. Shneidman & N. L. Farberow (Eds.), *Clues to Suicide*. New York: McGraw-Hill, 1957, pp. 170–187.
9. Hatton, C. L., Valente, S. M., & Rink, A. Assessment of suicidal risk. In C. L. Hatton & S. M. Valente (Eds.), *Suicide: Assessment and Intervention*, 2nd ed. E. Norwalk, Conn.: Appleton-Century-Crofts, 1984.
10. Farber, M. *Theory of Suicide*. New York: Funk & Wagnalls, 1968, p. 7.
11. Stengel, E. *Suicide and Attempted Suicide*. Baltimore: Penguin, 1964.
12. Motto, J. A., Heilbron, D. C., & Juster, R. P. Development of a clinical instrument to estimate suicide risk. *American Journal of Psychiatry*, 1985, 142, 680–686.
13. Shneidman, E. S., & Farberow, N. L. (Eds.) *Clues to Suicide*. New York: McGraw-Hill, 1957, pp. 119–130.
14. Ibid.
15. Shneidman, E. S., & Mandelkorn, P. *How to Prevent Suicide*, Public Affairs Pamphlet No. 406. New York: [N.Y. City Department of Public Affairs], 1967. (381 Park Avenue South, New York 10016.)
16. Freud, S. Mourning and melancholia. In S. Freud, *The Standard Edition of Complete Psychological Works of Sigmund Freud* (Vol. 14). London: Hogarth Press, 1957, pp. 243–258.
17. Shneidman, E. S. *On the Nature of Suicide*. San Francisco: Jossey-Bass, 1969, pp. 1–30.
18. Allen, J. R., & Allen, B. A. *Guide to Psychiatry*. New York: Medical Examination Publ. Co., 1978.
19. Ibid.
20. Beck, A. T. *Cognitive Therapy and the Emotional Disorders*. New York: International Universities Press, 1976.
21. Ibid.
22. Cain, A., & Fast, I. Children's disturbed reactions to parent suicide. *American Journal of Orthopsychiatry*, 1966, 36, 873.
23. Wallace, S. *After Suicide*. New York: Wiley, 1973.

24. Herzog, A., & Resnick, H. A clinical study of parental response to adolescent death by suicide. In N. Farberow (Ed.), *Proceedings of the 4th International Conference on Suicide Prevention.* Los Angeles: Delmar, 1967.

25. Henslin, J. Strategies of adjustment. In Cain, A. (Ed.), *Survivors of Suicide.* Springfield, Mass.: Bannerstone House, 1972.

26. Schuyler, D. Counseling suicide survivors: Issues and answers. *Omega*, 1973, 4, 313–321.

27. Ibid., pp. 313–314.
28. Ibid., p. 315.
29. Ibid., pp. 318–320.
30. Ibid., pp. 318–321.
31. Ibid., pp. 319–320.
32. Junghardt, D. Z. A program in postvention. In C. L. Hatton & S. M. Valente (Eds.), *Suicide: Assessment and Intervention*, 2nd ed. E. Norwalk, Conn.: Appleton-Century-Crofts, 1984, [p. 124].
33. Ibid.

Chapter 48

The Combative Patient

Ann Wolbert Burgess

Chapter Objectives

The students successfully attaining the goals of this chapter will be able to:

- Identify assessment areas of combative behavior.
- Assess the nature of aggressive behavior.
- Write a nursing care plan for an aggressive patient.

Mental health professionals must deal daily with individuals for whom aggression and violence is a serious problem both to themselves as well as to others.[1] Violent and aggressive behaviors are prevalent among psychiatric patients and often result in institutionalization or other severe disruptions of occupational, societal, familial, or other social functions.[2] Among patients in a New York State psychiatric hospital for longer than one month, 7 percent physically assaulted other persons at least once within a 3-month period.[3]

Aggressive behavior is not confined to institutions. The alarming levels of interpersonal violence seen in our society is of grave concern. Each year the number of homicides exceeds the combined number of deaths from bronchitis, emphysema, and asthma and now approaches 10.3 per 100,000 population.[4] Battery is a primary cause of injury to adult women, and child abuse statistics are increasing in many cities.

Aggressive behavior is defined by Eichelman as behavior that leads to, or appears to lead to, the damage or destruction of a target entity.[5] Violence can be defined as destructive aggression that inflicts physical damage on persons or property.[6] Widespread acceptance of these definitions does not alter the fact that aggressive behaviors represent a class of behaviors whose origin may be multifaceted.

The multifaceted nature of aggressive behavior is reflected in the theories that attempt to explain it. This characterization of human aggression is also reflected in the variable and diverse nosology contained in the *DSM-III-R*. For example, an adolescent who demonstrates violent behavior might generate a diagnosis of conduct disorder. An adult who displays the same behavior might be categorized as having an explosive disorder. In other examples, child abuse could be coded as a "V" code parent–child problem, not a mental disorder at all. Violent behavior might be considered a symptom of other psychiatric disorders including dementia, schizophrenia, drug intoxication, depression, mania, personality disorders, mental retardation, or an attention deficit disorder.[7]

This chapter reviews nursing interventions and case examples for the combative patient in a hospital setting and the aggressive patient who is brought to the hospital via the emergency department.

THE HOSPITALIZED COMBATIVE PATIENT

The trend to a more humane, least restrictive environment for the care of psychiatric patients has been a positive step in mental health care delivery. However, the issue of providing a safe and least restrictive environment for all while caring for combative patients creates a serious dilemma for nurses. In addition to helping patients cope with their aggressive feelings and behavior, nurses must also deal with violence directed toward them by their patients.[8]

Assessing Aggressive Behaviors

Four categories of aggressive behaviors have been outlined by Yudofsky et al. in the form of the Overt Aggression Scale (OAS) to help in the assessment step.[9] These four categories are outlined as follows.

Verbal Aggression

_____ Makes loud noises, shouts angrily.
_____ Yells mild personal insults, e.g., "You're stupid!"
_____ Curses viciously, uses foul language in anger, makes moderate threats to others or self.
_____ Makes clear threats of violence toward others or self ("I'm going to kill you") or requests to help control self.

Physical Aggression Against Objects

_____ Slams doors, scatters clothing, makes a mess.
_____ Throws objects down, kicks furniture without breaking it, marks the wall.
_____ Breaks objects, smashes windows.
_____ Sets fires, throws objects dangerously.

Physical Aggression Against Self

_____ Picks or scratches skin, hits self, pulls hair (with no or minor injury only).
_____ Bangs head, hits fist into objects, throws self onto floor or into objects (hurts self without serious injury).
_____ Small cuts or bruises, minor burns.
_____ Mutilates self, causes deep cuts, bites that bleed, internal injury, fracture, loss of consciousness, loss of teeth.

Physical Aggression Against Other People

_____ Makes threatening gesture, swings at people, grabs at clothes.
_____ Strikes, kicks, pushes, pulls hair (without injury to them).
_____ Attacks others, causing mild-to-moderate physical injury (bruises, sprain, welts).
_____ Attacks others, causing severe physical injury (broken bones, deep lacerations, internal injury).

The OAS can be used to assess a patient during each shift or during a 24-hour period. Each aggressive incident can be recorded as to the time the incident began and its duration. The intervention(s) used can also be indicated and are as follows.

Intervention (check all that apply)

_____ None
_____ Talking to patient
_____ Closer observation
_____ Holding patient
_____ Immediate medication given by mouth
_____ Immediate medication given by injection
_____ Isolation without seclusion (time out)
_____ Seclusion
_____ Use of restraints

_____ Injury required immediate medical treatment for patient

_____ Injury required immediate treatment for other person.

Crisis Management Protocol

The following crisis management protocol, prepared by Michael Sclafani, emphasizes behavior control techniques aimed at preventing a crisis from occurring or dealing with its escalation. Five major areas are outlined.

Therapeutic Environment

Factors within the therapeutic environment constitute the triggering precipitants for aggressive behaviors in patients. Thus, the environment is prepared, as much as possible, to minimize the potential for disruptive behaviors. Attention is given to temperature, noise control, lighting, furniture, etc., of the environment with the goal to have routines and attitudes conducive to peaceful and calm conditions.

Interventions at this level include visual observation of patients and their interactions with other patients, with family, visitors, and staff.

Verbal Intervention

Verbal interaction by staff with patients should be based on knowledge and skills concerning psychosocial interaction, information processing, caring, energy and assertion levels, as well as the step-by-step analysis of prevention of, intervention in, and resolution of various behavioral disorders.

Team Approach

When individual patients do not respond to individual verbal interventions, it is important that team members be coordinated and present a "show of concern" to the patient. Any show of concern should be made in a nonthreatening manner using a code name to alert the staff that team members should assemble. Verbal threats should not be used with patients. The strategy and goal are to convey to the patient that his impulses will be self-controlled in a safe environment. It is critical to have the team prepared before the patient's behavior escalates out of control. Once the team members arrive and are told the circumstances of the intervention, they are physically placed so that they are visible but not threatening to the patient. The team presence acts as a security blanket and conveys to the patient that physical acting out is not appropriate, it will not be tolerated, and that self-control is of prime concern. However, the first team approach is through a "talk down" and should take precedence over any form of physical contact.

Pharmacological Intervention

When individual and team efforts are only partially effective or fail completely, and physical danger is imminent, the use of rapid tranquilization is generally required. Rapid tranquilization is treatment intervention in which doses of antipsychotic medication are titrated against symptoms. Oral medications can be as effective as intramuscular injections if the patient will cooperate.[11] This approach is used after a physician trained in rapid tranquilization techniques has evaluated the patient. If the patient does not cooperate with oral or intramuscular medications, the team will (upon the physician's order) use team intervention strategies for additional behavior control techniques. The four-point personal control technique is a suggested tactic. It is cautioned that at no time should only one or two staff members try to make physical contact with a patient; rather, five staff members should be used, one for each limb and one to protect the head of the patient.

Mechanical Restraint

Mechanical restraints are the last resort, to be used when it becomes apparent that the patient will be harmful to self or others, if the agitation increases, or compliance with the first four interventions is not achieved. Patients should not be threatened with mechanical restraints, but when restraints are inevitable, only approved selected ones should be used, e.g., well-padded wristlets and anklets.

A patient in mechanical restraints is a psychiatric emergency and once restraints are employed, there must always be a staff person in the physical presence of the patient in a one-to-one situation to monitor the patient's response and progress.

Use of Physical Restraints to Limit, Contain, and Control Patients' Behavior.

Physical restraints are prescribed by the clinician in situations in which the patient has demonstrated an inability and unwillingness to control

Specific discipline: _____   Personnel responsible: _____

Date Entr/ Updte	Prob. Num.	Problem Description in Behavioral Terms	Measurable Outcome Objectives	Specific Treatment Approach	Targ. Date	Date Reslvd
		Potential for Violence Related to	**Long-term:** By discharge patient will identify warning signs that indicate loss of control and will begin to use constructive verbal and physical outlets to manage out-of-control behavior. By discharge patient will identify therapist or community resources for follow-up care. **Short-term:** Patient will not harm self or others while hospitalized. Will identify factors, internal signals of escalating anger, agitation by _____ (date).	A. Help patient to identify changes in his behavior as well as internal changes that lead to building anger or agitation. B. Encourage patient to seek out help when beginning to have difficulty maintaining control. C. Encourage patient to verbalize feelings rather than acting out physically. Encourage use of appropriate physical outlets. D. Help patient to identify support systems and areas for further work after discharge. E. Institute suicide or homicide precautions. F. Assess patient's ability to maintain control and encourage this ability. G. Communicate to patient expectation that he will		

951

Potential for Violence Related to	Will identify a plan to avoid reacting violently by _____ (date).	remain in control and get written or verbal contract from patient to alert staff when beginning to lose control.
(cont'd)		H. Provide external controls (e.g., remove patient from stimulating environment).
		I. Remove harmful items that patient can use to harm self or others.
		J. Develop plan with patient for unpredictable violence: 1) 2) 3) 4)
		K. Point out behaviors, signs of agitation and reinforce effective coping skills. Teach patient new or additional methods of coping.
		L. Develop plan with patient to deal with increasing agitation and stress management: 1) 2) 3)

Figure 48-1. Hanna Pavilion Interdisciplinary Treatment Plan. (*Source:* University Hospitals of Cleveland, Hanna Pavilion Nursing Diagnosis Care Plan Subcommittee. Reprinted with permission.)

his own behavior and where such behavior is considered to present a threat to his own safety or the safety of others. Limitation of activity and movement can be accomplished by (1) mechanical restraints, that is, devices that restrain the patient to a bed or stretcher (four-point leather restraints or muslin restraints such as a Posey body restraint made out of cotton muslin material that goes around the trunk of the body and restrains the upper half of the body and attaches to a bed or stretcher); (2) person restraints, that is, establishing control and authority through numbers and physical presence of hospital personnel in professional uniform, including nurses, security guards, and doctors; and (3) room restraints, that is, limiting mobility to a room with safety features such as a small area, padding, plexiglass windows and doors, and little or no furniture or objects. In most instances, a patient will be put into restraints against his will and may put forth a verbal or physical protest. However, most patients who are unable to control their behavior are extremely frightened and terrified, and they usually feel tremendously reassured and relieved when someone else "takes charge" and provides them with the controls they are unable to mobilize for themselves.

The nurse's role in the application and management of restraints includes: (1) assessing the need for restraints and the type to be used, securing the necessary authorization, and period-ically reevaluating the need for their continued use; (2) directing and assisting in the safe application and removal of restraints; (3) accurate recording of the time and reason for the application of restraints and their removal—describing activities and behaviors; and (4) monitoring and observing the patient in restraints so as to ensure that normal body functions are not interfered with and that the patient is physically comfortable and safe (i.e., checking respirations, vital signs, circulation, color of extremities and tightness of restraints, eliminatory functions (offering bedpan or taking person to the bathroom), and offering something to drink. Nurses should be familiar with and follow the State Mental Health standards in their state for the application and use of restraints as well as the hospital policy and protocol and legal guidelines.

Nursing Intervention

One North American Nursing Diagnosis Association (NANDA) nursing diagnosis is the potential for violence. The protocol used for this diagnosis at University Hospitals of Cleveland, Hanna Pavilion Nursing Department (Fig. 48-1), is shown as well as a case example to illustrate the nursing intervention with a combative patient.

--- CASE EXAMPLE* ---

The following case comes from an inpatient unit of a high-security forensic unit in a state hospital setting.

This is the eighth psychiatric hospitalization for Jack Chaney, a 29-year-old Caucasian male. His first hospitalization was in his junior year of college, after a car accident that was believed to be a self-destructive act. Jack Chaney's use of street drugs, specifically PCP, marijuana, and cocaine, during his college years was quite frequent. He was sent home to the care of his parents between hospitalizations but was rehospitalized yearly for episodes of violent behavior and paranoid thought patterns. He was placed in the high-security unit after strangling a male staff member to the point of unconsciousness. Currently, his content of speech is loose with many paranoid delusions expressed. His attention span is limited, with poor insight and judgment and concrete comprehension.

* This case is contributed by Nancy A. Orzechowski.

NURSING CARE PLAN

DSM-III-R DIAGNOSIS

- Axis I. 295.32 Schizophrenia, Paranoid Type, Chronic
- Axis II. V71.09
- Axis III. Physical disorders: None
- Axis IV. Psychosocial stressors: 5-extreme (enduring circumstance)
- Axis V. Current GAF: 20
      Highest GAF past year: 28

CLIENT STRENGTHS

- Completed two years of college
- Supportive family

NURSING DIAGNOSES

- Alterations in thought processes and perception related to paranoid delusions.
- Potential of violence directed towards staff and other patients.
- Alteration in self-care and self-interest.

GOALS

Short-Term
1. Patient's safety will be maintained.
2. Patient will be able to spend 30 minutes in the dayroom when others are present without requiring structuring of behavior.
3. Patient will regain his ability to perform ADLs with minimal assistance.
4. Patient will identify two personal strengths.
5. Patient will be able to verbalize feelings of anxiety and loss of control.

Long-Term
1. Patient will verbalize realistically oriented feelings about the future.
2. Patient will spontaneously initiate appropriate interactions with others.
3. Patient's episodes of violence will subside and he will develop the ability to deal with tension and aggressive feelings in a non-acting-out manner.

INTERVENTIONS

1. Remove potentially hazardous objects and extraneous stimuli from the environment.
2. Reinforce patient's appropriate behaviors.
3. Set strict limits for inappropriate behaviors, using quiet room and medication as necessary.
4. Reorient to person, place, and time.
5. Encourage patient to talk about feelings rather than act on them.
6. Spend 30 minutes per shift with patient, encourage interactions with others in dayroom:
   a. Use open-ended communication
   b. Focus on concrete events, feelings, and behavior
   c. Be simple, direct, and concise in directions
   d. Talk about concrete things, avoiding ideological or theoretical discussions.
7. Initiate social-skills training program.
8. Escort patient to unit activities including group therapy.
9. Encourage attendance in group therapy program:
   a. Base group on support and understanding, rather than insight;
   b. Begin therapy at a basic level of here and now, i.e., "This is how I see your behavior";
   c. Gradually move into other levels;
   d. Support emotional expression with accompanying reality testing for corrective emotional experience to occur.

PSYCHIATRIC EMERGENCY ADMISSIONS

Behavior That Threatens the Life of Others

Behavior that threatens the life of others includes assaults, homicide, attempted acts of violence, threats of violence, and impulsive and aggressive behavior. This type of behavior is most frequently clinically associated with (1) drug use (drugs that decrease inhibitions, such as alcohol, barbiturates, and amphetamines); (2) the presence of psychosis, regardless of etiology, accompanied by impairment in reality testing and judgment; (3) an acutely paranoid patient who is hallucinating and feels frightened and desperate; (4) chronic and acute organic states such as senile dementia, acute delirium, and acute alcohol intoxication (conditions sometimes accompanied by hallucinations and paranoia—the patient may become frightened and disorganized and may act on violent impulses); (5) neurological disease, such as seizure disorders, epilepsy, and structural brain disease; and (6) retardation.

It is important to note that violence is *more* prominent in persons who *are not* emotionally ill. In fact, less than 5 percent of all major crimes are committed by people with overt psychosis or mental retardation.

EXAMPLE ONE

A 20-year-old college dropout who had become increasingly withdrawn, suspicious, and isolated over the past 2 months since his return from out-of-state college is brought to the emergency room. His family reports that he has been looking at them strangely as if he didn't know them, refusing to talk to anyone, spending a lot of time in his room alone, refusing all help. The father brought the patient to the hospital against his will following a verbal argument in the course of which the patient had attempted to stab the father with a kitchen knife. The father had successfully subdued him and had removed the weapon. On arrival at the emergency room, the patient was agitated and exhibiting acutely psychotic and paranoid behavior.

EXAMPLE TWO

A 56-year-old male sometime day laborer came to the emergency department via the police department where he had been taken following an episode in which he had singly destroyed *all* the furniture in his house in the presence of his wife. He threw the pieces onto the street and threatened his wife, saying that she would be next if she didn't "shape up." The police were requesting psychiatric observation and evaluation. Upon arrival at the emergency department, the patient was neatly dressed, calm, and cooperative, with no evidence of thought disorder. The patient stated he broke the furniture so his wife would finally listen to him and so that he could show her who was boss. "I wanted to show her I wasn't playing and meant business." The patient stated he was angry and enraged over what he perceived as his wife's complete sexual withdrawal and lack of interest in him for the past 6 months.

The psychiatric nurse should consider the following factors in evaluating the potential for violence and homicidal behavior.

1. Degree of pathological family history.
2. Previous psychiatric history and treatment.
3. Previous history of violence, e.g., temper tantrums, and aggressive and impulsive behavior.
4. Detail and nature of homicidal plan and understanding of consequences of such behaviors.
5. Nature and severity of psychopathology.
6. Degree of self-esteem and positive self-image.
7. Interest in weapons.
8. Violent fantasies and daydreams.

The two basic principles that should guide nurses in dealing with this group of patients are[12]:

1. They should deal with the healthy ego; establish firm limits but treat the patient with honesty, dignity, and respect, calmly offering reassurance and explanations as to where he is, what is being done and why, and answering questions honestly and directly regarding restraints and controls.
2. They should establish control of the patient and the situation and create a safe environment for other patients and staff.

Intervention is geared toward controlling immediate behavior through a show of force (and use of security personnel if necessary), verbal communication, physical restraints, and chemical restraints (medications); and evaluating the potential for violence and the etiology of such behavior.

The staff in the emergency department will look toward the psychiatric nurse practitioner for leadership, authority, and direction. Therefore, it is imperative that the clinician convey an attitude of confidence, assurance, decisiveness, and composure. Since this type of patient behavior is perhaps one of the most difficult and anxiety-provoking situations for the psychiatric nurse, such an attitude may not be easy to accomplish. Often the psychiatric nurse will experience feelings of fear, anger, rejection, and retaliatory violence; and these feelings will spread quickly throughout the entire staff. Therefore, it is essential for the nurse in dealing with this situation (1) to enlist the support of other team members to share the responsibility of decision making and management; (2) to remove herself from the situation and allow others to take over if she is feeling overwhelmed; and (3) to ventilate and share feelings and experiences with peers both during the emergency and after it has been dealt with.

CLINICAL EXAMPLE*

Assessment

Mr. Allen was a 29-year-old, medium-built, casually dressed black man who was referred to the crisis clinic by another agency. The patient came to the clinic alone. The nurse working Mr. Allen collected the following data.

The patient worked in a large steel-making company. The company was laying off many workers and reassigning others. One month before, Mr. Allen was temporarily assigned to an area where he had had difficulty 2 years ago. The foreman, the patient believed, was now harassing him as he had previously. Two weeks ago the patient got angry at the foreman and had thoughts of wanting to kill him. Instead of taking violent action, Mr. Allen became dizzy, and his head ached. He requested medical attention but was refused. He then "passed out" and was taken by ambulance to the dispensary.

Since that time Mr. Allen had a comprehensive physical examination and was found to be in excellent health. His physician prescribed diazepam on an as-needed basis, but this was only slightly helpful. The patient returned to work for 2 days but felt "sick" again. The agency to which Mr. Allen registered a complaint against his foreman was the agency that referred him to the clinic.

Mr. Allen complained of being depressed, nervous,

* This case is contributed by Helen Pinkney.

and tense. He was not sleeping well, was irritable with his wife and children, and was preoccupied with angry feelings toward his foreman. He had paranoid feelings about his foreman harassing him. Mr. Allen denied suicidal thoughts while admitting to homicidal thoughts. He felt the homicidal thoughts were under control. At one point during the initial interview the patient was tearful despite strong attempts at control. He demonstrated adequate comprehension, above-average intelligence, a good capacity for introspection, an adequate memory, an affect more of anxiety than depression, and paranoid ideation in regard to the foreman at work. His thought processes were organized, and there was no evidence of a perceptual disorder. Ego boundary disturbance was evident in the patient's paranoid thoughts. It seemed that the foreman was, in fact, a difficult man to get along with. However, the description of personal harassment seemed distorted. There were no depressive symptoms.

Mr. Allen was raised by his parents. His father was "boss" and beat him and siblings often. His mother was quiet and always agreed with his father. Mr. Allen's parents were Jehovah's Witnesses, and he was Baptist. The patient had a younger brother, a younger sister, and an older sister. The patient and his brother had always been close. The two of them had stopped their father's beatings by ganging up on him and "psyching him out." As a child Mr. Allen hung around with a "tough crowd" and fought frequently. He stated he believed that he could physically overpower others but tried to keep out of trouble by talking to people rather than fighting and by working hard.

Mr. Allen had never before sought aid from a mental health facility. His physical health, as stated, was excellent. He was taking no medication at the time of his first interview. Mr. Allen had a tenth-grade education and had always achieved above-average grades. His work record up until this time was good. His interests included bowling and other sports. He also periodically took courses at a local community college for his own personal growth rather than in preparation for a degree.

Mr. Allen had been married for 9 years. His wife was 2 years younger than he. They had three daughters ages 9 and 7 years and 9 months. Mr. Allen stated that his relationship with his wife and daughters were satisfactory. Both his wife and his brother were strong supports at this time.

Mr. Allen's usual means of coping were talking calmly with the threatening party and working hard on his job, in school, and in leisure activities. These coping mechanisms failed to work for him at this time but had been successful in the past. Other strengths the patient exhibited were good work record under the other foreman and only mild impairment in spheres of his life outside work. He had no arrest record and showed the ability to not act impulsively but rather to think through his actions. Mr. Allen showed strong motivation for working on his problem. He was reaching out for help, and the beginning of a therapeutic relationship was developing.

Environmental supports seemed strong. The patient's wife and brother were supporting, but the patient saw his problem as not involving them. It was therefore decided that the patient would be seen alone for the sessions. The patient felt no supports at work.

Planning

Mr. Allen was in a situational crisis, an internal disturbance that resulted from a perceived threat. The threat or precipitating stress in this case was the transfer to a new boss. The patient's need for sexual role mastery was not being met, since he was not attaining vocational role success. Soon after the transfer Mr. Allen's usual means of coping became ineffective and he experienced increased anxiety. Symptoms that appeared included attacks of dizziness, headache, passing out, and paranoid thinking. There was no suicidal intent, but feelings toward the foreman contained some homicidal ideation. The patient demonstrated enough control over his impulses that hospitalization was believed to be unnecessary. Memories and themes in the patient's verbalizations emphasized his feelings of being harassed. He had had difficulty with his new boss before. Difficulty with his boss was speculated to be a repetition of an earlier conflict, that is, the patient's feelings toward his father, another harassing boss.

The overall goal of treatment would be for the patient to return to at least his precrisis level of functioning. If possible, he could reach a level above, having learned new methods of problem solving. A crisis intervention approach was decided on that considered the patient's needs and desires, the presenting problem, and the limitations of the clinic. The patient demonstrated a good potential for problem solving and the nurse made a contract with him for crisis intervention on a weekly basis.

Possible solutions were mutually explored:

1. It was believed that the patient should remain away from work temporarily so that his rage would not be likely to explode.
2. The patient's intellectual understanding of the crisis would be sought. By understanding what had happened to cause his anxiety, the patient would be able to see more clearly ways of solving the problem. Intellectual understanding rather than affective understanding was sought because of the time limitations and goals of crisis intervention. Affective understanding involves long-term treatment with much emphasis on unconscious processes.
3. Old constructive ways of handling anger would be reinforced. These included submitting a formal complaint at work and ventilating his feelings both to the nurse during the sessions and to his family and friends at other appropriate times.
4. New ways of coping would be taught. These included seeking support at work and following several official avenues of protest.
5. Because of the strength of the patient's feelings toward his boss, it was possible that new ways of handling anger would not suffice and that a transfer to another department might be a better solution.

Intervention

The level of intervention used by the nurse was the individual approach, which is the most sophisticated approach and includes general support and environmental manipulation. The individual approach was chosen because the patient's crisis was not one for which a known course could be mapped. Also, since there was a homicidal component to the patient's symptoms, it was believed to be the safest approach. With a clear understanding of psychodynamics, the nurse geared the intervention to aid the patient to achieve an adaptive resolution to his crisis.

Environmental manipulation was achieved by having the patient remain home from work temporarily. Letters were written by the nurse to his employer explaining his absence in general terms. The patient was encouraged to talk to his wife about his difficulties so that she could understand his anxiety and be emotionally supportive.

General support was given by the nurse, who provided an atmosphere of reassurance, nonjudgmental caring, warmth, empathy, and optimism. The patient was encouraged to talk freely about the problem without having his feelings judged as good or bad. The nurse offered reassurance that the problem was one that could be solved and that the patient would be feeling better. The nurse let the patient know that she understood his feelings and would help him overcome his crisis.

The generic approach was used to decrease the patient's anxiety and guide him through the various steps of problem solving common to all crises. Levels of anxiety were assessed and means of reducing anxiety or helping the patient tolerate moderate anxiety were employed. The patient was encouraged to use his anxiety consciously and constructively to solve his problem and develop new coping mechanisms.

The individual approach was used in assessing Mr. Allen's specific problems and treating those specific problems. An understanding of the patient's individual psychodynamics was sought and dealt with by the nurse and patient. The patient was reexperiencing harassment from a male authority figure as he had experienced with his father during his youth. Because of the repetition of harassing experiences, Mr. Allen perceived his treatment by his boss in a personal and paranoid way. In other words, he was strongly sensitive to unfair treatment and overreacted as a result of early repetitive childhood experiences. His emotional response was to strike out physically, as his father had struck out at him. Intellectually, Mr. Allen knew this would be a disastrous action, and his conflict was solved by becoming sick and passing out so that he could not assault his boss. Mr. Allen's intense anger was recognized and a high priority was placed on channeling the anger in a positive direction.

The first two interviews were used for data gathering and establishing a positive therapeutic relationship. Through the use of abreaction the patient ventilated angry feelings but did not concentrate on wanting to kill his boss. The nurse used clarification to help the patient begin to attain an intellectual understanding of the precipitating event and its effect on him. Suggestion was used by influencing the patient to see the nurse as one who can help. The nurse told the patient the problem could be worked out by the two of them and that he would soon be feeling better. The patient decided to contact several people at work to obtain information about transferring to another department or being laid off. The patient and nurse therefore were exploring solutions. The nurse reinforced the patient's use of problem solving by telling him his ideas about alternative solutions were good ones well worth his looking into. Throughout these and other sessions the nurse raised his self-esteem by communicating her confidence that he could participate actively in finding solutions to his problems. She also listened to and accepted work in his pursuits, the patient found some supportive individuals at work.

During the third session the patient described an incident in which he became furious at a worker at an automobile repair shop. The repairs on the patient's car were never right and the patient kept returning the car there. The patient shoved the worker but limited his physical assault to that. He then felt nervous and jittery. The patient had previously expressed pride in his ability to control his angry feelings and not physically strike out at others. Manipulation was used by telling the patient he showed control in stopping the assault before it had become a full-blown fight and it seemed apparent he could continue to exhibit this ability. During this session, also, the patient spoke of old angry feelings toward his father. Some of this ventilation was allowed, but soon thereafter the focus was guided back to the present crisis.

In the fourth session the patient reported no episode of uncontrollable anger. He still put much emphasis, however, on being harassed by others. The nurse questioned the fact that others were out to intentionally harass the patient. Mr. Allen's defenses were not attacked, but his gross use of projection was discouraged. In the fifth session the patient reported that a car tried to run him off the road. At a red traffic light the patient spoke calmly to the driver and the driver apologized. The nurse reinforced this behavior and supported his use of sublimation as a defense. Discussion of termination of the therapy was begun.

In the sixth session the patient told of his plans to return to work the following week. He would be going to a different department even though it seemed he would be laid off. He also talked about a course he had begun at a community college. He showed no evidence of anxiety or paranoia. Termination of the therapeutic relationship was further discussed. Only a few of the techniques of crisis intervention are described here. It should be kept in mind that the techniques, in actuality, are repetitively used in all sessions to be effective.

Evaluation

The intervention resulted in the desired effect, an adaptive resolution of the crisis. The changes that occurred were discussed with the patient. The patient's need for sexual role mastery was being met. He was returning to work in a department in which he felt comfortable and successful. His symptoms of anxiety, paranoia, dizziness, headaches, passing out, and homicidal thoughts had ended. He no longer felt harassed. His original coping mechanisms were again effective. He was talking calmly to people he was having difficulty with, and now was again working hard in a goal-oriented way (i.e., a college course). He had learned new methods of coping, which included talking about his feelings to significant others, following administrative or official avenues of protest, and seeking support. The patient and nurse discussed how Mr. Allen could use the methods of problem solving he had learned from the experience to help cope with future problems. The goal, return to the precrisis level of functioning, had been attained.

It was also recommended to the patient that he engage in long-term psychotherapy so that he could deal with the old angers that interfered with his present life. The patient refused the recommendation at this time and stated he would contact the clinic if he changed his mind.

The *DSM-III-R* diagnosis is 309.82 Adjustment Disorder with Physical Complaints. The primary NANDA nursing diagnosis is ineffective individual coping related to return to old area of working and old means of coping with distress surfacing leading to the patient's need for sexual role mastery (Fig. 48-2).

Specific discipline: _____

Personnel responsible: _____

Date Entr/ Updte	Prob. Num.	Problem Description in Behavioral Terms	Measurable Outcome Objectives	Specific Treatment Approach	Targ. Date	Date Reslvd
		Ineffective Individual Coping Related to	**Long-term:** By discharge patient will identify at least two effective ways to deal with stressors. By discharge patient will identify warning signs that indicate loss of control and will begin to use constructive verbal and physical outlets to manage out-of-control behavior. By discharge patient will identify support systems that are available in the community. **Short-term:** Patient will identify specific stressors _____ (date). Patient will demonstrate two skills for dealing with stressors on the unit by ___ (date). Patient will identify at least two personal responses to stress by ___ (date).	A. Teach effective problem-solving techniques. B. Teach relaxation techniques and use of physical exercise as ways of coping with stress. C. Encourage patient to verbalize feelings rather than acting out physically. Encourage use of appropriate physical outlets. D. Inform patient of appropriate support resources in the community (e.g., mental health clinics, hotlines, support groups, etc.) E. Help patient identify and list current existing stressors. F. Assess possible causes of stress. G. Use situations that occur in the milieu as a way to help patient solve methods of dealing with the specific situations. H. Assess patient's present coping skills. I. Support effective coping mechanisms. J. Teach patient his own personal responses to stress and help patient to recognize these when they occur (e.g., physiological or emotional responses).		

Figure 48-2. Hanna Pavilion Interdisciplinary Treatment Plan. (*Source:* University Hospitals of Cleveland, Hanna Pavilion Nursing Diagnosis Care Plan Subcommittee. Reprinted with permission.)

Summary

Nurses need to know how to deal with both aggressive and combative behaviors in order to protect both their patients and themselves. This chapter presents assessment criteria and crisis management protocols for reducing and containing aggressive behaviors. Case examples illustrate nursing diagnoses and nursing interventions.

Questions

1. Identify the types of verbal and physical behaviors for the assessment of aggression.
2. Cite examples of intervention categories for management of aggressive behaviors.
3. Autognose your feelings regarding an aggressive patient you have encountered in your nursing practice.
4. Review the nursing and legal journals for cases involving patient assault to nurses.
5. How would you deal with a combative patient if you were alone and help was not available?

REFERENCES AND SUGGESTED READINGS

1. Sclafani, M. Violence and behavior control. *Journal of Psychosocial Nursing*, 1986, 24(11), 9.
2. Yudofsky, s. C., Silver, J. M., Jackson, W., Endicott, J., & Williams, D. The overt aggression scale for the objective rating of verbal and physical aggression. *American Journal of Psychiatry*, 1986, 143, 35–39.
3. Tardiff, K., & Sweillam, A. Assaultive behavior among chronic inpatients. *American Journal of Psychiatry*, 1982, 139, 212–215.
4. Vital Statistic Report 33 (Suppl). Washington, D.C.: National Center for Health Statistics, June 1984, p. 27.
5. Eichelman, B. Toward a rational pharmacotherapy for aggressive and violent behavior. *Hospital and Community Psychiatry*, 1988, 39(1), 31.
6. Daniels, D. N., Gilula, M. F., Ochberg, F. M. (Eds.). *Violence and the Struggle for Existence*. Boston: Little, Brown, 1970.
7. Ibid., pp. 31–32.
8. Sclafani, op. cit.
9. Yudofsky, Silver, Jackson, Endicott, & Williams, op. cit., p. 37.
10. Sclafani, op. cit., pp. 11–12.
11. Dubin, W. R. The violent patient emergency evaluation and treatment. *Carrier Foundation Letter*, 1984, 1–4.
12. Salamon, I. Violence and aggressive behavior. In I. Salamon (Ed.), *Psychiatric Emergencies*. New York: Grune & Stratton, 1976, p. 113.

Chapter 49

Child Abuse, Neglect and Sexual Victimization

Maureen P. McCausland and Ann Wolbert Burgess

Chapter Objectives

The students successfully attaining the goals of this chapter will be able to:

- Identify the stages that countries go through while learning to address policy issues related to child maltreatment.
- Define child abuse and neglect as described in Public Law 93-247.
- Identify indicators of child abuse, neglect, and sexual abuse.
- Define sex ring crimes against children.
- Conduct an interview with a child or family in which there is suspected child maltreatment.
- Identify three ways in which nurses can participate in preventing child maltreatment.
- Identify nursing diagnoses associated with child maltreatment.

Child abuse and neglect have been discussed by authors for centuries.[1] Until recently, however, little attention has been focused on the right of children to be protected and nurtured. Health care providers and government agencies have been reticent to "interfere with family problems" in this area. It was only in the 1960s that we became aware of the extent of child maltreatment in the Western countries.

Nurses are in key positions to deal with the issues of child abuse, neglect, and sexual victimization. The wide variety of practice sites of nurses provide many areas for nursing prevention, case finding, and treatment of these issues.

Psychiatric–mental health nurses have a unique opportunity to work with abuse victims across the life cycle in settings ranging from child pyschiatric inpatient units to halfway houses for the deinstitutionalized chronically mentally ill.

SCOPE OF THE PROBLEM

Kempe has identified five developmental stages that countries go through in addressing the problem of child abuse.[2] In stage one, the problem is denied. In stage two, the more sensational and lurid aspects of abuse are recognized. In stage three, physical abuse is dealt with effectively and attention is given to issues such as failure to thrive. Emotional abuse and neglect are recognized in stage four. In stage five, sexual abuse is addressed. This framework provides an explanation for the length of time that elapsed before the United States began to systematically address issues of child abuse, neglect, and sexual victimization. Only recently has a national perspective on the problem of child victimization emerged. Because of the difficulty in collecting dependable statistics on the incidence and types of child maltreatment, data have been scarce. But in 1975, at the direction of the National Center on Child Abuse and Neglect, a National Incidence Study was initiated at nearly 600 community agencies, in 26 counties, across 10 states. Consistent definitions focused on relatively clear-cut and serious maltreatment situations in which children had experienced, during the study period, clearly avoidable injury, illness, or emotional and behavioral impairment resulting from purposive acts or inattention by guardians or parents.

At the study's completion in 1980, it was determined that 652,000 children annually are abused or neglected in the United States. The researchers noted that this number was a minimum; they suggested that as many as 1 million children annually are victimized. Of the study's six categories of child maltreatment, sexual exploitation ranked sixth, with 44,700 children estimated at risk yearly.[3]

Parents often seek health care for their maltreated children during crisis periods in the family. This "cry for help" may be a function of their guilt feelings, fear of serious damage to the child, or an indirect request for intervention in their familial or personal conflicts.

An understanding of the complexities of the manifestations of child abuse and neglect is essential for agencies to mobilize a multidisciplinary team to approach this problem. Such an approach will, it is hoped, provide the opportunity for crisis intervention and treatment to prevent further abuse or death.

DEFINITIONS

The Federal Child Abuse Prevention and Treatment Act (Public Law 93-247) uses the following definition:

Section 3. The term child abuse and neglect means the physical or mental injury, sexual abuse, negligent treatment or maltreatment of a child under the age of 18 by a person who is responsible for the child's welfare under circumstances which indicate that the child's health or welfare is harmed.

Physical Abuse

R. E. Helfer and C. H. Kempe define physical abuse as nonaccidental physical injury or injuries as a result of acts or omissions on the part of parents or guardians.[4] Included in this definition should be child-care lapses, such as poor environmental control and repetitive accidental poisonings.[5,6] Also included is sexual victimization, which involves either forced or pressured sexual contact between adult and child.

Neglect

There are four major types of neglect as delineated by the 1972 National Symposium on Child Abuse conducted by the American Humane Association, Children's Division.[7]

1. Physical neglect: The child's needs for food, shelter, or clothing are neglected.
2. Emotional neglect: The nurturing qualities necessary for sound personality development are denied.
3. Medical neglect: Parents or guardians do not provide the usual and locally accepted minimum levels of preventive, diagnostic, or therapeutic health care services.
4. Educational neglect: A child is not provided with the education ensured by law because of a failure on the parent's or guardian's part.

LEGAL RESPONSIBILITIES FOR PROFESSIONALS

The recent upsurge of interest and concern for the rights of children led to the passage of laws mandating reporting of suspected or documented cases of child abuse or neglect. Nurses, therefore, are required by law to report cases to the appropriate state agency. There is a legal protection built into this mandated reporting system. Any professional who reasonably suspects maltreatment of a child is specifically protected against countersuit in a case when abuse or neglect is not proven.

THEORETICAL FORMULATIONS OF CHILD ABUSE

The question "How can a parent hurt a child?" is frequently asked by mental health professionals new to the field of child abuse and neglect. Early reports in the literature focused on defining the clinical syndrome, estimating the incidence, and developing child protection services.[8–10]

More recently, theoretical formulations about the cause of child abuse and neglect have been based on social learning theory, psychoanalytic theories, social exchange theory, and crisis intervention theory.[11–14]

Social learning theory is a conceptual schema that postulates that the development of aggressive behavior is part of the socialization process.[15]

Psychoanalytic theory views the development of aggressive behavior as a process of displacement that redirects the self-destructive death instinct away from the individual and outward toward others.[16] Psychoanalytic theorists believe that child-abusing behavior is related to unresolved anxiety-provoking experiences that are repressed into the unconscious.

Social exchange theorists examine the power base within the family as a possible explanation of family violence.[17] Adults are viewed as having substantially more power than children. Abuse of this power can result in violent behavior aimed at the children.

Crisis theory examines the internal and external stressors that may precipitate child abuse and neglect in the family.[18]

Many experts in the field believe that child abuse and neglect constitute a complex, multidimensional phenomenon, one that requires further research to shed light on the patterns of factors related to violence against children.[19–21] Nurses must have a theoretical base from which to conceptualize the problem and to plan treatment for families suffering from abuse or neglect of children.

DIAGNOSING CHILD ABUSE OR NEGLECT OR SEXUAL VICTIMIZATION

Typically there is a discrepancy between the historical account of the mechanism of injury and the physical manifestations. Inconsistency or inappropriateness should alert the nurse to the possibility of abuse and the need for an especially careful history and evaluation. The following case example illustrates this situation:

Eric was an 18-month-old child brought to the pediatric emergency room by ambulance. His father, a 36-year-old laborer, stated the chief complaint was "mattress fell on leg."

The child's left thigh was swollen and painful. Radiological examination revealed a fractured femur.

The inconsistency between the history of the accident and the extent of the injury prompted the pediatrician and nurse to request a family consultation by the child-abuse team.

Nurses work in a variety of settings that place them in key positions to detect child sexual victimization. School nurses are especially valuable because they have an opportunity to see the child in day-to-day activities and can note any changes in behavior from one day to the next. Especially in incest situations, the nurse may be a primary ally to the child because the parent will not be protective in this case. If there are special classes or education modules that deal with personal safety and human sexuality or family life issues, children may more easily be able to turn to the nurse to discuss concerns that they are discouraged from discussing at home.

Indicators of Child Abuse

A systematic approach to identifying indicators of child abuse is crucial. The examples given here are not intended as all-inclusive but are a suggested framework for further investigation. There are various signs of physical abuse, psychological abuse, neglect, and sexual victimization.

Physical Signs

The nurse should be alert to considering child abuse when observing any injury in an infant under 12 months of age; gross or multiple injuries in a child of any age; repeated injuries; fractures in various stages of healing; intracranial injuries; unexplained cuts, bruises, abrasions, burns, rope or strap marks; hematomas; inability to move certain body parts; undue irritability; neurological signs of brain damage; convulsions; coma; abdominal distention; bleeding from any body orifice; venereal disease; and report by the child or signs of excessive corporal punishment.

Psychological and Behavioral Signs
The nurse should consider child abuse when observing any of the emotional indicators such as extreme fright, apathy, blunting of affect, whimpering, attempting to hide, or expressions of helplessness. The nurse should consider child abuse when hearing reports of or observing "acting out" behaviors such as truancy from school, running away from home, and drug and alcohol use.

Signs of Neglect
The nurse should consider child abuse when observing or detecting any of the following indicators: unexplained weight loss; severe malnutrition or failure to thrive (especially in very young children); dehydration under unusual circumstances; signs of poor care as evidenced by severe hunger, diaper rash, inappropriate clothing, poor hygiene, or abandonment for days or weeks, or for shorter periods of time repeatedly.

Signs of Abuse in the Care Giver

Research and knowledge about signs of abuse in the care giver are imprecise.[22] However, certain "red flags" should alert the observer to potential abuse situations.

Observation of interaction with the child may show evidence of inappropriate demands and expectations of a child. The following example illustrates a potential problem area:

The 24-year-old single mother reported on her second postpartum day: "She's just like her father. Isn't she pretty? Look at her; I can tell she loves him more than me."

Discipline may be unreasonable or inappropriate. For example, a toddler may be beaten for being impolite.

Other inappropriate types of behavior on the part of the care giver may include impulsive, angry gestures. The child might be belittled, kicked, or slapped. Professionals in any setting may notice such behavior.

The hospital pharmacist in the ambulatory care center

requested an evaluation of a mother after he noticed her banging her 2-year-old son against a brick wall and repeatedly yelling, "Stop it, do you hear me?" to the child.

Observation and assessment of other children in the family may help with the identification of high-risk families. The children may be in poor physical condition, perform poorly in school, be victims of "many accidents," or have been targets of suspected or documented abuse.

The parents' current behavior in relation to the child's condition during any encounter may also provide important data. Three indicators that might alert the nuse to the situation are described as: (1) inappropriate affect in the care giver; (2) inadequate or conflicting history of the injury; and (3) failure to seek health care promptly.[23]

Inappropriate Affect in the Care Giver
The emotional response shown by the care giver does not match the usual affect or emotional response shown by care givers in a similar situation. For example, a major injury such as a head concussion is viewed as minor or unimportant by the child's parent or guardian or care giver.

Inadequate or Conflicting History of the Injury
The care giver may be unable to explain an injury or will give different accounts of who was present at the time of the injury.

An 18-year-old mother brought her 3-month-old daughter to the pediatric emergency room. "Irritable and cranky" was the chief complaint voiced by the mother. A skull radiological series revealed a linear skull fracture. The child-abuse team was consulted, and the clinician interviewed the mother, who then stated, "the baby did roll off the bed last night."

Failure to Seek Health Care Promptly
Parents may not bring the child to the clinic or emergency room for days or weeks following an injury.

John, a 5-year-old, was brought to the pediatric emergency room by his mother and grandmother. The major concern was "a burn of the arm and back." Physical examination revealed an extensive second-degree burn of the left arm and trunk. Portions of the burn appeared infected, and the entire area required debridement. When questioned about the age of the injury, the mother reported, "It happened a week and a half ago. Sure he cried, but I thought it would get better."

OVERVIEW OF CHILD SEXUAL ABUSE

In the decade of the 1980s, the sexual exploitation of children has been identified as a major public health and criminal justice problem. Tremendous strides have been made in shifting the traditional balance of the criminal justice system in this country from an offender orientation focusing on the apprehension, prosecution, punishment, and rehabilitation of wrongdoers to concerns of victims, witnesses, and their extended families. Although previously it was acknowledged that the justice system could not function without the assistance and cooperation of victims and witnesses, little recognition was given to their rights and little effort was made to assist them in overcoming the frustrations and economic sacrifices that involvement in criminal proceedings caused. This attitude began to change in the past decade with the emergence of a strong national victim and witness assistance movement, which achieved success in establishing programs to assist victims and witnesses and in increasing the public's awareness of their problems and rights. At the national level, President Ronald Reagan appointed a Task Force on Victims of Crime on April 23, 1982, and the Congress enacted the Federal Victim and Witness Protection Act of 1982.[24]

When the President's Task Force on Victims of Crime studied the experience of crime victims in America, it recognized that family violence is often much more complex in causes and solutions than are crimes committed by unknown attackers. Because of this realization, the Task Force recommended that a separate study be undertaken to give this social problem individualized consideration. Thus, the Attorney General's Task Force on Family Violence was appointed in September 1983.

Important outcomes in the form of recommendations resulted from testimony provided to the Task Force on Family Violence. Recommendations related to child sexual victimization called for judges to consider treating incest and molestation as serious criminal offenses and to adopt special court rules and procedures for child victims, such as the use of hearsay evidence at preliminary hearings, the appointment of a special volunteer advocate for children when appropriate, the presumption that children are competent to testify, the allowing of children's trial testimony to be presented on videotape with agreement of counsel, flexible courtroom settings and procedures, and carefully managed press coverage. The Task Force recommendations also called for development of more effective prosecution techniques for cases of child sexual assault in order to minimize the additional trauma for the victim created by court procedures; development of law enforcement techniques to investigate sex crimes against young victims; and determination of how child molesters select victims, what strategies they use to entice victims to cooperate, and what circumstances they consider favorable for proceeding with an assault.

In October 1984, a national symposium on child molestation was sponsored by the Department of Justice's Office of Justice Assistance, Research and Statistics.[25] This gathering of dedicated leaders caring both about and for sexually abused children had two specific goals: (1) to share experiences and ideas in order to produce better strategies for addressing child sexual abuse throughout the country; and (2) to sound a loud, clear signal that child molestation is a serious criminal offense and will be treated as such.

In one of the symposium presentations, FBI Supervisory Special Agent Kenneth V. Lanning outlined child sexual victimization as involving three major areas. The first area, *sexual abuse of children*, involves sexual activity between the adult and the child. This activity can involve nonviolent sexual abuse, in which the child is pressured into sexual acts through attention, affection, and bribery. The cooperation of the child is gained through seduction techniques. Alternatively, the sexual activity can be violent, such as when the child is physically forced to engage in sexual activity. A certain amount of this sexual abuse activity involves incestuous relationships. The second major area of child sexual victimization is the *sexual exploitation of children* and includes *child pornography*, defined as the permanent record of sexual abuse of a child, and *child sex rings*, defined as involvement of multiple children in sexual abuse for either commercial (with money exchanged) or noncommercial (no exchange of money) purposes. The third major area, *missing children*, includes runaways and the abduction of children by strangers or parents.[26]

Concurrent with these criminal justice efforts, C. Everett Koop, the Surgeon General of the United States, planned and sponsored a workshop to study violence as a public health issue. Following the Final Report of this Leesburg, Virginia, conference he encouraged miniconferences in major cities on the subject, emphasizing that the health professions use an interdisciplinary approach to the problem of interpersonal violence.[27]

What Have We Learned About Child Sexual Abuse?

The sexual abuse of children is not a rare event. Law enforcement officials, social workers, clinicians, nurses, and survey researchers have amassed considerable evidence documenting both the common occurrence of child sexual abuse and serious disorders associated with its victims. Estimates of yearly rates of child sexual abuse cases range from 50,000 to over 1 million.[28] In a review of 19 studies of the prevalence of child sexual abuse, rates varied from 6 to 62 percent for females and from 3 to 31 percent for males.[29] Both researchers and clinicians in the child abuse field agree that the majority of child sexual abuse cases remain undetected.[30,31] When exploited children are not acknowledged, they fail to receive any special help or treatment. A parallel problem is that undetected child abusers continue to molest children. In a study of 200 nonincarcerated child molesters, it was found that child molesters involve themselves not only in child molestation, but also in various deviant sexual behaviors. Molesters with the greatest incidence of molestation are those who molest boys. Offenders who commit incest and have never been involved with other sex crimes are rare; most are involved with children outside their homes.[32] Both men and women can be offenders, but men are most commonly reported.

The adverse effects of child sexual abuse are numerous. Both controlled and uncontrolled retrospective studies of sexually exploited children indicate a variety of long-term emotional, behavioral, social, and sexual problems.[33-36] Symptoms include physical problems of headaches, stomachaches, sleeping and eating disorders; psychological reactions of fears and anxiety, depression, mood changes, guilt, and shame; social problems of school truancy and failure and of quarreling and fighting with family members and peers; and sexual problems, such as heightened sexual activity, compulsive masturbation, self-exhibition, and preoccupation with sex and nudity. Running away from home, adolescent prostitution, suicide attempts, substance abuse, gender identity confusion and sexual dysfunction, and socially deviant behaviors also have been identified as possible aftermaths of untreated childhood sexual abuse.[37-39]

Given this clinical background, what have we learned from a sociological view of the problem of child sexual abuse? One of our most pressing tasks, argue researchers David Finkelhor and Larry Baron, is to identify any group of children who may be at high risk. Such an identification will help focus prevention efforts and provide new clues about the causes of sexual abuse. Toward that goal, these sociologists carefully reviewed a number of surveys that provide information about the relative risk of persons from various backgrounds of experiencing sexual abuse during childhood. Interestingly, the surveys are fairly consistent in failing to find differences in rates according to social class or race. However, several other factors have emerged from community studies as being associated consistently with higher risk of abuse: (1) when a child lives without one of the biological parents; (2) when the mother is unavailable to the child either as a result of employment outside the home or disability and illness; (3) when the child reports that the parents' marriage is unhappy or conflictual; (4) when the child reports having a poor relationship with the parents or being subject to extremely punitive discipline or child abuse; and (5) when the child reports having a stepfather.[40]

The study of child sexual abuse is incomplete without information about the offender. One research consensus area suggests that responsibility for abuse lies with offenders.[41] Exploring this perspective, Finkelhor suggests that four preconditions must exist for sexual abuse to occur: (1) there must be an offender with the motivation to sexually abuse; (2) the offender must overcome internal inhibitions against abusing; (3) the offender must overcome external obstacles against abusing; and (4) the offender must overcome resistance by the child.[42]

Of particular concern is the area of boys as victims of child sexual abuse. Although virtually all studies have found higher abuse rates for girls, a substantial number of boys are sexually abused. The average rates of child sexual abuse from eight random community surveys indicated that about 70 percent of the victims were girls and 30 percent boys.[43] In a study of 148 child molesters, 51 percent selected only girls as victims, 28 percent selected only boys, and 21 percent selected both boys and girls as victims.[44] Nevertheless, researchers and clinicians believe that boys are less likely to report sexual abuse than girls. Possible reasons for not reporting are (1) that boys are taught to be self-reliant and to keep complaints of injuries to themselves; (2) that the stigma of engaging in homosexual activities prevents boys from reporting sexual abuse by men; (3) that since boys are socialized to seek sexual experiences with females, they are inhibited in reporting unwanted sexual experiences initiated by females; (4) that boys would lose their access to greater independence and unsupervised activities if they reported their sexual victimization experiences; (5) that since boys are socialized to enjoy sexual interactions, their victimization clashes with their perceptions of masculinity and they are discouraged from reporting their sexual abuse; and (6) that the news media has focused attention primarily on the abuse and vulnerability of girls rather than boys.[45]

Recent studies of special populations indicate that the sexual abuse of boys is not uncommon. In a sample of almost 3,000 male college students, 216 reported a sexual experience before the age of 14 that was classified as abusive by the researchers.[46] A study of 41 incarcerated serial rapists revealed that 56 percent had experienced sexual abuse as children and a study of incarcerated child molesters revealed over 50 percent had childhood histories of abuse.[47,48] In a Canadian sample of 89 male runaways seeking shelter, 38 percent reported having been sexually abused.[49]

Studies have also identified special characteristics of molesters of boys. Compared with molesters of girls, abusers of boys are more likely to continue their molestation, to start their offenses at an earlier age, to refrain from sexual activity with adults, and to confine their sexual interests to male children.[50] Thus, research, prevention, and treatment programs need to be concerned with the sexual abuse of boys as well as girls.

Addressing Child Sexual Abuse

The number of cases of child sexual abuse appears to be increasing. This prompts questions as to whether this is due to better reporting by victims, to a more responsive criminal justice system, to more sexual deviance, or to children who are making up stories. To deal with this, we need good information about what is occurring, what are the consequences, and what efforts we can make to address not only the victims of sexual abuse, but the behavior and continual abusive nature of offenders. The public needs to refuse to tolerate sexual exploitation; therapists need to evaluate victims and follow them over time to ensure that the victims have the resources and support to move on with their lives. At the same time, offenders need to be monitored.

OFFENDER AND VICTIM IN SEXUAL VICTIMIZATION OF CHILDREN

Sexual misuse of children can range from inappropriate fondling to lust murders. However, the majority of sexual abuse occurs within the child's family unit or by someone known to the child or family.

In adult relationships, sexual access generally occurs in three ways: (1) by negotiation and consent; (2) by pressure and exploitation; or (3) by force and assault.* The first way is considered the healthy, mature manner of relating sexually to another person; that is, there is mutual consent for sexual activity. In the second method, one adult takes advantage of another usually through a position of dominance, and the subordinate person agrees to the sexual activity in exchange for another nonsexual reason or need. The third method, legally termed rape, involves threat of physical injury or harm and the assault is usually life-threatening in nature. The second method is dishonorable, and the third method is pathological. Only through negotiation and consent can sexual contact properly be established. However, negotiation and consent are precluded in encounters between an adult and a preadolescent or underage person because a child has not developed sufficient knowledge or wisdom to be able to negotiate such an encounter on an equal basis with an adult. Although the child may be sexually mature, she or he is not physically or psychologi-

---

* This section, through page 969, is reprinted with permission from Groth, A. N. *Men Who Rape*, New York: Plenum, 1979.

cally equipped to deal with sexual situations on an equal basis with an adult and can, therefore, be easily taken advantage of by an adult without regard for the impact of such victimization on the child's psychosocial development, that is, on her or his sexual values, attitudes, and mores. By definition children are immature in their bio-psychosocial development. Thus, offenders can capitalize in self-serving ways on the naiveté of the child and in this manner can exploit the child in a variety of ways: physical, social, psychological, and emotional.

Gaining Access to the Child

There are two basic ways in which the offender gains sexual access to the child, one is by pressuring the child into sexual activity through enticement or encouragement, and the other is by compelling the child into the sexual activity through force or intimidation.

Pressure Situation

In the pressured situation, the offender initially establishes a nonsexual relationship with the child in which the child comes to trust and feel comfortable with the offender. Then, through the offer of some type of reward, such as candy or money, or by misrepresenting moral standards, such as telling the child, "All boys and girls do this; it's fun," or through trickery and deception, such as saying, "This is going to be a game; we're going to wrestle," the offender engages the child in inappropriate sexual activity. The most commonly used technique of luring the child into this pressured sexual activity is by capitalizing on a child's need for attention and human contact. In these situations the offender does pay a lot of attention to the child and makes the child out to be special or a favorite. In this context the child cooperates and goes along with the sexual demands of the offender in order to secure the promised rewards, or the child agrees because he is somewhat confused and does not fully appreciate the ramifications of the situation, or he does it for approval and recognition.

In sex-pressured situations the offender appears to be highly invested in the victim and uses the child to gratify unmet affiliation needs in his own life. The offender talks about his attraction to children as an expression of his need for affection, and describes feeling important or special to the child or of being loved and looked up to by the child. In essence, the offender states that the child makes him feel good. He does not find satisfaction for these needs in his adult relationships but in his encounters with children, and the sexual activity serves to validate his worth as a person.

When this is the dominant motive, the offense is characterized by a relative lack of physical force in the commission of the assault; in fact, the offender generally behaves in counter-aggressive ways. He entices the child into the sexual activity. This offender makes efforts to persuade his victim to cooperate and to acquiesce or consent to the sexual relationship, oftentimes by bribing or rewarding the child with attention, affection, approval, money, gifts, treats, and good times. But he is usually dissuaded if the child actively refuses or resists, and he does not resort to physical force. His aim is to gain sexual control of the child by developing a willing or consenting sexual relationship. At some level, he cares for the child and is emotionally involved with him or her.

The pedophiliac interest can be understood as the result of a projected identification on the part of the offender with the child. In sex-pressure situations, sexuality appears to serve the need for physical contact and affection. Such offenders typically describe the victim as innocent, loving, open, affectionate, attractive, and undemanding. They feel safer and more comfortable with children. Very often victim and offender know each other prior to their sexual involvement, and sometimes they are related. This involvement can be continuing and fairly consistent over time. The following case illustrates sex-pressure by enticement:

Fred is a 51-year-old married man convicted of eight charges of indecent assault on a child under 14. Over a 6-year period, Fred enticed several of the neighborhood male children ages 10 to 12 in sexual activity involving fondling and fellatio. He owned a swimming pool, and the children could come over to swim and would change into bathing suits in the basement of his home. At times Fred would suggest they not wear swimsuits, and horseplay would lead to sexual contact.

The sex-pressure offenders constitute the vast majority of child molesters.

Forced Situation

In the forced situation the offender gains access to the child through intimidation in the form of verbal threats; for example, "Do what I say and you won't get hurt"; or by physical gestures, such as grabbing the child; or through the use of a weapon, for example brandishing a knife; or the offender resorts to physical force to overcome the child's resistance and, in some cases, finds pleasure in hurting the child. Here we are dealing with situations that are comparable to rape. In these sex-force offenses, the motivational intent is a combination of power and anger. The offender's modus operandi is either one of intimidation, in which he exploits the child's helplessness, naiveté, and awe of adults, or one of physical aggression, in which he attacks and overpowers his victim.

The exploitive offender essentially forces himself upon the victim. He typically employs verbal threats, restraint, manipulation, intimidation, and physical strength to overcome any resistance on the part of his victim. He may strike the child, but whatever aggression exists is always directed toward accomplishing the sexual act. It is usually not the intent of the offender to hurt his victim, and he will normally only use whatever force is necessary to overpower the child. The physical risk to the victim is inadvertent rather than deliberate. This offender uses the child as an object for sexual relief. He makes no attempt to engage the child in any emotional way. Instead he sees the child as an outlet solely for his self-gratification. The child is regarded as a disposable object, one to be used and then discarded. The sex act constitutes the extent and duration of the relationship, and thus typically it is a temporary and unstable involvement.

This offender relates to his victim in an opportunistic, exploitive, and manipulative way. Self-entitlement characterizes his orientation toward the child, and sexuality appears to be in the service of a need for power. Such offenders describe the victim as weak, helpless, unable to resist, easily controlled, and manipulated. They feel stronger and more in charge with children.

The majority of child offenders intend no actual injury to their victim, submission being their objective, but at the same time they exhibit no strong reluctance about hurting the child if necessary. This type of offender exhibits a lack of concern for the consequences or cost to others of his sexual activity; he experiences his motivation to be strong sexual needs that he is incapable of delaying or redirecting. Children are objects of prey: they are stalked and hunted; and any resistance on their part can quickly release

anger and hostility in this offender. He will not take "no" for an answer and will enforce his sexual demands through coercion, often employing physical force or the use of a weapon or intimating that the victim will be harmed if he or she does not want to cooperate. A case illustration of a sex-assult, exploitive type follows.

Roger is a 30-year-old white male convicted of sexual contact in the first degree and given a sentence of 3 to 10 years. He is divorced and has a son 8 years old. Since adolescence Roger has been attracted to prepubescent girls between the ages of 8 to 12. In his last offense, Roger was driving home from work when he saw an 8-year-old girl get off the school bus. "As she proceeded down the road I approached her and told her I would walk her home because there was a man in the area with a gun. She was not facing me so I dropped my trousers to expose myself and began masturbating. She turned around and screamed and I pushed her to the ground and fell on top of her. In the excitement I ejaculated. Although I never had intercourse with any of the victims, I would fantasize about it."

There are a small number of sex-assault offenders who derive pleasure in actually hurting the child. Sexuality and aggression become components of a single psychological experience: sadism. The sadistic child offender inflicts sexual abuse on his victim, who serves as a target for his rage and cruelty. Physical aggression is eroticized. Consequently, the physical and psychological abuse and degradation of the child are necessary for the experience of sexual excitement and gratification in the offender. The victim is attacked or assaulted. He or she is generally beaten, choked, tortured, and sexually abused. It is the intention of the offender to hurt or punish the child in some way.

More force is used in the assault than would be necessary simply to overpower the victim. Instead the victim is brutalized. The offender finds pleasure in hurting the child, and typically the assault has been planned out, thought about, and fantasized for some time prior to its actual commission. In this respect it is not an impulsive act; it is premeditated. Sexuality becomes an expression of domination and anger. At some level the child symbolizes everything the offender hates about himself and thereby becomes an object of punishment. The victim's fear, torment, distress, and suffering are important and exciting to the sadistic pedophiliac, because only in this context is sexual gratification experienced. The complete domination, subjugation, and humiliation of the victim are desired, and typically a weapon such as a gun, knife, rope, chain, pipe, or belt is used for this purpose in the commission of the offense. The offender relates to the victim in a brutal, violent, and sadistic fashion. His intention is to hurt, depreciate, defile, or destroy the child. The extreme of this condition results in the "lust murder" of the victim.

There are a wide variety of types of sexual acts performed or demanded by offenders in their offenses. In some cases, such as in exhibitionism, there is no actual physical contact between the offender and his victim. Such offenders confine their activity to simply exposing their genitals in full view of the child. In other cases there is physical contact with the external surface of the victim's body. This would include hugging, kissing, fondling, sucking, and masturbating against the child. In still other sexual contacts the offender sexually penetrates the body of the victim in some fashion; orally, anally, or vaginally. And in still other cases, some offenders progress over time from fondling to intercourse. The child's reaction to such contact is often dependent on the type of acts the offender performs.

Children usually describe the experience in terms of whether or not it hurts. It is important to realize that not all sexual contacts between adults and children are considered negative or painful by the child. Some contacts may be pleasurable, especially in hand–genital contact.

As aggression and violence increase, there is an inverse relationship between the amount of violence exhibited in the offense and the incidence of such offenses. The most common sexual encounter between an adult and a child is one in which the adult exposes himself to the child; the rarest type of sexual offense is when the child is murdered.

SEX RING CRIMES AGAINST CHILDREN

The study of the sexual victimization of children has previously focused on incest or family-member abuse of female children. Recently, reports have indicated a growing number of abusers who are outside to the family and who abuse both males and females. Furthermore, reports from both the United States and the United Kingdom emphasize the need for health professionals and law enforcement to increase their efforts concerning sex ring cases involving multiple victims of the same offender.[51,52] A study reporting on 11 child sex rings throughout the United States included 14 adult male perpetrators and 84 identified child victims ages 8 to 15. A United Kingdom study reported details of 11 child sex rings in which there were 14 adult male perpetrators and 175 child victims ages 6 to 15. These studies indicate a need for increased attention to the child sex ring problem.

Sex ring crimes is a term describing sexual victimization in which there are an adult offender(s) and several children who are aware of each other's participation. Different types of child sex rings have been noted. The solo sex ring involves one adult perpetrator and several children. There is no exchange of photographs, materials, or activities with other adults. By contrast, a syndicated ring involves a number of adults, a number of child victims, and a wide range of exchange items including child pornography, types, and sexual activities. At a level between these two types of rings is the transition ring where the children or pictures are exchanged between adults and there is a testing of the child for monetary exchange (e.g., child prostitution). These three types of rings will be described with case illustrations.

Solo Sex Rings

Solo sex rings are distinguished by the involvement of a number of children in sexual activities with one adult, usually male, who recruits the victims into his illegal behavior by legitimate means. This offender can be assessed by his methods for access to and sexual entrapment of the children, for control of the children, and for maintaining the isolation and secrecy of the sexual activity and by the particulars of ring activities. The disclosure of the ring and the victims' physical symptoms are also important elements. Victims are both male and female and the ages can range from infancy to adolescence. Victims are found in nursery schools, baby sitting, youth groups, day care, and camps.

Access and Entrapment
The sexual abuse of a child is a consciously planned, premeditated behavior. The adult is usually someone known both to the child and

to the parent and who has ready access to the child. The offender has a relationship of dominance over the child, exploiting the child's vulnerability to suggestion and authority. After gaining access to the child, the adult engages the child in the illicit activity through the abuse of adult power as well as through the misrepresentation of moral standards.

In our first case, the adult offender was an authority figure not only because of his position as a youth-group leader but also because of the high esteem in which he was held by many parents as a result of his community service. So highly regarded was he that parents strongly encouraged their sons to stay in the youth group with this leader even when faced with their children's resistance to attending group meetings.

Control of the Children

In order to maintain sexual activity, the offender needs to control the children in some way. The children are manipulated and coerced into keeping the abuse secret, compelled to continue in the abusive relationship, and discouraged from acting against the abuser. The abuser selects strategies particular to each child and attempts to place the burden of guilt and blame for the abuse on the child. In this case, the boys ranged in age at introduction to the ring from 8 to 12. The boys were controlled both by offender threats if they told and other boys from the ring watching them in the community and through the photographs. The ring was in operation for at least 12 years as noted from testimony at the criminal trial.

Isolation and Secrecy

When an offender is successful in abusing his victim, he must try to conceal his deviant behavior from others. More likely than not, he will try to pledge the victim to secrecy in several ways. Secrecy strengthens the adult's power and control over the child and helps perpetuate the sexual activity. It is important to understand that the technique is usually successful; some children never tell anyone about sexual abuse. There are many reasons why the abuse is kept secret. The child is afraid of encountering disbelief, blame for the activity, or punishment for disclosure. The child may fear that the adult will carry out his threats, or the child may even wish to protect the abuser.

In case 1, the young boy usually was warned not to tell anyone ("This is our secret");

it was clearly implied that telling would be disastrous ("We'll both be in big trouble."). For many of the boys, this message meant they too were responsible for the sexual activity, and the stage was set for their feelings of guilt when the ring was disclosed. The power of the adult was tested when one boy told a parent about the abuse. Authorities who were notified by the parents discouraged any criminal action: "It is your boy's word against the word of an esteemed adult."

There were several ways that secrecy of the ring activity was ensured. First, the offender used bodily response level. Physical sensation and excitement helped to bind the boys to the ring. The fact that this excitement involved homosexual activity, however, made the boys fearful of exposure. Second, the abuser used threat of retaliation. The boys believed they would be held accountable for the ring activities if they revealed these activities, since part of the "membership" process involved recruiting younger boys into the ring and having sex with other boys. Fear and intimidation was a third method for maintaining secrecy. Several of the children who were abused and controlled by older boys felt they were being watched and would be beaten if they told as they had been threatened with bodily harm. Blackmail was a fourth way; the boys were introduced into other adult activities (cigarette smoking and liquor consumption) that could be used as blackmail. They also were photographed in the nude, performing sexual acts and using alcohol and cigarettes.

Ring Activities

There are a wide range of sexual behaviors that may occur between adults and children in combination with psychological pressure or physical force. There may be a slow progression of advancing sexual acts characteristic of sexual seduction, or the acts may be forceful and sudden (rape).

In the case discussed, the sexual abuse is best characterized as rape. Several of the boys independently reported their first experience with the adult. The offender would take the boy into the bedroom where he would see nude boys engaged in sex, reading pornographic magazines, and using vibrators to sexually stimulate themselves. As the boy watched this, he was chided by the other boys into the activity. The adult then performed fellatio on the boy, who was caught unaware by the attack, becoming immobilized, frightened, and confused. The adult offender sexually abused the boys quickly and directly, often on the first or second meeting. The boys described being caught unaware by the attack, becoming frightened and confused.

Disclosure

Disclosure of child sexual abuse can be accidental or purposeful. In accidental disclosure, a third party may note symptoms of the abuse in the child. In purposeful disclosure, a child consciously decides to tell a parent or trusted person about the abuse. More often than not, the first attempts at disclosure include only parts of the activity and not the full story. When disclosure occurs, the child must deal with the reactions of people (parents, friends, authorities) to the discovery of the abuse. It becomes important that these trusted persons believe the child, understand the confusion and fear that permeates the experience, and take protective action on behalf of the child.

Disclosure of the ring in case 1 occurred gradually. One of the boys told a parent and police were notified; yet the boy was not believed. Subsequently, a father telling his son about sex found the boy revealing he had already learned about sex from his youth-group leader. Gradually, parents began to discover the ring activities, and authorities could no longer ignore the complaints. Investigation of the allegations led to the arrest of the abuser and a second adult.

The boys were terrified of disclosure and of people knowing of the activity. Part of the disclosure phase in case 1 is the immediate reactions of the boys to the fact that other people suspected or knew of the ring activity. They had a wide range of responses including denial, withdrawal, physical symptoms, and risk-taking behaviors. Thus, when some of the boys were interviewed by detectives, they initially denied any knowledge or participation in the sex ring.

However, there were signs that some boys had tried to break away from the ring. Some of the boys acted up at home (avoiding chores or homework, fighting and arguing), and for punishment parents restricted their youth-group participation. Other boys would attend large group activities but not interact individually with the leader.

Symptoms

There were clear signs of the severe distress experienced by the boys in case 1 both before and after public disclosure of the ring through the arrest of the leader. The boys and their parent described physical symptoms of stomachaches, headaches, changes in appetite. Psychological symptoms included difficulty sleeping, nightmares, flashbacks, mood swings, phobias, and depression. Social symptoms were noted in their avoidance of school, declining school grades, increased peer fighting, running away, and fear of adult males. Behavioral symptoms included abusive or sexualized language, withdrawal, suicide attempts, sexual activity with other boys as well as with animals and younger children, antisocial acts such as lying and stealing, and sexually aggressive behaviors. These symptoms have been noted in boy victims where there is combined sex ring abuse, pornography, and an extended length of time in the ring.

Transition Sex Rings

In the transition sex ring, multiple adults are involved sexually with children, and the victims are usually adolescents. The children are tested for roles as prostitutes and thus are high risks for advancing to the next level of sex ring, the syndicated ring. The organizational aspects of the syndicated ring are absent in transition rings.

It is speculated that children enter transition sex rings by one of several routes. They may be initiated into solo sex rings by *pedophiles* (those with sexual interest, thoughts, urges and preferences for children under age 13) who lose sexual interest in the child as he or she approaches puberty and who may try, through an underground network, to move the vulnerable child into sexual activity with *pederasts* (those with sexual preferences for pubescent youth). The victims may be incest victims who have run away from home and who need a peer group for identity and economic support, or they may be abused children who come from families in which parental bonding has been absent and neglect and abuse are present. Finally, victims may be missing children who have been kidnapped and forced into prostitution.

It is difficult to identify clearly this type of ring because its boundaries are blurred and because the child may be propelled quite quickly into prostitution. Typically the adults in these transition rings do not interact sexually with each other but instead have parallel sexual interests and involvements with the adolescents, who exchange sex with adults for money as well as for attention or material goods.

In case 2, a male prostitution ring illustrates the connection between the solo ring and the transition ring. In the apartment of a man who had an extensive history of convictions for child molesting, investigators found numerous photos of naked youths as well as pornographic films. Sixty-three of the depicted youths were located and interviewed, and 13 agreed to testify before a grand jury. It was believed that the ring had been in operation for at least 5 years. From this testimony, additional men (many with professional and business credentials) were indicted on counts of rape and abuse of a child, indecent assault, sodomy, and unnatural acts.

At the trial of the first defendant, testimony from four prosecution witnesses revealed the linkages between the two types of rings. According to news reports, the first witness, a man who was serving a 15- to 25-year term after pleading guilty to charges related to a solo sex ring, admitted to having sexual relations with boys as young as 10 during the years he had rented his apartment. He testified that he could be considered a "master male pimp" and that he became involved in the sex-for-hire operation after meeting one of the other defendants. He said that initially no money was involved, but after a few months expenses increased. As a result, the men were charged, and the boys were given $5 to $10 for sexual services.

Newspapers reported that another prosecution witness admitted visiting the apartment more than 40 to 50 times over a 5-year period. He denied being a partner in a scheme to provide boys for hire but admitted taking friends, who paid for having sex with the boys, with him to the apartment. A third witness, a 17-year-old, testified to being introduced into homosexual acts by the first witness, who had told the boys they could make all the money they wanted. "All we had to do was lay there and let them do what they wanted to us," he said.

The fourth witness testified that at age 12 he had met the third witness through friends. He received gifts of clothes and money for going to the defendant's apartment. While there, he would drink beer, smoke pot, and watch stag movies. He brought his younger brother to the apartment, and they both had sex with the man. At age 14, he was charging $10 for oral sex and $20 for anal sex. At that point he met the defendant. The jury, sequestered for the 19-day trial, deliberated $2\frac{1}{2}$ days before reaching a verdict of guilty.

Syndicated Sex Rings

Syndicated sex rings consist of a well-structured organization involving the recruitment of children, the production of pornography, the delivery of direct sexual services, and the establishment of an extensive network of customers. The solo ring or the transition ring may, depending on various factors, constitute different stages in the evolution of a syndicated child prostitution ring, or they may represent only a loosely organized association of adults exploiting small groups of children. The ages and numbers of victims that might be involved in a syndicated ring generally range from 11 to 16. The geographical range may be wide; the victims may be transported across state lines.

The organizational components of the syndicated ring include the items of trade, the circulation mechanisms, the supplier of the items, the self-regulating mechanism, the system of trades, and the profit aspect.

Items of Trade
These include the children, photographs, films, and tapes. The degree of sexual explicitness and activities may vary. For example, photographs can range from so-called innocent poses of children in brief clothing to child subjects in graphic sexual activities. In the films, the child is often following cues provided by someone standing off camera. Also, in audiotapes the children may be heard conversing with age-appropriate laughter and noise as well as using language that is highly sexual and suggestive of explicit behaviors.

Circulation Mechanisms
Various circulation mechanisms for child pornography include the mail, tape cassettes, CB radio, telephone, beepers, and computers. The mail is a major mechanism for the circulation of child pornography and often facilitates the laundering process for money transactions. Buyers send their requests to another country; the mail, received by the overseas forwarding agent, is opened, and cash or checks are placed in a foreign bank account; the order is remailed under a different cover back to the United States. This procedure ensures that the subscriber is una-

ware of the operation's origin and inhibits law-enforcement investigation.

Suppliers

Suppliers of child pornography include pedophiles, professional distributors, and parents. Pedophiles with economic resources and community status may organize their own group to have access to children and to cover their illegal intentions, or they may work within the framework of existing youth organizations.

Professional distributors may include the pornographer with access to an illegal photographer who owns a clandestine film laboratory. While these photo laboratories can provide services to many illegal operations, they also present some problems to the professional pornographer, who may be purchasing photographs or films already released to someone else. The professional procurers who supply children also provide photographs and films through wholesale distributors and adult bookstores.

Another source of professional distribution is the photographic processing facility. A photographic development laboratory often has a storefront business that handles legitimate orders, while its mail order business is advertised in magazines. One such facility had a mail order division that promised, through its advertisements in "adult" magazines, confidential photofinishing. These advertisements were also found in periodicals catering to readers with special sexual interests.

Parental figures who supply children for pornographic and prostitution purposes include natural parents, foster parents, and group home workers. The supplier may operate a foster home, as in the case of a self-proclaimed clergyman, who by his own estimates sold approximately 200,000 photos per year with an income from this operation in excess of $60,000. The technique he used was to force older boys to engage younger boys in sex acts. If the child did not submit, he was beaten and abused by the older youth. After the child submitted, he was photographed in the sexual acts, and the man would then use the boys for his own sexual purposes. In order to ensure secrecy, the pornographer often keeps a blackmail file on each child victim.

Self-Regulating Mechanism

Syndicated child pornography operations do not have recourse to law enforcement or civil remedies for settling disputes that arise in matters of theft, unauthorized duplication of photographs, or resources of supply. Thus, a self-regulating mechanism develops for the elimination of members guilty of actions deemed unfair or against the best interests of the syndicate. Subscribers to classified ads are screened carefully through the grade of paper, typewriter keys, and number of letters as well as by the sincerity and insistence of their correspondence. Letters are kept as a security measure. Disputes between syndicate members can become extremely bitter, and fellow members are urged to chastise the guilty party through correspondence. Members of the syndicates remain alert to law-enforcement efforts against sex rings in general or their syndicate in particular.

System of Trades

One rule in trading pornography is that members of the syndicate assist each other in finding items of interest to other collectors. Through a system of trades, photographs held by syndicate members are evaluated and exchanged.

Profit Motive

The profit motive of child pornographers appears to be a highly individual one. Some collectors trade items only for their personal use, and others trade items for commercial as well as personal use. To some the financial lure is great. Frequently, collectors sell duplicate copies of items in their collections, thereby increasing their income to purchase additional photographs from other sources.

The following factors are essential to the operation of syndicated rings: time, storage, dual identity, sexual preference for children, camaraderie, and child erotic and pornography collections. *Time* is needed for the syndicate member to develop numerous contacts and extensive child erotica and pornography collections. Syndicated members need large blocks of time for maintaining correspondence with 20 to 30 other members who write on a constant basis, for reading, and for record keeping.

Storage space is needed for the correspondence and child erotic and pornography collections. People living alone devote large amounts of residential space to housing their collections. Highly sophisticated record keeping and data retrieval systems are often discovered, including file cabinets containing cross-indexed files coded to secondary files, which hold information about the identity of the contributor.

Pornography collectors and syndicate members often lead dual lives. The threat of discovery encourages the use of *dual identities*, fictitious names, and post-office boxes. Usually only first names or false names are used in correspondence with other syndicate members.

There is a strong need for collectors of child pornography to express their *sexual interest in children* and to relate their sexual activities to other sympathetic adults. This sense of *camaraderie* and mutual secret interest has been noted in other deviant behaviors.

Collectors are also obsessed with increasing the size of their *pornography and erotica collections*. No matter how large or sophisticated the collection, the collector wants additional photographs. It appears that until collectors are personally threatened by discovery, they will maintain and increase their collections by whatever means available. When they are discovered, the loss of the collection is experienced psychologically as a traumatic event.

Our third case illustrates syndicated sex rings. More than 300 girls had been enticed, over a 7-year period, into posing for photographs on the promise that they would become movie stars. The posing, however, turned into nude photo sessions.

The technique used a 55-year-old businessman who would meet young girls in fast-food restaurants and ask them to come, with their mothers, for a sitting. The mothers would accompany the girls; gradually, the girls would become accustomed to the modeling session, and the mothers would stop attending. Older girls would be present and, after being given drugs, the younger girls would pose nude.

Police investigation uncovered boxes of photographs featuring children in sexual positions as well as a diary in which the offender detailed his sexual activity with the girls and the customers. Among the six additional men indicated were an interior decorator, a gift-store proprietor, a restaurant owner, a lawyer, and a business manager.

The defendant claimed he was the victim of a discriminatory prosecutor whose reelection campaign was sagging. The trial had a change of venue, and the defendant eventually was sentenced to life in prison. One year later, a district court judge suspended the sentence, credited the offender with the 7 months he had served, and placed him on 5 years' probation.

This reversal of a penalty can impact on the victim's family who is unaware that this situation is common. The family needs additional support to adjust to the new judicial ruling and the reality of the defendant returning to society.

INTERVIEWING AND ASSESSMENT OF THE FAMILY

Careful interviewing and assessment of the child and family are major tasks after a potential case of abuse or neglect has been identified. The interview may be conducted by the pediatrician, nurse, or social worker, depending on the agency protocol.

It is essential that first-contact people in key agencies (e.g., hospital emergency rooms, clinics, schools, crisis centers, and mental health walk-in clinics) understand the principles of interviewing and assessing these families.

The Atmosphere

The setting for the interview, along with the manner in which the interviewer introduces herself, sets the tone for the interaction. Privacy, quiet, and a period without interruptions are basic prerequisites. Because this type of setting is not always available, the interviewer must be flexible and must be able to interview under difficult conditions, for example, in between procedures in the emergency room.

The Introduction

The clinician should begin by introducing herself to the family. This ensures the family's right to understand who is dealing with them. If the interviewer is a member of a child-abuse team, the family should be told this, but the clinician may decide the most appropriate manner in which to share this information.

It is helpful to negotiate with the family at the beginning of the interview. The clinician has an agenda, and the family has sought assistance with some issue. It is important to discuss all areas of concern so that the family has a clear understanding of the situation and is given an opportunity to share its wishes and concerns. A typical introduction might be structured like this:

"Hello, I am Ms. Smith. I am a nurse in the pediatric department of the hospital. Dr. Jones has called me because he has some concerns about Joanne's injury. I thought we could talk while the tests on Joanne are being completed.

I would like to know how we can help you and Joanne. Did you have any major worries when you brought her in to see the doctor?"

It is important that the atmosphere be warm and be conducive to establishing a trusting relationship. Overtones of interrogation and judgment should be avoided. An alliance of support and concern is helpful in gaining entry into the family system for investigation and treatment purposes.

The clinician should interview the child and care givers separately. This will provide an opportunity for all members of the family to share their concerns privately and will also reveal discrepancies between the child's version of the incident and that presented by the parents.

The Working Phase of the Interview

There is a substantial amount of past history to be obtained before the clinician discusses the most recent history. The clinician should begin with the family composition, the prenatal history of the child in question, the child's history of growth and development, the family's current situation, and then progress toward the history of the present injury.

The Family Composition

The interviewer should obtain a list of all those who live in the home, including extended family, foster children, natural children, and common-law partners. It is sometimes helpful to state that this information will not be forwarded to assistance-payment workers in the welfare department. The ages of all members of the household, the schools attended by the children, and sources of health care for everyone should be noted. In a tactful way, the clinician should get information on the heritage of the children—i.e., do they share the same father, and who assumes the father-figure role with the children.

A second area that can be assessed in the general family context is that of availability of support persons for the parents or guardians. Is there extended family support, significant others, or is the parent all alone?

The Prenatal History

The assessment of the child at risk begins with a prenatal history for two reasons. First, it gives the clinician a sense of the parents' initial reaction to the coming of this child. Second, it gives important information for the basis of the child's developmental history.

Because abused children are often viewed as "different" from their siblings, it is useful to ask how this pregnancy and the parents' reaction to it compared with earlier or subsequent ones.

The interviewer should ask the mother to discuss what she remembers about her initial reaction to the pregnancy, her family's reaction to the news, and the child's father's reaction. A discussion of the mother's physical condition during the pregnancy also provides valuable data. For example, was she physically ill, more tired than during other pregnancies, and did she obtain prenatal care?

The mother's emotional status during her pregnancy will tell the clinician about the mother's initial acceptance or rejection of the child. The interviewer should assess the amount of support the mother received during the pregnancy from key people in her life. For example, was she well cared for or abandoned by the child's father? The comparison she makes between this and other pregnancies must be listened to carefully.

History of the Child's Growth and Development

Beginning with the labor and delivery experience, the interviewer should obtain a history of the child's growth and development. This should be compared with other siblings in the family. It is important to assess whether this child is viewed as "different," "special," or "bad" by the parents.

The mother should be asked about initial bonding to the infant. Did she feel close to this child or did she feel the infant rejected her?

A review of developmental milestones and school performance will provide additional data about the child's development. A health history and review of any "accidents" or recurrent physical problems should be discussed. While conducting this segment of the interview, the clinician should be particularly attentive to any clues that point to the parents' unrealistic expectations of the child that can often increase their frustration. For example, do they expect the child to be toilet-trained before the child is developmentally capable of learning this? The following case describes an extreme situation of this nature:

A 3-year-old was brought by ambulance to the pediatric emergency room. He was in cardiac and respiratory arrest and resuscitation efforts failed. When interviewing the father, the clinician learned that he had beaten the boy repeatedly in the abdomen because he was not learning how to buckle his belt correctly. This child did not possess the fine motor skills to accomplish this expected task because of his age.

The Family's Current Situation

Five areas of the current family status should be assessed, as described below. The discussion of the past history will, it is hoped, facilitate enough rapport with the family to lead into this area of the interview.

Crisis History. Has the family experienced any major crises in the past year such as the death of a loved one, a major illness of a family member, or a sexual assault?

Living Conditions. What type of housing does the family have? This will shed some light on the amount of distance and relief available from the children. Does the mother have a chance to escape to another part of the house or apartment? Is she essentially with the children 24 hours a day?

Financial Status. What is the family's source and level of income? Has there been a recent change in the family's financial status that may have precipitated a crisis?

Social Network Supports. What kinds and amounts of support are available to the parents? Is there a supportive extended family? Can the parents use a babysitter or neighbors to enable them to go out? Is the parent lonely or isolated?

Stressors. It is helpful to directly ask the parents about the kinds of stressors and the amount of frustration they experience. This should be followed with a discussion of their coping mechanisms for handling the frustrations and stressors.

History of Present Injury

The professional should begin to obtain a history of the injury in the parents' own words. It is important to do this in a low-key, nonjudgmental manner that will foster frankness, so more can be learned and an approach to the whole problem can be initiated.[53] The following points should be covered during this portion of the interview.

The Circumstances of the Injury. What was the child doing before the injury? Who was with the child when the injury happened?

The Nature of the Injury. How was the injury sustained or inflicted? How was the injury discovered?

Events After the Injury. What type of action was initiated and by whom? When did the care giver seek medical assistance?

What Are the Parents' Concerns? Do the parents have any immediate concerns? How can the clinician be of help to them? Do they have any worries or fears that other clinicians in the agency can answer or address for them?

Discussion of the Report to the Child Protective Agency

Professionals often ask whether parents should be told of the decision to report suspected child abuse. Experts in the field feel that this is crucial. It facilitates the parents' understanding of the reasons for reporting and what will happen next, based on as clear an explanation as the clinician can give. Telling a parent about an abuse report means treating him or her with respect, often the first time the parent has been treated with respect in a very long time.[54]

INTERVIEW AND ASSESSMENT OF THE CHILD

The child should be interviewed by the clinician in the least stressful manner possible. It is imperative that the child be interviewed alone, to facilitate obtaining a history of his own words, if the child's physical condition permits.

The setting for the interview is usually in the clinic, emergency room, or school. It should have an atmosphere that is nonthreatening and warm. The interviewer's tone should be as nonthreatening as possible. Various techniques are useful in engaging the child in the interview. The clinician should introduce herself and explain that she is going to be talking with the child about why he was brought to the agency. It is necessary for the clinician to be friendly, relaxed, and unhurried.[55] Although the child's history of the "accident" or injury is of utmost importance, the interviewer may gain more data by discussing general issues with the child, such as school and playmates, and then gradually proceeding toward specific questions concerning the abuse.

Observations

Throughout the session the interviewer should assess the child's general appearance and ability to relate with the clinician. The following variables are also important:

1. Appearance. The child's size, appearance, and manner of dress should be noted. Such things as obesity, obvious handicaps, and mannerisms such as tics or speech disturbances are also important.
2. Mood or affect. What is the predominant feeling displayed by the child? How does this mood change from topic to topic? Is the child apprehensive at the beginning of the interview but relaxed toward the middle of it? Does the child appear frightened at the mention of a certain adult's name? How does the child respond to questions about the injury?
3. Coping mechanisms. How does the child handle the anxiety generated by the injury and the interview? Does the child cry, or use avoidance or evasion of the issue? Is the conversation disrupted as the interview approaches certain topics, for example, previous injuries?
4. Concept of self. Does the child see himself as good or bad, handsome or ugly, in comparison with siblings or others? How does the child approach the interviewer? Is he easily engaged or extremely ready to please the clinician?

Conclusion of Interview

The child should be given every opportunity to express his wishes, concerns, or questions. As the interview nears an end, the clinician should explain that the child will receive the necessary health care of the injury. It is also helpful to state clearly that the family and clinician will meet to discuss future plans for treatment before discharge. The clinician should never make promises to the effect that the child will not be admitted to the hospital or that the child will definitely be permitted to return home with his parents. The clinician must give an honest answer to any question if a sense of trust is to be developed in the vulnerable or abused child.

NURSING INTERVENTION

Nurses are key health professionals to conduct early case finding for child abuse. The early warning signs are part of a nursing diagnosis.

Diagnosis of Early Warning Signs of Child Abuse

The prevention of abuse is a major concern of many voluntary social service agencies, federally funded demonstration projects, and state-funded public welfare departments.

Some possible early warning signs include: severe developmental lag in a child, the signs of neglect discussed previously, and most importantly, the "cry for help" made by the family member. A mother who brings her child to the clinic repeatedly, listing what appears to be a trivial complaint or stating that he is ill when physical findings are negative, must be listened to carefully. This parent is telling us that she is unable to cope at home and is worried that she will harm the child. When professionals ignore this warning, it increases the child's danger and the parent's despair.

It is often necessary to admit children to the hospital when there is a high index of suspicion for being at risk from abuse or neglect.[56] The purpose of admission is to remove the child from a hazardous environment, to treat his injuries, and to evaluate and treat the family as a unit to facilitate the development of the home as a healthy and safe place for the child.

Treatment should only be undertaken with the full realization that it requires far more than words.[57] Experts in the field concur that traditional methods that leave initiation of requests for help and responsibility for following through with recommended treatment to patients, to families do not work; persistent outreach is necessary.[58]

Many agencies are faced with decisions of how to handle the immediate situation. The following decisions must be made during the initial meeting:

1. Should the child be separated from the family for safety reasons? Separation may be accomplished by hospital admission or emergency foster placement.
2. Is this a situation that requires immediate legal intervention? If the parents or caretakers refuse to cooperate with the agency, refuse to permit the child to be admitted to the hospital, or refuse foster placement, a temporary restraining order may be obtained from the local juvenile court justice. This type of legal order permits the agency to forcibly retain the child against the parents' wishes. All parties—parents, child, and professionals—must appear in court during the next working day. The case is presented to the judge after attorneys are assigned to the child and parents. A temporary disposition of the child's custody is arranged for by the judge.
3. Community assessment. It is a well-known fact that abusive parents use many health care agencies for treatment.[59] A thorough assessment of community agencies that know the family is helpful in planning treatment. Contact with the primary health care provider, the school, day-care centers, and the like will alert the agencies to a potential abuse situation and, it is hoped, will mobilize the systems that are viewed by the parents as supportive. This also provides the necessary linking of services for the family.
4. Follow-up treatment. If the child is returning home with the parents, it is important to assess what type of follow-up is being arranged until the child protective agency is able to assign a worker. A package of services such as day care, health care, visiting nurse, and outpatient psychiatric evaluation of the child and family may be necessary.

Interagency Cooperation and Use of a Multidisciplinary Team

The treatment of child abuse and neglect is difficult and complicated. Each agency has a responsibility to identify the potential for, as well as the actual abuse and neglect, and to report suspected cases.[60] Further activity will depend on a number of factors including interagency cooperation and the degree of involvement each agency wishes to undertake. It is crucial that every agency have a clear plan for handling those cases and a clearly identified staff with the responsibility for responding to families.

The use of a multidisciplinary team is suggested as a means of allowing the staff to share responsibility and to support each other in their different work. The core members of such a team are the physician, nurse, social workers, and agency legal counsel.

Comprehensive Treatment Program

A comprehensive treatment program includes the following services:

1. Home evaluation. This provides an additional perspective to the family life-style and living conditions. The general atmosphere of the home must be assessed. Variables to be considered include: cleanliness, availability of food, sleeping accommodations for family members, and mood of the home. Mood addresses the amount of light in the home, use of colors, and general tone, i.e., is the apartment dark, disorganized, and are all the shades drawn in the middle of the day? Or is it neat, bright, and decorated with pleasant colors? The first example describes a somewhat depressing mood; the second has a tone of cheerfulness.
2. Early diagnosis of parenting ability, with planning based on the diagnosis. This preventive approach to parenthood attempts to diagnose high-risk families and to provide appropriate intervention.
3. Group support for the therapist. Work with high-risk families is stressful and demands a clear, objective approach by therapists. Support for workers is often achieved through a team approach, which provides peer supervision and mutual support.
4. Group and individual treatment for the parents.
5. Group and individual treatment for the child.

In December 1973, the Early Childhood Task Force of the Education Commission of the States

(ECS) published its first model legislation for child abuse and neglect. Since then, a number of states have adopted in part or in total its suggested language.

In January 1974, the federal government enacted Public Law 93-247, which outlined certain requirements each state must meet to be eligible for federal funding. Model legislation was then drafted to meet the requirements of the new federal guidelines for states to consider in drawing up their own legislation.

Today, all 50 states and Washington, D.C., Puerto Rico, and the Virgin Islands have statutes requiring that physical abuse of children be reported to some state agency. Many of these laws, however, are limited in scope and, consequently, also limited in impact. Child abuse continues to be a major unresolved national problem. Hundreds of children die at the hands of their parents each year. If the definition of child abuse is expanded to include sexual molestation, neglect, and emotional abuse, the estimates of child abuse will increase even more significantly.

Child abuse is seldom a single assault, but usually repeated assaults on the same child, growing more severe the longer the abuse continues. The damage, both physically and psychologically, is cumulative. The longer the abusive behavior continues unchecked, the greater the chance of serious and permanent disability to the child.

Child abuse and neglect are multidimensional problems that must be confronted from a multidisciplinary point of view. All community services and all community treatment programs must be fully utilized. Communication, coordination, and cooperation among all community resources must be encouraged and fostered. Nurses are in key positions to be able to do this type of liaison. Specifically, nurses should be pressuring their states for legislation to address the following purposes[64]:

1. To encourage complete reporting of suspected child abuse and neglect cases by all persons who have contact with young children.
2. To encourage a therapeutic and treatment-oriented approach to child abuse and neglect, rather than a punitive approach.
3. To enable each state to meet the requirements of Public Law 93-247.

Investigating Suspected Sexual Victimization

There are several essential points to remember in investigating any suspected sexual victimization of a child. Physician Suzanne M. Sgroi identifies these key areas.[65]

1. Overall approach involves keeping an open mind, keeping cool, and staying alert to the situation as a potentially dangerous one.
2. The investigation should include medical examination by a physician or nurse-practitioner who is knowledgeable regarding sexual victimization, a credible witness in court, and unafraid to participate in this area.
3. The medical examination should follow specific guidelines.
4. The interviewing should be for facts and be within therapeutic parameters. The child should be interviewed alone, and the language and techniques should be appropriate to the developmental age of the child.

Approach Toward Child Protection

The investigation of suspected sexual victimization should include an approach toward child protection. Dr. Sgroi's guidelines regarding this component of the total investigation are as follows.

Reporting. Be prepared to report all cases of child sexual assault to:

1. Child protective services.
2. The sex crimes analysis unit. (Even if the facts of the case do not warrant or permit prosecution, a report should be made for statistical purposes if such an investigative and research unit exists.)

Confrontation. Avoid confrontation between the child victim and the alleged perpetrator whenever the alleged perpetrator is a family member. Never confront the alleged perpetrator with the child's own accusation against him or her in an intrafamily situation unless you are certain that the child or alleged perpetrator can and will be removed from the home. To permit or initiate this type of confrontation in the absence of an effective plan to protect the child from possible retribution by the perpetrator is to risk serious bodily injury or even death of the victim.

Offender–Child Relationship. Don't presuppose that the relationship between the child and perpetrator will be negative if sexual assault occurred. On the contrary, a warm relationship may exist. Observation of affection between child and offender neither supports nor disproves the allegation of sexual assault and should not be cited or treated as such.

Sex Bias Concerning Targets. Because females are traditionally regarded as the most common targets of sexual assault, it is easy to harbor a built-in bias that the only *child* victims of sexual assault are little girls. Do not overlook the very real possibility that little boys may be targets of sexual assault as well, in both intrafamily and extrafamily situations. All too often, attention is focused on female children in a situation in which male children are equally or perhaps at greater risk, depending on the circumstances. Whenever child sexual assault is being investigated, both male and female children should be considered possible targets and interviewed and examined accordingly.

Continuum of Exposure. In general, the incident of intrafamily child sexual assault that comes to community or professional attention is rarely the first incident that has occurred within the family. Be aware that the incest phenomenon usually proves to be a continuum of exposure to sexual contact experienced by the child victim over a long period of time. A continuum of exposure should therefore be presupposed by the investigator unless specifically proved otherwise, and examinations should proceed accordingly, regardless of how long ago the alleged incident is said to have occurred.

Irresolution. Every professional who is called upon to assist child victims of sexual assault must learn to live with irresolution of many cases. Frequently the total facts elicited by investigation will neither support nor disprove the allegation. Do not automatically regard all unproved cases as unfounded. Child victims of unproved cases are often more needy of professional support and assistance than are proved victims of sexual assault.[66]

Prevention of Rape: Education and Coordination

A word needs to be said about the prevention of sexual assault.[67] Families are concerned about this problem and very often will ask: How can we teach our children about sexual assault before it happens? Two suggestions can be made. First, parents and school can help, and second, interagency program planning is important. The need for everyone to work together on this issue of prevention is essential. We emphasize that we do not have good data on how people successfully avoid sexual assault. But we realize we must raise issues regarding prevention and thus offer the following issues for discussion:

1. Parents should be encouraged to talk with their children before anything happens. In these talks:
   a. Assess how much the child already knows about the subject. Some junior highs and high schools are beginning to implement rape education programs in their curricula.
   b. Talk about encountering dangerous situations in general. What do children identify as dangerous? What dangerous situations have they already encountered? How have they handled them?
   c. Role-play some dangerous scenes with the children. Ask them what they would do if a stranger asked them to get in his car or if a man told them he would give them money if they did something for him. Also ask the children what they would do if confronted with a gun or knife, or if they were grabbed and pushed into a car. Talking it over and suggesting tactics they might think of provides an opportunity for parents to assess their children's reactions and points out alternatives that might be helpful.
2. Parents can discuss with their children issues concerned with sexual assault. Parents can also reinforce previously taught general safety rules:
   a. Protection in the home. Certain rules should be observed, such as children reporting all strange telephone calls to parents: they should not let any strangers in the house; and they should telephone the police if they suspect any emergency and a parent is not available.

b. Protection of self. Children should always travel with a friend or adult; they should avoid dark, deserted areas when outdoors; and they should ask for directions only from authorized persons, such as a police officer.

c. Psychological self. Children should keep their mind alert and watch where they are going; they should rehearse in their mind what they would say if a stranger asked them a question or stopped them.

d. High-risk areas. Parents should talk with school officials and police officers about dangerous areas known in the community; they should be knowledgeable regarding teen-agers who hurt or pick on children and should impart this information to their children.

3. Parents can discuss with their children what they should do if they are threatened or actually assaulted.

a. If threatened, children should keep calm and try to talk their way out of the situation. They should try to get out of the situation in as safe a way as possible.

b. If attacked, they should try to keep a clear head and observe the perpetrator for any identifying features. They should focus their mind on survival and remember everything that they can that will enable them to identify the person afterward. For example, they should memorize the make of the car or license number, what the offender says, and any scars or distinguishing marks.

c. After the attack, children should escape and report to parents, police, or the hospital. Many agencies have victim services that can help the child and the family. Parents should be sure to get follow-up care for their children to decrease any chance of long-term symptoms.

4. The schools have a part to play in educating children to the laws of the society. History or social studies classes are excellent for having children study state laws that are de-

signed to protect them. Such study would help children to know the legal terminology as well as the reporting laws. Schools can teach the legal definitions of rape, incest, and more general child abuse so that children have the knowledge to know when someone is breaking the law.

a. If schools do teach the laws in class and children are aware that they can report themselves, school nurses and police officers need to be prepared to work with children when they do report. Also, services, both immediate and follow-up, should be available.

Gelles and Cornell report that researchers have used five approaches to gathering and presenting data on child abuse[68]: position papers, survey research, case-control designs, clinical case studies, and literature reviews. Nurses have the opportunity to add to each of these approaches.

In addition, nurse researchers offer a unique perspective to research in the area of abuse, neglect, and sexual victimization. Current nursing research reports have investigated the longitudinal effects of sexual victimization with pornography, the effectiveness of Parents Anonymous, and the coping strategies of women sexually abused as children.[69–71]

Nursing Research

There are several nursing research projects underway on the subject of child abuse. One federally funded project now being conducted at the University of Washington is studying indicators of potential for child abuse and neglect.

There are many areas of inquiry that nurses could initiate. All research that begins to look at the problem and produces new ways to aid the abused child and his or her family is to be encouraged.

Summary

The problems of child abuse, sexual victimization, and neglect are becoming visible. Nurses are in key positions to make a strong united front to deal with the subject. This chapter has identified the problem and has described the ways in which child abuse, sexual abuse, and neglect may be diagnosed, the interviewing techniques, and a comprehensive treatment plan with a multidisciplinary focus. The importance of rape education, community coordination, and nursing research is emphasized.

Questions

1. Why are child abuse and neglect and sexual victimization hidden problems?
2. What focus can be brought to bear on exposing these problems, and what is the nurse's role in such an endeavor?
3. Autognose your feelings about child abuse, sexual abuse, and neglect.
4. What stalls would you anticipate in conducting an interview with an abusing parent or an abused child?
5. Why is a multidisciplinary team approach needed in working with child abuse, sexual abuse, and neglect?
6. Identify two areas for nursing research in child maltreatment.
7. Give an example of a sex-pressure assault and a sex-force assault on a child.
8. What type of prevention programs exist in your community regarding child sexual victimization?

REFERENCES AND SUGGESTED READINGS

1. Helfer, R. E., & Kempe, C. H. The Battered Child. Chicago: University of Chicago Press, 1968.
2. Kempe, C. H. Recent developments in the field of child abuse. Child Abuse and Neglect, 1978, 2, 261–267.
3. Burgdorf, K., & Edmonds, J. National Study of the Incidence and Severity of Child Abuse and Neglect: Technical Report Number 1 (DHHS Publication No. (OHDS) 81-30326). Washington, D.C.: U.S. Government Printing Office, 1981.
4. Helfer & Kempe, op. cit., p. 20.
5. Gregg, G. S., & Elmer, E. Infants' injuries: Accidents or abuse? Pediatrics, 1969, 44, 434.
6. Dine, M. S. Tranquilizer poisoning: An example of child abuse. Pediatrics, 1965, 36, 782.
7. American Humane Association. Symposium on Child Abuse. Denver, Colo.: American Humane Association, 1972.
8. Caffey, J. Multiple fractures in the long bones of infants suffering from chronic subdural hematoma. American Journal of Roentgenology, 1946, 56, 163–173.
9. Gil, D. Physical abuse of children: Findings and implications of a nationwide survey. Pediatrics, (Suppl.), 1969, 44, 857.
10. DeFrancis, V. The Fundamentals of Child Protection. Denver, Colo.: American Humane Society, 1955, p. 71.
11. Kempe, C. H., & Helfer, R. E. Helping the Battered Child and His Family. Philadelphia: Lippincott, 1972, pp. 4–5.
12. Fraiberg, S., Adelson, E., & Shapiro, V. Ghosts in the nursery: A psychonanalytic approach to the problems of impaired infant–mother relationships. Journal of the American Academy of Child Psychiatry, 1975, 14, 338–421.
13. Skolnick, A. The Intimate Environment: Exploring Marriage and the Family, 3rd ed. Boston: Little, Brown, 1983, pp. 304–305.
14. Kempe & Helfer, op. cit., p. xv.
15. Roberts, T., Mock, L., & Johnstone, E. Psychological aspects of violence. In J. Hays, T. Roberts, & K. Solway (Eds.), Violence and the Violent Individual. New York: Spectrum, 1981.
16. Baron. R. Human Aggression. New York: Plenum, 1977, p. 17.
17. Skolnick, op. cit., pp. 304–305.
18. Hoff, L. A. People in Crisis: Understanding and Helping. Menlo Park, Calif.: Addison-Wesley, 1978, p. 173.
19. Kempe & Helfer, op. cit.
20. Gelles, R., & Cornell, C. International Perspectives on Family Violence. Lexington, Mass.: Lexington Books, 1983, pp. 13–18.
21. U. S. Health Services Administration, Child Abuse and Neglect, 1977, p. 5.
22. Ibid.
23. Reece, R. M., & Chamberlain, J. W. Manual of Emergency Pediatrics. Philadelphia: Saunders, 1978, p. 51.
24. President's Task Force on Victims of Crime. Final Report (No. 82-24146). Washington, D.C.: U.S. Government Printing Office, 1982.

25. *Final Report, A National Symposium on Protecting Our Children: The Fight Against Molestation* (No. 84-20124). Washington, D.C.: U.S. Government Printing Office, 1984.

26. Lanning, K. V. *Child Molesters: A Behavorial Analysis.* Washington, D.C.: National Center for Missing and Exploited Children, 1986.

27. Surgeon General's Workshop on Violence and Public Health. *Report* (DDHS Publ. No. HRS-D-MC 86-1). Washington, D.C.: Health Resources and Services Administration, U.S. Public Health Service, 1986.

28. Eve, R. A. Empirical and theoretical findings concerning child and adolescent sexual abuse: Implications for the next generation of studies. *Victimology: An International Journal,* 1985, *10,* 97–109.

29. Finklehor, D. *A Sourcebook on Child Sexual Abuse.* Beverly Hills, Calif.: Sage, 1986.

30. Russell, D. *Intrafamily Child Sexual Abuse, Final Report to the National Center on Child Abuse and Neglect.* Washington, D.C.: U.S. Government Printing Office, 1983.

31. Berliner, L., & Wheeler, R. Treating the effects of sexual abuse on children. *Journal of Interpersonal Violence,* 2(4) 415–435, 1987.

32. Abel, G. G. *The Evaluation of Child Molesters* (Final report to the Center on Antisocial and Violent Behavior, National Institute of Mental Health). Washington, D.C.: U.S. Government Printing Office, 1985.

33. Conte, J. *The Impact of Sexual Abuse on Children.* (Final Report to the National Institute of Mental Health) November 1986.

34. Briere, J. *The Long-Term Clinical Correlates of Childhood Sexual Victimization.* Paper presented at New York Academy of Sciences Conference on Human Sexual Aggression: Current Perspectives, New York City, January 1987.

35. Gelinas, D. The persisting negative effects of incest. *Psychiatry,* 1983, *43* 312–332.

36. Meiselman, K. *Incest.* San Francisco: Jossey-Bass, 1978.

37. Janus, M. D., McCormack, A., Burgess, A. W., & Hartman, C. R. *Adolescent Runaways.* Lexington, Mass.: Lexington Books, 1987.

38. Weisberg, D. K. *Children of the Night: A Study of Adolescent Prostitution.* Lexington, Mass.: Lexington Books, 1985.

39. Burgess, A. W., Hartman, C. R., & McCormack, A. Abused to abuser: Antecedents of socially deviant behaviors. *American Journal of Psychiatry,* 1987, *144*(11) 1431–1436.

40. Finkelhor, D., & Baron, L. Risk factors for child sexual abuse. *Journal of Interpersonal Violence,* 1986, *1*(1), 43–72.

41. Abel, G. G., op. cit.

42. Finkelhor, D. *Child Sexual Abuse: New Theory and Research.* New York: Free Press, 1984.

43. Finkelhor, D., op. cit. (1986).

44. Groth, A. N. *Men Who Rape.* New York: Plenum, 1979.

45. Ibid.

46. Risin, L. I., & Koss, M. P. The sexual abuse of boys: Prevalence and descriptive characteristics of the childhood victimizations. *Journal of Interpersonal Violence,* 1987, 2(3) 309–323.

47. Burgess, A. W., Hazelwood, R. R., Rokous, F., Hartman, C. R., & Burgess, A. G. *Serial Rapists: Reenactment and Repetition.* Paper presented at the New York Academy of Sciences Conference on Human Sexual Aggression, New York City, January 1987.

48. Seghorn, T. K., Prentky, R. A., & Boucher, R. J. Childhood sexual abuse in the lives of sexually aggressive offenders. *Journal of the American Academy of Child Psychiatry,* 1987, *26*(2), 262–267.

49. Janus, McCormack, Burgess, & Hartman, op. cit.

50. Groth, op. cit.

51. Burgess, A. W., Hartman, C. R., McCausland, M. P., & Powers, P. Response patterns in children and adolescents exploited through sex rings and pornography. *American Journal of Psychiatry,* 1984, *141,* 656–662.

52. Wild, N. J., & Wynne, J. M. Child sex rings. *British Medical Journal,* 1986, *293* (July), 183–185.

53. U.S. Health Services Administration, op. cit., p. 8.

54. Simmons, J. E. *Psychiatric Examination of Children,* 2nd ed. Philadelphia: Lea & Febiger, 1974, pp. 5–6.

55. Reece & Chamberlain, op. cit., p. 53.

56. U.S. Health Services Administration, op. cit., p. 10.

57. Ibid.

58. Ibid.

59. Reece & Chamberlain, op. cit., p. 55.

60. Fraiberg, Adelson, & Shapiro, op. cit., pp. 338–421.

61. Ibid.

62. Hunka, C. D., O'Toole, A. W., & O'Toole, R. Self-help theory in Parents Anonymous. *Journal of Psychosocial Nursing,* 1985, *23*(7), 24.

63. Hill, W. G. *Child Abuse and Neglect: Model Legislation for the States* (Report Number 71, Child Abuse and Neglect Project). Denver, Colo.: Education Commission of the States, pp. 1–3.

64. Ibid.

65. Sgroi, S. M. Comprehensive examination for child sexual assault: Diagnostic, therapeutic, and child protection issues. In A. W. Burgess, (Ed.), *Sexual Assault of Children and Adolescents.* Lexington, Mass.: Lexington Books, 1978, pp. 155–156.

66. Ibid.

67. Burgess, A. W., Holmstrom, L. L., & McCausland, M. P. Counseling young victims and their families. In A. W. Burgess, (Ed.), *Sexual Assault of Children and Adolescents.* Lexington, Mass.: Lexington Books, 1978, pp. 200–202.

68. Gelles, R. J., & Cornell, C. P., op. cit., p. 10.

69. Burgess, A. W., Hartman, C. R., McCausland, M. P., & Powers, P. Impact of child pornography and sex rings on child victims and their families. In A. W. Burgess (Ed.), *Child Pornography and Sex Rings*. Lexington, Mass.: Lexington Books, 1984.

70. Hunka, C. D., O'Toole, A. W., & O'Toole, R. op. cit., pp. 24–32.

71. Crockett, M. S. Surviving child abuse: Self-reported coping histories of fourteen women. *Health Care for Women International*, 1984, 5, 49–75.

Chapter 50

Victims of Rape

Ann Wolbert Burgess

Chapter Objectives

The students successfully attaining the goals of this chapter will be able to:

- Define crisis counseling for the rape victim in terms of: the short-term model, crisis request, coping behavior, crisis techniques, and rape trauma syndrome.
- Describe the phases of the working interview with the rape victim.
- Define *accountability* in rape counseling.

Rape and sexual assault are public health issues that impact on the psychosocial and biologic health of the nation. Sexual assaults against women and children (the most visible targets) are costly in terms of lost psychic energy, decreased productivity in work and school, and deterioration in social relationships. In addition, the consequences of rape may include problems such as substance abuse, mental illness, criminal behavior, and personality disorders. These relationships are just beginning to be understood.

Victims of rape and sexual assault include females and males of all ages, social classes, educational levels, and occupations. Rape creates disruption in normal life activities in the immediate crisis period and continues to cause life-pattern upheavals for months and years afterwards.

Research on sexual aggression has ex-

panded from the traditional pathological model to include sociological and physiological factors, as well as attempts to better understand the offender's perspectives. Empirically based typologies can facilitate investigation into the causes, courses, and prediction of sexual violence, leading to differential intervention techniques for rehabilitation of the sex offender.

The lot of the rape victim remains a difficult one. And rape remains a prevalent form of violence, directed primarily against females. Feminists, scholars, clinicians, criminal justice personnel, crisis center workers, legislators, and others have increasingly turned their attention to this problem during the past few years. Rape is now openly discussed and recognized as a problem, but much work remains to be done.

The chances for continued change depend a great deal on how the issue of rape is perceived. Rape has occurred for centuries, but only recently has it been transformed into a social and public health problem.

Rape as a serious social issue needs to be approached from many perspectives: social, cultural, legal, health, economic, political, and educational. What is to be addressed in this chapter is the clinical perspective. This does not mean that the clinical perspective is the most important, but it is an essential component and can offer some guidelines for nurses whose work brings them into contact with the victim.

It is important for nurses to keep in mind the historical development of aid to rape victims. The first wave of help to rape victims came from outside the standard institutional structure. Victims and potential victims created rape crisis centers on their own because established institutions such as hospitals and police at that time were unwilling to do so.[1] These centers typically operate on a very limited budget and have mainly nonprofessional volunteer staffs, but such crisis centers remain crucial to the full complement of victim services.

This chapter presents material from a research study that had two major goals and foci—a psychiatric nursing counseling goal and a sociological research goal. The major research findings are applied to a case illustration to emphasize the counseling points important to nurses. In addition to the diagnostic category that resulted from this research—the rape trauma syndrome—two further diagnostic categories were identified and will be discussed here: the silent rape trauma and the compounded reaction to rape.

CASE ILLUSTRATION

It started out an ordinary day. I had been shopping in Cambridge and was going home to make an apple pie. It was about 3 P.M. I had the keys to my apartment out. . . . I heard footsteps behind me; they came up the steps and this man grabbed me. I thought he was just trying to pick me up. I said, "I'm busy and can't talk to you now." I continued into my apartment and he followed . . . backed me against the apartment buttons and asked me for money. I told him I didn't have any, that I had spent it all. He hit me across the face. I pulled out my purse and gave him $37 and he said I must have more. . . . He asked me if I had keys. I said I was living with someone. He said he would kill him.

He held one arm over my mouth and one arm behind my back. I opened the door and he looked around the apartment. I said, "There's the TV—take it and go." He said that wasn't what he wanted. He grabbed a knife from my kitchen and told me he was a gangster and that he had raped three other women and killed them and that was what was going to happen to me. He waved the knife around and told me to undress and said, "If you don't hurry, I'll kill you. If you're not quiet, I'll kill you."

For the next 3 hours this 23-year-old woman was forced to have oral, anal, and vaginal penetration and endured physical beatings to her head and body and knife lacerations to her face, eye, and arm. The assailant then took her to a strange neighborhood, showing her off as "my woman." After several abortive attempts, she finally was able to free herself from him and sought protection in a firehouse.

The conceptual framework for the counseling of this victim developed from counseling 146 child, adolescent, and adult victims of sexual assault who were admitted to the Boston City Hospital emergency services over a one-year period.[2] These concepts have been useful in teaching hospital staff as well as interdisciplinary groups who work with victims in the hospital and in the community.

CONCEPTUAL FRAMEWORK FOR VICTIM COUNSELING

Short-Term, Issue-Oriented Model— Rape: The External Crisis

Victim counseling is an issue-oriented crisis treatment model. The focus of the initial interview and follow-up is on the rape incident, and the goal is to aid victims to return to their previous life-style as quickly as possible. Previous problems that are not associated with the rape are not considered priority issues for discussion in counseling. This would include individual or family problems, academic problems, and drinking and drug-abuse problems. Victim counseling is not considered psychotherapy. When other issues of concern are identified by the victim that indicate another treatment model, referrals are generally offered to the victim if so requested.

Crisis Request of the Victim

The victim is considered "normal"—that is, as an individual who was managing adequately in her life-style prior to the crisis situation. In this context, the victim is viewed as a customer of emergency services who has an immediate crisis request—that is, seeking a particular service from the professional.[3] A study of the crisis requests of the 146 sexual assault victims admitted to Boston City Hospital revealed five categories:

1. Police intervention: "I need police help."
2. Medical intervention: "I need medical care."
3. Psychological intervention: "I need to talk to someone."
4. Control: "I need control."
5. Uncertain: "I'm not sure I need anything."

Referring back to the case example, the victim had serious physical injuries to her face, arm, and body when she was admitted to the emergency floor. Her eye was severely swollen and bruised, and there was a question of injury to the cornea; her clothes were disheveled; and she was physically exhausted. It was very clear that her immediate crisis request at the hospital was for medical intervention. The police had been called by the firemen and had provided aid at the immediate scene and then brought her to the hospital.

Her comment following the medical examination expresses her relief to be free of the assailant and the circumstances.

I feel so safe here. I wish I could stay forever. He can't get me here—too many layers of concrete; too many people who care.

The crisis request is the common ground of communication between victim and counselor. For the counselor, being able to identify the request at the initial interview and to understand the request reduces and contains the sense of helplessness and powerlessness that she (or he) may feel in dealing therapeutically with the victim. Something *can* be done for the victim provided that the counselor first, jointly with the victim, figures out what needs to be done and what the priorities are.

Assessing Coping Behavior

Assessment of the coping behavior and strategies used in the three time phases of before, during, and after the rape is an essential step in crisis intervention.[4] This assessment can be used as a supportive measure. Counselors, in listening to the victim recount the rape, can identify the coping behavior and acknowlege this information to the victim. This support tells victims that they have coped as a positive adaptive mechanism in the service of surviving a life-threatening situation.

The above case example illustrated early awareness of danger ("I heard footsteps behind me"). The victim tried to verbally cope with the assailant. He used physical force and she complied by giving him the money when she realized the seriousness of the situation (phase two of prerape). Still not aware that the man also intended to rape as well as rob, she tried verbal bargaining ("Take the TV and go"). The assailant now bragged about his previous violent behavior. The victim thought of ways to escape and attempted action (almost got to her apartment door) following the first rape. The victim was unsuccessful in the coping task of escaping and complied with his order to go with him out of the apartment. She tried to calm him verbally, and tried to elicit help from people she passed (a bus driver, friend of the assailant, store woman). She complied with his demand for oral penetration in the service of survival ("If you don't get it up, I'll kill you"). She verbally convinced him to leave an especially frightening isolated area that he had taken her to, and finally physically escaped by fleeing to a fire station, telling the firemen of the rape and her fears and then hiding until the assailant was gone.

Crisis Intervention

In the Boston-based counseling program, telephone counseling was used as a primary intervention tool after seeing the victim for the initial interview at the hospital.[5] There are several reasons why telephone counseling is effective. It provides relatively quick access to the victim; it places the burden on the counselor to seek out the victim rather than on the victim to seek help at a time when she is in crisis and having difficulty making decisions; it allows the victim considerable power in the situation; it encourages the victim to resume a normal life-style as quickly as possible; it is cost-effective; and it provides an alternative way to discuss difficult issues rather than face to face.

In this case, telephone counseling was quite effective because the victim moved several times in the first few months and found it useful to be able to talk with the counselor about the changes that were occurring. There were landlord problems regarding breaking a lease and decisions to make about where and with whom to live, as well as her thoughts and feelings about identifying the assailant and then continuing through the court process.

Negotiating the Counseling Request

Negotiating the follow-up counseling request is a key factor in the clinical work as the counselor states what services are available to meet the request.[6] In studying the counseling requests of the 146 victims on telephone follow-up—that is, what services they were asking from the crisis counselor—five categories were identified:

1. Confirmation of concern: "It's nice to know you are available."
2. Ventilation: "It helps to get this off my chest."
3. Advice: "What should I do?"
4. Clarification: "I want to think this through."
5. Wants nothing: "I don't need the counseling services."

By learning what the victim wants in terms of follow-up, an important alliance is made because the victim has been listened to carefully and with respect. The term *respect* is used in the sense of paying attention to, observing carefully, and appreciating the worth and dignity of the person. The counselor communicates this to the victim by taking her seriously, by being honest, by listening well, and by regarding the victim as a person instead of an object.

In the previous example, the victim requested both ventilation and advice. She was concerned and anxious about the court process such as whether she needed a lawyer and her ability to identify the assailant. She asked many questions, which she herself had to make decisions about, but which the counselor could still listen to objectively and point out the various alternatives as data points for her to consider.

Rape Trauma Syndrome

Assessing, understanding, and evaluating the reactions and feelings of the victim following a rape are essential skills of the nurse. A rape experience triggers a two-phased reaction: an acute, highly confusing, and disorganized state, followed by a long-term period in which the victim attempts to put her or his life back into the order it had before the rape. This syndrome of behavioral, somatic, and psychological reactions is an acute stress reaction to a life-threatening situation. In the acute phase, the victim may experience such somatic reactions as physical trauma, skeletal muscle tension, gastrointestinal irritability, and genitourinary disturbance, as well as a wide range of emotional reactions such as fear, humiliation, embarrassment, anger, and self-blame. The long-term effects of the rape generally consist of an increase in motor activity such as changing residence or telephone. Victims may also turn to family members for support. Dreams and nightmares can be especially upsetting, and the development of fears and phobias, usually about the specific details of the assault, are common reactions. The recovery tasks include regaining control over physical, psychological, social, and sexual life-style disruptions.[7]

To refer back to the case illustration, the young woman experienced moderate symptoms of rape trauma syndrome. She had difficulty eating and said, "I'm getting a hole in my stomach because I can't eat." She had pain from the lacerations to her face, especially her eye, and needed additional medical consultation. She had fear of seeing the assailant again and said, "I just expect him to be everywhere." She experienced minor mood swings such as bursting out crying when a man came around a corner fast at work and scared her. She was fearful of returning to work because the neighborhood reminded her of the places she was forced to go with the assailant. She said she could hardly walk the two blocks from the trolley to work: "I never thought I would make it . . . panting when I got to work . . . had to talk to myself to calm down and cool it . . . just sheer panic walking that far in broad daylight."

She had to change residence, stating she would never be able to return to her apartment alone. She experienced further trauma from the landlord, who said she would have to sublet. "He seemed to think it was my personal problem . . . said it happens every day."

The court process reactivated the original crisis. The victim had difficulty identifying the assailant. She felt confident in selecting his picture from police photos, but when confronting him in court, was confused "because he seemed so cowed . . . not bragging and boasting as he was before." After court she was concerned that all his friends now knew where she worked, and she was "always looking around to see if they were around." The mother of the defendant had been observed walking around the hallway before court to find out who was "the one out to get my son." The victim counselor intervened and took the victim into a private interviewing room. However, after court when everyone was walking out, the mother came right up to the victim, and pointing her finger in her face, said, "You bitch, you're going to suffer." This was said in a very intimidating manner. The victim's reaction was "another face to memorize."

Compounded Reaction to Rape Trauma

There will be some victims who also have a history of past or current psychiatric, social, or physical difficulties in addition to acute rape trauma. This group may develop additional symptoms such as psychotic behavior, depression, psychosomatic disorders, suicidal behavior, and "acting out" behavior associated with drug use, alcoholism, and marked change in sexual behavior. This victim should be referred to her therapist for treatment in addition to crisis counseling. Prognosis in such cases is guarded and contingent upon the relationship of the rape and its meaning to the previous psychiatric or social problem.[8]

Silent Rape Trauma

Since a significant proportion of women still do not report a rape, nurses should be alert to a syndrome called *silent rape trauma*. This reaction occurs in the victim who had not told anyone of the rape, who has not settled her feelings and reactions on the issue, and who is carrying a tremendous psychological burden.[9] Very often, a second sexual trauma or crisis will reactivate the person's reaction to the prior experience. Because the probability for unresolved sexual trauma is so high in any given population, it is recommended that every person be routinely asked the following question on intake interview regardless of the reasons for seeking psychiatric assistance: "Have you ever been pressured or forced to have sexual activity of any kind?"

A diagnosis of silent reaction to rape trauma should be considered when the nurse observes any of the following symptoms during an evaluation inteview:

1. Increasing signs of anxiety as the interview progresses, such as long periods of silence, blocking of associations, minor stuttering, and physical distress.
2. The patient reports sudden marked irritability or actual avoidance of relationships with men or marked change in sexual behavior.
3. History of sudden onset of phobic reactions and fear of being alone, going outside, or being inside alone.
4. Persistent loss of self-confidence and self-esteem, an attitude of self-blame, paranoid feelings, or dreams of violence or nightmares.

When a diagnosis of silent reaction to rape or unresolved sexual trauma is made, the patient has three therapeutic tasks: (1) to discuss the previous assault in considerable detail and with a full range of feelings; (2) to identify the reasons as to why the assault was never revealed; and (3) to talk of the current traumatic situation and look at similarities and differences. The prognosis for resolving an unresolved sexual trauma is favorable if the patient is able to spend several sessions fully reviewing the experience and putting it into perspective.[10]

NURSING INTERVENTION

The initial encounter between helper and client in any crisis situation can be a vital force in either aiding victims or contributing to their further distress. All crisis workers need to view the initial encounter as crucial in terms of setting the scene for the future well-being of the victim. The interview provides the helper with important information that is needed by various disciplines working for the victim, and it is also the place where the victim can determine whether she wishes additional help.

The formalities of introduction are important. The victim has a right to be told who the interviewer is and the purpose of the interview. The interviewer's professional or work status should be clearly identified.

Establishing an Alliance

The purpose of establishing an alliance is to help the victim understand that the meeting between herself and the crisis worker is designed to help her (the victim). In order for the victim to trust the helper, she has to first see that there is something beneficial in the meeting for her.

Next, the interviewer should make the victim feel as relaxed and comfortable as can be expected in such a situation. This task requires being prepared for the fact that the victim may express any one of a whole gamut of emotions. The victim may be sobbing, sitting quietly, uncontrollably upset, smiling anxiously, or furious at being in the interview setting. The counselor's ability to remain calm no matter what emotions the victim expresses will have a calming effect on the victim.

Third, the counselor should stress that the concern in the counseling interview is with discussing the victim's emotional reactions and her thoughts and feelings about what had happened. Beginning with this counseling approach gets the victim in the habit of mentioning her feelings throughout the interview.

Fourth, the counselor should pay particularly close attention to the first words that the victim utters and the language that is used. Listening to the language used by a victim in describing an assault is one way to begin to assess the meaning of the assault to the victim.

Working Phase of the Interview

The Goal

The goal of the interview should guide the development of the working phase. The goal for crisis intervention is to understand as much of the incident as possible and to learn the reactions of the victim to it. The counselor should try to get as complete a picture of the event and its aftermath as possible. The areas that are most important to discuss with the victim in order to assess coping behavior follow.

The Assault

Circumstances. When and where was the victim approached? What was happening just before the encounter with the assailant?

The Assailant(s). Who did it? Was he known to the victim? As one victim described it:

He was so strong. I said "Stop!" And he said, "No!" I realized then. Before he was handsome, angelic. I couldn't believe it. Now his face was like granite, hard and glazed. I said, "You're going to rape me." He put his hand over my mouth and nose and said, "If you make a noise, I'm really going to hurt you."

Conversation. What kind of conversation occurred between victim and assailant prior to the rape? Did the assailant try to "charm" her or help her? Did he threaten her? Make humiliating comments? Did he talk during the rape? And what did she say back?

Sexual Details. The area of sexual details may be most difficult for the victim to discuss in terms of the type of sexual assault the assailant demanded and got and other degrading acts. It is generally the topic the victim wishes to forget, to *not* talk about. However, counseling has shown that the sexual details are apt to be the ones that will keep recurring in the victim's mind, and for the counseling process to be on-going, the intensity of the victim's reactions will need to be observed over a time period. Until the victim is able to talk about the details and is somewhat settled within herself when talking about the incident, the details will continue to haunt her and will influence her relationships with other men.

Physical and Verbal Threats. It is important to ask about threats and violence. Fear is one of the main reactions to the rape experience. Knowing the actual circumstances—Did the assailant have a weapon? Did he threaten the victim physically or verbally? What kind of violence was inflicted?—will help the counselor truly understand the intensity of the rape experience. Counselors need to discuss not only the victim's fears at the time of the incident but also what thoughts the victim had. A victim may often say, "I thought it was the end . . . that he would be the last person I would see alive." When the victim has a close encounter with death, the counselor should verbally acknowledge understanding this.

Struggle. It is important to find out not only how much the victim struggled but also how she feels about this action. At the time of the assault, many victims make a cognitive assessment that to struggle would increase their own danger. Confirming this strategy helps settle the guilt feeling the victim may get in terms of "I didn't do enough—I could have done more." Coping behavior is important to assess at the three time phases of before the rape, during the rape, and after the rape. The counselor should also go over the thoughts the victim has about her coping behavior during and after the attack.

Emotional Reaction. It is important to assess the victim's base-line reaction over time. How did the victim feel emotionally at the time and how does she feel emotionally now? What are the most painful parts to think about?

Part of settling the crisis involves the victim's being able to put her feelings into perspective about the rape. Thus, in addition to the comments she volunteers throughout the interview about her emotional reactions, it is worthwhile to ask questions that focus directly on this problem. As she talks about her feelings, she will thereby gain some control because she is verbalizing them. Discussing her feelings over a period of time also helps to lend some perspective and distance to the experience.

Sexual Reaction. What does the sexual assault mean to her? Was this a first sexual experience? What are her feelings about sex? Has she been raped or attacked before? Rape is a violent act in which sex is the weapon, and at some point the counselor wants to help the victim to be able to separate these two issues so that she can resume her normal sexual style.

Recovery from Rape Trauma

A favorable prognosis for treatment of acute rape trauma is most likely if the victim is seen immediately following the assault. In designing nursing intervention, therefore, consideration must be given to the speed in which the victim is seen. Crisis counseling may not be as effective when a nurse is not right on the scene, whether it be the emergency room or even the police station.

The majority of rape victims are able to reorganize their lives after the acute symptom phase, stay alert to possible threats to their lives, and focus on protecting themselves from further insult. However, the world is usually perceived as a traumatic environment after the assault. As one 21-year-old victim said, "On the exterior I am OK, but inside I feel every man is the rapist."

Rape victims are usually able to maintain a certain psychological equilibrium. The crisis that results from a rape is in the service of self-preservation. Victims feel that living is better than dying, and that is the choice that is made. The victims' reactions to the impending threat to their lives is the nucleus around which an adaptive pattern may be noted.

INSTITUTIONAL RESPONSE

Perhaps the most important statement about follow-up care for the rape victim is the need for cooperation between hospitals and mental health centers and other health care delivery agencies. Rape is a social problem that cuts across many discipline lines. Progress will never be made in terms of prevention and treatment unless disciplines work together and share their knowledge and approaches.

Accountability

Reporting a rape activates a complicated process. Several disciplines such as police, hospital staff, crisis workers, and court officials immediately become involved. These professionals generally work within a prescribed course of procedure, one that is to them routine and well structured. To the victim, however, the process is foreign, not completely understood, and at times bewildering. Although the victim may not actually disagree or refuse to cooperate with certain procedures, her rights as victim may well be ignored.[11] Victims also experience a wide range of emotional reactions as a result of going through this involved process. A key concept for all professionals working with rape victims is accountability.[12] Accountability may be defined by the following actions:

1. Defining one's role or practice to the victim.
2. Explaining the services or procedures to be provided to the victim.
3. Being competent in one's technical skills.
4. Negotiating the victim's request for services.
5. Accurately recording data for record keeping.
6. Assuming responsibility for one's practice.
7. Evaluating the results of one's practice.
8. Being answerable for the conclusions of one's practice.

Accountability by the professional is especially important in a crisis situation. Rape is experienced by victims as a life-threatening situation, and it thus triggers a gamut of responses. As a crisis situation, it makes them hypersensitive to the attitudes of those people to whom they turn for help and assistance.

Autognosis

A crucial factor in the treatment of sexual trauma is the nurse's own attitude toward the victim. If the nurse finds herself judging the victim rather than trying to understand the situation the victim has experienced, all therapeutic leverage will be lost. Nurses have to come to grips with their own self-identity and prejudices regarding sexuality and violence if they are to be effective in treating a victim of sexual assault in short-term or follow-up treatment. The problem of sexual assault raises issues involved with sexuality—what is consenting, negotiated, or forcible sex—and requires nurses to identify their own frames of reference for such situations.

Social Definition of Rape

The analysis of data on rape victims being processed through the criminal justice system shows that clearly what is rape to one person is not seen as a rape by another. Professionals who come into contact with victims often ask, "Is it a real rape?" Convictions for rape in court are few and far between. Those rape cases that approximate the "ideal case" are most likely to lead to convictions.[13]

One of the major findings from a sociological study of rape victims is that rape is currently seen as a legitimate act.[14] Thus, one of the recommendations from that study is stated as follows[15]:

The first and most important task . . . is to delegitimize rape—to make it be seen as unacceptable behavior. This task means changing the social definition of rape. It means seeing it as an act of aggression and violence, motivated primarily by power or anger, rather than by sexuality. And it means seeing that rape . . . can occur in many circumstances where people now will not acknowledge it. It means seeing, for example, that rape can occur when the victim initially accompanies the offender willingly, between people who are not strangers, when the victim is not a virgin, when there are no bruises because the victim did not dare to fight, and when both offender and victim are of the same race.

With the increasing reports of rape, this is not a private syndrome for the victim to endure. Rape should be a societal concern, and its treatment should be a public charge. Nurses will be called upon more and more to assist the victim of rape in the acute as well as the follow-up phase of treatment. If all professional and community-based groups bring pressure to bear on the problem, help will be more easily available to the victim.

Summary

This chapter presented a conceptual framework for rape victim counseling based on clinical nursing research and sociological projects that included: using a short-term, issue-oriented model; identifying crisis and counseling requests of the victim; assessing coping behavior before, during, and after the assault; and assessing and evaluating the degree of rape trauma experienced by the victim in the days and weeks following the assault. Establishing an alliance and using the initial interview to monitor victim reaction to the rape provide the nurse with important data for crisis counseling. Equally important in dealing with the rape victim is the accountability of the nurse, her ability to autognose feelings about violence and sexuality, and a knowledge of the social definition of rape.

Questions

1. How does rape counseling differ from other types of counseling situations?
2. What trauma reactions does a victim have following rape?

3. How does a victim cope with a rape?
4. How does the crisis request of a rape victim compare with the client's perspective?
5. What facilities does your community offer for rape victims?

REFERENCES AND SUGGESTED READINGS

1. Csida, J. B., & Csida, J. *Rape: How to Avoid It and What to Do About It If You Can't.* Chatsworth, Calif.: Books for Better Living, 1974.
2. Burgess, A. W., & Holmstrom, L. L. *Rape: Crisis and Recovery.* West Newton, Mass.: Awab, Inc., 1986.
3. Burgess, A. W., & Holmstrom, L. L. Crisis and counseling requests of rape victims. *Nursing Research*, 1973, 73(3), 196–202.
4. Burgess, A. W., & Holmstrom, L. L. Coping behavior of the rape victim. *American Journal of Psychiatry*, 1976, 133, 413–417.
5. Burgess & Holmstrom, op. cit. (1986).
6. Burgess & Holmstrom, op. cit. (1973).
7. Burgess, A. W., & Holmstrom, L. L. Rape trauma syndrome. *American Journal of Psychiatry*, 1974, 131, 982.
8. Ibid., p. 985.
9. Ibid.
10. Ibid.
11. Holmstrom, L. L., & Burgess, A. W. *The Victim of Rape: Institutional Reactions.* New York: Wiley, 1978.
12. Burgess, A. W., & Holmstrom, L. L. Accountability: A right for the rape victim. *Journal of Psychiatric Nursing and Mental Health Services*, 1975, 13 (May–June), 1–6.
13. Holmstrom & Burgess, op. cit.
14. Ibid., p. 253.
15. Ibid., p. 262.

Chapter *51*

Victims of Family Violence: Incest and Battering

Ann Wolbert Burgess

Chapter Objectives

The students successfully attaining the goals of this chapter will be able to:

- Identify the myths and stereotypes associated with family violence.
- Describe the concept of "divided loyalty" faced by families and the problem of dealing with the legal system.
- Describe how to explore with a woman whether she wants to leave her partner.
- Describe ways in which nurses can work within their community for the prevention of family violence.
- Identify ways to suspect incest.
- Describe the functions of shelters and safe homes for victims of family violence.

Over a decade has passed since the social problems of rape, battering, and incest were first addressed by small groups of women who gathered together to speak out on the abuse experienced in their lives. Prior to this action, these subjects had been cloaked by prudery, misunderstanding, and above all, silence. The subsequent years have seen progress in terms of positive institutional response to victims of rape, incest, and battering through the establishment of sex crime units by law enforcement agencies, victim advocates in crisis centers, victim specialists in prosecutor's offices, and victim counselors in emergency departments of general hospitals.

There has also been strong positive response to the plight of victims from the federal government through the Department of Justice. The chairwoman of the President's Task Force on Victims of Crime, Lois Haight Herrington, said, "If we take the justice out of the criminal justice system, we leave behind a system that serves only the criminal."[1]

TASK FORCE APPOINTED TO STUDY FAMILY VIOLENCE

In 1980 a Task Force on Victims of Crime was appointed by President Reagan to survey the problem and to report back recommendations. A report was filed in December 1982, and within 6 months, two thirds of the 60 recommendations had been implemented. One of these recommendations was the appointment of a task force to study the problem of family violence. In announcing the task force at a press conference in September 1983, Attorney General William French Smith included the following:

Family violence in America is a serious and complex crime problem. Reported cases of child victimization doubled from 1976 to 1981 to a total of more than 850,000 incidents. Battery is the single major cause of injury to women, exceeding rapes, muggings, and even automobile accidents. Also, as many as 5 percent of dependent elderly Americans may be abused. The reluctance of family violence victims to notify authorities and inadequate recording procedures prevent us from determining the true magnitude of these crimes.

The incalculable costs of these crimes in physical and emotional suffering, ruined lives, and future crimes are intolerable in our civilized society. Yet, violence within the family is still regarded by the public and many government officials, including criminal justice professionals, as a matter that should not be handled within the criminal justice system. A number of states barely address domestic violence. This problem has traditionally been seen as a private matter best resolved by the parties themselves without resort to the legal system.

Research in this area is also limited. Child abuse and molestation, incest, and elder abuse have never received adequate attention at the national level, and there has never been an organized effort to identify and document model programs developed by governments and private sector organizations at the local level.

New information is rapidly developing that contradicts long-standing popular belief and law enforcement practices. For example, a recent study by the National Institute of Justice indicates that arrest and overnight incarceration may be the most effective intervention in domestic violence cases. Studies such as this clearly point to the need to review basic assumptions and information that underpin the handling of family violence cases.

This chapter examines two types of family violence—incest and battering—by describing theoretical understandings, research reports, and the role of the nurse in dealing with the problem.

TYPOLOGY OF INCEST

Family Member Abuse

Incest has been a social issue and problem throughout civilization, and we can say that in the United States each generation sees increasing difficulty with it. Currently there are strong social forces giving it heightened perspective; these include the re-emergence of the women's movement, the new children-and-adolescent movement, and national attention to child abuse in general.

Historically clinicians have handled incest by denial; those professionals who were in the position of intervenors handled incest by supporting the adult, consequently playing into the adult's misuse of power, dominance, and authority, and minimizing the credibility of the child. Clinicians are being challenged to develop their skills and fulfill their clinical responsibility to children and to intervene in a positive supportive way for the child instead of avoiding or denying the problem.

Incest, like rape, is a legal term. Incest is proscribed in every state. The factor that distinguishes incest from child sexual abuse is that the offender shares a kin relationship to the victim; that is, as a parent, grandparent, uncle, sibling, etc.

Ambivalence in Social Attitude and Legal Definition

We can see the ambivalence in our societal attitude in the controversy about whether or not to involve some incest offenders in the criminal justice system. Armstrong documents the incredible reluctance of court systems to give voice to the abused child[2]; Berliner and Stevens note there are acts clearly agreed to be criminal and deserving of prosecution if committed by a stranger or acquaintance yet considered differently if committed by a family member.[3] That is, people have little conflict about criminal prosecution of a stranger for the rape of a child; yet let that child be raped by her father, and the criminal action issue becomes immensely blurred. Historically, there has been reluctance to intrude in the affairs of the family. As social scientists, especially feminists, have often observed, women and children have been considered property, and this usually has meant that the male adult family members could and perhaps still can do whatever they want to do with members of their own family.

Although statutes vary from state to state, incest usually refers to sexual intercourse between two persons so closely related that they are forbidden by law to marry. In that narrow sense, sexual intercourse between first cousins at age 20 could be legally termed incest, whereas oral copulation of a 4-year-old boy by his father would not be incest and could receive a different label of abuse.

Clinical Definitions

Clinical definitions are more helpful to consider. Herman and Hirschman differentiated incest (physical contact between parent and child that had to be kept secret) from seductive behaviors (peeping, exhibitionism, leaving pornographic materials visible for the child, and sharing detailed descriptions of the child's real or imagined sexual activities), those that were clearly sexually motivated but did not include secrecy and physical contact.[4]

Incidence of Incest

The incidence of incest is significantly underestimated by all reports, whether in psychiatric textbooks that report one case per million or official figures from court records on which textbooks base their figures.[5] Contemporary figures are best estimated from research surveys. Retrospective surveys of college-age females identify a 20 to 30 percent rate of child sexual victimization.[6–8] A consistent finding among the surveys that matches with clinical data is that 70 to 80 percent of offenders were known to the child, with about half of the molesters being relatives, 22 percent residing in the child's home, and 6 percent fathers or stepfathers.[9]

High-risk families show even higher rates. Surveys of foster children, runaways, drug addicts, and prostitutes find incestuous backgrounds in the 60 to 70 percent range. Mothers in treatment centers for child abuse are reporting 80 to 90 percent prevalence in incestuous abuse in their childhood, strongly suggesting the correlation between child sexual abuse, abusive parenting, and powerless protectors of their children.

Summit, using Finkelhor's data, gives a conservative estimate that some 5 million women in the United States were sexually victimized by a male relative.[10] This figure assumes approximately 10 percent of female children in incestuous relationships and assumes an adult female population of 50 million.

For this chapter we will focus on intergenerational incest between adult and child. Such incestuous offenses are not confined to sexual activity between a biological father and daughter but encompass any sexual relationship in which the male adult occupies an authority role in relation to the female or male child such as adoptive, step-, foster-, or common-law parent. We are concerned with age–power relationships and the betrayal of a trusted, caretaking role and less with the technicalities of penetration or genital touching and more with the child's sense that he or she has been sexually violated. Our position is unequivocally that sexualization of a child-caring relationship is a violation of ethics. As Finkelhor argues, a child is incapable of informed consent with a controlling adult because the child has no power to say no and has no information on which to base a decision.[11] Or as Summit points out, the child is just as powerless within the intimidating or ingratiating relationship as the adult rape victim would be at the point of a knife.[11]

INCEST: THEORETICAL UNDERSTANDINGS

It is a bit paradoxical that the incest issue, upon which the foundation of psychodynamic formulations originated, has been so neglected in terms of psychiatric research. The scant literature that existed prior to the 1960s viewed overt incest as an exotic but negligible phenomenon occurring between inadequate sociopathic fathers and seductive, retarded daughters.[13]

A major issue in incest, from a clinical perspective, is the magnitude of emotional impact of a childhood sexual trauma for adulthood. Early writings by Freud on hysteria stated that hysterical symptoms could be understood when traced to an early traumatic experience, and that the trauma was always related to the patient's sexual life. He said that the trauma manifested itself when revived later, usually after puberty, as a memory.[14]

However, Freud later reversed his belief and said that the sexual seductions his patients reported were not all reports of real events, and this created a major shift in the priorities of psychological investigation.[15] The external realistic trauma was replaced in importance by infantile sexual wishes and fantasies. Clinicians, as they understood the universality of those wishes and fantasies, began to focus attention on the person's reaction to the wishes and fantasies. This psychoanalytic view was challenged through the decades but with little success.

In 1932, psychoanalyst Ferenczi presented a paper at the Viennese Psychoanalytic Society, on the occasion of Freud's 75th birthday, titled "The Passions of Adults and Their Influence on the Sexual and Character Development of Children." This paper presented Ferenczi's belief that childhood trauma had been unjustly neglected over the years and that insufficient depth was afforded the exploration of external factors, resulting in premature interpretations and explanations. Ferenczi noted this response in his patients who were exhibiting symptoms ranging from attacks of anxiety, nightmares, and flashbacks of "almost hallucinatory repetitions of traumatic experiences" and he said:

I had to give free rein to self-criticism. I started to listen to my patients, when, in their attacks, they called me insensitive, cold, even hard and cruel, when they reproached me with being selfish, heartless, conceited. . . . I began to test my own conscience . . . for most of my patients energetically refused to accept such an interpretive demand although it was well supported by analytic material.[16]

Ferenczi's paper was later retitled and published as "Confusion of Tongues between the Adult and the Child" with a subtitle of "The Language of Tenderness and of Passion." The main message that apparently was lost through the years in the literature provided the corroborative evidence for Ferenczi's premise that the "trauma," especially sexual trauma, as the pathogenic factor cannot be valued highly enough. Ferenczi documented the following outcomes of early childhood trauma as: (1) the introjection of the guilt feelings of the adult; (2) the child's sexual life remains undeveloped or assumes perverted forms; (3) a traumatic progression of a precocious maturity; and (4) the terrorism of suffering.[17]

In a 1963 book, psychiatrist Bernard C. Glueck, Jr., raised the question of how much credence should be given to the evidence that unfolds in the treatment of schizophrenics suggesting childhood incest.[18] Glueck along with his resident colleagues had been taught to look skeptically upon incestuous material described by patients, particularly schizophrenic patients, and to interpret such material in the context of the patient's oedipal wishes and fantasies. Not to do so was scoffed at and viewed as naiveté and inexperience in appraising and understanding the unconscious. However, as a practicing and research psychiatrist using electroshock treatments with schizophrenics, he became increasingly aware of the reported incestuous experiences as patients recovered early memories as a result of the treatments. Inquiry was made to the families of these patients and the incestuous reports confirmed. Glueck then appealed to his colleagues to review their patient cases and to look critically at episodes suggestive of incest in schizophrenic patients rather than dismissing them as fantasies.

Dynamics of Incest

In 1932, Ferenczi stated his belief that the "real rape of girls who have hardly grown out of the age of infants, similar acts of mature women with boys, and also enforced homosexual acts are more frequent occurrences than has hitherto been assumed."[19] This observation led Ferenczi to further elaborate on the theory of identification or introjection of the aggressor as a major component of his hypothesis on the etiology of sexual trauma. This view is reviewed here for contemporary consideration.

Ferenczi believed that in the incestuous seductions, the child is psychologically paralyzed with anxiety. Children feel physically and morally helpless. Their personalities are not adequately organized to be able to protest, even if only in thought, because the overriding force and authority of the adult make them unaware of their senses. Ferenczi continues:

The same anxiety, however, if it reaches a certain maximum, compels them to subordinate themselves like automata to the will of the aggressor, to divine each one of his desires and to gratify these; completely oblivious of themselves; they identify themselves with the aggressor.[20]

It is through this identification or introjection of the aggressor that the aggressor disappears as part of the external reality and becomes intra- instead of extrapsychic. The intrapsychic is then subjected, in a dreamlike state as in a traumatic trance, to the primary process; i.e., according to the pleasure principle, the intrapsychic mechanism can be modified or changed by the use of positive or negative hallucinations. In any case, the attack as a rigid external reality ceases to exist, and in the traumatic trance the child succeeds in maintaining the previous situation of tenderness. The misused child changes into a mechanical, obedient automation or becomes defiant but is unable to account for the reasons for her defiance. The sexual life of the child remains undeveloped or assumes perverted forms. Ferenczi states his underlying assumption that the child's underdeveloped personality reacts to sudden distress not by defense but by anxiety-ridden identification and by introjection of the menacing person or aggressor.[21]

The cultural constructs of society must also be considered in the issue of incest. Herman and Hirschman comment on incest in a patriarchal society as follows:

A patriarchal society, then, most abhors the idea of incest between mother and even son, because this is an affront to the father's prerogatives. Though incest between father and daughter is also forbidden, the prohibition carries considerably less weight and is, therefore, more frequently violated. . . . This is in fact the case. Incest offenders are frequently described as "family tyrants": These fathers, who are often quite incapable of relating their despotic claim to leadership to their social efforts for the family, tend toward abuses of authority of every conceivable kind, and they not infrequently endeavor to secure their dominant position by socially isolating the members of the family from the world outside.[22]

These authors conclude and predict that the greater the degree of a male-oriented and male-dominated society, the greater the likelihood of father–daughter incest.[23]

Two Major Dilemmas for the Incest Victim

The literature cites two major dilemmas that the incest victim faces: role confusion and divided loyalty. In terms of the *role confusion*, Herman and Hirschman describe the situation as follows. A woman who has been raped by a nonfamily member can cope with the experience by reacting to it as an intentionally cruel and harmful attack. She is free to hate the rapist because she is not socially or psychologically dependent

upon him. But the daughter of incest is dependent on her perpetrator–father for additional parental tasks such as protection and care. Her mother frequently is not an ally, and thus she has no recourse. To quote the authors,

She does not dare express, or even feel, the depths of her anger at being used. She must comply with her father's demands or risk losing the parental love that she needs. She is not an adult. She cannot walk out of the situation (though she may try to run away). She must endure it, and find in it what compensation she can.[24]

The second issue of *divided family loyalty* arises if the incest is exposed.[25] As mentioned earlier, the child takes the risk of pressuring the family to place its loyalty either with her and against the perpetrator (another family member), or with the perpetrator and against her. It is highly improbable that a family can remain equally divided between two family members. Obviously, the closer the family relationship, the more difficult the family decision. The problem of divided loyalty is discussed in more detail in a case example on page 1000.

LONG-TERM EFFECTS ON THE VICTIM

There are several issues that need to be assessed in terms of long-term effects on young victims. Research is just beginning to provide data on this area of investigation. The work with sexual assault victims has helped to identify the following issues that appear to impact on the young person.

Relationship of Secrecy and Sexual Activity

Sexual activity that occurs over a period of time usually means that the child has been pressured into secrecy.

If the offender is successful with his victim, he tries to conceal the deviant behavior from others. In his attempt to achieve sexual control of the child, he will try to pledge the child to secrecy in several ways. The child may not be aware of the existence of the secret. The offender may say it is something secret between them, or in entrapment cases, he may threaten to harm the child if he or she does tell.

In most situations, the burden to keep the secret is psychologically experienced as fear. Victims have spontaneously described the following fears that bound them to the secret: fear of punishment, fear of repercussions from telling, fear of abandonment or rejection, and a communication barrier in knowing what words to use. The enforced silence may have some relationship with later behavior in which the child seeks nonverbal ways of dealing with stress. Such ways as alcohol and drug abuse have been noted in adults with a history of early sexual trauma.

Conflict in Feelings When the Offender is a Family Member

Psychologically to face the decision of having to side with one of two family members is experienced as a sense of divided loyalty. When the assailant is a family member, families are caught between two conflicting expectations. Should they be loyal to the child victim and treat the offender as they would treat any assailant, or should they be loyal to the offender and make an exception for him because he is a family member? They must choose and the choice may be a difficult one. Careful attention to the feelings of the child is important for conflict resolution when the offender is known to be a family member.

Vulnerability to Physical and Psychological Symptoms

Young victims are prone to express their distress through physical and psychological means. The issue of school problems and the potential for a school phobia are important to bear in mind.

Surveillance Issue

Children who have been pressured into secrecy over sexual activity often have been kept under surveillance by the adult authority figure. This enforced surveillance may have some relationship to the victim's feelings about herself or himself.

Sexuality

There are two components to the issue of sexuality and how it relates to the young victim.

The issue may include: (1) premature introduction into adult sexuality; and (2) learning to use sex in the service of nonsexual needs such as reward and approval.

CASE EXAMPLE OF CHILD RAPE BY FAMILY MEMBER: DIVIDED LOYALTY

Rape precipitates a crisis for the victim, for the family, and often for the community.* The areas of life-style that are disrupted by a rape generally include emotional, physical, social, and sexual. The main task in the reorganization phase of the crisis is to repair the disruption and to aid the victim back to the precrisis life-style, that is, to settle the four areas of her life.[26]

Settlement of the four disruptive areas is neither sequential nor predictable. A victim will usually have difficulty in settling at least one of the four areas. More often than not, a victim will have two areas that blur together and are difficult to settle. This occurs because the external crisis event (the rape) interacts with an internal maturational task (e.g., identity, intimacy, or generativity).[27]

An additional stress condition exists if a rape case goes to court. Analyses of data clearly show that the trial process recapitulates the original crisis and further traumatizes the victim.[28] In reviewing the areas of disruption in a child's life, it appears that a potential second crisis develops when the offender is a family member and a decision regarding pressing charges is faced.

THE ASSAULT

A 9-year-old girl was going to the neighborhood store at 6 P.M. Her 16-year-old cousin was with her and said, "If I had a girl, I'd rape her." The child said, "If you do that to me, I'll scream."

The cousin then grabbed her and took her to an alley and had forced vaginal intercourse. He threatened her by saying, "If you scream, I'll kick your bottom in . . . I'll kick your bottom in if you tell anyone!"

Following the assault, both cousins returned home. The nephew had blood on his hands and there was blood on the girl's pants. When questioned by the victim's parents, the nephew said he had cut himself

* This section, through page 1003, was written with the assistance of Lynda Lytle Holmstrom and Maureen P. McCausland.

and wiped his hands on his cousin's pants. The mother took her daughter into the bathroom thinking the girl had started her menstrual period. After about an hour of further questioning, the girl broke down and told her father what had happened.

The girl was then brought to the emergency ward of the hospital for examination. The mother did not tell the hospital admission clerk what had happened but told the nurse "My child's been attacked." At this time, the parents stated they were not going to press charges. The nephew begged the family not to tell his father.

The Initial Crisis

With child victims, just like adult victims, the disruption in life-style areas may be observed not only in the victim but in the family as a unit as well. In this case, in the first several weeks following the assault, the victim reported having nightmares and difficulty sleeping. The first several nights she slept with her mother, a common reaction in child victims. She remained at home following the assault until her mother said she had to return to school. She refused to go to the neighborhood store, did not play outside with other children, and was fearful her sister would tell the other children what had happened.

The mother reported being very upset and also had difficulty sleeping. There was tension in the marital relationship with the mother stating she was angry at her husband for "protecting the nephew." The father came to the hospital for the initial visit but refused for many weeks to talk with the nurse on the telephone for follow-up counseling. The 11-year-old brother of the victim, who also came to the hospital on the initial visit and who was known to the hospital as an asthmatic, was admitted as a patient to the hospital several days following the assault with an asthma attack. His reaction was as follows:

"Ever since he did that, all I can think about is kill, kill, kill when I get big enough."

This brother also had another asthma attack requiring hospitalization 5 weeks later.

Victim's Emotional Life-style
The disruption in the emotional life-style of the victim can be seen in minor mood swings, in the development of rape trauma symptoms that include phobias, social withdrawal, and night-

mares, and in an obsession with thoughts of the assault that seriously limits her ability to concentrate on regular life activities. The victim reported to the nurse:

"I still think about it . . . about what he did. I have dreams about it. My mom still wants him turned in to the police. I wake up crying sometimes. . . . I remember his saying he wished he had a girl and covering my mouth. . . . I don't like to wake up at night. There is something I didn't tell you. I was afraid. He did this before. He gave me some candy . . . then he put it in me. I kicked him and cried. My mind says I have to stand him, but it is hard. . . ."

Counseling helped this child to report a previous assault by the same cousin—an assault that had been kept secret.

Victim's Physical Life-style
The disruption in physical life-style is seen in the bruising and bleeding that occurred during the rape. On laboratory testing, it was also discovered that the child had a positive test for gonorrhea, presumably from the first sexual assault because there was no evidence she was sexually active. The penicillin medication required to treat the venereal disease was upsetting to the child as well as the follow-up laboratory tests that were required.

Victim's Social Life-style
The school-age child will show disruption in social life-style in the way she copes with formal organizations of school and church and the informal organizations of neighborhood and peer groups. In this case the victim had difficulty with school and was afraid that her playmates would find out. She said:

"I don't do my work at school. Sometimes I don't like it. That's why the teacher called my mother. I was thinking about it. Sometimes I just get mad . . . then I rip up my papers."

In this situation, the child was unable to explain to the teacher why she had ripped up her papers, and the teacher asked that the mother come in. The mother then told the teacher about the rape.

Victim's Sexual Life-style
One aspect of sexual assault peculiar to the victim with no prior sexual activity is that the victim

has nothing to compare it with. She does not know that sexual intercourse can be nonviolent. The prepuberty victim may not have had any sex education to know basic facts regarding pregnancy and venereal disease. About four weeks after the assault, the victim specifically telephoned the nurse to talk about sexual matters:

"Can I have a baby? . . . I'm going to adopt a baby. I know how my mother had me. She did the same thing he did. I'll never do that. I don't like that. It bothers me."

This victim also experienced a reaction similar to that of an adult woman in terms of having difficulty separating the behavior of the offender from that of all males. She says:

"I go outside to play. Sometimes the boys chase me and I get scared even though they're just friends. Sometimes it reminds me of it . . . sometimes I forget it and just play."

Decision to Press Charges or Not: A Potential Second Crisis

Victims and their families often find it very difficult to decide whether or not to press charges against an assailant. The agony of making this decision is frequently increased when the assailant is a family member.

Factors Influencing the Decision

Direct Action. The immediate reaction of the family was to deny the nephew access to the family. He was not allowed to visit. The mother instructed her children not to talk to any member of the extended family. The nephew's request not to have his parents told was denied, and his father was immediately contacted.

Betrayal within the Family. Feelings of betrayal happen when reciprocity between family members does not occur. For example, in this case the mother had treated her nephew well and expected the same in return:

"I treated him like my own. I gave him money, cooked him meals. He didn't love me. Look what he did. I don't care if his people get mad at me. Look what happened to my little girl."

The brother of the victim also felt betrayed

in terms of the cousin violating his trust. He saw his cousin as a friend. He said, "I thought I had a friend, but he came to see my sister, not me."

The betrayal of family ability to trust each other was cited when the mother said, "I tried to protect her from outsiders, and look what the family did." It becomes clear that as family members feel betrayed, this feeling will influence a decision regarding pressing charges.

Thinking through the Incident. Each member of the family struggled with his or her own thoughts about why the incident occurred and with his or her fears about the consequences of any decision that might be made. The fear of the nephew being sent away and incarcerated was a deterrent factor in making a decision to press charges. Being able to view the nephew as someone who needed help encouraged the family to make their decision.

The mother of the victim tried to rationalize her nephew's behavior by saying, "Maybe he had older girls in Florida. He didn't know any girls here." The father was unable to rationalize the nephew's behavior, saying, "How could he have done such a thing . . . messing around with a little girl like that?"

Family Members' Position. Each family member takes a position on the decision to be made. The victim stated to her parents and to the nurse that she wanted "something done." She said she was afraid of her cousin and asked that her parents call the police. The mother wanted to call the police and admitted that the situation scared her too. The brother wanted to take direct physical action on the cousin. It is to be noted that the increase in his hospitalizations for asthma attacks coincided with crisis points for the family—after the rape and just prior to making the decision to press charges 5 weeks later.

Key Decision Person. One person is the key in the final decision, and it is often the person who has the closest ties with the offender. The issue of divided loyalty will be heaviest to bear for this person. In this case, it was the victim's father. The crucial deciding point came during his son's hospitalization for asthma, when the father had a chance to talk with the nurse. He had avoided talking with her up to this point but finally was able to present some of his conflicts he was deliberating on.

He first identified with his brother: "I kept

thinking if my son did this." He was upset with his daughter's reactions and symptoms: "I think about this when I look at her. She's afraid to go to the store. I won't force her but it upsets me." He thought of the age of his nephew: "If he were older, I don't know what I would do." Then the father made a judgment on the nephew's behavior: "He was *wrong* to do it." Following this comment the father said to the nurse, "Yes, I think we need to tell the police." The nurse agreed to meet with the family at their home the next day. At that time, the family requested that the nurse intervene on their behalf and call the police: "Maybe they will come quicker for you." The mother later stated her reaction to the decision:

"I'm nervous, shaky. I'll never get over this. I don't want to hurt anyone. Why are they hurting me? I hope no one else goes through this. . . . I don't want anyone else's child to go through this."

Consequences of the Decision

The results of a decision to press charges have consequences to more than just the victim. In this case, the consequences of the decision may be viewed in terms of the resultant behavior of the extended family (offender's family).

After the decision is made, pressure may be exerted on the decision-making family members to try to change their minds. Family members may be contacted by mail, telephone, or in person by the extended family. In this case, the mother heard indirectly that the nephew's father was "going to get us." The mother also felt intimidated with the report that the family was going to "put a spell on us if it takes forever." She was concerned enough about this to ask the nurse whether she believed in spells.

Both parents were approached by other family members and were threatened. The father sought advice from the nurse.

"Is there any way to get a permit to carry a gun? I wouldn't hurt anyone but I've got to protect myself and the family. My cousin said to me, 'You don't know what you're doing. You're going to get hurt.' He has a gun. Back in '69 he shot at me during a falling out. I don't want to scare the Mrs., but I don't want to get hurt."

The victim coped with her fears of repercussions from the extended family by direct action ("I go to church to keep the danger away") and by praying ("I talk to God"). She also made a protective device for herself combining a fantasy and reality object:

"I have something in my purse to protect me. It's not a knife but a telecopter phone. I call 911 on it."

Carrying this telecopter phone in her purse helped desensitize her to fears of walking alone in the neighborhood. She said that each time she met a big boy on the street she would hold the purse and start to pray. Within a few weeks she was able to walk to church and in the neighborhood without her purse and telecopter phone.

The mother settled her feelings about the decision by focusing on her role as a mother:

"I'm doing what any other mother would do."

The brother's behavior was described by the mother as being more protective and cautious:

"He stopped bringing home friends and locks his windows on the third floor."

Summary of Crisis Resolution

This case illustrates how an external crisis of rape disrupts the victim's as well as the family's life-style and how a decision regarding pressing charges against a family member significantly taxes the family's coping and adaptive capacity. The data suggest that the presence of a nurse who is part of the health care system and has knowledge of the legal process may be of support to the family in thinking through family loyalty issues.

As health professionals become more involved in family crisis counseling involving legal matters, additional techniques may be necessary to deal with the cumulative crisis that may develop after the initial crisis. The staff of the various institutions that work with the same clients—in this case, the nurse, police, and prosecutor—will need to clearly identify the crisis issue of the individual and family to implement a plan of procedure that facilitates family homeostasis and minimizes the psychological trauma.

HISTORY OF A SURVIVOR

There are adult women who are making courageous efforts to break through the barriers of childhood silence on incest. One outstanding "survivor," as ex-incest victims prefer to be called, began facing her "14-year ghost" after recovering from an adult rape experience with the assistance of her psychologist–therapist. As is often noticed in cases of chronic or multiple incest victims, this woman had to be hypnotized to recall the past. The following is her memory of her experiences:

It started when I was 4 years old. He put his fingers inside me; I went into the closet and stayed there. All I remember is bleeding on my sister's blue shoes. I had vaginal pain until this incident was totally recalled and also woke in the night sitting in the closet.

Then I remembered being deprived of water at night because I was a bed-wetter. Mother would hang the sheets outside my window for people to see; couldn't drink anything after supper; was beaten with a belt. She assumed I did it on purpose and she was punishing me. (I stopped bed-wetting when I moved away from home at 17.) My brother offered me water if he could touch me. One night, Mom caught him coming out of my room (I was 8), and she beat me severely with a belt because I was a wicked, sinful little girl. She used hot-water enemas and douches to cleanse the devil out. After that, I *never* said anything. If my parents didn't help me, who would? So, the fondling went on till I was 14. Then my brother went away to college.

I was wild and sexually active as a teen-ager. I just didn't care about sex. Sex was a way of getting what I wanted: as a child: water, food, peace from my mother. As a teen-ager: gifts, learned how to drive a car, money, and most important, freedom to be by myself. Another problem I had as a child: I was very hard to wake—so much so that my parents took me to many doctors. I always felt something was wrong with me.

The night before my high-school graduation, my brother and his new wife came home for the ceremonies. That night while I was sleeping, he came into my room and raped me. I remember mother's good washcloth stuffed in my mouth but nothing else till a few hypnosis sessions. I didn't move or cry out— why would anyone help me now? I moved away from home then, but 2 months later found out I was pregnant and had to have an abortion. Under hypnosis I went through the labor and delivery for 45 minutes. Psychosomatic pain *always* starts before the actual memory of a trauma. Back to the abortion. There were no sedatives. I was made to look at the fetus. I've lost nearly 25 pounds through all this memory, and the sadness is so overwhelming it almost suffocates me. The anger is so intense, I'm afraid of it. Revenge is what I feel the most and loneliness.

My poetry is my outlet and provider of some peace of mind. The reason I am writing this is because I wish more people, especially professionals, knew or understood what it can feel like when a child realizes that he/she was not protected by their parents, and how it feels when there does not seem to be a safe place anywhere. Some people knew about my brother and didn't do anything because my father was rich and influential and they were afraid. I found this out a few months ago by asking old neighbors, friends, and relatives. Right now, I feel I'll never forgive them and I'm so angry and hurt and most of all wonder why I wasn't *worth* it! My parents were both alcoholics. Mother died on my birthday in 1977 and father is still alive but ill. My older brother and I have no communication except I sent him my poetry on incest a few weeks ago, but no reply yet.

One of the poems sent to her brother follows.*

MEMORIES OF THE RAIN

Older brother, oldest lover,
like a blackened banana I
feel rotted through and through.
How it started I don't recall.
Concealing feelings of helplessness,
dreaming of daylight freedom
that never came; only the rain.
So often I'm thrown into the past.
Night after night he'd call my name,
so I'd stare out the window
counting the rain.
I still wake in the night hoping
he won't be there, and I'm surrounded
alone wrapped in me; no torment there.
Remembering years ago possessed
by pain, always staring out the
window at the rain. Now, he's out
of reach and I sleep so peacefully.
Putting the past and distance behind me,
he no longer is the enemy, just sad memories
of the rain.
    K. Amanda

BATTERING

Battering—forcible physical assault—up until the late nineteenth century was considered a "necessary aspect of a husband's marital obligation to control and chastise his wife."[29] This behavior, in the twentieth century, is now proscribed by law. However, cultural attitudes continue to endorse such practice, and legal efforts to enforce the laws have failed to lend much aid.

---

* Reprinted with permission by K. Amanda.

The neglect of this problem in the professional literature was documented by O'Brien's finding that the index of the *Journal of Marriage and the Family* contained no references to "violence" from its inception in 1939 through the review of 1969.[30] The traditionally held view of wife abuse—similar to that of rape—was presented as an intrapsychic phenomenon in which violence was viewed as "fulfilling masochistic needs of the wife and necessary for the marital equilibrium."[31] Hilberman outlines the implications that follow from such explanations of causality: First, when wife abuse is viewed as occurring in deviant relationships, it will be defined as a private rather than public problem; second, if the victim is viewed as provoking the abuse, then the clinician can focus on the meaning of the "violence" rather than on the fact of the violence per se; and third, since women also believe these assumptions, they are reluctant to reveal the abuse and thus stay a silent victim. In summary, there has been a covert alliance, argues Hilberman, between victims and clinicians in which treatment of symptoms is offered as the preferred method of treatment rather than direct intervention and protection of the woman.[32]

Hilberman presents persuasively the societal attitudes that normalize the use of family violence as well as attitudes about women, men, and sex roles that leave women vulnerable to assaults by significant other men.[33] In a 1977–1978 study by Hilberman and Munson with 60 battered women in a general medical clinic setting, the following findings were reported[34]:

Lifelong violence was a frequent pattern for many abused wives. Half of the women reported violence between parents, paternal alcoholism, and their own physical or sexual abuse; many of the husbands had early exposure to emotional deprivation, alcoholism, lack of protection, and violence; suicides and homicides among family members and neighborhood acquaintances were common occurrences.

Most women left home at an early age to escape from violent, jealous, and seductive fathers; marriage during teen-age years was the norm for these women; many were teen-age mothers.

Drinking was noted in 93 percent of the sample as an association between alcohol use by the batterer and marital violence.

The marital relationship is characterized by extraordinary intensity. The cycle of violence is three-phased: (1) tension builds; (2) the violence erupts; and (3) there is relief from the tension. In this third phase the husband is often kind, loving, and remorseful and the woman is hopeful the husband will stop the violence.

Extreme jealousy characterizes the abuser. Wives are discouraged from social networks due to the extreme jealousy.

Violence erupted any time a husband did not immediately get his way. A common pattern described by the woman would be for the husband to come home late after being with another woman and to goad his wife into an argument that ended in violence. Some women were assaulted daily; others intermittently.

Assault weapons included hands, feet, fists, rocks, bottles, telephones, iron bars, knives, and guns. Scratching, slapping, punching with fists, throwing down, and kicking were prevalent with faces and breasts the most frequently mentioned sites of assault. These assaults led to multiple bruises, black eyes, fractured ribs, subdural hematomas, and detached retinas.

In a third of the families there was concurrent physical or sexual abuse of the children. All children were deeply affected by the family violence with a high incidence of somatic, psychological, and behavioral dysfunction being described in the children.

A Stress-Response Syndrome to Battering

The women studied by Hilberman and Munson exhibited paralyzing fear that was reminiscent of the rape trauma syndrome except that the stress was unending and the threat of assault ever-present.[35,36] Agitation and anxiety bordering on panic were almost always present. Sleep disturbance was also present with accompanying nightmares with themes of violence and danger. The waking lives of the women were characterized by overwhelming passivity and inability to act. They were fatigued, numb, and without energy to do the normal household tasks. Loss of control of aggression was a possibility and did occur in some cases. Some women became homicidal and others fantasized detailed plans for murdering their husbands as a way of coping with their anger.

Special Report on Family Violence Study

A five-year study was conducted at the Yale–New Haven Hospital and was funded by the National Institute of Mental Health. The major conclusions were reported as testimony by Evan Stark and Anne Flitcraft at the U.S. Attorney

General's Task Force on Family Violence during the first hearing site in New York City on December 2, 1983. Drs. Stark and Flitcraft reported the following:

The objective of the study was to determine the impact of battering on medicine, identify the appropriateness of the current clinical response, and assess the interrelationship between physical abuse and other problems. The study population involved a random sample of 3676 female patients using our emergency service for injury during a single year; a comparison within this group of approximately 650 battered and 650 nonbattered women; all suicide attempts presented by women during a year; and all instances of child abuse or neglect identified during a year. The full medical records for each group of patients were reviewed and every injury ever presented was classified using a methodology specifically developed to identify abuse for this study. Thus, although abuse is rarely noted by clinicians, this special classification scheme allows us to approximate the actual prevalence of abuse in a medical population and to distinguish it psychosocially, demographically, and as a cause of other major ills such as suicide attempt, child abuse, rape, and female alcoholism.

The major conclusion of this study is that under present conditions, almost 20 percent of all women using an emergency medical service for injuries develop a "battering syndrome" that includes, in addition to escalating and multiple injury, a range of psychosocial and behavioral problems. Although the syndrome is evoked by a deliberate assault by an intimate male, though not necessarily a "husband," the inappropriate response from medicine is clearly implicated in the subsequent development of injury and multiple psychosocial problems.

The battering syndrome appears to be a major precipitant and in some instances *the* major precipitant of multiple assaults, rape, female alcoholism, drug abuse among women, attempted suicide, child abuse, situational disorders, and psychoses.

A second major conclusion of the study is that the abuse of women and *not* "family violence" as such is the major precipitant of a range of family problems, including other forms of violence and neglect, e.g., child abuse.

A third major conclusion involves the origins of violence against women. It appears as if existential conflict explains abuse and *not* predisposing psychological or background factors. In other words, assault on women is a deliberate act, although aggravated by the usual combination of racial discrimination, economic poverty, and unemployment.

The fourth major conclusion is that the helping response provided by largely untrained clinicians appears to aggravate the problem, not to resolve it.

The findings represent the most complete evidence of a longitudinal kind on battering to date.

Although our study confirms that battering is far more widespread than many people suspect, it also indicates that as much as 75 percent of its prevalence may be the result of cases that have been brought to the attention of professionals—in this case physicians, psychiatrists, nurses, and social workers—and left unresolved. In addition, though the study confirms a long-suspected relationship between deliberate assault on women and a range of problems that impact the criminal justice system in addition to assault, it also indicates that the excess risk of these problems among victims of physical abuse arises only after the initial incident is reported to helping professionals. Combining these facts with the fact that no substantial evidence supports the belief that battering is the inevitable product of "poverty," psychopathology of a family predisposition provides a basis for optimism regarding the potential impact of comprehensive intervention designed to treat the battering syndrome at the federal, state, and local levels.

Whatever may motivate an individual man to beat his wife or girl friend, in general, abuse appears to be a deliberate criminal act aimed at subduing the will of another and by so doing exacting favors (often of a sexual kind), obedience, and/or dependence. Thus, whatever therapeutic alternatives may be developed to "treat" batterers or to help women who have been battered regain their self-confidence and social status, the need is clear that victims, and in this case women, need protection.

NURSING'S RESPONSE TO FAMILY VIOLENCE

Hospital-based programs also exist for battered women and their children.* One such program is described along with the use of the nursing process in working with battered women.

A Program for Battered Women at Boston City Hospital

The 1980s provided a springboard for innovative treatment programs to be planned, implemented, and researched throughout the United States. One such example is the work that occurred at Boston City Hospital. A victim counseling program was originally implemented here in 1972 as a first step toward dealing with the victims of violence. At that time, the victim counseling services were directed primarily to-

---

* This section through page 1011 was written by Shelia Levenseler.

ward rape victims. After the successful design of this program, the services were expanded to include victims of battering. The following discussion will focus on the nurse-directed program at Boston City Hospital and its work with battered women.

At Boston City Hospital, there is 24-hour coverage in the emergency room by the psychiatric emergency nursing team and the victim counseling service. These services, in cooperation, interview battered women, provide crisis counseling and follow-up, and make referrals to crisis hotlines, self-help groups, and shelters. With the increased awareness of the problem of battered women, the emergency department in general and psychiatric nurses in particular have become key people in identifying this population and responding to their needs.

The Nursing Process in Working with Battered Women

The use of the nursing process in working with battered women provides a useful practice framework. The key steps of the process include eliciting the crisis request, assessing the woman and family, making a nursing diagnosis, and negotiating a treatment plan.

Crisis Request

The clinical work in the emergency room with the battered victim is based on the concept of eliciting the crisis request.[37] Often the nurse will ask the woman, "How do you wish us to help you and your children?" By eliciting the crisis request from the woman, the staff are better able to help her and support the notion that she has some control over what happens to her and her children. The woman needs to be reassured that her treatment plan will be jointly decided upon by her and the nurse and in compliance with her initial request.

Eliciting the crisis request may require the nurse acting in an advocate role. The advocacy role of the nurse is crucial in situations in which the woman may not be able to readily express her request. The following case illustrates how this advocacy role was implemented by a triage nurse whose task was to determine which cases were seen by the psychiatric nurses in the emergency department and which cases would be routinely handled by emergency department staff.

A triage nurse noticed a man and a woman sitting in the waiting room of the emergency room. The woman was waiting to be seen for bruises of her face and some possible fractures. The nurse noticed that the man was holding onto the woman's arm and seemed to be angry with her. The nurse, suspecting something was wrong, decided to separate the couple and interview them separately. Once the woman was alone, she stated that her husband had caused her injuries and he did not want her to disclose the nature of her bruises.

Assessment

The following assessment areas are important in identifying situations of abuse. It is important that the nurse acknowledge the abuse in a tactful, nonthreatening manner. It is essential to obtain the victim's permission and cooperation regarding the history of abuse. The victim needs to be assured of confidentiality. Often, the partner of the victim has threatened her life if she discloses the source of abuse. Such threats are extremely difficult for a woman to bear psychologically.

The interview questions should be carried out in a supportive and sensitive manner. For women who openly discuss their abuse, we have found the following questions useful:

1. Inquire about any suspicious-looking injuries, how the injuries occurred, whether a partner inflicted the injuries, whether the abuse was disclosed, and how the disclosure was handled. In the nurse's physical assessment of the victim's injuries, any bruises, lacerations, or tenderness that are the result of the physical abuse should be documented. If the injuries are visible, the nurse can ask the woman for her written consent to have photographs taken of the injury. If the victim goes to court, the photographs can be used as evidence to verify the extent of her injuries.
2. Is the woman currently living with the abuser? If not, how did (does) he force entry into her living area?
3. If the woman is living with the abuser, has she ever left him? If not, has she wanted to leave? Is she afraid to leave? Often the woman has left in the past only to return because of lack of financial resources, or threats, or promises by the partner that he will reform.
4. Are there children at home? Does the woman feel they are in danger? Has the

abuser ever beaten or abused them? Have the children ever been investigated for suspected abuse?

5. Was the abuser taking drugs or drinking alcohol at the time of the abuse?

6. Does the woman need a safe place to go—with friends or relatives? Would she like to go to a shelter? Many women may not be aware of potential resources, which staff can be helpful in identifying.

7. Has the woman ever gone to the police or courts? If she does want to go to court, it might be helpful to identify a support person who can accompany her to file a complaint. Finding a support person can make the difference between pressing or dropping charges. It is important for the nurse to document in the medical record what the victim reports has happened to her in her own words. This type of information may be of help to the woman if she decides to go to court and press charges. Thus, this type of record can help to corroborate the woman's story of abuse if she goes to court.

8. Has the woman or her children received any prior counseling services? Are they interested?

Nursing Diagnosis of Battering

There are two ways a nursing diagnosis of battering may be made: (1) the battered victim explicitly tells the nurse that she has been abused by her partner; or (2) the nurse suspects an unreported battering. In the first method, the nurse should document the diagnosis with the patient's report of the battering and the assessment data. In the second method, the nurse needs to be knowledgeable about the signs and symptoms of silent battering syndrome and be able to evaluate assessment data regarding a nursing diagnosis of unreported battering.

Because many women and children try to keep the battering a secret, nurses are in key positions to case-find for such victim situations. From our clinical work with both adult- and child-abuse client populations, we recommend that the nurse maintain a high index of suspicion for unreported battering whenever she observes the following signs and symptoms:

1. The woman may describe agitation, anxiety, or nightmares. The nightmares may be aggressive, in which the woman describes herself as killing or assaulting her partner.

2. There are suspicious-looking bruises or lacerations that the woman may not discuss. Vague comments about being "roughed up" are made.

3. A woman may present with multiple somatic complaints: i.e., headaches, abdominal complaints, chest pain, back pain, gastrointestinal problems. She may present herself to the clinic frequently. Also, she may be dependent on tranquilizers.

4. Children may come to the emergency room or clinic with somatic complaints such as insomnia, nightmares, enuresis, and fearfulness about going to bed.

5. Teen-agers may present to the clinic in the following way:

Males   Complaints of fighting in school or with siblings, truant from school, poor concentration level, or temper tantrums.
Females Headaches, withdrawn, fighting with siblings, and sexual abuse.

6. The husband or boyfriend is described as jealous or possessive.

7. The husband or boyfriend is described as drinking or using drugs too much.

8. Victim may indicate that she or partner observed violence at home as children or were victims of sexual abuse.

9. The woman has an impaired self-concept and chronic depression.

10. Injuries in a pregnant woman (which may represent the partner's attempt to induce a miscarriage).

The Nursing Plan

The victim needs to be made aware of the variety of resources that are available to her. These may include crisis hotlines, community groups for women who have been abused, shelters, a variety of counseling opportunities (i.e., couples, individual, or group), and information regarding the victim's rights in the civil and criminal justice system. After the different resources are reviewed, the woman will be able to decide what choices she will make for herself. A nursing plan should be negotiated with the patient, paying careful attention to her individual needs and requests.

Staff Reaction to Working with Battered Victims

Autognosis is an important therapeutic tool in victim intervention. Abused victims frequently evoke strong thoughts, feelings, and actions in the nurse that have the potential to stall the therapeutic process. Some of the common reactions include thoughts of increased awareness of violence; feelings of helplessness, frustration, anger; and actions aimed at rescuing, labeling, or offering false reassurance. The nurse's awareness of these common reactions can serve to sensitize as well as optimize a therapeutic stance in relation to working with battered victims.

Increased Awareness of Violence

Nurses who work with battered victims quickly become aware of the amount of violence that occurs in our society. This increased awareness sensitizes nurses to the violence in the media such as television as well as in reality situations between people. Through working with battered women, the staff may identify with the impact of violence and their own vulnerability to becoming a victim. Members may voice this concern as, "If I help her, he may come after me too." The fear of retaliation and revenge, which is part of the violence cycle in partnerships, can easily transfer over to staff members who do not openly discuss their thoughts and fears after working with victims of violence.

Subjective Feelings

Working with battered women stirs up many feelings in staff members. Consider the following case in terms of the subjective feelings one might feel for the victim.

The victim, a 36-year-old woman, had been involved in a dating relationship with a boyfriend for the past 2 years. She said that before this violent episode, she had made the decision to see less of the boyfriend: "I started to feel closed in—he isolated me. . . . If I couldn't account for every minute of my time, he would make accusations that I had another boyfriend. He didn't want me to visit with my female friends."

On this particular evening, the boyfriend asked her if they could have a drink at a place near her home. She agreed to meet him at 8:30 P.M. and said she had to be home by 10:30 P.M.

She said they talked for several hours, "sort of chit-chat." Finally, she said she had to leave. They walked out together and crossed the street. She said, "I didn't see anything but felt something hard hit me in the face and I remember falling to the ground and being kicked repeatedly. Then I don't remember anything until I woke up in the ambulance."

The woman was treated for her injuries, which included black eyes, fractured nose, and facial fractures. After hospital treatment, the woman took a cab home. However, she told the cab driver to wait for her because she was concerned that the boyfriend might be waiting for her at home. Indeed he was, and as she approached the hallway of the building, she saw the boyfriend coming toward her with a bat in his hand, saying, "I've come back to finish the job." She said, "Haven't you done enough damage already?" Then she fled back to the cab and went directly to the police station. Officers then accompanied her back to her apartment. When she opened the door, her three daughters were crying and screaming, "Chris has been raped by Brian (the boyfriend)."

In the interim period that the woman had sought medical assistance, the boyfriend had broken into the apartment expecting to find the woman in her bedroom. Instead, he found her little girl who had fallen asleep. He awakened the girl, tied her up with vacuum wire, and sexually assaulted her.

The nurse providing counseling services to this woman found the experience emotionally draining and later discussed her subjective feelings in the team meeting:

"I looked at the mother. She looked terrible. Her face was already swollen. I can't imagine how she must have looked the next morning. She was in shock. I got so upset and felt such outrage at the boyfriend and felt very sad for the family."

Feelings of Helplessness. Staff members may experience feelings of helplessness in working with battered victims. Consider the following example:

"The phone rang . . . I was asleep . . . my husband came charging into our bedroom and pulled me up by the hair, then knocked me to the floor. He asked me to get up, but I couldn't move, I was so stunned . . . so he pulled me up again by the hair, pulling muscles in my neck and bruising my arm and shoulder. Later I tried to use the phone to get help, but he stopped me by wrapping the telephone cord around my neck and hitting me in the head with the phone. I thought I was going to pass out. I was scared. I really thought he was going to kill me."

This victim was unable to go to the hospital until the next day. She had a punctured eardrum and a number of bruises over her body. The victim decided to separate from her husband for a short time. After several months she went back with him. The last conversation that the nurse had with this victim ended as follows: "I can't talk with you . . . he's here."

Feelings of Frustration and Anger.

When there are known and repeated serious injuries to the victim, the staff's response can be one of frustration and anger. They want to ask:

- "Why does she stay with him?"
- "Why doesn't she just leave?"
- "Why doesn't she go to the police?"

It is advised that such questions be asked in peer support groups and not directly to the victim. Questions that begin with "why" are perceived as accusatory and may undermine any therapeutic leverage the nurse hopes to gain with the client.

One of the nurses said, "You see battered women and you hear what has happened to them. . . . You feel like you can offer some options or provide answers but she won't leave. . . . In my head I know she will leave when she is ready, but I feel so helpless trying to help her."

In fact, nurses have to acknowledge how difficult it is to work with abused people. Also, many women are not ready to move out of a situation. Therefore, as alternatives, the staff should have the names of hotlines and self-help groups for the women to turn to for help.

Nontherapeutic Staff Actions

There are several nontherapeutic actions that staff members may take in response to thoughts and feelings they have toward working with battered women. Three staff actions commonly observed include: (1) rescue actions; (2) labeling the victim; and (3) offering false reassurance.

Rescue Actions.

When staff members believe they have the magical ability to improve the situation, rescue actions emerge. Consider the following case:

The victim is a 25-year-old woman who was brought to the hospital via ambulance after receiving a severe beating to her head and face with a pool stick. Although she was stuporous on arrival, she did respond to painful stimuli. She was in the intensive care unit for 4 days and then was transferred to a medical unit. She remained unconscious for 9 days and would respond only to painful neurological stimuli.

The husband had called the police and reported that his wife had been beaten and raped. However, the police, arriving on the scene, arrested the husband because of his disorderly conduct and the suspicion that he had beaten his wife.

As the woman became conscious and oriented, she could not believe her husband had beaten her. Staff members noted old healed scars on her body and wondered if they were the results of previous beatings by the husband. When the husband did visit, he told his wife that he did do the beatings. Later, the victim told the staff that she could not believe he had done all the damage by himself. On further follow-up, while still in the hospital, the victim said:

"If I go back, things will be different. He'll have to change. He has already said he would."

For many women, the hope that the partner will stop his violent ways holds them in the relationship. The staff, who care for these women and believe they will be able to magically intervene and correct the situation, find it difficult to understand why these couples stay together. They (the staff) become defensive and angry at the women. A more useful focus for their anger would be to pressure clinicians to work with the abuser and to develop programs to intervene more effectively in the alcohol-aggression cycle.

Labeling the Victim.

The labeling of battered women may represent the clinicians' response to their own frustration in dealing with the issue. Two examples follow:

EXAMPLE ONE

The couple had been separated. The husband came into the house and started an argument with his wife. She said to her mother who was visiting, "Let's go," and they left the house and got into the mother's car. The husband followed them to the car and smashed the windshield of the car with his fist saying, "I'm going to kill you if you don't get into that house, and no one will stop me."

Two police officers were passing and stopped to see what the problem was. The husband said, "Shoot me. I have nothing to live for." They decided to take the man to the state hospital for an evaluation. He was seen briefly for a psychiatric evaluation, and then the psychiatrist asked to see the wife. He ended the interview by saying, "You must have liked being beaten. Otherwise you wouldn't have stayed all those years."

EXAMPLE TWO

In a recent staff meeting, the staff were discussing their care of a battered woman. The clinician present asked the staff if they would be interested in a psychoanalytic explanation of why the woman was masochistic. The clinician proceeded to give the explanation. When he realized his comments were not well received, in rebuttal to their views he stated that men may be masochistic also.

Such indiscriminate labeling is invariably based on flimsy data, is motivated by frustration with and anger at the patient, and serves no purpose in helping the patient.

Offering False Reassurance. Staff members may respond to their helplessness in dealing with battered women by offering false reassurance. The woman may be expressing her fear that the abuser will come back and kill her. The nurse should guard against denying this reality with a statement such as, ''Don't worry about that. He won't hurt you.'' The fact is that the abuser may return, may beat her again, and the end result may be a homicide.

A more therapeutic response is to help the woman express her feelings of fear and to help her take some concrete steps to protect herself. This allows the victim to talk about her concerns and to consider alternatives. This approach will help to increase her power and control in the situation and thus decrease her helplessness.

PREVENTION OF ABUSE

Spouse abuse is not a new phenomenon, but only recently has intrafamilial violence been defined as a social problem. There is a growing concern about intrafamilial violence with different health providers supporting services that will help prevent domestic violence.

One area of prevention that nurses are actively engaged in is clinical nursing research. The project at Boston City Hospital is just one example of how a program was implemented to provide services to a target population group. Data will continue to be collected on the battered women seen in the program in an attempt to further identify and clarify issues and concerns regarding the abuser and the abused.

Legislation regarding domestic violence may be reintroduced in both houses of Congress to provide federal support to state and local activities for the prevention of domestic violence and for assistance to its victims. In many states, there have been changes in state legislation pertaining to domestic violence. Major provisions regarding civil remedies have been instituted to assist battered women and their families.

A goal of the women's movement has been to identify the injustices toward the female sex in our society and to implement strategies to equalize the balance of power. Women's groups have been instrumental in providing services to help battered women alleviate some of the difficulties they have had to face in receiving services. Battered women now have alternatives such as support groups and shelters. Rather than remaining in a violent relationship, these women now have some viable options for themselves and for their children.

Many community groups are providing the public with information about spouse abuse. Their goals have been to identify the social myths and attitudes regarding abuse. In addition, they have acted as resource people by providing information about the different types of services for victims that are available in the area.

Summary

The sexual victimization of children is an issue of increasing concern. Nurses are in key positions both to identify and to assist the child who is the target of such abuse. Interagency cooperation is necessary in such situations, and nurses can take leadership roles in this enterprise for the protection of children.

The incidence of spouse abuse is becoming an increasingly visible issue.

The problem of domestic violence was the focus of a 1983–84 U.S. Attorney General's Task Force. Materials related to this problem are included in the chapter.

As the reporting of violence increases in our society, mental health professionals must be responsive to these demands by providing services to the victims and their families.

Questions

1. What are some similarities and some differences between incest and family violence?
2. Identify the theoretical issues in the clinical literature on incest.
3. What role does secrecy play in child sexual assault and how can this lead to symptom formation?
4. How can a nurse help a child and her family work on the issue of divided loyalty?
5. What is the relationship between the women's movement and battered victims?
6. How is autognosis a useful nursing tool in working with battered victims?
7. Why do nurses identify with battered victims and feel helpless in the therapeutic process?
8. What preventive measures can be taken in the area of battering?
9. What is the role of the staff nurse in working with battered victims?

REFERENCES AND SUGGESTED READINGS

1. President's Task Force on Victims of Crime. *Final Report*. Washington, D.C.: U.S. Government Printing Office, 1982, p. 1.
2. Armstrong, L. *Kiss Daddy Goodnight: A Speakout on Incest*. New York: Hawthorne, 1978.
3. Berliner, L., & Stevens, D. Special techniques for child witnesses. In L. G. Schultz (Ed.), *The Sexual Victimology of Youth*. Springfield, Ill.: Chas. C. Thomas, 1979.
4. Herman, J., & Hirschman, L. Father–daughter incest. *Signs: Journal of Culture and Society*, 1977, *2*, 1–22.
5. Henderson, D. J. Incest. In A. M. Freeman, H. I. Kaplan, & B. J. Sadock (Eds.), *Comprehensive Textbook of Psychiatry*, 2nd ed. Baltimore: Williams & Wilkins, 1975.
6. Landes, J. Experiences of 500 children with adult sexual deviants. *Psychiatric Quarterly Supplement*, 1956, *30*, 91–109.
7. Gagnon, J. H. Female child victims of sex offenses. *Social Problems*, 1965, *13*, 176–192.
8. Finkelhor, D. *Sexually Victimized Children*. New York: Free Press, 1970.
9. Ibid.
10. Summit, R. Beyond belief: The reluctant discovery and incest. In M. Kirkpatrick (Ed.), *Women in Context*. New York: Plenum, 1981.
11. Finkelhor, op. cit.
12. Summit, op. cit.
13. Summit, R., & Kryso, J. Sexual abuse of children: A clinical spectrum. *American Journal of Orthopsychiatry*, 1978, *48*, 237–251.
14. Freud, S. The aetiology of hysteria. In *Collected*

Papers (Vol. 1). London: Hogarth Press, 1953, p. 203.
15. Freud, S. On the history of psychoanalytic movement. In *Collected Papers* (Vol. 1). London: Hogarth Press, 1953, p. 300.
16. Ferenczi, S. Confusion of tongues between the adult and the child. *International Journal of Psychoanalysis*, 1949, *30*, 225–229.
17. Ibid., pp. 228–229.
18. Glueck, B. G., Jr. Early sexual experiences in schizophrenia. In H. Biegel (Ed.), *Advances in Sex Research*. New York: Harper & Row, 1963, pp. 248–255.
19. Ferenczi, op. cit., p. 227.
20. Ibid., p. 228.
21. Ibid., pp. 228–229.
22. Herman & Hirschman, op. cit., p. 741.
23. Ibid.
24. Ibid., p. 748.
25. Burgess, A. W., Holmstrom, L. L., & McCausland, M. P. Child sexual assault by a family member. *Victimology*, 1977, *2*, 236–251.
26. Burgess, A. W., & Holmstrom, L. L. Rape trauma syndrome. *American Journal of Psychiatry*, 1974, *131*, 981–986.
27. Burgess, A. W., & Holmstrom, L. L. *Rape: Crisis and Recovery*. Bowie, Md.: Brady, 1986.
28. Holmstrom, L. L., & Burgess, A. W. *The Rape Victim: Institutional Reactions*. New York: Wiley, 1978.
29. Dobash, R. E., & Dobash, R. P. *Violence Against Wives*. New York: Free Press, 1979.
30. O'Brien, J. E. Violence in divorce-prone families. *Journal of Marriage and the Family*, 1971, *33*, 692–698.
31. Snell, J. E., Rosenwald, R. J., & Robey, A. The wife-beater's wife. *Archives of General Psychiatry*, 1964, *11*, 107–112.

32. Hilberman, E. Overview: The "wife-beater's wife" reconsidered. *American Journal of Psychiatry*, 1980, *137*, 1336–1347.
33. Ibid.
34. Hilberman, E., & Munson, M. Sixty battered women. *Victimology*, 1977–78, *2*, 460–471.
35. Ibid.
36. Burgess & Holmstrom, op. cit. (1974), pp. 981–986.
37. Lazare, A., Eisenthal, S., & Wasserman, L. The customer approach to patienthood. *Archives of General Psychiatry*, 1975, *32*, 553–558.

Chapter 52

The Chronically Mentally Disabled

Nancy Worley

Chapter Objectives

The students successfully attaining the goals of this chapter will be able to:

- Explore the various types of chronic mental illness.
- Compare various treatment modalities.
- Relate treatment to type of illness.
- Assess public policy issues relating to the chronically mentally ill.

Because of advances in psychopharmacology, psychotherapy, and early case finding, approximately one third of those who suffer from a major mental illness will recover and go on to lead normal lives. The remaining two thirds, however, will suffer severe and persistent mental and emotional disorders that will interfere with their functional capacities in relation to such primary aspects of daily life as self-care, interpersonal relationships, and work or schooling and will necessitate prolonged hospital care or short, frequent hospitalizations. These persons constitute the group known as the chronically mentally disabled. Our concern for this group is relatively recent and results principally from the social policy change in mental health known as deinstitutionalization.

The number of residents in public mental hospitals has declined from 600,000 in 1955 to less than 100,000 today. This astounding change in the locus of care for the chronically mentally disabled from public institutions to the community is termed deinstitutionalization. New psychoactive drugs, concern about the civil rights of psychiatric patients, and the passage of the Community Mental Health Centers Act of 1963, coupled with a philosophical conviction that the mentally ill receive better and more humanitarian treatment in the community, have contributed to this change. This policy of deinstitutionalization affects not only former long-term residents of public mental hospitals but also a younger population who may either be admitted for the short term to these institutions though spending the majority of their time in the community or, as has become more common, are treated entirely in community facilities. A severe shortage of supportive and rehabilitative programs in the community to meet the needs of persons discharged (the long-term institutionalized) or diverted (the younger chronically mentally ill) has led to public concern not only about these two groups but also about a third population of persons, the homeless mentally ill, who, in addition to mental illness, suffer the hardships and indignities of life on the streets.

Clearly, the chronic mentally ill are not a homogeneous group. At least three distinct populations with different needs have been identified. This chapter will present patient characteristics, special needs, and intervention techniques for:

1. The mentally disabled who have spent much of their lives in public mental hospitals.
2. The young chronically mentally disabled who before deinstitutionalization might have resided in public institutions but now must be cared for in the community.
3. Homeless persons who are mentally disabled.

THE DEINSTITUTIONALIZED MENTALLY DISABLED PATIENT

It is estimated that 500,000 patients, nearly all of whom had been long-term residents of psychiatric hospitals, were discharged between 1955 and 1975. While approximately one third returned to their families, those without family support faced an uncertain future. Because of a lack of community-based facilities to care for these multiproblem patients, many were transferred directly from public mental hospitals to nursing homes.[1,2] Many moved into welfare hotels, which proliferated in many areas of the country to absorb the increased burden on housing created by the release of chronic psychiatric patients who had no place to go.[3] Board-and-care homes multiplied in deteriorated areas of cities where community objection to the influx of former mental patients was less vociferous than it was in more affluent areas. "Psychiatric ghettos" formed in areas adjacent to large public mental hospitals as former patients who no longer had family or social ties to the communities in which they had resided before hospitalization sought to remain close to the institutions that had been their homes for many years.

The inadequacy of community facilities for these formerly institutionalized patients has led to a phenomenon known as the "revolving door" in which patients are discharged from the hospital, live in the community for weeks or months, and then are readmitted for a short period of time before being discharged to the community to begin the cycle again.

Patient Characteristics

Although patients vary in the severity and course of their illness, their life circumstances, and in the makeup of their premorbid personality, certain characteristics are common to this group of patients. Generally, they have an underlying major mental illness. Approximately 70 percent have been diagnosed as having schizophrenia, the majority of the remaining 30 percent have a major affective disorder, a small percentage have a severe personality disorder, and a few suffer from more than one disorder. The course of these illnesses is generally one of acute exacerbations of the illness with florid psychotic symptoms, followed by periods of remission in which the overtly psychotic behavior subsides but milder, less disruptive symptomology, such as social isolation and dependency, remains. In addition to the illness itself, long-term residents of mental hospitals often exhibit symptoms that can be attributed to the interaction of the disease process and the effects of institutionalization. Goffman eloquently documented the effects that unstimulating environments have in dulling affect, initiative, and in promoting stereotyped behavior.[4] Life in mental hospitals differs from life in the community in ways that promote dysfunctional behavior. The institutional breakdown of the work, play, and sleeping spheres of life is not normal in outside society. Many human needs (eating, sleeping, showering, recreation) are handled through the beaurocratic organization of whole blocks of people. There is a basic split between patients and supervising staff in which there is a tendency for each group to stereotype the other. Social mobility between the two groups is restricted. Patients have restricted contact with the outside world while staff members are socially integrated into their communities, further pointing out the differences between the two. Under these circumstances, patients rapidly lose their conception of self. Their role in the outside world of worker, friend, and family member is replaced with the role of patient. Possessions, privacy, autonomy, and freedom of action are lost. Most people who suffer from chronic mental illness enter the hospital with an already-weak sense of self and a tendency to behave in dependent ways. Hospitalization often exacerbates these symptoms. Most of the social problem-solving skills that the patient might have had prior to hospitalization atrophy as a result of disuse, reinforcement of a sick role, and loss of motivation. The result is a passive "institutionalized" patient poorly prepared to function in the community.

Intervention

Neuroleptic drugs are effective in reducing such positive symptoms of schizophrenia as delusions and hallucinations. They are less effective in reducing negative symptoms, such as withdrawal and apathy, and have no effect on social and vocational handicaps. Numerous investigations have shown that there is a direct relationship between social competency and length of tenure in the community for former hospital patients.[5–7] Moreover, one of these studies found that more than 50 percent of a sample of chronic psychiatric patients had major deficits in many areas of basic human functioning such as socialization, grooming, and personal hygiene.[8] Until recently, little attention has been paid to changing public hospital environments in ways that will make them effective training centers for the retention of skills that patients had on entering the hospital and for the teaching of additional skills necessary for leading a satisfying life in the community. Currently, some public mental hospitals are experimenting with training patients in specific interpersonal skills through the use of highly directive behavioral techniques. Unlike traditional, nonspecific group activities that engage patients in socialization with the hope that incidental learning will take place, social skills training incorporates specific principles of human learning to promote the acquisition, generalization, and durability of skills needed in interpersonal situations.[9] Training uses role playing, modeling, prompting, feedback, reinforcement, and shaping. Videotaping is frequently used to present modeling performances and to provide feedback. An extensive assessment of the patient's present skill level is made, and target behaviors for change are identified. These might include affective expressions such as eye contact, voice volume

and intonation, and facial expression, or content behaviors such as asking for information or starting a conversation at an appropriate time and place. The following example illustrates the use of social skills techniques.

EXAMPLE

Tom is a 25-year-old patient with a diagnosis of chronic schizophrenia. This is his third admission to the state hospital in the past 6 years. His basic social skills are poor and he has been assigned to a social skills training group.

THERAPIST: Today we are going to practice starting a conversation. Yesterday we talked about the points to remember for performing this skill correctly. Tom, do you remember the first point?

TOM: Yes. You need to choose the right time and place.

THERAPIST: Excellent. And what is the next point to remember?

TOM: You greet the other person.

THERAPIST: Exactly. You remembered yesterday's lesson very well! And then?

TOM: And then you start to talk.

THERAPIST: That's right. You make small talk because you want to check something out. Do you remember what it is that you're checking out?

TOM: Well, I would want to know if the person was interested in continuing the conversation.

THERAPIST: How would you know that?

TOM: I don't remember.

THERAPIST: You would have to check if they were really listening to you, if they seemed interested in continuing the conversation. Let's try all of this out. I'll be your friend Bob, and we'll pretend that you came into the dayroom and found me watching TV. What would you do?

TOM: I'd say "Hi, Bob, how are you today?"

THERAPIST (BOB): Hi, Tom, this is a really exciting show. Would you like to watch it with me?

TOM: No. Did you have fun at the dance last night?

THERAPIST (BOB): [keeps eyes on TV and mumbles] Mmmm.

TOM: I'll catch you later.

THERAPIST: Why did you stop the conversation?

TOM: Because Bob wanted to watch TV.

THERAPIST: Excellent. You remembered to check whether the person was interested in having a conversation. And you made plans to come back later at a better time.

This vignette demonstrates some of the ways in which social skills training is used to gradually shape the patient's behavior through role playing and social reinforcement. Recent studies have shown that patients who have been involved in social skills training are viewed as more socially adept in the community after discharge.[10]

Recognition that traditional hospital programs tend to perpetuate dependency, apathy, and loss of a sense of responsibility has led to the development of several model programs designed to change the traditional relationships between staff and patients and to make the hospital environment more challenging. One of the most successful of these model programs has been the Fairweather Lodge model, which was developed by George Fairweather at a veterans hospital in California in the 1960s. Stroul describes the lodge model as follows.[11] Small problem-solving groups of 10 to 15 are formed while the patients are still in the hospital. Each small group meets daily without staff and discusses and makes recommendations about the problem behaviors of individual members or the group as a whole. The problems might be identified by group members or might be brought to the group's attention by staff through a formalized communication system. Staff retain the right to accept or reject the group's recommendations and meet with the group once a week to review and evaluate the group's performance.

A step system with different degrees of responsibility and rewards is used to teach patients to assume increasing responsibility and to prepare for discharge. By the time a group member reaches the highest step, he is expected to be a leader, to help others, and to be ready to leave the hospital. As the group nears discharge, the group members become involved in the task of preparing their group home in the community. Issues to be addressed include determining the location of the lodge, planning the kind of business that the lodge will operate, and anticipating some of the problems the group might encounter, such as community resistance. Other structured learning experiences to prepare for the move to the community might include planning and preparing meals, laundering, and using public transportation. All members have meaningful work roles within the community lodge. Some cook, while others wash dishes, clean the house, or manage the household accounts. In addition the lodge manages its own business to provide employment opportunities for its members. Various lodges around the country are operating janitorial services, household cleaning services, shoe repairs, printing, and furniture building.[12]

Fountain House, in New York City, is the model for a somewhat different approach to providing a spectrum of services to the long-term mentally disabled. Fountain House and subsequent agencies that patterned themselves on it or slightly modified the Fountain House approach all belong to a psychosocial rehabilitation model. The psychosocial rehabilitation model adopted its philosophy from physical rehabilitation, which focuses on building client skills and modifying environments.[13] Although approaches to skill building and environmental resource development vary, a psychosocial program is characteristically organized as a clubhouse or center. Clients are called members and are participants in the running of the center. With the center as the hub of activity, the model offers a specific package of services, which fall into four major areas: social and recreational, vocational, residential, and educational.[14] As in physical rehabilitation, there is intensive effort devoted initially to establishing a psychiatric rehabilitation diagnosis. During the diagnostic phase, staff and client work together to gather information about the client's current level of skills relevant to the demands of the environment in which the client wants to function. The rehabilitation diagnosis is the basis for the development of the rehabilitation plan, which is designed to increase the client's skills and to develop an environment more helpful to the client's functioning.[15]

EXAMPLE

A 20-year-old client who enters a psychosocial rehabilitation program may have obtaining an associate degree as a goal. Assessment reveals that the client had good grades in high school but dropped out during his senior year because of prolonged psychiatric hospitalization. He is currently living in a large and noisy boardinghouse far from the college he would like to attend. His psychiatric symptoms are currently under good control on maintenance doses of medication. The client is ambivalent about continuing the medication because "I might get addicted to it." The psychiatric diagnosis would contain the client's goal (obtaining an associate degree) and current level of skills relevant to the environment in which the client wants to function (needs to finish high school). A rehabilitation plan is then formulated on the basis of this information. Obtaining a high school diploma might be accomplished by either enrolling in a local high school or in an adult education program and taking the examination for a high school equivalency diploma. The client decides that he would be uncomfortable enrolling in high school at his age and will join an adult education program instead. The therapist and the client decide that the client will take the responsibility for investigating the various adult education programs available in the city, choosing the one he wants to attend, and obtaining the application form. Therapist and client will then fill out the application together. The client voices concern about possible difficulty in being able to concentrate on studying in his present living arrangement, in which he shares a room in a group home that is noisy in the evening when all the clients return from their daily activities and want to "let off steam." Studying in the local library will be difficult because rules at the group home require everyone to be in the home by nine in the evening. Client and therapist work on solving the problems around this issue and list the options to be explored: obtaining special permission from the group home supervisor to extend the client's curfew by 2 hours; request that a quiet place be set aside in the home for those who want to study or read; if neither of these options work out satisfactorily, explore the possibility of moving to a less-restrictive setting. During their joint work on the rehabilitation plan the therapist engages the client in conversation about his ambivalence toward his medication. The client agrees that his worries about his medications may be based on misinformation and agrees to attend a medication class for clients that is being given at the community mental health center.

This case study illustrates the underlying philosophy of psychosocial rehabilitation, which emphasizes (1) wellness rather than illness; (2) client empowerment; (3) skills building; (4) environmental support; and (5) positive expectations and optimism.

THE YOUNG CHRONICALLY MENTALLY ILL PATIENT

Today, the 64 million babies born during the "baby boom" of post World War II are entering young to middle adulthood. They represent one-third of the population in the United States and are in the age range in which people are most at risk for developing schizophrenia and the major affective disorders. Sheer numbers alone might not have made the members of this group who suffer from chronic mental illness so visible to the general public and mental health professionals had it not been for the social and policy changes which have accompanied them into young adulthood. Many of today's young chronic mentally disabled adults represent that group of individuals who most probably would have been long term state mental hospital patients before deinstitutionalization but now must be cared for in the community. The increased acceptance of the use of recreational drugs and the greater mobility of this age group relative to its counterpart 20–30 years ago has contributed to the emergence of a large group of high profile chronic mentally ill young adults in the community.

Client Characteristics

The problem of mental illness in the young adult is complicated by the developmental tasks facing all persons in this age group. Attaining appropriate independence from one's family of origin, choosing and succeeding at a vocation, forming satisfying interpersonal relationships, attaining some degree of intimacy and acquiring a positive sense of identity are difficult tasks to complete even under the best of circumstances. The mentally ill individual who often lacks ego strength, the capacity to withstand stress, and the ability to form meaningful relationships has little capacity to negotiate these milestones into responsible adulthood. Repeated failures to "keep up" with peers often leads to increased anxiety, depression and retreat into psychosis.

Since the advent of deinstitutionalization, the multiple developmental and psychiatric needs of this population must be met by community agencies. Because these clients have frequently not been institutionalized or have had only short stays in community inpatient settings, they tend to deny their mental disabilities and therefore complicate the task of providing adequate services to them. Their reluctance to acknowledge their need for ongoing treatment results in high treatment drop out rates, rejection of partial hospital programs, discontinuity of service and heavy reliance on emergency psychiatric services in times of crisis. Their denial of mental illness also makes them reluctant to see themselves as especially vulnerable to alcohol, marijuana, and other mind-altering drugs used recreationally by their peers and as a result a high percentage of this group have mental illness complicated by drug and alcohol abuse. Poor impulse control and severely impaired judgment lead to involvement with the criminal justice system for low-level offenses such as minor property damage, petty theft and minor assault. Poor impulse control, drug and alcohol abuse, and depression due to their inability to master age-appropriate tasks contributes to the high suicide rate among this group. In summary, the young chronic mentally ill patient has been characterized as being one or more of the following: treatment resistant, predominately male, socially isolated, transient, unemployed, with poor impulse control, judgmentally impaired, one with a history of arrests for minor offenses, potentially suicidal, a poly drug and alcohol abuser.[16–18]

Intervention

The difficulties of treating a group of clients who have severe psychiatric and character defects in an environment of uncoordinated services and fiscal scarcity cannot be overemphasized. These clients require a wide range of treatment, rehabilitation and social services and given the pluralistic service delivery system in this country, these services must be located and negotiated within a vast network of agencies. Clients who are psychiatrically disorganized and have a low tolerance for frustration and stress simply cannot negotiate these systems on their own. The discontinuity of the service network coupled with the personality characteristics of the young mentally disabled adult has led many mental health experts to recommend the provision of case management services for this population.[19–21]

Case management is generally defined as involving a service integration function designed to overcome the gaps and obstacles in the fragmented social service system.[22] Case management functions, approaches and models differ by setting but all tend to have in common the functions of outreach, assessment of client needs, strengths and deficits, the development of a comprehensive treatment plan, linkage with necessary services, monitoring of service delivery and client advocacy. Two quite different philosophies underlie the various models of case management. Although which of these philosophies best serves the client has been the sub-

ject of controversy in the mental health literature, it is likely that each is effective when matched with the appropriate patient type.[23–24] One approach views case management as essentially an administrative function in which the case manager acts as a broker of services for the patient. One of the services the case manager might arrange for the patient is psychotherapy but the case manager does not act as therapist for the patient. The second approach is that of the case manager-therapist in which the therapist's role is expanded in order to assist the patient in maintaining a facilitative physical and social environment. Considering the characteristics of the young chronic adult, the case manager-therapist role is likely to be more effective although research in this area needs to be done. Intaglia argues that the most influential aspect of the case management process is the quality of the relationship that develops between manager and client.[25] Young adults who are socially isolated, lonely, and dependent on, yet suspicious of close relationships can benefit greatly from developing a healthy relationship with the therapist-case manager. Such relationships can teach the client that there is a form of dependency that is necessary, normal and constructive.[26]

THE HOMELESS MENTALLY ILL

Persons who are homeless and seriously mentally ill are among the most vulnerable and disfranchised clients of the health and welfare system.[26] The advent of deinstitutionalization and the scarcity of community facilities, especially housing, has resulted in a situation in which the most disorganized of the mentally ill, those who are unable to keep appointments at mental health clinics, follow medication regimens, and apply for disability benefits, find themselves without shelter and forced to live on the streets.

Population Characteristics

The homeless population has changed significantly over the past 20 years. Not only has there been an astounding increase in homelessness, but the demographics of the population have changed as well. Women and young men are appearing with increasing frequency. Deinstitutionalization has contributed to the number of mentally ill in the homeless population. Attempts to discover the number of mentally ill among the homeless have been complicated by the nature of homelessness. Homeless persons tend to distrust representatives of authority and to place great value on their autonomy. They may react to questioning by giving false information or refusing to cooperate with interviews. It is often difficult to locate them for follow-up information. One of the first studies that systematically investigated the prevalence of mental illness among the homeless in shelters was conducted by Arce, Tadlock, and Vergare in Philadelphia.[27] Using *DSM-III* criteria and formal, extended interviews conducted by psychiatrists, they concluded that 85 percent of those interviewed had diagnosable mental illnesses and that over half had schizophrenia or a major affective disorder. Basuk, Rubin, and Lauriat interviewed homeless residents of a shelter in Boston and found that 91 percent had a diagnosable mental illness.[28] Baxter and Hopper presented preliminary screening data from one shelter in New York City that indicated that as many as 84 percent of the men interviewed were mentally ill, although their figures included drug and alcohol problems.[29] Lipton, Sabatini, and Katz reviewed the records of 90 consecutive patients at New York's Bellevue Emergency Room who were registered as homeless.[30] Of these patients, 97 percent showed a history of previous psychiatric hospitalization; 72 percent of the patients had a history of schizophrenia.

A more general survey of characteristics and health problems of the homeless was conducted in Hennepin County, Minnesota, which includes the city of Minneapolis.[31] All eight shelters in the county were visited by teams of interviewers on the same night. The guests were interviewed randomly by choosing every third name on a daily census sheet; 69 guests were interviewed, 60 males and 8 females. Forty-nine percent were under age 31, 22 percent were between 32 and 40, and 29 percent were between 41 and 68. Fifty-eight percent of the sample had never married, 38 percent were divorced, and 4 percent were currently married.

When asked about their use of other emergency services, 93 percent reported that they used hot meal programs, 63 percent used clothing banks, 53 percent used drop-in centers, 34 percent used hospital emergency rooms, and 25 percent used food banks.

Thirty-eight percent of the interviewees re-ported that they had chronic health problems. Respiratory complaints were the single most frequently reported health problem. Only 23 percent of those reporting health problems reported that they were receiving medical care; 63 percent reported that they were in need of dental treatment.

Chemical dependency was high: 44 percent considered themselves alcoholics, 46 percent reported at least one admission to a detoxification center, 46 percent reported admission to a residential chemical dependency program, and 13 percent had received outpatient treatment for chemical dependency. Only 2 percent reported a chemical dependency other than alcohol.

Previous or current contact with the mental health system was reported by 41 percent; 18 percent of the sample reported previous psychiatric hospitalization.

Although there were obviously limitations to this study as the authors point out (no attempt at inter-rater reliability, no attempt to verify the information given by the guests), it is valuable information for planners in the city surveyed and allows the rest of us a glimpse at a life-style we would otherwise know little about.

Intervention

The generally recognized causes of homelessness are unemployment, cuts in public assistance programs, decline in the low-income housing supply, drug and alcohol abuse, deinstitutionalization, and serious personal crisis.[32] The construction of permanent low-cost housing would go a long way toward alleviating the problem of homelessness but this action would take massive federal intervention which seems unlikely in the short term. Instead, the public response has been the construction or use of short term emergency accommodations. This approach has been found to be costly and ineffective largely because it is aimed toward the short-term assistance of those who suffer solely from temporary economic misfortune which research has shown to be a small percentage of the homeless. Since emergency shelters will remain the most common housing for the homeless in the foreseeable future some mental health professionals who are attempting to make them a more therapeutic environment. Lauriat suggest that shelter staff conduct a thorough intake evaluation of each client and use this data to develop a service plan.[33] A worker familiar with the social service system should then coordinate the planning and delivery of services to the client. Modeled on the case manager approach, the shelter worker would work with the client to connect with the services needed. Although this approach will not substitute for more long term policy solutions to the problems of the homeless, it would be an improvement over the services now provided by most shelters.

Summary

The chronic mentally ill, those who suffer from severe and persistent mental disorders, are not a homogeneous group of patients. At least three different groups with different needs have been identified. Those who have spent much of their lives in institutions need interventions which focus on learning or relearning social and vocational skills. The young adult chronic mentally ill are quite a different population with different treatment needs. Since they have spent little time in institutions, they tend to deny their mental illness and therefore complicate the task of providing service to them. Currently, case management seems to be the best solution available for connecting them with needed services. Deinstitutionalization has contributed to the growth of a group of chronic mentally ill homeless patients who have a still different set of needs. Since most of these patients have contact with shelters for the homeless, making the shelters a more therapeutic environment may be the best short-term solution to the problems of the homeless mentally ill. Better and more long-term solutions await changes in social and fiscal policies.

Questions

1. What is meant by deinstitutionalization?
2. How does long-term institutionalization exacerbate symptoms of mental illness?
3. What are some of the general characteristics of the young chronic mentally ill?
4. What are some of the causes of homelessness?

REFERENCES AND SUGGESTED READINGS

1. Becker, A., & Schulberg, H. Phasing out state mental hospitals: A psychiatric dilemma. *New England Journal of Medicine*, 1976, *294*, 255.
2. Greenblatt, M., & Glazier, E. The phasing out of mental hospitals in the United States. *American Journal of Psychiatry*, 1975, *132*, 1135.
3. Kraus, J., & Slavinsky, A. *The Chronically Ill Psychiatric Patients in the Community.* Boston, Mass.: Blackwell Scientific, 1982.
4. Goffman, E. *Asylums.* Garden City, N.Y.: Anchor Books, 1961.
5. Presley, A., Grubb, A., & Semple, D. Predictors of successful rehabilitation in long-stay patients. *Acta Psychiatrica Scandanavica*, 1982, *66*, 83–88.
6. Goldstein, A., Sprafkin, R., & Gershaw, N. *Skill Training for Community Living.* New York: Pergamon Press, 1976.
7. Sylph, J., Ross, H., & Kedward, H. Social disability in chronic psychiatric patients. *American Journal of Psychiatry*, 1978, *134*, 1391–1394.
8. Ibid.
9. Liberman, R., Massel, H., Mosk, M., & Wong, S. Social skills training for chronic mental patients. *Hospital and Community Psychiatry*, 1985, *36*, 396–403.
10. Ibid.
11. Stroul, B. *Models of Community Support Services.* Boston: Center for Psychiatric Rehabilitation, 1986.
12. Ibid.
13. Anthony, W., & Jansen, M. Predicting the vocational capacity of the chronically mentally ill:

Research and implications. *American Psychologist*, 1984, *39*, 537–544.

14. Stroul, B., op. cit.

15. Anthony, W., Cohen, M., & Cohen, B. The philosophy, treatment process and principles of the psychiatric rehabilitation approach. In L. Bachrach (Ed.) *New Directions for Mental Health Services: Deinstitutionalization*, No. 17. San Francisco: Jossey-Bass, March 1983.

16. Lamb, R. *Treating the Long-term Mentally Ill*. San Francisco: Jossey-Bass, 1982.

17. Bachrach, L. Continuity of care for chronic mental patients: A conceptual analysis. *American Journal of Psychiatry*, 1981, *138*, 1449–1456.

18. Pepper, B., & Ryglewicz, H. Treating the Young Adult Chronic Patient: An Update. In B. Pepper & H. Ryglewicz (Eds.), *New Directions for Mental Health Services: Advances in Treating the Young Adult Chronic Patient*, No. 21. San Francisco: Jossey-Bass, 1984.

19. Intaglia, J. Improving the quality of care for the chronically mentally disabled: The role of case management. *Schizophrenia Bulletin*, 1982, *8*, 655–674.

20. Levine & Fleming, op. cit.

21. Kanter, J. Case management of the young adult chronic patient. In J. S. Kanter (Ed.), *New Directions for Mental Health Services: Clinical Issues in Treating the Chronic Mentally Ill*, No. 27. San Francisco: Jossey-Bass, 1985.

22. Friday, J. *Case Managers for the Chronically Mentally Ill: Assessing and Improving their Performance*. Atlanta: Southern Regional Education Board, 1986.

23. Lamb, op. cit.

24. Kanter, op. cit.

25. Intaglia, op. cit.

26. Levine & Fleming, op. cit.

27. Arce, Tadlock, & Vergare, M. A psychiatric profile of street people admitted to an emergency shelter. *Hospital and Community Psychiatry*, 1983, *34*, 812–817.

28. Bassuk, E., Rubin, L., & Lauriat, A. Is homelessness a mental health problem? *American Journal of Psychiatry*, 1984, *141*, 1546–1550.

29. Baxter, E., & Hopper, K. The new medicancy: Homeless in New York City. *American Journal of Orthopsychiatry*, 1982, *52*, 393–408.

30. Lipton, F., Sabatini, A., & Katz, S. Down and out in the city: The homeless mentally ill. *Hospital and Community Psychiatry*, 1983, *34*, 817–821.

31. Kroll, J., Carey, K., Hagedorn, D., Fire Dog, P., & Benavides, M. A survey of homeless adults in urban emergency shelters. *Hospital and Community Psychiatry*, 1986, *37*, 283–286.

32. Hartman, C. The house part of the homelessness problem. In E. Bassuk (Ed.) *New Directions for Mental Health Services: The Mental Health Needs of the Homeless Persons*, No. 30. San Francisco: Jossey-Bass, June 1986.

33. Lauriat, A. Sheltering homeless families: Beyond an emergency response. In E. Bassuk (Ed.) *New Directions for Mental Health Services: The Mental Health Needs of Homeless Persons*, No. 30. San Francisco: Jossey-Bass, June 1986.

Chapter 53

Aging and Mental Health

Marcia A. Ullman

Chapter Objectives

The students successfully attaining the goals of this chapter will be able to:

- Identify stressors affecting older people.
- Recognize age-specific psychiatric symptoms.
- Understand the use of psychiatric and nursing diagnoses with the elderly.
- Plan care for the aging person who has a psychiatric diagnosis.
- Identify the reasons why the older adult population is underserved by the mental health system.

Americans are living longer. In 1985, one of every eight Americans (12 percent of the population) was 65 years or older. By 2030 the number of older adults will increase to 65 million (two and one half times their number in 1980) for a total of 21.2 percent of the population.[1] Although aging is a normal developmental process, adults experience a variety of stressors. Older adults have the potential either to adapt to this life process or to fail to meet the demands of this last stage of life. To provide quality mental health care to this population, nurses need accurate information about older people, the aging process, and the effects of aging on mental health.

The content in this chapter is organized ac-cording to the nursing process model and uses a stress/adaptation model throughout.

ASSESSMENT

Stressors Affecting Older Adults

There are a variety of stressors that complicate the older adult's life and challenge his adaptability. Some of these stressors are similar to those experienced by younger adults; others are age-specific and usually take the form of losses. Losses accumulate in later life, necessitating that the older person "... expend enormous amounts of physical and emotional energy in grieving and resolving grief, adapting to changes that result from loss, and recovering from the stresses inherent in these processes."[2] Losses, according to Butler and Lewis, can be either extrinsic (coming from outside the individual) or intrinsic (coming from within). Examples of extrinsic losses are:

- Death of marital partner.
- Death of significant others.
- Status losses as a result of cultural devaluation.
- Decrease in income.
- Forced retirement.
- Forced isolation.
- Marital problems.
- Relocation.

Examples of intrinsic losses are:

- Disease of any organ system.
- Sensory loss.
- Sexual losses leading to sexual problems.
- Decreased flexibility.
- Changes in physical appearance.
- Change in body size and shape.
- Decrease in response time.
- Decrease in mental acuity.
- The knowledge that death is inevitable.

Intrinsic losses are often the result of disease and are not the inevitable outcome of aging. The physiological factors such as exercise tolerance, maximal breathing rate, cardiac reserve, reaction time, physical strength, short-term memory, intelligence as measured by intelligence tests, ambulatory abilities, and social abilities, according to Fries and Crapo, can be maintained and even improved with advancing age.[3]

Before the nurse can make a nursing diagnosis or provide data for a psychiatric diagnosis of mental illness she needs to assess the emotional reactions and defense mechanisms commonly seen in older adults.

Emotional Reactions

Although most older adults are able to experience a full range of human feelings, the characters of such feelings are filtered according to the person's life events.[4]

Grief

Grief and mourning accompany the many losses experienced by older adults and should be considered a normal adaptive process unless prolonged for an inordinate amount of time or expressed in an aberrant way. Bereavement as a loss is hypothesized by Butler and Lewis to be a key factor in predicting a breakdown in either physical or emotional functioning.[5]

Guilt

Guilt may surface as older adults reflect on their past lives and recall past decisions and behaviors. Some older adults feel guilty about no longer working, whereas others feel guilty about outliving their contemporaries.

Loneliness

A variety of circumstances can cause older adults to be lonely, such as: (1) death of significant others; (2) death of a beloved pet; (3) language barriers (foreign language, aphasia, etc.) that prevent the older adult from participating actively in relationships; (4) pain; and (5) relocation to unfamiliar surroundings.[6]

Anxiety

Free-floating anxiety intensifies as individuals age, partly as a result of the increased adaptation demands but also as a result of the realization of one's vulnerability. Anxiety, however, may be difficult to identify in older adults, especially if it is expressed indirectly.[7]

Burnside identifies several behavioral cues to recognizing anxiety in both ambulatory and bedridden elderly clients.[8] Elderly people who are ambulatory show behaviors of pacing, wandering, excessive smoking, somatic complaints, insomnia, general complaining, fatigue, hostile remarks, excessive requests, fantasizing, and isolating themselves.

Those elderly who are bedridden may show the following behaviors: turning head away, closing eyes, looking out the window, or watching television—all in an attempt to avoid eye contact; fidgeting with bedclothes, fingers, hands, and jewelry; acting confused; or talking incessantly.

Anger

There are numerous causes of anger in older adulthood. Some older adults feel anger at growing older and at having to face death. Others get angry in response to forced retirement or decreased income.

According to Butler and Lewis many older adults manifest rage ". . . at the seemingly uncontrollable forces that confront them as well as the indignities and neglect of the society that once valued their productive capacities."[9]

Use of Defense Mechanisms

Defense mechanisms are attempts to deal with the anxiety caused by the stressors. When an individual's familiar coping mechanisms fail and he is unable to employ effective new ones, stress increases and mental illness may ensue.

The defense mechanisms of denial, projection, fixation, and displacement and selective memory are used in varying degrees by older adults, as summarized below by Butler and Lewis.[10]

Denial
The older adult may pretend to be young and refuse to deal with the aging process and its effects. He may ignore limitations such as a decrease in strength or hearing. Nurses are familiar with the patient who denies having a hearing problem in the face of overwhelming contravening evidence. Denial can help an individual to deal with anxiety. However, when the denial prevents a person from getting the help he needs (as in denying a hearing loss), the defense mechanism no longer accomplishes a protecting purpose but instead becomes maladaptive.

Projection
The older person, in an attempt to cope with the anxiety that accompanies certain negative feelings, may attribute these feelings to someone or something else. He may become suspicious and fearful (e.g., "They are doing that to me").

Fixation
The older person may reach a certain level of adaptation and then be unable to go further. For example, one older woman adjusted well to the death of her husband but was unable to accept help from anyone when her physical strength declined.

Regression
The term regression is often used to explain an older person's behavior. Much of the stress seen in older adults is believed to be caused by external forces rather than by internal psychological factors. The regressive behavior seen in older adults may need to be viewed as adaptive rather than pathological.

Displacement
The mechanism of displacement is used by individuals to reassure themselves that they are okay and may be used by older adults who are undergoing considerable change. The problems are seen to be outside themselves: "The world is going to pot." "What's wrong with the youth of today?" "These nurses don't know what they're doing!"

Selective Memory
Butler and Lewis suggest that the propensity of the older adult to remember distant past events with greater clarity than recent events (a condition usually thought to be caused by an organic disorder) may, at times, be a psychological attempt to turn away from the painfulness of the present.

PSYCHIATRIC AND NURSING DIAGNOSIS IN THE ELDERLY

According to the Federal Council on the Aging, 15 to 25 percent of the elderly who live in the community experience significant symptoms of mental illness.[11] Another 5 to 6 percent have senile dementia, and 10 percent have a clinically diagnosed depression. In nursing homes, 16 percent of the elderly residents have a primary diagnosis of mental disorder or "senility." Although the elderly constitute only 11 percent of the population, they account for 15 percent of known suicides.

As nurses, we work in a variety of settings (both medical and psychiatric) where we encounter the elderly. We are, therefore, in an excellent position to identify troubled older adults and to intervene on their behalf. In order to do this effectively we must be cognizant of certain age-specific variations in the causes, symptoms, and treatment of the organic and functional illnesses most common in older adults. This section outlines both psychiatric and nursing diagnosis of conditions specific to the elderly population.

Alterations in Cognitions

There is considerable disagreement in the literature as to the terminology used to describe alterations in thinking and perception and the symptoms of paranoia, delusions, and hallucinatory states in the elderly. Some case examples of typical symptoms are given below.

The Suspicious Elderly

Older adults do not suddenly develop delusional beliefs; rather there is a gradual preoccupation with auditory sounds or with imagined changes in their domestic arrangements. Certain persons in their environment (such as neighbors) are suspected of being their persecutors. Individuals with simple paranoid illnesses frequently go undetected. It is only when their delusional beliefs begin to interfere with their functioning or with the lives of others that they come to the attention of law enforcement officers or health professionals. A change in environment will frequently alter or stop the delusional content.[12]

CASE EXAMPLE

Mrs. Jeffrey, a 76-year-old, hearing-impaired widow, was admitted to the psychiatric inpatient unit from the emergency room. She had been brought there by the police who had been summoned to Mrs. Jeffrey's apartment by concerned neighbors. Mrs. Jeffrey had been banging on the adjoining wall between these apartments, yelling at them to "leave her alone" and to stop "tormenting her." During the admission interview, Mrs. Jeffrey stated that she was fed up with her neighbors bothering her. She said that she could hear their voices ridiculing her, threatening her, and shouting obscenities at her through the radiators and walls of her apartment. Aside from her paranoid behavior, Mrs. Jeffrey seemed to be quite well-adjusted.

The primary nurse and a psychiatric aide visited Mrs. Jeffrey's apartment, which was located in an old building. They discovered that a variety of sounds (knocking, hissing, running of water) emanated from the radiators in her room. In addition muffled voices and sounds could be heard through the walls from the apartments on both sides and above and below. The nursing diagnosis of increased suspiciousness was based on the hypothesis that Mrs. Jeffrey's hearing loss, combined with the isolation and loneliness

she experienced, had caused her to misinterpret these sounds. The plan was to have her hearing checked and to have her fitted with a new hearing aid. Mrs. Jeffrey and her family agreed that she would live with her daughter and her family. Periodically over the next two years, Mrs. Jeffrey was seen for follow-up visits. Although no new paranoid or delusional content was observed, Mrs. Jeffrey insisted that the experiences she had related about her old apartment actually occurred. She would not accept the idea that she might have misinterpreted the sounds.

The Lonely Elderly

Loneliness may make a person prone to altered mental states. The following case illustrates a delusion.

CASE EXAMPLE

Mr. Aldo, a 67-year-old, single retiree, came to the Mental Health Center because he believed that the people who were trying to "drive him crazy" would ease up if "they" believed "they" had been successful and he was in therapy. During the course of the evaluation, he told the interviewer that "they" had been after him most of his adult life, but that lately "they" had been "hitting below the belt." He stated that over the years "they" had poisoned his food and water, tapped his telephone, photographed him with his female friends, and generally had been a nuisance. The last straw occurred during a routine eye exam. He was convinced that the doctor was "one of them" and had shot a laser beam into his eye, causing him to see a perpetual spot before his eye. "Now, that's playing dirty!" The staff spoke with the physician and ascertained that it had been a routine exam and no laser had been used.

As therapy progressed, it became apparent that Mr. Aldo was a lonely individual whose self-esteem was low. One day he said, "I don't know who 'they' are, but I must be pretty important the way 'they' keep pestering me." By believing that "they" would stop bothering him, or at least ease up, if he sought help, Mr. Aldo made it possible for himself to seek the human contact he so badly needed. Despite the delusional system, or perhaps because of it, Mr. Aldo was able to function independently. When his coping mechanisms began to cause more anxiety than they relieved, he sought help.

Mood Disorders

Mood disorders are a serious mental health problem for persons 65 years of age and older. The incidence of depression, especially in older persons, has been reported to be in the range of 10 to 65 percent in many communities and hospitals.[13]

Why do some scholars estimate that only one tenth of older Americans suffer from affective disorders, while others estimate two thirds? According to Raskin, (1) the rates drop if you use a psychiatric diagnosis instead of a symptom pattern; (2) psychiatrists and other mental health professionals often differ on whether to label depressive episodes that last a few hours to a few days and are precipitated by external events as transient depressive attacks or as true depressive episodes; (3) psychiatrists, in at least one study, had an apparent bias toward diagnosing older adults as suffering from chronic organic brain syndrome, while overassigning the diagnosis of depression to clients 35 to 39 years of age.[14]

Waxman sheds additional light on this phenomenon.[15] He cites a National Institute of Mental Health study that reports a low prevalence rate of all types of mental disorders for the over-65 group. He raises the question of whether or not the unique nature and presentation of geriatric mental disorders (especially depression) was adequately addressed in the design and interpretation of this study. Waxman's own research indicates that depression is often difficult to diagnose in older adults because their clinical profile is different from the one we frequently see in younger adults. He concludes that depressed older adults, i.e. those scoring highest on the Geriatric Depression Scale, report four times the number of somatic complaints as those older adults scoring lowest on the scale. Older adults will frequently see general practice physicians for relief of these somatic complaints. However, these general practice physicians frequently do not recognize, diagnose, or treat depression in the elderly, nor do they refer the depressed elderly for mental health treatment. This finding certainly helps to explain the reported lower incidence of depression in older adults.

Late-Life Depression

According to Meyers and Mei-Tal, depression is the most frequent, nonorganic cause for admission of the elderly to psychiatric hospitals.[16] Salzman and Shader describe the circumstances under which late-life depression occurs.[17] Based on Erikson's work they suggest that the older adult needs to accept his life and to claim responsibility for his own actions. The adult's task is to try to integrate this final stage of life in the context of declining function, limited coping defenses, loss of social support relationships, and stress, such as disease, over which he has little control. It is within this complex relationship of acceptance of a past life with the acknowledgment of decline and an inability to correct past errors, note Salzman and Shader, that late-life depression most commonly evolves.

What factors can precipitate depression in older adults? Phifer and Murrell's investigation found that the two strongest predictors of depression in older adults are weak social support and poor physical health.[18] Social support has both a stress-buffering effect and a direct ameliorative effect on depressive symptoms. Poor physical health strongly influences the development of depression. A combination of poor physical health and a weak social support system places the older adult at great risk for developing depressive symptoms.

While older adults may become depressed in response to poor physical health, certain illnesses have depression as part of the clinical picture. These include: neurological conditions (e.g., Parkinson's disease, amyotrophic lateral sclerosis, brain tumors, multiple sclerosis, meningitis, and strokes); endocrine conditions (e.g., hypothyroidism, hyperthyroidism, hypoparathyroidism, hyperparathyroidism, Addison's disease, and Cushing's disease); pernicious anemia, diseases of the pancreas, urinary tract disease, chronic lymphoid leukemia, systemic lupus erythematosis, and early congestive heart failure.[19] Certain drugs may cause depression: digitalis, antihypertensives, antiparkinsonian drugs, female hormones, corticosteroids, antituberculosis agents, anticancer drugs, psychotropic drugs, neuroleptics, antidepressants, antianxiety agents, and hypnotics and sedatives.[20]

Clinical Picture of Depression in Older Adults.

Although older adults can experience all the signs and symptoms of depression listed in *DSM-III-R* there seem to be certain age-specific manifestations as well.[21] While there is little research that describes these differences, several authors have identified age-specific symptoms. Gerner's research review finds that depressed older adults seem to[22]:

1. Exhibit more physical symptoms and complaints than younger depressed people. (This finding is supported by Waxman's study.[23])

2. Express less guilt.
3. Report feeling depressed to a lesser extent than younger people.
4. Display more apathy than younger people.
5. Express more paranoid symptoms such as suspiciousness, irritability, and delusions.

Addington and Fry review their findings and designate the following as symptoms of depression in older adults: agitation, listlessness, self-depreciation, volitional difficulties, and somatic complaints.[24] Table 53-1 by Salzman and Shader is included to help the nurse to assess the older adult who presents with depressive symptoms and to make a differential diagnosis.

Suicide. According to Osgood:

Available statistics clearly demonstrate that the elderly are more prone to commit suicide than other age groups in the United States. . . . Males, the unmarried, whites, those in lower socioeconomic classes and low-status occupations or who have experienced "occupational skidding" and the lonely and isolated in urban areas are the most susceptible to suicide.[25]

Stenback has identified five main factors that contribute to suicidal behavior in older adults.[26]

1. General and age-specific losses and failures, which trigger depression with hopelessness and despair.
2. Self-centered or excessively individualistic personality.
3. Lack of family bonds, community interest groups, or supporting social services for an individual.
4. Pattern of resolving problems by impulsive action.

TABLE 53-1. CLINICAL EVALUATION OF DEPRESSION

Common Signs or Symptoms of Depression	Differential Diagnosis
Insomnia (early morning awakening)	Normal in the elderly, particularly if daytime napping; dyspnea secondary to congestive heart failure; pain; many medical illnesses.
Constipation	Normal in elderly; secondary to decreased autonomic innervation of gastrointestinal tract; dehydration; secondary to anticholinergic effects of drugs.
Anorexia	Many medical diseases such as failure to thrive, chronic infection, malignancy, diabetes.
Hopelessness, despair, gloom, sadness, apathy, withdrawal of interest	Many physical diseases such as cancer of pancreas, pernicious anemia, hypo- and hyperendocrine function; reaction to severe or chronic physical disease; secondary to sedating drugs; secondary to antihypertensive drugs such as L-dopa.
Memory loss	Mild forgetfulness is normal; pseudodementia; true early dementia; secondary to medical drugs, e.g., cardiac glycosides.
Multiple somatic complaints and pains	Many medical diseases such as hyperparathyroidism, Addison's disease, rheumatoid arthritis.
Withdrawal, mutism, retardation of affect and movement	Idiopathic parkinsonism; drugs, e.g., akinetic mutism secondary to phenothiazines; apathetic thyrotoxicosis; antihypertensives; early congestive heart failure.
Irritability	Secondary to benzodiazepine drugs, alcohol, and other disinhibitors; secondary to amphetamines; hyperadrenal function or cortisol drugs; drug withdrawal states (barbiturates, benzodiazepines, antipsychotics, antidepressants); many medical diseases; reaction to chronic illness.
Decreased libido	Some decrease is normal; secondary to physical illness; secondary to drugs, e.g., phenothiazines, antihypertensives.
Weight loss, pallor, increasing frailty	Failure to thrive; chronic infection; diabetes; advanced metastic cancer.

From: Salzman, C., 1979, p. 44, with permission.[17]

5. A suicide-promoting environment, either personal (e.g., suicides in the family) or cultural (e.g., acceptance or idealization of suicide).

Assessment is of paramount importance in preventing suicide. Three fourths of the elderly white men who commit suicide see a physician within 1 month before death.[27]

Waxman's finding, reported earlier in this chapter, that general practice physicians are not skilled in recognizing, diagnosing, or treating depression, sheds light on this pattern of suicidal behavior.[28] Nurses and physicians alert to the signs and symptoms of depression in the elderly and skilled in conducting a suicide assessment can be instrumental in preventing suicides and in helping the individual to get the help he needs.

—— CASE EXAMPLE ——

Mr. Randall, a 76-year-old widower, had been admitted to a nursing home after fracturing his hip. The staff described him as cantankerous and extremely difficult to get along with. He was rude to the nurses whenever they tried to help him get up in his wheelchair or tried to help him perform his daily activities. He refused to eat. He also refused to take the digoxin that had been prescribed for his cardiac condition. Many of the staff, in return, became very angry with him. Suspecting that Mr. Randall was depressed, the nurse decided to spend time with Mr. Randall. She accepted his anger. She reflected that he seemed to have given up on life. He started to cry and, in a very emotional diatribe, blurted out all his pent-up anger, frustration, and hopelessness. "If I had a gun, I'd end it all right now." A liaison psychiatric nurse specialist was consulted, and Mr. Randall agreed to therapy with her. Before his hospitalization Mr. Randall had been a very independent man. He managed his own apartment. He felt helpless and out of control in the nursing home. The only way he could obtain any sense of control was to refuse to eat and to refuse to take his pills.

The care plan offered is an initial one. Once Mr. Randall's suicidal risk and his depression were assessed and treatment was initiated, the nurse would revise the care plan to include the following nursing diagnoses:

1. Ineffective family coping: disabling.
2. Ineffective coping (individual).
3. Diversional activity deficit.
4. Grieving, dysfunctional.
5. Impaired physical mobility.
6. Alteration in nutrition (inadequate food intake).

The student is referred to Schultz and Dark's, *Manual of Psychiatric Nursing Care Plans.* It includes a comprehensive care plan for nursing the depressed client.[29]

NURSING CARE PLAN
Potential For Violence (Suicidal Ideation) Related to Depression

GOALS

Long-Term
Patient will achieve and maintain his optimal level of functioning.

Short-Term
1. Patient will not injure himself:
   a. Patient will take the digoxin.

  b. Patient will gradually increase his food intake.
  c. Patient will not make any other suicidal gesture.
2. Patient will verbalize his feelings.
3. Patient will agree to participate in therapy with a psychiatric liaison nurse.

INTERVENTIONS

1. Assess potential for suicide by means of the following questions:
   a. Has patient attempted suicide in the past?
   b. Has patient experienced recent losses?
   c. Does patient have support systems (family, community ties, friends)?
   d. Has patient resolved past problems by impulsive action?
   e. Is there a suicide-promoting environment?
   f. Does patient have a plan?
   g. Is patient able to carry out this plan?
   h. Does patient have the energy to carry out plan?
   i. How old is the patient?
2. Provide for patient's safety based on the nursing assessment of the suicidal risk:
   a. Remove sharp objects from room (e.g., razor blades).
   b. Be with the patient during meals.
   c. Establish a schedule for checking on patient. (The frequency depends on the degree of suicidal intent.)
   d. If suicidal risk is low, concentrate your efforts on helping the patient to decrease his depression.
3. Establish a therapeutic relationship with the patient:
   a. Use therapeutic communication techniques.
   b. Spend time with patient.
   c. Be an "active listener."
   d. Use silence appropriately.
   e. Use touch.
   f. Express empathy.
   g. Encourage ventilation of feelings.
   h. Provide for the physical needs of the patient. This conveys several important messages to the patient:
      i. "You are a person who is worthy of my time and efforts."
      ii. "Your well-being is important to me."
      iii. "I care about you."

SUMMARY OF SUICIDAL ASSESSMENT

Patient is suicidal. He is not able to carry out his plan to use a gun but is able to endanger his life by refusing the digoxin and by reducing his food intake. Patient believes suicide is a "sin" and became very angry when the nurse suggested that his refusal to take the digoxin and to eat were indeed suicidal gestures. His religious beliefs may act as a deterrent to his using other means to hurt himself (such as cutting his wrists).

Patient was not in imminent danger of hurting himself by means other than the refusal to take the digoxin and the decrease in the quantity of food he consumed.

The nurse Ms. Stein met with Mr. Randall when she helped another nurse turn Mr. Randall onto his side. During this procedure, Mr. Randall experienced a considerable amount of pain and verbally attacked Ms. Stein. Recognizing that Mr. Randell's anger was not a personal attack, Ms. Stein expressed her sorrow that the turning hurt him and offered to give Mr. Randall a back rub. He accepted but continued to berate her throughout the procedure. Ms. Stein determined that Mr. Randall was severely depressed and decided to spend time with him at intervals throughout the day. Each time she saw Mr. Randall she did something for him (e.g., offering him a drink of juice). Mr. Randall began to express feelings other than anger. He stated how lonely he was, how he had messed up his life, and how he just wanted to die. He frequently cried. The nurse listened in silence as he related many unhappy events from his past. She frequently held Mr. Randall's hand during these conversations. Ms. Stein told Mr. Randall that she could see how unhappy and desperate he was and suggested that he might benefit from talking to a psychiatric liaison nurse. Mr. Randall agreed and after the first visit, he resumed taking the digoxin and began to eat.

Organic Mental Disorders

Although this topic is discussed at length in Chapter 36, one point about organic mental disorders deserves further emphasis here. Depression in older adults is often accompanied by a mild to severe reversible dementia that can be extremely difficult to distinguish from Alzheimer's disease.[30] Furthermore, depression frequently accompanies progressive dementia. The individual becomes depressed when he realizes that his mental capacities are diminishing. If these conditions are considered irreversible or untreatable by health professionals, the prognosis for the older adult is poor. He may accept the "hopeless" label and the behavior accompanying it. It is within the nurse's capabilities to try to motivate the older adult and to try to improve his health status to the optimal level of functioning. Lucas, Steele, and Bognanni's article, "Recognition of Psychiatric Symptoms in Dementia," discusses several psychiatric conditions that accompany dementia and summarizes the signs and symptoms of these syndromes.[31]

Alcohol Abuse in the Older Adult

It is estimated that 10 to 15 percent of the elderly in the United States (over 2 million people) suffer from alcoholism.[32] Although there are many theories that attempt to explain the etiology of alcoholism, the exact cause is still unknown. The role that age-related stressors (such as retirement, loss of spouse and friends, decreased income, ageism, etc.) play in the development of alcoholism in older adults needs to be investigated further.

Older adults can and do benefit from intervention. Price and Andrews cite several authors who support the view that older alcoholics respond more favorably to treatment than do younger alcoholics.[33] When elderly alcoholics, like other age groups, are dealt with, it is the alcoholism and not the suspected causes that should be treated first. That is, the individual must be encouraged not to drink. All too often health professionals inadvertently support the alcoholic's continued consumption of alcohol. The alcoholic is encouraged to "work on his problems," with the hope that once he has solved the problems, he will stop drinking. In the meantime, he continues to consume alcohol, using his problems as an excuse to continue drinking. Many of the problems thought to be the cause of excessive drinking are, in fact, the result of excessive drinking (or at least they are magnified as a result of drinking).

Informed nurses can: (1) help to educate the public about the signs and symptoms of alcoholism; (2) identify older adults with drinking problems; and (3) intervene with the elderly alcoholic and his family and help to support them as they attempt to deal with alcoholism. The reader should consult the article by Price and Andrews for a list of suggested methods the nurse can use to alleviate problems in elderly alcoholics.[34]

INTERVENTIONS

Disproportionate Use of Mental Health Services by the Elderly

A 1978 report by the National Institute of Mental Health (NIMH) states: "While emotional distress and mental illness are more prevalent among the elderly than in the general population, the elderly are served at less than one fourth the rate of the 25- to 44-year-old group."

The explanations offered in the literature to account for this disproportionate use of mental health services by the elderly include inadequate transportation, insufficient funding of programs specifically designed to meet the needs of the elderly, shortage of professionals educated to work with older adults, failure to coordinate the various services available for the elderly, and an overriding belief that mental health services are "wasted" on older adults. In addition to these sociocultural barriers, Hagebak and Hagebak identify psychological barriers in views held by therapists and by older adults themselves that prevent the distressed older adult from seeking and receiving the necessary help.[35] These "barrier" views, if held by nurses, may act as stalls in the communication process and may interfere with the development of a therapeutic relationship.

The barriers for the nurse therapist are identified as follows[36]:

1. The "can't teach an old dog" syndrome, in which the therapist holds the attitude that a lifetime of learning one set of behaviors can be overcome only with the greatest difficulty, even though those learned behav-

iors work to handicap the elderly patient in coping with the pressure of modern life.

2. The "my God, I'm mortal too" syndrome, in which the therapist, through work with the elderly, comes face to face with the unpleasant realities of his own mortality and the effects of the aging process in his own life, fearing or resenting this forced personal awareness.

3. The "why bother?" syndrome, in which the therapist sees little value in working with persons who have a relatively short life expectancy and may even see the elderly as having little potential to become productive members of society in the conventional sense.

4. The "I'm the child" syndrome, in which a role reversal occurs in therapy due to the differences in age between helper and "helpee." The therapist's response to the elderly patient is as though to a parent. It is difficult to help a parent in therapy, or to be a parent to your therapist.

5. The "patient is a child" syndrome, in which the therapist holds that older people are "just like children" and treats the elderly in that manner, failing to recognize that while dependency needs may be similar, the lifetime of experience and accumulated knowledge of the elderly patient make this a particularly erroneous analogy.

6. The "senility is natural" syndrome, in which the therapist believes that virtually all of us become senile as we grow older and that forgetfulness is a natural part of the aging process. As a result, many organic problems that might be successfully treated are not.

Hagebak and Hagebak identify psychological barriers for the elderly as follows[37]:

1. The "senility is natural" syndrome, in which the elderly person believes that virtually everyone becomes senile as he grows older, a common attitudinal barrier held by the therapist as well. In this case, however, it works to block the elderly person from seeking services that have an excellent prognosis for successful treatment.

2. The "who/why am I?" syndrome, in which the elderly person has lost most meaningful life roles: work roles, parenthood roles, marital roles. Without these roles to hang the self-concept on, with no role except

"me," the elderly person may experience such reduced feelings of self-worth that no effort is exerted to seek help. This is a corollary of the "why bother?" syndrome sometimes found among therapists.

3. The "do for yourself" syndrome, in which the elderly person adopts a fiercely independent stance, particularly with regard to the services provided by public agencies. Public service is, in this case, equated with "welfare" and is therefore rejected.

4. The "I'm distrustful and afraid" syndrome, in which the elderly client holds an image of mental health services accurate enough a generation ago but hardly in keeping with the active deinstitutionalization programs in vogue today.

5. The "doing what's expected" syndrome, in which some elderly clients may very well display behaviors in therapy that reinforce the role of child or parent played by the therapist, or support stereotypes held by the public. It's as if the client were saying, "I'm getting old, and old age is depressing; therefore I'm depressed," or "You want me to be this way; therefore I am this way."

Waxman's research also identified negative attitudes, both on the part of the care giver and the older adult, as an important deterrent to the older adult's use of mental health services.[38] In order to remedy this situation, he suggests that we launch an immediate educational and public relations initiative directed at general practice physicians, potential patients, and their families.

These "barriers" reflect the ageism that is prevalent in our society. Ageism is a term coined by Robert Butler to describe ". . . the prejudices and stereotypes that are applied to older people sheerly on the basis of age."[39]

General Treatment Principles for Health Professionals

Butler and Lewis offer several treatment principles that are applicable to all members of the health team[40]:

Principle 1
When in doubt, treat and see if improvement occurs. The cause of confusion in the elderly is often difficult to assess. Indeed, many times it

is assumed to be irreversible when in fact it is reversible. If there is any possibility that it is reversible, the individual should be treated. If the mental confusion clears up with the administration of an antidepressant, a diagnosis of depression, rather than one of an organic mental disorder, can be made. This principle has important implications for nursing care. It should never be assumed that a patient is at his highest level of functioning. Instead, nursing care should be aimed at helping each person to perform at his optimal level.

Principle 2
Treatment is a collaboration between the older person, his family, and the mental health personnel. Whenever possible, the older adult should be consulted. The best of treatment plans can fail if the older person involved is not in agreement with it. Families usually want and need to be included in planning and treatment. Families can be a great source of support to their older members. There are times when physical or mental incapacity may prevent the older person from being involved in planning, and in such cases, health personnel, together with family members, must make the decision.

Principle 3
Full attention must be paid to physical complaints. Because of the close relationship between psyche and soma, relief from physical discomfort will often bring relief from emotional discomfort as well. Many of the afflictions of older adulthood such as varicose veins, constipation, senile vaginitis, dry and itchy skin, cold extremities, and pain are treatable. Nursing measures to relieve pain and discomfort convey caring and concern to the older adult and help to establish and maintain the therapeutic relationship.

Phifer and Murrell's findings, presented earlier in this chapter, are significant for nurses who work in general hospitals as well as those who work in psychiatric settings.[41] Because physical problems tend to increase as a person ages and because, according to Phifer and Murrell, they increase the risk of depression, nurses need to be hypervigilant in identifying and meeting the physical needs of older adults to prevent depression. Furthermore, nurses need to assess for concomitant signs of depression in organic disorders and to initiate nursing measures to alleviate the depression should it exist.

Because a strong social support system helps to prevent depression and to alleviate depressive symptoms should they occur, nurses also need to identify, explore and strengthen the older adult's social support system.

Principle 4
What we call someone often defines how we will treat him, or, at least, how we view him. Older adults should be respectfully addressed as Mr., Mrs., Miss, or Ms. unless they specifically ask to be called by their first names. Terms such as *gramps*, *granny*, and *honey* are condescending and should not be used. Derogatory terms such as *old crock* and *old biddy* have no place in a therapeutic environment. The term *older person* is perhaps the simplest and most dignified one in terms of how to refer to people over age 65. For people in advanced old age the term *elderly* is acceptable. The student is referred to Emma Elliot's poignant account of her mother's battle with ageism in a large teaching hospital. It's entitled, "My Name is Mrs. Simon."[42]

Types of Treatment

Age alone does not determine the applicability or advisability of any specific treatment. Older adults can and do benefit from a variety of treatment modalities. The choice of therapy depends on the needs of the individual and the strength of his ego. Several forms of therapy, along with age-related considerations, are discussed here.

Psychotherapy
Individual and group, supportive, insight-oriented, and psychoanalytic therapy are all feasible. Because older adults suffer so many losses, the aim of therapy is frequently, but not always, to help the client to grieve.

Psychopharmacology
There is a general trend, as the human organism ages, for drugs to stay in the body longer, to have more prolonged biologic activity, and hence generally to have more powerful clinical and toxic effects on the organism. Therefore, starting and maintenance doses should generally be one third to one half those for younger adults, and increases should be made gradually. Salzman, van der Kolk, and Shader recommend that any older adult who is to receive psycho-

pharmacologic agents should have, in addition to a careful psychiatric evaluation, a complete physical, including blood pressure (supine and erect), complete blood count, total protein and albumin and globulin ratios, urinalysis, electrocardiogram, and a brief neurological exam. After a patient has been started on a neuroleptic or antidepressant medication, he should be followed carefully for 6 weeks. The follow-up should include biweekly checks of complete blood count and daily recordings of pulse and blood pressure. Long-term administration of these drugs necessitates making a brief neurological examination at regular intervals.[43]

Electroconvulsive Therapy (ECT)

Butler and Lewis suggest that, in the presence of serious suicidal risk, ECT should be administered initially instead of waiting out a drug trial.[44] A 1985 study by Meyers and Mei-Tal compared the efficacy of tricyclic antidepressants (TCAs) and ECT in the treatment of 70 depressed psychogeriatric patients.[45] They found that ECT proved to be a more effective treatment for depression than TCAs. Although the sample size is small, their findings add credence to Butler and Lewis assertions.

Psychodrama

This author once worked in a day-treatment program that included psychodrama in the treatment regimen. Each week a different patient would ask to be the "star" and would "act out" various emotional conflicts. Everyone was surpised when a depressed older man, Mr. Deming, asked to be the star. He had been attending the center for several weeks after a suicide attempt and had been exceptionally quiet in the groups. The staff questioned whether or not this was the best form of treatment for him. In the warm-up session before the actual psychodrama, he told this story:

He had grown up on a farm. His father had been an alcoholic who physically and mentally abused Mr. Deming, his mother, and his six brothers and sisters. One day when Mr. Deming was 15, his father, who had been drinking, got into a heated argument with him and they exchanged blows. Mr. Deming told his father that he hated him and that he was going away and never coming back. He left with only the clothes on his back and went to a friend's house, 2 miles away. The next day his younger brother found him and said that his father was missing and that his mother needed his help in finding him. Mr. Deming

acquiesced and returned home. After hours of searching he found his father hanging in an abandoned barn. Mr. Deming felt responsible for his father's death and bore that guilt for 50 years.

Until the psychodrama, Mr. Deming had not disclosed his "secret" to anyone. During the final scene of the drama he told his "father" (played by a staff member) how responsible he felt for his death and how angry and hurt he had been most of his life. His "father" accepted full blame for his actions and his suicide. He also told Mr. Deming that he loved him and that he wished he could have stopped drinking. After the psychodrama, other clients and staff crowded around Mr. Deming, hugging him and expressing their concern and caring. Mr. Deming became an active participant in the program and was discharged 2 months later, a much happier man. He began to do woodworking again and to visit friends.

The staff, as well as the younger clients, had not considered Mr. Deming a potential candidate for psychodrama, primarily because of his age. Mr. Deming reminds us that the potential for growth and healing is not limited to the young. Because of his therapy, Mr. Deming's older adulthood promised to be the first stage of his life in which he would be truly happy and guilt-free.

Activity and Recreation Therapy

Purposeful activities and recreation are beneficial to both the well and ill older adult because they help him to: (1) maintain present skills; (2) regain previous skills; (3) develop new skills; and (4) share expertise and experiences.

Therapeutic Dance and Movement. The use of dance movement therapy with older patients is advocated by Raymond Harris because it has the following benefits[46]:

1. The dance movements help to maintain and improve mobility, balance, coordination, rhythm, endurance, strength, and flexibility.
2. The music can calm, soothe, and stimulate feelings.
3. The group participation inherent in such activities helps to develop outlets for both positive and negative emotions. Meaningful relationships with others can be developed as well.

4. In addition, the creative activity helps to develop a greater sense of personal identity, wider resources, and an awareness of community relations.
5. The nonverbal aspects (touching, feeling, and moving) stimulate greater sensory awareness and help to establish new neural patterns.

In one television program a segment describing a wheelchair ballet was presented. It featured a dance therapist working with several wheelchair-bound older adults, all of whom reported feeling happier and "more alive" when they were dancing. This videotape is a testimony to the effectiveness of this form of therapy.

Poetry Writing. Koch relates his experiences teaching elderly nursing home residents to write poetry in *I Never Told Anybody*.[47] Once they overcame their initial reticence, the participants enjoyed writing and sharing their poems. The poetry writing sessions were designed so that success was ensured. As the participants' skill in writing poetry increased, so did their self-esteem. Many memories were evoked and shared, and a sense of camaraderie developed.

Nursing Intervention

Nurses spend a considerable amount of time with older adults in a variety of settings and are, therefore, able to have a positive influence on their lives. To do this, nurses need to be familiar with the various treatments and services available to older adults. In particular, nurses should be aware of nursing actions that will help the older adult to adjust to the many stressors inherent in the aging process.

Butler and Lewis suggest that health professionals, in their interventions with older adults, should seek to[48]:

1. Increase the individual's restitution capacity. That is, the ability to compensate for and recover from deeply felt losses.
2. Provide opportunities for growth and renewal, i.e., to help the patient to discover and use his innate potential.
3. Assist the older adult in gaining perspective by assisting him in life review, recalling past experiences including unresolved conflicts.

To meet these goals, the nurse has to establish a therapeutic relationship with the older adult and use effective communication skills. The ability to "actively listen" is one of the most important skills a nurse can possess. The nurse should also examine her attitudes to determine if any of them act as psychological barriers to care. As stated earlier, these barriers can act as stalls in the communication process and need to be addressed.

Nursing Actions to Promote Restitution

How can nurses help older adults to cope with losses? Initially the nurse needs to support the older person through the grieving process (see Chapter 39). Once this has been accomplished, there are numerous things that the nurse can do to help the older person compensate for losses. Here are some suggestions:

1. Decrease or Loss of Hearing
   a. Encourage patient to wear a hearing aid.
   b. Make sure the batteries are working.
   c. Always speak slowly and distinctly.
   d. Do not shout.
   e. Face the individual to whom you are speaking.
   f. Keep a pad of paper and a pencil near the person so that staff can write messages if necessary.
2. Decreased Ability to Read because of Loss of Vision
   a. Make sure patient's glasses are clean.
   b. Suggest magnifying lenses or sheets that fit over a page and magnify the print to improve reading.
   c. Obtain books with extra-large print.
   d. Obtain audio recordings of patient's favorite books.
   e. Encourage friends and relatives to read to client.
   f. Arrange lighting for maximum benefit.
3. Decreased Feelings of Usefulness
   a. For the client who enjoyed gardening but is no longer able to do it, suggest growing things on a smaller scale. A small vegetable garden, a window box, or houseplants can be acceptable substitutes for larger gardens.
4. Loss of Meaningful Relationships
   a. Provide opportunities for the older person to meet other people. Group activities such as poetry writing and dance and movement therapy can help in this endeavor.

b. Encourage the older person to "help others." Several years ago a picture appeared in the Brockport (N.Y.) *Post* that showed "foster grandparents" being greeted by their "foster grandchildren." The children, who were developmentally disabled, had been corresponding with their "foster grandparents" for some time and had invited them to come to school and enjoy a lunch that they had prepared. According to the *Post* story, both the children and the older adults benefited from this special relationship.

c. Encourage older adults to share their talents and skills with others.

CASE EXAMPLE

Mrs. Reyes, an elderly woman on a psychiatric unit, sat by herself every day. She stated that she was lonely and that there wasn't any purpose to her life anymore. During one conversation, Ms. Crawford, a student nurse, learned that Mrs. Reyes used to give sewing classes. Ms. Crawford brought in the materials necessary for doing embroidery and encouraged Mrs. Reyes to teach her the basic stitches. Several young patients on the unit subsequently became interested and became Mrs. Reyes' students. Both Mrs. Reyes and the young people enjoyed these "classes," which took on the flavor of a social hour.

Nursing Actions to Promote Growth and Renewal

Older adulthood can be an exciting and interesting time. Individuals may get to do things they have always wanted to do but just never got around to.

CASE EXAMPLE

Ms. Defev, a woman in her 70s, volunteered to participate in a panel discussion on aging. She explained that she might be a little late for this event because the wine-making class she was taking did not end until 10 minutes before the discussion was scheduled to begin. This same woman reported that the receptionist at the local exercise salon was shocked when she stated her age during the registration process. "She gave me a look that said, "What are you doing here?"

Many of the older adults that nurses work with are incapacitated because of physical or emotional illness. Nevertheless, there are many ways in which the nurse can facilitate growth and renewal.[49] Some examples are listed below:

1. Talking with patients to ascertain what activities they have always wanted to do.
2. Discussing which things are feasible and making plans to carry them out. The possibilities here are limitless—college courses; classes in such things as arts and crafts, music, poetry writing, cooking, and woodworking; trips; concerts, etc.
3. If frailties prevent clients from leaving the facility, classes and entertainment can be brought to them.

Nursing Activities to Promote Perspective

Perhaps the most effective means the older adult has in gaining perspective on his life is reminiscence. Ryden believes that time spent in reminiscing may be a behavioral indication that the older adult is coping with the tasks of Erik Erikson's eighth and final stage of development, Ego Integrity versus Despair, and that the individual may benefit greatly from nursing intervention in support of reminiscence. However, if the individual is in Erickson's extended stage of Generativity versus Stagnation, nursing actions suggested under restitution and growth and renewal would be more appropriate.[50]

To intervene effectively, nurses must have an understanding of the purpose of reminiscence and a high level of interpersonal skills as cited here by Ryden[51]:

The literature suggests that the purpose of reminiscence is to maintain self-esteem, to stimulate thinking, and to enhance and support the natural healing process of life review so that the client can find meaning, worth, and an acceptance of what life has been.

Ryden suggests various ways in which the nurse can increase the effectiveness of reminiscing behavior in older adults.[52] The nurse can:

1. Initiate reminiscing behavior.
2. Reinforce reminiscing behavior.
3. Help the individual to deal with the feelings associated with reminiscing.
4. Help family members to deal with reminiscing behavior.

The following activities can facilitate the reminiscing process:

1. Using open-ended questions to stimulate discussion of the past.
2. "Active listening."
3. Looking at old photographs together.
4. Helping the patient to put photographs or memorabilia in albums.
5. Encouraging the patient to record memories by either writing (prose or poetry) or taping them.
6. Using a "time line" to stimulate discussion. (A "time line" is a list of past events and the dates when they occurred.)
7. Accepting both the positive and negative feelings that are expressed during reminiscence.

Reminiscing has one more important function: Reactions to death are closely related to a resolution of life's experiences and problems as well as a sense of one's contributions to others. The process of working through one's feelings about death begins with a growing personal awareness of the eventual end of life and the implications of this for one's remaining time alive.[54]

It is hypothesized that older adult parents and their adult children undergo a termination process not unlike that experienced by therapist and client.[55] This is the final developmental task for the older adult and there are benefits for both the older adult and the adult child.

Termination gives parents an opportunity to:

1. Discuss their feelings and views about death, dying, and afterlife.
2. Express thoughts and feelings about the child and the child's accomplishments.
3. Work through any problems in the relationship and heal old wounds.
4. Reminisce with the child.
5. Pass along the family history.
6. Express their wishes about the distribution of their personal belongings.
7. Help the adult child to accept the inevitability of the parent's death.

8. Face and accept the reality of their own death.
9. Achieve what Erikson calls "a sense of integrity as far as the parent–child relationship is concerned."[56]

This process gives adult children an opportunity to:

1. Recognize, express, and resolve feelings about the parents with them.
2. Reminisce with parents and thereby acquire a sense of history and closure.
3. Plan for the eventual death of the parents.
4. Experience anticipatory grieving.[57]

By offering support, encouragement, and compassion to parents and children as they say good-bye to each other, nurses can function in a very important primary prevention role.

To be able to help an individual to find meaning to his life and ultimately to accept death can be one of the most challenging and rewarding nursing experiences. Nurses are in an excellent position to facilitate this adaptive process.

The profession has made great strides in overcoming ageism and in responding to the needs of older adults. However, much remains to be done. According to Burnside, the shortage of adequately prepared geropsychiatric nurses is severe.[58] She suggests that geropsychiatric content be included in all levels of nursing education.

Further research on graduate and student nurses' knowledge and attitudes about older adults is necessary. Additional methods of altering negative attitudes need to be devised and tested. In order to work effectively with older adults, nurses have to recognize and cope with their own fears about aging and dying.

We are all born, we flower, we fade, and we die and in the act of our dying we replenish the earth and a great created order continues. All creatures age.[59]

CASE STUDY*

Mrs. Rowley, a 73-year-old widowed mother of four came to the arthritis clinic because of exacerbation of her rheumatoid arthritis symptoms. The following history was obtained:

Age 1½   Mother ill. Raised by mother's closest friend.

---

* Sources: J. M. Schultz & S. L. Dark, pp. 97–100.[29]; M. C. Townsend, *Nursing Diagnoses in Psychiatric Nursing, A Pocket Guide For Care Plan Construction.* Philadelphia: Davis, 1988, pp. 205–207.

Age 7   Mother died. Patient returned home and took on major household responsibilities including helping to look after her three younger sisters, the youngest of whom was 1 year of age. Patient cried throughout the account of her mother's death and the subsequent years.

Age 17   Completed high school and entered nursing school.

Age 20   Married.

Age 23   Her husband deserted her when she was 3 months pregnant and their first child was slightly over 1 year of age.
Worked private duty to support family.

Age 26   Started her own nursing home. Reported that this was one of the happiest periods in her life.

Age 32   Remarried and had two more children.

Age 37   Sold business so that she could devote all her time and energy to her family. Mrs. Rowley reported becoming extremely depressed following the sale of the nursing home. Tearfully she stated, "I should never have given up the business."

Age 47   Two grandchildren died in a fire.

Age 54   Rheumatoid arthritis diagnosed.

Age 67   Husband of 35 years suffered a severe heart attack. Mrs. Rowley nursed him at home for 5 months until he died. Reports experiencing a severe depression after his death.

Age 68   Sold family home, to "get rid of the memories," but states she regrets having done so. Reports strained relationships with all her children. "I'm a failure as a mother."

Summary of losses suffered by patient:

- Separation from family
- Death of mother
- Loss of carefree childhood
- Desertion by first husband
- Loss of financial security
- Sale of nursing home
- Death of grandchildren
- Death of second husband
- Sale of family home
- Alteration in health status
- Loss of satisfying relationships with children

Because of the severity of her physical and psychological problems, Mrs. Rowley was admitted to the inpatient unit of the clinic. The clinic used a health team approach and addressed the psychological as well as the physical aspects of her illness.

The nursing staff identified the following diagnoses and listed them in order of priority.

1. Chronic pain and loss of mobility related to rheumatoid arthritis.
2. Dysfunctional grieving related to bereavement overload.
3. Impaired family relationships related to patient's unmet dependency needs.
4. Disturbance in self-concept (role performance) related to rheumatoid arthritis and aging.
5. Impaired social relationships related to limitations imposed by rheumatoid arthritis.

The following is an excerpt from the care plan.

DIAGNOSIS #2

Dysfunctional grieving related to bereavement overload (cumulative grief from multiple unresolved losses).

GOALS

Short-Term
The patient will

1. Recognize the losses she has suffered as losses to be grieved for.
2. Express feelings about the losses both verbally and nonverbally.

Long-Term
1. Grieve over each and every loss.
2. Verbalize acceptance of the losses.
3. Demonstrate initial integration of the losses into her life.
4. Demonstrate changes in life-style and coping mechanisms incorporating the fact of loss.
5. Verbalize realistic future plans integrating the losses.
6. Demonstrate physical recuperation from the stress of loss and grieving.

INTERVENTION WITH RATIONALE

1. Establish rapport with patient before bringing up losses. The nurse–client relationship is the vehicle by which the nurse and client can work together to achieve the goals they have identified.
2. Bring up the losses in a supportive manner. The nurse's emotional support will make it easier for Mrs. Rowley to face and express uncomfortable and painful feelings.
3. Point out to the patient that this is a nurturing time, a time for growth and learning from which to gather strength to go forward. Grieving allows the patient to adjust to the changes brought about by the losses and to move forward.
4. Talk with patient in realistic terms concerning each of her losses. Discuss concrete changes that have occurred in her life as a result of each of her losses. Discussing the loss on this level may help to make it more real for the patient and gives her the opportunity to recognize and express her feelings.
5. If patient appears frightened by the feelings, explain that although the feelings are uncomfortable, they are a necessary part of the grieving process and that she can withstand them. The patient may fear the intensity of her feelings and may need reassurance that she can withstand them.
6. Reassure patient that all feelings, both ''positive'' and ''negative'' are acceptable.
7. Offer patient a variety of ways to express her feelings (e.g., talking, writing, crying and drawing). Convey your acceptance of whatever feelings the patient expresses and of the way the patient chooses to express them. By expressing her feelings, Mrs. Rowley will identify them and will begin to accept them.
8. Use reminiscing techniques to help patient recall experiences and to talk about her relationships with the people she has lost (her mother, first husband, grandchildren and second husband) and the lost objects (her house, nursing home, health and youth). Discussing the lost person or object can aid the patient in identifying the loss and its significance in her life and the feelings she is experiencing as a result of the loss.
9. Encourage patient to make plans to deal with the effects of the losses on the various aspects of her life (financial, housing, social interactions, recreational, etc.). Engage other health team members to help in this process. Making future plans will help patient to integrate the losses into her life and to move on to the next phase of her life.
10. Encourage Mrs. Rowley to join a ''grief and grieving'' group. Sharing her feelings with others who are experiencing similar feelings will help Mrs. Rowley feel ''normal'' in grieving. Talking about her grief in social interactions may make Mrs. Rowley's friends feel uncomfortable. They may avoid her.
11. Inform patient that physical stress is an integral part of any loss. Encourage Mrs. Rowley to eat a balanced diet, to exercise as tolerated, and to get sufficient rest and sleep.

Summary

As the elderly population in American continues to increase, nurses will be called upon to provide health teaching, assessment, and diagnosis in mental health and mental illness conditions. This chapter conceptualizes the aging process, identifies stressors affecting older adults, and outlines the assessment process. The psychiatric and nursing diagnosis section includes alterations in cognitions, mood disorders, organic disorders, alcohol abuse, and suicidal behavior. General treatment principles for health professionals and types of treatment are included with case examples and a nursing care plan.

Questions

1. Give an example of an aging person for whom you have cared in a general hospital setting and who had a mental health problem.
2. How are the elderly treated in your community when there is a psychiatric diagnosis?
3. Devise a nursing care plan integrating psychiatric and nursing diagnoses for an elderly patient in your agency.

REFERENCES AND SUGGESTED READINGS

1. Fowles, D. G. American Association of Retired Persons (AARP) and the Administration on Aging (AOA), U.S. Department of Health and Human Services. *A Profile of Older Americans: 1986.*
2. Butler, R. N., & Lewis, M. I. *Aging and Mental Health.* St. Louis: Mosby, 1982, p. 43.
3. Fries, J. F., & Crapo, L. M. *Vitality and Aging.* San Francisco: Freeman, 1981, p. 110.
4. Butler & Lewis, op. cit., p. 50.
5. Ibid., p. 52.
6. Burnside, I. M. *Nursing and the Aged.* New York: McGraw-Hill, 1981, pp. 66–67.
7. Butler & Lewis, op. cit., p. 53.
8. Burnside, op. cit., pp. 63–64.
9. Butler & Lewis, op. cit., p. 54.
10. Ibid., pp. 54–58.
11. The Federal Council on the Aging. What is the mental health status of the elderly? In *The Need for Long Term Care* (DHHS Publication No. (OHDS) 81-20704). Washington, D.C.: U.S. Government Printing Office, 1981, p. 32.
12. Post, F. Paranoid schizophrenia-like and schizophrenic states in the aged. In J. E. Birrin & R. B. Sloane (Eds.), *Handbook of Mental Health and Aging.* Englewood Cliffs, N.J.: Prentice-Hall, 1980, pp. 596–597.
13. Raskin, A. Signs and symptoms of psychopathology in the elderly. In A. Raskin & L. F. Jarvik (Eds.), *Psychiatric Symptoms and Cognitive Loss in the Elderly.* New York: Wiley, 1979, p. 3.
14. Ibid., pp. 3–4.
15. Waxman, H. M. Community mental health care for the elderly—A look at the obstacles. *Public Health Reports*, 1986, *101*(3), 294–299.
16. Meyers, B. S., & Mei-Tal, V. Empirical study on an inpatient psychogeriatric unit: Biological treatment in patients with depressive illness. *International Journal of Psychiatry in Medicine*, 1985–86, *15*(2), 12.
17. Salzman, C., & Shader, R. I. Clinical evaluation of depression in the elderly. In A. Raskin & L. F. Jarvik (Eds.), *Psychiatric Symptoms and Cognitive Loss in the Elderly.* New York: Wiley, 1979, pp. 39–40.
18. Phifer, J. F., & Murrell, S. A. Etiologic factors in the onset of depressive symptoms in older adults. *Journal of Abnormal Psychology*, 1986, *95*, 282–291.
19. Salzman & Shader, op. cit., pp. 50–56.
20. Ibid., pp. 58–63.
21. *DSM-III-R*, pp. 213–215.
22. Gerner, R. H. Depression in the elderly. In O. J. Kaplan (Ed.), *Psychopathology of Aging.* New York: Academic Press, 1979, pp. 100–101.
23. Waxman, op. cit., pp. 294–299.
24. Addington, J., & Fry, P. S. Directions for clinical-psychosocial assessment of depression in the elderly. In J. Addington & P. S. Fry, (Eds.) *Clinical Gerontology, A Guide to Assessment and Intervention.* New York: Hawthorne, 1986, p. 100.
25. Osgood, N. J. *Suicide in the Elderly.* Rockville, Md.: Aspen Systems Corporation, 1985, p. x/iii.

26. Stenback, A. Depression and suicidal behavior in old age. In J. E. Birrin & R. B. Sloane (Eds.), *Handbook of Mental Health and Aging*. Englewood Cliffs, N.J.: Prentice-Hall, 1980, p. 645.

27. Miller, M. Toward a profile of the older white male suicide. *Gerontologist*, 1978, 80.

28. Waxman, op. cit., pp. 294–299.

29. Schultz, J. M., & Dark, S. L. *Manual of Psychiatric Nursing Care Plans*. Boston: Little, Brown, 1986, pp. 79–86.

30. LaPorte, H. J. Reversible causes of dementia: A nursing challenge. *Journal of Gerontological Nursing*, 1982, *8*(2), 77.

31. Lucas, M. J., Steele, C., & Bognanni, A. Recognition of psychiatric symptoms in dementia. *Journal of Gerontological Nursing*, 1986, *12*, 11–15.

32. Price, J. H., & Andrews, P. Alcohol abuse in the elderly. *Journal of Gerontological Nursing*, 1982, *8*(1), 16.

33. Ibid., p. 18.

34. Ibid., p. 19.

35. Hagebak, J. E., & Hagebak, B. R. Serving the mental health needs of the elderly. *Community Mental Health Journal*, 1980, *18*(4), 264.

36. Ibid., p. 263–266.

37. Ibid., p. 267.

38. Waxman, op. cit., pp. 294–299.

39. Butler & Lewis, op. cit., p. 175.

40. Ibid., pp. 137–141.

41. Phifer & Murrell, op. cit.

42. Elliot, E. My name is Mrs. Simon. *Ladies Home Journal*, August 1984.

43. Salzman, C., van der Kolk, B., & Shader, R. I. Psychopharmacology and the geriatric patient. In R. I. Shader (Ed.), *Manual of Psychiatric Therapeutics*. Boston: Little, Brown, 1978, pp. 172–173.

44. Butler & Lewis, op. cit., p. 255.

45. Meyers & Mei-Tal, op. cit., p. 111.

46. Harris, R. Foreword. In E. Caplow-Lindner, L. Horpoz, & S. Samberg (Eds.), *Therapeutic Dance Movement*. New York: Human Sciences Press, 1979, pp. 15–18.

47. Koch, K. *I Never told Anybody, Teaching Poetry Writing in a Nursing Home*. New York: Vintage Books, 1977.

48. Butler & Lewis, op. cit., pp. 193–194.

49. Schultz & Dark, op. cit., pp. 97–102.

50. Ryden, M. B. Nursing intervention in support of reminiscence. *Journal of Gerontological Nursing*, 1981, *7*(8), 46.

51. Ibid.

52. Ibid.

53. Ibid., pp. 462–463.

54. Butler & Lewis, op. cit., p. 49.

55. Ullman, M. A. Termination: The final developmental tasks. *Clinical Gerontologist*, 1986, *4*(4), 50–53.

56. Ibid., p. 52.

57. Ibid., p. 52.

58. Burnside, I. Some do not fly over the cuckoo's nest. *Journal of Gerontological Nursing*, 1986, *12*(1), 5.

59. Kuhn, M. *Aging in America*. Minneapolis: University of Minnesota, 1980. (Audio recording)

Chapter 54

The Psychosocial Issues Concerning Acquired Immune Deficiency Syndrome (AIDS)

Janis Davidson

Chapter Objectives

The students successfully attaining the goals of this chapter will be able to:

- Understand the impact of the diagnosis of AIDS.
- Formulate a plan of nursing care for the person with AIDS.
- Discuss the quality-of-life issues persons with AIDS face.
- Discuss dying and bereavement that AIDS patients and their families face.

The medical idiosyncrasies of the acquired immune deficiency syndrome (AIDS) have made it the primary American public health problem of the 1980s. These idiosyncrasies include its nearly uniform fatality, its rapid spread, its debilitating and dementing course, and the lack of vaccine, cure, or definitive treatment for it. The epidemiologic association with homosexual men and intravenous (IV) drug users has given rise to new discrimination toward groups who have been traditionally ostracized by society. The association with the causal retrovirus HIV, or human immunodeficiency virus, has raised widespread fear of contagion while presenting the American public with a mandate for radical change in sexual behavior and recreational drug use.

Because of these converging factors, the potential for psychosocial distress in AIDS is enor-

mous. The diagnosis of AIDS carries with it the combined psychological liabilities that belong to life-threatening illness on the one hand and to minority group discrimination on the other. AIDS frequently forces catastrophic social change on its patients. Increased dependency imposed by the sick role requires adaptation. Disability and prohibitive medical expenses often require application for Medicaid and public assistance.

IV drug users face comparable social ostracism in American society. The diagnosis of AIDS may force them to confront the difficult process of detoxification—which may include physiological withdrawal, residential treatment, and abrupt disruption of drug-related friendships.[1]

As a result of these converging factors, the person with AIDS is vulnerable to reactive psychiatric symptoms, consisting of the triad of depression, anxiety, and preoccupation with illness. Diagnosis or progression of AIDS elicits a full range of existential depressive symptoms. These include: dysphoric mood; hopelessness and helplessness; anhedonia; and abandonment or rejection sensitivity. Both suicidal ideation and suicidal plans or attempts are common.

THE PROBLEM

In late 1980, T-cells were discovered as the key components of the immune system. There are two types of T-lymphocyte cells: the T-helper cells that activate the specific disease-fighting cells and give chemical instructions for creating the antibodies that destroy microbial invaders, and the T-suppressor cells that tell the immune system when the threat ended. In patients seen in 1980 with overwhelming infections of usual body microbes, T-helper cells were not present in their blood. Researchers sought to find what disease sought and killed such specific blood cells.

Since identification of the HIV in 1985, the scope of research worldwide has broadened dramatically. AIDS is the most discussed subject in the United States, yet some of its most important characteristics are not understood. From the beginning it was thought of as a homosexual's disease, created by "promiscuity." Then with the isolation of the virus in blood, transmission was found to be occurring in people who received blood and blood products before blood was screened for the virus in May 1985. Now the transmission was seen in people who were intravenous drug abusers because they were sharing needles.

AIDS is transmitted by intimate sexual contact and by exposure to contaminated blood. Normally the body's protective barrier, the skin, prevents infection by agents like HIV; if the barrier is broken by injury or by needle puncture, fluid containing the virus may enter the body. HIV is transferred from one person to another in sexual activities that involve exchange of body fluids, especially if minor breaks in the skin barrier are involved.

What is AIDS?

AIDS is an infectious disease characterized by an impairment of the immune system that leaves the affected individual susceptible to certain types of cancer and a number of opportunistic diseases. The profound loss of normal cellular and humoral immune function leads to laboratory data definitive of infection, with T-4 counts as low as $400/mm^3$ (normal value 40 to 58,000/mm^3) and reverse T-4:T-8 ratio less than 1.0 (normal 2.0) and pancytopenia. The condition was first diagnosed in the United States in 1981. However, as we learn more about the virus, evidence leads researchers to data that suggest the retrovirus has been infecting Americans since 1967. The virus has been documented in Africa since 1955.

AIDS is believed to be caused by a variant form of the human T-cell lymphotrophic virus, called HTLV-III. Researchers of the virus have used lymphadenopathy associated virus (LAV), AIDS-associated retrovirus (ARV), and HIV. The mortality rate of AIDS is extremely high: 80 percent of people diagnosed before 1985 are now dead.

The increasing incidence of AIDS and its concentration among certain groups (male homosexuals, intravenous drug users, recipients of blood transfusions, and hemophiliacs) have stirred great concern among these groups and the general population, spurred a growing number of research and epidemiologic studies, and raised a number of public policy issues.

Social Isolation

There is cause for concern about AIDS. The acute condition generally causes death; the virus can also travel through the barrier in the body between the blood and the nervous system and settle in the brain, causing meningitis, dementia, and other forms of neurological damage; there will not likely be a cure for AIDS soon; and a vaccine will be very hard to make. In addition to some 50,000 cases (in 1987) in the United States, growing numbers are seen in 90 countries.

Much of this information has been reported in the press, and public reaction has been clear. We have seen parents demanding that children who are HIV seropositive not go to school and that even healthy children who live with other children with AIDS be excluded as well. A major airline banned AIDS patients from flying on the carrier; apparently it felt that AIDS patients posed a danger to other passengers by using the

1044   SPECIAL POPULATIONS

same toilet seats; an actress refused to have kissing scenes with a male actor who had not passed an AIDS blood test; prospective jurors have asked to be dismissed from a trial in which the defendant had the disease; some Christian worshipers have expressed fears that drinking from the same communion cup would spread the disease; and some police departments are keeping lists of known AIDS patients so they will screen calls for responding to people in specific areas of the city.

Such response is not confined to the United States. In countries where homosexuality is a legal offense, the courts may order compulsory psychiatric treatment because AIDS might result from "genetic mutations" caused by "mixed marriages."

Any serious disease that is contagious is likely to cause fear and demands for precise and certain knowledge about how it spreads—demands that are usually impossible to fulfill. Not only has public apprehension about AIDS intensified, but many people seem to cling to private fears about the illness and question what public health officials report.

The Public Health Service, which governs five central agencies including the Center for Disease Control, the Food and Drug Administration, and the National Institutes of Health (NIH), is a section of the Department of Health and Human Services. Most of the government research on AIDS has been done by the NIH. The epidemic was clearly foreseen in March of 1981, and research at NIH began in 1983. Most of the researchers who saw and treated some of the first cases of AIDS say that it will probably prove to be the plague of the millenium. Research reports are issued periodically.

PSYCHOSOCIAL IMPACT OF AIDS: SITUATIONAL DISTRESS MODEL[2]

Stage	Characteristic Symptoms	Interaction Approach
Crisis	Shock, denial, guilt	Attempt to establish ongoing support system; seek effective communication without challenging denial.
Transitional state	Denial superseded by anger, anxiety, depression, guilt; social disruption and withdrawal common (work, family, living arrangements)	Peer support, group counseling may become important; psychiatric intervention and medication may be necessary. Help patients with restructuring of social relationship.
Deficiency state and acceptance	Acceptance of limitations, formation of new sense of self; often marked by interest in altruistic or community activities (coinciding with losses in health, energy, independence)	Encourage group and community involvement.
Preparation for death	Fear of dependency	Encourage completion of unfinished business; address family and next-of-kin issues as helpfully as possible.

Alteration in Quality of Life

The major concerns of 30 people diagnosed with AIDS were surveyed by researchers from NIH and Massachusetts General Hospital in the summer of 1987. The findings revealed the following:

1. Talking with patients about the impact of AIDS on their lives was seen as therapeutic by patients interviewed.
2. Patients expect nurses to be knowledgeable and to share this information with them.
3. Patients consistently asked for acceptance,

a nonjudgmental attitude, and concern about them as interesting persons.

4. Patients expressed great concern about confidentiality.
5. A diagnosis of AIDS should not be given over the telephone and should be given with counseling and with crisis intervention services made available.
6. Emotional support and referrals to agencies that provide support should be a high priority for those without readily available support systems.
7. Health care workers should never take away patients' hope and should find ways to foster hope.[3]

The effect of HIV on the nervous system results in disorganization in thinking and daily habits. Patients are often too tired to work and feel too well not to work. They describe experiencing "bankruptcy" of life.

The diagnosis of AIDS sets into motion a crisis period for the person. Disruption and disorganization in thinking and daily habits become the daily routine. They suffer the infections that AIDS presents. What were manageable illnesses of living become catastrophic events for patients. The HIV destroys the body's ability to fight infections; thus common organisms are a disastrous threat to the person.

People with AIDS have altered energy levels. They may have 2 good hours in the morning or afternoon to do something enjoyable, yet, their fatigue limits vocational and social participation.

Patient Teaching

HIV-infected persons are instructed about transmission routes of the virus through intercourse—anal, oral, and vaginal—and through sharing of needles. They are instructed to use condoms for intercourse. IV drug users are instructed how to wash needles in household Clorox that is diluted to kill the virus. They are told to inform their sexual partners and to abstain from unprotected intercourse and needle sharing.

Infection Control

There has been much concern over the possibility of the transmission of HIV to health care workers caring for patients with AIDS. However, the risk of transmission of HIV after a needle stick or other parenteral exposure has been estimated to be significantly less than 1 percent; the risk of transmission of hepatitis B, another blood-borne infection, ranges in such circumstances from 6 percent to 30 percent, with 300 deaths from hepatitis B in health care workers in 1987. This led to the development of recommendations based on the familiar precautions for preventing hepatitis B; because the hepatitis B virus is more easily transmitted, through similar routes, similar measures should prevent HIV exposure in health care and workplace settings.[4]

Health care providers do not have a high risk of getting AIDS as a result of their work with patients even when they regularly care for people with full-blown AIDS in hospitals. The risk is associated with unprotected care giving of infected patients and needle stick injuries. Guidelines for prevention of transmission of AIDS virus to health care providers are: use enteric precautions, that is, wear gloves when handling bodily fluids.

NEUROLOGICAL ABNORMALITIES OF HIV

Sixty percent of patients hospitalized with AIDS will have neurological symptoms of headache, confusion, dementia, or hallucinations. The neurological complications are being recognized with increasing frequency in persons infected with HIV. The incidence suggests that HIV itself is responsible for the subacute encephalopathy, polyneuropathy, and vacuolar myelopathy seen in patients with AIDS.

The presence of the virus in cerebrospinal fluid and not concurrently in the serum suggests that HIV may at times replicate preferentially in the brain and that its presence may not immediately cause neurological signs or symptoms.

Psychological distress in AIDS is seen in

1. Anxiety symptoms
   a. Uncertainty about disease and treatment
   b. Anxiety about any new physical symptoms
2. Depressive symptoms
   a. Sadness
   b. Helplessness
   c. Lowered self-esteem

d. Guilt
e. Worthlessness
f. Hopelessness
g. Suicidal thoughts
h. Social withdrawal
i. Anticipatory grief
3. Social isolation and reduced support
4. Anger
   a. Suspiciousness of attitudes of others[5]

Clinical experience and neuropathologic data indicate that neurological complications occur in most patients with AIDS. Although infections from toxoplasma and lymphoma produce well-defined lesions in the brain, the most common dysfunction of the central nervous system is a nonfocal encephalopathy, which includes dementia as the dominant feature. First identified by Snider and associates it is a form of subcortical dementia.[6] This diffuse disorder is the most frequent form of neurological dysfunction.

The early clinical picture of this encephalopathy resembles depression and is often indistinguishable without neuropsychiatric testing. Usual symptoms are, initially, forgetfulness and poor concentration. Psychomotor retardation, gait disturbance ataxia, decreased alertness, apathy, withdrawal, diminished interest in work, and loss of libido develop soon after. Over several months, frank confusion, disorientation, seizures, myoclonus, mutism, profound dementia, coma, and death ensue.[7] The progression of symptoms may be extremely rapid over a few weeks, but more typically the decline is over several months.

Management of the person with AIDS who has neuropsychiatric complications is to rule out treatable central nervous system diseases, such as toxoplasma infection or lymphoma. No definitive treatment exists for the AIDS dementia at present; supportive interventions are crucial in management, as well as a supervised living situation.

ILLNESS CARE MANAGEMENT OF AIDS

At present there is no known cure for AIDS. Three different approaches are being used in treatment: (1) treatment of the opportunistic infection or cancer from which the patient is suffering; (2) treating the AIDS virus itself; and (3) stimulating the patient's immune system. The first approach is palliative, that is, designed to make and keep the patient comfortable, since it does not eliminate the underlying cause of the patient's disease. Certain drugs have had limited success in reducing or eliminating Kaposi's sarcoma lesions and in treating the other forms of cancer and some of the opportunistic infections that affect these patients. Since the treatment process does not improve the immune system, the infections will eventually recur. These infections are particularly difficult to treat.

The second approach attempts to make use of antiviral drugs to inhibit the AIDS virus. HIV contains an enzyme, reverse transcriptase, which is necessary for viral replication. Several antiviral agents are capable of inhibiting this enzyme and are being investigated for their usefulness in the treatment of HIV infections. Although new drugs are continuing to be developed, the small number that are currently available have severe side effects because they act on the host cell that is infected with the virus.

The HIV incorporates its genetic material into that of the infected host cell, making it indistinguishable from the host. Each time the host cell divides, the viral genes are reproduced. Drug therapy may never be able to eliminate the virus from the patient, and therefore the patient must be treated for the rest of his life in order to control the virus.

On September 19, 1986, the Public Health Service along with Burroughs Wellcome Company announced the decision to allow more AIDS patients access to the drug azidothymidine, or AZT. A thymidine analogue with potent antiviral activity against HIV, AZT can be administered orally or intravenously. This agent is able to cross the blood–brain barrier. It seems relatively safe of serious side effects and is virustatic and provides partial immunologic reconstitution in some patients.[8] AZT does not provide a cure for AIDS, but it does seem to decrease the mortality rate of some patients with AIDS. Patients receiving the drug have fewer serious medical complications and an improved sense of well-being.

Treating the patient early in the course of the disease, before the immune system has been destroyed, may offer the best hope for recovery. However, since the incubation period of the disease may be as long as 10 years and is often asymptomatic, it may be difficult to determine when treatment should begin and for how long it should be continued.

Framework for Nursing Care

The nursing diagnosis labels for the patient with AIDS include[9]:

- Activity intolerance
- Adjustment, impaired
- Airway clearance, ineffective
- Coping, ineffective family: Disabled
- Coping, ineffective individual
- Diversional activity, deficit
- Family processes, altered
- Fear
- Fluid volume deficit
- Gas exchange, impaired
- Grieving, dysfunctional
- Home maintenance management, impaired
- Hopelessness
- Infection: Potential for
- Knowledge deficit
- Mobility, impaired physical
- Nutrition, altered: Less than body requirements
- Powerlessness
- Role performance, altered
- Self-care deficit: Bathing/hygiene, dressing/grooming, feeding, toileting
- Self-concept, disturbance in: Body image
- Self-concept, disturbance in: Self-esteem
- Sexuality, altered patterns
- Skin integrity, impaired: Actual/potential
- Social interaction, impaired
- Social isolation
- Spiritual distress
- Thought processes, altered
- Violence, potential for: Self-directed

Disturbance in the estimate one places on oneself, including one's self-worth, self-approval, self-confidence, and self-respect, is seen as a sequela to the stigma of AIDS. AIDS as a sexually transmitted disease leads patients to feel guilty and dirty for loving. The internal dialogue is "What did I do to deserve this?" Surfacing the internalized homophobia leads to "I have AIDS because I am gay"; bargaining, "I'll go straight, if only I am cured"; and self-condemnation concerning "life in the fast lane."

One nursing diagnosis for an AIDS patient could be formulated as follows[10]:

DISTURBANCE IN SELF-CONCEPT: SELF-ESTEEM FRAMEWORK

Related to

- Situational crisis AIDS
- Psychological impairment AIDS
- Unmet expectations for life
- Terminal illness AIDS

Patient Outcomes

- To identify personal strengths.
- To acknowledge impact of situation on existing personal relationships, life-style, role performance.
- To maintain close personal relationships.
- To verbalize willingness to consider life-style change.
- To express willingness to use suggested resources on discharge.
- To adapt to changes in body and thinking.

Nursing Intervention

Presence of the nurse will demonstrate unconditional positive regard in acceptance of the patient. The nurse engages herself in communications that reward feedback from the patient. The congruent behavior and time spent in genuine interest and concern for what the patient is experiencing and how the patient is feeling will encourage the patient to identify strengths and potentials. Problem solving established as a mutual goal of the nurse–patient relationship will encourage the patient to explore and design outcomes for living his life.[11]

SPECIFIC INTERVENTIONS[12]

Symptom	Etiology	Intervention
Memory loss	Lymphoma	Instruct care givers in neurological symptoms; help them to understand and cope with these changes.

Symptom	Etiology	Intervention
Confusion	Meningitis	Talk to patient in simple, short sentences; keep calendar at bedside with appointments to minimize confusion; use large clock in room.
Weakness	Encephalopathy	Arrange for 24-hour care as mental status deteriorates to ensure a safe environment.
	Toxoplasmosis	Lorazepam (Ativan) 2 × 6 mg p.o. QID

CASE EXAMPLES

Example One

Marc was a 38-year-old gay white man with no psychiatric history except episodic binge drinking and a 2-month history of AIDS (*Pneumocystis carinii* pneumonia). He was admitted after he became disruptive in an alcohol treatment program. Clinically, he appeared to be suffering an episode of bipolar (mania) disorder and exhibited insomnia, hyperactivity, pressured speech, flight of ideas, lability, grandiose and religious delusions, auditory and visual hallucinations, markedly impaired judgment, and complete denial of his AIDS diagnosis. It was unclear if his symptoms were directly caused by HIV infection of his brain or were part of a reactive or "functional" disorder. A negative CT scan and lumbar puncture suggested the latter was the case. Marc improved moderately after treatment with antipsychotic medication; lithium was not used as Marc had recent renal complications of AIDS. He was released 10 days after admission, following a successful challenge of his mental health held in Superior Court.

Marc was readmitted 10 days later after increasing fatigue and severely impaired judgment rendered him unable to provide food, clothing, and shelter. Treatment with antipsychotic medication was reinstituted. At first he continued to exhibit manic symptoms. On one occasion he became threatening and required seclusion. He repeatedly abused the telephone, calling 911 so the police would rescue him, badgering friends, and trying to order everything from plane tickets to brass bands.

After a few weeks, Marc's clinical status began to change. Many of his "manic" symptoms diminished or disappeared; for the most part, he maintained his grandiose denial of his prognosis although this was punctuated by periodic lucidity and acknowledgment of his illness. He began to show signs of dementia: decreased attention to grooming and common etiquette, disorientation, failing short-term memory, wandering, and visual spatial recognition deficits. He had a number of medication complications although he was able to tolerate a neuroleptic and gradually required less of this. His dementia progressed rapidly and he grew weaker and more in need of nursing assistance with basic activities.

Marc was placed in permanent conservatorship and no longer required acute psychiatric hospitalization after approximately 2 months, although he remained on the unit for nearly 6 months until he could be placed in a residential program with 24-hour care. He died 10 days after discharge.

Example Two

Ben was a 39-year-old businessman who lived with his lover of 8 years. Following his first episode of pneumocystosis, Ben's attitude toward his illness was marked by an intense belief that he "was going to beat this disease." Ben essentially withdrew from any discussion about his illness or the possibility that he might get sick again. He embarked on a strict diet of natural foods, placed himself on a regular regimen of light exercise, and practiced visualization techniques daily. He led an active though restrained social life, refusing to tell others, including his elderly mother, about his illness.

Ben did well for 10 months. He and his lover were on a month's vacation in Europe when Ben began to notice increasing fatigability. They returned to the United States where Ben was hospitalized with his second bout of pneumocystosis. He also complained of difficulty swallowing, and Kaposi's sarcoma lesions were found in his throat and esophagus. He began to lose weight rapidly as eating was increasingly painful and hampered by his esophageal lesions.

Ben was referred for psychiatric consultation for depression and social withdrawal. At first Ben was resistant, but after repeated crying spells and intense, uncomfortable anxiety attacks appeared, he relented. His anxiety symptoms, including a racing heartbeat, sweaty palms, and an intense fear of "going crazy" prompted him to seek treatment.

A prescription for alprazolam in increasing doses was successful in blunting Ben's anxiety attacks. While the medication never fully stopped the attacks, the symptoms were brought under sufficient control so that Ben no longer found them intolerable. He became increasingly interested in his psychotherapy and began to "unload" his fears and worries about his illness. With his anxiety symptoms under control, he entered a period of profound sadness as he began to face the reality of his failing health. He began to open up to his lover and their friends as he realized how important each had been to him. Through psychotherapy, he grew to understand aspects of his relationship with his mother that facilitated their being able to communicate about his illness.

Finally, several joint sessions with Ben and his lover were helpful in clarifying issues around power of attorney and planning for funeral arrangements—issues that previously had been too difficult to confront.

Treatment issues commonly encountered with patients in this phase of illness largely consist of reassuring patients that they will not be abandoned and that they will be given adequate pain medication. The use of antidepressants as an adjunct to pain management is sometimes indicated. Often patients will begin to withdraw emotional investment in others as they begin to turn away from the living and focus more on themselves and their approaching death. Understanding this is a common development and communicating this to family and friends often can be very comforting to them. The patient is often relieved by the opportunity to discuss his fears and concerns about dying with the nurse. The patient is encouraged to take care of any business he feels is left to finish and is supported in permission to let go of life with the understanding that the nurse will do all she can to see that the patient's wishes are followed after his death.

THE PATIENT DYING OF AIDS*

The needs of patients with known fatal diseases differ from other healthy individuals only with respect to the intensity and urgency. Time takes on a much greater import when it is known to be "running out," and consequently the dying person becomes acutely aware of how time is used. Frustration may result readily when delays occur due to "complications in plans," complications that interfere with events taking place precisely as planned or scheduled. Waiting to

* This section through page 1053 is adapted from pp. 664–671 of A. W. Burgess, Psychiatric Nursing in the Hospital and the Community, 4th ed., Englewood Cliffs: Prentice Hall, 1985.

see physicians, waiting for treatments, or waiting for the results of diagnostic studies may become a source of increased anxiety and anger for the patient who is acutely aware that his life expectancy is severely limited.

Another important aspect of caring for terminally ill patients is that of recognizing their need for time to discuss their personal feelings, needs, and concerns with at least one trusted person in their environment. Patients with terminal illnesses are often denied such time by the busy schedules of hospital personnel or the anxiety generated by such encounters. Health care professionals who deal with dying patients must confront (at least unconsciously) the reality of their own mortality in order to be supportive to the dying patient.

The patient who has a fatal illness needs to feel useful, worthwhile, and productive for as long as this is possible. Such patients should be permitted and encouraged to retain as many opportunities for decision making as possible and should be afforded maximum flexibility in routines for nursing care and treatment. The nurse needs to be cognizant of the patient's need to finish whatever "unfinished" business is important to him and should assist the patient with such endeavors whenever this is appropriate.

Furthermore, family members and friends may require support in order to prevent a dramatic shift from occurring in their attitudes, responses, and reactions to a family member who is dying. Alterations in family and friends' reactions to the dying patient may result in the deprivation of the patient's basic human need to be needed and thus can cause diminished feelings of self-esteem. Also, alterations in reactions can result in the establishment of an environment that is new, forlorn, and unpredictable to the patient at a time when he is being faced with multiple adjustments in life-style and circumstances. Rosenthal's own response to dying underscores the impact that the reaction of others can have on the dying patient. He states:

As frightened as I thought I should be, or might be, everybody else expressed feelings in striking contrast to my own. I never really saw what fear was until I looked at everybody else looking at me. And I didn't reciprocate. . . . It just made me nervous. And I realized that I wasn't frightened at all.[13]

In addition to the dying person's need for time and for continued normalcy in his life is the increased need for meaningful relationships with other people involved in his life situation.

The Nurse's Role as Patient Advocate

The patient with a fatal illness should be afforded whatever measures are necessary to promote physical comfort and reduce suffering. Nurses may find their role as patient advocate to be greatest in this area since it is the nurse who is in an ideal position to assess the patient's level of comfort and response to medication. In addition, nurses who deal with patients who are dying should not underestimate the comfort afforded by simply being present to such patients in a compassionate and caring way. Maximal benefit can be afforded from the nurse's presence if: (1) she is able to accept the patient at whatever state the patient is at in the dying process; (2) if she can allow the patient to progress through this process at his own pace; and (3) if she does not try to force the patient to move through this process quickly or prematurely.

The Hospice movement offers another option for dealing with the needs and issues specific to dying patients and their families. The goals of Hospice include helping the dying patient achieve maximum freedom from physical and emotional pain; keeping him functioning at a maximum level until death comes; and meeting any special needs of the patient and members of the family that arise from the stresses associated with the final stages of illness, dying, and bereavement. Nurses, because of their ongoing contact with the public, are in a prime position to provide information and education about Hospice as an alternative to conventional forms of care for the dying.

AUTOGNOSIS: STAFF REACTIONS TO DYING AND DEATH

Effective management of dying patients and their survivors first requires that the health care professionals examine their own personal anxiety, fears, concepts, and attitudes regarding this human experience. Interrelated with the professionals' need to come to grips with their own finiteness is the importance of developing a flexible conceptual framework for the care and management of those with whom they will in-

teract in such situations. This framework is of particular importance since during their professional education, the majority of health care professionals still receive generally inadequate preparation to deal with encounters involving the dying and their survivors, in spite of recent recognition of the need for such preparation and the proliferation of the articles and books on this subject.

Although most nursing programs have progressed to the point of including some content relative to these issues in their curriculum, the scope and quality of such information continue to vary from school to school, and no specific standardized guidelines exist with regard to what should be taught or how these concepts should be presented. Reports in the literature still suggest that death is an area that is laden with anxiety, fear, avoidance, and denial; that such programs can influence nurses' attitudes in a positive way; and that nurses who lack confidence in their ability to care for dying patients also have difficulty in dealing with the family members of these patients.

The lack of support, preparation, and understanding that nurses receive with regard to their difficulties in dealing with dying patients and their survivors is not a phenomenon that is restricted or unique to academia. Mandel notes that:

There appears to be little awareness of the psychological impact that dealing with the chronically and terminally ill can have on the staff. At least little is done to help relieve the tension that can result. For example, individuals in the helping professions do not have the freedom to express the negative or difficult aspects of their work. Instead, these feelings are usually expressed by acting tired at work, being ill, or through voicing grievances against the institution in which they work.[14]

Nurses who work with terminally ill and patients dying from AIDS on a regular basis must recognize that such work is emotionally demanding and that it involves continual loss and separation experiences.

Need for Multidisciplinary Team and Realistic Goals

It should be recognized that the complex care that is called into play when dealing with the dying and the bereaved cannot be single-hand-edly and effectively managed by one person but requires the skill and efforts of a multidiscipli-nary team. Such a team of professionals must form a network of mutual support and sharing that allows for the expression of anger, frustra-tion, and grief, which the team members as well as family members experience.[15] In addition, setting realistic goals can reduce the sense of failure that so often is experienced by health care professionals, who traditionally have focused their efforts on "saving lives," even when death was inevitable, rather than on helping those pa-tients facing death to do so in as good a con-dition—physically, emotionally, and spiritu-ally—as possible.

The patient with an AIDS diagnosis strug-gles with many thoughts and feelings. There are two specific feelings that a nurse may be able to help the person bear: these are the feelings of loss and sadness.

Helping the Patient Bear the Feelings of Loss and Sadness

One of the essential therapeutic tasks in the gen-eral hospital setting for the nurse is to help pa-tients bear their painful feelings, especially the feeling of sadness. Since sadness is a healthy emotion and since its avoidance leads to medical and psychiatric pathology including depression, it is important to look at some of the ways in which the nurse may be therapeutic to the pa-tient in dealing with loss and the subsequent feeling of sadness.

In the hospital setting the patient is reach-ing out. He may be searching for the slightest cue from the nurse to confirm that what he feels is acceptable to talk about. He begins to discuss his personal life or his feelings about his illness. It is at this point that the nurse may easily stall the process of the patient's expressing his feel-ings. An example is when the patient cries. The nurse may cut the patient off in several ways: She may directly state that the patient should not cry and that he should be brave; she may quickly reassure the patient that everything will be fine; she may change the subject or busy her-self with straightening the patient's room; she may refer the patient to a psychiatric nurse cli-nician; or she may dismiss the patient in her own mind as "feeling sorry for himself."

There are many understandable reasons

why nurses stall this process and wish to avoid the patient's sadness.

1. It is painful to listen to someone's psycho-logical distress.
2. The nurse, as she sees the outflow of tears and affect-laden thoughts, is afraid of opening Pandora's box. Can she handle what she fears will come next?
3. The nurse's own discomfort may be further exaggerated because some unresolved sad-ness in her own life is reawakened by the patient's experience.
4. When loss is related to a medical procedure (surgery, for example), the patient's sense of loss and sadness is often accompanied by feelings of anger toward the hospital and staff. It is very difficult for the nurse to be understanding toward someone who is angry with her.
5. The nurse feels helpless as she listens. She wants to do something and has not yet had the experience of knowing that listening is doing something.

In order to prevent the stall from occurring, the nurse must realize that there is a great deal that she can do to help to bear the patient's feel-ing of sadness. The nurse should assume that the patient who experiences serious illness has feelings of sadness over the loss of function or change in body image. For example, the patient with an AIDS diagnosis may have to give up otherwise normal activities. The patient needs understanding and encouragement to talk with someone about these feelings. If the patient ap-pears upset, tense, sad, or tearful, the nurse should call his attention to these feelings by say-ing: "You seem troubled today. . . ." The pa-tient may correctly perceive the statement and the expectant pause as a show of interest and a willingness to listen on the part of the nurse. When the patient does not appear to be upset or strained, the nurse might then be more direct: "What does having an AIDS diagnosis mean to you?" "How do you feel about your new symp-toms?" The patient then thinks: "The nurse is perceptive enough to know I am suffering and she can bear to hear me talk about how I feel." Sometimes expressions such as "Your heart is heavy," "Your heart is aching," "Your heart is full of tears," or "You hurt inside" may seem appropriate for a particular patient and situa-tion. These phrases, sincerely expressed, may elicit a great outpouring of feeling.[16] The patient needs to know that it is natural to have these feelings. And the nurse needs to learn how to cope and bear with the intensity of the emotion.

The Dying Patient

One of the most difficult situations for the staff is caring for the dying AIDS patient. The nursing process involved in caring for this person provokes a variety of reactions in the nurse.

People may need to talk about the "letting go" of life. As one patient said,

I don't want to die. It is hard to go. . . . The letting go of life. I just don't want to let go.

The nurse may be asked to talk with the family after there has been a death. The nurse helps the family members begin the grieving process by letting them know that it is all right to feel and express sadness. Her presence communicates that what was done for the patient was done with respect. The nurse can bear to face and talk with the family. The reality of what has happened is present. People are grateful to be acknowledged in such a respectful manner.

If nurses are able to minimize their feelings of helplessness, deal with their own reactions to death, and find the active as well as the passive ways to be therapeutic with the dying patient, they have achieved a high degree of competence. Being physically present and attending to the physical comfort of the patient are essential. But whether or not nurses are able to increase their sensitivity in helping the dying person depends on how they autognose their own feelings about dying, about the disease of AIDS, and on how therapeutic they are to the patient.

It is not always necessary to have a specific nurse care for the patient in his dying process, but it may be helpful for the staff to be able to call upon the psychiatric nursing services in difficult situations. We believe that caring for the dying person is a vital part of every nurse's credo.

The psychiatric nurse may help the staff with their feelings about caring for the dying patient and thus help them avoid potential stalls. These stalls occur because of nurses' feelings about caring for the dying AIDS patient.

Stall Situation One

One stall situation develops from the feeling of helplessness experienced by the nurses. They say, "I can't help the patient to live; therefore I am helpless." What has to be understood is that the nurse need not feel helpless to the point that the patient is abandoned as he is dying. Nurses cannot stop the actual dying process and to that extent they are helpless. But they can be therapeutic in helping the person to be comfortable as he dies. The presence and caring of another person during this very difficult life experience are some of the most human aspects of all nursing.

Stall Situation Two

A second common stall situation in the patient's dying process is staff identification with the illness. Staff members who are close in age to terminally ill patients may experience feelings of identification with them. These patients are difficult to care for if the staff members are unable to express their own feelings of anxiety and fear over the possibility of this illness in themselves.

Other factors heighten the identification process of staff with AIDS patients. Sometimes the gender preference or lifestyle factors affects this reaction. The similarities between the patient and staff all contribute. The staff person thinks, "This could be me and I wonder how I would react if it were me? What would I do?" These factors can be explored in staff meetings in order to help sift out the feelings and thus enable the staff to care appropriately for the patient and not to withdraw because of a conflict of feelings.

Stall Situation Three

A third stall situation may occur when the patient asks something the nurse feels cannot be answered. Nurses say they fear that the patient will request something they would not know how to handle. Or they say, "I might give something away or tell something the doctor should tell." All that these excuses do is keep the nurse from the patient. Other evasive methods used by the nurse in dealing with the patient are to send other staff in, to keep busy with the records or reports, or to be in staff meetings. The nurse has to work through her feelings of discomfort and insecurity when talking with patients about troublesome subjects.

The stall warning should sound when the nurse feels herself withdrawing from the dying patient, or when she finds herself reacting personally to the patient's expressed feeling. For example, the patient will often feel angry and sad when he realizes he is dying. He may tell the nurse to leave him alone or to go away. He may turn his back on staff members or turn the radio up loudly when they enter the room.

The therapeutic task is to help the patient bear the painful feelings he is having: those feelings of having to let go and leave this world alone.

After the death of the patient, family members may or may not be allowed to spend time with the patient's body. Whenever possible, time should be provided, especially if the body is to be cremated. If the nurse assesses that the family may have difficulty coping after the death, a referral to a community agency should be made.

CASE EXAMPLE OF ORGANIC MENTAL DYSFUNCTION WITH AIDS

History

A 26-year-old, single, Hispanic male was admitted to a state hospital after a brief psychotic episode in which he started a stove fire in his girl friend's apartment in an attempt to burn down the apartment. The patient also made threats to his girl friend and her three young children.

His admitting psychiatric diagnoses were:

Axis I   Organic Mental Disorders with Delusions and Mixed Substance Abuse
Axis II   Antisocial Personality Disorder
Axis III AIDS with organicity

The patient had an 8-year history of substance abuse, admitting to the regular use of alcohol, marijuana, amphetamines, barbiturates, mainlining heroin and cocaine, and free-basing cocaine. The diagnosis of AIDS was made 18 months previously, with the intravenous use of drugs identified as the cause of the disease.

Hospital Course

Over a 6-month hospitalization, the patient's mental status remained relatively stable although he was very depressed and withdrawn. He suffered from occasional episodes of confusion with delusional ideation and attempted suicide by hanging 3 months after admission. Physically, he had become progressively weaker. He was anemic and plagued by various somatic complaints and associated symptoms ranging from intermittent fevers as high as 105°F, nausea, vomiting, abdominal pain, and severe headache.

Family History

The patient was the second oldest of five children ranging in age from 28 to 13. The father was deceased, having died of a stroke at the age of 67. The mother was alive and living locally. The only interested family were the patient's mother and girl friend who visited approximately once to twice each month. Both parties were unable to take the patient home because he required a great deal of care and medical supervision. The patient had no contact with his siblings since his admission.

Nursing Diagnosis

Coping, ineffective.

Nursing Intervention

The patient occasionally verbalized his feelings of loneliness and isolation but did not develop a trusting relationship with any staff member. The nurse planned to try to establish a relationship of trust and support, communicating an empathetic understanding of his present situation. The patient isolated himself within his room and the staff who cared for him had fears concerning contagion. Efforts were made to help staff autognose their feelings regarding his disease and his care.

The patient was viewed within his social context, that context being the hospital environment where he was expected to reside until his death. Interventions were directed at assisting the patient to adapt to the hospital environment and at accepting his disease. A major goal was to preserve individuation, the client being a human being first and a patient with AIDS second, and to support mutuality.

Summary

AIDS is a syndrome with profound medical and psychosocial consequences. When persons with AIDS have either been referred for or have requested psychiatric intervention, the therapist should bear in mind the relationship between the patient's presenting complaints and his medical status. A series of psychiatric consultants with persons with AIDS reveal that the management of mood disorders and dementia are the most frequent reasons for intervention. Medications will play an important role, and psychotherapy will be essential for the persons experiencing depression. Working with persons with AIDS, especially over time, can be an emotionally charged and draining experience for the care giver. Nonetheless, the relationship with the care giver can provide immeasurable comfort to the patient in need, and the willingness of the care giver to be available can add significantly to the patient's quality of life.

Nurses deal daily with the reality of death and dying. This chapter describes the process of dying and ways of integrating mental health concepts to assist the dying patient and his or her family, the grieving process for the bereaved, diagnosis of uncomplicated grief, and autognosis of staff reactions to dying patients, death, and AIDS.

Questions

1. Autognose your feelings about AIDS.
2. Describe the grieving process and cite a clinical example.
3. What are the criteria for diagnosing uncomplicated grief response?
4. Describe a clinical situation in which the multidisciplinary concept was used effectively in managing the bereavement process.

REFERENCES AND SUGGESTED READINGS

1. Des Jarlais, D. C., Friedman, S. R., & Hopkins, W. Risk reduction for the acquired immunodeficiency syndrome among intravenous drug users. *Annals of Internal Medicine*, 1985, *103*, 755–759.
2. Nichols, S. E. Psychosocial reactions of persons with the acquired immunodeficiency syndrome. *Annals of Internal Medicine*, 1985, *103*, 765–767.
3. Grady, C. Concerns of people with AIDS. *FOCUS, a Guide to AIDS Research*, 1987, *2*(9), 2.
4. Martin, L. S., et. al. Prevention of workplace transmission of HTLV-III/LAV infection. *Journal of Infectious Diseases*, 1985, *152*, 400.
5. Holland, J. C., & Tross, S. The psychosocial and neuropsychiatric sequelae of the acquired immunodeficiency syndrome and related disorders. *Annals of Internal Medicine*, 1985, *103*, 760–764.
6. Snider, W. D., Simpson, D. M., et. al. Neurological complications of acquired immune deficiency syndrome: Analysis of 50 patients. *Annals of Neurology*, 1983, *14*, 403–418.
7. Ibid.
8. Yarchoan, R., Klecker, R. W., Weinhold, K. J., et al. Administration of 3'-Azido-3'-Deoxythymidine, an inhibitor of HTLV-III/LAV replication, to patients with AIDS or AIDS-related complex. *Lancet*, 1986, 575–580.
9. Lederer, J. R., et. al. *Care Planning Pocket Guide; A Nursing Diagnosis Approach*. Menlo Park, Calif.: Addison-Wesley, 1988.
10. Ibid.
11. Zderad, L. T. *Theory Development: What, Why, How?* (15-1708). New York: National League for Nursing, 1978, pp. 35–48.
12. Durham, J. D., & Cohen, F. L. *The Person with AIDS: Nursing Perspective*. New York: Springer, 1987.
13. Rosenthal, T. *How Could I Not Be Among You?* New York: Braziller, 1973, p. 26.
14. Mandel, H. R. Nurses' feelings about working with dying patients. *American Journal of Nursing*, 1975, *75*, 1194.
15. Gyulay, J.-E. The forgotten grievers. *American Journal of Nursing*, 1975, *75*, 1474.
16. Lazare, A. The difference between sadness and depression. *Medical Insight*, 1970, *2*(23), 26.
17. Engel, G. L. Grief and grieving. *American Journal of Nursing*, 1964, *64*, 93–96.
18. Ibid.
19. Parkes, C. M. *Bereavement: Studies of Grief in Adult Life*. New York: International Universities Press, 1972.
20. Ibid.

DSM-III-R Classification: Axes I and II Categories and Codes

All official *DSM-III-R* codes are included in ICD-9-CM. Codes followed by a * are used for more than one *DSM-III-R* diagnosis or subtype in order to maintain compatibility with ICD-9-CM.

Numbers in parentheses are page numbers.

A long dash following a diagnostic term indicates the need for a fifth digit subtype or other qualifying term.

The term *specify* following the name of some diagnostic categories indicates qualifying terms that clinicians may wish to add in parentheses after the name of the disorder.

NOS = Not Otherwise Specified

The current severity of a disorder may be specified after the diagnosis as:

mild ⎤
moderate ⎬—— currently meets diagnostic criteria
severe ⎦

in partial remission
   (or residual state)
in complete remission

DISORDERS USUALLY FIRST EVIDENT IN INFANCY, CHILDHOOD, OR ADOLESCENCE

DEVELOPMENTAL DISORDERS
Note: These are coded on Axis II.

Mental Retardation (28)

317.00	Mild mental retardation
318.00	Moderate mental retardation
318.10	Severe mental retardation
318.20	Profound mental retardation
319.00	Unspecified mental retardation

Pervasive Developmental Disorders (33)

299.00	Autistic disorder (38)
	Specify if childhood onset
299.80	Pervasive developmental disorder NOS

Specific Developmental Disorders (39)

Academic Skills Disorders

315.10	Developmental arithmetic disorder (41)

315.80 Developmental expressive writing disorder (42)
315.00 Developmental reading disorder (43)

Language and Speech Disorders
315.39 Developmental articulation disorder (44)
315.31* Developmental expressive language disorder (45)
315.31* Developmental receptive language disorder (47)

Motor Skills Disorder
315.40 Developmental coordination disorder (48)
315.90* Specific developmental disorder NOS

Other Developmental Disorders (49)

315.90* Developmental disorder NOS

Disruptive Behavior Disorders (49)

314.01 Attention-deficit hyperactivity disorder (50)
        Conduct disorder (53),
312.20   group type
312.00   solitary aggressive type
312.90   undifferentiated type
313.81 Oppositional defiant disorder (56)

Anxiety Disorders of Childhood or Adolescence (58)

309.21 Separation anxiety disorder (58)
313.21 Avoidant disorder of childhood or adolescence (61)
313.00 Overanxious disorder (63)

Eating Disorders (65)

307.10 Anorexia nervosa (65)
307.51 Bulimia nervosa (67)
307.52 Pica (69)
307.53 Rumination disorder of infancy (70)
307.50 Eating disorder NOS

Gender Identity Disorders (71)

302.60 Gender identity disorder of childhood (71)
302.50 Transsexualism (74)
        Specify sexual history: asexual, homosexual, heterosexual, unspecified
302.85* Gender identity disorder of adolescence or adulthood, nontranssexual type (76)
        Specify sexual history: asexual, homosexual, heterosexual, unspecified
302.85* Gender identity disorder NOS

Tic Disorders (78)

307.23 Tourette's disorder (79)
307.22 Chronic motor or vocal tic disorder (81)
307.21 Transient tic disorder (81)
        Specify: single episode or recurrent
307.20 Tic disorder NOS

Elimination Disorders (82)

307.70 Functional encopresis (82)
        Specify: primary or secondary type
307.60 Functional enuresis (84)
        Specify: primary or secondary type
        Specify: nocturnal only, diurnal only, nocturnal and diurnal

Speech Disorders not Elsewhere Classified (85)

307.00* Cluttering (85)
307.00* Stuttering (86)

Other Disorders of Infancy, Childhood, or Adolescence (88)

313.23 Elective mutism (88)
313.82 Identity disorder (89)
313.89 Reactive attachment disorder of infancy or early childhood (91)
307.30 Stereotypy/habit disorder (93)
314.00 Undifferentiated attention-deficit disorder (95)

ORGANIC MENTAL DISORDERS (97)

Dementias Arising in the Senium and Presenium (119)

Primary degenerative dementia of
the Alzheimer type, senile onset,
(119)
290.30　　with delirium
290.20　　with delusions
290.21　　with depression
290.00*　uncomplicated
(Note: code 331.00 Alzheimer's
disease on Axis III)

Code in fifth digit:
1 = with delirium, 2 = with delusions, 3 = with
depression, 0* = uncomplicated
290.1x　Primary degenerative dementia of
the Alzheimer type, presenile
onset, ＿＿＿ (119)
(Note: code 331.00 Alzheimer's
disease on Axis III)
290.4x　Multi-infarct dementia, ＿＿＿ (121)
290.00*　Senile dementia NOS
Specify etiology on Axis III if known
290.10*　Presenile dementia NOS
Specify etiology on Axis III if known
(e.g., Pick's disease, Jakob-
Creutzfeldt disease)

Psychoactive Substance-Induced Organic Mental Disorders (123)

Alcohol

303.00　　intoxication (127)
291.40　　idiosyncratic intoxication (128)
291.80　　Uncomplicated alcohol withdrawal
(129)
291.00　　withdrawal delirium (131)
291.30　　hallucinosis (131)
291.10　　amnestic disorder (133)
291.20　　Dementia associated with alcoholism
(133)

Amphetamine or Similarly Acting Sympathomimetic

305.70*　intoxication (134)
292.00*　withdrawal (136)
291.81*　delirium (136)
292.11*　delusional disorder (137)

Caffeine

305.90*　intoxication (138)

Cannabis

305.20*　intoxication (139)
292.11*　delusional disorder (140)

Cocaine

305.60*　intoxication (141)
292.00*　withdrawal (142)
292.81*　delirium (143)
292.11*　delusional disorder (143)

Hallucinogen

305.30*　hallucinosis (144)
292.11*　delusional disorder (146)
292.84*　mood disorder (146)
292.89*　Posthallucinogen perception disorder
(147)

Inhalant

305.90*　intoxication (148)

Nicotine

292.00*　withdrawal (150)

Opioid

305.50*　intoxication (151)
292.00*　withdrawal (152)

Phencyclidine (PCP) or Similarly Acting Arylcyclohexylamine

305.90*　intoxication (154)
292.81*　delirium (155)
292.11*　delusional disorder (156)
292.84*　mood disorder (156)
292.90*　organic mental disorder NOS

Sedative, Hypnotic, or Anxiolytic

305.40*　intoxication (158)
292.00*　uncomplicated sedative, hypnotic,
or anxiolytic withdrawal (159)

292.00*   withdrawal delirium (160)
292.83*   amnestic disorder (161)

Other or Unspecified Psychoactive Substance (162)

305.90*   intoxication
292.00*   withdrawal
292.81*   delirium
292.82*   dementia
292.83*   amnestic disorder
292.11*   delusional disorder
292.12   hallucinosis
292.84*   mood disorder
292.89*   anxiety disorder
292.89*   personality disorder
292.90*   organic mental disorder NOS

Organic Mental Disorders Associated with Axis III Physical Disorders or Conditions, or Whose Etiology is Unknown (162)

293.00   Delirium (100)
294.10   Dementia (103)
294.00   Amnestic disorder (108)
293.81   Organic delusional disorder (109)
293.82   Organic hallucinosis (110)
293.83   Organic mood disorder (111)
          Specify: manic, depressed, mixed
294.80*   Organic anxiety disorder (113)
310.10   Organic personality disorder (114)
          Specify if explosive type
294.80*   Organic mental disorder NOS

PSYCHOACTIVE SUBSTANCE USE DISORDERS (165)

Alcohol (173)

303.90   dependence
305.00   abuse

Amphetamine or Similarly Acting Sympathomimetic (175)

304.40   dependence
305.70*   abuse

Cannabis (176)

304.30   dependence
305.20*   abuse

Cocaine (177)

304.20   dependence
305.60*   abuse

Hallucinogen (179)

304.50*   dependence
305.30*   abuse

Inhalant (180)

304.60   dependence
305.90*   abuse

Nicotine (181)

305.10   dependence

Opioid (182)

304.00   dependence
305.50*   abuse

Phencyclidine (PCP) or Similarly Acting Arylcyclohexylamine (183)

304.50*   dependence
305.90*   abuse

Sedative, Hypnotic, or Anxiolytic (184)

304.10   dependence
305.40*   abuse
304.90*   Polysubstance dependence (185)
304.90*   Psychoactive substance dependence NOS
305.90*   Psychoactive substance abuse NOS

SCHIZOPHRENIA (187)

Code in fifth digit: 1 = subchronic, 2 = chronic, 3 = subchronic with acute exacerbation, 4 = chronic with acute exacerbation, 5 = in remission, 0 = unspecified.

Schizophrenia

295.2x   catatonic, _____
295.1x   disorganized, _____

295.3x	paranoid, _____
	Specify if stable type
295.9x	undifferentiated, _____
295.6x	residual, _____
	Specify if late onset

DELUSIONAL (PARANOID) DISORDER (199)

297.10	Delusional (Paranoid) disorder
	Specify type: erotomanic
	grandiose
	jealous
	persecutory
	somatic
	unspecified

PSYCHOTIC DISORDERS NOT ELSEWHERE CLASSIFIED (205)

298.80	Brief reactive psychosis (205)
295.40	Schizophreniform disorder (207)
	Specify: without good prognostic features or with good prognostic features
295.70	Schizoaffective disorder (208)
	Specify: bipolar type or depressive type
297.30	Induced psychotic disorder (210)
298.90	Psychotic disorder NOS (Atypical psychosis) (211)

MOOD DISORDERS (213)

Code current state of Major Depression and Bipolar Disorder in fifth digit:

1 = mild
2 = moderate
3 = severe, without psychotic features
4 = with psychotic features (*specify* mood-congruent or mood-incongruent)
5 = in partial remission
6 = in full remission
0 = unspecified

For major depressive episodes, *specify* if chronic and *specify* if melancholic type.

For Bipolar Disorder, Bipolar Disorder NOS, Recurrent Major Depression, and Depressive Disorder NOS, *specify* if seasonal pattern.

Bipolar Disorders

	Bipolar disorder (225)
296.6x	mixed, _____
296.4x	manic, _____
296.5x	depressed, _____
301.13	Cyclothymia (226)
296.70	Bipolar disorder NOS

Depressive Disorders

	Major Depression (228)
296.2x	single episode, _____
296.3x	recurrent, _____
300.40	Dysthymia (or Depressive neurosis) (230)
	Specify: primary or sercondary type
	Specify: early or late onset
311.00	Depressive disorder NOS

ANXIETY DISORDERS (OR ANXIETY AND PHOBIC NEUROSES) (235)

	Panic disorder (235)
300.21	with agoraphobia
	Specify current severity of agoraphobic avoidance
	Specify current severity of panic attacks
300.01	without agoraphobia
	Specify current severity of panic attacks
300.22	Agoraphobia without history of panic disorder (240)
	Specify with or without limited symptom attacks
300.23	Social phobia (241)
	Specify if generalized type
300.29	Simple phobia (243)
300.30	Obsessive–compulsive disorder (or Obsessive–compulsive neurosis) (245)
309.89	Post-traumatic stress disorder (247)
	Specify if delayed onset
300.02	Generalized anxiety disorder (251)
300.00	Anxiety disorder NOS

SOMATOFORM DISORDERS (255)

300.70*   Body dysmorphic disorder (255)
300.11   Conversion disorder (or Hysterical
          neurosis, conversion type) (257)
          Specify: single episode or recurrent
300.70*   Hypochondriasis (or
          Hypochondriacal neurosis) (259)
300.81   Somatization disorder (261)
307.80   Somatoform pain disorder (264)
300.70*   Undifferentiated somatoform
          disorder (266)
300.70*   Somatoform disorder NOS (267)

DISSOCIATIVE DISORDERS (OR HYSTERICAL NEUROSES, DISSOCIATIVE TYPE) (269)

300.14   Multiple personality disorder (269)
300.13   Psychogenic fugue (272)
300.12   Psychogenic amnesia (273)
300.60   Depersonalization disorder (or
          Depersonalization neurosis) (275)
300.15   Dissociative disorder NOS

SEXUAL DISORDERS (279)

Paraphilias (279)

302.40   Exhibitionism (282)
302.81   Fetishism (282)
302.89   Frotteurism (283)
302.20   Pedophilia (284)
          Specify: same sex, opposite sex, same
          and opposite sex
          Specify if limited to incest
          Specify: exclusive type or
          nonexclusive type
302.83   Sexual masochism (286)
302.84   Sexual sadism (287)
302.30   Transvestic fetishism (288)
302.82   Voyeurism (289)
302.90*   Paraphilia NOS (290)

Sexual Dysfunctions (290)

Specify: psychogenic only, or psychogenic and
          biogenic (Note: If biogenic only, code on
          Axis III)

Specify: lifelong or acquired
Specify: generalized or situational

Sexual Desire Disorders (293)

302.71   Hypoactive sexual desire disorder
302.79   Sexual aversion disorder

Sexual Arousal Disorders (294)

302.72*   Female sexual arousal disorder
302.72*   Male erectile disorder

Orgasm Disorders (294)

302.73   Inhibited female orgasm
302.74   Inhibited male orgasm
302.75   Premature ejaculation

Sexual Pain Disorders (295)

302.76   Dyspareunia
306.51   Vaginismus
302.70   Sexual dysfunction NOS

Other Sexual Disorders

302.90*   Sexual disorder NOS

SLEEP DISORDERS (297)

Dyssomnias (298)

          Insomnia disorder
307.42*   related to another mental disorder
              (nonorganic) (300)
780.50*   related to known organic factor
              (300)
307.42*   Primary insomnia (301)
307.44   Hypersomnia disorder
              related to another mental disorder
              (nonorganic) (303)
780.50*   related to a known organic factor
              (303)
780.54   Primary hypersomnia (305)
307.45   Sleep-wake schedule disorder (305)
          Specify: advanced or delayed phase
              type, disorganized type, frequently
              changing type
          Other dyssomnias
307.40*   Dyssomnia NOS

Parasomnias (308)

307.47   Dream anxiety disorder (Nightmare
         disorder) (308)
307.46* Sleep terror disorder (310)
307.46* Sleepwalking disorder (311)
307.40* Parasomnia NOS (313)

FACTITIOUS DISORDERS (315)

         Factitious disorder
301.51   with physical symptoms (316)
300.16   with psychological symptoms (318)
300.19   Factitious disorder NOS (320)

IMPULSE CONTROL DISORDERS NOT ELSEWHERE CLASSIFIED (321)

312.34   Intermittent explosive disorder (321)
312.32   Kleptomania (322)
312.31   Pathological gambling (324)
312.33   Pyromania (325)
312.39* Trichotillomania (326)
312.39* Impulse control disorder NOS (328)

ADJUSTMENT DISORDER (329)

         Adjustment disorder
309.24   with anxious mood
309.00   with depressed mood
309.30   with disturbance of conduct
309.40   with mixed disturbance of
            emotions and conduct
309.28   with mixed emotional features
309.82   with physical complaints
309.83   with withdrawal
309.23   with work (or academic) inhibition
309.90   Adjustment disorder NOS

PSYCHOLOGICAL FACTORS AFFECTING PHYSICAL CONDITION (333)

316.00   Psychological factors affecting
         physical condition
         Specify physical condition on Axis III

316.00   Psychological factors affecting
         physical condition
         Specify physical condition on Axis III

PERSONALITY DISORDERS (335)
Note: These are coded on Axis II.

Cluster A

301.00   Paranoid (337)
301.20   Schizoid (339)
301.22   Schizotypal (340)

Cluster B

301.70   Antisocial (342)
301.83   Borderline (346)
301.50   Histrionic (348)
301.81   Narcissistic (349)

Cluster C

301.82   Avoidant (351)
301.60   Dependent (353)
301.40   Obsessive compulsive (354)
301.84   Passive aggressive (356)
301.90   Personality disorder NOS

V CODES FOR CONDITIONS NOT ATTRIBUTABLE TO A MENTAL DISORDER THAT ARE A FOCUS OF ATTENTION OR TREATMENT (359)

V62.30   Academic problem
V71.01   Adult antisocial behavior

V40.00   Borderline intellectual functioning
         (Note: This is coded on Axis II.)

V71.02   Childhood or adolescent antisocial
         behavior
V65.20   Malingering
V61.10   Marital problem
V15.81   Noncompliance with medical
         treatment
V62.20   Occupational problem
V61.20   Parent–child problem
V62.81   Other interpersonal problem
V61.80   Other specified family circumstances

V62.89   Phase-of-life problem or other life
         circumstance problem
V62.82   Uncomplicated bereavement

| V71.09* | No diagnosis or condition on Axis II |
| 799.90* | Diagnosis or condition deferred on Axis II |

ADDITIONAL CODES (363)

300.90   Unspecified mental disorder
         (nonpsychotic)
V71.09* No diagnosis or condition on Axis I
799.90* Diagnosis or condition deferred on
         Axis 1

MULTIAXIAL SYSTEM

Axis I   Clinical Syndromes
          V Codes
Axis II   Developmental Disorders
          Personality Disorders
Axis III Physical Disorders and Conditions
Axis IV   Severity of Psychosocial Stressors
Axis V   Global Assessment of Functioning

SEVERITY OF PSYCHOSOCIAL STRESSORS SCALE: ADULTS

| Code | Term | Examples of Stressors | |
		Acute Events	Enduring Circumstances
1	None	No acute events that may be relevant to the disorder	No enduring circumstances that may be relevant to the disorder
2	Mild	Broke up with boyfriend or girl friend; started or graduated from school; child left home	Family arguments; job dissatisfaction; residence in high-crime neighborhood
3	Moderate	Marriage; marital separation; loss of job; retirement; miscarriage	Marital discord; serious financial problems; trouble with boss; being a single parent
4	Severe	Divorce; birth of first child	Unemployment; poverty
5	Extreme	Death of spouse; serious physical illness diagnosed; victim of rape	Serious chronic illness in self or child; ongoing physical or sexual abuse
6	Catastrophic	Death of a child; suicide of spouse; devastating natural disaster	Captivity as hostage; concentration camp experience
0	Inadequate information, or no change in condition		

SEVERITY OF PSYCHOSOCIAL STRESSORS SCALE: CHILDREN AND ADOLESCENTS

| Code | Term | Examples of Stressors | |
		Acute Events	Enduring Circumstances
1	None	No acute events that may be relevant to the disorder	No enduring circumstances that may be relevant to the disorder
2	Mild	Broke up with boyfriend or girl friend; change of school	Overcrowded living quarters; family arguments
3	Moderate	Expelled from school; birth of sibling	Chronic disabling illness in parent; chronic parental discord
4	Severe	Divorce of parents; unwanted pregnancy; arrest	Harsh or rejecting parents; chronic life-threatening illness in parent; multiple foster home placements

(Continued)

(Continued)

SEVERITY OF PSYCHOSOCIAL STRESSORS SCALE: CHILDREN AND ADOLESCENTS

Code	Term	Examples of Stressors	
		Acute Events	*Enduring Circumstances*
5	Extreme	Sexual or physical abuse; death of a parent	Recurrent sexual or physical abuse
6	Catastrophic	Death of both parents	Chronic life-threatening illness
0	Inadequate information, or no change in condition		

Global Assessment of Functioning Scale (GAF Scale)

Consider psychological, social, and occupational functioning on a hypothetical continuum of mental health–illness. Do not include impairment in functioning due to physical (or environmental) limitations.

Note: Use intermediate codes when appropriate, e.g., 45, 68, 72.

Code

90
|
81
Absent or minimal symptoms (e.g., mild anxiety before an exam), **good functioning in all areas, interested and involved in a wide range of activities, socially effective, generally satisfied with life, no more than everyday problems or concerns** (e.g., an occasional argument with family members).

80
|
71
If symptoms are present, they are transient and expectable reactions to psychosocial stressors (e.g., difficulty concentrating after family argument); **no more than slight impairment in social, occupational, or school functioning** (e.g., temporarily falling behind in schoolwork).

70
|
61
Some mild symptoms (e.g., depressed mood and mild insomnia) **OR some difficulty in social, occupational, or school functioning** (e.g., occasional truancy, or theft within the household), **but generally functioning pretty well, has some meaningful interpersonal relationships.**

60
|
51
Moderate symptoms (e.g., flat affect and circumstantial speech, occasional panic attacks) **OR moderate difficulty in social, occupational, or school functioning** (e.g., few friends, conflicts with coworkers).

50
|
41
Serious symptoms (e.g., suicidal ideation, severe obsessional rituals, frequent shoplifting) **OR any serious impairment in social, occupational, or school functioning** (e.g., no friends, unable to keep a job).

40
|
|
31
Some impairment in reality testing or communication (e.g., speech is at times illogical, obscure, or irrelevant) **OR major impairment in several areas, such as work or school, family relations, judgment, thinking, or mood** (e.g., depressed man avoids friends, neglects family, and is unable to work; child frequently beats up younger children, is defiant at home, and is failing at school).

30
|
|
21
Behavior is considerably influenced by delusions or hallucinations OR serious impairment in communication or judgment (e.g., sometimes incoherent, acts grossly inappropriately, suicidal preoccupation) **OR inability to function in almost all areas** (e.g., stays in bed all day; no job, home, or friends).

20   **Some danger of hurting self or others** (e.g., suicide attempts without clear expectation of death, frequently violent, manic excitement) **OR occasionally fails to maintain minimal personal hygiene** (e.g., smears feces) **OR gross impairment in communication** (e.g., largely incoherent or
11   mute).

10   **Persistent danger of severely hurting self or others** (e.g., recurrent violence) **OR persistent inability
1   to maintain minimal personal hygiene OR serious suicidal act with clear expectation of death.**

GLOSSARY

Abnormal behavior Behavior may be labeled *abnormal* when it is unusual, causes distress to others, and makes it difficult for a person to adjust to his environment.

"Acting out" Expressing certain kinds of unconscious conflicts through behavior.

Adaptation Dynamic process by which an individual responds to the environment and the changes that occur within it. Ability to modify one's behavior to meet changing environmental requirements. Adaptation to a given situation is influenced by one's personal characteristics and the type of situation.

Addiction Physical or psychological dependence on alcohol or drugs.

Adjustment Ability to harmonize with the environment to conform to new conditions.

Adolescence A time of passage from childhood to adulthood; extends from about age 12 to the late teens.

Adrenalectomy Surgical removal of the adrenal glands.

Adversary Antagonist, opponent, enemy, foe.

Affect Emotion, feeling, or mood—pleasant or unpleasant, intense or mild. Tone of feeling accompanying a thought.

Affective disorder One of a group of disorders of which the most important feature is a primary disturbance of mood or emotions. Disturbance may be episodic or chronic.

Affiliation motive Motive or desire to associate with or be around other people.

Aggression A feeling or action that may be self-assertive, forceful, or hostile.

Agitation Marked restlessness and excitement.

Agoraphobia Pathological fear of open spaces.

Alarm reaction First stage of the General Adaptation Syndrome. Pattern of bodily changes that occur in reaction to stress.

Alcoholics Anonymous Organization of people devoted to the rehabilitation of alcoholics.

Alcoholism Maladaptive behavior associated with the chronic or excessive consumption of alcoholic beverages.

Alienation Condition characterized by the lack of meaningful relationships with others. May result in depersonalization and estrangement from others.

Alzheimer's disease Chronic brain disorder, occurring as early as the fourth decade of life and involving a progressive destruction of nervous tissue, which results in slurring of speech, involuntary muscular movements, and gradual intellectual deterioration with growing lapses of memory.

Ambivalence Simultaneous conflicting feelings or attitudes toward a person or object.

Amnesia A dissociative experience in which the person's recollection is lost or split off from conscious recall. May be functional or organic.

Anaclitic Characterized by dependence; a leaning on.

Androgen Male hormone.

Anorexia nervosa Prolonged loss of appetite with consequent weight loss.

Anoxia Lack of sufficient oxygen.

Antabuse Drug that interacts with alcohol to produce unpleasant physical sensations. Used as a therapeutic measure to treat alcoholism.

Antianxiety drugs Commonly called *tranquilizers*. Used to calm anxious people.

Antidepressant drugs General term for a number of drugs used to relieve depression and to elevate mood.

Antipsychotic drugs A group of chemical compounds used in the treatment of individuals who show severely disturbed behavior and thought processes, especially in cases of schizophrenia.

Antisocial Exhibiting attitudes and overt behavior contrary to accepted customs, standards, and moral principles of a society.

Anxiety An affect with both a psychological and physiological side. Generally, an unpleasant emotional state accompanied by physiological arousal and the cognitive elements of apprehension, guilt, and a sense of impending disaster. Distinguished from fear, which is an emotional reaction to a specific or identifiable object.

Anxiety disorder Formerly called *neurosis* or *neurotic disorder*; characterized by anxiety as the most prominent symptom. Includes panic disorder, phobic disorder, obsessive–compulsive disorder, and post-traumatic stress disorder.

Apathy A state of indifference.

Aphasia Loss of previously possessed speech.

Arteriosclerosis Thickening or hardening of the walls of the arteries, as in old age.

Asphyxia Lack of oxygen to the brain.

Assailant A person who attacks someone.

Assault An attack that may be physical or verbal.

Assessment Information gathering aimed at the description and prediction of behavior.

Association Connecting one thought or feeling with another.

Attention Focusing on certain features of a stimulus pattern while simultaneously ignoring others.

Attitude The position taken on an issue.

Attribution process The way in which an individual analyzes cause and effect.

Audit Process of evaluation and examination of events.

Autism An absorption in fantasy to the complete exclusion of reality and understood only by the individual.

Autoerotic Sensual self-gratification as through thumb-sucking, stroking, masturbation.

Autoeroticism Self-stimulation of the genitals.

Autognosis The process by which the nurse can understand a clinical situation by paying attention to subjective reactions.

Aversion Fear or phobic reaction.

Behavior The actions of an individual or persons.

Behavioral assessment Use of observation of specific characteristics of patient behavior as a record for psychosocial assessment.

Bisexuality Sexually oriented to both sexes.

Blunting A dulling of emotional response.

Borderline personality disorder Disorder characterized by impulsive and unpredictable behavior and marked shifts in mood. Areas of instability may include personal relationships, behavior, mood, and images of self.

Castration anxiety Psychoanalytic term for apprehensiveness over fear of loss of the genital function. Symbolically, a state of powerlessness or psychological impotence.

Catalepsy Trance-like state and immobility.

Celibacy Abstaining from various degrees of sexual activity.

Cerea flexibilitas Waxy flexibility in which a person holds his body in one position for long periods of time.

Character The personality traits or behavioral style of an individual.

Child abuse Serious mistreatment of a child by an adult.

Cognition Denoting the mental processes of thinking, memory, comprehension, and reasoning.

Coitus Genital sexual intercourse.

Community A population within a geographic area engaging in social interaction and having common ties.

Community mental health center Community-based facility or complex of facilities for the prevention and treatment of mental illness.

Complex A group of associated ideas that have a strong emotional tone and generally are unconscious.

Compulsion Irresistible and repetitive act or behavior that an individual recognizes as irrational but cannot easily cease. Often viewed as a defense against obsessive thoughts.

Concreteness Style of thinking in which there is an overemphasis on specific detail.

Concussion Head injury that does not cause lasting structural damage. Rate of recovery is proportional to the severity of the injury.

Condensation Unconscious compression of several experiences, locations, or individuals into one idea. Mental mechanism characteristic of the dream state.

Confabulation Type of thinking characterized by the filling of memory gaps with false irrelevant information and details. The person believes the stories to be true.

Confidentiality Responsibility of the agency and professional to keep all information, records, and correspondence confidential, allowing access to records only under specific circumstances.

Conflict Condition of opposition between responses, impulses, needs, or desires that are mutually exclusive.

Conformity Behavior that is conventional and in agreement with social rules, norms, and customs.

Confusion A state of disordered orientation.

Congenital Inherent at birth.

Consciousness Process or state of being aware of or comprehending what is happening around one.

Constitution The psychological and physical endowment of an individual; the potential or physical inheritance from birth.

Consumer One who uses services.

Conversion disorder Type of somatoform disorder in which there is a loss or change in physical functioning that suggests a physical disorder, but there seems to be a direct expression of a psychological conflict.

Coping Problem-solving efforts in a stressful situation.

Correlation Degree of correspondence between two variables; a statistical index of covariation that varies from $+1.00$ to -1.00.

Countertransference Psychoanalytic term that refers to the therapist's emotional reactions to the patient.

Crime Conduct that is in violation of the law.

Crisis A crucial situation that causes a disequilibrium in an individual's life-style.

Crisis intervention Short-term treatment that attempts to assist the patient in the settlement of a crisis.

Culture General values, attitudes, achievements, and behavior patterns shared by members of the same society.

Cunnilingus Mouth and tongue stimulation of the female genitals.

Customer One who purchases some commodity or service.

Data Factual evidence from which conclusions can be inferred.

Daydreaming Reverie; free play of thought or imagination.

Defendant The person required to make answer in a suit of law or in a criminal action; as opposed to the plaintiff.

Defense mechanisms Processes by which the mind seeks relief from emotional conflict.

Deinstitutionalization Movement whose purpose is to remove patients from large mental hospitals and to obtain treatment and sheltered living conditions for them in the community.

Déjà vu A feeling of familiarity with a place or situation that one has never actually been to or seen.

Delinquent child A person under a specific age who has violated the law.

Delirium A state of mental disturbance caused by organic conditions and characterized by disorientation, confusion, and often hallucinations.

Delirium tremens Delirium induced by prolonged and excessive use of alcohol.

Delusion Incorrect belief maintained despite clear evidence to the contrary.

Dementia An irreversible deterioration of mental capacities.

Dementia praecox An obsolete term for schizophrenia.

Denial A defense mechanism by which the mind refuses to acknowledge a thought, feeling, wish, need, or reality factor.

Dependency needs Essential needs for mothering, love, affection, shelter, protection, security, food, and warmth that begin at birth.

Dependent personality disorder Disorder characterized by an inability to make major decisions and a belittling of a person's own abilities and assets. Intense discomfort is experienced if the person remains alone for more than a brief period.

Dependent variable Aspect of behavior that changes according to manipulation of the independent variable in an experiment.

Depersonalization The experiencing of feelings of unrealness about the self or the environment.

Depression Pervasive feelings of sadness, dejection, or melancholy that may begin after some loss or stressful event but continue long afterwards.

Deprivation, sensory Lack of adequate perceptual stimuli, such as may occur to a confined prisoner.

Descriptive psychiatry A system of psychiatry based on the study of observable phenomena; to be differentiated from dynamic psychiatry.

Deterioration A progressive decline.

Developmental stages Divisions of the lifespan, representing periods during the individual's life that are typically characterized by specific clusters of behavior.

Developmentally disabled A person whose adaptive ability has been compromised in one or more areas of functioning, occurring during childhood.

Deviant behavior Behavior that differs from some norm or standard.

Diagnosis A careful examination of evidence to determine an opinion as to the nature of a traumatic, injured, or diseased condition. In nursing, the act or process of determining the human response to stress.

Discrimination To separate one person or group from another by the use of preferential characteristics.

Disengaged family Family members isolated from each other.

Disfranchise To deprive of a right, privilege, or power. Also *disenfranchise*.

Disorientation Loss of awareness of the position of self in terms of time, space, or other people.

Displacement A defense mechanism whereby a feeling is transferred to a more acceptable substitute object.

Dissociation A mental defense of separating one item from another item.

Dissociative disorder Sudden, temporary alteration in the functions of consciousness, identity, or motor behavior in which some part of one or more of these functions is lost.

Double bind Type of conflict created when a person is confronted with contradictory messages and demands.

Dream Mental activity during sleep that is dissociated from the self and consciousness of the waking state.

Drive Motivation or basic urge in humans; to be distinguished from the purely biologic concept of drive.

Dynamic Forceful and active.

Dynamic psychiatry The study and interpretation of emotional processes and the changing factors in human behavior and its motivation.

Dynamics of behavior The understanding and significance of a person's behavior.

Dysfunction Disturbance or impairment in normal functioning.

Dysmnesia An impairment in the ability to retain and recall information.

Dyspareunia Type of sexual dysfunction in which persistent and recurrent genital pain is associated with coitus.

Ecchymosis A bruise; extravasation of blood into the tissues.

Echolalia Meaningless repetition of words.

Echopraxia Pathological repetition by imitation of the movements of another person.

Eclectic Selecting from various systems.

Edema An abnormal accumulation of fluid in cells and tissues.

Ego That part of the psychic structure that deals with reality.

Egocentric Concern with self.

Ego ideal That part of the psychic structure that represents the ideal aims and goals of the individual.

Egomania Preoccupation with self.

Electroconvulsive therapy Electric treatments to produce a grand mal convulsion in an individual.

Electroencephalogram A tracing by an electroencephalograph to record electrical discharges in the brain.

Emotion Consciously perceived states such as anxiety or anger.

Empathy The capacity for participating in, or a

vicarious experience of, another's feelings, volitions, or ideas.

Empirical Based on experience or observation. Capable of being confirmed, verified, or disproved by observation or experiment.

Encopresis Fecal soiling.

Enmeshed family An excess of communication and concern between members resulting in emotional overload.

Enterprise An undertaking that involves activity, energy, and courage.

Enuresis Incontinence of urine; bed-wetting.

Epilepsy A neurological disorder of consciousness that is often accompanied by a convulsion.

Erectile dysfunction (impotence) Type of sexual dysfunction in which the male is occasionally or chronically unable to achieve or maintain a penile erection. The condition may have physical or psychological causes.

Erotomania Preoccupation with erotic activities.

Erythema Redness of skin due to irritation and dilation of capillaries.

Etiology Assignment of a cause. Scientific study of causes and origins of maladaptive behavior.

Euphoria Intense feelings of self-contentment.

Exhibitionism Exposure of the genitals in public for purposes of obtaining sexual pleasure and gratification.

Extroversion Behavior, thoughts, and feelings that are directed outward from the self.

Fabrication Made-up events to fill in gaps of memory.

Fainting Temporary loss of consciousness.

Family A subsystem within a larger community.

Fantasy A sequence of imagined events as in daydreaming.

Fear An emotional response to perceived danger; to be distinguished from anxiety, which does not necessarily identify the danger.

Feedback Communication to the sender concerning the effect his original message had on those to whom it was relayed.

Fellatio Taking the penis into the mouth.

Feminist counseling Counseling that addresses personal, social, and political aspects of a problem.

Feminist movement A social movement organized on the behalf of women's rights.

Fetishism Sexual deviation in which sexual interest is centered upon some body part or inanimate object that becomes capable of stimulating sexual excitement.

Fixation Inappropriately strong attachment for someone or something. Often refers to an abnormal attachment developed during infancy or childhood that persists into adult life.

Flight of ideas The rapid succession of ideas that are not necessarily related to each other.

Forensic Legal aspect.

Free association A psychoanalytic technique whereby the patient says whatever comes into his mind.

Fugue state A dissociative state characterized by amnesia and actual physical flights from an intolerable situation.

Functional disorder Maladaptive behavior having no demonstrable organic basis and precipitated primarily by psychological and social factors.

Fusion Blurring of boundaries.

Gay Liberation Homosexual movement.

Gender Sex identification of male or female.

General adaptation theory Concept proposed by Selye. Three-stage reaction of an organism to excessive and prolonged stress, including (1) an alarm or mobilization reaction; (2) a resistance stage; and (3) a final stage of exhaustion.

General paresis A psychosis caused by a chronic syphilitic infection in the central nervous system.

Genetic Pertaining to hereditary factors.

Genitalia The reproductive organs; generally, the external reproductive organs.

Genogram Structured technique of drawing a family map.

Geriatrics Study of the health problems of aging.

Ghetto A section of a city in which members of a social group are segregated.

Gigolo Males who sell sexual services to females.

Globus hystericus A symptom in which there is a sensation of having a ball in the throat; a hysterical spasm of the esophagus.

Goal Any object, position, or state toward which the individual strives.

Grandiose A term referring to delusions or feelings of power, fame, splendor, magnificence.

Grief A normal emotional response to recognized loss; self-limiting and gradually subsiding within a reasonable time.

Group dynamics The study of the process of small groups.

Habit Acquired activity that has become relatively fixed and consistent as a result of repeated performances.

Hallucination An imaginary sense perception.

Health State of complete physical, mental, and social well-being; not merely the absence of disease or infirmity.

Herpes Chronic sexually transmitted viral disease.

Heterosexual Sexual attraction between members of the opposite sex.

Hierarchy Arrangement or ordering on the basis of importance.

Histrionic personality disorder Disorder characterized by overly reactive behavior of a histrionic, exhibitionistic type with traits of egocentricism.

Holistic Viewing a human being as a unified biologic, psychological, and social organism whose total configuration must be studied.

Homeostasis Maintenance of equilibrium and constancy among the bodily processes.

Homosexual Sexual attraction between members of the same sex.

Hostility Personality trait disposing the individual toward aggressiveness, negativism, and a generalized tendency to evaluate experience in a negative manner.

Human That which is characteristic of people.

Humanistic approach Theories characterized by an emphasis on self-fulfillment and social systems in which everyone has an equal opportunity to become fully human through realizing his individual potential.

Hyperactive Abnormally active.

Hyperkinesis Increased muscular movement.

Hypnosis An induced dissociative state.

Hypochondriasis A strong and abnormal preoccupation with one's state of health.

Id A psychoanalytic term to identify that part of the psychic structure that is unconscious, contains primitive drives, and operates on the pleasure principle.

Ideas of reference The incorrect interpretation of incidents as having direct reference to the self.

Identification Emotional tie unconsciously causing a person to think, feel, and act as he imagines the person with whom he has the tie does. Viewed both developmentally and as a mental defense.

Identity Generally refers to the constellation of traits, values, and attitudes that form a person's relatively stable perception of "self."

Illusion The misinterpretation of an actual sensory experience.

Implosive therapy Behavior technique whereby the patient is repeatedly presented with strongly anxiety-provoking stimuli until he no longer reacts in an anxious manner.

Impotence Difficulty in achieving or maintaining a penile erection.

Impulsivity Tendency to act without thinking or planning.

Incest Sexual activity or intercourse between close family members.

Incorporation A psychological mechanism whereby a person symbolically takes in a part of another person to be part of his self. For example, the infant fantasizes that the mother's breast is part of him.

Infertility Inability to conceive a pregnancy after 1 year of sexual relations without contraception; the inability to carry a pregnancy to a live birth.

Informed consent Requirement that patients must be given adequate information about the benefits and risks of planned treatment before they agree to the procedure.

Inhibition Restraint or control exercised over an impulse, drive, or response tendency.

Insanity Legal term connoting mental incompetence, inability to distinguish "right from wrong," and inability to care for oneself.

Insight Self-knowledge and a major goal of psychotherapy. This includes the individual's understanding of the nature, origin, and mechanisms of his thoughts, feelings, and behaviors.

Instinct Inborn drive; present without being learned.

Insulin shock A somatic treatment in which a coma is induced by the injection of insulin.

Intellectualization Defense mechanism related to isolation. Emotional bond or link between symbols and their emotional charge is broken by this process.

Intelligence Generally includes three concepts: (1) the ability to deal with abstractions; (2) the ability to learn; and (3) the ability to cope with new or novel situations.

Interpretation Explanation of the actual or deep meaning of behavior or fantasy as opposed to the surface meaning.

Interview To question or have a conversation with someone, especially in order to obtain information.

Intrapsychic That which takes place in the mind.

Introjection A mental mechanism in which one incorporates and accepts patterns, attitudes, and ideals of others.

Introspection Process of trying to gain knowledge by the study of one's own thoughts.

Introversion Preoccupation with one's self; the opposite of extroversion.

Isolation Defense mechanism by which inconsistent or contradictory attitudes and feelings are walled off from each other in consciousness. Similar to repression, except that in isolation, the impulse or wish is consciously recognized but is separated from the present behavior; in repression, neither the wish nor its relation to action is recognized. Intellectualization is a special form of isolation.

Issue A matter on which there exist two or more points of view.

Juvenile delinquency A legal classification of children's behavior that violates the law.

Korsakoff's syndrome (psychosis) Chronic brain disorder precipitated by a vitamin deficiency stemming from alcoholism. Characterized by marked disorientation, amnesia, and falsification of memory.

Labeling Cognitive device by which a person classifies his own emotional responses as a way of controlling behavior, especially in stress-producing situations; a way of stereotyping.

Labile Rapidly shifting emotions.

Law Rules of conduct formally recognized as binding by authority.

Learned helplessness Acquired belief in helplessness. First developed by Seligman in dogs who were subjected to an inescapable noxious stimulus.

Learning General term for a relatively enduring change in behavior produced directly or indirectly by experience.

Lesbianism Female homosexuality.

Lesion An injury. Brain lesions can cause a multiplicity of behavioral disorders.

Libido Psychoanalytic term referring to the general instinctual drives of the id; psychic energy.

Litigation A suit of law.

Maladaptive behavior Behavior that is deficient or excessive and hinders successful interacting with the environment and dealing with stress; responses that are inappropriate to environmental circumstances.

Malingering A deliberate endeavor to use an illness to avoid an uncomfortable situation.

Mania Euphoric, hyperactive state in which the individual's judgment is impaired.

Manic episode Distinct period when the individual's mood is expansive and euphoric or irritable.

Mannerism Habitual and stereotyped movement or gesture.

Masochism Deviation in which sexual pleasure is attained from pain inflicted on oneself, from being dominated, or from being mistreated.

Masturbation Self-stimulation of the genitals.

Maturation Growth processes in the individual that result in orderly changes in behavior.

Megalomania A psychiatric syndrome characterized by delusions of great self-importance, wealth, or power.

Melancholia Alternate term for severe depression.

Mental Pertaining to the mind.

Mental mechanisms Specific intrapsychic defensive processes that relieve a person from uncomfortable or intolerable situations; also called *defense mechanisms*.

Mental retardation Level of intellectual functioning significantly below average, apparent early in life, characterized by behavioral deficiencies over a wide range of abilities.

Milieu The people and factors within an environment with which a person interacts.

Molest To annoy or disturb; to unjustifiably meddle with sexually.

Motivation The force within the individual that impels him to act.

Multiple personality Dissociative disorder characterized by the development and existence of two or more relatively independent and coexisting personality systems within the same individual.

Mutism The inability to speak.

Narcissism A psychoanalytic term meaning self-love.

Narcissistic personality disorder Disorder characterized by a sense of self-importance and a preoccupation with fantasies of unlimited success.

Narcolepsy A condition in which the individual is overcome by an uncontrollable desire to sleep.

Necromania Preoccupation with the dead.

Negativism Aggressive withdrawal that includes the refusal to cooperate or obey orders, usually expressed by behavior exactly the opposite of what is expected, appropriate, or desired.

Negotiate A discussion whereby an agreement is reached.

Neologism The formation or development of a new word from parts of existing words.

Nervous breakdown A popular term for decompensation in the face of stress; nonspecific term for emotional illness.

Neurasthenia A collection of symptoms including fatigue, feelings of physical and mental weakness, aches, and pains.

Neurosis Older term for what is now called *anxiety disorder*.

Nightmare A frightening dream, often accompanied by a sensation of helplessness and impending doom.

Nosological Classification or list of diseases.

Object A psychoanalytic term meaning *person*.

Object relationship The emotional bonds that exist between one individual and another.

Obsession Persistent and uncontrollable thoughts.

Obsessive–compulsive disorder Reaction characterized by persistent and repetitive thoughts, often of an anxiety-provoking nature (obsessions), and by uncontrollable and repetitive acts (compulsions).

Oedipus complex A psychoanalytic term whereby the child has feelings of attachment for the parent of the opposite sex and feelings of envy and aggression toward the parent of the same sex.

Oophorectomy Surgical removal of the ovaries.

Operant conditioning A technique of behavior therapy in which the desired behavior is rewarded and the undesired behavior is either ignored or acknowledged by punishment.

Oppositional behavior Actions that go contrary to prescribed behavior.

Organic mental illness A mental illness caused by organic brain changes.

Orgasmic dysfunction Inability to achieve orgasm.

Overcompensation A defense mechanism whereby a physical or psychological deficit produces exaggerated correction.

Overt Observable; refers to behaviors, actions, and verbalizations.

Panic Acute, intense, and overwhelming anxiety.

Paranoid Feelings of persecution or suspicion; may develop into delusions.

Paraphilia Sexual deviation that involves choice of inappropriate sex partners or inappropriate goals for the sex act. Pedophilia, sadism, and voyeurism are examples.

Passive–aggressive personality Personality disorder usually characterized by aggressive behavior exhibited in passive ways (e.g., pouting).

Pathology Disease or abnormal physical condition.

Pedophilia Sexual deviation in which an adult desires or engages in sexual relations with a child. May be either homosexual or heterosexual in nature.

Peer group Social group composed of members of approximately equivalent ages and social status.

Perseveration Rigid repetition of an activity or thought pattern.

Personality The sum total of the behavioral style and patterns of the individual.

Personality disorder Deeply ingrained, inflexible, maladaptive patterns of thought and behavior that persist throughout a person's life.

Perversion A deviation from socially acceptable patterns of sexual gratification.

Pharmacology Study of the preparation, qualities, uses, and effects of drugs.

Phobia An obsessive, persistent, and unrealistic fear of an external object or situation. Common phobias are: *acrophobia* (heights), *agoraphobia* (open spaces), *aquaphobia* (water), *claustrophobia* (closed spaces), *mysophobia* (dirt), *myctophobia* (dark), *pyrophobia* (fire).

Physical abuse Nonaccidental physical injury.

Physical dependence Bodily state that manifests itself by intense physical disturbances (withdrawal symptoms) when the use of a drug is stopped.

Pica Abnormal craving for substances that have no nutritional value, such as paper, paint, or soil.

Pick's disease Type of progressive dementia caused by atrophy of organ systems within the body.

Play therapy A treatment approach used with children to establish interaction between the nurse and child and to foster the thoughts of the child more directly.

Pleasure principle Psychoanalytic term for the regulatory mechanism of mental life that functions to reduce tension and gain gratification.

Posey belt Type of body restraint made of cotton muslin material that secures the trunk of the body and restrains the upper half of the body and attaches to bed or stretcher.

Postvention Activities following a suicide that assist the bereaved survivors.

Preapism Prolonged and painful erection.

Preconscious That part of the psychic structure in which thoughts are not in immediate awareness but can be recalled by conscious effort.

Prediction Statement about the probability that an event not yet observed will occur.

Prevention, secondary Early detection of illness and prompt treatment.

Prevention, tertiary Rehabilitative efforts to minimize the effects of an illness.

Primary health care A system that provides a framework for organizing the dimensions of health care and emphasizes continuity and first contact.

Primary prevention The promotion of health and the prevention of illness.

Prognosis Forecast; probable course and outcome of a disorder.

Projection A defense mechanism whereby thoughts, attitudes, and motivations are directed out into the environment; attributing characteristics that belong to but are not acceptable to onseself.

Psychiatric emergency Sudden appearance of unusual disordered behavior needing immediate attention.

Psychiatric nursing A specialty within the nursing profession in which efforts are directed to diagnosing and planning interventions for human response to stress involving psychiatric–mental health issues.

Psychiatric social work Field of social work in which the worker specializes in maladaptive behavior in a clinical setting.

Psychiatrist Physician with postgraduate training in the diagnosis and treatment of psychiatric disorders.

Psychoanalysis A theory of human development, human behavior, and a form of psychotherapeutic treatment developed by Sigmund Freud and his followers.

Psychoanalyst A psychiatrist or a lay therapist who has had additional training in psychoanalysis and who practices the techniques of psychoanalytic therapy.

Psychodynamics The systematized knowledge and theory of human behavior, its motivation, and principles.

Psychogenesis The causation of symptoms by mental or emotional factors, as opposed to organic causes.

Psychological autopsy Review of all factors related to the death of a person in order to speculate on motivation.

Psychologist A health professional who specializes in psychology and has earned a graduate degree in it.

Psychology A science and a profession that deals with knowledge of the psyche in relation to problems of mind and behavior.

Psychopharmacology Study of the effects of drugs on psychological functioning and behavior.

Psychosis Disorder that includes any of the following: delusions, hallucinations, incoherence, repeated derailment of thought, marked poverty of thought content, marked illogicality, and grossly disorganized or catatonic behavior.

Psychotherapy A form of treatment using verbal interchanges with patients as a means for resolving their inner conflicts and modifying their behavior.

Pyromania Compulsive fire setting.

Racism A belief in the inherent superiority of a given race and its right to dominate others; a political or social system based on racism.

Rape Forced sexual activity, without a person's consent.

Rape trauma The resulting symptomatology to the act of rape.

Rationalization A defense mechanism by which logical, socially approved reasons for one's behavior are presented that, although plausible, do not represent the real reasons or motives behind the action.

Reaction formation A defense mechanism that allows the person to express an unacceptable impulse by transforming it into the opposite.

Recidivism Repeated or habitual commission of criminal or delinquent behavior.

Regression A defense mechanism whereby the individual reverts to earlier patterns of behavior.

Rejection The state of refusing to accept.

Repression A defense mechanism that keeps unpleasant experiences and thoughts from conscious awareness.

Requests The wishes or hopes of a person for a desired service or item.

Residential care Live-in situation with some professional support and supervision.

Resistance An individual's reluctance to bring repressed thoughts or impulses into awareness.

Role A set of expectations that is associated with a position in a social system and that determines behavior within specified limits regardless of the personality of the incumbent.

Rorschach test A psychological test designed to disclose conscious and unconscious traits and emotional conflicts. The person being tested tells what is suggested to him when viewing a series of standard inkblot patterns.

Sadism Pleasure derived from inflicting pain on others.

Sadomasochism A condition of inflicting and receiving pain.

Schizoid Used as an adjective to describe traits of introversion, withdrawal, aloofness.

Schizophrenia Group of disorders that always involves at least one of the following at some time: delusions, hallucinations, or certain characteristics of thought disorder.

Self Integrating core of the personality.

Sex All the characteristics that distinguish between the female and the male.

Sex role Different patterns of attitudes and behavior in a given society that are deemed appropriate to one sex or the other.

Sex therapy Therapy aimed at overcoming sexual dysfunctions.

Sexual assault An attack on an individual that has sexual connotations.

Sibling Brother or sister.

Social support Presence of interested, helpful, caring people or of community agencies that may make it possible for a person to be less affected by stress-producing situations.

Sociology The scientific study of social institutions and social relationships, especially the study of the development, structure, and function of human groups, conceptualized as processes of interaction or as organized patterns of collective behavior.

Soma The physical aspect of humans as distinguished from the psyche.

Somatic Physical.

Somatization Emotion exhibited in maladaptive physical response.

Somatoform disorders Disorders characterized by physical symptoms that suggest a physical disorder but for which there are (1) no organic findings to explain the symptom; and (2) strong evidence or suggestion that the symptoms are linked to psychological factors or conflicts.

Stall A loss in the amount of forward progress necessary to maintain the therapeutic process.

Statutes Laws.

Stress Feeling or reaction when faced with a situation that demands action from an individual.

Stressor The incident or event that provokes the stress.

Style The distinctive and characteristic mode of one's behavior.

Subconscious A lay term for that part of the mind not in awareness.

Sublimation A defense mechanism in which libido energy is diverted into socially acceptable avenues.

Substitution A defense mechanism in which one attitude or emotion is replaced by another.

Superego A psychoanalytic term to represent that part of the psychic structure that is the individual's standard of values, ethics, and conscience.

Supervision In psychiatric nursing, a teaching or educative process by which the therapy is managed.

Suppression A defense mechanism in which conscious effort is made to overcome unpleasant thoughts or experiences.

Surrogate One who takes the place of another; a substitute.

Symbiosis A relationship between two people who are totally dependent on each other.

Symbolization A defense mechanism in which an abstract representation is made of an actual object.

Symptom Form of behavior that indicates the presence of a psychopathological condition according to psychodynamic theories. Sign or indicator of an underlying maladaptive process.

Syndrome Pattern or grouping of symptoms that characterize a particular disorder or disease.

Testify To give evidence under oath in court.

Therapeutic Serving to assist or heal.

Tranquilizer Medication prescribed to calm an individual.

Transference Feelings and attitudes of the patient toward a therapist that are a displacement of the patient's feelings toward other people in his life.

Transsexualism Intense desire or need to change one's sexual status, including anatomic structure.

Transvestism Sexual deviation in which the individual derives gratification from wearing clothing of the opposite sex.

Trauma The result of an injury or wound violently produced; in mental health, the result of an emotional wound that is long-term in effect.

Triage The sorting of injured people preliminary to treatment and care, in terms of type and degree of injury and the subsequent care to be provided.

Triangle An organizing principle in patterns of family relationships.

Unconscious Out of awareness. Mental contents that can only be brought to awareness with great difficulty.

Undoing Defense mechanism aimed at negating or atoning for some disapproved act or impulse.

Vaginismus Painful intercourse produced by spastic involuntary constriction of vaginal muscles.

Victim Someone who is harmed, injured, killed, destroyed, or sacrificed, whether it be by ruthless design or incidentally or accidentally.

Victimology The study of the victim.

Voyeurism Attaining sexual gratification from observing the sexual behavior of others. Synonymous with the term *peeping tom*.

Vulnerability Tendency to react maladaptively; to be insufficiently defended.

Waxy flexibility Response exhibited by some catatonic schizophrenics. They may retain a position imposed upon them for many hours.

Withdrawn A form of behavior that implies a retreat from reality.

Word salad Incoherent jumble of words and neologisms.

Index